Textbook of
Traumatic Brain Injury

Editorial Board

Textbook of Traumatic Brain Injury

Edited by

Jonathan M. Silver, M.D.
Thomas W. McAllister, M.D.
Stuart C. Yudofsky, M.D.

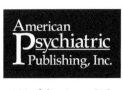

American Psychiatric Publishing, Inc.

Washington, DC
London, England

Manufactured in the United States of America on acid-free paper
09 08 07 06 05   5 4 3 2 1
First Edition

Typeset in Adobe's Janson and Frutiger.

American Psychiatric Publishing, Inc.
1000 Wilson Boulevard
Arlington, VA 22209-3901
www.appi.org

**WL
354
T355
2005**

Library of Congress Cataloging-in-Publication Data
Textbook of traumatic brain injury / edited by Jonathan M. Silver, Thomas W. McAllister,
  Stuart C. Yudofsky.--1st ed.
      p. ; cm.
  Includes bibliographical references and index.
  ISBN 1-58562-105-6 (hardcover : alk. paper)
    1. Brain damage. I. Silver, Jonathan M., 1953- II. McAllister, Thomas W.
III. Yudofsky, Stuart C.
    [DNLM: 1. Brain Injuries--complications. 2. Mental Disorders--etiology. 3. Brain
Injuries--rehabilitation. 4. Mental Disorders--diagnosis. 5. Mental Disorders--therapy.
WL 354 T355 2005]
RC387.5.T46 2005
617.4'81044--dc22

2004050262

British Library Cataloguing in Publication Data
A CIP record is available from the British Library.

To the courage of our patients:

"Who can foresee what will come?…
Do with all your might whatever you are able to do."
—Ecclesiastes

To the devotion of our families:
Orli, Elliot, Benjamin, and Leah
Jeanne, Ryan, Lindsay, and Craig
Beth, Elissa, Lynn, and Emily

"A fruitful bough by a well;
Whose branches run over the wall."
—Genesis 49:22

Contents

Contributors xiii

Foreword. xvii
    Sarah and James Brady

Preface. xix

PART
I
Epidemiology and Pathophysiology

1 Epidemiology 3
    Jess F. Kraus, M.P.H., Ph.D.
    Lawrence D. Chu, M.S., M.P.H., Ph.D.

2 Neuropathology 27
    Thomas A. Gennarelli, M.D.
    David I. Graham, M.B.B.Ch., Ph.D.

3 Neurosurgical Interventions. 51
    Roger Hartl, M.D.
    Jamshid Ghajar, M.D., Ph.D.

4 Neuropsychiatric Assessment 59
    Kimberly A. Arlinghaus, M.D.
    Arif M. Shoaib, M.D.
    Trevor R. P. Price, M.D.

5 Structural Imaging 79
    Erin D. Bigler, Ph.D.

6 Functional Imaging. 107
    Karen E. Anderson, M.D.
    Katherine H. Taber, Ph.D.
    Robin A. Hurley, M.D.

7 Electrophysiological Techniques 135
    David B. Arciniegas, M.D.
    C. Alan Anderson, M.D.
    Donald C. Rojas, Ph.D.

8 Issues in Neuropsychological Assessment 159
    Mary F. Pelham, Psy.D.
    Mark R. Lovell, Ph.D.

9 Delirium and Posttraumatic Amnesia 175
    Paula T. Trzepacz, M.D.
    Richard E. Kennedy, M.D.

10 Mood Disorders 201
    Robert G. Robinson, M.D.
    Ricardo E. Jorge, M.D.

11 Psychotic Disorders 213
    Cheryl Corcoran, M.D.
    Thomas W. McAllister, M.D.
    Dolores Malaspina, M.D.

12 Posttraumatic Stress Disorder and Other Anxiety Disorders 231
    Deborah L. Warden, M.D.
    Lawrence A. Labbate, M.D.

13 Personality Disorders 245
    Gregory J. O'Shanick, M.D.
    Alison Moon O'Shanick, M.S., C.C.C.-S.L.P.

14 Aggressive Disorders 259
    Jonathan M. Silver, M.D.
    Stuart C. Yudofsky, M.D.
    Karen E. Anderson, M.D.

15 Mild Brain Injury and the Postconcussion Syndrome 279
    Thomas W. McAllister, M.D.

16 Seizures 309
    Gary J. Tucker, M.D.

17 Cognitive Changes 321
    Scott McCullagh, M.D.
    Anthony Feinstein, M.D., Ph.D.

18 Disorders of Diminished Motivation 337
    Robert S. Marin, M.D.
    Sudeep Chakravorty, M.D.

19 Awareness of Deficits 353
Laura A. Flashman, Ph.D.
Xavier Amador, Ph.D.
Thomas W. McAllister, M.D.

20 Fatigue and Sleep Problems 369
Vani Rao, M.D.
Pamela Rollings, M.D.
Jennifer Spiro, M.S.

21 Headaches 385
Thomas N. Ward, M.D.
Morris Levin, M.D.

22 Balance Problems and Dizziness 393
Edwin F. Richter III, M.D.

23 Vision Problems 405
Neera Kapoor, O.D., M.S.
Kenneth J. Ciuffreda, O.D., Ph.D.

24 Chronic Pain 419
Nathan D. Zasler, M.D.
Michael F. Martelli, Ph.D.
Keith Nicholson, Ph.D.

25 Sexual Dysfunction 437
Nathan D. Zasler, M.D.
Michael F. Martelli, Ph.D.

PART
IV

Special Populations and Issues

26 Sports Injuries 453
Jason R. Freeman, Ph.D.
Jeffrey T. Barth, Ph.D.
Donna K. Broshek, Ph.D.
Kirsten Plehn, Ph.D.

27 Children and Adolescents 477
Jeffrey E. Max, M.B.B.Ch.

28 Elderly 495
Edward Kim, M.D.

29 Alcohol and Drug Disorders 509
Norman S. Miller, M.D.
Jennifer Adams, B.S.

PART
V
Social Issues

30 The Family System 533
    Marie M. Cavallo, Ph.D.
    Thomas Kay, Ph.D.

31 Systems of Care 559
    D. Nathan Cope, M.D.
    William E. Reynolds, D.D.S., M.P.H.

32 Social Issues. 571
    Andrew Hornstein, M.D.

33 Ethical and Clinical Legal Issues. 583
    Robert I. Simon, M.D.

PART
VI
Treatment

34 Psychopharmacology 609
    Jonathan M. Silver, M.D.
    David B. Arciniegas, M.D.
    Stuart C. Yudofsky, M.D.

35 Psychotherapy 641
    Irwin W. Pollack, M.D., M.A.

36 Cognitive Rehabilitation 655
    Wayne A. Gordon, Ph.D.
    Mary R. Hibbard, Ph.D.

37 Behavioral Treatment 661
    Patrick W. Corrigan, Psy.D.
    Patricia A. Bach, Ph.D.

38 Alternative Treatments 679
    Richard P. Brown, M.D.
    Patricia L. Gerbarg, M.D.

PART
VII
Prevention

39 Pharmacotherapy of Prevention **699**
   Saori Shimizu M.D., Ph.D.
   Carl T. Fulp, M.S.
   Nicolas C. Royo, Ph.D.
   Tracy K. McIntosh, Ph.D.

40 Prevention **727**
   Elie Elovic, M.D.
   Ross Zafonte, D.O.

Index **749**

Contributors

Jennifer Adams, B.S.
Michigan State University, East Lansing, Michigan

Xavier Amador, Ph.D.
Adjunct Professor, Columbia University College of Physicians and Surgeons, New York, New York

C. Alan Anderson, M.D.
Associate Professor of Neurology, Psychiatry, and Emergency Medicine, University of Colorado Health Sciences Center; Staff Physician, Denver Veterans Affairs Medical Center, Denver, Colorado

Karen E. Anderson, M.D.
Assistant Professor, Departments of Psychiatry and Neurology, University of Maryland School of Medicine, Baltimore, Maryland

David B. Arciniegas, M.D.
Assistant Professor of Psychiatry and Neurology and Director, Neuropsychiatry Service, University of Colorado Health Sciences Center, Denver, Colorado

Kimberly A. Arlinghaus, M.D.
Associate Professor of Psychiatry and Physical Medicine and Rehabilitation, Baylor College of Medicine; Senior Consultant for Psychiatry and Director, Psychiatry Consultation/Liaison Program, Michael E. DeBakey VA Medical Center, Houston, Texas

Patricia A. Bach, Ph.D.
Assistant Professor of Psychology, Illinois Institute of Technology, Institute of Psychology, Chicago, Illinois

Jeffrey T. Barth, Ph.D.
Director, Brain Injury and Sports Concussion Institute, University of Virginia School of Medicine, Charlottesville, Virginia

Erin D. Bigler, Ph.D.
Professor, Departments of Psychology and Neuroscience, Brigham Young University, Provo, Utah; Adjunct Professor, Departments of Psychiatry and Radiology, University of Utah School of Medicine, Salt Lake City, Utah

Donna K. Broshek, Ph.D.
Assistant Professor and Associate Director, Brain Injury and Sports Concussion Institute, University of Virginia School of Medicine, Charlottesville, Virginia

Richard P. Brown, M.D.
Associate Professor of Clinical Psychiatry, Columbia University College of Physicians and Surgeons, New York, New York

Marie M. Cavallo, Ph.D.
Assistant Director, Adult Day Services Department, and Director, TBI Services, Association for the Help of Retarded Children, New York, New York

Sudeep Chakravorty, M.D.
Assistant Professor of Psychiatry, University of Pittsburgh School of Medicine, Pittsburgh, Pennsylvania

Lawrence D. Chu, M.S., M.P.H., Ph.D.
Assistant Professor in Biostatistics and Epidemiology, Department of Health Sciences, California State University–Northridge, Northridge, California

Kenneth J. Ciuffreda, O.D., Ph.D.
Distinguished Teaching Professor, Chair, Department of Vision Sciences, SUNY State College of Optometry, New York, New York

D. Nathan Cope, M.D.
Chief Medical Officer, Paradigm Health Corporation, Concord, California

Cheryl Corcoran, M.D.
Assistant Professor of Clinical Psychiatry, New York State Psychiatric Institute, New York, New York

Patrick W. Corrigan, Psy.D.
Professor of Psychiatry and Psychology, Northwestern University, Center for Psychiatric Rehabilitation at Evanston Northwestern Healthcare, Evanston, Illinois

Elie Elovic, M.D.
Associate Professor, Department of Physical Medicine and Rehabilitation, University of Medicine and Dentistry of New Jersey–New Jersey Medical School, Newark, New Jersey; Director, Traumatic Brain Injury Laboratory, Kessler Medical Rehabilitation Research and Education Corporation, West Orange, New Jersey

Anthony Feinstein, M.D., Ph.D.
Professor, Neuropsychiatry Program, University of Toronto, Sunnybrook and Women's College Hospital, Toronto, Ontario, Canada

Laura A. Flashman, Ph.D.
Associate Professor of Psychiatry, Department of Psychiatry, Division of Neuropsychiatry, Dartmouth Medical School, Lebanon, New Hampshire; New Hampshire Hospital, Concord, New Hampshire

Jason R. Freeman, Ph.D.
Associate Director, Brain Injury and Sports Concussion Institute, University of Virginia School of Medicine, Charlottesville, Virginia

Carl T. Fulp, M.S.
Predoctoral Fellow, Traumatic Brain Injury Laboratory, Department of Neurosurgery, University of Pennsylvania School of Medicine, Philadelphia, Pennsylvania

Thomas A. Gennarelli, M.D.
Professor and Chair, Department of Neurosurgery, Medical College of Wisconsin, Milwaukee, Wisconsin

Patricia L. Gerbarg, M.D.
Assistant Professor of Clinical Psychiatry, New York Medical College, Valhalla, New York

Jamshid Ghajar, M.D., Ph.D.
President, Brain Trauma Foundation, New York, New York

Wayne A. Gordon, Ph.D.
Jack Nash Professor, Department of Rehabilitation Medicine, Mount Sinai School of Medicine, New York, New York

David I. Graham, M.B.B.Ch., Ph.D.
Professor and Head of Neuropathology, Institute of Neurological Sciences, Southern General Hospital, Glasgow, Scotland

Roger Hartl, M.D.
Assistant Professor of Neurosurgery, Department of Neurological Surgery, Joan and Sanford I. Weill Cornell Medical College, Cornell University, New York, New York

Mary R. Hibbard, Ph.D.
Professor, Department of Rehabilitation Medicine, Mount Sinai School of Medicine, New York, New York

Andrew Hornstein, M.D.
Assistant Clinical Professor of Psychiatry, Columbia University College of Physicians and Surgeons, New York, New York; Attending Psychiatrist, Head Injury Services, Helen Hayes Hospital, West Haverstraw, New York

Robin A. Hurley, M.D.
Associate Professor, Departments of Psychiatry and Radiology, Wake Forest University School of Medicine, Winston-Salem, North Carolina; Clinical Associate Professor, Department of Psychiatry, Baylor College of Medicine, Houston, Texas; Associate Chief of Staff/Mental Health, Hefner VAMC, Salisbury, North Carolina

Ricardo E. Jorge, M.D.
Assistant Professor of Psychiatry, Roy J. and Lucille A. Carver College of Medicine, University of Iowa, Iowa City, Iowa

Neera Kapoor, O.D., M.S.
Associate Clinical Professor, Department of Clinical Sciences and Director, Raymond J. Greenwald Rehabilitation Center, SUNY State College of Optometry, New York, New York

Thomas Kay, Ph.D.
Assistant Clinical Professor, Department of Rehabilitation Medicine, New York University School of Medicine; Rusk Institute of Rehabilitation Medicine, New York, New York

Richard E. Kennedy, M.D.
Assistant Professor, Departments of Psychiatry and Physical Medicine & Rehabilitation, Virginia Commonwealth University School of Medicine, Richmond, Virginia

Edward Kim, M.D.
Associate Professor of Psychiatry, University of Medicine and Dentistry of New Jersey–Robert Wood Johnson Medical School, Piscataway, New Jersey

Jess F. Kraus, M.P.H., Ph.D.
Professor of Epidemiology, University of California, Los Angeles, School of Public Health; Director, Southern California Injury Prevention Research Center, Los Angeles, California

Lawrence A. Labbate, M.D.
Professor of Psychiatry and Behavioral Sciences, Medical University of South Carolina, Charleston, South Carolina

Morris Levin, M.D.
Associate Professor of Medicine (Neurology) and Associate Professor of Psychiatry, Dartmouth Medical School, Lebanon, New Hampshire

Mark R. Lovell, Ph.D.
Director, Sports Medicine Concussion Program, University of Pittsburgh Medical Center, Pittsburgh, Pennsylvania

Dolores Malaspina, M.D.
Professor of Clinical Psychiatry, New York State Psychiatric Institute, New York, New York

Robert S. Marin, M.D.
Associate Professor of Psychiatry, University of Pittsburgh School of Medicine, Western Psychiatric Institute and Clinic, Pittsburgh, Pennsylvania

Michael F. Martelli, Ph.D.
Clinical Associate Professor, Department of Physical Medicine and Rehabilitation, University of Virginia, Charlottesville, Virginia; Clinical Assistant Professor, Departments of Psychology and Psychiatry, Virginia Commonwealth University Health System, Richmond, Virginia; Concussion Care Centre of Virginia, Ltd., Tree of Life, L.L.C., Glen Allen, Virginia

Jeffrey E. Max, M.B.B.Ch.
Professor, In-Residence, Department of Psychiatry, University of California, San Diego, School of Medicine; Director of Neuropsychiatric Research, Children's Hospital and Health Center, San Diego, California

Thomas W. McAllister, M.D.
Professor of Psychiatry, Department of Psychiatry, Section of Neuropsychiatry, Dartmouth Medical School, Lebanon, New Hampshire

Scott McCullagh, M.D.
Assistant Professor, Neuropsychiatry Program, University of Toronto, Sunnybrook and Women's College Hospital, Toronto, Ontario, Canada

Tracy K. McIntosh, Ph.D.
Professor of Neurosurgery and Director, Traumatic Brain Injury Laboratory, Department of Neurosurgery, University of Pennsylvania School of Medicine, Philadelphia, Pennsylvania

Norman S. Miller, M.D.
Professor of Psychiatry and Medicine, Department of Psychiatry, Michigan State University College of Human Medicine, East Lansing, Michigan

Keith Nicholson, Ph.D.
Comprehensive Pain Program, Toronto Western Hospital, Toronto, Ontario, Canada

Alison Moon O'Shanick, M.S., C.C.C.-S.L.P.
Center for Neurorehabilitation Services, Midlothian, Virginia

Gregory J. O'Shanick, M.D.
Medical Director, Center for Neurorehabilitation Services, Midlothian, Virginia; National Medical Director, Brain Injury Association of America, McLean, Virginia

Mary F. Pelham, Psy.D.
Neuropsychologist, Moss Rehab, Elkins Park Hospital, Elkins Park, Pennsylvania

Kirsten Plehn, Ph.D.
Fellow in Clinical Neuropsychology, Department of Psychiatric Medicine, University of Virginia School of Medicine, Charlottesville, Virginia

Irwin W. Pollack, M.D., M.A.
Emeritus Professor of Psychiatry, University of Medicine and Dentistry of New Jersey–Robert Wood Johnson Medical School, Piscataway, New Jersey

Trevor R. P. Price, M.D.
Private Practice of General Adult Psychiatry, Geriatric Psychiatry, and Neuropsychiatry, Bryn Mawr, Pennsylvania

Vani Rao, M.D.
Assistant Professor, Division of Geriatric Psychiatry and Neuropsychiatry, Department of Psychiatry and Behavioral Sciences, Johns Hopkins University School of Medicine, Baltimore, Maryland

William E. Reynolds, D.D.S., M.P.H.
Public Service Professor, School of Social Welfare, and Clinical Associate Professor, School of Public Health, State University at Albany, Albany, New York

Edwin F. Richter III, M.D.
Associate Clinical Director, Rusk Institute of Rehabilitation Medicine, New York, New York

Robert G. Robinson, M.D.
Paul W. Penningroth Professor and Head of Psychiatry, Roy J. and Lucille A. Carver College of Medicine, University of Iowa, Iowa City, Iowa

Donald C. Rojas, Ph.D.
Associate Professor of Psychiatry, University of Colorado Health Sciences Center, Denver, Colorado

Pamela Rollings, M.D.
Adult Psychiatry, Wellspan Behavioral Health, Division of Neurosciences, Behavioral Health Services, Wellspan Health–Delphic Office, York, Pennsylvania

Nicolas C. Royo, Ph.D.
Postdoctoral Fellow, Traumatic Brain Injury Laboratory, Department of Neurosurgery, University of Pennsylvania School of Medicine, Philadelphia, Pennsylvania

Saori Shimizu, M.D., Ph.D.
Postdoctoral Fellow, Traumatic Brain Injury Laboratory, Department of Neurosurgery, University of Pennsylvania School of Medicine, Philadelphia, Pennsylvania

Arif M. Shoaib, M.D.
Clinical Assistant Professor, Department of Psychiatry, University of Texas Health Science Center at Houston, Houston, Texas

Jonathan M. Silver, M.D.
Clinical Professor of Psychiatry, New York University School of Medicine, New York, New York

Robert I. Simon, M.D.
Clinical Professor of Psychiatry and Director, Program in Psychiatry and Law, Georgetown University School of Medicine, Washington, D.C.

Jennifer Spiro, M.S.
Research Coordinator, Division of Geriatric Psychiatry and Neuropsychiatry, Department of Psychiatry and Behavioral Sciences, Johns Hopkins University School of Medicine, Baltimore, Maryland

Katherine H. Taber, Ph.D.
Research Health Scientist, Research and Education Service Line, Hefner VAMC, Salisbury, North Carolina; Research Fellow, School of Health Information Sciences, University of Texas Health Science Center at Houston, Houston, Texas

Paula T. Trzepacz, M.D.
Clinical Professor of Psychiatry, University of Mississippi School of Medicine, Jackson, Mississippi; Adjunct Professor of Psychiatry, Tufts University School of Medicine, Boston, Massachusetts; Medical Director, U.S. Neurosciences, Lilly Research Laboratories, Indianapolis, Indiana

Gary J. Tucker, M.D.
Emeritus Professor, Department of Psychiatry, University of Washington School of Medicine, Seattle, Washington

Thomas N. Ward, M.D.
Associate Professor of Medicine, Section of Neurology, Dartmouth-Hitchcock Medical Center, Lebanon, New Hampshire

Deborah L. Warden, M.D.
Associate Professor of Neurology and Psychiatry, Uniformed Services University of the Health Sciences, Bethesda, Maryland; National Director, Defense and Veterans Brain Injury Center, Walter Reed Army Medical Center, Washington, D.C.

Stuart C. Yudofsky, M.D.
D.C. and Irene Ellwood Professor and Chairman, Menninger Department of Psychiatry and Behavioral Sciences, Baylor College of Medicine; Chief, Psychiatry Service, The Methodist Hospital, Houston, Texas

Ross Zafonte, D.O.
Professor and Chair, Department of Physical Medicine and Rehabilitation, University of Pittsburgh School of Medicine, Pittsburgh, Pennsylvania

Nathan D. Zasler, M.D.
Clinical Associate Professor, Department of Physical Medicine and Rehabilitation, University of Virginia, Charlottesville, Virginia; Concussion Care Centre of Virginia, Ltd., Pinnacle Rehabilitation, Inc., Tree of Life, L.L.C., Glen Allen, Virginia

Foreword

TRAUMATIC BRAIN INJURY (TBI) is a major public health problem in the United States, yet it is hardly recognized and receives little support or attention from the media and policy makers. As a family, we have lived with the consequences of TBI for many years. We know from firsthand experience the suffering and pain, the frustration and disappointment, and the anger and grief families go through after TBI.

Information is the key to understanding TBI and bringing about the support that people with TBI need. The cost in terms of dollars is staggering, more than $48 billion per year; the costs to families and individuals with TBI are overwhelming.

We decided to write this foreword for the new *Textbook of Traumatic Brain Injury* because it is comprehensive and addresses the key problems of psychosocial and psychological deficits, which are the major sources of disability after TBI. We believe that a major part of the reason TBI is not recognized as a major health problem is the lack of scientific, understandable information on the neuropsychological sequelae of TBI. There has been a lack of appropriate education in this area for psychiatrists, for other mental health professionals, and for those involved in the rehabilitation of persons with TBI. This text goes a long way in fulfilling this educational need.

This text will help in the understanding of the complex nature of TBI and in the education of professionals, who often are not trained in treating TBI. The authors are all well known in the field, and the topics covered provide a rich source of information and material all in one text.

There are 40 chapters divided into seven sections covering everything from epidemiology, aggressive disorders, cognitive changes, fatigue and sleep problems, chronic pain, mood disorders, family systems, and pharmacological therapy to prevention. In other words, this text is so full of data-based information and useful material that it is a must read for everyone involved in the care and treatment of TBI, as well as for those concerned about training and prevention.

We are grateful to Professor Jonathan M. Silver, M.D., Professor Thomas W. McAllister, M.D., and Professor Stuart C. Yudofsky, M.D., for editing and organizing this text.

Sarah and James Brady

Preface

EACH YEAR IN the United States, more than three million people sustain a traumatic brain injury (TBI). In this population, the psychosocial and psychological deficits are the major source of disability to the patient and of stress to the family. Patients may have difficulties in many vital areas of functioning, including family, interpersonal, work, school, and recreational activities. Many have extreme personality changes. Unfortunately, the psychiatric impairments caused by TBI often are unrecognized because of the deficiency of appropriate education in this area for psychiatrists and other mental health professionals. Most clinicians lack experience in treating and evaluating patients with TBI and are, therefore, unaware of the many subtle but disabling symptoms.

In 1994, we edited the book *Neuropsychiatry of Traumatic Brain Injury* as a comprehensive data-based text to serve as a clinically relevant and practical guide to the neuropsychiatric assessment and treatment of patients with TBI. Since that time, there has been an explosion of information in this area. We have greatly expanded our previous book and decided to change the title to *Textbook of Traumatic Brain Injury*. The emphasis remains on the neuropsychiatric aspects of traumatic brain injury, and we recognize that this edition does not address all aspects of acute management, neurosurgical interventions, and rehabilitation interventions. Whereas in the initial volume there was one chapter on neuropsychiatric assessment, that chapter has been divided into separate chapters that cover structural imaging, functional imaging, and electrophysiologic techniques. The first volume also included a chapter on neuropsychological assessment. We realized that readers can find many chapters and texts on this issue. Therefore, we have decided to include a chapter that specifically addresses issues relevant to TBI that arise during neuropsychological assessment. All chapters covering neuropsychiatric disorders have been revised. To address the multiple neuropsychiatric sequelae experienced by our patients, but not encompassed by the usual psychiatric syndromes, we included chapters reviewing apathy, awareness of deficits, fatigue, pain, headaches, balance problems, visual difficulties, and sports injuries. New chapters on social issues and systems of care are included. The full range of treatment modalities is discussed, including a chapter on alternative therapies.

As before, we have endeavored to assemble a group of authors who are authoritative and renowned in their areas. We hope that this book will be used by psychiatrists, neuropsychologists, clinical psychologists, physiatrists, neurologists, and other professionals, including residents and trainees, involved in brain injury rehabilitation.

We have learned from readers' comments in our other books, such as *The American Psychiatric Press Textbook of Neuropsychiatry*, that few people read a textbook from cover to cover. Most read only one or several chapters during any particular period. Consequently, we tried to ensure that each chapter would be complete in itself. As a result, there is some unavoidable overlap among chapters, but we have judged that this was necessary from an information-retrieving standpoint and to prevent readers from having to "jump" from section to section while reading about a particular subject.

This book would not have been possible without the help and support of many people. First, we thank the many chapter authors who labored diligently to produce contributions that we consider unique, scholarly, and enjoyable to read. We spent countless hours on the telephone with the authors reviewing their chapters and providing suggestions, usually agreed on but occasionally disputed. Their continued willingness to answer our calls and letters was greatly appreciated. We also added a distinguished international and multidisciplinary editorial board, which served as a final review for many of the chapters. We appreciate as well the efforts of the staff at American Psychiatric Publishing, Inc.

Last, and most important, we thank our patients with TBI and their families, who have been our greatest source of inspiration to further our knowledge on presentation, assessment, and effective treatment of the psychiatric symptoms and syndromes associated with TBI. We hope that the efforts of all who have participated in this book will result in reducing your suffering and enhancing your recovery.

Jonathan M. Silver, M.D.
Thomas W. McAllister, M.D.
Stuart C. Yudofsky, M.D.

PART I

Epidemiology and Pathophysiology

1

Epidemiology

Jess F. Kraus, M.P.H., Ph.D

Lawrence D. Chu, M.S., M.P.H., Ph.D

THIS CHAPTER SUMMARIZES the epidemiological literature of the last 15–20 years and examines five fundamental characteristics of brain injuries: 1) the occurrence or incidence of new cases of medically attended brain injury in the population, 2) the prevalence of traumatic brain injury (TBI) in the population, 3) the characteristics of high-risk groups and high-risk exposures, 4) the types and severity of brain injuries, and 5) the consequences or results of brain injury at hospital discharge or posthospital follow-up. The literature on brain injury expands annually, but most of the published information is specific to hospitalized patients. Although the clinical literature has inherent value for the practitioner, the epidemiological literature provides a broader and more accurate assessment of the occurrence, characteristics, and consequences of brain injury in the community.

The epidemiological literature on brain injury is limited to a handful of studies conducted primarily in the late 1970s and early 1980s and a few published in the 1990s in the United States (Annegers et al. 1980; Centers for Disease Control and Prevention 1997; Cooper et al. 1983; Gabella et al. 1997; Guerrero et al. 2000; Jagger et al. 1984; Kalsbeek et al. 1980; Klauber et al. 1981; Kraus et al. 1984; Thurman and Guerrero 1999; Thurman et al. 1996; Whitman et al. 1984). In assessing the literature, including studies cited in this chapter, the reader should be mindful that there are many methodological differences among the research papers, making direct comparisons of their results problematic. Studies differ on parameters such as how brain injury is defined, methods of case ascertainment, and how the exposure and outcome information is collected and categorized. A major definition difficulty in many studies is that brain injuries often are subsumed under the term *head injury*. Although it is clear that many of the authors intended to study only neurological trauma, some case definitions (e.g., Annegers et al. 1980; Gabella et al. 1997; Thurman and Guerrero 1999; Whitman et al. 1984) allow the inclusion of nonneurological head injuries such as fractures of the skull or face and damage to soft tissues of the head or face.

Case definitions and inclusion criteria vary from one study to another (Table 1–1). In some studies (e.g., Auer et al. 1980; Bruce et al. 1979; Rimel 1981), the research populations were composed of patients who were referred to neurosurgical intensive care units. In other studies (e.g., Gronwall and Wrightson 1974; Plaut and Gifford 1976), patients treated in emergency departments and released for outpatient observation were included in the study base. And in still other studies (e.g., Jennett et al. 1979), persons with immediate death or death on arrival at the emergency department were excluded. Therefore, it is important to understand case definition and information collection across studies before comparing their results.

Various methods have been used over the past decade to measure amounts of brain damage (see Table 1–1), including a newer proposal to classify severe brain injury using

Some information in this chapter derives from the San Diego County cohort study of brain injury of the early 1980s. Special thanks to David Watson for editorial review. Work on this chapter was supported by the Southern California Injury Prevention Research Center (Centers for Disease Control and Prevention, grant R49: CCR903622).

TABLE 1–1. Case identification, source, and brain injury severity criteria and scoring: selected United States incidence studies

Study	Location and years	Case definition and source	Severity criteria/scoring
Annegers et al. 1980	Olmsted County, Minnesota, 1965–1974	Head injury with evidence of presumed brain involvement (i.e., concussion with LOC, PTA, or neurological signs of brain injury or skull fracture.	1) Fatal (<28 days) 2) Severe: intracranial hematoma, contusion, or LOC >24 hours, or PTA >24 hours 3) Moderate: LOC or PTA 30 minutes to 24 hours, skull fracture or both 4) LOC or PTA <30 minutes without skull fracture
Klauber et al. 1981	San Diego County, California, 1978	ICD A-8 Codes 800, 801, 804, 806, and 850–854 with hospital admission diagnosis or cause of death with skull fracture, LOC, PTA, neurological deficit or seizure (no gunshot wounds).	GCS (3, 4–5, 6–7, 8–15)
Rimel 1981	Central Virginia, 1977–1979	CNS referral patients with significant head injury admitted to neurosurgical service.	GCS (3–5, 6–8, 9–11, 12–15) Severe=≤8; moderate=9–11; mild=12–15
Kraus et al. 1984	San Diego County, California, 1981	Physician-diagnosed physical damage from acute mechanical energy exchange resulting in concussion, hemorrhage, contusion, or laceration of brain.	Modified GCS Severe= ≤8; moderate=9–15 plus hospital stay of 4–8 hours and brain surgery, or abnormal CT, or GCS 9–12; mild=all others, GCS 13–15
Whitman et al. 1984	Chicago area, 1979–1980	Any hospital discharge diagnosis of ICD-9-CM 800–804, 830, 850–854, 873, 920, 959.0. Injury within 7 days before hospital visit and blow to head/face with LOC, or laceration of scalp or forehead.	1) Fatal 2) Severe=intracranial hematoma, LOC/PTA >24 hours contusion 3) Moderate=LOC or PTA 30 minutes to <24 hours 4) Mild=LOC to PTA <30 minutes 5) Trivial=remainder
MacKenzie et al. 1989	Maryland 1986	ICD-9-CM codes 800, 801, 803, 804, 850–854.	ICDMAP—converts ICD codes to AIS scores (Association for the Advancement of Automotive Medicine [1990]) of 1–6
Thurman et al. 1996	Utah 1990–1992	Discharge data from all 40 acute care hospitals using ICD-9-CM codes 800.0–801.9, 803.0–804.9, and 850.0–854.1 in any primary or secondary data fields.	1) Initial GCS: severe=≤8; moderate=9–12; mild=13–15 2) Demonstrated intracranial traumatic lesions 3) Focal abnormalities on neurologic examination
Centers for Disease Control and Prevention 1997	Colorado, Missouri, Oklahoma, Utah, 1990–1992	Discharge data from all state hospitals or health care providers.	No severity data reported.
Gabella et al. 1997	Colorado 1991–1992	Colorado surveillance system of hospitalized and fatal TBI using ICD-9-CM codes 800, 801, 803, 804, and 850–854.	ICDMAP using as many as five ICD discharge diagnoses Severe TBI=fatal or ISS ≥9

TABLE 1–1.   Case identification, source, and brain injury severity criteria and scoring: selected United States incidence studies (continued)

Study	Location and years	Case definition and source	Severity criteria/scoring
Sosin et al. 1996	United States 1991	Self-reported data from U.S. National Health Interview Survey Injury Supplement for mild and moderate brain injury defined as loss of consciousness in previous 12 months.	Severity not evaluated
Thurman and Guerrero 1999	United States 1980–1995	All hospital discharge records with one or more ICD codes of 800.0–801.9, 803.0–804.9, or 850.0–854.1 from the National Hospital Discharge Survey.	ICDMAP used to convert ICD codes to approximate AIS scores: 1–2 = mild; 3 = moderate; 4–6 = severe
Jager et al. 2000	United States 1992–1994	Same ICD codes as Thurman et al. 1996; identified from U.S. National Hospital Ambulatory Medical Care Survey.	Severity not evaluated
Guerrero et al. 2000	United States 1995–1996	All visits to emergency departments with same ICD codes as Thurman et al. 1996; identified from U.S. National Hospital Ambulatory Medical Care Survey.	Severity not evaluated

Note.   LOC = loss of consciousness; PTA = posttraumatic amnesia; GCS = Glasgow Coma Scale (Jennett and Teasdale 1981); ICD = International Classification of Diseases; ICD-9-CM = International Classification of Diseases, 9th Revision, Clinical Modification (World Health Organization 1986); CNS = central nervous system; CT = computed tomography; TBI = traumatic brain injury; AIS = Abbreviated Injury Scale; ISS = Injury Severity Score.

computed tomography (CT) (Marshall et al. 1991). The Glasgow Coma Scale (GCS; Jennett and Teasdale 1981) is commonly used for the initial assessment of severity. The GCS, a clinical prognostic indicator, is an important contribution to standardizing early assessment of the severity of brain injury (Table 1–2). Although its application was intended to be repeated, typical current practice generally consists of a single observation. Herein lies one of the major difficulties in the application of the GCS: not knowing in various studies when the GCS was administered during the early stages of treatment. In some studies, the GCS was administered at the scene of the injury or during emergency transport, whereas in others it was done on arrival at the emergency department or just before hospital admission; in still others, the time of assessment was not reported.

Obviously, GCS results during the hospital course change according to patient improvement or deterioration. For proper comparison of research findings, the GCS should be administered at approximately the same time postinjury. Assessment on arrival at the emergency department is recommended.

An inherent weakness of the GCS is its limited relevance to some patients with brain injuries. The GCS is

TABLE 1–2.   Glasgow Coma Scale

Eye opening (E)	Spontaneous	4
	To speech	3
	To pain	2
	Nil	1
Best motor response (M)	Obeys	6
	Localizes	5
	Withdrawn	4
	Abnormal flexion	3
	Extensor response	2
	Nil	1
Verbal response (V)	Oriented	5
	Confused conversation	4
	Inappropriate words	3
	Incomprehensible sounds	2
	Nil	1

Coma score (E + M + V) = 3–15

Source.   Adapted from Jennett B, Teasdale G: *Management of Head Injuries*. Philadelphia, PA, FA Davis, 1981.

difficult or impossible to apply to young children, patients with significant facial swelling from blunt trauma, patients under the influence of alcohol or other substances, and patients who are not able to respond to the verbal component because of language differences or an inability to comprehend. The current emergency department practice of immediate intubation or sedation may further invalidate (or restrict) GCS measurements. Regardless of these restrictions, the GCS remains one of the most consistently used measures of brain injury severity.

Epidemiological studies of patients with brain injuries are infrequently undertaken, and in the past 10 years, more reliance has been placed on administrative data sets to estimate the incidence and features of persons with TBI. Such data sources include the U.S. National Health Interview Survey (NHIS), U.S. National Hospital Ambulatory Medical Care Survey (NHAMCS), U.S. National Hospital Discharge Survey (NHDS), and equivalent data sets from individual states and groups of states (see Table 1–1).

In discussing the nature and severity of injury, we have drawn some information from a large brain injury cohort study conducted in San Diego County, California, during the early 1980s (Kraus et al. 1984). For the purposes of this chapter, we focus on the specifics of diagnosis, considering skull fracture status as an important confounding factor. In addition, we provide basic information on the relationship between demographic characteristics such as age, sex, and socioeconomic status (SES) and the severity and type of brain injury. Finally, we develop a predictive model for outcome at hospital discharge.

All epidemiological studies involving people hospitalized with brain injury indicate that a large majority of patients treated in emergency departments and admitted to hospitals (for observation or treatment) have sustained what has been termed *mild traumatic brain injury* (MTBI)—that is, one with a GCS score of 13–15. Because this injury occurs so often and the information on the injuries and outcomes is so incomplete, a Consequences of Mild TBI section addressing the nature of the available data and selected aggregate findings on outcome parameters has been included toward the end of this chapter.

Estimates of Occurrence of Brain Injury

Incidence

Data summarized in Figure 1–1 show that brain injury occurrence rates range from a low of 92 per 100,000 population in seven states (Thurman and Guerrero 1999) to a high of 618 per 100,000 population in a United States national survey (Sosin et al. 1996). Caution must be taken

in interpreting these findings because brain injury definitions, criteria for diagnoses, and sources were not the same in all studies (see Table 1–1). In addition, the precision of population-at-risk estimates varied considerably (i.e., some rates were based on catchment area population estimates in noncensus years).

Nevertheless, a current average rate of fatal plus nonfatal hospitalized brain injuries reported in all United States studies is approximately 150 per 100,000 population per year. If the highest and lowest estimates are excluded from consideration, the estimated rate is approximately 120 per 100,000 per year, which is the estimate used in this chapter for purposes of disability estimation.

Brain Injury Death and Death Rates

In 2001, 157,078 people died from acute traumatic injury—approximately 6.5% of all deaths in the United States (Centers for Disease Control and Prevention 2002). The exact percentage of deaths involving significant brain injury is not precisely known, but data from Olmsted County, Minnesota (Annegers et al. 1980), and San Diego County, California (Kraus et al. 1984), suggest that approximately 50% are caused by trauma to the brain. National Center for Health Statistics multiple-cause-of-death data indicate that an average of approximately 28% of all injury deaths involve significant brain trauma (Sosin et al. 1995). This percentage is probably incorrect because, as the investigators pointed out, the case-finding process relied on a limited set of specific injury diagnoses. Furthermore, the actual death certificates were not examined—a crucial problem when "massive multiple trauma" is recorded on the death certificate but specific body locations and types of trauma are not recorded. Sosin et al. (1989) reported a possible underestimate in the actual proportion of fatal brain injury of 23%–44%.

The reported brain injury fatality rate varies from 14 to 30 per 100,000 population per year (Figure 1–2). The range in rates probably reflects a lack of specificity of diagnosis on some death certificates.

Nonfatal Brain Injury

National estimates of nonfatal brain injury for the United States have been derived from the National Health Interview Survey (NHIS; Sosin et al. 1996), the National Hospital Ambulatory Medical Care Survey (NHAMCS; Jager et al. 2000), the National Hospital Discharge Survey (NHDS; Thurman and Guerrero 1999), and the National Center for Injury Prevention and Control (NCIPC; Thurman et al. 1999). The NHIS reported that approxi-

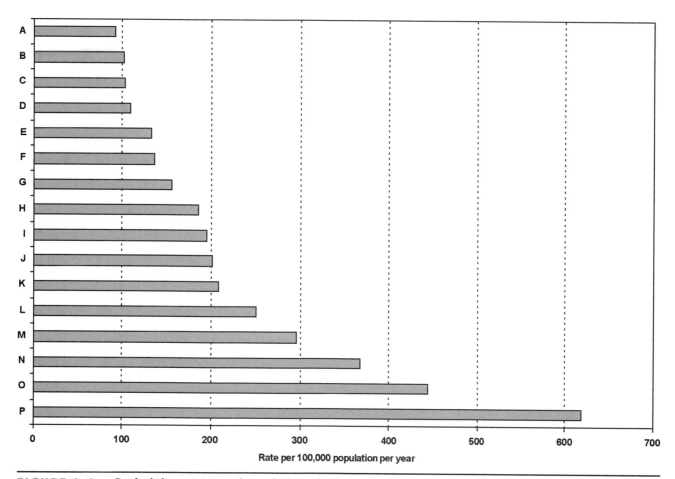

FIGURE 1–1. **Brain injury rates: selected United States studies.**

A=United States estimate 1980–1995 (Thurman and Guerrero 1999); *B*=Colorado 1991–1992 (Gabella et al. 1997); *C*=Colorado, Missouri, Oklahoma, Utah 1990–1992 (Centers for Disease Control and Prevention 1997); *D*=Utah 1990–1992 (Thurman et al. 1996); *E*=Maryland 1986 (MacKenzie et al. 1989); *F*=United States estimate 1981 (Fife 1987); *G*=Rhode Island 1979–1980 (Fife et al. 1986); *H*=San Diego County, CA, 1981 (Kraus et al. 1986); *I*=Olmsted County, MN, 1965–1974 (Annegers et al. 1980); *J*=United States estimate 1974 (Kalsbeek et al. 1980); *K*=Virginia 1978 (Jagger et al. 1984); *L*=Bronx, NY, 1980–1981 (Cooper et al. 1983); *M*=San Diego County, CA, 1978 (Klauber et al. 1981); *N*=Chicago area 1979–1980 (Whitman et al. 1984); *O*=United States estimate 1992–1994 (Jager et al. 2000); *P*=United States estimate 1991 (Sosin et al. 1996).

mately 1.5 million head injuries occur per year (Sosin et al. 1996). However, this estimate includes self-reported concussions and skull fractures, as well as a mixture of different types of intracranial injuries requiring professional medical care, some with and some without neurological trauma. The extent of emergency department and non–emergency department diagnosis and treatment of brain injury is unknown. The Centers for Disease Control and Prevention (CDC) reported to Congress in 1999 that more than 5 million Americans, or 2% of the nation's population, were living with TBI-related disabilities (Thurman et al. 1999).

A large number of TBI cases are caused by sports and physical activity. From July 2000 to June 2001, an estimated 350,000 persons were treated in emergency departments for sports- and recreation-related head inju-

ries; of these persons, 200,000 were diagnosed with a brain injury (Gotsch et al. 2002). Countless sports-related TBIs go unreported because the majority are MTBI cases—for example, concussions without loss of consciousness (Collins et al. 1999). Identification of these cases is vital for proper treatment and prevention of long-term deleterious effects.

On a reexamination of the NHIS database for 1985–1986, Fife (1987) concluded that only 16% of all head injuries resulted in an admission to a hospital. Hence, only one of six people with head (not necessarily brain) injury require hospitalization. As expected, findings from NHIS, NHAMCS, and NHDS vary widely (see Figure 1–1) because the data sources are so different from one another.

An estimate derived from published sources (summarized in Figure 1–3 and Table 1–3) suggests that approxi-

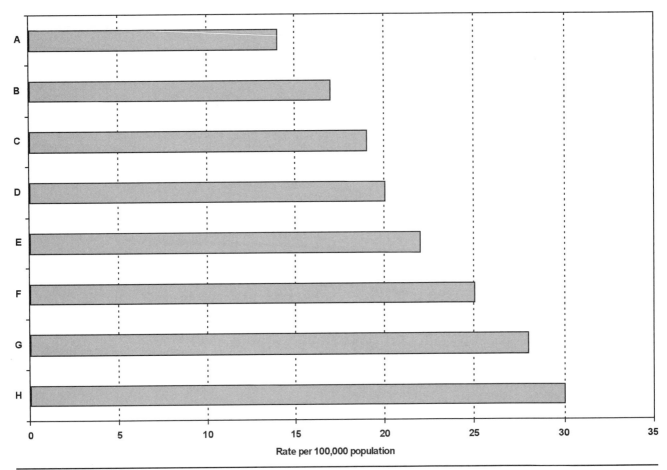

FIGURE 1–2.   Brain injury fatality rates: selected United States studies.

A=Virginia 1978 (Jagger et al. 1984); *B*=United States estimate 1981 (Fife 1987); *C*=United States estimate 1992 (Sosin et al. 1995); *D*=Olmsted County, MN, 1965–1974 (Annegers et al. 1980); *E*=San Diego County, CA, 1978 (Klauber et al. 1981); *F*=Chicago area 1979–1980 (Whitman et al. 1984); *G*=Bronx, NY, 1980–1981 (Cooper et al. 1983); *H*=San Diego County, CA, 1981 (Kraus et al. 1984).

mately 234,000 people were discharged from hospitals in the United States in 1998 with a brain injury diagnosis; based on 1998 census estimates of 270 million persons, a hospital admission rate of approximately 87 per 100,000 population per year is deduced. The hospital discharge rate is useful for estimating the annual disability rate from injury (discussed later in Estimation of Number of New Disabilities). The difference in estimates obtained using average incidence values in aggregate United States studies versus data from hospital discharges or visits is because of definitional variation. The actual United States incidence rate is presumed, therefore, to range from 100 to 150 per 100,000 population per year.

The relative importance of brain injury discharge frequencies is illustrated in Table 1–3. As seen, the brain injury discharge rate is the third highest compared with other major central nervous system (CNS) diagnoses. The hospital discharge count (or rate) shown in Figure 1–3 and Table 1–3 is not the true figure, because not all cases

are found within the International Classification of Diseases discharge diagnoses used to identify brain injury cases (see Table 1–1). The purpose of gathering information on brain injury occurrence rates is threefold: to monitor changes in incidence in the population, to evaluate the effects of specific countermeasures, and to identify high- (or low-) risk groups and exposure circumstances.

Characteristics of High-Risk Groups

Age

All studies of brain injury occurrence in the United States show that people ages 15–24 years are at the highest risk. Patterns in age-specific rates (Figure 1–4) illustrate at least two high-risk age groups: those ages 15–24 years and those older than age 64 years. It is noteworthy that rates for people younger than age 10 years (and particularly

TABLE 1–3. Frequency of selected first-listed diagnoses for inpatients discharged from short-stay, nonfederal hospitals, 1998

ICD-9-CM code[a]	Diagnosis	Number of discharges (× 1000)	Discharge rate (per 100,000 population)
Multiple[b]	Brain injury	234	86.6
191	Malignant neoplasm of brain	32	11.8
295	Schizophrenic disorders	256	94.7
331	Cerebral degeneration (nonchildhood)	64	23.7
331.0	Alzheimer's disease	43	15.9
332	Parkinson's disease	26	9.6
340	Multiple sclerosis	26	9.6
345	Epilepsy	52	19.2
346	Migraine	43	15.9
430	Subarachnoid hemorrhage	19	7.0
431, 432	Intracerebral and intracranial hemorrhage	87	32.2
434	Occlusion of cerebral arteries	309	114.3
436, 437	Other cerebrovascular disease	195	72.2

Note. Brain injuries include *any* listed diagnoses.
[a]International Classification of Diseases, 9th Revision, Clinical Modification (ICD-9-CM; World Health Organization 1986).
[b]Includes ICD-9-CM codes 800, 801, 803, 804, 850, 851, 852, 853, 854, 905, 907. These codes may not include all admissions with brain injuries but include diagnoses such as skull fracture with and without concussion, contusion, or hemorrhage and late effects of skull fracture or intracranial injury.
Source. Reprinted from Popovic JR, Kozak LJ: "National Hospital Discharge Survey: Annual Summary, 1998." *Vital and Health Statistics* 13:1–194, 2000. Used with permission.

those younger than age 5 years) are high in some studies reporting age-specific data. The age-related risk distribution reflects differences in exposure, particularly to motor vehicle crashes.

Gender

All incidence reports published worldwide indicate that brain injuries are far more frequent among men than women, and United States studies have found a rate ratio of approximately 1.6–2.8 (Figure 1–5). Variation in rate ratios cannot be attributed solely to reporting differences. The differences in rate ratios may reflect different exposure levels. For example, there may be a higher proportion of injuries connected with motor vehicle crashes (which involve more males) as compared with injuries connected with falls in the home (which involve more females).

Race or Ethnicity

Some studies show higher brain injury incidence in nonwhites compared with whites, but there is justifiable concern over the quality of the data used to derive the rates. Because hospital reporting practices vary widely in recording ethni-

city or race in medical records, racial or ethnic differences in brain injury rates have yet to be determined accurately.

Alcohol

The positive association between blood alcohol concentration (BAC) and risk of injury is well established for all external causes of injuries, including motor vehicle crashes, general aviation crashes, drownings, and violence (Smith and Kraus 1988). Less studied is the role of alcohol and the outcome of specific kinds and anatomical locations of injuries such as CNS trauma and burns. Although animal studies demonstrate a variety of physiological effects of alcohol on CNS injuries, human data are unequivocal. In one study (Kraus et al. 1989), 56% of adults with a brain injury diagnosis had a positive BAC test result. It is noteworthy that 49% of those adults tested had a BAC that was at or above the legal level (0.10%). The prevalence of a positive BAC varied by severity of brain injury; the highest prevalence was among those with MTBI compared with those with moderate or severe brain injury (71% vs. 49%, respectively). However, selection bias may occur in emergency department BAC testing of injured people with different severities or types

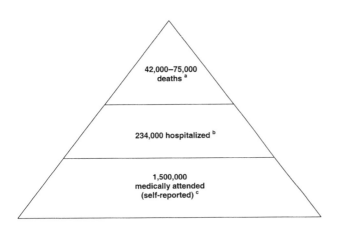

FIGURE 1–3. **Estimated annual brain injury frequency.**

[a]*Source.* Sosin et al. (1995) and Kraus et al. (1994).
[b]*Source.* National Hospital Discharge Survey, 1995–1996 (Thurman and Guerrero 1999).
[c]*Source.* National Health Interview Survey, 1991 (Sosin et al. 1996).

of injuries or different inherent sociodemographic or external-cause features. For example, blood testing was less frequent for males, young adults, people with mild brain injuries, and those injured from falls. Despite this potential bias, Kraus et al. (1989) found that the BAC level was positively associated with physician-diagnosed neurological impairment and length of hospitalization.

Recurrent TBI

Annegers and associates (1980) were the first to measure the relative risk (RR) of recurrent TBI in their epidemiological study of head injuries in Olmsted County, Minnesota. They estimated the RR of a second TBI among those with an earlier TBI at approximately 2.8–3.0 times that of the general noninjured population. The RR of recurrent TBI given an initial head injury increased with age, and the RR of a third TBI given a second head injury was between 7.8 and 9.3 times that of an initial head injury in the population. Salcido and Costich (1992) reviewed the published

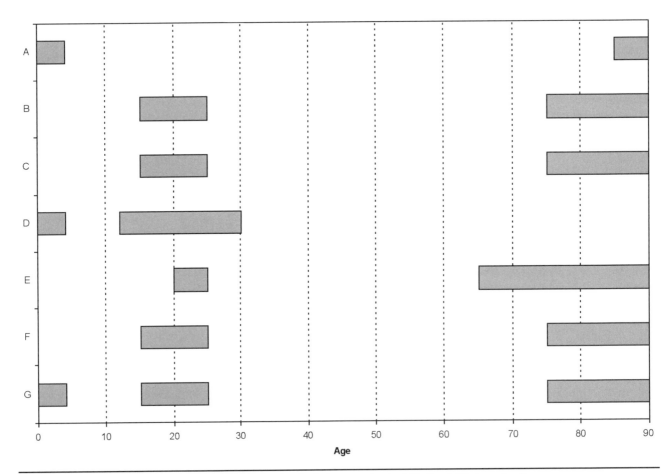

FIGURE 1–4. **Peak age groups at risk for brain injury: selected United States studies.**

A=United States estimate 1992–1994 (Jager et al. 2000); *B*=United States estimate 1991 (Sosin et al. 1996); *C*=San Diego County, CA, 1981 (Kraus et al. 1986); *D*=Virginia 1977–1979 (Rimel 1981); *E*=Colorado 1991–1992 (Gabella et al. 1997); *F*=Colorado, Missouri, Oklahoma, Utah 1990–1992 (Centers for Disease Control and Prevention 1997); *G*=Utah 1990–1992 (Thurman et al. 1996).

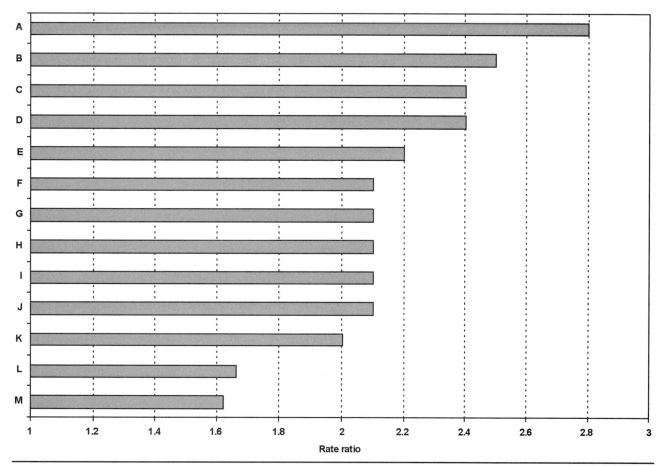

FIGURE 1–5. Male/female brain injury rate ratios: selected United States studies.

A=Virginia 1978 (Jagger et al. 1984); *B*=Rhode Island 1979–1980 (Fife et al. 1986); *C*=San Diego County, CA, 1981 (Kraus et al. 1986); *D*=Maryland 1986 (MacKenzie et al. 1989); *E*=United States estimate 1974 (Kalsbeek et al. 1980); *F*=Bronx, NY, 1980–1981 (Cooper et al. 1983); *G*=Chicago area 1979–1980 (Whitman et al. 1984); *H*=Colorado 1991–1992 (Gabella et al. 1997); *I*=Colorado, Missouri, Oklahoma, Utah 1990–1992 (Centers for Disease Control and Prevention 1997); *J*=Utah 1990–1992 (Thurman et al. 1996); *K*=Olmsted County, MN, 1965–1974 (Annegers et al. 1980); *L*=United States estimate 1992–1994 (Jager et al. 2000); *M*=United States estimate 1991 (Sosin et al. 1996).

literature on recurrent TBI in 1992 and concluded that repetitive injury may be due to three possible causes: repeated exposure to an external or environmental factor (e.g., alcohol abuse), some internal factor that gives rise to increased vulnerability, or a combination of external or environmental factors and internal vulnerability. The literature has established a strong association between recurrent TBI and alcohol abuse (Kreutzer et al. 1990; Ruff et al. 1990). Effective interventions after TBI must incorporate alcohol cessation even for those with the less serious forms of injury.

Recurrent TBI has been the subject of many reports in the area of head injury in sports. Case reports (Cantu and Voy 1995; Kelly et al. 1991; Saunders and Harbaugh 1984) and case series studies (Jordan and Zimmerman 1990) have highlighted the need to carefully mentor the concussed player before permitting his or her return to sporting exposures. There is no evidence that repeated brain injuries in sports lead to unusual risk of TBI in non-sports–associated exposures.

Socioeconomic Status

The NHIS for 1985–1987 (Collins 1990) showed that the estimated average annual number of injuries and the rates per 100 people per year are highest in families at the lowest income levels. This finding was also observed by Kraus et al. (1986) in San Diego County, California; by Whitman et al. (1984) in two socioeconomically different communities in Chicago; and by Sosin et al. (1996) in the United States. In the Kraus et al. (1986) study, the surrogate for individual SES was median family income per census tract, and, in the report by Sosin et al. (1996), family income was the variable used for SES. Multivariate analysis by Kraus et al. (1986)

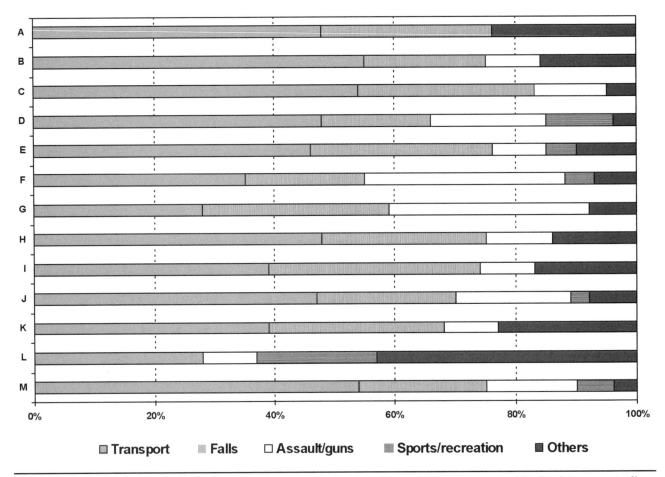

Transport **Falls** **Assault/guns** **Sports/recreation** **Others**

FIGURE 1–6.   **Percentage distribution of brain injuries by external cause: selected United States studies.**
A=United States estimate 1974 (Kalsbeek et al. 1980); *B*=Virginia 1978 (Jagger et al. 1984); *C*=San Diego County, CA, 1978 (Klauber et al. 1981); *D*=San Diego County, CA, 1981 (Kraus et al. 1984); *E*=Olmsted County, MN, 1965–1974 (Annegers et al. 1980); *F*=Chicago area 1979–1980 (Whitman et al. 1984); *G*=Bronx, NY, 1980–1981 (Cooper et al. 1983); *H*=Maryland 1986 (MacKenzie et al. 1989); *I*=Rhode Island 1979–1980 (Fife et al. 1986); *J*=Colorado, Missouri, Oklahoma, Utah 1990–1992 (Centers for Disease Control and Prevention 1997); *K*=United States estimate 1992–1994 (Jager et al. 2000); *L*=United States estimate 1991 (Sosin et al. 1996); *M*=Utah 1990–1992 (Thurman et al. 1996).

and Sosin et al. (1996) suggested that using race and/or ethnicity as a proxy for SES may be inappropriate. Other aspects of exposure nested within the socioeconomic environment should be explored, such as low income and living alone (Sosin et al. 1996).

Characteristics of High-Risk Exposures

Published studies use inconsistent classifications of external cause of injury, which restricts any meta-analysis of cause of brain injury. Broad groupings of external causes (Figure 1–6) can be used to make general statements about the nature of the exposures associated with brain injury.

Despite the limitations of the categorization of external cause, available data suggest that the most frequent type of exposure associated with fatal and nonfatal brain injury is transport. Transport includes automobiles, bicycles, motorcycles, aircraft, watercraft, and others (e.g., farm equipment). The most common transport-related external cause is motor vehicle crashes (Figure 1–7).

Falls are the second leading cause of brain injury and are associated most frequently with older age (see Figure 1–6). Assault-related brain injury, most frequently involving the use of firearms, is an important factor in penetrating brain injuries (Centers for Disease Control and Prevention 1997; Cooper et al. 1983; Kraus et al. 1984; Sosin et al. 1995; Thurman et al. 1996; Whitman et al. 1984). It is not possible to identify brain injuries related to sports or recreation in some studies because they have been grouped into an "other" category. In at least four studies (Annegers et al. 1980; Kraus et al. 1984; Sosin et al. 1996; Whitman et al. 1984), sports were identified as a significant exposure for brain injury. A

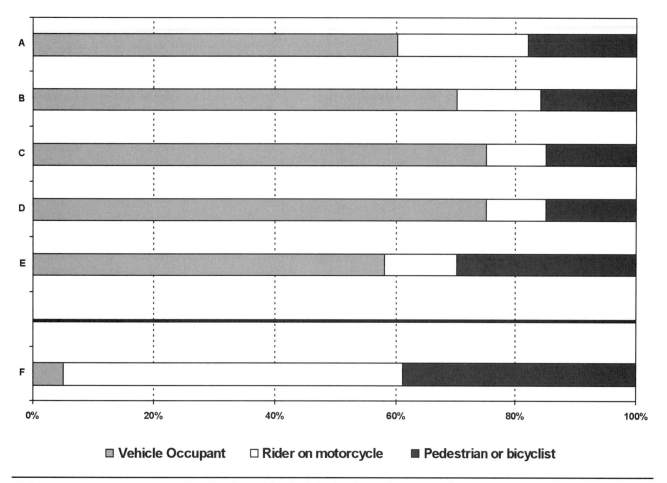

FIGURE 1-7. Percentage distribution of brain injuries for subcauses of motor vehicle–related exposures: selected studies.

A=San Diego County, CA, 1981 (Kraus et al. 1986); *B*=San Diego County, CA, 1978 (Klauber et al. 1981); *C*=Olmsted County, MN, 1965–1974 (Annegers et al. 1980); *D*=Virginia 1978 (Jagger et al. 1984); *E*=Seattle 1981 (Gale et al. 1983); *F*=Taiwan 1977–1987 (Lee et al. 1990).

major caveat in this discussion is that in some studies all bicycle-related exposures have been classified as transportation related. Kraus et al. (1987) found that approximately two-thirds of the brain injuries related to bicycles are not because of collisions with motor vehicles. The dominant form of exposure in motor vehicle crashes is as an occupant of a road vehicle. Classification difficulties across studies do not allow for characterization of occupant location (i.e., driver vs. passenger), but it is possible to categorize motor vehicle–related exposures into three general groups: vehicle occupants, riders on motorcycles, and pedestrians or bicyclists. Brain injuries are most frequent in the vehicle occupants group. Motorcyclists also frequently sustain brain injuries. There are no data on the actual number of people who are occupants or riders on motorcycles; hence, data on specific rates of occurrence cannot be derived. Special note should be made of the report from Taiwan (Lee et al. 1990), where motorcyclists, including scooter

riders, form the largest portion of the motor vehicle–related brain injury problem in the population.

Severity and the Types of Brain Injury

All studies published before 1996 showed that the greatest proportion of brain injuries were "mild" (i.e., generally, a GCS score of 13–15). The distribution of the severity of brain injury, as assessed by the GCS, is shown in Figure 1–8. In terms of emergency department visits and hospital admissions, the majority of brain injuries in people who were hospitalized over the past 25 years were of mild severity. Among those people admitted to a hospital alive, the severity distribution is approximately 80% mild (GCS score of 13–15), 10% moderate (GCS score of 9–12), and 10% severe (GCS score of 8 or less). The lower proportion of mild brain injuries (and higher proportion of moderate and severe injuries) found in the Virginia

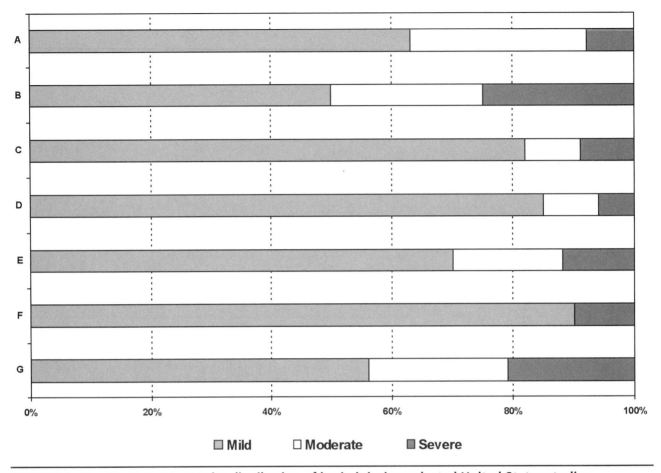

FIGURE 1–8.   Percentage severity distribution of brain injuries: selected United States studies.

A=Olmsted County, MN, 1965–1974 (Annegers et al. 1980); *B*=Virginia 1978 (Jagger et al. 1984); *C*=San Diego County, CA, 1981 (Kraus et al. 1986); *D*=Chicago area 1979–1980 (Whitman et al. 1984); *E*=Maryland 1986 (MacKenzie et al. 1989); *F*=San Diego County, CA, 1978 (Klauber et al. 1981); *G*=United States estimate 1980–1995 (Thurman and Guerrero 1999).

study (Jagger et al. 1984) reflects the nature of the referral institution (i.e., serious injuries were more likely to be referred to the University of Virginia Hospital from the surrounding catchment area).

Reports published over the past 5–7 years show that the severity of TBI in hospitalized patients is more equally divided among mild, moderate, and severe categories of injury (Thurman and Guerrero 1999; Thurman et al. 1996). Changes in hospital admission practices may be the reason underlying the dramatic decline in proportions of patients admitted with MTBI. The effect of these practices in short- or long-term outcomes is unknown and should be the focus of current research.

Hospital Discharges and Diagnoses

Information on people discharged from short-stay non-federal hospitals in the United States in 1998 is available

through the NHDS (Popovic and Kozak 2000). This data source provides information on any listed diagnosis of brain injury coded according to the International Classification of Diseases, 9th Revision, Clinical Modification (ICD-9-CM; World Health Organization 1986). Data on discharge rates with any listed brain injury diagnosis are summarized in Figures 1–9 and 1–10. The rate for those discharged with a brain injury from short-stay hospitals during 1998 was approximately 87 per 100,000 population. The rate for males was twice as high as that for females. Figure 1–10 shows that most people discharged from a hospital with a brain injury were diagnosed as having a hemorrhage, contusion, or laceration without fracture of the skull. Approximately 18% of the discharges involved "other intracranial injury" without skull fracture, and intracranial injury with fracture represented approximately 22% of all hospital discharges.

The only age-specific national data on hospital discharges are grouped into four generally heterogeneous age

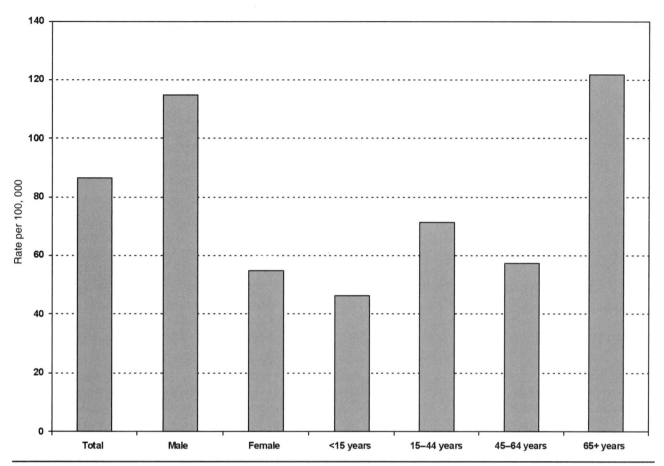

FIGURE 1–9. Sex- and age-specific (in years) brain injury hospital discharges per 100,000 population: United States 1998. All listed diagnoses.

Source. Reprinted from Popovic JR, Kozak LJ: "National Hospital Discharge Survey: Annual Summary, 1998." *Vital and Health Statistics* 13:1–194, 2000. Used with permission.

groups (see Figure 1–9). Those younger than age 15 years (showing the lowest discharge rates in Figure 1–9) include infants, toddlers, young children, and adolescents; each group has various types of exposures. The 15- to 44-year-old group combines people in their late 20s, 30s, and early 40s with those who are generally at highest risk of brain injury (i.e., those ages 15–24 years), thus dramatically reducing the incidence shown in Figure 1–9 for this larger age range. It should be noted that the aggregate age-specific injury incidence rates (reported in Figure 1–4) are considerably higher than the age-specific discharge rates from the NHDS (see Figure 1–9). One possible explanation for the high brain injury rate among hospital discharges for infants is "birth trauma," a diagnosis that is excluded from most brain injury databases. Patients who died at the scene of injury, during emergency transport, or in the emergency facility are not included in the estimates.

In evaluating these data, it should be noted that NHDS data are based on *discharges* from short-stay hospitals, but some injured people may have been admitted to multiple hospitals or to the same hospital on multiple occasions for

the same injury. Hence, the discharge does not represent a mutually exclusive occurrence, and a patient who had one or more admissions to one or more hospitals during the observation period is counted multiple times. Independent information from our experience suggests that multiple hospital admissions are relatively common, particularly in today's climate of different payment requirements for public versus private institutions.

Types of Brain Lesions

Although the literature is replete with reports describing brain trauma, each report typically is based on a clinical series from a single institution. Few epidemiological studies have addressed the question of the nature and severity of brain lesions, and for this purpose, specific data were retrieved from the 1981 San Diego County cohort study (Kraus et al. 1984). In this study, clinical information was uniformly recorded from the physician's notes in the medical record. The reader should be aware that these

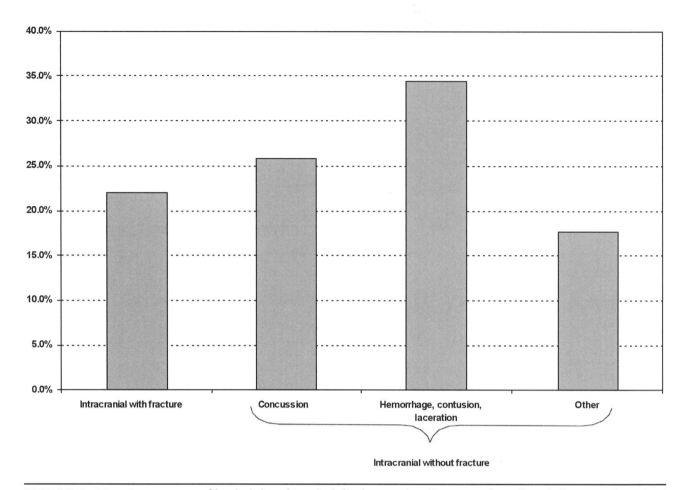

FIGURE 1–10. Percentage of brain injury hospital discharges by diagnoses (any listed diagnoses): United States 1998. All listed diagnoses.

Source.   Reprinted from Popovic JR, Kozak LJ: "National Hospital Discharge Survey: Annual Summary, 1998." *Vital and Health Statistics* 13:1–194, 2000. Used with permission.

data refer to a single time period from all hospitals in the region and, hence, are population based. Also, the data reported in Figure 1–11 represent only adults age 15 years and older. The information on pediatric brain injury can be found elsewhere (Kraus et al. 1990).

The distribution of types of fractures associated with focal and diffuse lesions of the brain is shown in Figure 1–11. In all four major brain lesion categories, at least one-half of the cases do not have a concurrent fracture of the skull. Fracture is much less common among patients with concussion or other cranial injury than among those with contusion, laceration, or hemorrhage.

ICD-9-CM allows for a classification of "other intracranial injury." This nosological category is nonspecific and serves as a catch-all for other and unspecified brain injuries. This coding must be refined to enhance the specificity of the nature of the brain lesion, which will lead to better epidemiological studies. Our clinical colleagues may need to record more specific detail on the nature of the lesions to provide hospital medical record reviewers

and coders with sufficient information to accurately code the injuries.

Consequences of Brain Injury

Immediate Outcomes: Case Fatality Rates

One immediate outcome after brain injury is death. Whereas the fatality rates (see Figure 1–2) provide an idea of the level or magnitude of severity in the general population, the case fatality rates after hospital admission measure the immediate gross consequences of the trauma.

Case fatality data are available from eight United States population-based incidence studies and one estimate based on the NHDS for 1994–1995 (Figure 1–12). Case fatality rates range from approximately 3 per 100 hospitalized cases in Rhode Island (Fife et al. 1986) to approximately 8 per 100 hospitalized cases in the Bronx, New York (Cooper et al. 1983). However, these case fatal-

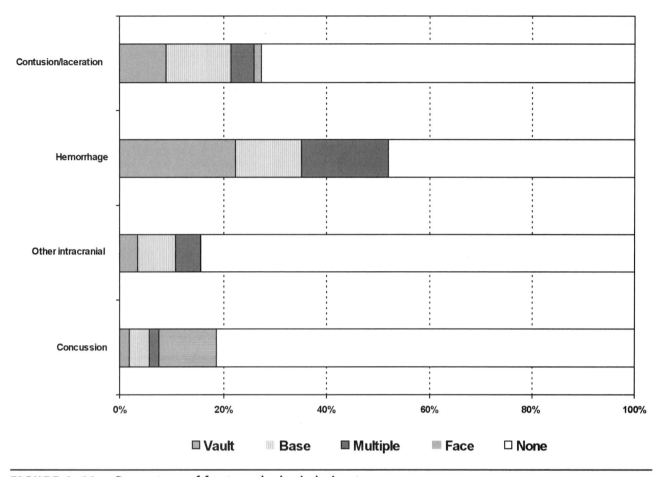

FIGURE 1–11. **Percentage of fractures by brain lesion type.**

ity rates were not severity adjusted, which precludes adequate comparison across studies. Hospitals that admit a high proportion of patients with severe or moderate brain injury would be expected to have higher case fatality rates compared with those admitting a large proportion of patients with MTBI, who sustain fewer deaths. Figure 1–12 also shows a case fatality rate from a report from Taiwan (Lee et al. 1990). This high case fatality rate illustrates further the difficulties in comparing rates across study centers where severity mixes in patient populations have not been standardized. For this reason, it is not appropriate to suggest that differences in outcome after hospitalization relate to differences in quality of care.

Measurement of Long-Term Consequences

One widely used scale in assessing outcome of acute brain injury is the Glasgow Outcome Scale (GOS; Jennett and Teasdale 1981). The GOS is a crude indicator of medical (neurological) complications or residual effects at time of discharge from the primary treatment center. The major classifications of the GOS are 1) death, 2) persistent vegetative state (i.e., no cerebral cortical function as judged

behaviorally), 3) severe disability (conscious but dependent on 24-hour care), 4) moderate disability (disabled but capable of independent care), and 5) good recovery (mild impairment with persistent sequelae but able to participate in a normal social life).

The major difficulty with the GOS is the inability to properly classify patients because of the lack of specific objective criteria that separate severe from moderate or moderate from good recovery. Good recovery does not mean, nor was it intended to mean, complete recovery. Hence, it is important to assess GOS findings with some degree of caution.

Consequences of Mild TBI

Understanding the outcomes of MTBI is complicated by the many differences among research investigations. Study differences include how the sample was identified and drawn, how MTBI was defined, the length of follow-up, and what outcome measures were used. As shown in Figures 1–13 and 1–14, in research reports from 1984 to early 1991, definitions for MTBI in children, adolescents, and adults encompassed broad ranges of the length of loss of consciousness (from none to 60 minutes) and the GCS scores (from 15

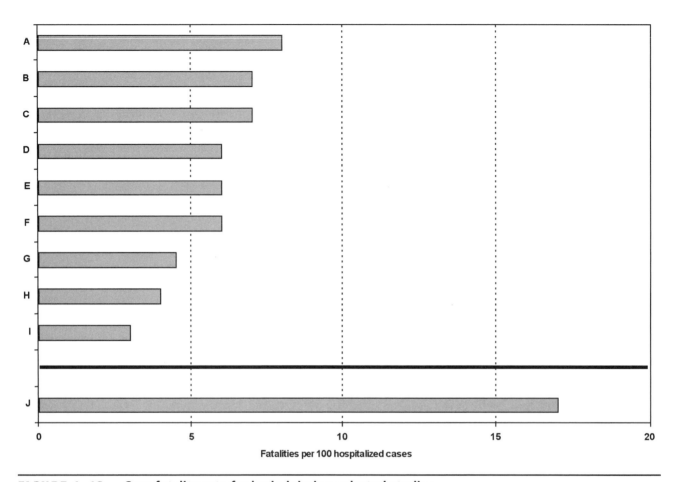

Fatalities per 100 hospitalized cases

FIGURE 1–12. **Case fatality rate for brain injuries: selected studies.**

A=Bronx, NY, 1980–1981 (Cooper et al. 1983); *B*=Virginia 1978 (Jagger et al. 1984); *C*=Utah 1990–1992 (Thurman et al. 1996); *D*=San Diego County, CA, 1981 (Kraus et al. 1986); *E*=Maryland 1986 (MacKenzie et al. 1989); *F*=Colorado, Missouri, Oklahoma, Utah 1990–1992 (Centers for Disease Control and Prevention 1997); *G*=United States estimate 1980–1995 (Thurman and Guerrero 1999); *H*=San Diego County, CA, 1978 (Klauber et al. 1981); *I*=Rhode Island 1979–1980 (Fife et al. 1986); *J*=Taiwan 1977–1987 (Lee et al. 1990) (case series).

only to a range of 8–15). Injury severity varied considerably across these studies of "mild" brain injury. The variation is regrettable, given that the severity of the injury appears to be a primary factor in long-term recovery. It is hoped that the CDC National Center for Injury Prevention and Control Expert Working Group on Mild Traumatic Brain Injury will arrive at a consensus definition of MTBI for surveillance and clinical purposes.

Evidence on the frequency and nature of negative cognitive outcomes after MTBI is far from clear. As shown in Figure 1–15, most reports have assessed motor skills or a combination of learning and motor skills. A review of 13 outcome studies (Bassett and Slater 1990; Bawden et al. 1985; Costeff et al. 1988; Dennis and Barnes 1990; Ewing-Cobbs et al. 1985, 1987; Gulbrandson 1984; Hannay and Levin 1988; Jordan and Murdoch 1990; Jordan et al. 1988; Levin et al. 1987, 1988; Tompkins et al. 1990) indicated that children with MTBI

scored worse than their noninjured counterparts on measures of general intelligence, language, and a combination of learning and motor skills. In contrast, most studies indicated that adults with MTBI did not differ from noninjured individuals on measures of motor and spatial skills. Also, results were not consistent for mental functioning among skills as diverse as language, learning and memory, motor skills, and spatial skills. Furthermore, these studies are plagued by a common threat to validity—all assessments were made postinjury, so the groups may have differed on the variables of interest before the brain injury occurred. In addition, preinjury information on inherent host factors (e.g., behavior) compromise the ability to ascertain postinjury changes in function.

The current scientific literature contains studies with small numbers of subjects, retrospective study designs, and inadequate control or comparison groups. Small numbers of study subjects and many different outcome

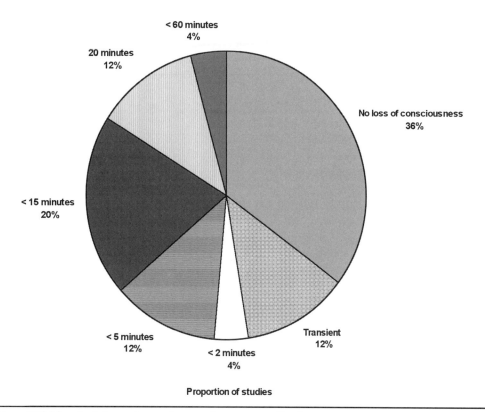

FIGURE 1–13. Mild brain injury: loss of consciousness criterion.

measures compromise the researcher's ability to detect differences in risks or outcomes. Almost no studies were designed to adequately identify differences between people who had sustained MTBI and those who had not. Given that there is not a sufficient body of literature from which to draw conclusions with confidence about the negative consequences of MTBI, the task of future research is to use sufficiently sophisticated research methods to detect these consequences if they exist. It is hoped that the work of the International Task Force on Mild Traumatic Brain Injury (source: H. von Holst, Stockholm, Sweden) will synthesize the world's literature to give the best insights yet on these issues.

Predicting Initial Consequences of Brain Injury

It would be useful to know which factors predict unfavorable consequences after acute brain injury. Not all of the potential predictive factors from the moment of injury through emergency transport, emergency department treatment, and definitive care have been adequately measured or evaluated. A few factors, however, are available to help predict severe outcome after trauma. For this discussion, we divide outcomes into three general categories: 1) death; 2) an unfavorable GOS score of moderate disability, severe disability, or persistent vegetative state; and 3) presence of any neurological deficit or limitation on discharge. As mentioned in the section Consequences of Mild TBI, it is difficult to evaluate all variables in cross-

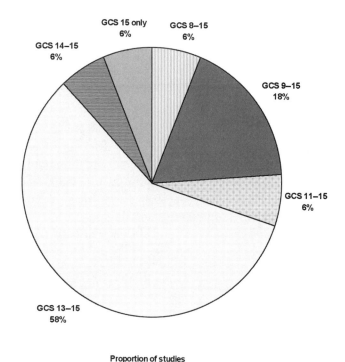

FIGURE 1–14. Mild brain injury: Glasgow Coma Scale (GCS) criterion (Jennett and Teasdale 1981).

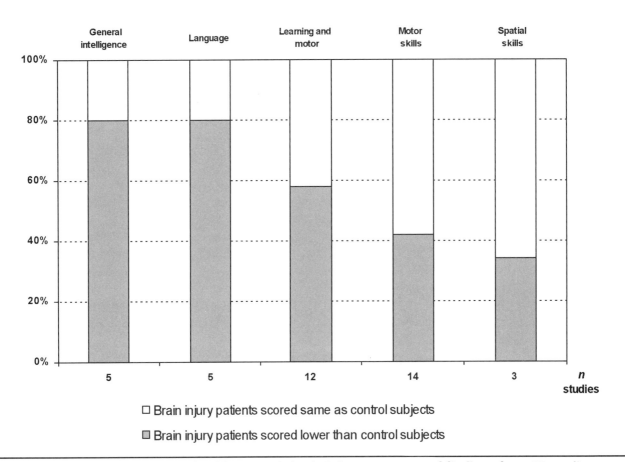

FIGURE 1–15. **Consequences of mild traumatic brain injury: summary of findings from 13 studies.**
Source.   Bassett and Slater 1990; Bawden et al. 1985; Costeff et al. 1988; Dennis and Barnes 1990; Ewing-Cobbs et al. 1985, 1987;
Gulbrandson 1984; Hannay and Levin 1988; Jordan and Murdoch 1990; Jordan et al. 1988; Levin et al. 1987, 1988; Tompkins et al. 1990.

institutional comparisons because they have not been assessed in a similar way. Hence, for this discussion, we use the information from the 1981 San Diego County brain injury cohort study (Kraus et al. 1984). Variables which were confirmed in the hospital record include age, sex, GCS score, Maximum Abbreviated Injury Scale (MAIS; Association for the Advancement of Automotive Medicine 1990) for non-head injury, fracture status, and type of brain lesion (i.e., concussion, hemorrhage, contusion, laceration, or other intracranial injury).

Figures 1–16 and 1–17 provide adjusted odds ratios (the ratio of unfavorable outcome [e.g., death] to a favorable outcome when injury severity, age, sex, etc., are controlled) for an unfavorable outcome (see preceding paragraph). The adjusted odds ratios show that hemorrhage and fracture are important predictive factors for all unfavorable outcome measures. Increasing age (in 10-year increments), low GCS score, and high MAIS score are other factors that independently predict an unfavorable outcome. Although these data are not likely to apply to all brain injury populations, they illustrate the potential for

using patient descriptive and diagnostic measures to assist in identifying factors that need increased clinical attention in the effort to improve current outcomes for brain injury.

Published guidelines for treatment of severe TBI (Bullock et al. 1996) have concluded, based on the published evidence, that older age, hypotension, CT scan irregularities, abnormal pupillary responses, and GCS score of 3–5 are reasonably predictive of a poor outcome after TBI. However, the specific cutoff points in age and level of hypotension are not known. Information on other factors is incomplete, and data for predictive factors for moderate and mild forms of TBI are not available.

Estimating Brain Injury Disability in the Population

Estimation of the Number of New Disabilities

Several assumptions are necessary to devise an estimate of the number of new disabilities (i.e., neurological deficits or limitations) each year after brain injury (the incidence

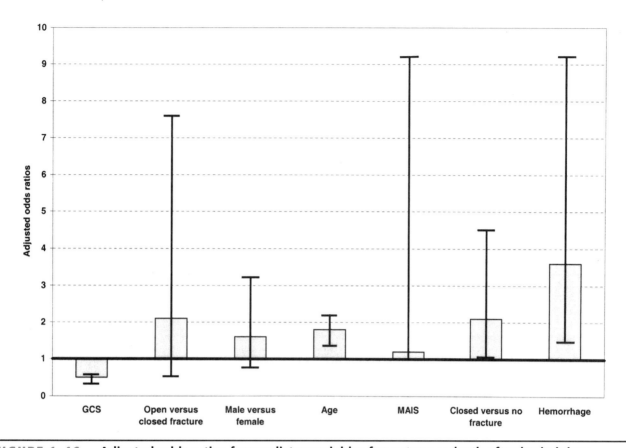

FIGURE 1–16.   **Adjusted odds ratios for predictor variables for outcome: death after brain injury.**

MAIS=Maximum Abbreviated Injury Scale (Association for the Advancement of Automotive Medicine 1990); GCS=Glasgow Coma Scale (Jennett and Teasdale 1981).
Source.   Unpublished data from the San Diego County Brain Injury Cohort Study (see Kraus et al. 1984).

rate was based on a pooled estimate from all incidence studies reported earlier in this chapter):

1. Brain injury incidence=120/100,000
2. United States population size, 2000=280 million
3. Total new cases in 2000=(120 × 2,800)=336,000
4. Prehospital brain injury deaths=(0.0001 × 280,000,000)=28,000
5. Total cases admitted to hospital alive=308,000
6. United States hospital admissions by severity:
   Mild: 50% × 308,000=154,000
   Moderate: 30% × 308,000=92,400
   Severe: 20% × 308,000=61,600
7. Discharge rate (alive) (Kraus et al. 1984; Levin et al. 1987; MacKenzie et al. 1989) by severity of brain injury:
   Mild=100%
   Moderate=93%
   Severe=42%

If 50% of all new hospital-admitted patients have mild injuries, 154,000 (100% × 154,000) are discharged alive.

If 30% of all new hospital-admitted cases have moderate injuries, 92,400 (30% × 308,000) are admitted to a hospital, and 85,932 (93% × 92,400) are discharged alive. If 20% of all brain injuries are severe, 61,600 (20% × 308,000) are admitted to a hospital annually, but only 25,872 (42% × 61,600) are discharged alive. Hence, the total pool of people discharged alive from a hospital by severity of admission is 265,804 (154,000 [mild] + 85,932 [moderate] + 25,872 [severe]).

The disability rate varies by severity of brain injury. If we assume that 10% of those with MTBI have some neurological limitation, then 15,400 people are afflicted. Also, if two-thirds of those with moderate brain injury are disabled, 57,288 have some disability. Finally, if 100% of severely injured patients have residual effects, 25,872 can be expected to have some form of disability. The total number of new disabilities from brain injuries for 2000 is approximately 98,560, a rate of approximately 35 per 100,000 population.

This estimating procedure can be summarized as follows (model, Figure 1–18):

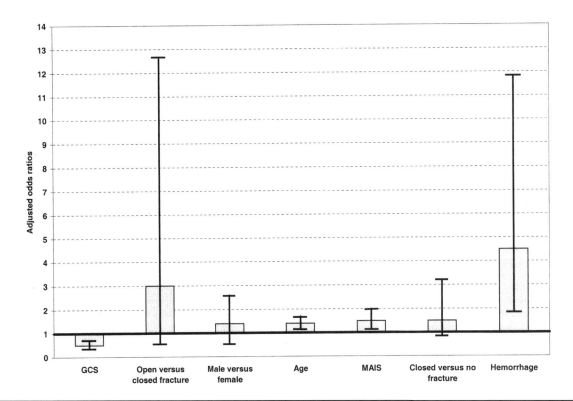

FIGURE 1–17. **Adjusted odds ratios for predictor variables for outcome: Glasgow Outcome Scale (Jennett and Teasdale 1981) less than good recovery.**

MAIS=Maximum Abbreviated Injury Scale (Association for the Advancement of Automotive Medicine 1990); GCS=Glasgow Coma Scale (Jennett and Teasdale 1981).

Source.   Unpublished data from the San Diego County Brain Injury Cohort Study (see Kraus et al. 1984).

Let BID equal the number of brain-injured patients who are discharged alive from hospitals each year with disability

n=size of population (i.e., United States 2000, 280,000,000)

H=hospitalization admission rate of brain injury patients in the population (i.e., 0.0011/year)

p_i=proportion of brain injury patients in the i-th severity group

(i=1...k, where k=3), where p_1=0.50, p_2=0.30, p_3=0.20

F_i=cumulative hospital fatality for the i-th group where

F_1=0, F_2=0.07, F_3=0.58

P_i=posthospital prevalence of disability in the i-th group where

P_1=0.1, P_2=0.667, P_3=1.0

Hence

$$BID = Hn\sum_{i=1}^{k} p_i(1 - F_i)P_i$$

that is,

BID=0.0011 (280,000,000) [0.5(1 – 0)(0.1) + 0.3(1 – 0.07)(0.667) + 0.2(1 – 0.58)(1)]=98,560

Cost of Head Injury

Almost no information was available on the cost of head injuries until Max et al. (1991) provided the first insights into the financial impact of head injuries in the population. The data show that the average lifetime cost for head injury was approximately $85,000 per person during 1985. Max et al. pointed out that the lifetime costs for minor, moderate,

If

BID = n brain injury patients with disability

n = population

H = hospital admission rate

p_i = proportion in severity groups

   (mild, moderate, severe)

F_i = hospital case fatality rate for severity groups in p_i

P_i = posthospital prevalence of disability in each

   severity group

Then

$$BID = Hn\sum_{i=1}^{k} p_i (1 - F_i) P_i$$

FIGURE 1–18.   **Estimating model.**

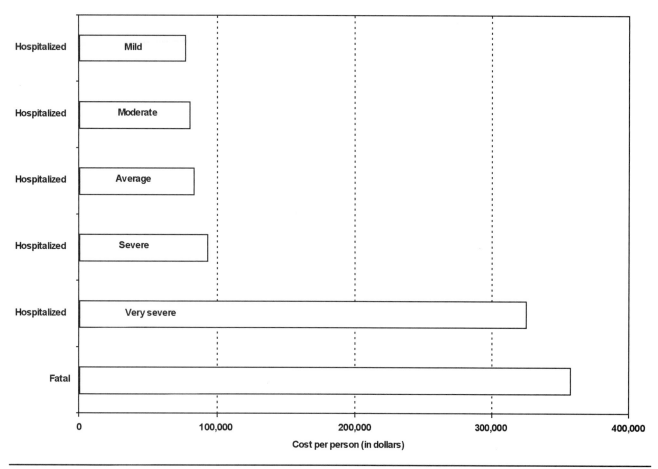

FIGURE 1–19. Lifetime cost of head injury, 1985 (by severity of injury).

Source.   Reprinted from Max W, MacKenzie E, Rice D: "Head Injuries: Costs and Consequences." *The Journal of Head Trauma Rehabilitation* 6:76–91, 1991. Used with permission.

and severe head injury are surprisingly close, ranging from approximately $77,000 to $93,000 (Figure 1–19). This finding illustrates the problem associated with mild head injury, namely, that specific treatment costs are nearly as high as those for moderate and severe brain injury because the mild injury incurs other associated treatment costs and affects full-time employment. The lifetime cost for a brain injury fatality is approximately $357,000, a figure not much higher than the $325,000 for a very severe nonfatal brain injury.

The lifetime costs of head injury by age (Figure 1–20) are much higher for people between the ages of 15 and 44 years than for those in younger or older age groups. Although the data have not been severity adjusted, they reflect costs associated with loss of productivity (and physical, as well as psychosocial, limitations) during the middle, most productive years.

Total costs for all 328,000 head injuries that occurred in 1985 were estimated to be $37.8 billion (Max et al. 1991). Approximately 65% of the total costs were accrued among those who survived a head injury; the remainder were associated with head injury deaths.

Miller and associates (1995) gave additional information on comprehensive costs in 1989 dollars for hospital and nonhospital costs per case. The costs were approximately $337,000 and $53,000 per case, respectively. The total comprehensive costs per year in 1989 dollars were $4.1 billion and $154.9 billion for hospital and nonhospital, respectively.

Another estimate provided by Lewin-ICF (1992) found direct and indirect costs of TBI in the United States (in 1991 dollars) totaled more than $48 billion per year, with $32 billion for survivors and $16 billion for fatal brain injuries. Average medical and nonmedical costs for each fatal TBI case ($450,000) were three times higher than for TBI survivors ($150,000). The lifetime costs for one person surviving a severe TBI, however, can be as high as $4 million (National Institute of Neurological Disorders and Stroke 1989).

Summary and Conclusion

The current brain injury research literature should be read cautiously because of the wide differences in the research

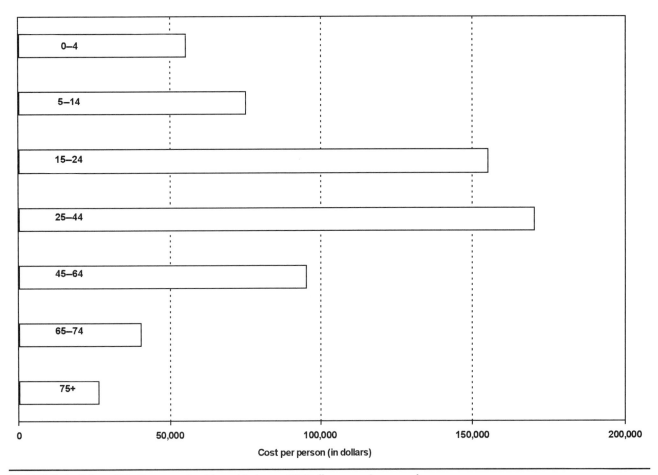

FIGURE 1–20.   Lifetime cost of head injury, 1985 (by age, in years).

Source.   Reprinted from Max W, MacKenzie E, Rice D: "Head Injuries: Costs and Consequences." *The Journal of Head Trauma Rehabilitation* 6:76–91, 1991. Used with permission.

methods and interpretation of clinically based, as opposed to epidemiologically based, data. This is especially important in the consideration of the definition of brain trauma and the ways in which injury severity is measured. The results of these methodological inconsistencies (points of interpretation) make cross-study comparisons extremely difficult, if not impossible. The epidemiological literature is far less prevalent than the clinical literature. Since the mid-1970s, there have been only a handful of studies that incorporated sound epidemiological methods in case definition, case ascertainment, severity definition, incidence measurement, and risk-marker or risk-factor evaluation. There are even fewer studies that address the long-term sequelae of brain injury that are population based and have standardized and rigorous cohort follow-up.

Despite these limitations, there are some findings that can be summarized from the available literature. Aggregate average incidence values are approximately 120 per 100,000 population per year, which includes fatal and nonfatal hospitalized brain injuries reported in all United States studies. The estimates based solely on hospital discharge data may

be an undercount of the true incidence because of difficulties in definition and ascertainment of repetitive admission of patients to a single institution. The epidemiological data suggest that the age of highest occurrence is in the late teens and early 20s, with a second period of high frequency after age 65 years. Males have approximately two to three times the frequency of brain injury experienced by females. Most studies show that transport-related causes are a dominant form of exposure. Almost all population-based incidence studies show that approximately 80% of brain injuries (the average of all hospital-admitted cases) are mild, approximately 10% are moderate, and approximately 10% are severe. Later studies, however, show a declining proportion of hospital-admitted patients with mild traumatic brain injury.

The most frequent diagnosis category in hospitalized cases is hemorrhage, contusion, or laceration. Less than 30% of all cases have concurrent fracture of the vault or base of the skull. Case fatality rates vary considerably across different studies, with a range of 3–8 per 100 patients admitted to a hospital. The literature is inconclusive with regard to the long-term effects in patients with short-time loss of consciousness and a Glasgow Coma Scale (GCS) score of 13–15. Methodological difficulties hamper a scientific assessment of this question. Available data suggest that hemorrhage, closed versus open head injury, absence of fracture, high Maximum Abbreviated Injury Scale score, and increased age are independent predictors of unfavorable outcome after brain injury. Hemorrhage is the most important of all outcome predictive factors. A GCS score of 3–5, abnormal computed tomography scan, abnormal pupillary response, and hypotension are also important predictors of a poor outcome in severe traumatic brain injury.

An algorithm used to estimate brain injury disability suggests that approximately more than 98,000 individuals each year who sustain a brain injury will have neurological deficit or disability. This cumulative prevalence is noteworthy because of the current pressures for effective delivery of long-term health care, as well as because of the impact on the patient, family, and community.

References

Annegers JF, Grabow JD, Kurland LT, et al: The incidence, causes, and secular trends in head injury in Olmsted County, Minnesota, 1965–1974. Neurology 30:912–919, 1980

Association for the Advancement of Automotive Medicine: The Abbreviated Injury Scale, 1990 Revision. Des Plaines, IL, 1990

Auer LM, Gell G, Richling B, et al: Predicting lethal outcome after severe head injury: a computer-assisted analysis of neurological symptoms and laboratory values. Acta Neurochir 52:225–238, 1980

Bassett SS, Slater J: Neuropsychologic function in adolescents sustaining mild closed head injury. J Pediatr Psychol 15:225–236, 1990

Bawden HN, Knights RM, Winogron HW: Speeded performance following head injury in children. J Clin Exp Neuropsychol 7:39–54, 1985

Bruce DA, Raphaely RC, Goldberg AI, et al: Pathophysiology, treatment and outcome following severe head injury in children. Childs Brain 5:74–191, 1979

Bullock R, Chestnut RM, Clifton G, Ghajar J, et al: Guidelines for the management of severe head injury. J Neurotrauma 11:639–734, 1996

Cantu RC, Voy R: Second impact syndrome: a risk in any sport. Physician Sports Med 23:27–36, 1995

Centers for Disease Control and Prevention: Traumatic brain injury—Colorado, Missouri, Oklahoma, and Utah, 1990–1993. MMWR 46:8–11, 1997

Centers for Disease Control and Prevention: 1998, United States, All Injury and Adverse Effects Deaths and Rates per 100,000, E800–E999. Available at: http://webapp.cdc.gov/sasweb/ncipc/mortrate9.html. Accessed February 20, 2002

Collins JG: Types of Injuries by Selected Characteristics: United States, 1985–1987 (Vital and Health Statistics, Series 10: Data From the National Health Survey, No 175) (DHHS Publication No PHS-91-1503). Hyattsville, MD, U.S. Department of Health and Human Services, 1990

Collins MW, Grindel SH, Lovell MR, et al: Relationship between concussion and neuropsychological performance in college football players. JAMA 282:964–970, 1999

Cooper JD, Tabaddor K, Hauser WA: The epidemiology of head injury in the Bronx. Neuroepidemiology 2:70–88, 1983

Costeff H, Abraham E, Brenner T, et al: Late neuropsychologic status after childhood head trauma. Brain Dev 10:381–384, 1988

Dennis M, Barnes MA: Knowing the meaning, getting the point, bridging the gap, and carrying the message: aspects of discourse following closed head injury in childhood and adolescence. Brain Lang 39:428–446, 1990

Ewing-Cobbs L, Fletcher JM, Landry SH, et al: Language disorders after pediatric head injury, in Speech and Language Evaluation in Neurology. Edited by Darby JK. New York, Grune & Stratton, 1985, pp 71–89

Ewing-Cobbs L, Levin HS, Eisenberg HM, et al: Language functions following closed-head injury in children and adolescents. J Clin Exp Neuropsychol 9:575–592, 1987

Fife D: Head injury with and without hospital admission: comparisons of incidence and short-term disability. Am J Public Health 77:810–812, 1987

Fife D, Faich G, Hollenshead W, et al: Incidence and outcome of hospital-treated head injury in Rhode Island. Am J Public Health 76:773–778, 1986

Gabella B, Hoffman RE, Marine WW, et al: Urban and rural traumatic brain injuries in Colorado. Ann Epidemiol 7:207–212, 1997

Gale JL, Dikmen S, Wyler A, et al: Head injury in the Pacific Northwest. Neurosurgery 12:487–491, 1983

Gotsch K, Annest JL, Holmgreen P, et al: Nonfatal sports- and recreation-related injuries treated in emergency departments—United States, July 2000–June 2001. MMWR 51:736–740, 2002

Gronwall SL, Wrightson P: Delayed recovery of intellectual function after minor head injury. Lancet 2:605–609, 1974

Guerrero J, Thurman DJ, Sniezek JE: Emergency department visits association with traumatic brain injury: United States, 1995–1996. Brain Inj 14:181–186, 2000

Gulbrandson GB: Neuropsychological sequelae of light head injuries in older children 6 months after trauma. J Clin Exp Neuropsychol 6:257–268, 1984

Hannay HJ, Levin HS: Visual continuous recognition memory in normal and closed-head-injured adolescents. J Clin Exp Neuropsychol 11:444–460, 1988

Jager TE, Weiss HB, Coben JH, et al: Traumatic brain injuries evaluated in U.S. emergency departments, 1992–1994. Acad Emerg Med 7:134–140, 2000

Jagger J, Levine J, Jane J, et al: Epidemiologic features of head injury in a predominantly rural population. J Trauma 24:40–44, 1984

Jennett B, Teasdale G: Management of Head Injuries. Philadelphia, PA, FA Davis, 1981

Jennett B, Murry A, Carlin J, et al: Head injuries in three Scottish neurosurgical units. BMJ 2:955–958, 1979

Jordan BD, Zimmerman RD: Computed tomography and magnetic resonance imaging comparisons in boxers. JAMA 263:1670–1674, 1990

Jordan FM, Murdoch BE: Linguistic status following closed head injury in children: a follow-up study. Brain Inj 4:47–54, 1990

Jordan FM, Ozanne AE, Murdoch BE: Long-term speech and language disorders subsequent to closed head injury in children. Brain Inj 2:179–185, 1988

Kalsbeek WD, McLauren RL, Harris BSH, et al: The national head and spinal cord injury survey: major findings. J Neurosurg 53 (suppl):S19–S31, 1980

Kelly JP, Nichols JS, Filley CM, et al: Concussion in sports. Guidelines for prevention of catastrophic outcome. JAMA 266:2867–2869, 1991

Klauber MR, Barrett-Connor E, Marshall LF, et al: The epidemiology of head injury: a prospective study of an entire community: San Diego County, California, 1978. Am J Epidemiol 113:500–509, 1981

Kraus JF, Black MA, Hessol N, et al: The incidence of acute brain injury and serious impairment in a defined population. Am J Epidemiol 119:186–201, 1984

Kraus JF, Fife D, Ramstein K, et al: The relationship of family income to the incidence, external causes and outcome of serious brain injury, San Diego County, California. Am J Public Health 76:1345–1347, 1986

Kraus JF, Fife D, Conroy C: Incidence, severity and outcomes of brain injuries involving bicycles. Am J Public Health 77:76–78, 1987

Kraus JF, Morgenstern H, Fife D, et al: Blood alcohol tests, prevalence of involvement, and outcomes following brain injury. Am J Public Health 79:294–299, 1989

Kraus JF, Rock A, Hemyari P: Brain injuries among infants, children, adolescents, and young adults. Am J Dis Child 144:684–691, 1990

Kreutzer JS, Doherty KR, Harris JA, et al: Alcohol use among persons with traumatic brain injury. J Head Trauma Rehab 5:9–20, 1990

Lee S, Lui T, Chang C, et al: Features of head injury in a developing country: Taiwan (1977–1987). J Trauma 30:194–199, 1990

Levin HS, Mattis S, Ruff RM, et al: Neurobehavioral outcome following minor head injury: a three-center study. J Neurosurg 66:234–243, 1987

Levin HS, High WM, Ewing-Cobbs L, et al: Memory functioning during the first year after closed head injury in children and adolescents. Neurosurgery 22:1043–1052, 1988

Lewin-ICF: The Cost of Disorders of the Brain. Washington, DC, The National Foundation for Brain Research, 1992

MacKenzie EJ, Edelstein SL, Flynn JP: Hospitalized head-injured patients in Maryland: incidence and severity of injuries. Md Med J 38:725–732, 1989

Marshall L, Marshall S, Klauber M, et al: A new classification of head injury based on computerized tomography. J Neurosurg 75 (suppl):S1–S66, 1991

Max W, MacKenzie E, Rice D: Head injuries: costs and consequences. J Head Trauma Rehabil 6:76–91, 1991

Miller TR, Pindus NM, Douglass JB, et al: Data Book on Nonfatal Injury. Washington, DC, Urban Institute Press, 1995, p 89

National Institute of Neurological Disorders and Stroke: Interagency Head Injury Task Force Report. Bethesda, MD, 1989

Plaut MR, Gifford RRM: Trivial head trauma and its consequences in a perspective of regional health care. Milit Med 141:244–247, 1976

Popovic JR, Kosak LJ: National hospital discharge survey: annual summary, 1998. Vital Health Stat 13:1–194, 2000

Rimel RW: A prospective study of patients with central nervous system trauma. J Neurosurg Nurs 13:132–141, 1981

Ruff RM, Marshall FL, Klauber MR, et al: Alcohol abuse and neurologic outcomes of the severely head injured. J Head Trauma Rehab 5:21–31, 1990

Salcido R, Costich JF: Recurrent traumatic brain injury. Brain Inj 6:293–298, 1992

Saunders RL, Harbaugh RE: The second impact in catastrophic contact-sports head trauma. JAMA 252:538–539, 1984

Smith GS, Kraus JF: Alcohol and residential, recreational and occupational injuries: a review of the epidemiologic evidence. Am J Public Health 79:99–121, 1988

Sosin D, Sacks J, Smith S: Head injury-associated deaths in the United States from 1979 to 1986. JAMA 262:2251–2255, 1989

Sosin DM, Sniezek JE, Waxweiler RJ: Trends in death associated with traumatic brain injury, 1979 through 1992. JAMA 273:1778–1780, 1995

Sosin DM, Sniezek JE, Thurman DJ: Incidence of mild and moderate brain injury in the United States, 1991. Brain Inj 10:47–54, 1996

Thurman DJ, Guerrero J: Trends in hospitalization associated with traumatic brain injury. JAMA 282:954–957, 1999

Thurman DJ, Jeppson L, Burnett CL, et al: Surveillance of traumatic brain injuries in Utah. West J Med 165:192–196, 1996

Thurman DJ, Alverson C, Browne D, et al: Traumatic Brain Injury in the United States: A Report to Congress. Centers for Disease Control and Prevention, 1999

Tompkins CA, Holland AL, Ratcliff G, et al: Predicting cognitive recovery from closed head injury in children and adolescents. Brain Cogn 13:86–97, 1990

Whitman S, Coonley-Hoganson R, Desai BT: Comparative head trauma experiences in two socioeconomically different Chicago-area communities: a population study. Am J Epidemiol 119:570–580, 1984

World Health Organization: International Classification of Diseases, 9th Revision, Clinical Modification. Ann Arbor, MI, Commission on Professional and Hospital Activities, 1986

2 Neuropathology

Thomas A. Gennarelli, M.D.
David I. Graham, M.B.B.Ch., Ph.D.

VARIOUS PROCESSES THAT may damage the brain after trauma, singly or in combination, are referred to in the literature as *traumatic brain injury* (TBI), with the increasing belief that what separates mild, moderate, and severe categories of injury is not so much the nature of brain lesions as their multiplicity, amount, and distribution. If correct, then there is likely to be a continuum from mild to severe brain damage, the structural basis of which can be inferred from postmortem studies of patients who have died with varying degrees of disability after brain injury.

Classification and Mechanisms of Brain Damage

Any classification of brain damage after trauma to the head must take into account the full spectrum of clinical presentation and outcome—from the patient who remains in coma from the moment of injury until death, to the patient who is apparently healthy after the initial injury but who, as a result of a complication, subsequently relapses into fatal coma. Given that some structural damage is likely in all forms of TBI, an important determinant of outcome is the preinjury condition of the brain. In other words, a good recovery is more likely in a healthy individual with no preexisting brain disorders who experiences TBI than in an individual with a similar level of injury who, either because of preexisting developmental or acquired disorders, had abnormal brain function before injury. The outcome, even after relatively mild brain injury, in an individual who has already experienced cerebrovascular disease or brain injury is likely to be worse than if such premorbid conditions were not present (Jennett and Teasdale 1981).

Earlier classifications based on clinicopathological correlations helped identify potentially preventable complications in patients after brain injury and, in particular, in those who "talked and died" (Reilly et al. 1975) or "talked and deteriorated" (Marshall et al. 1983). The fact that a patient had initially talked after TBI only to deteriorate or subsequently die was taken as evidence that the initial structural damage was mild, although the brain injury had initiated a progressive sequence of events that led to a fatal outcome or persisting disability. TBI was therefore considered to be either primary (induced by mechanical forces), which occurred at the moment of injury, or secondary/delayed (not mechanically induced), which was superimposed on an already mechanically injured brain. Such secondary damage could be due to complications either initiated via or independent of the primary damage (Graham and Gennarelli 2000). These pathophysiological processes are not unique to the brain-injured patient but are commonly found in other types of intracranial disease (Table 2–1).

Although the circumstances by which the brain can be injured after trauma are diverse and complex, major advances have been made in understanding the mechanisms by which brain damage occurs after head injury. In the

Kishor Malavade, M.D., provided editorial assistance in the preparation of this chapter.

TABLE 2–1. Classification of traumatic brain injury

Primary	Secondary
Injury to scalp	Hypoxia-ischemia
Fracture of skull	Swelling/edema
Surface contusions/ lacerations	Raised intracranial pressure and associated vascular changes
Intracranial hematoma	Meningitis/abscess
Diffuse axonal injury	
Diffuse vascular injury	
Injury to cranial nerves and pituitary stalk	

main, it has been determined that there are two principal mechanisms of brain injury: contact and acceleration/deceleration (Gennarelli 1983). The conditions extant at the time of injury in large measure determine the associated pathology, reflecting, among other things, the amount of mechanical loading, the way in which it is distributed, and the time over which it has been applied (Gennarelli and Thibault 1985) (Table 2–2).

Brain lesions due to contact, therefore, tend to result from either an object striking the head or contact between the brain and the skull. Brain injury due to acceleration/deceleration results from unrestricted movement of the head that leads to shear, tensile, and compressive strains, the principal structural consequences of which are acute subdural hematomas (SDHs) from tearing of bridging veins and widespread damage to axons or blood vessels.

Yet another classification has been derived based on the clinical and neuroradiological appreciation that structural brain damage after trauma can be categorized as focal or diffuse (multifocal) (Graham et al. 2002) (Table 2–3).

TABLE 2–2. Mechanisms of brain damage after brain injury

Contact	Acceleration/deceleration
Injury to scalp	Tearing of bridging veins with formation of subdural hematoma
Fracture of skull with or without an associated extradural hematoma	Diffuse axonal injury, tissue tears, and associated intracerebral hematomas
Surface contusions and lacerations and associated intracerebral hematomas	Diffuse vascular injury

TABLE 2–3. Classification of damage after brain injury

Focal	Diffuse (multifocal)
Injury to scalp	Diffuse axonal injury
Fracture of skull	Hypoxic-ischemic damage
Surface contusions/lacerations	Meningitis
Intracranial hematoma	Vascular injury
Raised intracranial pressure and associated vascular changes	

From these considerations it should be clear that in any given patient the outcome is determined by many factors. However, it is generally agreed that the focal pathologies associated with contact are likely to be sustained as a result of a fall, whereas the diffuse pathologies are more commonly associated with acceleration/deceleration after traffic accidents or a fall from a height. It is only with an understanding of the biomechanical, molecular, and cellular events associated with brain injury after trauma that it is possible to target specific mechanisms in the hope of improving outcome (Graham et al. 2000, 2002; McIntosh et al. 1998; Teasdale and Graham 1998).

The account of the pathology of brain damage after trauma that follows is based on autopsy studies, the full benefit of which can only be appreciated if the brain has been properly fixed before dissection and appropriate histological studies have been carried out (Adams et al. 1980). This applies to blunt injuries, which are by far the more common in civilian practice (an account of which follows), and to missile injuries, which are not considered further in this chapter. However, in the future, such detailed studies may not be possible or may be particularly difficult to undertake, at least in the United Kingdom. Recent events have necessitated an urgent assessment of the way in which human autopsy tissues are accrued and for what purpose (Royal College of Pathologists 2001). Considerable distress has been experienced by relatives of the deceased in relation to organ retention, especially in pediatric practice (Bristol Royal Infirmary Inquiry, 2000; Royal Liverpool Children's Inquiry, 2000). Procedures are in place to obtain fully informed consent for the use of organs and tissues beyond diagnostic purposes, to inform patients and family about the benefits of research and medical education to society, and to provide information on limits and safeguards to prevent any future use not covered by the consent form (Medical Research Council 2001).

Brain Damage in Fatal Blunt Head Injury

Focal Injury

Lesions of the Scalp, Skull, and Dura

Lesions of the scalp, skull, and dura often provide a clue to the site and nature of the injury and alert the clinician to potential complications. For example, bruising at the back of the scalp is often associated with severe contusions of the frontal lobes, whereas bruising of the mastoid process may be associated with traumatic subarachnoid hemorrhage. A bruise in the temple may be associated with a fracture and the subsequent development of an extradural hematoma. In many instances, the laceration of the scalp is not of any great significance, but, if there is severe bleeding, the patient may become hypotensive, thereby adding a secondary insult to the already damaged brain. Furthermore, if there is an associated open, depressed fracture of the skull, a laceration of the scalp may be a potential route for intracranial infection.

In general, the more severe the brain injury, the greater the frequency of a fracture of the skull. For example, the frequency of skull fracture is 3% in those patients who present to emergency departments, 65% in patients admitted to a neurosurgical unit, and 80% in fatal cases (Jennett and Teasdale 1981). Fractures of the skull may be limited to the vertex, the base of the skull, or may affect both (Table 2–4). The majority of skull fractures are linear, affecting the vault of the skull in 62% of cases, with extension into the base of the skull in 17%.

A fracture of the skull is not necessarily associated with underlying brain damage. For example, injury due to crush may result in extensive fractures of the skull with little underlying brain damage, with the patient often remaining conscious. More localized injury, as, for example, after an assault with a blunt object, may produce brain damage limited to the site of impact. Even under these circumstances, the fracture may be depressed, but brain function remains intact, there being only brief or limited loss of consciousness.

As a corollary, the absence of a skull fracture does not necessarily mean that the brain has not been injured. Indeed, a skull fracture is absent in some 20% of fatal cases. This is particularly true in pediatric patients because the capacity of the skull to bend in children may prevent the development of fracture but nevertheless be associated with a considerable amount of underlying structural brain damage.

There is a strong association between the presence of a skull fracture and the development of an intracranial hematoma (Cooper 2001; Mendelow et al. 1983), particularly if, after the injury, the patient has a depressed level of consciousness. For example, it has been determined that only 1 in 6,000 patients presenting to emergency departments who did not have either a depressed level of consciousness or a skull fracture subsequently developed an intracranial hematoma, whereas the risk becomes 1 in 4 if these clinical features are present. The site of the fracture is also important given that if it affects the squamous part of the temporal bone there is a possibility that an extradural hematoma may develop.

Surface Contusions and Lacerations of the Brain

By definition, the pia-arachnoid is intact over surface contusions and is torn in lacerations. Contusions have been considered to be the hallmark of brain damage due to head injury (Table 2–5), and they have a characteristic distribution affecting the poles of the frontal lobes; the inferior aspects of the frontal lobes, including the gyri recti; the cortex above and below the operculum of the Sylvian fissures; the temporal poles; and the lateral and inferior aspects of the temporal lobes (Figure 2–1). Less commonly, they are seen on the underaspects of the cerebellar hemispheres. They may extend into white matter, comprising a mixture of hemorrhage and necrosis at the margin of which is an area of swelling (Figure 2–2). Particularly where there has been extensive damage, an actual hematoma may develop within the affected gyrus, and, if laceration of the pia-arachnoid has taken place, then there may be bleeding into the subdural space. The combination of extensive contusion and an associated SDH is referred to as a *burst lobe*. Depending on the location of the lesion, there may or may not be an associated sensorimotor neurological deficit.

TABLE 2–4.   Types of fracture of the skull

Linear or fissure

Depressed if fragments of the inner table are displaced inward by at least the thickness of the diploe

Compound if depressed fracture is associated with laceration of scalp, and penetrative if there is also a tear in the dura

Hinge if fracture extends across the base of the skull

Coup at site of injury

Contre coup if fracture is located a distance from the point of injury

Growing fractures occur in infancy and are due to interposition of soft tissue between the edges of the fractures that may prevent healing

TABLE 2–5.   Surface contusion and lacerations

Found in 96% of fatal adult brain injury, they are the most common source of bleeding into the subarachnoid space.

Characteristically affect crests of gyri.

Appear as punctate or streaks of hemorrhage at right angles to the cortical surface.

At vertex, are related to fractures and inferiorly correspond to irregular bony contours at base of skull.

In early infancy, they appear as tears in the subcortical white matter and in the inner layers of the cortex of the frontal and temporal lobes.

Healed contusions are found incidentally in 2%–5% of adult autopsies.

The surface contusions/lacerations and associated swelling may be sufficient to act as a mass lesion, with the subsequent sequelae of raised intracranial pressure (ICP). Indeed, such a sequence of events was attributed to contusional injury alone in 6 of 66 patients who "talked and died," 25% of whom did not have significant intracranial hematoma (Reilly et al. 1975).

Various types of contusion have been described. Reference has already been made to fracture contusions that occur at the site of a fracture and are particularly severe in the frontal lobes and in association with fractures of the anterior fossae; coup contusions occur at the site of contact in the absence of a fracture, and contrecoup contu-

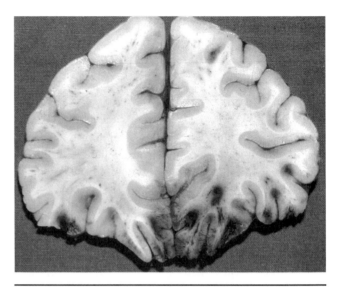

FIGURE 2–2.   Acute contusions: 48-hour survival.
Coronal section through frontal lobes to show distribution and extent of contusions.

sions occur in brain tissue diametrically opposite the point of contact (Adams 1992).

The development of a contusion index has allowed the depth and extent of contusions in different parts of the brain to be expressed quantitatively (Adams et al. 1985). This index has shown that severe contusions are present in some 10% of fatalities, moderately severe contusions in 78%, and mild contusions in 6%. The index has confirmed that contusions occur most commonly in the frontal and the temporal lobes, are more severe in patients with a fracture of the skull than in those without a fracture, are less common in patients with diffuse brain injury than in those with focal brain injury, and are more severe in patients who do not experience a lucid interval than those who do. More recently, a hemorrhagic lesion score has been derived that provides a finer discrimination of the distribution and severity of injury by including hemorrhagic lesions involving the corpus callosum and deep grey and white matter (Ryan et al. 1994).

Intracranial Hematoma

Intracranial hematoma is the most common cause of clinical deterioration and death in patients who experience a lucid interval, the group who "talk and die" or talk and deteriorate after injury (Bullock and Teasdale 1990; Klauber et al. 1989; Reilly et al. 1975; Rockswold et al. 1987). Indeed, it is the late recognition and treatment of intracranial hematoma that constitutes one of the most, if not the most, important avoidable factors in the management of TBI. Regardless of the severity of the brain injury, there is always the possibility that an intracranial hema-

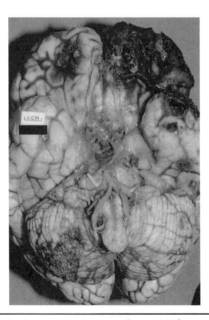

FIGURE 2–1.   Acute contusions: 18-hour survival.
Base of brain to show hemorrhagic defects and associated subarachnoid hemorrhage on underaspects of frontal lobes and in relation to temporal poles.

TABLE 2–6.   Types and frequency of intracranial hematoma

Type	Frequency (%)
Extradural (epidural)	4
Intradural	56
Subdural	13
Subarachnoid	3
Discrete intracerebral or intracerebellar hematoma not in continuity with the surface of the brain	15
The "burst" lobe—an intracerebral or intracerebellar hematoma in continuity with the related subdural hematoma.	25

TABLE 2–7.   Extradural (epidural) hematoma

Present in 5%–15% of fatal brain injury.

There is an associated skull fracture in 85% of adults; fracture is commonly absent in children.

There is a fracture in the squamous part of the temporal bone in 70% of cases; in remaining cases, fractures are frontal or parietal or even occur in the posterior fossa.

The hematoma reliably indicates the site of a fracture.

Hematoma is most common in young adults and is rarer in children.

In 5%–10% of patients, an extradural hematoma coexists with an intradural hematoma.

toma may complicate the injury. The bleeding usually begins at the time of injury, and, by the time of admission to hospital some 3 to 4 hours later, there is a hematoma in between approximately 30% and 60% of patients admitted who are in a coma.

If the injury is mild, then loss of consciousness may be limited to a few minutes, but a secondary loss of consciousness may develop due to an expanding intracranial hematoma. This classical textbook description of a lucid interval followed by coma occurs in only a minority of cases, there being many more patients who are in a coma from the time of injury and in whom a hematoma progressively develops.

Traumatic intracranial hematomas are usually classified according to the anatomical compartment in which they develop (Table 2–6).

Extradural (epidural) hematoma.   An extradural (epidural) hematoma consists of an ovoid mass of clotted blood that lies between the bone of the vault or the base of the skull and the dura (Table 2–7) (Freytag 1963; Jamieson and Yelland 1968; Maloney and Whatmore 1969).

In two-thirds of cases, the extradural hematoma is caused by a fracture in the squamous part of the temporal bone; in the remaining cases, the hematoma may develop in relation to the frontal and parietal parts of the brain or even within the posterior fossa (Lewin 1949; McKissock et al. 1960), and, occasionally, they are multiple. Because the source of the bleeding is usually arterial, the hematoma enlarges fairly rapidly, gradually stripping the dura from the scalp to form a circumscribed ovoid mass that progressively indents and flattens the adjacent brain. In many cases, there is little associated underlying brain damage (Figure 2–3).

Small hematomas may become completely organized, although larger ones may undergo partial organization,

with their centers becoming cystic and filled with dark viscous fluid. After approximately 2 weeks, the hematomas become smaller and, in the majority of patients, are completely resolved by the fourth to sixth week after the injury (Bullock et al. 1985).

Intradural hematomas.   *Subarachnoid hematoma.*   Some degree of subarachnoid hemorrhage occurs in any serious brain injury. Most occur in association with surface contusions. In many cases, there is a thin layer of blood clot over the lateral and inferior aspects of the frontal and temporal lobes, but in approximately 10%–15% of patients, the amounts are larger and may constitute a subarachnoid hematoma. Under these circumstances, there may be associated constriction (vasospasm) of the cerebral arteries, and, if large amounts of subarachnoid hemor-

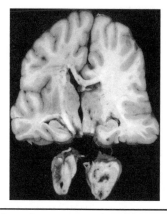

FIGURE 2–3.   Acute extradural hematoma: 23-hour survival.

Coronal section through cerebral hemispheres at level of anterior thalamus. Note absence of acute contusions but considerable distortion of right side of brain, with development of supracallosal and tentorial herniae, asymmetry of ventricles, and secondary hemorrhage in the brainstem.

TABLE 2–8. Acute subdural hematoma

In 70% of cases, injury is produced by a fall or an assault.

Approximately 70% of patients have a skull fracture, but in approximately 50% of these cases, the fracture is contralateral to the side of the hematoma.

Peak incidence of intradural hematoma is in the fifth and sixth decades of life.

Only 2%–3% of traumatic hematomas are in the posterior fossa, where intradural hematomas are as common as extradural.

An acute hematoma is associated with swelling of an ipsilateral cerebral hemisphere; such swelling often persists after the hematoma has been evacuated.

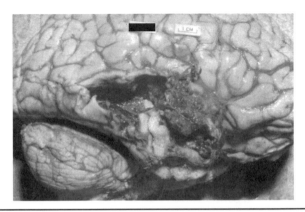

FIGURE 2–4. "Burst" temporal lobe: 37-hour survival.

Note extensive contusional injury to temporal lobes that at surgery was associated with a large acute subdural hematoma.

rhage are present in the posterior fossa, acute obstructive hydrocephalus may develop. The entity of traumatic subarachnoid hemorrhage is well recognized as a result of damage to blood vessels in the posterior fossa (Harland et al. 1983) often in association with a fracture of the base of the skull (Vanezis 1979, 1986).

Subdural hematomas. A small amount of hemorrhage within the subdural space is common in fatal brain injury. Because this blood can spread freely throughout the subdural space, it tends to cover the entire hemisphere, with the result that an SDH is usually larger than an extradural hematoma. The great majority of SDHs are due to rupture of veins that bridge the subdural space where they connect the upper surface of the cerebral hemisphere to the sagittal sinus. Occasionally, they are arterial in origin (Table 2–8).

SDHs large enough to act as significant mass lesions have been variously reported in between 26% and 63% of blunt head injuries (Freytag 1963; Maloney and Whatmore 1969) (see Figure 2–3). In approximately 8%–13% of cases, the hematomas are pure with little evidence of other brain damage. However, most are associated with considerable brain damage, and, therefore, the mortality and morbidity are greater in subdural than in extradural hematomas. This is particularly true in cases with a "burst" frontal or temporal lobe (Figure 2–4).

The current literature classifies SDH as acute when it is composed of clot and blood (usually within the first 48 hours after injury), subacute when there is a mixture of clotted and fluid blood (developing between 2–14 days after injury), and chronic when the hematoma is fluid (developing more than 14 days after injury) (Bullock and Teasdale 1990). Chronic SDH occurs weeks or months after what may appear to have been a trivial head injury. However, a history of head injury is present in 25%–50% of cases (Fogelholm and Waltimo 1975; Marshall et al.

1983). The hematoma becomes encapsulated and slowly increases in size, and may become sufficiently large to produce distortion and herniation of the brain (see Brain Damage due to Raised Intracranial Pressure). Chronic SDH is more common in older than in younger patients, in patients who are alcoholic, and in patients taking anticoagulation therapy.

Intracerebral and intracerebellar hematomas. Intracerebral and intracerebellar hematomas are present in approximately 16%–20% of fatal brain injury cases. They are often multiple and occur most commonly in the frontal and temporal lobes (Bullock and Teasdale 1990). Less commonly, they occur in the cerebellum. Sometimes, traumatic intracerebral hematomas develop several days after the injury, and recognition of this possibility may have important medicolegal implications if the patient dies (Elsner et al. 1990; Nanassis et al. 1989). There is greater recognition of relatively small hematomas deeply seated in the brain as a result of computed tomography (CT) scanning and magnetic resonance imaging (MRI): many hematomas are often rather small and centered on midline structures, including parasagittal white matter (a so-called gliding contusion), the corpus callosum, the structures in the walls of the third ventricle, and in the striatum (so-called basal ganglia hematomas). In the majority of these cases, the patients are in a coma, and the small hematomas are part of the clinicopathological entity of diffuse (traumatic) axonal injury (Adams et al. 1986; Macpherson et al. 1986).

Sometimes, patients present with a history of possible brain injury so that the finding of a solitary hematoma requires consideration that it may be due to either a nontraumatic hypertensive bleed or the rupture of a saccular aneurysm. Interpretation of the autopsy findings can be difficult, and much depends on the site of the hematoma.

For example, if the hematoma is in the subfrontal or temporal region, it is more likely to be traumatic than not. There are a number of risk factors for the development of intracerebral hematoma that include tumor, vascular malformation, and substance abuse. Patients receiving thrombolytic therapy are also at risk, and those receiving anticoagulants are at particular risk of developing intracerebral hemorrhage related to contusions.

Burst lobe. The term *burst lobe* describes an intracerebral or an intracerebellar hematoma that is continuous with a SDH. It is presumed to be due to damage to or laceration of superficial brain tissue. It is present in approximately 25% of fatal cases of brain injury and occurs most commonly in the frontal and temporal lobes.

Brain Damage due to Raised Intracranial Pressure

ICP is frequently elevated in patients after brain injury due to the mass effects of contusions/lacerations, intracranial hematomas, and brain swelling occurring in what is essentially an enclosed space.

In a healthy adult, the ICP is usually in the range of 0 to 10 mm Hg. Pressures greater than 20 mm Hg are abnormal, and when the ICP is greater than 40 mm Hg, there is neurological dysfunction and impairment of brain electrical activity. As the ICP continues to rise, the ability of the cerebral circulation to maintain autoregulation and the normal cerebral perfusion becomes compromised. An ICP greater than 60 mm Hg is invariably fatal, and there is increasing evidence that even pressures between 20 and 40 mm Hg may be associated with increased morbidity.

If unchecked, an increase in the ICP is likely to kill the patient as a result of deformation of tissue, shift of the midline structures, the development of internal herniae, and secondary damage to the upper brainstem. This mechanism is the most common cause of death in the neurosurgical intensive care unit, being present in approximately 75% of brain-injured patients who die (Graham et al. 1987).

A unilateral mass lesion causes distortion of the brain, a reduction in the volume of cerebrospinal fluid (CSF), and, in the closed skull, the formation of internal herniae. Principal among these herniae are the displacement of the cingulate gyrus under the free edge of the falx (a subfalcine or supracallosal hernia) and the medial temporal gyrus downward through the incisura (a tentorial hernia). A mass lesion in the posterior fossa may result in herniation of the cerebellar tonsil through the foramen magnum (a tonsillar hernia). As these herniae develop, CSF spaces are obliterated, and pressure gradients begin to develop between the various intracranial compartments. Further progression is likely to mechanically deform blood vessels sufficiently to cause vascular complications, such as hemorrhage and/or infarction in the upper brainstem and variable degrees of ischemic damage within the territories of one or both posterior cerebral arteries. Less commonly, there is infarction of brain tissue supplied by the anterior cerebral, anterior choroidal, and the superior cerebellar arteries (Graham et al. 1987). Infarction has also been recorded in the anterior lobe of the pituitary gland in approximately 45% of cases (Harper et al. 1986).

Other Types of Focal Brain Injury

In accidents causing hyperextension of the head on the neck, traumatic separation of the pons and medulla is a well-recognized cause of death (Lindenberg and Freytag 1970; Simpson et al. 1989). In many cases, there is an associated ring fracture at the base of the skull or dislocation and/or fracture of the first or second cervical vertebra. Although complete tears are immediately fatal, patients with small or incomplete tears at the pontomedullary junction may survive for some time after injury (Britt et al. 1980; Pilz 1980; Pilz et al. 1982).

Almost any of the cranial nerves may be damaged at the time of injury. The frequency of injury to the cranial nerves has been underestimated, as demonstrated by MRI, which provides a much more sensitive means of identifying damage than was previously possible with CT (Gean 1994).

Damage can also occur to the hypothalamus and pituitary gland. Occasionally, the pituitary stalk is torn at the time of brain injury, but, more frequently, the stalk is intact, although there is infarction in the anterior lobe of the pituitary. A number of potential mechanisms have been suggested to explain this type of damage, including a fracture at the base of the skull that extends into the sella turcica; elevation of the ICP, leading to distortion and compression of the pituitary stalk; and hypotensive shock analogous to the situation occurring in postpartum necrosis of the pituitary.

Damage to blood vessels may also occur. It is possible to identify various vascular lesions by angiography, including dissection or occlusion of the internal carotid or vertebral arteries, traumatic pseudoaneurysm, traumatic arteriovenous fistula, and venous thrombosis and an assessment of vasospasm.

Imaging techniques after brain injury have shown that in many patients there are multiple lesions in the brain, some of which are hemorrhagic. MRI is particularly useful in the detection of these lesions, the principal neuropathological correlates of which are lesions in lobar white matter, in the corpus callosum, and in the dorsolateral sector(s) of the rostral brainstem adjacent to the superior cerebellar peduncles. These areas have become known as the *shearing injury triad*. However, such lesions are not restricted to these areas, being found also in periventricular structures, the hippocampal formation, the internal capsule, and, occasionally, deep within the cerebellar hemispheres.

Multiple petechial hemorrhages are not uncommonly found when patients die from severe brain injury. Although many of these may indeed have histological evidence of diffuse axonal injury (DAI) (see Diffuse Axonal Injury section), there are many others, including diffuse vascular injury (see Diffuse [Multifocal] Vascular Injury section), in which the hemorrhages can be ascribed to a number of causes that include ischemic damage in the territory supplied by the pericallosal arteries—usually secondary to a supracallosal hernia, fat embolism, and a host of vascular and hematological abnormalities that constitute some of the medical complications of head injury.

Diffuse Brain Injury

Diffuse brain injury describes a number of pathologies, some of which are a consequence of acceleration/deceleration applied to white matter, whereas others are vascular in nature, and yet others are secondary to hypoxia. Although it is true that these pathologies are widely distributed and in some instances are diffuse, the overall generic term *diffuse brain injury* is somewhat of a misnomer, because in the majority of cases the pathology is multifocal.

Diffuse Axonal Injury

DAI is a type of brain damage that has many synonyms and was first described under the heading of *diffuse degeneration of white matter* (Strich 1956). Since then, a variety of terms have been used that have helped to further characterize DAI (1) by mechanism (e.g., shearing injury) (Peerless and Rewcastle 1967; Strich 1961), (2) by location of the underlying pathology (e.g., inner cerebral trauma) (Grcevic 1988), or (3) by combination of mechanism and the location of the principal pathology (e.g., diffuse damage of immediate impact type [Adams et al. 1977] and diffuse white matter shearing injury [Zimmerman et al. 1978]). There was international recognition for the term *diffuse axonal injury* (Adams et al. 1982; Gennarelli et al. 1982), but this has been superseded by the term *traumatic axonal injury* (TAI).

In severe cases of DAI (Table 2–9), the hemorrhages in midline structures, including the brainstem, can usually be seen at the time of brain cutting (Figure 2–5). This is in contrast to the widespread damage to axons that can only be identified microscopically. The histological appearances of the lesions depend on the length of survival after injury (Table 2–10). If the patient survives for only a

TABLE 2–9. Pattern and frequency of hemorrhages and tissue tears in severe cases of diffuse traumatic axonal injury

Pattern	Frequency (%)
Dorsolateral sector of upper brainstem	95
Corpus callosum	92
Choroid plexus of third ventricle	90
Parasagittal (gliding) contusion	88
Hippocampus	88
Periventricular (third ventricle)	83
Interventricular septum	80
Cingulate gyrus	61
Thalamus	56
Basal ganglia	17

few days, midline structure lesions are usually hemorrhagic, but over time these result in shrunken, often cystic, scars. However, the appearance of the important axonal lesions changes considerably over time. Thus, if survival is short (days), there are numerous axonal swellings and axonal bulbs that can be readily identified either as argyrophilic swellings in silver-stained preparations or by immunohistochemistry (Figure 2–6). The swellings and bulbs are most commonly seen in deep structures and, in particular, in the white matter of the parasagittal cortex, the corpus callosum, the internal capsule, and the

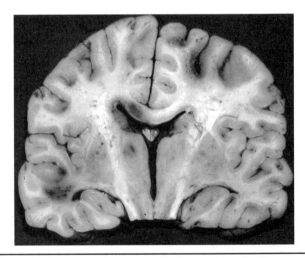

FIGURE 2–5. **Traumatic diffuse axonal injury (DAI): 5-day survival.**

Note absence of surface contusions and midline hemorrhages in the corpus callosum and in the left thalamus. Hemorrhages were also seen in the dorsolateral sector of the upper brainstem. Microscopy revealed widely distributed axonal damage, with a severity grading of DAI 3.

TABLE 2–10. Diffuse traumatic axonal injury: histological appearances and their time course

Time	Histological appearance
Hours	Hemorrhages and tissue tears
	Axonal swellings
	Axonal bulbs
Days or weeks	Clusters of microglia and macrophages; astrocytosis
Months to years	Wallerian degeneration

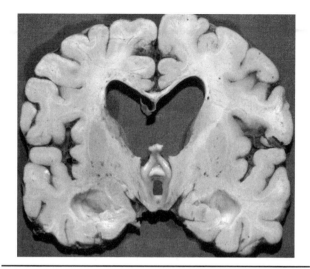

FIGURE 2–7. Traumatic axonal injury: 17-month survival in a vegetative state.

There is marked symmetrical dilatation of the ventricular system, thinning of the corpus callosum, reduction in the amount of each centrum semi ovale, overall preservation of the cortical ribbon and subcortical grey matter, and an absence of surface contusions.

long tracts of the brainstem. If survival extends to a number of weeks, the bulbs become less prominent, their site of formation now being characterized by the development of clusters of microglia and macrophages. With even longer survival (months and years) neither bulbs nor microglia clusters can be seen, and axonal damage is recognized by the identification of the breakdown products of myelin. Therefore, in those patients who survive in a severely disabled or vegetative state, abnormalities in the brain may be limited to small, healed, superficial contusions and extensive degeneration in the white matter. Coronal sections of specimens from such patients reveal the characteristic features of relatively intact grey matter, a greatly reduced amount of central white matter, and compensatory enlargement of the ventricular system (Figure 2–7). In most cases, it is still possible to identify the telltale focal lesions in the corpus callosum and in the rostral brainstem.

Clinical and pathological grades of diffuse traumatic axonal injury. With increasing experience, it is apparent that TAI forms a distinct clinicopathological entity and probably is the principal pathological substrate that produces a continuum of neurological deficit from mild up to severe brain injury. The entity was originally described in a series of patients in whom there was diffuse brain injury without an associated intracranial mass lesion, which accounted for approximately 35% of all deaths after head injury (Gennarelli 1983). Such patients were usually deeply comatose from the time of injury, with abnormal motor function consisting most frequently of extensive posturing of both the upper and lower limbs occurring spontaneously or in response to painful stimulation. The patient remained in this state for many weeks, during which time spontaneous eye opening returned, though in general the patient did not show an organized response to environment and recovery was limited to severe disability or a vegetative state. Under these circumstances, death was usually attributed to intercurrent infection. Evidence for a continuum was suggested in the late 1960s when it was shown that occasional clusters of microglia can be found in patients dying from some unrelated cause soon after mild brain injury (Oppenheimer 1968). These findings were confirmed by Clark (1974), who also drew attention to the frequent occurrence of clusters of microglia in the white matter of patients dying as a result of brain injury, and Pilz (1980), who described the occurrence of axonal swellings in human brain injuries of vary-

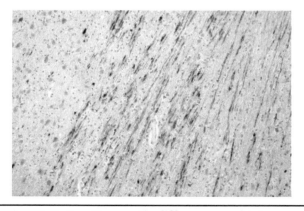

FIGURE 2–6. Traumatic diffuse axonal injury (DAI): 5-day survival.

Same case as in Figure 2–5. There are abnormal axons—swellings and bulb formation—throughout the white matter of the neuro-axis. Immunohistochemistry: β-amyloid precursor protein × 320.

ing severity. Further support for the concept of varying degrees of TAI has been provided by Blumbergs et al. (1989). In 1989, Adams et al. (1989) introduced a new grading system. In grade 1, abnormalities were limited to histological evidence of axonal damage throughout the white matter without any focal accentuation in any of the midline structures. Patients were designated grade 2 if, in addition to the widely distributed axonal injury, there was also a focal lesion in the corpus callosum. Grade 3 TAI, which represents the most severe form of the spectrum, was characterized by diffuse damage to axons in the presence of focal lesions in both the corpus callosum and the brainstem. Further refinement of this grading system introduced subdivisions of grades 2 and 3 in which "M" indicated that the focal midline lesion could be seen macroscopically and "m" indicated that it could only be identified histologically. Associated clinicopathological correlations indicated that the lesser degrees of axonal injury could be associated with either a complete or partial lucid interval. Indeed, of the 122 patients studied by Adams et al. (1989), there were 2 patients with a complete lucid interval who had grade 1 injury and 15 with grade 2 TAI who had experienced a partial lucid interval. In contrast, none of the patients with grade 3 TAI talked. The use of immunohistochemistry has further clarified the situation. By using antibodies against amyloid precursor protein, evidence of axonal damage has been found in a small series of patients who died from causes other than those associated with a previously sustained mild brain injury (Blumbergs et al. 1994). Immunohistochemistry has also provided greater insight into the distribution of axonal damage after brain injury, and Blumbergs et al. (1995) have derived a sector scoring method, the sensitivity of which allows the identification of variable amounts of axonal injury (and other pathologies) in patients with a wide range of results on the Glasgow Coma Scale.

It takes between 15 and 18 hours for axonal bulbs to be identified with certainty using silver impregnation techniques in the human brain after brain injury, which limits the testing to patients who survive at least that long. However, as revealed by the more sensitive immunohistochemistry technique, the incidence of DAI is likely higher than the published figures would suggest. Indeed, in a recent study it has been shown that axonal injury of varying amounts is almost a universal finding in cases of fatal brain injury (Gentleman et al. 1993, 1995), and, furthermore, damage to axons can now be identified in those patients whose survival has been as short as 2 hours (Blumbergs et al. 1989; McKenzie et al. 1996; Sherriff et al. 1994). However, in patients who survive for less than 3 hours, although TAI may be strongly suspected, particularly if there are focal lesions in the corpus callosum and

in the brainstem, a definitive diagnosis cannot be made at present.

It is apparent that a pattern of β-amyloid precursor protein immunoreactivity, similar to that first described as TAI, may be seen in association with brain swelling (Kaur et al. 1999) after global ischemia (Dolinak et al. 2000a) and after hypoglycemia (Dolinak et al. 2000b). There are, of course, many conditions in which it is possible to identify abnormal axons, but in medicolegal settings it is particularly important that due attention is paid to the circumstances surrounding death and that large numbers of blocks from appropriate brain areas are taken in a standardized way (Geddes et al. 1997, 2000). Because a degree of confusion and uncertainty exists in the literature about TAI, it is recommended that TAI be referred to as *diffuse traumatic axonal injury*.

Mechanisms of axonal injury.   There have been considerable advances in the understanding of the nature and time course of axonal injury since the early 1990s (Maxwell et al. 1993; Povlishock 1992; Povlishock and Christman 1995). The classical view was that axons are torn at the moment of injury (i.e., primary axotomy [immediate axonal disruption]); this does not appear to be true in most cases, although it does occur under conditions of high mechanical loading (e.g., a pontomedullary rent [see Other Types of Focal Brain Injury section]). In contrast, in conditions of mild to moderate brain injury, it is apparent that there are processes of delayed axotomy, in which the affected axons become lobulated between 6 and 12 hours after injury, and secondary axotomy, which occurs 24–72 hours after injury. Recent experimental work suggests that the time course of secondary axotomy is influenced by the species, the injury model, and the intensity of the injury (Erb and Povlishock 1988; Povlishock and Jenkins 1995; Povlishock et al. 1983; Yaghmai and Povlishock 1992). In general, the time taken for secondary axotomy to occur in cats and pigs is longer than in the rat and is longest in humans.

A well-recognized feature of axonal injury is that of wallerian degeneration. The importance of deafferentation of various target sites has been recognized (Erb and Povlishock 1991), one consequence of which is a phase of excitation (Faden et al. 1989; Hayes et al. 1988, 1991; Jenkins et al. 1988). Such changes might provide a possible explanation, not only for the immediate morbidity, but for subsequent adaptive plasticity and associated recovery.

It has been suggested that physical stretch, or mechanoporation at the time of injury, results in damage to the axolemma and related axoplasm at the injured node of Ranvier (Adams et al. 1991; Gennarelli 1996). This change in membrane structure disrupts the capability of axons to maintain physiological ionic gradients and results in changes in concentrations of calcium, potassium, sodium, and chloride within the axoplasm. These changes in ion concentration in certain fibers may activate neutral proteases, which in turn denature the axonal cytoarchitecture. However, this hypothesis has not been universally accepted (Smith et al. 1999), an alternative view being that TBI can either mechanically or functionally disturb the neurofilament subunits, thereby impairing axoplasmic transport (Povlishock and Jenkins 1995; Stone et al. 2000). Although changes in all three neurofilament subunits were identified, it was found that antibodies to the 68-kd subunit were particularly useful, in that within 60 minutes of brain injury there was a highly localized degradation of this subunit. These views are not necessarily incompatible or irreconcilable, because it is increasingly apparent that the changes are complex, that there are both direct and indirect consequences of mechanical loading, and that ensuing functional impairment is a product of many factors (Maxwell et al. 1997) that may not include morphological abnormality (Tomei et al. 1990).

The anatomical origins of posttraumatic coma have been explored in a pig model of inertial brain injury induced by head rotational acceleration in the axial and coronal planes (Gennarelli 1994). It was found that immediate and prolonged coma was produced by head rotation in both planes. However, extensive damage to axons in the brainstem was limited to animals subjected to axial rotation. Furthermore, the severity of coma correlated with both the extent of axonal damage in the brainstem and the applied kinetic loading conditions. There was no relationship between coma and the extent of axonal damage in other regions. This study had two major conclusions: 1) injury to axons in the brainstem plays an important role in the induction of immediate posttraumatic coma, and 2) TAI can occur without coma.

Hypoxic-ischemic brain damage. Neuropathological studies in the 1970s suggested that irreversible brain damage due to hypoxia-ischemia was not only common after fatal blunt head injury, but in large measure could be attributed to a critical reduction in regional cerebral blood flow (CBF) and, therefore, was potentially avoidable. In the initial study, it was shown that irreversible damage was present in more than 90% of patients and was classified as severe in 27%, moderately severe in 43%, and mild in 30% (Graham et al. 1978). The lesions occurred more frequently within the hippocampus (more than 80% of patients) and in the basal ganglia (approximately 80%) than in the cerebral cortex (46%) and in the cerebellum (44%). Clinicopathological correlations reported associations with episodes of hypoxia and raised ICP.

Because much of this damage was considered to be avoidable or preventable, this finding led to the reappraisal of the management and organization of patient care, with increased attention to the recognition and treatment of hypoxia and hypotension at the scene of the accident, during interhospital transfer, and in critical care units, and with increased attention to the detection and release of brain compression by traumatic intracranial hematoma. Reappraisal of the amount of hypoxic-ischemic damage in a second cohort of fatal blunt head injury was carried out 10 years later in which it was found that hypoxic-ischemic brain damage was still common (occurring in 88% of patients), and there was no statistical difference in the amount of moderately severe and severe damage between the two groups of patients—55% (1968–1972) and 54% (1981–1982), respectively (Graham et al. 1989b)—although there was an increase in the proportion of cases with diffuse damage in the cortex of the type seen in global cerebral ischemia. This was rather surprising, because it would have been expected that the greater use of resuscitative measures would have reduced this type of brain damage at least to some extent. Likely explanations included that the critical events responsible for these changes may have occurred almost immediately after the injury before first admission to the hospital and even before the arrival of any skilled personnel at the scene of the accident. Also, admission policies for the department of neurosurgery had changed in the 10 years between studies, meaning that more patients with intracranial mass lesions were being admitted than previously for investigation and treatment, some of whom would probably have died either in the emergency department or primary surgical ward under previous admission guidelines.

Early clinical studies of acute brain injury had failed to demonstrate any evidence of cerebral ischemia (Muizelaar 1989). However, subsequent work showed that CBF was reduced to threshold levels (equal to or less than 18 mL/100 g/minute) in 33% of patients within the first 6 hours of injury, and that a significant correlation existed between motor score and CBF in the first 8 hours after injury (Bouma et al. 1992). Further work using xenon-CT CBF measurements showed that during the first 4 hours after brain injury, patients without a surgical mass lesion showed a trend toward low initial flow, with subsequent increases in CBF at 24 hours, and that CBF in the first 24 hours after injury was significantly correlated with a low initial Glasgow Coma Scale score. Such studies suggest that reductions in either regional or global CBF with subsequent ischemia may occur within the first hours after severe injury and that a decreased perfusion might have important effects on brain viability and the subsequent outcome.

Although the suggested presence of true ischemia in the acute posttraumatic period remains rather controversial, it seems likely that the early postinjury period is associated with concomitant alterations of brain metabolism that may create a relative ischemia in vulnerable brain areas (Doberstein et al. 1993; Hovda 1996; Hovda et al. 1995; Jones et al. 1994; Miller 1993). Under these conditions, it is postulated that there is an acute increase in glucose utilization and energy demand coupled with a global hypoperfusion or oligemia and that this may therefore reflect a state of relative ischemia that may adversely affect ion homeostasis, membrane function, and neuronal survival.

Several mechanisms may contribute to posttraumatic reduction in CBF that may ultimately lead to cerebral ischemia and infarction. These include the stretching and distortion of brain vessels as a result of mechanical displacement of brain structures (e.g., brain shift or herniation caused by an intracranial mass lesion [see above]), arterial hypotension in association with multiple injuries, vasospasm of blood vessels in the circle of Willis, and posttraumatic changes in small blood vessels (Dietrich et al. 1994; Maxwell et al. 1988, 1991). The role of vasospasm as a potential mechanism underlying the development of posttraumatic hypoperfusion has been emphasized through the use of transcranial Doppler ultrasonography (Chan et al. 1992, 1993; Weber et al. 1990).

Secondary Insults

There is little doubt that primary traumatic damage to the brain may be made worse by the superimposition of so-called secondary insults that may occur soon after the injury, during transfer to the hospital, and during the subsequent treatment of the brain-injured patient. Such insults may be of either intracranial or systemic origin and may actually arise during initial management or later in the intensive care unit. The full extent of these secondary insults became apparent between 1970 and 1985 when a number of authors reported that in severely brain-injured patients hypoxia was found in 30% and arterial hypotension in 15% of them on arrival in the emergency department. Largely because of better onsite resuscitation and transport arrangements, there has been a reduction in these early insults, with attention now being directed toward the increasing awareness that such events after brain injury may actually occur within the intensive care unit. This awareness has been due largely to continuous monitoring during intensive care and the correlations that exist between the adverse influences of these secondary insults and the clinical outcome. Current experience suggests that secondary insults occur more frequently and last longer than previously had been thought and that the duration of these insults matters as much as their severity.

Even the lowest grade of severity of insult has been shown to have an adverse impact on outcome, although apparently the most relevant predictors of mortality at 12 months postinjury have been the durations of hypotension, pyrexia, and hypoxemia (Marshall 2000).

Diffuse (Multifocal) Vascular Injury

Diffuse (multifocal) vascular injury is a form of acute brain injury after trauma that is characterized by a series of multiple, small hemorrhages that are particularly conspicuous in the white matter of the frontal and temporal lobes, in and adjacent to the thalamus, and in the brainstem. Small hemorrhages may also be seen in parasagittal white matter and in the corpus callosum. This pattern of brain damage is seen in patients who die either instantly or at the scene of the accident, although a number may survive for up to 24 hours. It is thought to represent a severe form of brain injury in which, as a result of acceleration/deceleration, tearing has occurred in small blood vessels. The relationship between this entity and that of TAI has yet to be defined.

Brain Swelling

Brain swelling may be either localized or generalized and may occur alone or in combination with other pathologies. In general, brain swelling is due to an increase in the cerebral blood volume (congestive brain swelling) or in the water content of the brain tissue (cerebral edema). Brain swelling may contribute to an elevation of the ICP and death from secondary damage to the brainstem.

Swelling of the Brain Adjacent to Contusions, Lacerations, or an Intracerebral Hematoma

As a result of damage to the blood-brain barrier, water, electrolytes, and protein leak into brain tissue and spread into the adjacent white matter to form vasogenic edema readily detected within 24–48 hours of injury by CT or MRI. In many cases, the swelling reaches its peak between 4 and 8 days after injury, but it is largely due to a combination of vascular damage, inadequate cerebral perfusion, and retention of fluid within the extracellular space. Therefore, this type of swelling is easy to understand when it occurs adjacent to contusions and lacerations (Figure 2–8).

Swelling of One Cerebral Hemisphere

Swelling of one cerebral hemisphere is most often seen in association with an ipsilateral acute SDH. When the hematoma is evacuated, the brain expands to fill the space (Figure 2–9). The pathogenesis of this entity has not been fully determined, but it is likely due to reperfusion of a

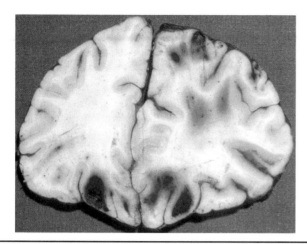

FIGURE 2–8. **Swelling associated with contusion: 17-hour survival.**

There is swelling of the right frontal lobe in close association with contusional injury.

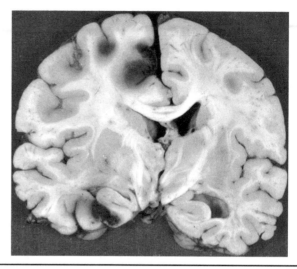

FIGURE 2–9. **Unilateral swelling of the cerebral hemisphere: 49-hour survival.**

An acute left-sided subdural hematoma was evacuated. At autopsy, the space previously occupied by the clot has been filled by an expanded cerebral hemisphere. Note the resultant displacement of midline structures, internal herniae, and distortion of the ventricles. There was also compression of the brainstem and secondary hemorrhages.

vascular bed that has lost its physiological tone as a result of the mass effect of an SDH. When this vascular bed is reperfused, the blood vessels dilate, the blood-brain barrier becomes leaky, and there is diffuse swelling of one cerebral hemisphere that in large measure is a consequence of vasogenic edema.

Diffuse Swelling of Both Cerebral Hemispheres

Diffuse swelling of both cerebral hemispheres is a feature of children and young adults. If fatal, the brain is swollen diffusely, and the ventricles are small and symmetrical. In a detailed neuropathological study of 63 fatally brain-injured children aged between 2 and 15 years, diffuse brain swelling was found in 17% of patients (Graham et al. 1989a). In a few patients, the swelling was associated with widespread hypoxic-ischemic brain damage, secondary to posttraumatic status epilepticus or cardiorespiratory arrest. In most cases, it was idiopathic, with the assumption that, as with diffuse swelling of one cerebral hemisphere, the main etiology was reperfusion of a vascular bed that had become unresponsive to physiological stimuli after brain injury. At first, vasodilation induces a defective blood-brain barrier, leading to true vasogenic edema. However, neuroimaging has produced inconsistent results.

Brain Injury in Infancy and Childhood

Brain injuries in infancy and childhood are common in practice, are predominantly mild, and are therefore of little consequence. However, TBI is the single most common cause of death and new disabilities in childhood (Luerssen 1991), especially in children younger than 12

months (Adelson and Kochanek 1998; Duhaime et al. 1992; Weiner and Weinberg 2000). Injuries from child abuse account for almost 25% of all hospital admissions for children younger than 2 years. The majority of hospital admissions in children between the ages of 2 and 4 years are caused by injuries from falls, whereas most older children are admitted because of injuries from bicycling and motor vehicle accidents.

Fracture of the skull in infancy is not common because the skull is relatively thin and breaks easily after impact. Skull fracture in infancy can be associated with subepicranial hygroma when a dural tear is involved, allowing CSF to dissect beneath the periosteum (Epstein et al. 1961). Furthermore, a growing skull fracture may develop that results from the herniation of contused and swollen brain through the dura mater, thereby separating the bones along the line of the fracture. Scarring at the junction between the brain and dura mater prevents secondary closure of the dura, thereby perpetuating the growing fracture (Scarfo et al. 1989).

Extra (epi) dural hematomas rarely result from injury to the middle meningeal artery: venous bleeding from the bone is the usual cause. Chronic SDHs occur most commonly at 6 months of age and are rare after 12 months (Weiner and Weinberg 2000).

Child abuse is a major cause of TBI in infants—resulting in the so-called battered child. The term *shaken baby syndrome* has been used to describe the acute SDH and subarachnoid hemorrhage, retinal hemorrhages, and periosteal new bone formation attributed to the to-and-fro shaking of a child's body, producing a whiplash motion of the child's head on the neck (Caffey 1974). The term *shaken baby* has been questioned because inertial forces generated by shaking alone were insignificant compared with those caused by impact (Duhaime et al. 1987, 1998). The consensus view is that brain-injured infants undergo shaking followed by sudden inertial injury from impact.

In an autopsy series of 87 children (Geddes et al. 2001a, 2001b), the principal finding was similar to those found in adults. The main exception was the increased frequency of bilateral hemispheric swelling, which was attributed in 27 of 45 children to hypoxia-ischemia, contusions, or intracranial hematomas, or a combination of these factors: in the remaining 18 patients, the underlying cause could not be found.

Recent clinicopathological studies (Geddes et al. 2001a, 2001b) involving 53 cases of nonaccidental pediatric TBI, of which 37 were infants aged 20 days to 9 months and 16 were children aged between 13 months and 2 years 6 months, showed that TAI of the type seen in adults was only present in children older than 12 months. In infants younger than 12 months, hypoxic-ischemic damage was the principal finding. Therefore, contrary to some literature (Gleckman et al. 1999; Hahn et al. 1988; Shannon et al. 1998), TAI is not a feature of nonaccidental TBI in infants in whom structural damage that results from hypoxia-ischemia is thought to be consequent to respiratory distress and/or apnea due to axonal injury at the craniocervical junction.

Neurochemical Changes

It is likely that posttraumatic neurochemical alterations may involve changes in the synthesis and/or release of both endogenous "neuroprotective" and "autodestructive" compounds. The identification of these compounds from the timing of the pathological cascade after brain injury provides a window of opportunity for treatment with pharmacological agents designed to modify gene expression, synthesis and release of transmitters, and receptor binding, or the physiological activity of these factors with subsequent prevention or attenuation of neuronal damage. Some of the more important changes are as follows.

Acetylcholine

An increase in the concentration of acetylcholine in the brain has been reported after experimental TBI. Other studies have shown a decrease in the binding of cholinergic receptors, and fluid percussion brain injury in the rat significantly decreases the affinity of muscarinic and cholinergic receptor binding in both the hippocampus and brainstem, changes that may last as long as 15 days postinjury (Jiang et al. 1994; Lyeth et al. 1994). These and other data have led to the suggestion that activation of muscarinic cholinergic systems in the rostral pons mediates behavioral suppression associated with TBI, whereas lasting behavioral deficits result from pathological excitation of forebrain structures induced by the release of acetylcholine. More recently, it has been shown that controlled cortical impact in the rat causes an impairment of cholinergic neurons that produces enhanced vulnerability to disruption of cholinergically mediated cognitive function, and previous studies have shown that the administration of the anticholinergic compound scopolamine reduces neurobehavioral dysfunction after experimental brain injury in rats. In a recent study of pre- and postsynaptic markers of cholinergic transmission in human postmortem brains from patients who died after brain injury and matched controls, the mean value of choline acetyltransferase activity was reduced by approximately 50% in the brain-injured group. In contrast, there was no difference between the brain-injured and control groups in the levels of M_1 or M_2 receptor binding (Dewar and Graham 1996). Given the involvement of acetylcholine in cognitive function, it is possible to speculate that reduced cholinergic acetyltransferase activity may be associated with cognitive impairment in patients who survive a brain injury (Murdoch et al. 2002).

Arachidonic Acid Cascade

Damage to the cell membrane by calcium-activated proteases and lipases induces the production of a variety of potentially pathogenic agents from a breakdown of endogenous intracellular fatty acids. The formation of compounds such as arachidonic acid–activated phospholipase A_2 lipooxygenase, cyclooxygenase, and leukotrienes; thromboxanes; free-fatty acids; and other breakdown products with arachadonic acid cascade have been associated with neuronal death and poor outcome in models of experimental brain injury (DeWitt et al. 1988; Ellis et al. 1989; Hall 1985; Nakashima et al. 1993; Shohami et al. 1987; Wei et al. 1982; Yergey and Heyes 1990).

Catecholamine and Monoamine Neurotransmitters

Laboratory studies have shown that circulating levels of epinephrine and norepinephrine increase with increasing severity of injury and that there are regional changes in the tissue concentration of them and of dopamine after experimental fluid percussion and controlled cortical impact brain injury in rats (McIntosh et al. 1994b; Prasad et al. 1992; Prasad et al. 1994). Changes in α_1-adrenergic receptor binding in damaged cortex and hippocampus after experimental lateral fluid percussion in the rat have also been described (Prasad et al. 1994).

Activation of the serotonergic (5-HT) system has also been suggested to play a role in TBI, and an increase in 5-HT has been shown to be closely associated with the depression of local cerebral glucose utilization in regions showing extensive histological damage (Pappius 1981; Prasad et al. 1992; Tsuiki et al. 1995).

Cytokines

There is an increased number of immunocompetent cells in the plasma of brain-injured patients, and it is possible that such cells, because the blood-brain barrier is opened, often for long periods, may enter the injured brain and exert a neurotoxic effect. Polymorphonuclear leucocytes accumulate within 24 hours in injured brain (Biagas et al. 1992; Zhuang et al. 1993), and this correlates with the onset of posttraumatic brain swelling in rats (Schoettle et al. 1990). However, experimentally induced neutropenia does not appear to influence the development of posttraumatic edema or reduce cortical lesion volume, although a decrease in volume after occlusion of the middle cerebral artery in immunosuppressed (neutropenic) rats has been described (Chen et al. 1993). Macrophages undoubtedly play an important role in wound healing, and many of them secrete soluble factors, including cytokines that may influence posttraumatic neuronal survivability and outcome. Moreover, injured neuronal and nonneuronal cells within the central nervous system (CNS) can synthesize and secrete inflammatory cytokines that may mediate further brain damage. Among the cytokines implicated in this additional damage are tumor necrosis factor (TNF) and the interleukin family of peptides. For example, after mechanical trauma to the brain, there is a large increase in the regional brain concentration of interleukin-1, -6, and TNF, suggesting that the CNS-derived cytokines may play a role in the pathophysiological cascade of brain damage after trauma (Fan et al. 1995; Mocchetti and Wrathall 1995; Shohami et al. 1994). Studies have documented the beneficial effects of pharmacological blockade of interleukin-1β and TNF, suggesting that the release and/or upregulation of these pathways may be either pathogenic (Woodroofe et al. 1991) or protective (Dietrich et al. 1996).

Although many compounds have been measured after TBI, the identification of neuron-specific enolase and the

S-100 protein in the CSF or serum indicate nerve cell or glial damage (Herrmann et al. 2000; McKeating et al. 1998; Ogata and Tsuganezawa 1999; Singhal et al. 2002).

Endogenous Opioid Peptides

There is an increase in the regional immunoreactivity of the endogenous opioid dynorphin after a fluid percussion brain injury that has been shown to correlate with structural brain damage and reductions in regional CBF (McIntosh et al. 1987a, 1987b). Furthermore, both the intracerebroventricular and intraparenchymal microinjection of dynorphin and other kappa-agonists worsens neurological injury, suggesting that, indeed, dynorphin has a pathogenic effect after brain injury (McIntosh et al. 1994a). However, pharmacological studies would suggest that the effect is indirect and that it may be mediated by other neurotransmitter or neurochemical systems, including the excitatory amino acids (EAAs) glutamate and aspartate, an effect that can be reversed by both competitive and noncompetitive N-methyl-D-aspartate (NMDA) antagonists (Isaac et al. 1990). Although the mechanisms by which dynorphin induces NMDA receptor–mediated activity remain speculative, some studies suggest that opioids may modulate the presynaptic release of EAA neurotransmitters, thereby contributing to regional neuronal damage during the acute posttraumatic period (Faden 1992).

Excitatory Amino Acids

There is a marked increase in the extracellular EAAs glutamate and aspartate after TBI (Jenkins et al. 1988; Katayama et al. 1990; Nilsson et al. 1990; Palmer et al. 1993). Although the amount varies in different models of TBI, there is a close association between the increased intracellular concentration and total tissue concentrations of sodium and calcium (Olney et al. 1987; Rothman and Olney 1995). The exact mechanisms underlying EAA-mediated cell death are not well understood, but it has been postulated that the sustained release of glutamate with prolonged postsynaptic excitation causes the early accumulation of intracellular sodium, which in turn leads to acute neuronal swelling and delayed calcium influx that causes a cascade of metabolic disturbances within neurons that may lead eventually to cell death. These findings have suggested that posttraumatic cognitive deficits may result in part from excitotoxic events specifically targeting the hippocampus, inducing overt neuronal cell loss, cellular stress, and/or dysfunction, thereby disrupting normal synaptic transmission (Smith and McIntosh 1996).

Laboratory evidence for the glutamate hypothesis is good, particularly in models of focal cerebral ischemia in which treatment is started either immediately before or after the procedure. Cerebral ischemia is common after TBI, and because there is good evidence both in animal models of neurotrauma (Chen et al. 1991; Gordon and Bullock 1999; Landolt et al. 1998; Smith and McIntosh 1996) and in human TBI (Zauner and Bullock 1995) that glutamate is released in large amounts, it is logical to hypothesize that antagonists directed toward the NMDA receptor might be effective. However, the initial clinical trials have been disappointing (Narayan et al. 2002).

Growth Factors

The potential of neurons and glial cells to recover after TBI depends both on the posttraumatic ionic/neurotransmitter environment and on the presence of neurotrophic substances (growth factors). They support nerve cell survival, induce the sprouting of neurites (plasticity), and facilitate the guidance of neurites to their proper target sites. The most well-characterized neurotrophic factors include nerve growth factor (NGF), basic fibroblast growth factor (FGF), brain-derived neurotrophic factor, glial-derived neurotrophic factor, and NT-3. Some studies have suggested that these factors are synthesized or released after traumatic CNS injury and that their concentration increases during the first few days after a number of experimental procedures (Conner et al. 1994; Varon et al. 1991). Relatively little is known about the neurotrophic factor response in experimental TBI (Leonard et al. 1994), but NGF- and FGF-like neurotrophic activity has been observed to increase in the CSF of brain-injured patients (Patterson et al. 1993). The intraparenchymal infusion of NGF over 14 days postinjury has also been reported to reduce septohippocampal cellular damage and improve neurobehavioral motor and cognitive function after fluid percussion brain injury in the rat (Sinson et al. 1995). A neuroprotective effect of FGF has also been found in a rodent model of cortical contusion (Dietrich et al. 1996).

Ion Changes

The principal ion changes in TBI are in calcium, magnesium, and potassium. Changes in calcium ion homeostasis are believed to be pivotal in the development of neuronal cell death. For example, total brain tissue calcium concentrations have been found to be significantly elevated in injured areas after both experimental fluid percussion brain injury and cortical contusion in rats (Shapira et al. 1989a, 1989b). Furthermore, there is a significant increase in regional calcium accumulation that has been shown to persist for at least 48 hours after fluid percussion

brain injury in the rat (Hovda et al. 1991). In support of this hypothesis is the finding of increased expression of some of the immediate early genes after fluid percussion injury, because they are known to be activated by an increase in intracellular calcium (Raghupathi et al. 1995; Yang et al. 1994).

Magnesium is involved in a number of critical cellular processes, and alterations in its tissue amounts impair maintenance of normal intracellular sodium and potassium gradients. After traumatic injury to the CNS, there is a reduction in brain magnesium that is hypothesized to impair glucose utilization, energy metabolism, and protein synthesis, thereby reducing both oxidative and substrate phosphorylation (Vink and McIntosh 1990; Vink et al. 1990). Because magnesium has an important regulatory role with respect to calcium transport and accumulation and cerebrovascular contractility, changes in intracellular magnesium could potentially contribute to posttraumatic calcium-mediated neurotoxicity and/or the regulation of regional posttraumatic blood flow.

After experimental brain injury, there is a rapid and massive increase in the release of potassium into the extracellular space that can be associated with burst discharges, depolarization, and spreading depression (Siesjo and Wieloch 1985). The increase in extracellular potassium has been thought to contribute to disruption of energy homeostasis, cerebral vasoconstriction, changes in cerebral glycolysis, and loss of consciousness (Siesjo and Wieloch 1985). The excess extracellular potassium is rapidly taken up by astrocytes: this may result in astrocytic edema, which in turn may impair neuronal oxygen transport.

Oxygen-Free Radicals and Lipid Peroxidation

Hypoperfusion of brain tissue may stimulate the generation of oxygen-free radicals, principal amongst which is superoxide. Superoxide may arise from a number of sources that include the arachidonic acid cascade, the autooxidation of amine neurotransmitters, mitochondria leakage, xanthine oxidase activity, and the oxidation of extravasated hemoglobin (Hall 1996; Kontos and Povlishock 1986). Additional sources, at least in the first few hours and days after trauma, may be activated microglia, infiltrating neutrophils, and macrophages. Within the injured brain where pH is lowered, conditions are also favorable for the potential release of iron, which may then participate in the formation of hydroxy radical. Iron also promotes the process of lipid peroxidation. Multiple studies have shown that in cats subjected to fluid percussion injury there is early generation of superoxide radicals in injured brain, and the generation of these radicals occurs in parallel with secondary injury to the brain and its microvasculature, including the formation of vasogenic edema (Hall 1996; Kontos and Povlishock 1986; Siesjo and Wieloch 1985).

Cellular Changes

After fluid percussion–induced brain injury (Bramlett et al. 1997; Hall 1996; Kontos and Povlishock 1986; Pierce et al. 1998; Raghupathi et al. 1995; Siesjo and Wieloch 1985; Smith et al. 1997a; Vink and McIntosh 1990; Vink et al. 1990) and controlled cortical impact (Dixon et al. 1999) in the rat, the volume of cortical contusion and the ventricles increased with lengthening survival. Such findings, combined with clinical and neurological observation, suggest that, in addition to any cellular necrosis induced at the time of injury (Graham et al. 1978; 1989b), there may also be a series of cellular events with a more protracted time course. One such process is programmed cell death (PCD) the first evidence of which after experimental TBI was demonstrated by TUNEL histochemistry, gel electrophoresis, and electron microscopy (Rink et al. 1995). It was found that TUNEL+ cells could be detected for up to 72 hours after initial injury, the longest time for which the animals were allowed to survive. More recent studies have confirmed that PCD and the nuclear changes of apoptosis can occur at 2 months after experimental TBI (Clark et al. 1997; Colicos et al. 1996; Conti et al. 1998; Newcomb et al. 1999; Yakovlev et al. 1997). The findings of PCD in experimental models have been replicated in clinical studies (Clark et al. 1999; Shaw et al. 2001; Smith et al. 2000). Recent work has identified TUNEL+ cells predominantly in white matter in patients surviving up to 12 months after TBI (Williams et al. 2001). Although the exact nature of the TUNEL+ cells in these studies was not established by morphological and immunohistochemical criteria, they were considered to be predominantly macrophages occurring in association with wallerian degeneration.

Experimental Models of Focal and Diffuse TBI

Although the understanding of TBI has been greatly enhanced by the use of physical, computer, and cell culture models, it has been necessary to provide biological validation of them by parallel animate models in which the studies are designed to replicate certain aspects of human brain injury. Such models have been used extensively to investigate precise mechanisms leading to the various sequelae of brain injury that may have an origin in

either focal or diffuse, or both, types of brain injury. However, there is an increasing appreciation that, although the various pathologies may be described and characterized as either focal or diffuse, there is considerable overlap between them, although pure examples of each exist in clinical practice.

Models of Focal TBI

In general, there are three techniques that are used commonly to produce experimental focal brain injury: 1) weight drop (Feeney et al. 1981; Shapira et al. 1989a), 2) fluid percussion (Dixon et al. 1987; McIntosh et al. 1989; Toulmond et al. 1993), and 3) rigid indentation (Dixon et al. 1991; Smith et al. 1995; Soares et al. 1992). In all three models, the head is held rigidly in one position during the experimental procedure. In weight drop models of brain injury, weights are dropped through a guiding apparatus to impact the closed cranium, a metal plate fixed to the cranium, or through a craniectomy directly onto the brain. In models of fluid percussion, there is a rapid injection of fluid through a sealed port into the closed cranial cavity. In rigid indentation, typically there is a pneumatically driven impactor to deform brain tissue through a craniectomy at a specific velocity and depth. Each of the three techniques may be adjusted to generate a reproducible spectrum of injury severity (Gennarelli 1994).

All three models typically produce focal contusion of the cortex, which histologically appears as hemorrhagic foci of necrosis that undergo changes characterized by absorption of the dead tissue, scarring, and the development of a cavity. A further feature of the contusion is local disruption of the blood-brain barrier, but change is also seen well beyond the immediate vicinity of the contusion. This disruption facilitates the formation of vasogenic edema, a decrease in regional CBF, and an increase in glucose metabolism. Although blood flow adjacent to the contusion may not be at critical levels, it is apparent that oligemia, when occurring in association with a hypermetabolic response to trauma, creates an injury-induced vulnerability after traumatic injury in which the brain may be at risk to even minor changes in CBF, increases in ICP, or apnea (see section Hypoxic-Ischemic Brain Damage).

With survival, there is a cellular response to the traumatic injury. For example, neutrophil polymorphs increase in number by 24 hours after injury and migrate into the necrotic tissue. This is followed by activation of microglia and the development of macrophages, which are particularly prominent at the sites of contusion. However, activation of microglia is also present throughout regions demonstrating disruption of the blood-brain barrier, including the hippocampus and thalamus. The cellular changes herald expression of cytokines and other markers of injury, including heat shock protein and immediate early genes. There is also a rapid and florid astrocytic response that defines the margins of the contusion with the establishment of a glial limitans.

In many of the models, there is also evidence of more widely distributed pathology. Such changes include tissue tears in the dentate gyrus of the hemisphere and evidence of axonal swellings and bulb formation in the white matter of both the ipsi- and contralateral hemispheres.

Reference was made in the section Classification and Mechanisms of Brain Damage to the concept of primary and secondary brain damage, with the implication that the latter is not restricted to head injury but is the consequence of a further insult to an already damaged brain. Additional evidence for this concept is the identification of changes in various neuronal populations that are remote from the site of contusion. There are a number of mechanisms that might account for these lesions, and their importance has been demonstrated by the finding that lesions in the CA-3 subfield and hilus of the dentate gyrus correlate with the severity of posttraumatic memory dysfunction (Smith et al. 1995).

Models of Diffuse TBI

Typically, models of diffuse traumatic brain injury attempt to replicate the human clinicopathological entity of TAI, in which there is widespread microscopical evidence of damage to the axons. Damage to axons under these conditions has been shown to be produced primarily by high-strain rotational or angular acceleration, not necessarily associated with impact. Until relatively recently there was only one animal model that replicated all of the clinical features of TAI. This was the Penn-2 Hyge model using nonhuman primates, in which it was possible to induce a pattern and type of damage that paralleled the features seen in humans (Adams et al. 1982; Gennarelli et al. 1982). Nonhuman primates were originally chosen for this experimental model due to their large brain mass, which allows the development of high strain between regions of tissue. As the brain size decreases, the forces necessary to induce similar strains increase exponentially. To exemplify this point, the Penn-2 device is capable of producing 18,000 kg of thrust, just enough to generate sufficient forces to cause TAI in a 50- to 75-g nonhuman primate brain. In this model, it was possible to induce a spectrum of pathology, the exact nature of which depended on the biomechanical profile of the injury. For example, rapid rotation acceleration in the sagittal plane produced SDHs, whereas a slower acceleration in the coronal plane produced DAI (Gennarelli and Thibault 1982).

More recently, a porcine model of rotational acceleration brain injury has been developed using young adult miniature swine that have a brain mass of approximately 60–70 g (Meaney et al. 1993). To date, although axonal injury has been produced in subcortical white matter in the porcine model, it has not been possible to induce tissue tears or gliding contusions, and axonal injury is associated with only brief loss of consciousness (Smith et al. 1997b).

A model of impact acceleration brain injury in rats has been shown to produce widely distributed axonal damage. In this model, a weight is dropped onto a plate fixed to the cranium of a rat (Marmarou et al. 1994). Unlike most brain injury models, the head is not fixed in place and is allowed to rotate downward. It has been suggested that it is this motion, in combination with impact, which results in the overt widespread damage to axons.

Models have also been developed to mimic closed head injury in infants and children. These include the use of immature rats (Adelson et al. 1996) and juvenile pigs (Duhaime et al. 2000; Madsen and Rejke-Nielsen 1987). A more recent study using the Hyge apparatus in the immature pig has demonstrated that nonimpact, inertial brain trauma induced SDH and TAI, with a characteristic distribution (Raghupathi and Margulies 2002).

References

Adams JH: Head injury, in Greenfield's Neuropathology. Edited by Adams JH, Duchen LW. London, Edward Arnold, 1992, pp 106–152

Adams JH, Mitchell DE, Graham DI, et al: Diffuse brain damage of immediate impact type. Brain 100:489–502, 1977

Adams JH, Graham, DI, Scott G, et al: Brain damage in fatal non-missile head injury. J Clin Pathol 33:1132–1145, 1980

Adams JH, Graham DI, Murray LS, et al: Diffuse axonal injury due to non-missile head injury in humans: an analysis of 45 cases. Ann Neurol 12:557–563, 1982

Adams JH, Doyle D, Graham DI, et al: The contusion index: a reappraisal in human and experimental non-missile head injury. Neuropathol Appl Neurobiol 11:299–308, 1985

Adams JH, Doyle D, Graham DI, et al: Deep intracerebral (basal ganglia) haematomas in fatal non-missile head injury in man. J Neurol Neurosurg Psychiatry 49:1039–1043, 1986

Adams JH, Doyle D, Ford I, et al: Diffuse axonal injury in head injury: definition, diagnosis and grading. Histopathology 15:49–59, 1989

Adams JH, Graham DI, Gennarelli TA, et al: Diffuse axonal injury in non-missile head injury. J Neurol Neurosurg Psychiatry 54:481–483, 1991

Adelson PD, Kochanek PM: Head injury in children. J Child Neurol 13:2–15, 1998

Adelson PD, Robichaud P, Hamilton RL, et al: A model of diffuse traumatic brain injury in the immature rat. J Neurosurg 85:877–884, 1996

Biagas KV, Uhl MW, Schidine JK, et al: Assessment of post-traumatic polymorphonuclear leukocyte accumulation in rat brain using tissue myeloperoxidase assay and vinblastine treatment. J Neurotrauma 9:363–371, 1992

Blumbergs PC, Jones NR, North JB: Diffuse axonal injury in head trauma. J Neurol Neurosurg Psychiatry 52:838–841, 1989

Blumbergs PC, Scott G, Manavis, J, et al: Staining of amyloid precursor protein to study axonal damage in mild head injury. Lancet 344:1055–1056, 1994

Blumbergs PC, Scott G, Manavis J, et al: Topography of axonal injury as defined by amyloid precursor protein and the sector scoring method in mild and severe closed head injury. J Neurotrauma 12:565–572, 1995

Bouma GJ, Muizelaar JP, Stringer WA, et al: Ultra-early evaluation of regional cerebral blood flow in severely head-injured patients using xenon-enhanced computerized tomography. J Neurosurg 77:360–368, 1992

Bramlett HM, Dietrich WD, Green EJ, et al: Chronic histopathological consequences of fluid percussion brain injury in rats: effects of post-traumatic hypothermia. Acta Neuropathol 93:190–199, 1997

Bristol Royal Infirmary Inquiry: The inquiry into the management of care of children receiving complex heart surgery at the Bristol Royal Infirmary, 2000. Available at: http://www.bristolinquiry.org.uk. Accessed July 28, 2004.

Britt RH, Herrick MK, Mason RT, et al: Traumatic lesions of the pontomedullary junction. Neurosurgery 6:623–631, 1980

Bullock R, Teasdale G: Surgical management of traumatic intracranial hematomas, in Handbook of Clinical Neurology, Vol 15: Head Injury. Edited by Brackman R. Amsterdam, Elsevier, 1990, pp 249–298

Bullock R, Smith RM, van Dellen JR: Nonoperative management of extradural hematoma. Neurosurgery 16:602–606, 1985

Caffey J: The whiplash shaken infant syndrome—manual shaking by the extremities with whiplash—induced intracranial and intaocular bleeding linked with residual permanent brain damage and mental retardment. Paediatrics 54:396–403, 1974

Chan KH, Miller JD, Dearden NM: Intracranial blood flow velocity after head injury: relationship to severity of injury, time, neurological status and outcome. J Neurol Neurosurg Psychiatry 55:787–791, 1992

Chan KH, Dearden NM, Miller JD: Transcranial Doppler sonography in severe head injury. Acta Neurochir Suppl (Wien) 59:81–85, 1993

Chen H, Chopp M, Schultz L, et al: Sequential neuronal and astrocytic changes after transient middle cerebral artery occlusion in the rat. J Neurol Sci 118:109–116, 1993

Chen MH, Bullock R, Graham DI, et al: Ischemic neuronal damage after acute subdural hematoma in the rat: effects of pre-treatment with a glutamate antagonise. J Neurosurg 74:944–950, 1991

Clark JM: Distribution of microglial clusters in the brain after head injury. J Neurol Neurosurg Psychiatry 37:463–474, 1974

Clark RSB, Chen J, Watkins SC, et al: Apoptosis-suppressor gene: Bcl -2 expression after traumatic brain injury in rats. J Neurosci 17:9172–9182, 1997

Clark RSB, Kochanek PM, Chen M, et al: Increases in Bcl-2 and cleavage of caspase-1 and caspase-3 in human brain after head injury. FASEB J 13:813–821, 1999

Colicos MA, Dixon CE, Dash PK: Delayed selective neuronal death following experimental cortical impact injury in rats. Possible role in memory deficits. Brain Res 739:111–119, 1996

Conner JM, Fass-Holmes B, Varon S: Changes in nerve growth factor immunoreactivity following entorhinal cortex lesions: possible molecular mechanism regulating cholinergic sprouting. J Comp Neurol 345:409–418, 1994

Conti AC, Raghupathi R, Trojanowski JQ, et al: Experimental brain injury induces regionally distinct apoptosis during active and delayed post-traumatic period. J Neurosci 18:5663–5672, 1998

Cooper PR: Post-traumatic intracranial mass lesions, in Head Injury. Edited by Cooper PR, Golfinos JG. New York, McGraw-Hill, 2001, p 293

Dewar D, Graham DI: Depletion of choline acetyltransferase activity but preservation of M_1 and M_2 muscarinic receptor binding sites in temporal cortex following head injury: a preliminary human postmortem study. J Neurotrauma 13:181–187, 1996

DeWitt DS, Kong DL, Lyeth BG, et al: Experimental traumatic brain injury elevates brain prostaglandin E_2 and thromboxane B_2 levels in rats. J Neurotrauma 5:303–313, 1988

Dietrich WD, Alonso O, Halley M: Early microvascular and neuronal consequences to traumatic brain injury: a light and electron microscopic study in rats. J Neurotrauma 11:289–301, 1994

Dietrich WD, Alonso O, Busto R, et al: Posttreatment with intravenous basic fibroblast growth factor reduces histopathological damage following fluid-percussion brain injury in rats. J Neurotrauma 13:309–316, 1996

Dixon CE, Lyeth BG, Povlishock JT, et al: A fluid percussion model of experimental brain injury in the rat: neurological, physiological, and histopathological characteristics. J Neurosurg 67:110–119, 1987

Dixon CE, Clifton G, Lighthall JW, et al: A controlled cortical impact model of traumatic brain injury in the rat. J Neurosci Methods 39:1, 1991

Dixon CE, Kochanek PM, Yan HQ, et al: One year study of spatial memory performance. Brain morphology and cholinergic markers after moderate controlled cortical impact in rats. J Neurotrauma 16:109–122, 1999

Doberstein CE, Hovda DA, Becker DP: Clinical considerations in the reduction of secondary brain injury. Ann Emerg Med 22:933–937, 1993

Dolinak D, Smith C, Graham DI: Global hypoxia per se is an unusual cause of axonal injury. Neuropathol Appl Neurobiol 100:553–560, 2000a

Dolinak D, Smith C, Graham DI: Hypoglycaemia is a cause of axonal injury. Neuropathol Appl Neurobiol 26:448–453, 2000b

Duhaime AC, Gennarelli TA, Thibault LE, et al: The shaken baby syndrome: a clinical, pathological and biochemical study. J Neurosurg 66:409–415, 1987

Duhaime A, Alario AJ, Lewander WJ, et al: Head injury in very young children: mechanisms, injury types, and ophthalmologic findings in 100 hospitalised patients younger than 2 years of age. Paediatrics 90:179–185, 1992

Duhaime AC, Christian CW, Rorke LB, et al: Nonaccidental head injury in infants in the "shaken-baby" syndrome. N Engl J Med 338:1822–1829, 1998

Duhaime AC, Margulies SS, Durham SR, et al: Maturation-dependent response of the piglet brain to scaled cortical impact. J Neurosurg 93:455–462, 2000

Ellis EF, Police RJ, Rice LY, et al: Increased plasma PGE2, 6-keto-PGF1a and 12-HETE levels following experimental concussive brain injury. J Neurotrauma 6:31–37, 1989

Elsner H, Rieamonti D, Corradino G, et al: Delayed traumatic intracerebral hematomas. J Neurosurg 72:813–815, 1990

Epstein JA, Epstein BS, Small M: Subepicranial hygroma: a complication of head injuries in infants and children. J Pediatr 59:562–566, 1961

Erb DE, Povlishock JT: Axonal damage in severe traumatic brain injury: an experimental study in the cat. Acta Neuropathol 76:347–358, 1988

Erb DE, Povlishock JT: Neuroplasticity following traumatic brain injury: a study of GABAergic terminal loss and recovery in the cat dorsal lateral vestibular nucleus. Exp Brain Res 83:253–267, 1991

Faden AI: Dynorphin increases extracellular levels of excitatory amino acids in the brain through a nonopioid mechanism. J Neurosci 12:425–429, 1992

Faden AI, Demediuk P, Panter SS, et al: The role of excitatory amino acids and NMDA receptors in traumatic brain injury. Science 244:798–800, 1989

Fan L, Young PR, Barone FC, et al: Experimental brain injury induces expression of interleukin-1β mRNA in the rat brain. Mol Brain Res 30:125–130, 1995

Feeney DM, Boyeson MG, Linn RT, et al: Responses to cortical injury, I: methodology and local effects of contusions in the rat. Brain Res 211:67–77, 1981

Fogelholm R, Waltimo O: Epidemiology of chronic subdural haematoma. Acta Neurochir (Wien) 32:247, 1975

Freytag E: Autopsy findings in head injuries from blunt forces: statistical evaluation of 1,367 cases. Arch Pathol 75:402–413, 1963

Gean AD: Imaging of Head Trauma. New York, Raven Press, 1994

Geddes JF, Vowles GH, Beer TW, et al: The diagnosis of diffuse axonal injury: implications for forensic practice. Neuropathol Appl Neurobiol 23:339–347, 1997

Geddes JF, Whitwell HL, Graham DI: Traumatic axonal injury: practical issues for diagnosis in medicolegal cases. Neuropathol Appl Neurobiol 26:105–116, 2000

Geddes JF, Hackshaw AK, Vowles GH, et al: Neuropathology of inflicted head injury in children, I: patterns of brain damage. Brain 124:1290–1298, 2001a

Geddes JF, Vowles GH, Hackshaw AK, et al: Neuropathology of inflicted head injury in children, II: microscopic brain injury in infants. Brain 124:1299–1306, 2001b

Gennarelli TA: Head injury in man and experimental animals: clinical aspects. Acta Neurochir Suppl (Wien) 32:1–13, 1983

Gennarelli TA: Animate models of human head injury. J Neurotrauma 11:357–368, 1994

Gennarelli TA: The spectrum of traumatic axonal injury. Neuropathol Appl Neurobiol 22:509–513, 1996

Gennarelli TA, Thibault LE: Biomechanics of acute subdural hematoma. J Trauma 22:680–686, 1982

Gennarelli TA, Thibault LE: Biological models of head injury, in Central Nervous System Trauma Status Report. Edited by Becker JP, Povlishock JT. Bethesda, MD, National Institutes of Health, 1985, p 591

Gennarelli TA, Thibault LE, Adams JH, et al: Diffuse axonal injury and traumatic coma in the primate. Ann Neurol 12:564–574, 1982

Gentleman SM, Nash MJ, Sweeting CJ, et al: β-amyloid precursor protein (β-APP) as a marker for axonal injury after head injury. Neurosci Lett 160:139–144, 1993

Gentleman SM, Roberts GW, Gennarelli TA, et al: Axonal injury: a universal consequence of fatal closed head injury? Acta Neuropathol 89:537–543, 1995

Gleckman AM, Bell MD, Evans RJ, et al: Diffuse axonal injury infants with non-accidental craniocerebral trauma; enhanced detection by beta-amyloid precursor protein immunohistochemical staining. Acta Pathol Lab Med 123:146–151, 1999

Gordon DJ, Bullock P: Fluid percussion brain injury exacerbates glutamate-induced focal damage in the rat. J Neurotrauma 16:195–201, 1999

Graham DI, Gennarelli TA: Pathology of brain damage after head injury, in Head Injury. Edited by Cooper PR, Golfinos JG. New York, McGraw-Hill, 2000, pp 133–153

Graham DI, Adams JH, Doyle D: Ischaemic brain damage in fatal non-missile head injuries. J Neurol Sci 39:213–234, 1978

Graham DI, Lawrence AE, Adams JH, et al: Brain damage in non-missile head injury secondary to a high ICP. Neuropathol Appl Neurobiol 13:209–217, 1987

Graham DI, Ford I, Adams JH, et al: Fatal head injury in children. J Clin Pathol 42:18–22, 1989a

Graham DI, Ford I, Adams JH, et al: Ischaemic brain damage is still common in fatal non-missile head injury. J Neurol Neurosurg Psychiatry 52:346–350, 1989b

Graham DI, McIntosh TK, Maxwell WL, et al: Recent advances in neurotrauma. J Neuropathol Exp Neurol 59:641–651, 2000

Graham DI, Gennarelli TA, McIntosh TK: Trauma, in Greenfield's Neuropathology. Edited by Graham DI, Lantos PL. London, Arnold, 2002, p 823

Grcevic N: The concept of inner cerebral trauma. Scand J Rehabil Med 25 (suppl 17):25–31, 1988

Hahn Y, Chyung GC, Barthel MJ, et al: Head injuries in children under 36 months of age: demography and outcome. Child Nerv Syst 4:34–40, 1988

Hall E: Beneficial effects of acute intravenous ibuprofen on neurologic recovery of head-injured mice: comparison of cyclooxygenase inhibition with inhibition of thromboxane A$_2$ synthetase or 5-lipoxygenase. J Neurotrauma 2:75–83, 1985

Hall ED: Free radicals and lipid peroxidation, in Neurotrauma. Edited by Narayan RK, Wilberger JE, Povlishock JT. New York, McGraw-Hill, 1996, p 1405

Harland WA, Pitts JF, Watson AA: Subarachnoid haemorrhage due to upper cervical trauma. J Clin Pathol 36:1335–1341, 1983

Harper CG, Doyle D, Adams JH, et al: Analysis of abnormalities in the pituitary gland in non-missile head injury. J Clin Pathol 39:769–773, 1986

Hayes RL, Jenkins LW, Lyeth BG, et al: Pretreatment with phencyclidine, an N-methyl-D-aspartate antagonist, attenuates long-term behavioral deficits in the rat produced by traumatic brain injury. J Neurotrauma 5:259–274, 1988

Hayes RL, Jenkins LW, Lyeth BG: Neuropharmacological mechanisms of traumatic brain injury: acetylcholine and excitatory amino acids. J Neurotrauma 8:S173, 1991

Herrmann M, Jost S, Kutz S, et al: Temporal profile of release of neurobiochemical markers of brain damage after traumatic brain injury is associated with intracranial pathology as demonstrated in cranial computerised tomography. J Neurotrauma 17:113–122, 2000

Hovda DA: Metabolic dysfunction, in Neurotrauma. Edited by Narayan RK, Wilberger JE, Povlishock JT. New York, McGraw-Hill, 1996, p 1459

Hovda DA, Yoshino A, Fineman I, et al: Intracellular calcium accumulates for at least 48 hours following fluid percussion brain injury in the rat. Proc Am Assoc Neurol Surg 1:452, 1991

Hovda DA, Lee SM, Smith ML, et al: The neurochemical and metabolic cascade following brain injury: moving from animal models to man. J Neurotrauma 12:903, 1995

Isaac L, Van Zandt O'Malley T, Ristic H, et al: MK-801 blocks dynorphin A (1–13)-induced loss of the tail-flick reflex in the rat. Brain Res 531:83–87, 1990

Jamieson KG, Yelland JD: Extradural hematoma: report of 167 cases. J Neurosurg 29:13–23, 1968

Jenkins LW, Lyeth BG, Lewelt W, et al: Combined pre-trauma scopolamine and phencyclidine attenuate posttraumatic increased sensitivity to delayed secondary ischemia. J Neurotrauma 5:275–287, 1988

Jennett BJ, Teasdale G: Management of Head Injuries. Philadelphia, Davis, 1981

Jiang JY, Lyeth BG, Delahunty TM, et al: Muscarinic cholinergic receptor binding in rat brain at 15 days following traumatic brain injury. Brain Res 651:123–128, 1994

Jones PA, Andrews PJD, Midgley S, et al: Measuring the burden of secondary insults in head-injured patients during intensive care. J Neurosurg Anesthesiol 6:4–14, 1994

Katayama Y, Becker DP, Tamura T, et al: Massive increases in extracellular potassium and the indiscriminate release of glutamate following concussive brain injury. J Neurosurg 73:889–900, 1990

Kaur B, Rutty GM, Timperley WT: The possible role of hypoxia in the formation of axonal bulbs. J Clin Pathol 52:203–209, 1999

Klauber MR, Marshall LF, Luerssen TG, et al: Determinants of head injury mortality: importance of the low risk patient. Neurosurgery 24:31–36, 1989

Kontos HA, Povlishock JT: Oxygen radicals in brain injury. Cent Nerv Sys Trauma 3:257–263, 1986

Landolt H, Fujisawa H, Graham DI, et al: Reproducible peracute glutamate induced focal lesions of the normal rat brain using microdialysis. J Clin Neurosci 5:193–202, 1998

Leonard JR, Maris DO, Grady SM: Fluid percussion injury causes loss of forebrain choline acetyltransferase and nerve growth factor receptor immunoreactive cells in the rat. J Neurotrauma 11:379–392, 1994

Lewin W: Acute subdural and extradural haematoma in closed head injury. Ann R Coll Surg Engl 5:240, 1949

Lindenberg R, Freytag E: Brainstem lesions of traumatic hyperextension of the head. Arch Pathol 90:509–515, 1970

Luerssen T: Head injury in children. Neurosurg Clin N Am 2:399–410, 1991

Lyeth BG, Jiang JY, Delahunty TM, et al: Muscarinic cholinergic receptor binding in rat brain following traumatic brain injury. Brain Res 640:240–245, 1994

Macpherson P, Teasdale E, Dhaker S, et al: The significance of traumatic haematoma in the region of the basal ganglia. J Neurol Neurosurg Psychiatry 49:29–34, 1986

Madsen FF, Reske-Nielsen E: A simple mechanical model using a piston to produce localized cerebral contusions in pigs. Acta Neurochir (Wien) 88:65–72, 1987

Maloney AF, Whatmore WJ: Clinical and pathological observations in fatal head injuries: a 5-year study of 173 cases. Br J Surg 56:23–31, 1969

Marmarou A, Foda MA, van den Brink W, et al: A new model of diffuse brain injury in rats. J Neurosurg 80:291–300, 1994

Marshall LF: Head injury, recent, past, present, and future. Head Surgery 47:546–561, 2000

Marshall LF, Toole BM, Bowers SA: The National Traumatic Coma Data Bank, part 2: patients who talk and deteriorate: implications for treatment. J Neurosurg 59:285–288, 1983

Maxwell WL, Irvine A, Adams JH, et al: Response of cerebral microvasculature to brain injury. J Pathol 155:327–335, 1988

Maxwell WL, Povlishock JT, Graham DI: A mechanistic analysis of nondisruptive axonal injury: a review. J Neurotrauma 14:419–440, 1997

Maxwell WL, Irvine A, Watt C, et al: The microvascular response to stretch injury in the adult guinea pig visual system. J Neurotrauma 8:271–279, 1991

Maxwell WL, Watts C, Graham DI, et al: Ultrastructural evidence of axonal shearing as a result of lateral acceleration of the head in non-human primates. Acta Neuropathol 86:136–144, 1993

Maxwell WL, Povlishock JT, Graham DI: A mechanistic analysis of non-disruptive axonal injury. J Neurotrauma 14:419–440, 1997

McIntosh TK, Hayes RL, DeWitt DS, et al: Endogenous opioids may mediate secondary damage after experimental brain injury. Am J Physiol 253:E565–E574, 1987a

McIntosh TK, Head VA, Faden AI: Alterations in regional concentrations of endogenous opioids following traumatic brain injury in the cat. Brain Res 425:225–233, 1987b

McIntosh TK, Vink R, Noble L, et al: Traumatic brain injury in the rat: characterization of a lateral fluid percussion model. Neuroscience 28:233–244, 1989

McIntosh TK, Fernyak S, Yamakami I, et al: Central and systemic K-opioid agonists exacerbate neurobehavioral response to brain injury in rats. Am J Physiol 267:R665–R672, 1994a

McIntosh TK, Yu T, Gennarelli TA: Alterations in regional brain catecholamine concentrations after experimental brain injury in the rat. J Neurochem 63:1426–1433, 1994b

McIntosh TK, Saatman KE, Raghupathi R, et al: The molecular and cellular sequelae of experimental traumatic brain injury: pathogenetic mechanisms. Neuropathol Appl Neurobiol 24:251–267, 1998

McKeating EG, Andrews PJ, Mascia L: Relationship of neuron specific enolase and protien S-100 concentrations in systemic and jugular venous serum to injury severity and outcome after traumatic brain injury. Acta Neurochir Suppl (Wien) 71:117–119, 1998

McKenzie KJ, McLellan DR, Gentleman SM, et al: Is β-APP a marker of axonal damage in short-surviving head injury? Acta Neuropathol 92:608–613, 1996

McKissock W, Taylor JC, Bloom WH, et al: Extradural haematoma: observations on 125 cases. Lancet 2:167–172, 1960

Meaney DF, Smith DH, Ross DT, et al: Diffuse axonal injury in the miniature pig: biomechanical development and injury threshold. ASME WAM 25:169–175, 1993

Medical Research Council: Human tissue and biological samples for use in research: operational and ethical guidelines, 2001. Available at: http://www.mrc.ac.uk.

Mendelow AD, Teasdale G, Jennett B: Risks of intracranial haematoma in head injured adults. BMJ 287:1173–1176, 1983

Miller JD: Head injury. J Neurol Neurosurg Psychiatry 56:440–447, 1993

Mocchetti I, Wrathall JR: Neurotrophic factors in central nervous system trauma. J Neurotrauma 12:853–870, 1995

Muizelaar J: Cerebral blood flow, cerebral blood volume, and cerebral metabolism after severe head injury, in Textbook of Head Injury. Edited by Becker DP, Gudeman SK. Philadelphia, WB Saunders, 1989, pp 221–240

Murdoch I, Nicoll JAR, Graham DI, et al: Nucleus basalis of Meynert: pathology in the human brain after fatal head injury. J Neurotrauma 19:279–284, 2002

Nakashima T, Takenaka K, Nishimura Y, et al: Phospholipase C activity in cerebrospinal fluid following subarachnoid hemorrhage related to brain damage. J Cereb Blood Flow Metab 13:255–259, 1993

Nanassis K, Frowein RA, Karimi A: Delayed post-traumatic intracerebral bleeding. Neurosurg Rev 12 (suppl 1):243–251, 1989

Narayan RK, Michel ME, et al: Clinical trials in head injury. J Neurotrauma 19:503–557, 2002

Newcomb JK, Zhao X, Pike BR, et al: Temporal profile of apoptosis like changes in neurons and astrocytes following controlled cortical impact injury in the rat. Exp Neurol 158:76–88, 1999

Nilsson P, Hillered L, Ponten U, et al: Changes in cortical extracellular levels of energy-related metabolites and amino acids following concussive brain injury in rats. J Cereb Blood Flow Metab 10:631–637, 1990

Ogata M, Tsuganezawa O: Neuron-specific enolase as an effective immunohistochemical marker for injured axons after fatal brain injury. Int J Legal Med 113:19–25, 1999

Olney JW, Price M, Salles K, et al: MK-801 powerfully protects against N-methyl aspartate neurotoxicity. Eur J Pharmacol 141:357–361, 1987

Oppenheimer DR: Microscopic lesions in the brain following head injury. J Neurol Neurosurg Psychiatry 31:299–306, 1968

Palmer AM, Marion DW, Botscheller ML, et al: Traumatic brain injury-induced excitotoxicity assessed in a controlled cortical impact model. J Neurochem 61:2015–2024, 1993

Pappius HM: Local cerebral glucose utilization in thermally traumatized rat brain. Am J Neurol 9:484–491, 1981

Patterson SL, Grady MS, Bothwell M: Nerve growth factor and a fibroblast growth factor-like neurotrophic activity in cerebrospinal fluid of brain injured human patients. Brain Res 605:43–49, 1993

Peerless SJ, Rewcastle NB: Shear injuries of the brain. Can Med Assoc J 96:577–582, 1967

Pierce JE, Smith DH, Trojanowski JQ, et al: Enduring cognitive neurobehaviour and histopathological changes persist for up to one year following severe experimental brain injury in rats. Neuroscience 87:359–369, 1998

Pilz P: Axonal injury in head injury. Acta Neurochir Suppl (Wien) 32:119–123, 1980

Pilz P, Strohecker J, Grobovschek M: Survival after pontomedullary tear. J Neurol Neurosurg Psychiatry 45:422–427, 1982

Povlishock JT: Traumatically induced axonal injury: pathogenesis and pathobiological implications. Brain Pathol 2:1–12, 1992

Povlishock JT, Christman CW: The pathobiology of traumatically induced axonal injury in animals and humans: a review of current thoughts. J Neurotrauma 12:555–564, 1995

Povlishock JT, Jenkins LW: Are the pathobiological changes evoked by traumatic brain injury immediate and irreversible? Brain Pathol 5:415–426, 1995

Povlishock JT, Becker DP, Cheng DLY, et al: Axonal change in minor head injury. J Neuropathol Exp Neurol 42:225–242, 1983

Prasad MR, Tzigaret CM, Smith D, et al: Decreased alpha-adrenergic receptors after experimental brain injury. J Neurotrauma 9:269–279, 1992

Prasad MR, Ramaiah C, McIntosh TK, et al: Regional levels of lactate and norepinephrine after experimental brain injury. J Neurochem 63:1086–1094, 1994

Raghupathi R, Margulies SS: Traumatic axonal injury after closed head injury in the neonatal pig. J Neurotrauma 19:843–853, 2002

Raghupathi R, McIntosh TK, Smith DH: Cellular responses to experimental brain injury. Brain Pathol 5:437–442, 1995

Reilly PL, Graham DI, Adams JH, et al: Patients with head injury who talk and die. Lancet 2:375–377, 1975

Rink A, Fung KM, Trojanowski JQ, et al: Evidence of apoptotic cell death after experimental traumatic brain injury in the rat. Am J Pathol 147:1575–1583, 1995

Rockswold GL, Leonard PR, Nagib ME: Analysis of management in thirty-three closed injury patients who 'talked and deteriorated.' Neurosurgery 21:51–55, 1987

Rothman SM, Olney JW: Excitotoxicity and the NMDA receptor—still lethal after eight years. Trends Neurosci 18:57–58, 1995

Royal College of Pathologists: Transitional guidelines to facilitate changes in procedures for handling "surplus" and archival material from human biological samples, 2001

Royal Liverpool Children's Inquiry: The report of the Royal Liverpool Childrens' Inquiry (The "Richard Report"), 2000. Available at: http://www.rlcinquiry.org.uk. Accessed July 28, 2004.

Ryan GA, McLean AJ, Vilenius AT: Brain injury patterns in fatally injured pedestrians. J Trauma 36:469–476, 1994

Scarfo GB, Mariottini A, Tomaccini D, et al: Growing skull fractures: progressive evolution of brain damage and effectiveness of surgical treatment. Child Nerv Syst 173:163–167, 1989

Schoettle RJ, Kochanek PM, Magargee MJ, et al: Early polymorphonuclear leukocyte accumulation correlates with the development of post-traumatic cerebral edema in rats. J Neurotrauma 7:207–217, 1990

Shannon P, Smith CR, Deck J, et al: Axonal injury and the neuropathology of shaken baby syndrome. Acta Neuropathol 95:625–631, 1998

Shapira Y, Shohami E, Sidi A, et al: Experimental closed head injury in rats: mechanical, pathophysiologic, and neurologic properties. Crit Care Med 16:258–265, 1989a

Shapira Y, Yadid E, Cotev S, et al: Accumulation of calcium in the brain following head trauma. Neurol Res 11:169–172, 1989b

Shaw K, MacKinnon MA, Raghupathi R, et al: TUNEL-positive staining in white and grey matter after fatal head injury in man. Clin Neuropathol 20:106–112, 2001

Sherriff FE, Bridges LR, Sivaloganathan S: Early detection of axonal injury after human head trauma using immunocytochemistry for β-amyloid precursor protein. Acta Neuropathol 87:55–62, 1994

Shohami E, Shapira Y, Sidi A, et al: Head injury induces increased prostaglandin synthesis in rat brain. J Cereb Blood Flow Metab 7:58–63, 1987

Shohami E, Novikov M, Bass R, et al: Closed head injury triggers early production of TNFα and IL-6 by brain tissue. J Cereb Blood Flow Metab 14:615–619, 1994

Siesjo B, Wieloch T: Brain injury: neurochemical aspects, in Central Nervous System Trauma Status Report. Edited by Becker DP, Povlishock JT. Bethesda, MD, National Institutes of Health, 1985, p 513

Simpson DA, Blumbergs PC, Cooter RD, et al: Pontomedullary tears and other gross brainstem injuries after ventricular accidents. J Trauma 29:1519–1525, 1989

Singhal A, Baker AJ, Hare GM: Association between cerebrospinal fluid interleukin-6 concentrations and outcome after severe human traumatic brain injury. J Neurotrauma 19:929–937, 2002

Sinson G, Voddi M, McIntosh TK: Nerve growth factor (NGF) administration attenuates cognitive but not neurobehavioral motor dysfunction or hippocampal cell loss following fluid-percussion brain injury in rats. J Neurochem 65:2209–2216, 1995

Smith DH, McIntosh TK: Traumatic brain injury and excitatory amino acids, in Neurotrauma. Edited by Narayan RK, Wilberger JE, Povlishock JT. New York, McGraw-Hill, 1996, p 1445

Smith DH, Soares HD, Pierce JS, et al: A model of parasagittal controlled cortical impact in the mouse: cognitive and histopathologic effects. J Neurotrauma 12:169–178, 1995

Smith DH, Chen XH, Pierce JE, et al: Progressive atrophy and neuronal death for one year following brain trauma in the rat. J Neurotrauma 14:715–727, 1997a

Smith DH, Shen XH, Xu BN, et al: Characterisation of diffuse axonal pathology and selective hippocampal damage following inertial brain trauma in the pig. J Neuropathol Exp Neurol 56: 822–834, 1997b

Smith DH, Wolf JA, Lusardi TA, et al: High tolerance and delayed elastic response of cultured axons to dynamic stretch injury. J Neurosci 19:4263–4269, 1999

Smith FM, Raghupathi R, MacKinnon MA, et al: TUNEL-positive staining of surface contusions after fatal head injury in man. Acta Neuropathol 100:537–545, 2000

Soares HD, Thomas M, Cloherty K, et al: Development of prolonged focal cerebral edema and regional cation change following experimental brain injury in the rat. J Neurochem 58:1845–1852, 1992

Stone JR, Singleton RH, Povlishock JT: Antibodies to the C-terminus of the β amyloid precursor protein (APP): a site specific marker for the detection of traumatic axonal injury. Brain Res 871:288–302, 2000

Strich SJ: Diffuse degeneration of the cerebral white matter in severe dementia following head injury. J Neurol Neurosurg Psychiatry 19:163–185, 1956

Strich SJ: Shearing of the nerve fibres as a cause of brain damage due to head injury. Lancet 2:443, 1961

Teasdale GM, Graham DI: Craniocerebral trauma and retrieval of the neuronal population after injury. Neurosurgery 43:723–737, 1998

Tomei G, Spagnoli D, Ducati A, et al: Morphology and neurophysiology of focal axonal injury experimentally induced in the guinea pig optic nerve. Acta Neuropathol 80:506–513, 1990

Toulmond S, Duval D, Serrano A, et al: Biochemical and histological alterations induced by fluid percussion brain injury in the rat. Brain Res 620:24–31, 1993

Tsuiki K, Takada A, Nagahiro S, et al: Synthesis of serotonin in traumatized rat brain. J Neurochem 64:1319–1325, 1995

Vanezis P: Techniques used in the evaluation of vertebral trauma at post mortem. Forensic Sci Int 13:159–165, 1979

Vanezis P: Vertebral artery injuries in road-traffic accidents: a post-mortem study. J Forensic Sci 26:281–291, 1986

Varon S, Hagg T, Manthorpe M: Nerve growth factor in CNS repair and regeneration. Adv Exp Biol Med 296:267–276, 1991

Vink R, McIntosh TK: Pharmacological and physiological effects of magnesium on experimental traumatic brain injury. Magnes Res 3:163–169, 1990

Vink R, McIntosh TK, Romhanyi R, et al: Opiate antagonist nalmefine improves intracellular free Mg2+, bioenergetic state and neurological outcome following traumatic brain injury in rats. J Neurosci 10:3524–3530, 1990

Weber M, Grolimund P, Seiler RW: Evaluation of post traumatic cerebral blood flow velocities by transcranial Doppler ultrasonography. Neurosurgery 27:106–112, 1990

Wei EP, Lamb RG, Kontos HA: Increased phospholipase C activity after experimental brain injury. J Neurosurg 56:695–698, 1982

Weiner HL, Weinberg JS: Head injury in the paediatric age group, in Head Injury. Edited by Cooper PR, Golfinos JG. New York, McGraw-Hill, 2000, pp 419–456

Williams S, Raghupathi R, MacKinnon MA, et al: In-situ DNA fragmentation occurs in white matter up to 12 months after head injury in man. Acta Neuropathol 102:581–590, 2001

Woodroofe MN, Sarna GS, Wadhwa M, et al: Detection of interleukin-1 and interleukin-6 in adult rat brain, following mechanical injury by in vivo microdialysis: evidence of a role for microglia in cytokine production. J Neuroimmunol 33:227–236, 1991

Yaghmai A, Povlishock J: Traumatically induced reactive change as visualized through the use of monoclonal antibodies targeted to the neurofilament subunits. J Neuropathol Exp Neurol 51:158–176, 1992

Yakovlev AG, Knoblach SM, Fan L, et al: Activation of CPP 32–like caspases contributed to neuronal apoptosis and neurological dysfunction after traumatic brain injury. J Neurosci 17:7415–7424, 1997

Yang K, Mu XS, Xue JJ, et al: Increased expression of c-fos mRNA and AP-1 transcription factors after cortical impact injury in rats. Brain Res 664:141–147, 1994

Yergey JA, Heyes MP: Brain eicosanoid formation following acute penetration injury as studied by in vivo microdialysis. J Cereb Blood Flow Metab 10:143–146, 1990

Zauner A, Bullock R: The role of excitatory amino acids in severe brain trauma: opportunities for therapy: a review. J Neurotrauma 12:547–554, 1995

Zhuang J, Shackford SR, Schmoker JD, et al: The association of leukocytes with secondary brain injury. J Trauma 35:415–422, 1993

Zimmerman RA, Bilaniuk LT, Gennarelli T, et al: Computed tomography of shearing injuries of the cerebral white matter. Radiology 127:393–396, 1978

3 Neurosurgical Interventions

Roger Hartl, M.D.

Jamshid Ghajar, M.D., Ph.D.

WITH APPROXIMATELY 52,000 deaths per year in the United States, traumatic brain injury (TBI) is the most common cause of death and disability in young people and accounts for approximately one-third of all trauma deaths. The costs of TBI to society are immense, and neurotrauma is a serious public health problem. Motor vehicle accidents are the major cause of TBI, particularly in young people. Falls are the leading cause of death and disability from TBI in people older than age 65 years. TBI is graded as mild, moderate, or severe based on the level of consciousness or the Glasgow Coma Scale (GCS) score after resuscitation (see Table 1–2 in Chapter 1, Epidemiology). Mild TBI is characterized by a GCS score between 13 and 15. Patients with moderate TBI are typically stuporous or lethargic, with a GCS score between 9 and 13. A comatose patient who is unable to open his or her eyes or follow commands and has a GCS score lower than 9 has a severe TBI by definition.

The prognosis for patients with severe TBI is not as hopeless as previously thought. It is now known that patients with TBI are susceptible to posttraumatic arterial hypotension, hypoxia, and brain swelling, and these may contribute significantly to the poor outcomes seen from TBI in the past (Table 3–1). All major advances in the care of these patients have been achieved by reducing the severity of these secondary insults on the injured central nervous system. Rapid resuscitation of trauma patients in the field, direct transport to a major trauma center, and improved critical care management in the hospital with intracranial pressure (ICP) monitoring have cut down mortality in severe TBI from up to 50% in the 1970s and 1980s to between 15% and 25% in most recent series.

Guidelines for the Management of Severe TBI

The development of scientifically based management protocols for the treatment of TBI holds considerable promise for further improvement in outcome. The guideline movement in neurosurgery began in 1995 when the first edition of the *Guidelines for the Management of Severe Traumatic Brain Injury* was published as a joint effort of the Brain Trauma Foundation and the American Association of Neurological Surgeons (Brain Trauma Foundation 2000b). These *Guidelines* are composed of 14 topics, ranging from trauma systems and prehospital resuscitation to monitoring and treatment of intracranial hypertension and other intensive care treatments. It is important to understand that all Brain Trauma Foundation *Guidelines* per se are not practical clinical tools but rather summaries and reviews of scientific evidence. They must be embedded into a comprehensive, multidisciplinary treatment protocol that comprises all different aspects of patient care as well as geographical and infrastructure-related characteristics of a particular trauma center. In this chapter, we refer to four recently published, evidence-based documents covering the prehospital and in-hospital surgical and medical management of patients with severe TBI and their prognosis (Brain Trauma Foundation 2000a, 2000b, 2000c, in press). These documents can be accessed via the Internet at http://www.braintrauma.org.

TABLE 3–1. Secondary insults that adversely affect outcome from traumatic brain injury (TBI)

Secondary insults in TBI	Main cause
Systolic blood pressure <90 mm Hg	Blood loss, sepsis, cardiac failure, spinal cord injury, brainstem injury
Arterial O_2 saturation <90%, PaO_2 <60 mm Hg, apnea, cyanosis	Hypoventilation, thoracic injury, aspiration
Sustained $PaCO_2$ <25 mm Hg	Induced or spontaneous hyperventilation
ICP >20–25 mm Hg	Mass lesion, brain swelling

Note. ICP=intracranial pressure; PaO_2=partial pressure of oxygen, arterial; $PaCO_2$=partial pressure of carbon dioxide.

Management of Severe TBI

Prehospital Management

The prehospital management of patients with severe TBI is outlined in *Guidelines for Prehospital Management of Traumatic Brain Injury* (Brain Trauma Foundation 2000c). Rapid and physiologic resuscitation is the first priority in these patients. After stabilization of airway, breathing, and circulation, the GCS score should be determined by direct verbal or physical interaction with the patient. Patients with a GCS score between 9 and 13 should be transported to a trauma center, and patients with a GCS score lower than 9 should be brought to a trauma center with 24-hour computed tomography (CT) scanning capability, 24-hour operating room availability, and prompt neurosurgical care.

Comatose patients with a GCS score lower than 9 should be intubated. Patients who respond to nail-bed pressure or axillary pinch with abnormal extension, are flaccid, or have asymmetric and/or dilated pupils are presumed to have high ICP and should be hyperventilated at a rate of 20 beats per minute. All patients should have their oxygenation and blood pressure assessed at least every 5 minutes. Their oxygen saturation should be maintained above 90%, and their systolic blood pressure should be kept above 90 mm Hg. In the prehospital phase, hypoxia and arterial hypotension have been shown to be the most significant secondary insults. A single hypotensive episode has been shown to be associated with increased morbidity and a doubling of mortality (Chesnut et al. 1993; Fearnside et al. 1993).

Typical Emergency Department Workup of Patients with TBI

A typical initial neurotrauma evaluation with possible critical findings is summarized in Table 3–2. The goals of emergency department (ED) management are to determine the severity of the primary TBI, identify patients at risk for deterioration, prevent secondary brain damage, and identify associated injuries. ED patients with TBI or suspected TBI must be followed closely for neurological deterioration. A complete trauma workup should be initiated if there is any suspicion of associated injuries. Nausea and/or vomiting, progressive headaches, restlessness, pupillary asymmetry, seizures, and increasing lethargy should be interpreted as signs of neurodeterioration, and a head CT scan should be obtained immediately. Blood alcohol level determination and urine toxicology screening should be considered in all patients presenting with TBI. Routine blood tests, including coagulation parameters, should be obtained in patients with moderate and severe TBI and in patients with associated injuries. Tetanus toxoid must be administered if there are any associated open wounds. Immobilization of the cervical spine using a hard collar is mandatory in all patients with TBI. Any complaint of neck pain should also lead to a radiographical assessment of the cervical spine, regardless of a patient's GCS score. All patients with moderate or severe TBI should undergo cervical spine imaging.

Maintaining brain perfusion is the guiding principle in managing comatose patients with severe TBI. The cornerstones of resuscitation of the patient with severe head injury are as follows:

- Primary survey with cervical spine control and brief neurological assessment
- Resuscitation (airway, breathing, circulation)
- Secondary survey with complete neurological examination and determination of the GCS score (see Table 3–2)

In-Hospital Management of Severe TBI

Computed Tomography Scan Assessment

As soon as possible after resuscitation, all stable patients with severe TBI should undergo a CT scan of the head. The CT scan can demonstrate a life-threatening mass lesion that requires surgical evacuation, evidence of raised ICP, and the degree of intracranial injury.

Approximately 10% of initial head CT scans in patients with severe TBI do not show any abnormalities (Lobato et al. 1986; van Dongen et al. 1983). The absence of abnormalities on CT scan at admission does not preclude increased ICP. Significant new lesions and increased ICP may develop in 40% of patients with an initially normal head CT scan.

TABLE 3–2. Initial assessment and clinical examination of patients with TBI

Resuscitation

Oxygenation/ventilation

Critical findings: Apnea, cyanosis, SaO$_2$ <90%

Intubation if hypoxemic despite supplemental O$_2$, keep PaCO$_2$ at 35 mm Hg

Blood pressure

Critical finding: Systolic blood pressure <90 mm Hg

Fluid resuscitation

Primary survey

Spinal stability

Critical findings: Pain, step-off, external signs of trauma to neck, mechanism

Immobilization with cervical collar, spine precautions, X rays

Postresuscitation GCS score

Critical finding: GCS score <9

Consider intubation, normoventilation, head CT

Motor examination, pupillary diameter, light reflex, direct orbital trauma

Critical findings: Flaccidity or motor posturing and asymmetric or fixed and dilated pupils suggest cerebral herniation

Short-term hyperventilation ± mannitol if herniation suspected

Placement of lines, urinary and gastric catheters, cervical spine, chest and pelvis X rays

Secondary survey

Detailed neurological examination

Critical findings: GCS score <9, cerebral herniation syndrome

Short-term hyperventilation ± mannitol if herniation suspected

Visual inspection, external signs of cranial trauma

Critical findings: Raccoon's eyes, Battle's sign, cerebrospinal fluid from ears and/or nose, hematotympanum, facial fractures, proptosis, direct orbital trauma, skull base fractures

Consider special computed tomographic imaging of skull base, ear, nose, and throat/oral and maxillofacial surgery service involvement, prophylactic antibiotics

Note. CT=computed tomography; GCS=Glasgow Coma Scale; SaO$_2$=arterial oxygen saturation.

Intracranial Pressure Monitoring and Treatment of Elevated Intracranial Pressure

Comatose TBI patients (GCS score of 3 to 8) with abnormal CT scans should undergo ICP monitoring. ICP monitoring helps in the earlier detection of intracranial mass lesions, limits the indiscriminate use of therapies that can be potentially harmful to control ICP, and helps in determining prognosis. There is substantial evidence that ICP monitoring may improve outcome. Elevated ICP is present in the majority of patients with severe head injury (Luerssen 1997). We prefer intraventricular devices using a fluid-coupled catheter with an external strain gauge for ICP monitoring. The ventricular catheter can be placed in the operating room or under sterile conditions in the ED or intensive care unit. It has the advantage of not only measuring ICP but also allowing therapeutic cerebrospinal fluid drainage.

Cerebral perfusion pressure (CPP) is defined as the mean arterial blood pressure minus ICP. This physiologic variable defines the pressure gradient driving cerebral blood flow and metabolite delivery and is therefore closely related to cerebral ischemia. A threshold CPP of 60 mm Hg for adults is currently recommended. Increased ICP or compromised CPP should be treated vigorously. The ICP management of the typical TBI patient at our institution is outlined in Table 3–3. Hyperventilation should not be used routinely in these patients because of the risk of further compromising cerebral perfusion. We use hyperventilation only for brief periods when there is acute neurological deterioration or intracranial hypertension is refractory to other treatment interventions. Glucocorticoids have not been shown to improve outcome from severe TBI.

Mannitol is effective for the control of raised ICP after severe TBI. Limited data suggest that intermittent boluses may be more effective than continuous infusion. Effective doses range from 0.25 to 1.00 g/kg body weight.

Studies have shown that not feeding patients with severe TBI by the first week after injury increases mortality. Therefore, it is our practice to initiate tube feedings within the first days after TBI.

Treatment of Seizures

Posttraumatic seizures (PTSs) are divided into early (less than 7 days after trauma) and late (more than 7 days after trauma) seizures. In recent TBI studies that followed high-risk patients up to 36 months, the incidence of early PTSs varied between 4% and 25%, and the incidence of late PTSs varied between 9% and 42% in untreated patients. Prophylactic use of phenytoin, carbamazepine, or phenobarbital is not recommended for preventing late PTSs. Anticonvulsants may be used to prevent *early* PTSs

TABLE 3–3. Treatment algorithm for patients with intracranial hypertension

In all patients with GCS score <9	Add if ICP >20 mm Hg	Add if ICP >25 mm Hg	Add for persistent ICP >25 mm Hg	Add for persistent ICP >25 mm Hg and/or pupillary abnormalities
ICP monitoring	Ventricular CSF drainage	Neuromuscular blockade: vecuronium, atracurium	Moderate hypothermia, core temperature 34–36°C	High-dose propofol infusion
Elevate head of bed 30 degrees				
Maintain euvolemia and hemodynamic stability	IV sedation with midazolam or lorazepam	Mannitol bolus infusions every 4–6 hours	Hyperventilation to $PaCO_2$ 30–35 mm Hg	Hyperventilation to $PaCO_2$ 25–30 mm Hg
PaO_2 >90 mm Hg	Analgesia: fentanyl or morphine			Consider hypertonic saline bolus infusion
$PaCO_2$ 35–40 mm Hg				Consider decompressive craniectomy
Systolic blood pressure >90 mm Hg	"CPP management": Inotropic and pressor support to maintain CPP			
CPP≈60 mm Hg	Repeat head CT to exclude operable mass lesion			

Note. CPP=cerebral perfusion pressure; CSF=cerebrospinal fluid; CT=computed tomography; GCS=Glasgow Coma Scale; ICP=intracranial pressure; $PaCO_2$=partial pressure of carbon dioxide; PaO_2=partial pressure of oxygen, arterial.

in patients at high risk for seizures after TBI. Phenytoin and carbamazepine are effective in this setting. However, the available evidence does not indicate that prevention of early PTSs improves outcome after TBI. Routine seizure prophylaxis for more than 1 week after TBI is therefore not recommended. If late PTSs occur, patients should be managed in accordance with standard approaches to patients with new-onset seizures.

Surgical Management of Acute TBI

The decision regarding whether an intracranial lesion requires surgical evacuation can be difficult and is based on a patient's GCS score, pupillary examination, comorbidities, CT scan findings, age, and—in delayed decisions—ICP. Neurological deterioration over time is also an important factor influencing the decision to operate. The surgical management of TBI has recently been addressed by the *Guidelines for the Surgical Management of Traumatic Brain Injury* (Brain Trauma Foundation, in press).

This discussion of the surgical management of acute TBI has been organized according to the traditional literature-based classification of posttraumatic mass lesions—namely, epidural hematoma (EDH), acute subdural hematoma (SDH), intraparenchymal lesions (e.g., contusion, intracerebral hematoma), acute posterior fossa mass lesions, and depressed fractures of the skull. In many patients with severe or moderate TBI, two or more of these lesions may

coexist. For this reason, the formulation of an optimal neurosurgical treatment plan requires individual management, more so than in other areas of TBI management.

Epidural Hematoma

An EDH is characterized as a biconvex, extraaxial, hyperdense mass on a head CT scan (Figure 3–1). The incidence of surgical and nonsurgical EDH among TBI patients is approximately 3%. Among patients in coma, up to 9% harbor an EDH requiring craniotomy. The peak incidence of EDH is in the second decade, and the mean age of patients with EDH is between 20 and 30 years. Traffic-related accidents, falls, and assaults account for the majority of all EDHs. EDHs usually result from injury to the middle meningeal artery but can also be due to bleeding from the middle meningeal vein, the diploic veins, or the venous sinuses. In patients with EDH, one-third to one-half are comatose on admission or immediately before surgery. The classically described "lucid interval" (i.e., a period during which a patient who was initially unconscious wakes up before secondarily deteriorating) is seen in approximately one-half of patients undergoing surgery for EDH.

Surgical indication. Clot thickness, hematoma volume, and midline shift (MLS) on the preoperative CT scan are related to outcome. Noncomatose patients without focal neurological deficits and with an acute EDH with a thickness of less than 15 mm, a volume less than 30 cc, and an MLS less

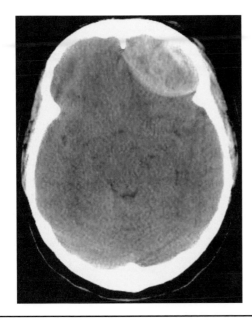

FIGURE 3–1.   Computed tomographic scan of the head of a patient with severe traumatic brain injury demonstrating a left frontal acute epidural hematoma with significant mass effect.

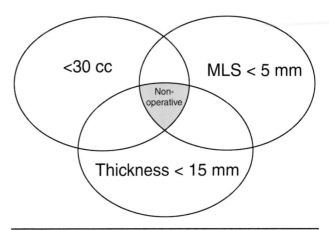

FIGURE 3–2.   Treatment option for epidural hematoma (EDH) in patients with a Glasgow Coma Scale score greater than 8.
Noncomatose patients with an EDH volume less than 30 cc and a thickness less than 15 mm with less than 5 mm midline shift (MLS) can be managed nonoperatively.

than 5 mm may be managed nonoperatively with serial CT scanning and close neurological evaluation in a neurosurgical center (Figure 3–2). The first follow-up CT scan in nonoperative patients should be obtained within 6–8 hours after TBI. Temporal location of an EDH is associated with failure of nonoperative management and should lower the threshold for surgery. Patients with a GCS score lower than 9 and an EDH volume greater than 30 cc should undergo surgical evacuation of the lesion. All patients, regardless of GCS score, should undergo surgery if the volume of their EDH exceeds 30 cc. Patients with an EDH volume less than 30 cc should be considered for surgery but may be managed successfully without surgery in selected cases. Time from neurological deterioration to surgery correlates with outcome. Therefore, surgical evacuation should be done as soon as possible.

Acute Subdural Hematoma

SDHs are diagnosed on a CT scan as extracranial, hyperdense, crescentic collections between the dura and the brain parenchyma (Figure 3–3). They can be divided into acute and chronic lesions. The incidence of acute SDH is between 12% and 29% in patients admitted with severe TBI. The mean age is between 31 and 47 years, and the vast majority of patients are men. Most SDHs are caused by motor vehicle–related accidents, falls, and assaults. Falls have been identified as the main cause of traumatic SDH in patients older than ages 75 and 80 years. Between 37% and 80% of patients with acute SDH present with an initial GCS score of 8 or less.

Surgical indication.   Clot thickness or volume and MLS on the preoperative CT scan correlate with outcome. Patients with SDH with a clot thickness greater than 10 mm or MLS greater than 5 mm should undergo surgical evacuation, regardless of their GCS score. Noncomatose patients with a clot thickness less than 10 mm and MLS less than 5 mm may undergo nonoperative management (Figure 3–4). Comatose patients (GCS score less than 9) with an SDH with a thickness less than 10 mm and MLS

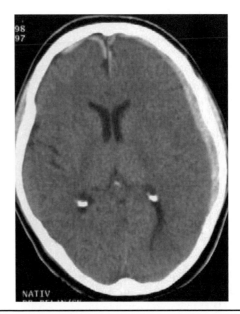

FIGURE 3–3.   Computed tomographic scan of the head of a patient with severe traumatic brain injury demonstrating left-sided acute subdural hematoma.

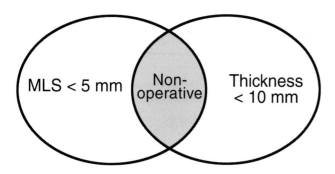

FIGURE 3–4.   Treatment option for patients with acute subdural hematoma (SDH) with a Glasgow Coma Scale score greater than 8.

Noncomatose patients with an SDH less than 10 mm thick and with less than 5-mm midline shift (MLS) can be managed nonoperatively.

less than 5 mm can be treated nonoperatively, providing that they undergo ICP monitoring, are neurologically stable, and have no pupillary abnormalities or intracranial hypertension (i.e., ICP greater than 20 mm Hg). A frequently observed complication with surgical evacuation of acute SDH is acute brain swelling, sometimes so dramatic that it is impossible to close the dura after evacuation of the hematoma. We use a surgical technique that avoids brain herniation by cutting multiple 2- to 3-cm slits in the dura. This allows rapid and complete removal of the blood clot and at the same time prevents the brain from protruding out of the craniotomy (Figure 3–5).

Traumatic Parenchymal Lesions

Traumatic parenchymal mass lesions occur in up to 10% of all patients with TBI and 13% to 35% of patients with severe TBI (Figure 3–6). Most small parenchymal lesions do not require surgical evacuation. However, the development of mass effect from larger lesions may result in secondary brain injury, placing the patient at risk of further neurological deterioration, herniation, and death. Parenchymal lesions tend to evolve, and timing of surgery affects outcome.

Surgical indication.   Patients with parenchymal mass lesions and signs of progressive neurological deterioration referable to the lesion, medically refractory intracranial hypertension, or signs of mass effect on CT scan should be treated operatively. Comatose patients with frontal or temporal contusions greater than 20 cc in volume with MLS of 5 mm or more and/or cisternal compression on CT scan, as well as patients with any lesion greater than 50 cc in volume, should be treated operatively. Patients with parenchymal mass lesions who do not show evidence of neurological compromise and have con-

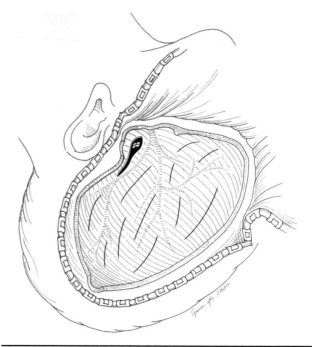

FIGURE 3–5.   Slit technique for evacuation of acute subdural hematoma in patients with traumatic brain injury.

The dura is incised at multiple sites to drain the subdural blood collection and prevent the brain from herniating out of the cranial opening.

trolled ICP and no significant signs of mass effect on CT scan may be managed nonoperatively.

Posterior Fossa Mass Lesions

Less than 3% of patients with TBI present with posterior fossa lesions. The vast majority of these lesions are posterior fossa EDHs. It is important to recognize these lesions early on, because patients can undergo rapid clinical deterioration due to the limited size of the posterior fossa and the propensity for these lesions to produce brainstem compression. Patients with fourth ventricular mass effect on CT scan or with neurological dysfunction or deterioration referable to the lesion should undergo a suboccipital craniectomy as soon as possible. Patients without significant mass effect on CT scan and without signs of neurological dysfunction may be managed by close observation and serial imaging.

Depressed Skull Fractures

Depressed skull fractures complicate up to 6% of head injuries, and the presence of skull fracture is associated with a higher incidence of intracranial lesions, neurological deficit, and poorer outcome. Patients with open skull fractures depressed greater than the thickness of the skull should undergo operative intervention to prevent infec-

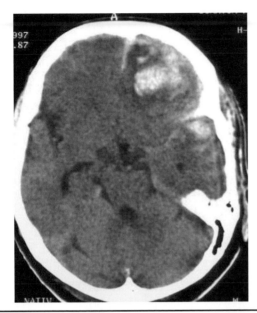

FIGURE 3–6.   Computed tomographic scan of the head of a patient with severe traumatic brain injury demonstrating left-frontal and temporal-parenchymal hemorrhages with swelling.

tion. Patients with open depressed fractures should be treated with antibiotic prophylaxis.

Decompressive Craniectomy for Control of Intracranial Hypertension

Decompressive procedures, such as subtemporal decompression, temporal lobectomy, and hemispheric decompressive craniectomy, are surgical procedures that have been used to treat patients with refractory intracranial hypertension and diffuse parenchymal injury. Decompressive craniectomy may be effective if it is done early after TBI in young patients who are expected to develop postoperative brain swelling and intracranial hypertension.

Prognosis After TBI

The most important factors for predicting outcome after severe TBI are age, GCS score, pupillary examination results, arterial hypotension, and certain CT scan findings (Brain Trauma Foundation 2000a). Studies show that the probability of poor outcome increases with decreasing admission GCS score in a continuous, stepwise manner. Increasing age is a strong independent factor in prognosis from severe TBI, with a significant increase in poor outcome for patients older than age 60 years. This circumstance is not explained by the increased frequency of systemic complications in older patients.

Several studies confirm that among comatose patients with acute SDH, no patient older than age 75 years who was preoperatively comatose and/or demonstrated signs of cerebral herniation made a good recovery (Cagetti et al. 1992; Jamjoom 1992; Kotwica and Jakubowski 1992). The pupillary diameter and the pupilloconstrictor light reflex can prognosticate outcome from severe TBI. Bilaterally unreactive pupils on admission are associated with a greater than 90% chance of poor outcome.

A posttraumatic systolic blood pressure lower than 90 mm Hg measured on the way to the hospital or in-hospital has been associated with an almost 70% likelihood of poor outcome. This likelihood increases to 79% when hypoxia is present. A single recording of arterial hypotension doubles mortality from severe TBI. Among these prognostic indicators of outcome, arterial hypotension is the only factor that can be significantly affected by therapeutic intervention. CT scan findings associated with poor outcome from severe TBI are compressed or absent basal cisterns, traumatic subarachnoid hemorrhage, MLS greater than 5 mm, and intracranial mass lesions.

Overall, mortality from severe TBI has been reduced from up to 50% in the 1970s and 1980s to between 15% and 25% in most recent series. In the absence of any pharmacological breakthrough, this improvement has to be attributed to more effective resuscitation in the field, rapid transport of TBI patients to trauma hospitals, more widely accepted ICP monitoring, and improvements in critical care management.

Do TBI Treatment Protocols Based on the *Guidelines* Make a Difference in Patient Outcome?

Three studies are available that examine the impact of TBI management protocols on patient outcome (Fakhry et al. 2004; Palmer et al. 2001; Vitaz et al. 2001). Their main results are summarized in Table 3–4. The design of these studies was based on a comparison of patients treated before and after implementation of a *Guidelines*-based treatment protocol. Details of the management protocols differed between institutions, but they were all based on the *Guidelines for the Management of Severe Traumatic Brain Injury*. All protocols emphasized rapid cardiopulmonary resuscitation, close hemodynamic monitoring, monitoring of ICP, and aggressive treatment of intracranial hypertension and compromised CPP. The introduction of treatment protocols was associated with a reduction of mortality from severe TBI and a decreased length of intensive care unit stay. In summary, multidisci-

TABLE 3–4. Effect of traumatic brain injury (TBI) management protocols based on the *Guidelines for the Management of Severe Traumatic Brain Injury* on mortality and length of stay in intensive care unit at three TBI centers

	Palmer et al. *N*=37/56	Vitaz et al. *N*=43/119	Fakhry et al. *N*=219/188 (high compliance group)
Mortality			
When determined	At 6 months	At discharge	At discharge
Before protocol (%)	43.24	39	17.8
With protocol (%)	16.07[a]	47 n.s.	11.2[a]
Intensive care unit days			
Before protocol	21.03	21.2	9.7
With protocol	22 n.s.	16.8[a]	7.2[a]

Note. *N*=number of patients in the groups before protocol implementation and after protocol implementation; n.s.=not significant.
[a]Significant difference when compared with results obtained before protocol implementation.

plinary, comprehensive clinical pathways based on scientifically based treatment guidelines for TBI streamline patient care, standardize critical care management, and hold the potential for significantly improving patient outcome and reducing hospital costs.

References

Brain Trauma Foundation, The American Association of Neurological Surgeons, The Joint Section on Neurotrauma and Critical Care: Early indicators of prognosis in severe traumatic brain injury. J Neurotrauma 17:535–627, 2000a. Available at: http://www2.braintrauma.org/guidelines/downloads/btf_guidelines_management.pdf. Accessed April 30, 2004.

Brain Trauma Foundation, The American Association of Neurological Surgeons, The Joint Section on Neurotrauma and Critical Care: Guidelines for the Management of Severe Traumatic Brain Injury. J Neurotrauma 17:449–554, 2000b. Available at: http://www2.braintrauma.org/guidelines/downloads/btf_guidelines_management.pdf. Accessed April 30, 2004.

Brain Trauma Foundation, The American Association of Neurological Surgeons: Guidelines for Prehospital Management of Traumatic Brain Injury. New York, Brain Trauma Foundation, 2000c. Available at: http://www2.braintrauma.org/guidelines/downloads/btf_guidelines_prehospital.pdf. Accessed April 30, 2004.

Brain Trauma Foundation, The American Association of Neurological Surgeons: Guidelines for the Surgical Management of Traumatic Brain Injury. Neurosurgery (in press). Available at: http://www2.braintrauma.org/guidelines/downloads/btf_guidelines_surgical.pdf . Accessed April 30, 2004.

Cagetti B, Cossu M, Pau A, et al: The outcome from acute subdural and epidural intracranial haematomas in very elderly patients. Br J Neurosurg 6:227–231, 1992

Chesnut R, Marshall S, Piek J, et al: Early and late systemic hypotension as a frequent and fundamental source of cerebral ischemia following severe brain injury in the Traumatic Coma Data Bank. Acta Neurochir Suppl (Wien) 59:121–125, 1993

Fakhry SM, Trask AL, Waller MA, et al: Management of brain-injured patients by an evidence-based medicine protocol improves outcomes and decreases hospital charges. J Trauma 56:492–499, 2004

Fearnside MR, Cook RJ, McDougall P, et al: The Westmead Head Injury Project outcome in severe head injury: a comparative analysis of pre-hospital, clinical and CT variables. Br J Neurosurg 7:267–279, 1993

Jamjoom A: Justification for evacuating acute subdural haematomas in patients above the age of 75 years. Injury 23:518–520, 1992

Kotwica Z, Jakubowski J: Acute head injuries in the elderly: an analysis of 136 consecutive patients. Acta Neurochir (Wien) 118:98–102, 1992

Lobato RD, Sarabia R, Rivas JJ, et al: Normal computerized tomography scans in severe head injury: prognostic and clinical management implications. J Neurosurg 65:784–789, 1986

Luerssen TG: Intracranial pressure: current status in monitoring and management. Semin Pediatr Neurol 4:146–155, 1997

Palmer S, Bader M, Qureshi A, et al: The impact on outcomes in a community hospital setting of using the AANS traumatic brain injury guidelines. J Trauma 50:657–664, 2001

van Dongen KJ, Braakman R, Gelpke GJ: The prognostic value of computerized tomography in comatose head-injured patients. J Neurosurg 59:951–957, 1983

Vitaz T, McIlvoy L, Raque G, et al: Development and implementation of a clinical pathway for severe traumatic brain injury. J Trauma 51:369–375, 2001

4 Neuropsychiatric Assessment

Kimberly A. Arlinghaus, M.D.

Arif M. Shoaib, M.D.

Trevor R. P. Price, M.D.

A TRAUMATIC BRAIN injury (TBI) is a significant event that may result in dramatic alterations in an individual's cognition, behavior, and emotions. The neuropsychiatric manifestations of such an injury depend on several factors: 1) preexisting variables such as the patient's personality and temperament before the injury, family psychiatric history, and previous psychiatric, medical, and neurological history; 2) the patient's psychosocial, economic, and vocational status at the time of injury; 3) the type, location, and severity of the brain injury; 4) the emotional and psychological responses of the individual to the TBI-mediated disturbances in cognition and behavior; and 5) the impact of such changes on personal and professional roles and relationships, especially those involving the family. The multiple variables that result in neurobehavioral disturbances subsequent to TBI require a comprehensive and integrated approach to data collection, diagnostic formulation, and treatment planning.

Clinical Assessment: The Biopsychosocial Approach

A useful conceptual framework for a comprehensive neuropsychiatric assessment is the biopsychosocial model. The biopsychosocial model integrates clinical data from three interrelated domains: 1) biological disturbances in brain function; 2) the patient's emotional and psychological reactions to impairments in cognition and disturbances of behavior, including his or her awareness and acceptance of the impairments; and 3) disruptions of interpersonal relationships, family interactions, and work capacities. A comprehensive, integrated clinical assess-

ment based on such a framework leads to the identification of specific problem areas, a multidimensional formulation of etiology, and development of treatment approaches that focus specifically, yet comprehensively, on the patient's problems.

History Related to the Brain Injury and Recovery Period

There are a number of questions that are relevant to the neuropsychiatric assessment of the patient with TBI (Table 4–1). Traditionally, the clinical database begins with the elicitation of the patient's chief complaint, which may or may not include a spontaneous report of a history of TBI. Gordon et al. (1998) describe "The Enigma of 'Hidden' Traumatic Brain Injury," noting that TBI may be "hidden" in three senses: 1) the diffuse axonal injury (DAI) of mild TBI is rarely detected by brain imaging, 2) the effects of TBI are usually not obviously physical, and 3) individuals with TBI are often unaware that significant problems have occurred as a result of the injury. Because TBI is often "the invisible injury," the history of TBI may elude both the examiner and the patient; therefore, the clinician must specifically inquire about events that may be associated with TBI such as motor vehicle accidents (MVAs), falls, assaults, and sports or recreational injuries.

Once a history of TBI is obtained, it is useful to delineate the type, severity, and location of the injury and when it occurred. Several parameters are commonly used to ascertain the severity of injury, including the Glasgow Coma Scale (GCS), duration of loss of consciousness (LOC), and posttraumatic amnesia (PTA)

TABLE 4–1. Sample questions for traumatic brain injury (TBI) assessment

Questions	Rationale
Have you ever hit your head? Have you ever been in an accident?	Probe for car/motorcycle/bicycle/other motor vehicle accidents, falls, assaults, sports or recreational injuries
(If so) Did you black out, pass out, or lose consciousness?	Establish LOC (verify LOC with witness, if possible)
What is the last thing you remember before the injury?	Establish extent of retrograde amnesia
What is the first thing you recall after the injury?	Estimate duration of LOC and begin to quantify posttraumatic amnesia (must ask further about when contiguous memory function returned)
(If no LOC) At the time of the injury, did you experience any change in your thinking or feel "dazed" or "confused"?	Establish change in mentation or level of consciousness
What problems did you have after the injury?	Delineate post-TBI symptoms (see Table 4–3)
Has anyone told you that you're different since the injury? If so, how have you changed?	Detect problems outside survivor's awareness or those he/she may be minimizing
Did anyone witness or observe your injury?	Identify source of collateral history
Many people who have injured their head had been drinking or using drugs; how about you?	Offer survivor greater "permission" to admit substance use
Have you had any other injuries to your head or brain?	Identify previous TBIs that may increase morbidity from current injury

Note. LOC=loss of consciousness.

TABLE 4–2. Classification of traumatic brain injury (TBI)

Type of TBI	Glasgow Coma Scale	Loss of consciousness	Posttraumatic amnesia
Mild	13–15	30 minutes or less (or none)	<24 hours
Moderate	9–12	30 minutes to 1 week	>24 hours to <1 week
Severe	≤8	>1 week	>1 week

(Table 4–2). Because the survivor of a TBI does not know whether he or she was rendered unconscious by the trauma, it is important to verify LOC with a witness, if possible. The survivor may believe that LOC occurred when, in actuality, he or she was conscious but in a state of PTA. Introduced by Teasdale and Jennett (1974), the GCS (see Table 1–2 in Chapter 1, Epidemiology) has become the standard for measuring the acute severity of a TBI. Estimating the severity of an acute TBI guides the physician in quantifying the signs and symptoms as-

sociated with mild, moderate, or severe TBI as well as the patient's likely prognosis. According to Asikainen et al. (1998), the GCS score and duration of LOC and PTA all have strong predictive value in assessing functional or occupational outcome for TBI patients. However, Lovell et al. (1999) question the predictive value of LOC based on the lack of statistical correlation between LOC and neuropsychological functioning in a large sample of patients with mild head trauma.

A temporal relationship should be established between the onset of current signs and symptoms and the occurrence of the traumatic injury. This information helps to differentiate the premorbid personality characteristics and psychiatric and behavioral symptoms from those arising after the brain injury. Any number of emotional and behavioral difficulties that existed in milder form before the brain injury can be accentuated after it. Careful consideration of temporal relationships also must address the phase of recovery and associated behavioral changes, because improvement after TBI tends to occur along a continuum, with certain sequelae generally resolving before others (e.g., confusion and disorientation generally resolve before short-term memory impairment). The clinician should also focus attention on the patient's psychological reactions and adjustment to injury-induced cognitive and emotional changes, as well as their impact on interpersonal relationships, family dynamics, and employment status.

In the assessment of TBI, it is helpful to categorize observed signs and symptoms into the broad domains of cognition, emotion, behavior, and physical symptoms (Table 4–3). This categorization permits more precise diagnosis of the patient's problems and assists in the formulation of an optimal treatment plan.

Importance of Collateral History

Because insight into disturbances of cognition, behavior, and emotional state are often compromised in patients

TABLE 4–3.   Traumatic brain injury symptom checklist

Cognitive	Emotional	Behaviorial	Physical
Level of consciousness	Mood swings/lability	Impulsivity	Fatigue
Sensorium	Depression	Disinhibition	Weight change
Attention/concentration	Hypomania/mania	Anger dyscontrol	Sleep disturbance
Short-term memory	Anxiety	Inappropriate sexual behavior	Headache
Processing speed	Anger/irritability	Lack of initiative	Visual problems
Executive function (planning, abstract reasoning, problem-solving, information processing, ability to attend to multiple stimuli, insight, judgment, etc.)	Apathy	"Change in personality"	Balance difficulties
			Dizziness
			Coldness
			Change in hair/skin
Thought processes			Seizures
			Spasticity
			Loss of urinary control
			Arthritic complaints

Source.   Adapted from Hibbard MR, Uysal S, Sliwinski M, et al: "Undiagnosed Health Issues in Individuals With Traumatic Brain Injury Living in the Community." *The Journal of Head Trauma Rehabilitation* 13:47–57, 1998.

with brain injury, it is incumbent on the clinician to verify from collateral sources the accuracy of the patient's account of his or her history and symptomatology. In cases of severe TBI, patients rarely recall the incidents surrounding the injury. This disturbance in recall of the incident itself, in conjunction with the patient's decreased awareness of his or her deficits, makes accessing collateral information essential. Collateral history may be obtained from a variety of sources (Table 4–4), including family and friends who can describe changes in behavior, cognition, personality, and general level of functioning since the brain injury.

Collateral history is also pivotal because survivors of TBI and their families and friends see the injuries through different lenses. For example, Sbordone et al. (1998) found that patients with TBI generally underreported cognitive, behavioral, and emotional symptoms as compared to those reported by significant others, regardless of the severity of injury. For example, 58.8% of significant others in the study noted emotional lability or mood swings in the patients with TBI, whereas only 5.9% of the patients reported such difficulties. Circumstantiality was observed by 29.4% of significant others; but none of the patients reported such problems. In those with severe TBI, none of the patients recognized problems with judgment, whereas 45% of their significant others identified this problem.

Hospital records related to the acute treatment of a TBI provide invaluable information about the traumatic event. This information includes the nature of the

trauma (e.g., MVA, fall, or blunt trauma); severity (GCS, period of unconsciousness, presence of traumatically related seizures, duration of retrograde amnesia and PTA, medical complications, and course of recovery); time of onset and types of neurobehavioral changes that occurred during the acute and postacute phases of recovery; and results of neuroimaging, electrophysiological, and neuropsychological testing delineating the location and extent of injury and pattern of cognitive and memory impairment associated with it. Medical and psychiatric records for the period before the trauma are also helpful in relating current signs and symptoms to past psychiatric disturbances and premorbid personality, and can assist in ascertaining the relative contributions of

TABLE 4–4.   Sources of collateral history

People	Documents
Family	Police reports
Friends	Emergency medical service reports
Co-workers	Medical records
Witnesses to injury	Educational history
Medical staff	Driving record
Allied health professionals (occupational, physical, and speech therapists, etc.)	

antecedent variables, the brain injury itself, and current psychosocial parameters to observed neurobehavioral changes.

If available, posttrauma psychiatric and/or rehabilitation records help delineate the course of the patient's recovery, including the acute versus chronic nature of presenting psychiatric complaints, and provide a source of additional behavioral observations. Relevant posttrauma records also should be reviewed for the emergence of subsequent medical problems, results of neurodiagnostic studies, and indications of the efficacy and adverse effects of various treatment interventions the patient may have received. Additional sources of collateral information that may prove helpful include police reports and emergency medical service records (to provide information about the accident and condition of the patient at the scene), educational records, and driving record (to provide a history of prior MVAs).

Current Neuropsychiatric Symptoms

Within days of a mild to moderate TBI, a significant number of patients experience headaches, fatigue, dizziness, decreased attention, memory disturbance, slowed speed of information processing, and distractibility (Levin et al. 1987b; McLean et al. 1983). Other symptoms that frequently occur within the first few days after such an injury include hypersensitivity to noise and light, irritability, easy loss of temper, sleep disturbances, and anxiety (Binder 1986). These symptoms, which are often referred to as "postconcussive" symptoms, are described in more detail in Chapter 15, Mild Brain Injury and the Postconcussion Syndrome.

Although there are some discrepancies in the results of available follow-up outcome studies, it is apparent that most patients experience substantial resolution of cognitive, somatic, and emotional symptoms within 1–6 months after a mild brain injury (Barth et al. 1983; Rimel et al. 1981). However, there is a significant subgroup of patients who continue to experience difficulties with reasoning, information processing, memory, vigilance, attention, and depression and anxiety (see Chapter 17, Cognitive Changes).

The symptom profile with moderate TBI is generally similar to that seen with mild TBI, but the frequency of symptoms is greater, and they tend to be more severe (Rimel et al. 1982). Severe TBI is associated with a large number of chronic neurobehavioral changes, acute as well as delayed in onset (Table 4–5). Recovery from severe TBI is typically marked by a number of stages that can be documented using the Rancho Los Amigos Cognitive Scale (Table 4–6).

TABLE 4–5. Neurobehavioral symptoms associated with severe brain injury

Symptoms	Relative frequencies during postinjury period (%)		
	6 months	12 months	2 years
Forgetfulness	—	—	54
Slowness	69	69	33–65
Tiredness	69	69	28–30
Irritability	69	53–71	38–39
Memory problems	59	69–87	68–80
Decreased initiative	—	53	—
Impatience	64	57–71	—
Anxiety	66	58	16–46
Temper outbursts	56	50–67	28
Personality change	58	60	—
Depressed mood	52	57	19–48
Headaches	46	53	23
Childishness	—	—	60
Emotional lability	—	—	21–40
Restlessness	—	—	25
Poor concentration	—	—	33–73
Lack of interest	—	—	16–20
Dizziness	—	—	26–41
Light sensitivity	—	—	25
Noise sensitivity	—	—	23

Source. Adapted from Jacobs 1987; Mauss-Clum and Ryan 1981; McKinlay et al. 1981; Thomsen 1984; and Van Zomeren and Van Den Berg 1985.

Severe TBI

A common sequence of stages has been identified in the recovery from severe TBI. It is important to note that not everyone follows this sequence. For example, one may reach a particular stage and fail to progress further, or one may demonstrate features of different stages simultaneously.

The first stage of recovery after a severe TBI is coma, which is characterized by LOC and unresponsiveness to the environment. A simple but useful measure of the depth of coma is the GCS. On emerging from deep coma, the patient enters the second stage of recovery, a state of unresponsive vigilance, marked by apparent gross wakefulness with eye tracking, but without purposeful responsiveness to the environment. The third stage of recovery is characterized by mute responsiveness, in which there

TABLE 4-6.	Rancho Los Amigos Cognitive Scale

I. No response: Unresponsive to any stimulus

II. Generalized response: Limited, inconsistent, and nonpurposeful responses—often to pain only

III. Localized response: Purposeful responses; may follow simple commands; may focus on presented object

IV. Confused, agitated: Heightened state of activity; confusion, and disorientation; aggressive behavior; unable to perform self-care; unaware of present events; agitation appears related to internal confusion

V. Confused, inappropriate: Nonagitated; appears alert; responds to commands; distractible; does not concentrate on task; agitated responses to external stimuli; verbally inappropriate; does not learn new information

VI. Confused, appropriate: Good directed behavior, needs cuing; can relearn old skills as activities of daily living; serious memory problems, some awareness of self and others

VII. Automatic, appropriate: Appears appropriately oriented; frequently robotlike in daily routine; minimal or absent confusion; shallow recall; increased awareness of self and interaction in environment; lacks insight into condition; decreased judgment and problem solving; lacks realistic planning for future

VIII. Purposeful, appropriate: Alert and oriented; recalls and integrates past events; learns new activities and can continue without supervision; independent in home and living skills; capable of driving; defects in stress tolerance, judgment, and abstract reasoning persist; may function at reduced levels in society

Source. Reprinted with permission from the Adult Brain Injury Service of the Rancho Los Amigos Medical Center, Downey, California.

are no vocalizations, but the patient responds to commands. Identification of this stage depends on demonstrating the patient's capacity to carry out simple commands that will not be confused with reflex activity and do not depend on intact language function, because the patient may have an aphasia or apraxia. Requesting that the patient carry out various eye movements is often the best task to use, and the movements can range from simple to complex (Alexander 1982).

The next phase of recovery is characterized by the return of speech and language function. During this stage, the patient begins to demonstrate a confusional state akin to delirium as indicated by fluctuating attention and concentration and an incoherent stream of thought (see Chapter 9, Delirium and Posttraumatic Amnesia). The confused or delirious patient usually displays distractibility, perseveration, and a disturbance in the usual sleep/wake cycle. Such

patients may become agitated and demonstrate increased psychomotor activity. This stage is also frequently associated with sensory misperceptions, hallucinations, confabulation, and denial of illness (Alexander 1982).

During the stage of confusion, the patient is not able to form new memories in a normal fashion and is disoriented. This stage is the period when posttraumatic anterograde amnesia is prominent. PTA is considered to be present until the patient is consistently oriented and can recall particulars of his or her environment in a consistent manner. The duration of PTA can be assessed with the Galveston Orientation and Amnesia Test (GOAT) (Levin et al. 1979a, 1979b) (see Figure 8–1 in Chapter 8, Issues in Neuropsychological Assessment), which monitors both the degree of orientation and recall of newly learned material. The length of PTA is one of the best indicators of the severity of injury and is a clinically useful predictor of outcome. Furthermore, the length of PTA may correlate with the occurrence of psychiatric and behavioral sequelae.

When the stage characterized by PTA resolves, attention and concentration improve, confabulation lessens, and the sleep/wake cycle normalizes, although problems often persist with daytime fatigue and insomnia. These changes mark a major transition from the acute to the subacute and chronic phases of recovery. This transition phase is characterized by persistent, though less severe, disturbances in attention, concentration, memory impairments, and limited awareness of the presence of other disturbances of cognitive function. Some patients also experience retrograde amnesia, which rapidly shrinks and is usually relatively short in duration.

As the chronic phase of recovery unfolds, changes in personality, behavior, and emotions may emerge and be superimposed on the cognitive disturbances. Many patients with severe TBI complain of forgetfulness, irritability, slowness, poor concentration, fatigue, and dizziness, in addition to headache, mood lability, apathy, depressed mood, and anxiety (Hinkeldey and Corrigan 1990; Thomsen 1984; Van Zomeren and Van Den Burg 1985).

Signs and Symptoms After TBI

The types of signs and symptoms that may occur after a TBI of any severity are, in part, related to the type of injury (diffuse or focal) and its anatomical location. Symptoms that are thought to be associated with DAI include mental slowness, decreased concentration, and decreased arousal (Alexander 1982; Gualtieri 1991).

Symptoms after TBI are often linked to lobar or regional areas of the brain (frontal lobe syndromes or temporal lobe syndromes). Although such models lend convenience and

TABLE 4–7.   **Traumatic brain injury (TBI)–related DSM-IV-TR disorders**

TBI sequelae	DSM-IV-TR disorders
PTA	Delirium due to TBI (293.0)
Persistent global cognitive impairments in context of intact sensorium (after resolution of PTA)	Dementia due to TBI, with or without behavioral disturbance (294.11 and 294.10, respectively)
"Postconcussive" syndrome	Cognitive disorder not otherwise specified (294.9) (research criteria specific for "postconcussional disorder" in Appendix B)
Isolated impairment of memory	Amnestic disorder due to head trauma (294.0)
Changes in personality	Personality change (apathetic, disinhibited, labile, aggressive, paranoid, other, combined, unspecified) due to TBI (310.1)
Persistent hallucinations, delusions	Psychotic disorder (with delusions or hallucinations) due to TBI (293.81 and 293.82, respectively)
Persistent depression, mania	Mood disorder (with depressive, major depressive-like, manic, or mixed features) due to TBI (293.83)
Persistent anxiety symptoms	Anxiety disorder (with generalized anxiety, panic attacks, or obsessive-compulsive symptoms) due to TBI (293.84)
Impaired libido, arousal, erectile dysfunction, anorgasmia, etc.	Sexual dysfunction due to TBI: female or male hypoactive sexual desire (625.8 and 608.89, respectively); male erectile disorder (607.84); other female or male sexual dysfunction (625.8 and 608.89, respectively)
Insomnia, reversal of sleep-wake cycle, daytime fatigue, etc.	Sleep disorder due to TBI (780.xx): insomnia type (.52); hypersomnia type (.54); parasomnia type (.59); mixed type (.59)

Note.   PTA=posttraumatic amnesia.

Source.   Adapted from American Psychiatric Association: *Diagnostic and Statistical Manual of Mental Disorders*, 4th Edition, Text Revision. Washington, DC, American Psychiatric Association, 2000.

order to the understanding of the sequelae of TBI, they may be too simplistic because individuals often present with symptoms from several regions. Neuropsychiatric symptoms may be more closely linked to circuits that connect a number of lobes and regions involved in similar functions. Although it may not be possible to link structural lesions with symptoms based on anatomical location alone, the following syndromes are classic.

Focal lesions involving the convexities of the frontal lobes (or, more likely, frontal lobe circuitry) are typically associated with decreased initiation, decreased interpersonal interaction, passivity, mental inflexibility, and perseveration. Focal lesions involving the orbitofrontal surfaces are associated with disinhibition of behavior, dysregulation of mood and anger, impulsivity, and sexually and socially inappropriate behavior (Cummings 1985; Gualtieri 1991; Mattson and Levin 1990).

Temporal lobe lesions are often associated with memory disturbances (left-sided lesions interfering with verbal memory and right-sided lesions with nonverbal memory), increased emotional expressiveness, uncontrolled rages, sudden changes in mood, unprovoked pathological crying and laughing, manic symptoms, and delusions (Gualtieri

1991). Bilateral temporal lobe injuries may cause a Klüver-Bucy–like syndrome, characterized by placidity, hyperorality, increased exploratory behavior, memory disturbance, and hypersexuality (Cummings 1985; Gualtieri 1991).

Some of the signs and symptoms of TBI result from the patient's emotional and psychological responses to having experienced a TBI and having to deal with its negative interpersonal and social consequences. Patients with TBI may experience frustration, anxiety, anger, depression, irritability, isolation, withdrawal, and denial in response to the losses they have experienced. The array of psychiatric and behavioral symptoms demonstrated by patients with TBI do not always cluster in a syndromically defined fashion (with the possible exception of the postconcussive syndrome in mild TBI), nor do they always allow for a specific diagnosis based on DSM-IV-TR criteria (American Psychiatric Association 2000). Table 4–7 shows common DSM-IV-TR diagnoses used in TBI-related neuropsychiatric sequelae.

According to a number of studies, TBI appears to be a risk factor for a number of psychiatric disorders, including major depression, dysthymia, obsessive-compulsive disorder, phobias, panic disorder, alcohol or substance abuse/dependence, bipolar disorder, and schizophrenia (Hibbard et al. 1998a; Silver et al. 2001), although the incidence of bipolar disorder and schizophrenia after TBI is much less frequent than depression and select anxiety disorders. Other psychiatric disorders commonly seen after TBI include generalized anxiety disorder (Jorge et al. 1993), posttraumatic stress disorder (Bryant and Harvey 1999; Hibbard et al. 1998a), psychosis (Fujii and Ahmed 2001), attention-deficit/hyperactivity disorder, conduct disorder, and oppositional defiant disorder (Max et al. 1998). The incidence of comorbidity is also high, especially for major depression, anxiety disorders, and substance use disorders, as noted by Hibbard et al. (1998a) in a study of 100 adults with TBI in which 44% of patients met criteria for two or more Axis I disorders. In another study of 100 individuals with TBI focused on identifying Axis II pathology, Hibbard et al. (2000) found that 66% of patients met criteria for at least one personality disorder, most commonly borderline, avoidant, paranoid, obsessive-compulsive, and narcissistic types. Given the significant burden of both Axis I and II pathology, it is not surprising that those patients with TBI have a greater lifetime prevalence of suicide attempts (nearly four times that of individuals without a history of TBI) and poorer quality of life, according to Silver et al. (2001).

Neurological Symptoms

Brain injuries cause a number of subtle as well as gross neurological disturbances, including visual and sensory disturbances, motor dysfunction, ataxias, tremor, aphasias, apraxias, and seizures. Inquiring about neurological symptoms and a careful neurological examination may shed light on the nature and extent of brain injury and associated focal neurological dysfunction. However, it is important to note that the neurological examination may be entirely normal despite the presence of a TBI because the examination focuses primarily on sensorimotor function.

The neurological examination (Table 4–8) should assess various aspects of motor function, such as strength, tone, gait, cerebellar function (ataxia), fine motor movements (speed and coordination), motor imitation, and reflexes. Vision should be tested to identify any field cuts or diminished acuity. Sensory function, including the sense of smell, should also be examined. Although infrequently detected, anosmia (the impairment of the sense of smell) is a common sequela of TBI often associated with negative functional outcomes related to orbitofrontal damage and executive function deficits (Callahan and Hinkebein 1999). Because the olfactory nerves are located in close proximity to the orbitofrontal cortex, anosmia may serve as a marker for frontal lobe deficits. Frontal lobe damage or dysfunction may also be indicated by the presence of frontal release signs, including the grasp reflex, glabellar

TABLE 4–8. Neurological examination after traumatic brain injury: key areas of assessment

Sensory	Motor	Other
Vision (look for field cuts)	Strength, tone, gait (r/o ataxia)	Aphasia, confabulation, perseveration
Smell (r/o anosmia)	Fine motor movements, speed, coordination (observe for tremor)	Seizures
Recognition (r/o agnosia)	Motor imitation (r/o apraxia)	Frontal release signs
	Reflexes	

Note. r/o=rule out.

blink reflex (Meyerson's sign), Hoffmann's sign, palmomental reflex, and suck, snout, and rooting reflexes.

In addition to focal neurological disturbances after TBI, there is growing concern that TBI may be a risk factor for the later development of neurological illnesses, including Alzheimer's disease (see Chapter 28, Elderly) and multiple sclerosis (MS). The association between trauma and MS has been debated in the literature for many years. Multiple studies have demonstrated that central nervous system (CNS) trauma disrupts the blood-brain barrier (BBB), allowing passage of blood components that deliver the instruments of inflammation to the brain (Poser 2000). Lehrer (2000) notes that cytokines released by TBI disrupt the BBB and precipitate exacerbation in MS. Other investigators disagree and suggest that brain inflammation may cause a secondary change in the BBB rather than the opposite (Cook 2000). Although Cook acknowledges the possibility of a slight adverse effect on the course of MS after trauma, he states that there is no convincing evidence that physical trauma causes MS. In addition, the preponderance of evidence reviewed by the Therapeutics and Technology Assessment Subcommittee of the American Academy of Neurology reveals no association between physical trauma and either MS onset or MS exacerbation (Goodin et al. 1999).

Patients with severe TBI may experience impairment in expressive speech and receptive language function (posttraumatic aphasias), which may be indicated by deficits in naming, repetition, and word fluency (Levin et al. 1976; Sarno 1980). Patients with frontal lobe lesions may produce speech that is simple in structure and poorly organized. Patients with orbitofrontal damage may demonstrate confabulation and digressive speech, whereas patients with left dorsolateral lesions may have linguistic deficits, marked perseveration, and difficulty initiating speech (Kaczmarek 1984).

Due to the vast array of neuropsychiatric symptoms that may occur in seizure disorders, it is essential that the physician carefully evaluate patients with TBI for post-traumatic seizures (see Chapter 16, Seizures).

Endocrine Symptoms

Endocrine disturbances may be seen subsequent to TBI (Table 4–9). These tend to appear during the acute phase of recovery, presumably secondary to DAI and shear-strain damage to the hypothalamus and pituitary stalk (Crompton 1971). Abnormalities in thyroid function, growth hormone release, and adrenal cortical function, as well as cases of hypopituitarism, hypothalamic hypogonadism, and precocious puberty, all have been described (Clark et al. 1988; Edwards and Clark 1986; Gottardis et al. 1990; Klingbeil and Cline 1985; Maxwell et al. 1990; Shaul et al. 1985; Sockalosky et al. 1987; Woolf et al. 1990). Patients also may experience CNS-mediated hyperphagia and temperature dysregulation (Glenn 1988). Complaints of feeling cold, without actual alteration in body temperature, may also be seen (Silver and Anderson 1999). Furthermore, TBI patients in the acute phase of recovery can develop the syndrome of inappropriate antidiuretic hormone, as well as diabetes insipidus (Bontke and Cobble 1991). In addition, women may experience menstrual irregularities subsequent to severe TBI, making inquiry about the menstrual cycle and reproductive function an important part of the history (Bontke and Cobble 1991). Patients who have sustained frontal lobe injuries may manifest behavioral disinhibition, hypersexuality, and new-onset sexual perversions, whereas those with temporal lobe injuries may be hyposexual, with decreased libido, and erectile dysfunction may be seen in men.

Other Physical Symptoms

In a self-reported study involving 338 individuals with TBI, Hibbard et al. (1998b) identified a high prevalence of neuroendocrine, neurologic, and arthritic complaints (see Table 4–3). Physical problems included headaches, seizures, balance difficulties, spasticity, sleep disturbances, loss of urinary control, and changes in hair/skin texture, body temperature, and weight. Prevalence of these ongoing health problems was related to duration of LOC.

History Before the Injury

Psychiatric Disorders

Although many neurobehavioral disturbances appear to result directly from damage to the brain, the contributions of premorbid personality features, temperament, and ante-

TABLE 4–9. Common endocrine disturbances after traumatic brain injury

Hypo/hyperthyroidism

Impaired growth hormone release

Impaired adrenal cortical function

Hypopituitarism

Hypothalamic hypogonadism

Precocious puberty

Hyperphagia

Temperature dysregulation

Syndrome of inappropriate antidiuretic hormone

Diabetes insipidus

Menstrual irregularities

Changes in sexual function

cedent psychiatric disturbances are also important in determining the nature of post-TBI psychiatric and behavioral syndromes, particularly in patients with mild to moderate brain injuries. In a review of mild TBI, Kibby and Long (1996) note several preinjury factors that influence recovery: alcohol abuse, age, level of education, occupation, personality, emotional adjustment, and neuropsychiatric history. Premorbid anxiety, depression, psychosis, personality disorder, attention deficit hyperactivity disorder, and alcohol and/or substance abuse may significantly influence the recovery from TBI. Individuals with certain personality disorders (antisocial and obsessive-compulsive) may experience greater post-TBI adjustment issues (Hibbard et al. 2000). Max et al. (1997) found that preinjury psychiatric history along with severity of injury and preinjury family function predicted the development of "novel" psychiatric disorders in children and adolescents during the second year postinjury. The presence of mental retardation or learning disabilities also may influence the presentation of TBI-associated neurobehavioral disturbances.

Neurobehavioral changes after recovery from TBI result from the interplay of temperament, underlying personality traits, premorbid coping mechanisms, TBI-induced alterations in brain function, and injury-related losses and psychosocial stressors. Because all of these factors may influence outcome, all must be carefully assessed in the development of a clinical database. Many recent studies of patients with TBI do not include patients with previous psychiatric disorders or substance abuse. However, clinical experience indicates that premorbid personality traits, whether normal or pathological, are often exaggerated after TBI, possibly due to damage to inhibitory frontal lobe circuits.

Drug and Alcohol Abuse

Alcohol use is estimated to be a contributing factor in at least 50% of all TBIs (Sparadeo et al. 1990). Among TBI patients with positive blood alcohol levels at the time of evaluation in the emergency department, 29%–56% were legally intoxicated (Sparadeo et al. 1990). Alcohol and some substances may artificially lower the GCS due to their sedative effects (see Chapter 29, Alcohol and Drug Disorders).

Alcohol use at the time of injury is associated with a more complicated recovery, as indicated by longer hospitalization, longer periods of agitation, and more impaired cognitive function on discharge (Sparadeo et al. 1990). Brooks et al. (1989) observed that TBI patients with higher blood alcohol levels at the time of injury demonstrated poorer verbal learning and memory function compared to those with lower blood alcohol levels. A history of excessive alcohol use before brain injury is associated with an increase in mortality at the time of injury, greater risk of space-occupying, intracranial lesions acutely, and poorer overall outcome (Ruff et al. 1990). Continued excessive use of alcohol in TBI patients may further compromise their functional capacities, interfere with their rehabilitation, and place them at greater risk for subsequent TBIs (Strauss and Sparadeo 1988). Therefore, attention to pre- and postinjury substance use and abuse is important in assessing current levels of functioning, prognosis for recovery, and perhaps most important, treatment planning that addresses the substance abuse problem. Fuller et al. (1994) found that the CAGE screen and the Brief Michigan Alcohol Screening Test are easy to administer and sensitive as well as specific for substance abuse in this population.

Medical History

A thorough medical history and a careful review of systems are important parts of the neuropsychiatric evaluation. Detailed knowledge of prior, as well as current, medical problems, both related and unrelated to the brain injury, allows the clinician to assess their impact on the patient's overall neurobehavioral status and to take them into account in making recommendations for safe and appropriate treatments. Any history of early childhood illnesses, particularly seizure disorders, previous TBIs, and/or attention deficit hyperactivity disorder, should be sought. A history of prior TBIs has been associated with a subsequent increased incidence of moderate TBI (Rimel et al. 1982), a longer duration of postconcussive symptoms (Carlsson et al. 1987), and a poorer overall outcome (Levin 1989). TBI patients who eventually develop dementia are more likely to have had multiple previous brain injuries, alcoholism, and atherosclerosis (Gualtieri 1991). Assessment of developmental milestones and previous levels of cognitive, intellectual, and attentional functioning also provide the clinician with valuable baseline information against which to compare postinjury cognitive capabilities and coping strategies.

A detailed history of preinjury, idiopathic, or posttraumatic seizure disorders, and associated treatment, is important in understanding the impact of seizures and anticonvulsants on current cognitive and behavioral functioning. Detailed knowledge of seizure disorders and their current treatment is particularly important to the clinician in choosing safe and efficacious psychotropic medications.

Medications

Obtaining a thorough history of past treatment trials with psychotropic drugs, as well as the current types and doses of such medications and their efficacy, is important in establishing the value of previous drug trials, the responsiveness of current neurobehavioral symptoms to medications, and the potential efficacy of pharmacotherapy in maintaining or enhancing current levels of functioning. Psychotropic agents, anticonvulsants, and many other kinds of medication can have important effects on cognition and behavior, and their contributions to the patient's current neurobehavioral status must be ascertained. Benzodiazepines can impair memory and interfere with coordination. Anticholinergic drugs can increase confusion. If a patient is being treated with anticonvulsants, the clinician needs to determine whether this is for prophylaxis (and the patient never had a seizure or had seizures only immediately after the TBI) or for a continuing seizure disorder. Patients treated with anticonvulsants for prophylaxis beyond 1 week may have sedating and cognition-impairing side effects without any actual seizure prophylaxis. A careful review of the patient's medication history should also reveal any drug allergies or drug intolerances.

Family Psychiatric and Medical History

Knowledge of the family psychiatric and medical history can help in differentiating the increased risk of psychiatric disturbance due to genetic predisposition from that due to current psychosocial stressors or the TBI itself. Familiarity with the family history of psychiatric disturbances, medical illness, deaths, and their causes, can provide a better understanding of the possible role these factors may be playing in current abnormalities of emotional and psychological functioning in a TBI patient.

Social History

Social history encompasses information on 1) family structure and other support systems; 2) social, school, occupational, and recreational functioning; and 3) data on legal problems and personal habits. The social history provides extremely important data on the patient's level of current functioning, the nature and severity of psychosocial stressors, characteristic patterns of adaptation to stress, and the adequacy of coping mechanisms and social support systems. Psychopathological reactions may result from severe stresses associated with the losses and disruptions in an individual's life that can be caused by a TBI.

TBI often has an enormous impact on the patient's family (Mauss-Clum and Ryan 1981), as illustrated by the high frequency of psychiatric symptoms reported by family members of patients with TBI (Table 4–10). The clinician must sensitively assess the level of distress experienced by the family and should attempt to understand the quality of the relationships between the TBI patient and his or her spouse, children, parents, and siblings. Families are generally more troubled by behavioral and personality changes that occur in TBI patients than they are by their physical disabilities (Brooks 1991). Understanding the nature of the stresses on the family and the family's concerns about the TBI patient enables the clinician to make appropriate referrals for family and/or couples therapy. In addition to the clinical interview, a number of self-report instruments, rater-administered scales, and structured interviews are available to assist in quantifying and monitoring family functions and adaptation over time (Bishop and Miller 1988).

It is important to evaluate the patient's level of social integration postinjury due to the frequent interruption in social relationships and subsequent loneliness encountered by persons with TBI. Patients with severe TBI have the greatest difficulty establishing new social contacts and pursuing leisure activities (Morton and Wehman 1995).

School Functioning

Children and adolescents with TBI may experience disturbances in cognition and behavior that interfere with school functioning. Thus, careful inquiries about learning difficulties and academic performance, social and interpersonal interactions with peers, and difficulties with school authorities or the law are important in understanding the role that the brain injury may be playing in neurobehavioral disturbances that are contributing to school difficulties. This information guides recommendations for neuropsychological and educational testing, counseling, behavioral and pharmacologic treatments, and possible alternative special educational programming.

Formal assessment of cognition and behavior should be carried out as close to the start of an educational intervention as possible to establish a baseline against which progress over time can be measured (Telzrow 1991). Assessment of cognitive function after TBI should be carried out only when a period of stability has been achieved—not during the phase of

TABLE 4–10. Symptoms reported by family members of patients with severe brain injury

Reported symptom	% Reporting	
	Mother	Wife
Frustration	100	84
Irritability	55	74
Annoyance	55	68
Depression	45	79
Decreased social contact	27	77
Anger	45	63
Financial insecurity	18	58
Guilt	18	47
Feeling trapped	45	42

Source. Adapted from Mauss-Clum N, Ryan M: "Brain Injury and the Family." *Journal of Neurosurgical Nursing* 13:165–169, 1981.

rapid recovery (Telzrow 1991). Periodic reassessments thereafter are helpful in adjusting continuing intervention programs to achieve optimal levels. Any child or adolescent presenting for evaluation of behavioral problems should be queried specifically about previous TBI, particularly when disturbances in attention or memory function, impulsive or aggressive behavior, mood lability, or impaired social skills are evident (Obrzut and Hynd 1987).

Occupational Functioning

TBI often has a significant impact on the ability of a patient to maintain gainful employment. A number of studies have investigated the percentage of TBI patients returning to work, and the reported rates vary from 12% to 96% (Ben Yishay et al. 1987). These authors suggest that the reasons for this wide degree of variability include the broad range of severity of the TBI patients sampled, the absence of uniform criteria for defining return to work, the lack of verification of actual work performance and occupational status, and the lack of sufficiently long follow-up periods to establish reliable data.

According to a review by Kibby and Long (1996), approximately 90% of patients with mild TBI and 80% with moderate TBI return to work by 1 year after the injury. The majority of individuals with mild TBI return to work by 3 months postinjury. Factors possibly adversely affecting return to work include older age, lower levels of motivation to work, lower levels of education, poor social support, or poor coping strategies.

Ben Yishay et al. (1987) cited a study of four comparable groups of 30–50 TBI patients with moderate to severe brain injury who had received extensive rehabilitation and were considered ready for vocational assessment and placement. When followed over time, less than 3% of the patients were able to achieve and maintain competitive employment for as long as 1 year. The high failure rate was attributed to cognitive impairments (deficits in attention, memory, and executive functioning complicated by distractibility and behavioral impersistence), problems with apathy and disinhibition, impaired interpersonal skills, lack of awareness and appreciation of the impact of the injury on functioning, and unrealistic expectations concerning the suitability of various types of employment. Clinicians can target these specific areas in an attempt to facilitate the patient's return to work by using a variety of modalities, including psychotropic medications, supportive psychotherapy, cognitive remediation, and vocational and occupational rehabilitation.

Physical Examination

Although history is the most critical source of information in diagnosing TBI, physical examination is also important, with particular emphasis on the neurological examination. Patients with moderate to severe TBI may have mental status and Mini-Mental State Examination (MMSE) abnormalities as well as focal neurologic findings that reflect the location and severity of the injury. However, because the majority of TBIs are mild, the neurological examination is nonfocal and the MMSE normal in most TBI patients. Frontal release signs may be elicited in TBI patients who have no focal findings.

Mental Status Examination and "Bedside" Cognitive Testing

Mental status and MMSE testing should always be carried out as part of a neuropsychiatric evaluation, keeping in mind that both may be relatively normal, particularly when deficits due to the TBI are subtle and involve frontal lobe functions. Although neuropsychological testing provides the most comprehensive "map" of the injury and its sequelae, the clinician may administer a few simple tests in the office or at beside to evaluate frontal lobe functions because the MMSE is inadequate for this purpose. Perhaps the most efficient test is clock drawing. This exercise provides information not only about the individual's executive function, but also attention, visuospatial function, registration of information, and recall. For a listing of additional tests of frontal lobe functions that the neuropsychiatrist can easily use, see Table 4–11.

Behavioral Assessment

There are numerous rating scales that can be used to quantify various aspects of cognition, memory function, emotion, and behavior (see other chapters for specific scales for depression, mania, aggression, delirium, agita-

---

TABLE 4–11. "Bedside" evaluation of frontal lobe function

Test	Description	Frequent findings
Clock-drawing test	Instruct the patient to draw a clock, including all of the numbers, setting the time at 10 past 11.	Poor planning (numbers inappropriately positioned; numbers don't fit inside clock; excess space inside clock, perseveration, etc.)
		Incorrect hand placement: hour and minute hands inappropriately placed; "stimulus-bound" (hands connecting 10 and 11), perseveration, etc.
Verbal fluency	Number of words that begin with the same letter or number of animals named in 1 minute	Unable to name 10 or more
		Perseveration
Set shifts and sequencing (verbal and written)	Verbal: 1A–2B–3C (ask the patient to continue the pattern)	Perseveration
	Written (Trails B): ask the patient to connect numbers and letters in a sequential and alternating manner (1A–2B–3C, etc.)	Inability to consistently shift sets (1A–2B–3C–4C–5C–6C, etc., or 1A–2B–3C–3D–3E–3F, etc.)
"Fist-palm-side"	Ask the patient to place his or her right fist into left palm, the right palm into left palm, then right side of hand into left palm in a sequential manner	Perseveration of movement
"Go–No Go" test	Ask the patient to say "two" when one finger is held up; "one" when two fingers are displayed	Inability to inhibit the visual stimulus (says "one" when one finger is displayed)

tion, and others). Several rating scales have particular utility in evaluating behavior and cognition during the various phases of recovery from TBI.

In the assessment of coma, the GCS described earlier (see Table 1–2 in Chapter 1, Epidemiology) is one of the most useful instruments for monitoring changes in levels of consciousness and the patient's emergence from coma. The GCS assesses eye movements, motor coordination, and verbal responses. The GCS severity index scores range from 3 to 15, with scores of 3–8 indicating severe, 9–12 moderate, and 13–15 mild injury.

After emergence from coma, the GOAT (see Figure 8–1 in Chapter 8, Issues in Neuropsychological Assessment) can be used to follow the course of improvement in PTA and establish the end of this period (Levin et al. 1979b). The GOAT is a 10-item, rater-administered questionnaire, which assesses orientation to person, place, and time, and recall of events before and after the injury. The score is calculated by subtracting error points from 100. A score of 65 or less is considered abnormal, whereas borderline abnormal scores range from 65 to 75 (Levin et al. 1979a, 1979b). GOAT scores correlate with the severity of injury, and, because this test provides an assessment of the duration of PTA, it is helpful in predicting long-term outcome.

Similar to and highly correlated with the GOAT is the Orientation Log (O-Log, Figure 4–1)—a scale introduced by Jackson et al. (1998) as a brief measure of orientation for patients undergoing rehabilitation. Health care providers may use the O-Log to plot a patient's recovery curve by assigning a score of 0–3 for each item, adding the scores, and graphing the sum on the orientation index. In addition to being brief, this scale has some advantages over the GOAT, including consistent scoring across items and the ability to evaluate a patient who is unable to respond (or who responds inaccurately). It can also be administered to individuals with speech impairment.

As the period of PTA ends, the patient enters the chronic phase of recovery, in which assessment of TBI-related neurobehavioral and neurocognitive changes becomes especially important. The previously mentioned Rancho Los Amigos Scale (see Table 4–6) is a useful tool in tracking cognitive and behavioral recovery. A more comprehensive instrument was developed by Levin et al. (1987a)—the Neurobehavioral Rating Scale (NRS)—which measures disturbances in behavior, cognition, emotion, thought content, and language function during the long-term recovery from brain injury. Levin et al. (1990) enhanced the reliability and content validity of the NRS, creating the Neurobehavioral Rating Scale—Revised (NRS-R, Figure 4–2). It consists of a 4-point scale on which ratings for each item range from absent to severe in regard to the impact of a particular behavior on the per-

son's social and occupational functioning. Administration of the NRS-R requires a 15- to 20-minute structured interview, which includes tests of orientation, attention, concentration, memory of recent events, delayed recall, proverb interpretation, and mental flexibility as well as questions about the emotional state and postconcussional symptoms. During the administration of the tests the interviewer observes the patient closely for fatigability, signs of anxiety, disinhibition, agitation, hostility, disturbance of mood, and difficulties with expressive and receptive communication. Approximately one-third of the item ratings are solely based on examiner's observation, whereas the rest of the items are rated according to the patient's performance on the tasks performed (McCauly et al. 2001). Early administration after severe TBI followed by serial assessments provide a means of quantifying change in the deficits over time. Vanier et al. (2000) found the NRS-R to be a useful tool for predicting psychosocial recovery and assessing neuropsychological factors related to social autonomy.

A thorough clinical neuropsychiatric evaluation requires careful assessment of cognitive functioning. The Neurobehavioral Cognitive Status Examination (NCSE), which can be completed in 5–20 minutes, is an extremely useful tool for rapid cognitive screening. Kiernan and colleagues developed the NCSE to assess attention, orientation, language, visuoconstructional skills, memory, calculation, abstract reasoning, and levels of consciousness (Kiernan et al. 1987; Schwamm et al. 1987). Most of the NCSE's assessment categories begin with a screening item that is a relatively demanding test of the skill involved. If the screening item is successfully completed, no further testing in that domain is required. This allows for rapid completion when there is little cognitive impairment. The NCSE generates a performance profile that reflects differentiated functioning and can be compared to group norms for various neuropsychiatric disorders. The NCSE is particularly useful as a screening tool in identifying patients for whom formal neuropsychological testing is indicated and is a valuable adjunct to other clinical neurodiagnostic studies when neuropsychological testing is not readily available. Scales for specific assessment of other psychiatric or behavioral problems are discussed elsewhere in this text (e.g., the Overt Aggression Scale [see Chapter 14, Aggressive Disorders] and the Hamilton Rating Scale for Depression).

Additional Assessment Tools

In addition to history, physical, mental status examination, MMSE, "bedside" cognitive testing, and behavioral assessment, one may incorporate additional evaluation tools to complete the neuropsychiatric evaluation. These diagnostic tools include neuropsychological testing, structural

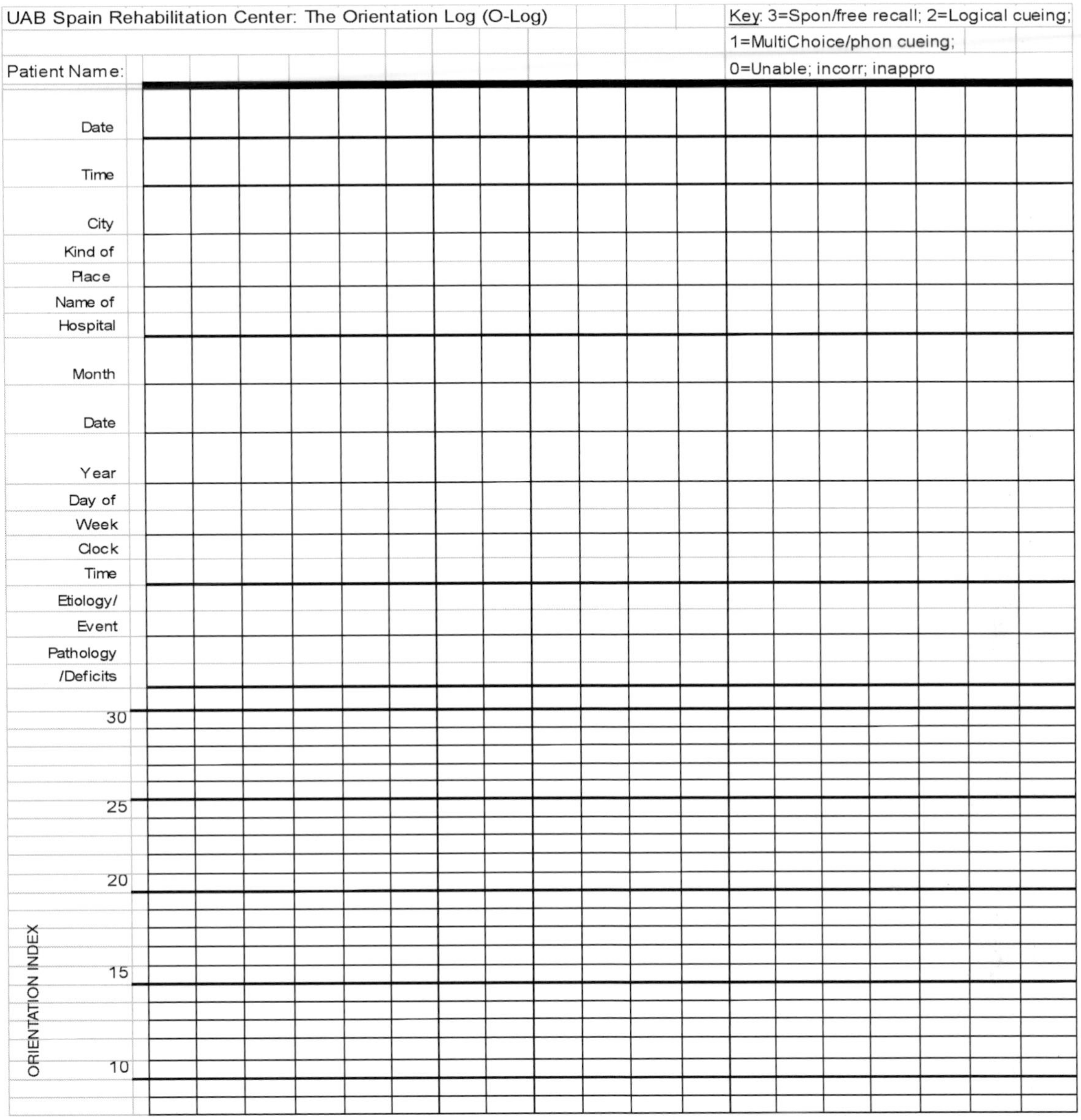

UAB Spain Rehabilitation Center: The Orientation Log (O-Log)									Key: 3=Spon/free recall; 2=Logical cueing;								
									1=MultiChoice/phon cueing;								
Patient Name:									0=Unable; incorr; inappro								
Date																	
Time																	
City																	
Kind of Place																	
Name of Hospital																	
Month																	
Date																	
Year																	
Day of Week																	
Clock Time																	
Etiology/ Event																	
Pathology /Deficits																	

ORIENTATION INDEX: 30, 25, 20, 15, 10

FIGURE 4–1.   The Orientation Log.

inappro=inappropriate; incorr=incorrect; MultiChoice=multiple choice; phon=phonetic; Spon=spontaneous.

Source.   Adapted from Jackson WT, Novack TA, Dowler RN: "Effective Serial Measurement of Cognitive Orientation in Rehabilitation: The Orientation Log." *Archives of Physical Medicine and Rehabilitation* 79:718–720, 1998.

and/or functional neuroimaging, electroencephalogram, and evoked potentials (see Chapters 5, Structural Imaging; 6, Functional Imaging; and 7, Electrophysiologic Techniques for more information).

Overview of Other Types of Brain Injuries

In addition to brain injury due to blunt or penetrating injuries or DAI, brain injury may be due to a number of other causes. These include metabolic factors such as hypoxia/anoxia; hypoglycemia, hypothyroidism, and certain vitamin deficiencies; exposure to CNS toxins such as heavy metals or other industrial/environmental toxins; drugs of abuse, including toxic inhalants and carbon monoxide poisoning; and passage of electrical current through the brain in electrocutions or lightning-related injuries. Another important and increasingly common kind of brain injury occurs as a complication of coronary artery bypass surgery. This kind of diffuse brain injury is believed to result, in part, from gaseous or particulate microemboli released into the cerebral circulation as a result of complications of the bypass procedure itself or

IDENTIFICATION

Patient name: _____ Gender: F__ M __ Date of accident: _____

Date of birth: _____   Date of evaluation: _____

Address: _____

Evaluator's name: _____

LIST OF THE VARIABLES

	Absent	Mild	Mod.	Severe			Absent	Mild	Mod.	Severe	
1.	____	____	____	____	Reduced alertness	16.	____	____	____	____	Guilt
2.	____	____	____	____	Hyperactivity and agitation	17.	____	____	____	____	Lability of mood
3.	____	____	____	____	Disorientation	18.	____	____	____	____	Blunted affect
4.	____	____	____	____	Attentional difficulties	19.	____	____	____	____	Irritability
5.	____	____	____	____	Difficulties in articulation	20.	____	____	____	____	Disinhibition
6.	____	____	____	____	Difficulties in oral expression	21.	____	____	____	____	Excitement
7.	____	____	____	____	Difficulties in oral comprehension	22.	____	____	____	____	Hostility
8.	____	____	____	____	Memory difficulties	23.	____	____	____	____	Suspiciousness
9.	____	____	____	____	Motor slowing	24.	____	____	____	____	Emotional withdrawal
10.	____	____	____	____	Exaggerated somatic concern	25.	____	____	____	____	Conceptual disorganization
11.	____	____	____	____	Self-appraisal difficulties	26.	____	____	____	____	Difficulty in mental flexibility
12.	____	____	____	____	Hallucinations	27.	____	____	____	____	Difficulty in planning
13.	____	____	____	____	Unusual thought content	28.	____	____	____	____	Decreased initiative or motivation
14.	____	____	____	____	Anxiety	29.	____	____	____	____	Mental fatigability
15.	____	____	____	____	Depressive mood						

FIGURE 4–2.   Neurobehavioral Rating Scale—Revised.

F=female; M=male; Mod.=moderate.

Source.   Adapted from Vanier M, Mazaux J-M, Lambert J, et al: "Assessment of Neuropsychologic Impairment After Head Injury: Interrater Reliability and Factorial and Criterion Validity of the Neurobehavioral Rating Scale—Revised." *Archives of Physical Medicine and Rehabilitation* 81:796–806, 2000. Used with permission.

surgical manipulations that occur during and immediately after the time the patient is on bypass. The kinds of neurological, cognitive, and behavioral sequelae that occur with these kinds of brain injury are similar to those seen with TBI, both with respect to the types and severity of deficits and the dysfunction and disability they may cause. As is the case with TBIs, the specific neurocognitive and behavioral sequelae that occur are dependent on the regions of the brain that have been damaged.

Anoxia/Hypoxia

Anoxia is defined as inadequate oxygenation of body tissues. Anoxic brain injury owing to a lack of oxygen in the ambient air is known as *anoxic anoxia*. Anoxia owing to acutely decreased blood volume or lowered hemoglobin concentration in the blood is referred to as *anemic anoxia*, and anoxia owing to insufficient cerebral blood flow because of cerebrovascular accidents, arrhythmias, or cardiac arrests is called *ischemic anoxia*. Finally, there is *toxic anoxia*, which is because of toxins or metabolites that may interfere with oxygen utilization.

In general, hypoxia with ischemia is more harmful than hypoxia alone because potentially toxic metabolic products such as lactic acid may contribute to tissue damage. The nature of hypoxic ischemic injury is neuropathologically different from traumatic injury, in that the former affects the neurons themselves, whereas the latter tends to be an axonal phenomenon. In addition to cardiac and respiratory arrest, anoxic brain injury occurs in cases of near drowning, strangulation, and anesthetic accidents (Wilson 1996).

Although the brain comprises only 2% of the body's total weight, it accounts for a disproportionate 20% of the total oxygen utilization and 65% of the glucose uptake. Approximately 15% of the cardiac output is directed to the brain to meet its energy needs (Kuroiwa and Okeda 1994; White et al. 1984). When disruption of the oxygen delivery system occurs, a series of cerebrovascular homeostatic mechanisms become activated to maintain adequate oxygen supply to the brain (Cohen 1976; Strandgaard and Paulson 1984). When there is a sustained disruption in oxygen supply (for a period of 4–8 minutes or longer), cerebral infarction and/or disseminated cellular death may occur (Bigler and Alfonso 1988; Caronna 1979; Cohan et al. 1989; Cohen 1976; Strandgaard and Paulson 1984; White et al. 1984).

The mechanism of anoxic brain damage comprises a complex cascade of time-dependent alterations in neuronal function, metabolism, and morphology (Haddad and Jiang 1993; Pulsinelli et al. 1982). The most important acute effect of hypoxia on the brain is the release of exci-

tatory neurotransmitters, leading to an influx of sodium, cellular edema, and consequent cellular injury (Hansen 1985; Kjos et al. 1983; Rothman and Olney 1986). Longer-term effects are due to an increase in neuronal excitability, which results in calcium influx, formation of oxygen-free radicals that injure cells, and eventual cell death (Ascher and Nowak 1987; Choi 1990; Gibson et al. 1988; Haddad and Jiang 1993; Hansen 1985; Maiese and Caronna 1989; Schurr and Rigor 1992; Siesjo 1981; White et al. 1984).

Whether a patient with hypoxia will develop neurological signs depends more on the severity and duration of the process causing hypoxia than its etiology (Berek et al. 1997). Two factors that determine the vulnerability of cells in a given brain region to hypoxia include distribution of the cerebral blood vessels and adequacy of their baseline perfusion and the specific metabolic and biochemical properties of the neural structures involved. The most vulnerable regions of the brain are the watershed areas of the cortex. That is because normal cellular metabolism in these areas is dependent on an adequate flow of normally oxygenated blood through the distal cerebral arterioles that perfuse them. Cellular and tissue damage occur first in these areas where inadequate oxygenation of the blood due to hypoxia fails to meet minimal metabolic requirements, especially when impaired perfusion is also present (Brierley and Graham 1984; Parkin et al. 1987). Cells in brain regions with higher metabolic demand are also more likely to be affected by oxygen deprivation (Moody et al. 1990; Myers 1979). In addition to these general principles, it has been shown that cells in various brain regions respond differentially to the degree and duration of hypoxia. For example, basal ganglia and cerebral cortical cells show signs of necrosis shortly after a cardiac arrest, whereas similar changes in the hippocampus may not be seen until 2–3 days after the event (Kuroiwa and Okeda 1994; Petito et al. 1987; Pulsinelli et al. 1982).

Coma is a frequent outcome of significant and sustained hypoxia. The three leading causes of coma in descending order of frequency are: trauma, drug overdose, and cardiac arrest (Shewmon et al. 1989). From a prognostic point of view, patients with traumatic coma have a better chance of recovery than those with nontraumatic coma. Among patients in the nontraumatic group, recovery generally occurs in the following descending order of frequency: metabolic causes, coma secondary to cardiac arrest, and coma from cerebrovascular causes (Berek et al. 1997). Clinical outcomes typically depend on the presence or absence of the prognostic factors listed in Table 4–12.

Neuropsychological deficits after anoxic brain damage may include memory and executive dysfunction, apperceptive

TABLE 4–12. Clinical parameters indicating unfavorable prognosis in patients with coma

Clinical parameters	Unfavorable prognosis
Duration of anoxia	>8–10 minutes
Duration of cardiopulmonary resuscitation	>30 minutes
Duration of postanoxic coma	>72 hours
Pupillary light reaction	Absent on day 3
Motor response to pain	Absent on day 3
Blood glucose on admission	>300 mg%
Glasgow Coma Scale score on day 3	<5

Source. Adapted from Berek K, Jeschow M, Aichner F: "The Prognostication of Cerebral Hypoxia After Out-of-Hospital Cardiac Arrest in Adults." *European Neurology* 37:135–145, 1999.

tive agnosia, and visual deficits. Most patients with anoxic brain damage have preserved attention and concentration abilities. Some patients who have sustained severe anoxic brain injury may remain in a persistent vegetative state with no observable cognitive functioning at all (Parkin et al. 1987; Wilson 1996).

Cognitive Problems After Coronary Artery Bypass Graft Surgery

Approximately 800,000 patients worldwide undergo coronary artery bypass graft (CABG) surgery per year (Selnes et al. 1999). CABG is associated with significant cerebral morbidity, manifested by cognitive decline or stroke (Roach et al. 1996; Van Dijk et al. 2002). The incidence of cognitive decline may vary from 3% to 50%, depending on patient characteristics, definition of decline, and the type and timing of neuropsychological assessment (Diegeler et al. 2000; Roach et al. 1996; Van Dijk et al. 2002). Intraoperative transcranial Doppler monitoring has clearly demonstrated that during cardiopulmonary bypass (CPB), microemboli are released into the brain. This release of microemboli is correlated with postoperative neurological deficits (Syliviris et al. 1998). A study comparing the neurocognitive effects of CABG with and without CPB surgery demonstrated that patients with their first CABG without CPB had less cognitive impairment at 3 months, but by 12 months the differences between the groups had become negligible (Van Dijk et al. 2002).

The emotional and cognitive state before CABG surgery is an important factor in the development of anxiety, depression, and cognitive deficits after the procedure (Adrian et al. 1988; Savageau et al. 1982). Even though a

high percentage of patients may exhibit neuropsychological deficits immediately or during the first few weeks after the surgery, most return to their premorbid level of neuropsychological functioning within several months after the procedure (Frank et al. 1972; Savageau et al. 1982).

Patients about to undergo CABG surgery should be screened for neurocognitive deficits and emotional disturbances before the procedure (Adrian et al. 1988). Asking patients about their expectations for the outcome of the procedure is also important because these expectations have an important bearing on the postoperative emotional state, cognitive deficits, and recovery from the surgery.

Electrical Injuries

Electrocution can cause brain damage in two ways—direct cellular damage due to passage of current through brain tissue and cardiac arrest induced by it. Electrical injuries occur as a result of exposure to live wires at work or home or lightning strikes during thunderstorms. The degree of damage is determined by the amount and type of current, duration of exposure, parts of the body affected, and the pathway of current through the body. Injuries acquired from exposure to electric current at home or work (low voltage injuries <1,000 volts) are different from those sustained from lightning or contact with high-voltage wires (high-voltage injuries >1,000 volts). Injuries due to alternating current are more serious in comparison to those from direct current (Browne and Gaasch 1992; Fish 1993). Patients who experience high-voltage electrical injury may initially show some cognitive deficits with confusion and memory loss, which usually clear within a few days. In cases in which these deficits persist, neuropsychological evaluation should be performed because some symptoms may be permanent, especially in cases of direct electrical injury to the brain (Table 4–13).

Looking Into the Future

There is still much to be learned about the molecular and cellular cascades that follow brain injury—no matter what the cause. Tracing these chemical and electrical derangements may lead to a better understanding of the origins of many neuropsychiatric illnesses. Recent investigations suggest that TBI may be linked to the later development of at least three neuropsychiatric conditions—MS, Alzheimer's disease, and schizophrenia. Perhaps future research will uncover common mechanisms of brain injury and disease states, reducing the gap between "neurologic" and "psychiatric" conditions and practice.

TABLE 4–13. Acute and delayed sequelae of electrical injury

Acute	Delayed
Confusion	Depression
Impaired concentration	Memory loss
Disorientation	Aphasia
Personality changes	Cerebellar dysfunction
Paralysis	Cataracts
Subdural hematomas	Delayed ascending paralysis
Suppression of respiratory center	Syndrome resembling amyotrophic lateral sclerosis
Seizures	Transverse myelitis
Loss of consciousness	Incomplete cord transection
Coagulation of the cortex	
Epidural hematoma	
Intraventricular hemorrhage	
Coma	

Source. Adapted from Browne and Gaasch 1992; Farrell and Starr 1968; and Fish 1993.

Summary

Comprehensive neuropsychiatric assessments of patients experiencing neurocognitive and neurobehavioral symptomatology and/or functional disability subsequent to brain injuries due to trauma as well as anoxia, hypoxia, and electrocution are essential and should assist the clinician in choosing optimal combinations of pharmacotherapy; individual, group, and family psychotherapy; and rehabilitation, occupational, and resocialization interventions. Such assessments should elicit and integrate clinical data from each of the three major biopsychosocial domains as they apply to patients with TBIs.

Optimal outcomes from neuropsychiatric treatment depend on careful elicitation of medical, neurological, psychiatric, and substance abuse histories, with special emphasis on premorbid functioning, details of the acute traumatic event, delineation of the nature and time course of development of posttraumatic neurocognitive and neurobehavioral problems, and precise descriptions of the patient's current psychiatric and behavioral symptomatology and functional disabilities. In addition to psychotherapeutic, behavioral, and rehabilitative interventions, psychotropic drug treatment is often beneficial if the clinician is aware that the patient may have residual symptoms due to brain trauma and prescribes lower-than-usual doses of psychotropic medications.

The more the neurophysiological effects of various kinds of brain injuries and diseases of the brain are understood, the more commonalities in their underlying pathophysiological mechanisms may be identified. Perhaps individuals who experience poor outcomes from TBI and/or later develop MS, schizophrenia, or dementia, are particularly vulnerable to free radicals, the excitotoxic cascade, calcium toxicity, N-methyl-D-aspartate activation, cytokines, and other neurocellular apoptotic processes. As future research defines the mechanisms of cellular damage and destruction after brain trauma, it may be discovered that many are identical to those found in a variety of primary neuropsychiatric diseases. Illuminating these shared pathophysiological mechanisms may then focus attention on promising treatments that might be effective in traumatic brain injury as well as other neuropsychiatric and neurodegenerative disease states.

References

Adrian J, Crankshaw DP, Tiller JWG, et al: Affective, cognitive and subjective changes in patients undergoing cardiac surgery—a preliminary report. Anesthesia and Intensive Care 16:144–149, 1988

Alexander MP: Traumatic brain injury, in Psychiatric Aspects of Neurologic Disease, Vol II. Edited by Benson DF, Blumer D. New York, Grune & Stratton, 1982, pp 219–249

American Psychiatric Association: Diagnostic and Statistical Manual of Mental Disorders, 4th Edition, Text Revision. Washington, DC, American Psychiatric Association, 2000

Ascher P, Nowak L: Electrophysiological studies of the NMDA receptors. Trends Neurosci 10:284–293, 1987

Asikainen I, Kaste M, Sarna S: Predicting late outcome for patients with traumatic brain injury referred to a rehabilitation programme: a study of 508 Finnish patients 5 years or more after injury. Brain Inj 12:95–107, 1998

Barth JT, Macciocchi SN, Giordani B, et al: Neuropsychological sequelae of minor head injury. Neurosurgery 13:529–533, 1983

Ben Yishay Y, Silver SM, Piasetsky E, et al: Relationship between employability and vocational outcome after intensive holistic cognitive rehabilitation. J Head Trauma Rehabil 2:35–48, 1987

Berek K, Jeschow M, Aichner F: The prognostication of cerebral hypoxia after out-of-hospital cardiac arrest in adults. Eur Neurol 37:135–145, 1997

Bigler E, Alfonso M: Anoxic encephalopathy: neuroradiological and neuropsychological findings. Arch Clin Neuropsychol 3:383–396, 1988

Binder LM: Persisting symptoms after mild head injury: a review of the postconcussive syndrome. J Clin Exp Neuropsychol 8:323–346, 1986

Bishop DS, Miller IW: Traumatic brain injury: empirical family assessment techniques. J Head Trauma Rehabil 3:16–30, 1988

Bontke CF, Cobble ND: Rehabilitation in brain disorders, II: clinical manifestations and medical issues. Arch Phys Med Rehabil 72 (suppl):S320–S323, 1991

Brierley JB, Graham DI: Hypoxia and vascular disorders of the central nervous system, in Greenfield's Neuropathology. Edited by Blackwood W, Corsellis JAN. London, Edwin Arnold, 1984, pp 125–207

Brooks DN: The head-injured family. J Clin Exp Neuropsychol 13:155–188, 1991

Brooks N, Symington C, Beattie A, et al: Alcohol and other predictors of cognitive recovery after severe head injury. Brain Inj 3:235–246, 1989

Browne BJ, Gaasch WR: Electrical injuries and lightning. Emerg Med Clin North Am 10:211–229, 1992

Bryant RA, Harvey AG: Postconcussive symptoms and post-traumatic stress disorder after mild traumatic brain injury. J Nerv Ment Dis 187:302–305, 1999

Callahan CD, Hinkebein J: Neuropsychological significance of anosmia following traumatic brain injury. J Head Trauma Rehabil 14:581–587, 1999

Carlsson GS, Svardsudd K, Welin L: Long term effects of head injuries sustained during life in the male populations. J Neurosurg 67:197–205, 1987

Caronna JJ: Diagnosis, prognosis and treatment of hypoxic coma. Adv Neurol 26:1–15, 1979

Choi DW: Cerebral hypoxia: some new approaches and unanswered questions. J Neurosci 10:2493–2501, 1990

Clark JDA, Raggatt PR, Edwards OM: Hypothalamic hypogonadism following major head injury. Clin Endocrinol 29:153–165, 1988

Cohan SL, Seong KM, Pellie J, et al: Cerebral blood flow in humans following resuscitation from cardiac arrest. Stroke 20:761–765, 1989

Cohen MM: Clinical aspects of cerebral anoxia, in Handbook of Clinical Neurology, Vol 27. Edited by Vinken PJ, Bruyn GW. Oxford, UK, North-Holland Publishing Co., 1976, pp 39–51

Cook SD: Trauma does not precipitate multiple sclerosis. Arch Neurol 57:1077–1078, 2000

Crompton M: Hypothalamic lesions following closed head injury. Brain 94:165–172, 1971

Cummings JL: Clinical Neuropsychiatry. New York, Grune & Stratton, 1985

Diegeler A, Hirsch R, Schneider F, et al: Neuromonitoring and neurocognitive outcome in off-pump versus conventional coronary bypass operation. Ann Thorac Surg 69:1162–1166, 2000

Edwards OM, Clark JDA: Post-traumatic hypopituitarism: six cases and a review of the literature. Medicine 65:281–290, 1986

Farrell DF, Starr A: Delayed neurological sequelae of electrical injuries. Neurology 18:601–606, 1968

Fish R: Electric shock, II: nature and mechanism of injury. J Emerg Med 11:457, 1993

Frank KA, Heller SS, Koenfeld DS, et al: Long-term effects of open-heart surgery on intellectual functioning. J Thorac Cardiovasc Surg 64:811–815, 1972

Fujii DE, Ahmed I: Risk factors in psychosis secondary to traumatic brain injury. J Neuropsychiatry Clin Neurosci 13:61–69, 2001

Fuller MG, Fishman E, Taylor CA, et al: Screening patients with traumatic brain injuries for substance abuse. J Neuropsychiatry Clin Neurosci 6:143–146, 1994

Gibson GE, Freeman GB, Myklyn V: Selective damage in striatum and hippocampus with in vitro anoxia. Neurochem Res 13:329–333, 1988

Glenn MB: Pharmacologic interventions in neuroendocrine disorders following traumatic brain injury, part I. J Head Trauma Rehabil 3:87–90, 1988

Goodin DS, Ebers GC, Johnson KP, et al: The relationship of MS to physical trauma and psychological stress. Neurology 52:1737–1745, 1999

Gordon WA, Brown M, Sliwinski M, et al: The enigma of "hidden" traumatic brain injury. J Head Trauma Rehabil 13:39–56, 1998

Gottardis M, Nigitsch C, Schmutzhard, et al: The secretion of human growth hormone stimulated by human growth hormone releasing factor following severe cranio-cerebral trauma. Intensive Care Med 16:163–166, 1990

Gualtieri CT: Neuropsychiatry and Behavioral Pharmacology. New York, Springer Verlag, 1991

Haddad GG, Jiang C: Oxygen deprivation in the central nervous system: on mechanisms of neuronal response, differential sensitivity and injury. Progress Neurobiol 40:227–318, 1993

Hansen AJ: Effect of anoxia on ion distribution in the brain. Physiol Rev 65:101–148, 1985

Hibbard MR, Uysal S, Kepler K, et al: Axis I psychopathology in individuals with traumatic brain injury. J Head Trauma Rehabil 13:24–39, 1998a

Hibbard MR, Uysal S, Sliwinski M, et al: Undiagnosed health issues in individuals with traumatic brain injury living in the community. J Head Trauma Rehabil 13:47–57, 1998b

Hibbard MR, Bogdany J, Uysal S, et al: Axis II psychopathology in individuals with traumatic brain injury. Brain Inj 14:45–61, 2000

Hinkeldey NS, Corrigan JD: The structure of head-injured patients' neurobehavioral complaints: a preliminary study. Brain Inj 4:115–133, 1990

Jackson WT, Novack TA, Dowler RN: Effective serial measurement of cognitive orientation in rehabilitation: the orientation log. Arch Phys Med Rehabil 79:718–720, 1998

Jacobs HE: The Los Angeles Head Injury Survey: project rationale and design implications. J Head Trauma Rehabil 2:37–50, 1987

Jorge RE, Robinson RG, Starkstein SE, et al: Depression and anxiety following traumatic brain injury. J Neuropsychiatry Clin Neurosci 5:369–374, 1993

Kaczmarek BL: Neurolinguistic analysis of verbal utterances in patients with focal lesions of the frontal lobes. Brain Lang 21:52–58, 1984

Kibby MY, Long CJ: Minor head injury: attempts at clarifying the confusion. Brain Inj 10:159–186, 1996

Kiernan RJ, Mueller J, Langston JW, et al: The Neurobehavioral Cognitive Status Examination: a brief but differentiated approach to cognitive assessment. Ann Intern Med 107:481–485, 1987

Kjos BO, Brant-Zawadzki M, Young RG: Early CT findings of global central nervous system hypoperfusion. Am J Radiol 141:1227–1232, 1983

Klingbeil GEG, Cline P: Anterior hypopituitarism: a consequence of head injury. Arch Phys Med Rehabil 66:44–46, 1985

Kuroiwa T, Okeda R: Neuropathology of cerebral ischemia and hypoxia: recent advances in experimental studies on its pathogenesis. Pathol Int 44:171–181, 1994

Lehrer GM: The relationship of MS to physical trauma and psychological stress: report of the Therapeutics and Technology Assessment Subcommittee of the American Academy of Neurology [Correspondence]. Neurology 54:1393–1395, 2000

Levin HS: Neurobehavioral outcome of mild to moderate head injury, in Mild to Moderate Head Injury. Edited by Hoff JT, Anderson TE, Cole TM. London, Blackwell Scientific Publications, 1989, pp 153–185

Levin HS, Grossman RG, Kelly PJ: Aphasic disorder in patients with closed head injury. J Neurol Neurosurg Psychiatry 39:1062–1070, 1976

Levin HS, O'Donnell VM, Grossman RG: The Galveston Orientation and Amnesia Test: a practical scale to assess cognition after head injury. J Nerv Ment Dis 167:675–684, 1979a

Levin HS, Grossman RG, Rose JE, et al: Long-term neuropsychological outcome of closed head injury. J Neurosurg 50:412–422, 1979b

Levin HS, High WM, Goethe KE, et al: The Neurobehavioral Rating Scale: assessment of the behavioral sequelae of head injury by the clinician. J Neurol Neurosurg Psychiatry 50:183–193, 1987a

Levin HS, Mattis S, Ruff RM, et al: Neurobehavioral outcome following minor head injury: a three-center study. J Neurosurg 66:234–243, 1987b

Levin HS, Mazaux J-M, Vaniér M, et al. Evaluation des troubles neurophysiologique et comportementaux des traumatizes craniens par le clinicien: proposition d'une echelle neuro-comportmentale et premiers resultants de sa version française. Annales de Readaptation et de Medecine Physique 33:109–112, 1990

Lovell MR, Iverson GL, Collins MW, et al: Does loss of consciousness predict neuropsychological decrements after concussion? Clin J Sport Med 9:193–198, 1999

Maiese K, Caronna JJ: Neurological complications of cardiac arrest, in Neurology and General Medicine. Edited by Aminof MJ. New York, Churchill Livingstone, 1989, pp 145–157

Mattson AJ, Levin HS: Frontal lobe dysfunction following closed head injury. J Nerv Ment Dis 178:282–291, 1990

Mauss-Clum N, Ryan M: Brain injury and the family. J Neurosurg Nurs 13:165–169, 1981

Max JE, Robin DA, Lindgren SD, et al: Traumatic brain injury in children and adolescents: psychiatric disorders at two years. J Am Acad Child Adolesc Psychiatry 36:1278–1285, 1997

Max JE, Lindgren SD, Knutson CS, et al: Child and adolescent traumatic brain injury: correlates of disruptive behaviour disorders. Brain Inj 12:41–52, 1998

Maxwell M, Karacostas D, Ellenbogen RG, et al: Precocious puberty following head injury. J Neurosurg 73:123–129, 1990

McCauley SR, Levin HS, Vanier M, et al: The Neurobehavioral Rating Scale—Revised: sensitivity and validity in closed head injury assessment. J Neurol Neurosurg Psychiatry 71:643–651, 2001

McKinlay W, Brooks D, Bowd M, et al: The short-term outcome of severe blunt head injury as reported by relatives of the injured persons. J Neurol Neurosurg Psychiatry 44:527–533, 1981

McLean A Jr, Temkin NR, Dikmen S, et al: The behavioral sequelae of head injury. J Clin Neuropsychol 5:361–376, 1983

Moody DM, Bell MA, Challa R: Features of the cerebral vascular pattern that predict vulnerability to perfusion or oxygenation deficiency: an anatomic study. Am J Neuroradiol 11:431–439, 1990

Morton MV, Wehman P: Psychosocial and emotional sequelae of individuals with traumatic brain injury: a literature review and recommendations. Brain Inj 9:81–92, 1995

Myers RE: A unitary theory of causation of anoxic and hypoxic brain pathology, in Advances in Neurology, Vol 26. Edited by Fahn S. New York, Raven, 1979, pp 195–213

Obrzut JE, Hynd GW: Cognitive dysfunction and psychoeducational assessment in individuals with acquired brain injury. J Learn Disabil 20:596–602, 1987

Parkin AJ, Miller J, Vincent R: Multiple neuropsychological deficits due to anoxic encephalopathy: a case study. Cortex 23:655–665, 1987

Petito K, Feldman E, Pulsinelli WA, et al: Delayed hippocampal damage in humans following cardiorespiratory arrest. Neurology 37:1281–1286, 1987

Poser CM: Trauma to the central nervous system may result in formation or enlargement of multiple sclerosis plaques. Arch Neurol 57:1074–1077, 2000

Pulsinelli WA, Brierley JB, Plum F: Temporal profile of neuronal damage in a model of transient forebrain ischemia. Ann Neurol 11:491–498, 1982

Rimel RW, Giordani B, Barth JT, et al: Disability caused by minor head injury. Neurosurgery 9:221–228, 1981

Rimel RW, Giordani B, Barth JT, et al: Moderate head injury: completing the clinical spectrum of brain trauma. Neurosurgery 11:344–351, 1982

Roach GW, Kanchuger M, Mangano CM, et al: Adverse cerebral outcomes after coronary bypass surgery. N Engl J Med 335:1857–1863, 1996

Rothman S, Olney J: Glutamate and the pathophysiology of hypoxic-ischemic brain damage. Ann Neurol 19:105–111, 1986

Ruff RM, Marshall LF, Klauber MR, et al: Alcohol abuse and neurological outcome of the severely head injured. J Head Trauma Rehabil 5:21–31, 1990

Sarno MT: The nature of verbal impairment after closed head injury. J Nerv Ment Dis 168:685–692, 1980

Savageau JA, Stanton BA, Jenkins CD, et al: Neuropsychological dysfunction following elective cardiac operation, II: a six-month assessment. J Thorac Cardiovasc Surg 84:595–600, 1982

Sbordone RJ, Seyranian GD, Ruff RM: Are the subjective complaints of traumatically brain injured patients reliable? Brain Inj 12:505–515, 1998

Schurr A, Rigor BM: The mechanism of cerebral hypoxic-ischemic damage. Hippocampus 2:221–228, 1992

Schwamm LH, Van Dyke C, Kiernan RJ, et al: The Neurobehavioral Cognitive Status Examination: comparison with the Cognitive Capacity Screening Examination and the Mini-Mental State Examination in a neurosurgical population. Ann Intern Med 107:486–491, 1987

Selnes OA, Goldsborough MA, Borowicz LM, et al. Neurobehavioral sequelae of cardiopulmonary bypass. Lancet 353:1601–1606, 1999

Shaul PW, Towbin RB, Chernausek SD: Precocious puberty following severe head trauma. Am J Dis Child 139:467–469, 1985

Shewmon DA, De Giorgio CM: Early prognosis in anoxic coma, in Ethical Issues in Neurological Practice, Neurologic Clinics, Vol 7. Edited by Bernat JL. Philadelphia, PA, WB Saunders, 1989, pp 823–843

Siesjo BK: Cell damage in the brain: a speculative synthesis. J Cereb Blood Flow Metab 1:155–185, 1981

Silver JM, Anderson K: Vasopressin treats the persistent feeling of coldness after brain injury. J Neuropsychiatry Clin Neurosci 11:248–252, 1999

Silver JM, Kramer R, Greenwald S, et al: The association between head injuries and psychiatric disorders: findings from the New Haven NIMH Epidemiologic Catchment Area Study. Brain Inj 15:935–945, 2001

Sockalosky JJ, Kriel RL, Krach LE, et al: Precocious puberty after traumatic brain injury. J Pediatr 110:373–377, 1987

Sparadeo FR, Strauss D, Barth JT: The incidence, impact, and treatment of substance abuse in head trauma rehabilitation. J Head Trauma Rehabil 5:1–8, 1990

Strandgaard S, Paulson OB: Cerebral autoregulation. Stroke 15:413–416, 1984

Strauss D, Sparadeo FR: The incidence, impact and treatment of substance abuse in head trauma rehabilitation: proceedings from the NHIF Task Force on Substance Abuse, White Paper, Southborough, MA, 1988

Syliviris S, Levi C, Matalanis G, et al: Pattern and significance of cerebral microemboli during coronary artery bypass grafting. Ann Thorac Surg 66:1674–1678, 1998

Teasdale G, Jennett B: Assessment of coma and impaired consciousness: a practical scale. Lancet 2:81–84, 1974

Telzrow CF: The school psychologist's perspective on testing students with traumatic brain injury. J Head Trauma Rehabil 6:23–34, 1991

Thomsen IV: Late outcome of very severe blunt head trauma: a 10–15 year second follow-up. J Neurol Neurosurg Psychiatry 47:260–268, 1984

Van Dijk D, Jansen EWL, Hijman R, et al: Cognitive outcome after off-pump and on-pump coronary artery bypass graft surgery. JAMA 287:1405–1412, 2002

Van Zomeren AH, Van Den Burg W: Residual complaints of patients two years after severe head injury. J Neurol Neurosurg Psychiatry 48:21–28, 1985

Vanier M, Mazaux J-M, Lambert J, et al: Assessment of neuropsychologic impairment after head injury: interrater reliability and factorial and criterion validity of the Neurobehavioral Rating Scale—Revised. Arch Phys Med Rehabil 81:796–806, 2000

White BC, Wiegenstein, JG, Winegar CD: Brain ischemic anoxia: mechanism of injury. JAMA 251:1586–1590, 1984

Wilson BA: Cognitive functioning of adult survivors of cerebral hypoxia. Brain Inj 10:863–874, 1996

Woolf PD, Cox C, Kelly M, et al: The adrenocortical response to brain injury: correlation with the severity of neurologic dysfunction, effects of intoxication, and patient outcome. Alcohol Clin Exp Res 14:917–921, 1990

5 Structural Imaging

Erin D. Bigler, Ph.D.

THE ADVENT OF computed tomography (CT) in the 1970s revolutionized the clinical assessment of traumatic brain injury (TBI). Even in the earliest stages of neuroimaging development, the crude views of the brain generated by CT imaging provided the first in vivo assessment of brain structure and permitted clinical evaluation of such abnormalities as hemorrhage, contusion, edema, midline shift, and herniation (Eisenberg 1992). The initial limitations of CT imaging due to slow speed of image processing and limited resolution rapidly gave way to technological improvements, such that current CT imaging can be completed in minutes and provides excellent detection of macroscopic abnormalities associated with trauma (Figure 5–1). Because CT imaging can be done quickly and on patients requiring life support or other medical equipment (e.g., heart pacemaker), CT is the method of choice for the acute assessment of the head-injured patient (Gean 1994; Haydel et al. 2000). Although magnetic resonance (MR) imaging has superior resolution and better anatomic fidelity than CT, it is often not used acutely because of its susceptibility to metal and motion artifact, incompatibility with certain life-support equipment within the MR environment, length of scan time, and decreased sensitivity (compared with that of CT) in detecting skull fractures.

Because of these factors, typically in the TBI patient the first scan performed is CT, and MR imaging is usually chosen for follow-up neuroimaging. Thus, much of the research and clinical information regarding CT imaging centers on acute injury characteristics, whereas the findings of MR imaging pertain to the subacute and chronic phases of recovery. When MR imaging is performed on the head-injured patient, there are various standard or common clinical imaging sequences typically done. However, new techniques involving image acquisition and analysis are being developed that may increase the sensitivity of MR detection of abnormalities associated with TBI, and part of the sensitivity of MR detection of any abnormality after TBI relates to the time postinjury when scanning is performed. Accordingly, the neuroimaging of TBI is typically broken down into acute imaging using CT, subacute and chronic imaging using MR imaging, and various experimental and clinical applications of MR imaging that permit more refined analyses to detect TBI neuropathology. These distinctions—CT imaging, MR imaging, and new techniques—serve as the guidelines in this chapter for discussing the use of structural imaging in TBI.

Computed Tomography Imaging

Indications and Relationships to Outcome

A number of studies have examined CT imaging associated with acute brain injury (Haydel et al. 2000; Marshall et al. 1991; Shiozaki et al. 2001; Wallesch et al. 2001). The consensus of such studies is that acute CT is

The technical expertise and assistance of Tracy Abildskov and the manuscript assistance of Jo Ann Petrie are gratefully acknowledged. Much of the research reported in this chapter was supported by a grant from the Ira Fulton Foundation.

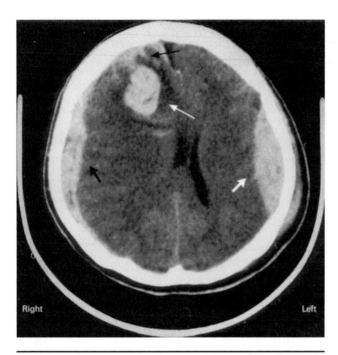

Right

Left

FIGURE 5–1. **The axial section of a computed tomography scan of the head at the level of the lateral ventricles.**

Obtained without the addition of contrast medium, this scan revealed four types of acute posttraumatic intracranial hemorrhages (left is on the reader's right side): an epidural hematoma (thick white arrow) and a squamous temporal fracture (not shown) on the left side, a laminate subdural hematoma (thick black arrow) on the right side, right-sided periventricular and frontal lobe contusions containing an intraparenchymal hematoma (thin white arrow), and a subarachnoid hemorrhage (thin black arrow) in the right frontal region. These injuries were sustained in a fall.
Source. Reproduced from Mattiello JA, Munz M: "Four Types of Acute Post-Traumatic Intracranial Hemorrhage." *New England Journal of Medicine* 344:580, 2001. Used with permission. Copyright 2001, Massachusetts Medical Society. All rights reserved.

an excellent clinical tool in determining the presence of treatable lesions, such as subdural hematoma (see Figure 5–1), and providing baseline information concerning the location and nature of pathological conditions such as cortical contusion, intraparenchymal hemorrhage, petechial hemorrhage, and localized or generalized edema. CT is also excellent in detecting skull fractures and associated pneumocephalus, which may require surgical intervention. There is a direct relationship between CT imaging findings and the acute clinical status of the TBI patient, based on the Glasgow Coma Scale (GCS) score and other characteristics such as pupillary abnormalities, loss of consciousness (LOC), and posttraumatic amnesia. There are also several CT rating scales available, but probably the most common is the Trauma Coma Data-

bank as outlined by Marshall et al. (1991) and presented in Table 5–1. What is important about this rating scale is that it provides a basis for evaluating the severity of injury during the acute stage. It also can provide a baseline for future monitoring of change over time (Vos et al. 2001), as is discussed in the section Relationship of Acute Computed Tomography Abnormalities to Rehabilitation Outcome. Additionally, this scale overviews the common injuries observed in CT imaging of the acute TBI patient.

Relationship of Acute Computed Tomography Findings to Severity of Injury

The most clinically important aspect of acute CT imaging is the initial management, monitoring, and surgical intervention for any treatable lesion(s). Additionally, acute CT imaging of the TBI patient often provides more clinical information than what comes from the physical examination of the acutely injured patient, particularly the patient with altered mental status. For example, the comatose patient may have no visible abnormalities on CT imaging, whereas the patient with only mild disorientation may be found to have significant CT abnormalities, some requiring emergent intervention. This is shown in Figure 5–2, which illustrates that the frequency of CT abnormalities, using the ratings outlined in Table 5–1, was associated with the GCS score (highest within 24 hours of injury) and LOC in 240 consecutively admitted rehabilitation patients (Bigler et al. 2004). As can be seen, the entire gamut of CT abnormalities was observed in this large sample of TBI patients who had injuries sufficient to require hospitalization, but the most common was a level II injury (see Table 5–1)—some mild edema; the presence of small, mostly petechial hemorrhages or contusions; and no mass effect. As for LOC, similar observations are made in Figure 5–2, which demonstrates that LOC of any duration was most likely to be related with a level II injury as well.

Relationship of Acute Computed Tomography Abnormalities to Rehabilitation Outcome

Despite the accuracy of CT in identifying gross structural pathology during the acute stage, such findings often do not relate well to the neurobehavioral outcome at the time of discharge from rehabilitation, which makes the accurate prediction of outcome from acute CT findings alone difficult (Dikmen et al. 2001; Temkin et al. 2003). The exception occurs with patients who have brainstem lesions, because the presence of brainstem pathology typically relates to poor outcome. Using both the Disability Rating

TABLE 5–1. Diagnostic categories of abnormalities visualized on computed tomography (CT) scan

Category	Definition
1: Diffuse injury I (no visible pathology)	No visible intracranial pathology seen on CT scan
2: Diffuse injury II	Cisterns present with midline shift 0–5 mm and/or:
	Lesion densities present
	No high- or mixed-density lesion >25 cc
	May include bone fragments and foreign bodies
3: Diffuse injury III (swelling)	Cisterns compressed or absent with midline shifts 0–5 mm, no high- or mixed-density lesion >25 cc
4: Diffuse injury IV (shift)	Midline shift >5 mm, no high- or mixed-density lesion >25 cc
5: Evacuated mass lesion V	Any lesion surgically evacuated
6: Nonevacuated mass lesion VI	High- or mixed-density lesion >25 cc, not surgically evacuated
7: Brainstem injury VII	Focal brainstem lesion, no other lesion present

Source. Adapted from Marshall LF, Marshall SB, Klauber MR, et al: "A New Classification of Head Injury Based on Computerized Tomography." *Journal of Neurosurgery* 75:514–520, 1991.

Scale (DRS)[1] and Functional Independence Measure (FIM)[2] discharge scores, Bigler et al. (2004) demonstrated that the 240 TBI patients with CT ratings from no visible abnormality to discernible major abnormalities had similar rehabilitation outcomes (i.e., diffuse injury category I to category IV; see Table 5–1). This means that outcome is poorly predicted by just the acute injury characteristics seen on CT imaging performed on the day of injury (DOI). This finding should come as no surprise, because it may take days to weeks to track the evolution of a lesion and months before stable degenerative patterns are established by neuroimaging findings ([Blatter et al. 1997; Shiozaki et al. 2001; Vos et al. 2001]; see section Relationship of Magnetic Resonance Imaging Findings to Outcome for better predictors of rehabilitation outcome). As is shown later in

this chapter, the better predictor of long-term outcome comes from quantitative analysis of MR imaging done after 3–6 months postinjury, and these relationships are often enhanced by tracking changes in neuroimaging using the DOI CT scan. Accordingly, instead of using CT as an absolute predictor of outcome, it is often better to consider CT as a tool for establishing the baseline at the acute stage of injury and then tracking the injury with either CT or MR imaging at follow-up intervals.

Day of Injury as Baseline

Because the DOI scan is typically one of the first diagnostic tests run on the acutely injured TBI patient, it is performed early in the injury process. Because the morphological consequences from trauma take time to evolve, the DOI scan

---

[1]*Disability Rating Scale (DRS).* The DRS consists of the following eight items and range of scores (0 = no disability): 1) eye opening, 0–3; 2) verbal response, 0–4; 3) motor response, 0–4; 4) cognitive ability in feeding, 0–3; 5) cognitive ability in toileting, 0–3; 6) cognitive ability in grooming, 0–3; 7) dependence on others, 0–5; and 8) employability, 0–3. A total DRS score is calculated by adding the scores for each of the eight items (see Rappaport et al. 1982). Hall et al. (1993) offered the following distinctions in considering the DRS score: 0 = no disability, 1 = mild disability; 2–3 = partial disability; 4–6 = moderate disability; 7–11 = moderately severe disability; 12–16 = severe disability; 17–21 = extremely severe disability; 22–24 = vegetative state; 25–29 = extreme vegetative state; and 30 = death. For the purposes of comparing DRS admission and discharge findings by ventricle to brain ratio outcome, DRS scores were combined as follows: 0 = no disability; 1–3 = mild disability; 4–11 = moderate disability; 12–21 = moderately severe disability; and 22+ = extremely severe-vegetative (see Figure 5–11).

[2]*Functional Independence Measure (FIM).* The FIM (State University of New York at Buffalo Department of Rehabilitation Medicine 1990) is an 18-item, 7-level ordinal scale that can be used to assess level of function at time of admission to and discharge from a rehabilitation unit. It is a general tool for all types of rehabilitation patients and has been successfully used in TBI (Hamilton et al. 1987). The version used in this study was the 3.1 version. By virtue of its ordinal scale, the lowest score is 7 and the highest is 126.

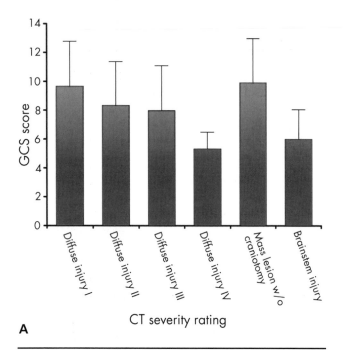

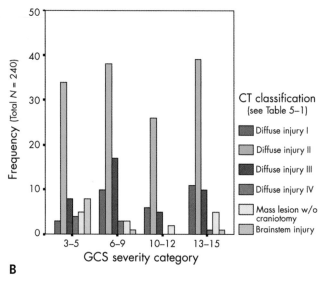

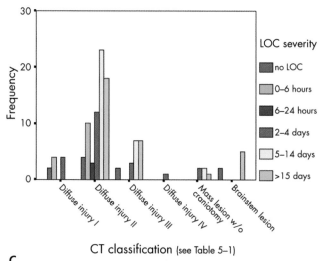

FIGURE 5–2. **Computed tomography (CT) overview of 240 patients with traumatic brain injury (TBI).** The charts presented in this figure overview the acute CT of 240 TBI patients admitted to an inpatient rehabilitation facility by average Glasgow Coma Scale (GCS) (A) and GCS frequency by CT classification (B), demonstrating that the most frequent CT abnormality was a diffuse injury II, which occurred with a near-similar frequency across all levels of severity; and loss of consciousness (LOC) by CT abnormality classification (C), demonstrating again that diffuse injury II was the most common classification wherein the majority of TBI patients experienced some LOC. Acute CT classification abnormalities are given in Table 5–1.

Source. Bigler ED, Ryser DK, Ghandi P, et al: "Day-of-Injury Computerized Tomography, Rehabilitation Status, and Long-Term Outcome as They Relate to Magnetic Resonance Imaging Findings After Traumatic Brain Injury." *Brain Impairment* 5:S122–123, 2004.

often provides important baseline information. This is demonstrated in Figure 5–3, which depicts a 3-year-old restrained passenger involved in a high-speed motor vehicle accident. The DOI scan demonstrates a right intraparenchymal hemorrhage in the region of the internal capsule-putamen. The anterior horns of the lateral ventricular system can be identified on the DOI scan, but cortical sulci are not well visualized, which can be a sign of generalized edema. By 2 days postinjury, there is definite generalized cerebral edema with obliteration of the ventricular system—a clear sign of massive cerebral edema. One year later, there is global atrophy manifested by generalized ventricular dilatation, prominent cortical sulci, and a large cavitation in the right basal ganglia area—a consequence of the focal hemorrhage. The hemorrhage likely resulted from shearing forces disrupting the deep vascular supply to the basal ganglia.

Limitations

The problem with all contemporary imaging methods is that they provide only a gross inspection of the macroscopically visible brain, whereas most of the critical functioning is at the microscopic (neuronal and synaptic) level. For structural imaging using CT or MR, detection of an abnormality is based on resolution measured in millimeters, whereas at the microscopic level the resolution of clinically significant abnormalities is measured at the micron level (Bain et al. 2001; Ding et al. 2001). Simply stated, a "normal" scan merely indicates that no visible macroscopic pathology was detected that reached a threshold of 1 mm or more. CT, or any other neuroimaging method, simply cannot answer the question of brain pathology below its level of detection. This circumstance is nicely demonstrated in Figure 5–4. The scan

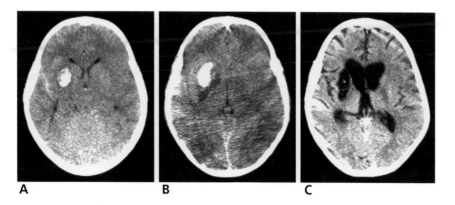

FIGURE 5–3. Computed tomography scans from a 3-year-old male traumatic brain injury patient injured in a high-speed motor vehicle accident.

Right is on the reader's left side. Day of injury (A). Note the right intraparenchymal hemorrhage and blood in the right Sylvian fissure. However, in addition to these acute injury factors, note the size of the anterior horns of the lateral ventricle, which offer a baseline from which to monitor atrophic changes over time. By 2 days postinjury (B), there is severe cerebral edema, manifested by obliteration of cortical sulcal patterns, loss of definition between gray and white matter, and delineation of the anterior aspect of the interhemispheric fissure, along with collapse of the ventricular system. By 7 months postinjury (C), there is extensive atrophy noted by generalized ventricular dilatation, prominent cortical sulci, and the right Sylvian fissure. Also note the large cavitation left by the intraparenchymal hemorrhage. By viewing these different scans, an excellent picture of how the brain changes over time after an injury can be objectively established.

represented in the middle of the figure is the acute DOI CT, interpreted as within normal limits, taken approximately 2 hours after injury (brief LOC, GCS score of 14 at the scene of a severe head-on high-speed motor vehicle accident; GCS score of 15 on hospital admission). The patient was also found to have a cervical fracture that was neurosurgically repaired, along with a large frontal scalp laceration. He was hospitalized for 4 days. He developed the typical constellation of postconcussive symptoms, including headache, fatigue, irritability, some depression, and mild cognitive problems, which gradually but not completely abated over the next several months. He was able to return to work on a part-time basis, but he complained of problems of mental inefficiency and feeling "dull." He was in excellent general health, but he unexpectedly experienced a spontaneous cardiac arrest while exercising and died 7 months postinjury, at which time a full brain autopsy was performed. Gross brain anatomy was normal, as shown Figure 5–4A, but histolog-

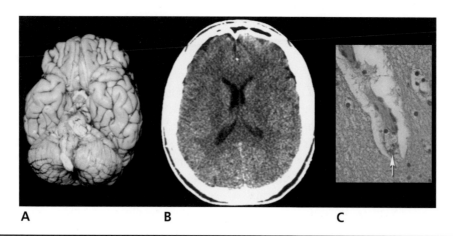

FIGURE 5–4. Findings in mild traumatic brain injury (TBI).

This patient sustained a mild TBI (admission Glasgow Coma Scale, 14) 7 months before an unexpected death from cardiac arrest. The ventral view of the intact brain at autopsy showed no cortical contusions or other gross abnormalities (A). Likewise, the computed tomography (CT) scan performed on the day of injury shows no abnormalities (B), again supporting the clinical view of no gross brain abnormalities. However, on microscopic examination, scattered hemosiderin (white arrow) deposits were observed, as shown in the histological section (C). These were most prominent in the white matter. This demonstrates microscopic abnormalities as a consequence of brain injury, even mild TBI, that are below detection by direct visual inspection of the brain using neuroimaging techniques (see Bigler et al. 2004).

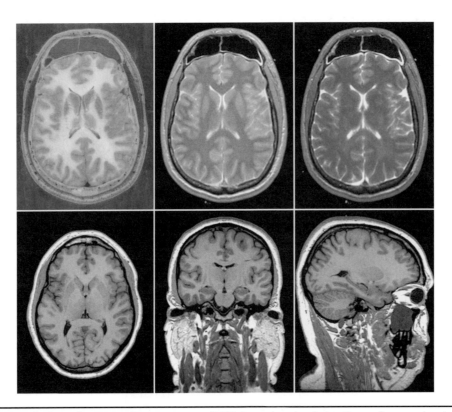

FIGURE 5–5. **The clarity of magnetic resonance (MR) imaging in detection of gross brain anatomy.**

The horizontal section on the top left was done at postmortem, whereas the two MR scans on the top right were performed antemortem and are at identical levels. The closeness with which the MR scans approximate actual anatomy is obvious. There are three different types of MR scans depicted in this figure, all with different properties in displaying underlying anatomy as well as pathology. The top middle MR scan is a proton density (PD), or mixed-weighted, scan in which excellent definition of white and gray matter can be visualized. The top right view represents a T2-weighted image, in which cerebrospinal fluid is readily identified. The bottom views are from a different subject and are all T1-weighted images. The bottom row demonstrates not only the clarity of gross brain anatomy depicted by MR imaging but also the different planes that can be viewed (bottom left—axial; middle—coronal, bottom right—sagittal).

ical examination demonstrated hemosiderin (a blood by-product)-laden macrophages and lymphocytes in the white matter (WM). Obviously, this finding suggests perturbation of brain microvasculature and WM injury that was well below the detection of the "normal" CT. Such microscopic lesions are undoubtedly the basis of many neurobehavioral sequelae associated with brain injury when imaging is "normal." This is further supported by the work of Gorrie et al. (2001) who examined 32 children at postmortem who succumbed to road accidents. With direct visual inspection, 17 of these TBI cases demonstrated no macroscopic abnormalities of the type that would be detected by CT imaging. However, when viewed at ×100 magnification, all cases readily demonstrated microscopic injury.

Magnetic Resonance Imaging

The anatomic specificity of MR imaging approximates gross brain anatomy and can be done in any plane (Figure 5–5). Because of this anatomic specificity, MR imaging is the pre-

ferred method for detailed investigations of structural changes in the brain that accompany trauma, particularly changes in WM and direction of atrophy. Strich's (1956) article is often referenced as the seminal contribution to the neuropathological literature on TBI; her discussion of the preponderance of WM damage and generalized cerebral atrophy that accompanies severe TBI is particularly important. MR imaging can be used to detect these gross changes.

In terms of neuropsychiatric sequelae, MR imaging is most useful in the late follow-up of a brain injury (see Jorge et al. 2004), because it is at this stage when structural MR imaging is excellent in its ability to detect TBI-induced cerebral atrophy, which is typically observed as ventricular dilatation (ventriculomegaly; Figure 5–6) coexistent with prominent cortical sulci (Bigler 2000, 2001a, 2001b). Likewise, thinning of the corpus callosum (CC) in conjunction with the expansion of the ventricle is usually apparent when these structures are viewed in the midsagittal plane in the chronic stage of TBI. Additionally, the MR-imaging method is well suited for quantitative image analysis, through which almost all major brain structures can be

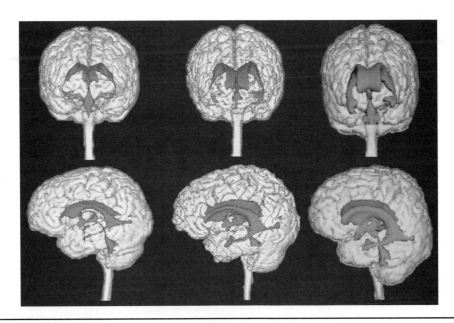

FIGURE 5–6. **Ventriculomegaly in traumatic brain injury (TBI).**

Hydrocephalus ex vacuo is a common sequela of brain injury and is often proportional to the severity of injury. The top row shows a frontal view based on three-dimensional magnetic resonance renderings of the brain, with the visible ventricular system depicted in black. The bottom row represents the lateral view: the image on the left is from a noninjured control subject, the image in the middle is from a moderately injured TBI patient, and the image on the right is from a subject with severe brain injury. It is important to note that it is the entire ventricular system that typically dilates, indicating the diffuse nature of impact brain injury. By taking the volume of the ventricular system, as shown in black, and dividing it by the volume of the brain, a ventricle to brain ratio (VBR) can be calculated. Increasing VBR is a sign of increasing cerebral atrophy. Typically, increased VBR is associated with worse outcome (see Figure 5–11 and Ariza et al. 2004).

readily identified, quantified (either as volumes or surface areas), and compared to a normative sample (Bigler 1999). The table in Appendix 5–1 summarizes regions that have been shown to exhibit atrophy in response to trauma. There is extensive clinical literature on the use of MR in the acute and subacute diagnosis and management of TBI (Atlas 2001; Gean 1994; Orrison 2000), but as indicated above, with regard to neuropsychiatric morbidity abnormalities identified in the chronic stage typically have better correlation with outcome than the acute or sub-acute findings (Henry-Feugas et al. 2000; Jorge et al. 2004; van der Naalt et al. 1999; Vasa et al. 2004; Wilson et al. 1988). Accordingly, the primary focus of the remainder of this chapter is MR imaging performed more than 45 days postinjury so that the more stable and chronic lesions can be related to neurobehavioral deficits, particularly those resulting in neuropsychiatric sequelae.

Indications

There is a multitude of reasons for performing MR imaging in the TBI patient, but typically the reasons center on monitoring the status of the patient, often during the subacute and more chronic phases of recovery. For example, because of its capacity for exquisite anatomic detail and detection of water, MR is suitable for monitoring edema, midline shift,

and the changing status of a hemorrhage and for evaluating lesions that may underlie posttraumatic epilepsy. It is also helpful in the clinical correlation of the patient's acute status, as depicted in Figure 5–7, and the structural imaging. The patient shown in this figure had normal CT reading on admission but was in a coma (GCS score of 5). MR imaging performed later on the DOI was also read as "normal"; however, the MR scan performed 4 days later clearly demonstrated the beginnings of significant degenerative changes, including areas of shearing that were not definitively observed on the DOI CT or MR scan. Another reason for MR imaging is to monitor changes over time, which is important because the degeneration often takes months to reach an endpoint. Blatter et al. (1997) demonstrated that the time that elapses between injury and brain volume stabilization equivalent to that expected with normal aging may be more than 3 years, although most pathological changes occur within the first 6 months. Thus, acute and subacute MR imaging is performed to assess potentially medically treatable abnormalities associated with brain trauma, track degenerative changes that occur with time, and relate imaging findings to neurobehavioral sequelae.

As indicated in the section Computed Tomography Imaging, often all early and subacute neuroimaging is done with CT, particularly with patients on life support, due to the incompatibility of life-support equipment with

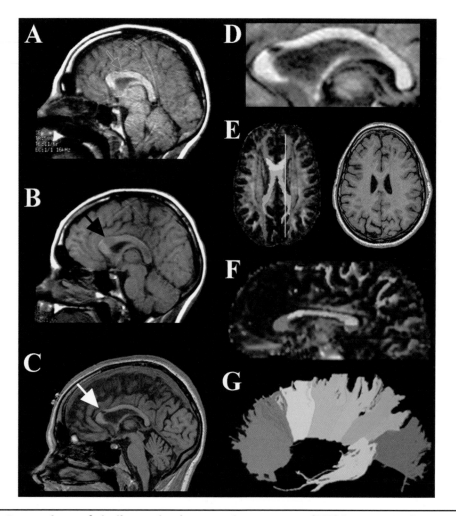

FIGURE 5–7. **Comparison of similar sagittal magnetic resonance (MR) images to demonstrate injury and subsequent atrophy to the corpus callosum at different stages postinjury.**

The midsagittal day-of-injury MR scan (A, top left) was taken on admission to the hospital after the patient sustained a severe TBI. Some movement artifact diminished the quality of the image but was interpreted as within normal limits. However, within 1 week postinjury (B), signal intensity changes are clearly visible in the corpus callosum both anteriorly (black arrow) as well as posteriorly. At 4 years postinjury (C), corpus callosum atrophy is clearly evident and is generalized including all aspects (compare the original size of the corpus callosum in A with that observed in C). Generalized atrophy is also noted by the dark signal, especially seen in the frontoparietal aspects of the midsagittal view of C, indicating increased cerebrospinal fluid (CSF) in the space of the interhemispheric fissure, a sign of reduced brain volume (note that brain parenchyma in A and B is light gray, but a dark signal covers the midsagittal surface in C because of increased CSF in these regions secondary to atrophy). Also, as clearly visible (white arrow in C), a major shear lesion is evident where most of this segment of the corpus callosum has been transected. For better clarification of this lesion involving the corpus callosum, the injured corpus callosum has been enlarged and highlighted in D. When viewing A (the day-of-injury scan) in retrospect, there is some signal change noted in the region that eventually shows the shear lesion. The colorized images in E, F, and G are all from diffusion-tensor imaging sequences in which tractography involving the projections of the corpus callosum in a noninjured subject is displayed (Lazar et al. 2003). The images are color-coded on the basis of their projection (i.e., red shows frontal projection). In E, the diffusion scan on the left is depicted in the axial plane, which shows the projections across the corpus callosum from this perspective. The scan to the right in E is from the injured patient. In F, the colorized projections are shown in the midsagittal view. Accordingly, by comparing the view of the location of the lesion in D with the view in F, one can see that this injury would result in disrupted projections in primarily the midfrontal region. G shows the tractography plots mapped through the corona radiata. The vertical line in E is the approximate location of these maps that depict the hemispheric projections of callosal white matter fiber tracks. *Source.* Diffusion-tensor imaging tractography color images courtesy of Mariana Lazar, Ph.D., and Andrew Alexander, Ph.D., University of Wisconsin, Madison.

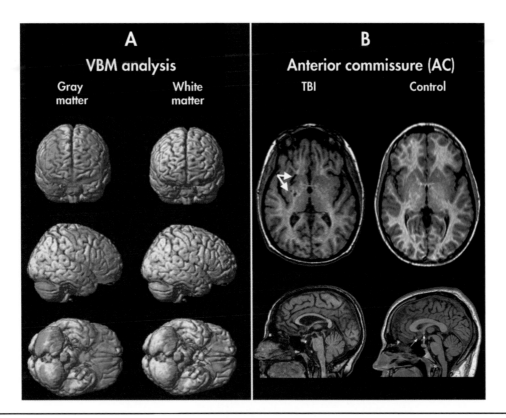

FIGURE 5–8.   Voxel-based morphometry (VBM) in traumatic brain injury (TBI).

VBM provides a method to simultaneously compare—voxel-by-voxel—where the major differences occur in subjects with TBI compared with age-matched control subjects without damage. In this figure, by using three-dimensional (3D) magnetic resonance (MR) imaging, the diffuseness of frontotemporal involvement can be more fully appreciated (shown in red) when TBI subjects who had sustained frontotemporal contusions are compared with control subjects by using VBM techniques; the differences (i.e., regions of reduced voxel density of either gray or white matter) are plotted on a standard 3D surface plot of the brain. VBM was applied to MR imaging performed on 6 subjects (mean age = 16; standard deviation = 5.1) with moderate-to-severe TBI (all had Glasgow Coma Scale scores at or below 8) compared with 18 control subjects (3 control subjects within 2 years per TBI patient). Young subjects were selected to minimize any long-term age effect that could potentially relate to volume reduction. The VBM findings (A) distinctly demonstrate extensive frontotemporal differences in the TBI subjects, particularly in the ventral frontal region, more so in gray matter than white. Given the ventral basis of the changes seen in this illustration, the basal forebrain (slanted white arrow, control subject, sagittal view, lower right)—including the region involving the anterior commissure (AC), a thin white matter band critical for white matter interhemispheric connections, as shown in B—was also quantified and compared with the control subjects. Quantitatively, the basal forebrain region demonstrated over a 15% reduction in volume in the TBI subjects, who also were found to have significantly reduced AC widths of 2.00 mm (SD = 0.44) compared with control subjects, in whom the mean width was 3.18 mm (SD = 0.40). In the TBI subject presented in B, the AC width was 1 mm compared with an age-matched control subject whose AC width was 3.5 mm. The blue arrow identifies the location of the AC, and the conjoined white arrows show where shear injuries occurred in the TBI subjects, leaving regions of cavitation in the basal ganglia and internal capsule. In the sagittal view, the control subject's AC (B, lower right) is clearly visible (vertical white arrow), whereas the AC is almost not discernible in the sagittal view of the TBI patient (lower left). Note also the thinness of the corpus callosum in the TBI patient, another reflection of generalized injury.

the MR imaging environment. It is helpful to compare baseline CT images with follow-up MR images, as demonstrated in Figures 5–3, 5–10, and 5–12.

Typical Lesions Identified by Magnetic Resonance Imaging

More details concerning the neuropathology of TBI are presented in Chapter 2, Neuropathology. For the purposes of this discussion, just a brief overview of the neuropathology observed in MR imaging of the brain in TBI is offered, but the reader should be aware that a multitude of pathologies exist that can be detected by MR imaging (Atlas 2001; Gean 1994; Orrison 2000). The typical lesions described below are the ones most commonly observed to relate to significant neuropsychiatric sequelae (Bigler 2001b) and most commonly occur because of the greater likelihood of frontotemporal damage (see Figure 5–8). Table 5–2 is

TABLE 5–2.   Appearance of magnetic resonance (MR) images based on the type of image sequence

	Typical MR imaging sequences for detecting TBI abnormalities				Additional MR imaging sequences for evaluating TBI	
	T1	T2	FLAIR	T2 GRE	PD	DW imaging
					See Figure 5–5	See Figure 5–13
Appearance of cerebrospinal fluid[a]	Low	High	Dark	Medium gray	Isointense	Dark
Appearance of edema[a]	Low	High	Bright	Light gray	High	Bright
General appearance of an abnormality[a]	Low to black	High	Bright unless CSF or hemosiderin	Bright or dark depending	High	Bright
Hemosiderin	Darker	Darker	Darker	Darkest	Dark	Darkest
Air	Signal loss	Signal loss	Signal loss	Signal loss	Signal loss	Signal loss

Note.   CSF=cerebrospinal fluid; DW=diffusion-weighted; FLAIR=fluid-attenuated inversion recovery; GRE=gradient recalled echo; PD=proton density.
[a]Compared with normal adult brain parenchyma.

offered as a guide to integrating MR imaging findings using standard imaging sequences (i.e., T1, T2, fluid-attenuated inversion recovery [FLAIR], gradient recalled echo [GRE]) in detecting abnormalities associated with TBI. The image sequences depicted in Table 5–2 based on one patient with severe TBI 1 year postinjury demonstrates how different image sequences identify structural pathology. Tong et al. (2004) and Goetz et al. (2004) have clearly demonstrated how certain clinical sequences may simply be insensitive in detecting structural pathology and reinforce the recommendation to use multiple sequences to increase the likelihood of detecting clinically significant abnormalities caused by brain injury. The key in integrating scans is to look for changes in symmetry or differences in signal intensity in comparison to normal tissue. By using Table 5–2, where normal appearance is summarized, detection of pathology can often be readily made. However, it must be emphasized that the information offered in Table 5–2 can change with certain scan parameters; therefore, these findings are not absolutes.

The traditional T1 image is most useful for establishing the presence of focal atrophy. The combination of T1 and T2 imaging is best in establishing ventricular and cerebrospinal fluid (CSF) changes. The GRE sequence is often excellent in detecting hemosiderin changes, whereas the FLAIR and proton density (PD) sequences

may be more sensitive to general WM pathology, as may different types of DW imaging. Because there is so much that can be done clinically with MR imaging, it is best that the clinician work closely with the neuroradiologist in attempting to identify clinically useful protocols for imaging patients with TBI.

Shear Injury

The CC is a structure in which shearing due to TBI frequently occurs (Johnson et al. 1994; Levin et al. 2000). In the patient shown in Figure 5–7, there is literally a tear in the anterior aspect of the CC. When shearing occurs outside of the CC, it is most frequently observed at the junction of WM and gray matter, particularly in the frontal and temporal regions. Because the tensile forces that are sufficient to shear axons are also sufficient to shear blood vessels, sites where axonal shearing is suspected are often also sites where hemosiderin deposits are detected. Detection of such abnormalities is also dependent on the image sequence, as shown in Figure 5–8.

Contusion

Contusion most commonly occurs where bony ridges (i.e., the sphenoid) or protuberances (i.e., crista galli) are located. Acutely, these lesions may also be associated

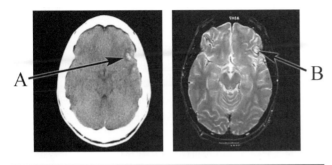

FIGURE 5–9. Cortical contusion as seen in the acute stage (A) and chronic stage (B).

The contusion developed around the sphenoid bone and was caused by the brain parenchyma's grating against the sphenoid ridges, shearing blood vessels as well as macerating tissue. The density changes in this posterior region of the frontal lobe on the day-of-injury (DOI) computed tomography (CT) scan show a mixture of blood and edema, which also extends into the peri-Sylvian region of the brain. The chronic lesion resulting from this focal injury is seen in B through the use of magnetic resonance (MR) imaging. The lesion shows an area of greater cerebrospinal fluid collection, which means loss of parenchymal integrity and atrophy as well as hemosiderin, the dark ring around the lesion site representing old, degraded blood by-products. Of interest is the fact that the temporal lobe contusion aspect of the lesion seen on the DOI scan does not clearly image on the MR scan. When such lesions "resolve," the clinician should not assume that surrounding tissue is not affected—the DOI CT scan suggests that it is likely that the temporal lobe is more generally damaged at this level but that damage is not detected by the MR imaging done during the chronic phase.

with focal edema. Acute contusions may resolve, leaving no detectable abnormality on MR imaging. This circumstance represents another case in which it is important to have the DOI information, because an acute contusion most likely results in damaged parenchyma, regardless of the MR imaging findings. As with shear injuries, sites of contusion often reveal hemosiderin deposits (Figure 5–9).

White Matter Signal Abnormalities

Due to the susceptibility of WM to injury in TBI, small, subtle, but nonetheless detectable WM abnormalities may show up as either WM hyperintensities and/or deposition of hemosiderin, as already mentioned in the section Shear. These areas of WM damage often correspond to areas where petechial hemorrhages have been noted on DOI CT imaging (see Table 5–2 and Figure 5–9). A simple WM-hyperintensity rating method, easily used by the clinician, is offered in the section Clinical Rating of Scans and Relationship to Neurobehavioral Changes at the end of this chapter.

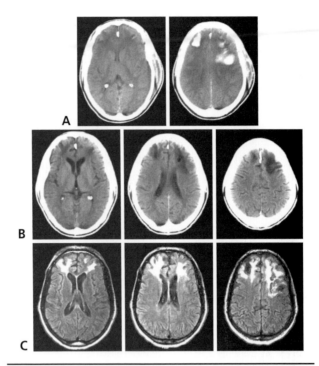

FIGURE 5–10. Demonstration of frontal contusions and intraparenchymal hemorrhaging that resulted in focal bifrontal atrophy after a high-speed motor vehicle–pedestrian accident.

The illustration also demonstrates the progression of pathology in brain injury from the day-of-injury computed tomography (CT) scan (A), to the CT scan at 4 months postinjury (B), to 2 years postinjury, as shown in magnetic resonance (MR) imaging findings (C). Note the ventricular expansion and the better definition and more extensive pathology identified by MR imaging during the chronic phases (2 years postinjury).

Focal Atrophy

A variety of trauma factors may coalesce to produce focal atrophy in particular regions of the brain, most commonly in the frontal and/or temporal lobes. This situation is demonstrated in Figure 5–10. A simple clinical rating method for establishing frontal and temporal lobe atrophy is offered in the section Clinical Rating of Scans and Relationship to Neurobehavioral Changes at the end of this chapter. This rating method can be quickly applied by the clinician; the presence of atrophy established by this method is associated with deficits in memory and executive function.

Quantitative Magnetic Resonance Neuroimaging

A most fortuitous circumstance exists at the gross structural level of brain parenchyma—it is comprised of two general tissue types, namely gray matter and WM. Gray matter, composed mostly of cell bodies and dendritic trees (where synapses are located)—the neuropil—and WM, composed mainly of myelinated axons, yield different signal characteristics on MR imaging. These dissimilar signal intensities permit their isolation, and therefore gray matter and WM can be "segmented" from one another (Laidlaw et al. 2000). Likewise, because CSF spaces are fluid filled, they too have different signal characteristics from brain parenchyma, as does bone. Once these different tissue-CSF compartments are segmented, accurate estimates of the volume of any region of interest can be made because the slice thickness of the scan and the distance between slices are known (Bigler and Tate 2001). Because contemporary MR imaging has resolution to approximately 1 mm, fine structural analysis can be achieved of any region that can be visualized with gross inspection of the brain. As already mentioned in the section Magnetic Resonance Imaging, numerous areas have been quantitatively analyzed and shown to degenerate in response to brain trauma (see Appendix 5–1 for a partial listing). In fact, inspection of this table demonstrates the nonspecific susceptibility of the brain to traumatic injury and, as discussed below, typically the generalized nature of TBI is in proportion to the severity of the injury. Even mild TBI may show qualitative and quantitative changes (Hofman et al. 2001; McGowan et al. 2000).

Global Atrophy Associated With TBI

Moderate-to-severe TBI, defined by a GCS score of 12 or lower, has been shown to be associated with nonspecific volume loss of brain parenchyma (see Appendix 5–1). Because the CSF housed within the ventricle is under pressure, any loss of brain volume results in a passive expansion of the ventricular system (i.e., hydrocephalus ex vacuo) (see Figure 5–6). A straightforward method to demonstrate this quantitatively comes through the use of the ventricle to brain ratio (VBR). This ratio is the total volume of the ventricles (lateral, III, and IV) divided by the total brain volume. Because there are inherent differences in head and body sizes (as well as types), the comparison of different patients with a single measure requires a correction for head-size differences. This is automatically accounted for by the VBR. VBR, or increasing atrophy, is directly related to the severity of injury, as manifested by duration of unconsciousness or posttraumatic amnesia.

Regardless of the method used to determine injury severity, increasing severity of injury results in greater brain volume loss and ventricular dilatation (see Figure 5–6). Increased VBR in the TBI patient is reflective of global changes but may disproportionately reflect WM volume loss compared to that of gray matter (Adams et al. 2000; Gale et al. 1995; Garnett et al. 2000; Strich 1956; Thatcher et al. 1997). This is particularly evident when viewing changes in the CC (see Figure 5–7). Figure 5–6 shows a three-dimensional comparison of the ventricular systems of a noninjured control, a patient with moderate TBI, and a patient with severe injury. It is obvious in viewing these figures that the ventricular dilatation is nonspecific, affecting all aspects of the ventricular compartment—a reflection of global atrophy induced by TBI.

Quick Guide to Visualizing Atrophy for the Clinician

Although neuroimaging is rapidly moving toward automated image analysis systems, another decade will likely pass before quantitative information is routinely included in the neuroimaging report. Likewise, the typical clinician is not equipped with the hardware and software for image analysis, so how can he or she visualize atrophy? As implied in the section Global Atrophy Associated With TBI, visually inspecting scans over time often permits the identification of cerebral atrophy by comparing the size of the ventricle; in particular, the DOI scan may be compared to scans done weeks or months later. Another way to examine atrophy, if sequential MR imaging has been performed, is to view the CC in midsagittal view. The CC is susceptible to atrophic change because it houses the long, coursing, interhemispheric WM-fiber pathways and often is directly injured by shearing action or secondary degeneration due to cortical injury, particularly contusions (see Figure 5–7). Because the CC is organized in an anterior-posterior fashion, when greater atrophy is noted regionally, that is often a sign of more atrophy in a particular lobe (i.e., atrophy of the genu associated with frontal atrophy). In contrast, degeneration of the entire length of the CC is most likely a sign of generalized, nonspecific WM change secondary to trauma. Several studies have shown modest relationships between CC atrophy and neurobehavioral sequelae, particularly changes in memory (Johnson et al. 1996; Levin et al. 2000). Last, simple rating methods for lobar atrophy and WM changes may be helpful in identifying MR-detected pathology. These methods are more fully discussed in the section Clinical Rating of Scans and Relationships to Neurobehavioral Changes at the end of this chapter, after additional MR pathology findings in TBI are discussed.

Relationship of Magnetic Resonance Imaging Findings to Outcome

There is no simple answer or review that can be offered on the topic of the relationship of MR imaging findings to outcome (Bigler 2000, 2001a, 2001b). There are multiple reasons for this complexity, including the very nature of what it means to be human and have a brain that

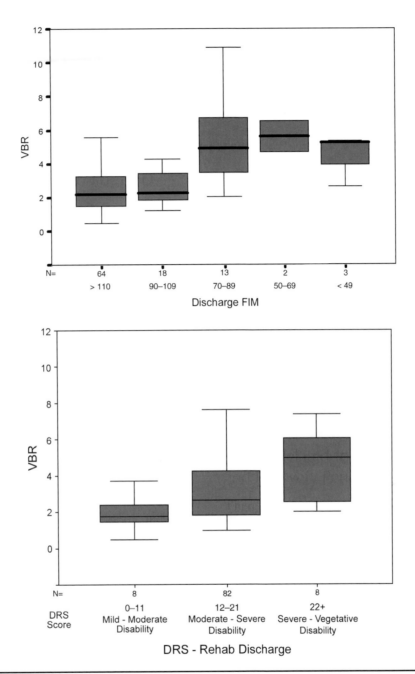

FIGURE 5–11. Box plots demonstrating the relationship between generalized atrophy measured by the ventricle to brain ratio (VBR) and discharge status from in-patient rehabilitation (Rehab) using the Functional Independence Measure (FIM) and the Disability Rating Scale (DRS).

Normal VBR is approximately 1.5. Clearly, presence of increased cerebral atrophy was associated with greater disability. See footnotes 1 and 2 (p. 81) for an explanation of the DRS and FIM.

controls and regulates all facets of human behavior. Accordingly, such individual factors as age, sex, education, individual differences in intellectual and cognitive abilities, health status at the time of injury, and trauma variables, including lesion location, diffuse injury effects, and presence of secondary injury effects (e.g., hypoxemia, edema, and systemic injury), all enter into the equation that predicts outcome from injury. Relating findings from brain imaging to neuropsychiatric outcome also depends on what outcome measurements are used and when during the postinjury time period assessments are made. Nonetheless, taking all these factors into consideration, there is the expected relationship that the greater the residual structural abnormality, the greater the potential for neuropsychiatric morbidity. This relationship can be seen in Figure 5–11, which demonstrates outcome assessed at the time of discharge from the rehabilitation unit after TBI (the modal patient had a moderate TBI with GCS score of approximately 8) compared to the late MR imaging findings. As can be seen from this figure, increasing cerebral atrophy, meaning increased nonspecific effects of the brain injury, was associated with greater disability at the time of discharge from the rehabilitation unit.

As for an even more long-term outcome, research suggests that the more prevalent the structural abnormalities, the greater the neuropsychiatric disability (Bigler 2001a; Jorge et al. 2004; Vasa et al. 2004). There is another factor that must be mentioned when discussing outcome: the relationship between significant head injury and the aging process. If brain injury results in atrophy and if brain volume loss also occurs with aging, then age effects in the injured brain may start from different baselines depending on the age of the patient. This combination may result in less-than-optimal aging (i.e., increased cognitive deficits with aging), increasing the likelihood of neurobehavioral sequelae, including affective disorder (Holsinger et al. 2002) and an earlier age of dementia onset (Guo et al. 2000; Plassman et al. 2000). Because the hippocampus is one of the structures more vulnerable to injury and is the limbic structure most often implicated in degenerative diseases, it seems reasonable that there is likely a connection.

Many of the studies listed in Appendix 5–1 examined the relationship of quantitative imaging to long-term outcome. Because one of the most frequent cognitive sequela to be associated with TBI is impaired memory, various quantitative studies (see Appendix 5–1) have examined temporal lobe structures and memory in TBI patients. In a detailed analysis of the temporal lobe, Bigler et al. (2002a) demonstrated that changes in WM integrity and volume loss of the hippocampus were the sequelae most related to memory deficits after TBI.

Small but Critical Lesions

There are dedicated pathways in the brain, such as the corticospinal pathway, that have little capacity for adaptation, rerouting, or functional reorganization after significant injury. Accordingly, a small but strategically placed lesion in the internal capsule may produce hemiplegia due to direct injury to the corticospinal tract. For example, the child shown in Figure 5–3 with a right internal capsule–basal ganglia hemorrhagic shear lesion had a dense hemiplegia, whereas the patient shown in Figure 5–10, who had massive hemorrhagic lesions bifrontally with concomitant focal frontal atrophy, did not have paralysis. Small but devastating lesions may also disrupt the integrity of the limbic

system, where a small lesion of the fornix or fornical atrophy may be responsible for significant memory deficits (Blumbergs et al. 1994; Tate and Bigler 2000). This situation is shown in Figure 5–7, in which it is clearly visible that the fornix progresses through various degenerative stages postinjury. The hippocampus—another relatively small structure and the origin of the majority of WM pathways that make up the fornix—is also particularly vulnerable to injury that also leads to memory impairment (Tate and Bigler 2000). Small temporal lobe lesions, including those of the hippocampus, may be the source of posttraumatic epilepsy (Diaz-Arrastia et al. 2000). It may also be that small, nonspecific lesions detected by MR imaging are the basis of the relationship between head injury and dementia, as even mild injury increases the risk ratio for dementia (Guo et al. 2000; Plassman et al. 2000).

Functional Lesion Likely Larger Than Structural Lesion

Figure 5–12 depicts the structural injuries sustained by a construction worker in a fall. Acute CT imaging demonstrated the presence of hemorrhagic lesions and midline shift that ultimately resulted in focal right frontal and temporal atrophy that was quite extensive (shown in red). However, when the structural MR imaging was integrated with single-photon emission computed tomography (SPECT), the physiological abnormality could be seen to extend far beyond the boundaries of the focal structural lesions observed on the MR scan; the MR-SPECT scan actually shows a left frontal defect with no concomitant structural abnormality (see Umile et al. 2002).

New Structural Imaging Techniques and Analyses

Considerable advances in MR technology have occurred over the past decade that will undoubtedly improve the detection and identification of structural pathology associated with acquired brain injury (Derdeyn 2001; Govindaraju et al. 2004; Levine et al. 2002; Makris et al. 1997; McGowan et al. 2000; Scheid et al. 2003; Sinson et al. 2001; Toga and Thompson 2001). The exciting possibilities are literally too numerous to elaborate in this chapter. However, there are several that are currently being used and will likely become standard methods in the evaluation of TBI. For example, DW-MR imaging capitalizes on the molecular motion of water, which may be pathologically altered in brain injury. This is depicted in Figure 5–13, in which a focal infarct is clearly demonstrated despite only the faintest appearance of an abnormality on CT imaging.

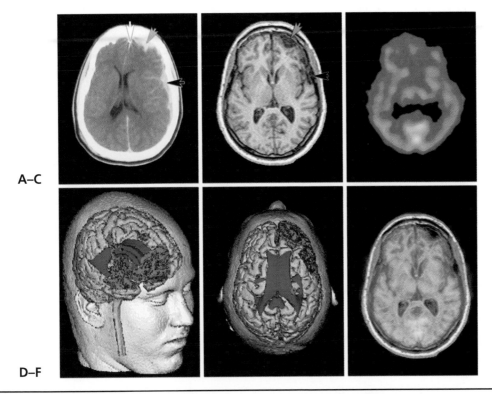

FIGURE 5–12.   Use of day-of-injury (DOI) computed tomography (CT).

DOI scan (A) showing right subdural hemorrhage, subarachnoid hemorrhage in peri-Sylvian fissure on the right, and significant (white arrow) right-to-left midline shift (B) (gray arrows in frontal region, dark arrows in temporal region). Magnetic resonance (MR) imaging performed 2.5 years later, demonstrating focal frontal and frontotemporal encephalomalacia as permanent sequelae to the DOI lesions observed in A. Single-photon emission computed tomography (SPECT) scan (C) demonstrating significant perfusion abnormalities, particularly in the frontal regions bilaterally and right frontotemporal areas. This can be best viewed in the MR-SPECT fused image (F). A three-dimensional image of the brain (D) outlines the extensive frontotemporal pathology from the right frontal oblique. The pathology from a dorsal perspective is illustrated in E. This figure demonstrates how using the DOI CT as a baseline permits the tracking of subsequent atrophy, how physiological abnormalities often exceed the focal structural pathology, and how all of this can be demonstrated in three dimensions.

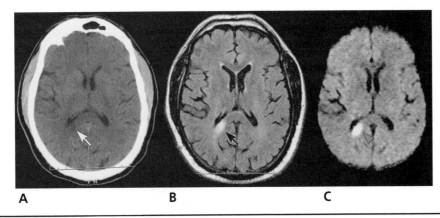

FIGURE 5–13.   The superiority of magnetic resonance (MR) techniques in detecting pathology.

The computed tomography (CT) scan (A) provides a faint hint of a density change in the corpus callosum. However, both MR images (B, a fluid-attenuated inversion recovery [FLAIR] image; C, a diffusion-weighted [DW] image) clearly demonstrate the abnormality. This figure shows the superiority of MR techniques in detecting pathology.

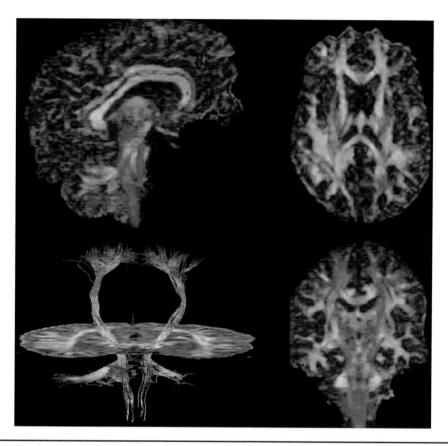

FIGURE 5–14.   RGB (red-green-blue) color diffusion-tensor imaging (DTI).

RGB color DTI images depict the major eigenvector of the diffusion tensor weighted by anisotropy degree. The fibers running from side to side (x-direction) appear red, the fibers running anteriorly to posteriorly appear green (y-direction), and the fibers running superiorly to inferiorly appear blue (z-direction). The fibers running in other directions than x, y, and z appear as a combination of the RGB colors. For example, in the axial image, the corpus callosum appears red at the midline and turns yellow (red plus green) when oriented in xy direction. In the sagittal image, the cingulum appears mostly green (running in the y-plane) and the corticospinal tract appears blue. Diffusion tensor approximates the diffusion profile of the water molecules existent in the tissue at each sampling point. The diffusion pattern is related to the microstructural properties of the tissue. One important observation is that in white matter fibers (or other fibrous tissues such as muscle), the water diffuses preferentially along the fiber direction. The image in the lower left shows the separation of the corticospinal tract, with an anterior-oblique-axial magnetic resonance view at the level of the temporal-occipital lobes showing the corticospinal tract descending through the cerebral peduncles. This technology will likely be used in studying traumatic brain injury to demonstrate pathway abnormalities produced by shearing and other pathological consequences of injury (see Jellison et al. 2004; Lazar et al. 2003).
Source.   Figure courtesy of Mariana Lazar, Ph.D., and Andrew Alexander, Ph.D., University of Wisconsin, Madison.

Diffusion-tensor imaging (DTI) is another technique that may provide refined detail concerning the integrity of WM in the brain and permit the tracking of aggregate groups of axons and their projection within the brain (Arfanakis et al. 2002; Jellison et al. 2004; Lazar et al. 2003; Wakana et al. 2004). Two examples of DTI technology are given in Figures 5–14 and 5–15. Figure 5–14 shows how DTI technology capitalizes on two simple biological principles of brain organization: 1) WM projections in the brain follow orderly projection routes, namely anterior-posterior, lateral, and inferior-superior projections; and 2) WM integrity can be assessed by applying the principle of anisotropy: the diffusion rates of water molecules are dependent on the direction of the WM pathway, which can

be determined by the physics and mathematics of vectors, or tensors (hence the name *diffusion-tensor imaging*). Using DTI, these dispersion differences define the orientation of pathways and can be easily color-coded using the red-green-blue color base (see Figure 5–14).

Such a color map provides in two dimensions what is actually occurring in the three-dimensional space of the brain. For example, as shown in Figure 5–14, green represents anterior-posterior pathways and red the lateral pathways across the CC; however, just outside the midpoint of the CC, the color turns yellow because the pathways there are coursing in a different direction, resulting in a different color combination. Some pathways, such as the corticospinal pathway, can be easily delineated and highlighted, as shown

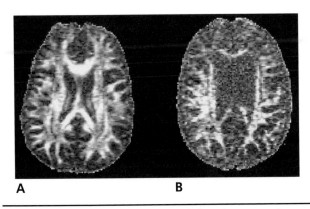

A B

FIGURE 5–15. **Diffusion-weighted magnetic resonance (MR) imaging.**

Diffusion-weighted MR imaging using fractional anisotropy (FA) mapping showing normal distribution of white matter noted by the bright signal, particularly in the genu of the corpus callosum (CC) in A. In comparison, the FA maps of the traumatic brain injury (TBI) patient in B demonstrate extensive loss of white matter coherence, particularly in the frontal area and anterior CC, 20 years postinjury. *Source.* Figure courtesy of Sterling C. Johnson, Ph.D., University of Wisconsin, Madison.

in Figure 5–14. The implications of such refined image analyses are obvious in studying the integrity and effects of TBI on motor, sensory, and language systems that have a known anatomical basis. It is likely that the use of such technology will make possible more refined image analysis of subtle perturbations associated with TBI. Although these applications are a bit futuristic, DTI has current application in TBI, as illustrated in Figure 5–15, which depicts a patient who sustained TBI 20 years before DTI. Using what is called *fractional anisotropy* (FA), FA maps of the brain can be created in which brighter voxels represent greater anisotropy and thus greater integrity, directionality, or coherence. As clearly seen in Figure 5–15, through the use of the DTI technique there is a general loss of integrity throughout the brain in severe TBI, particularly in frontal regions.

Last, there is a host of functional imaging methods, discussed in Chapter 6, Functional Imaging, that will be integrated with structural imaging in the future for the detection of objective abnormalities that can be related to the neuropsychiatric state of the patient after a brain injury.

Clinical Rating of Scans and Relationships to Neurobehavioral Changes

Much of the research discussed in this chapter deals with quantitative MR imaging. The difficulty and limitation of

quantitative analyses of scans are that they require the proper computer hard and software as well as expertise to do the analyses, some of which take considerable time. The clinician may not need the types of detailed analyses that are more suitable for research. Accordingly, simple rating scales used in conjunction with the clinical radiological report can provide an index of generalized as well as focal atrophy along with changes in WM integrity. As discussed throughout this chapter, WM is particularly vulnerable in TBI, and underlying WM pathology is at the basis of much of the volume loss and signal changes seen in MR imaging of TBI. The degree of ventricular dilatation has been related to the amount of WM volume loss (Gale et al. 1995a, 1995b); by comparing the DOI scan with follow-up scans, clinical estimates of the degree of generalized atrophy can be made. Because it takes time for the full spectrum of pathological effects to develop postinjury (Bramlett and Dietrich 2002), it is best if the comparison follow-up scan is performed at least several months postinjury. An example of how this technique can be used is presented in Figures 5–3 and 5–12, and a more in-depth example is presented in Figure 5–16. The case presented in Figure 5–16 is from a young adult who presented 7.5 years postinjury with persistent problems with memory. However, family members believed that problems with initiative and problem solving were just as significant as the memory impairments. Reviewing the DOI CT scan and using that information as a baseline made it obvious that generalized ventricular dilatation occurred in addition to residual focal lesions associated with the original TBI.

Lobular atrophy, particularly in the frontotemporal regions as shown in Figure 5–17, is commonplace in TBI, as is discussed throughout this chapter. In a study by Bergeson et al. (2004), a four-point atrophy rating scale (0=none, 0.5=minimal, 1.0=moderate, 2=severe) was applied to lobular atrophy on the basis of the methods outlined by Victoroff et al. (1994). Significant atrophy was found in both frontal and temporal regions in a group of TBI subjects compared with age-matched control subjects. Parietal atrophy was not observed in the TBI patients compared with controls, however. Bergeson et al. (2004) found that the degree of frontal and/or temporal atrophy was related to the level of impairment in memory and executive function. Figure 5–17 provides examples of these rating methods in the identification of frontal and temporal lobe atrophy that can be used by the clinician. This patient, who was a long-distance semitruck driver, sustained a severe TBI when he lost control of his tractor-trailer rig in poor weather. Imaging studies were done approximately 3 years postinjury and demonstrated significant frontal and temporal atrophy as well as gener-

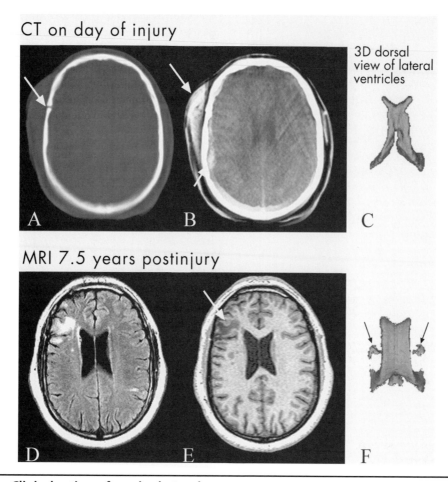

FIGURE 5-16.   Clinical rating of cerebral atrophy.

In these images, left is on left. This patient sustained a severe TBI caused by a fall from a roof. As shown in A, the day-of-injury (DOI) computed tomography (CT) bone window clearly shows the location of a linear skull fracture (arrow) just beneath where major extracranial trauma occurred (note swelling in both A and B) as a result of blunt impact associated with the fall. On admission, the patient had a Glasgow Coma Scale score of 5. B: The clinical DOI CT scan showing the location of an epidural hematoma (bottom arrow) and massive swelling about the head (top arrow). Parts D (fluid-attenuated inversion recovery image) and E (T1 image) show the chronic effects of this injury manifested by ventricular dilatation as well as other pathology. As shown in B, the left aspect of the lateral ventricle is effaced by expanding pressure over the left hemisphere because of the hematoma and lateralized intraparenchymal edema. Nonetheless, even though the ventricle is distorted and some cerebrospinal fluid is displaced to the right lateral ventricle, the original size of the lateral ventricle can still be assessed in this DOI scan. Comparing ventricular size in the DOI scan in B with that shown in D and E, the follow-up magnetic resonance imaging clearly shows ventricular dilatation. E clearly shows the asymmetry of the lateral ventricle on the left, which represents some degree of hydrocephalus ex vacuo affected by volume loss of the major frontal lesion, shown in both D and E. Part F depicts the three-dimensional dorsal view of the lateral ventricle, which clearly shows general dilatation of the ventricular system. Note that the ventricle is nonspecifically expanded in F, a reflection of global volume loss seen in TBI. Also, note in C that temporal horns of the lateral ventricle are not visualized. This is common in moderate to severe TBI because of bilateral temporal lobe edema. In F, the temporal horns (arrows) are visible and dilated, an indication of temporal lobe atrophy that occurred over time from the DOI scan. Last, note that in D–F the ventricle is slightly asymmetric in its enlargement, reflective of the more lateralized damage to the left hemisphere.

alized cerebral atrophy (note the ventricular dilatation and corpus callosum atrophy). Neuropsychologically, the patient manifested significant deficits in memory and executive function.

Examples of the susceptibility of WM pathology in TBI have been demonstrated throughout this chapter as well as

elsewhere (Goetz et al. 2004; Graham et al. 2002). When MR imaging detects WM pathology, characteristic signal differences are present depending on the image sequence used (see Table 5–2). WM pathology, regardless of its etiology, is the basis of a wide variety of neuropsychiatric disorders (Filley 2001; Litcher and Cummings 2001). Simple rat-

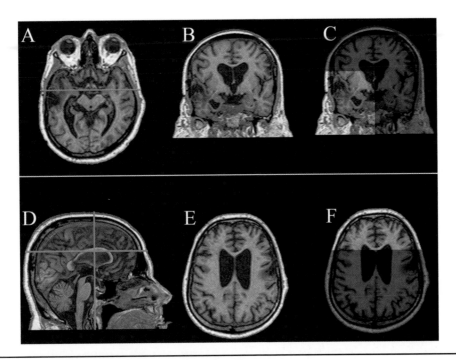

FIGURE 5–17.   Temporal and frontal lobe clinical rating.

These ratings are based on Victoroff et al.'s (1994) method of lobular rating, again using a 4-point scale (0 = no atrophy, 0.5 = mild, 1.0 = moderate, and 2.0 = severe). These are all T1 images obtained approximately 3 years postinjury. Part A represents an axial view in which the red line shows the plane of the coronal cut, which is also reflected in D (vertical red line). The coronal plane is used for rating temporal lobe atrophy, as shown in B. The temporal lobe region rated is highlighted in C. There is marked temporal horn dilation, increased cerebrospinal fluid signal, and volume reduction noted in the temporal lobe rated (temporal atrophy rating = 2). Frontal atrophy is rated in the axial plane as shown in E, focusing on the anterior region of the frontal lobe as highlighted in F. The horizontal line shown in D shows the level of the axial cut in E and F. Attention is directed to the width of the frontal gyri and prominence of the interhemispheric fissure. The frontal atrophy rating is 2. Increased ratings of frontal or temporal atrophy are associated with deficits in cognitive ability, particularly short-term memory, attention/concentration, and executive function (see Bergeson et al. 2004).

ing methods for WM pathology were first used in aging and dementia (Victoroff et al. 1994) as well as in disorders such as multiple sclerosis and anoxic brain damage (Parkinson et al. 2002) that more selectively damage WM. More recently, these methods have been applied to TBI (Hopkins et al. 2003). When WM abnormalities are identified, they are rated on a four-point scale (same categories as the atrophy ratings given in the preceding paragraph) on the basis of their location and size. Much of the WM literature shows that damage to the periventricular region tends to be more disruptive of neurobehavioral and neurocognitive function by interrupting long coursing tracts that participate in integration of function and speed of processing. Lesions more in the region of the centrum-semiovale may be more locally disruptive of function than productive of more global deficits (Bigler et al. 2002b, 2003). Figure 5–18 demonstrates a case of WM pathology and its rating and relationship to neuropsychological outcome in an older adolescent who sustained severe TBI in a head-on motor vehicle collision.

The last point to make is that in TBI, damage can occur anywhere in the brain and be manifested in numerous ways on neuroimaging studies. As a quick guide to the clinician, one should first view the brain for any differences in normal symmetry or obvious abnormalities or deviations from normal. Next, viewing the midsagittal view of the corpus callosum provides a quick reference regarding general WM integrity. Figure 5–5 provides a nice reference of how normal symmetry should look, and Figure 5–8 shows an atrophic corpus callosum contrasted with a normal-appearing one. Next, viewing the ventricular system and cortical sulcal widths offers a quick reference of the degree of generalized atrophy. The third ventricle is particularly susceptible to enlargement in TBI, and clinical rating methods for such enlargement have been published by Groswasser et al. (Groswasser et al. 2002; Reider-Groswasser et al. 2002). Temporal horn dilation is often not only a sign of temporal lobe atrophy but also of atrophy of the hippocampus and amygdala (Bigler et al. 2002a). By reviewing the location and degree of the structural imaging abnormality, the clinician may use that information in the neuropsychiatric assessment, care, and treatment of the patient with TBI.

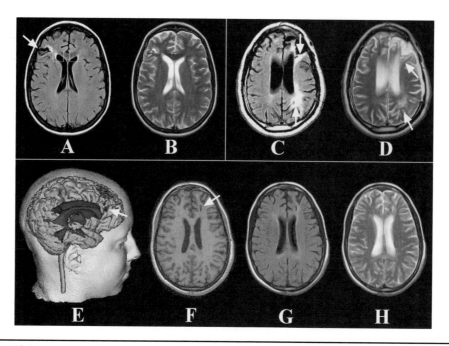

FIGURE 5–18.   White matter (WM) abnormalities and traumatic brain injury (TBI).

In these images, left is on left. As shown in the figures that are part of Table 5–3, different MR imaging sequences are sensitive to different aspects of WM damage. For clinical rating, the Victoroff et al. (1994) method is again used but is adapted to include fluid-attenuated inversion recovery image (FLAIR) and gradient recalled echo sequences. Lesions are "quantified" by their size and location. No lesion is rated as 0, small as 0.5, medium as 1.0, and large as 2.0. More explicit details for rating can be found in Parkinson et al. (2002). In the Victoroff et al. (1994) study, the WM lesions were hyperintense, or white, because they used T2- and proton density–weighted MR images. This is also true on the FLAIR sequence, but often these WM shear lesions are also associated with hemosiderin deposits, which classify oppositely as hypointense, or black. As shown in this illustration, the images at the top depict the boundaries for lesions within the periventricular (PV) area, defined by Victoroff et al. (1994) as hyperintensities hugging the ventricle. The image used (see A in the FLAIR sequence and B in the T2 sequence) is typically at the body of the lateral ventricle where the dorsal aspect of the head and body of the caudate nucleus can be visualized (partly identified by the white box). The centrum semiovale (CS) region is taken at a similar level to that for the lateral ventricle but is defined as residing outside the WM adjacent to the ventricle, which defines the PV region. The TBI patient in C (FLAIR) and D (T2) shows extensive white matter lesions in the CS region. Because the WM pathology seen in TBI may be more widely distributed than that observed in some other disorders, this rating method can be applied to any region of the brain or could be done lobe by lobe. The clinician using these rating methods should refer back to Victoroff et al.'s (1994) original for the standard comparisons as referenced for rating pathology. The Victoroff et al. (1994) method for rating WM hyperintensities can be adapted for use in rating WM pathology in TBI (Hopkins et al. 2003). The patient shown in A and B is an adolescent female (the same FLAIR and T2 scans appear in Table 5–3) who sustained a severe TBI in a high-speed rollover motor vehicle accident. There is an obvious large residual hemorrhagic cortical contusion in the frontal region (arrow) that represents a mixture of gliotic tissue, old blood (hemosiderin), and cerebrospinal fluid (CSF). Note the ventricular asymmetry, particularly the expansion toward the lesion. In rating PV lesions, the signal intensity involving the WM that "hugs" the ventricle is rated. The signal intensity is abnormal in the box on the left that highlights the anterior aspect of the lateral ventricle in comparison with the box on the right. Note that the FLAIR sequence better defines the abnormality than the T2 image of this subject. The WM rating abnormality is 1.0. The patient whose images are shown in C (FLAIR) and D (T2) also sustained a severe TBI after being ejected from a vehicle after impact. Extensive CS WM lesions are present that are rated as 2.0. A third patient is depicted in F–H who sustained a severe TBI as a consequence of a head-on collision. Initial CT imaging demonstrated numerous bilateral frontal petechial hemorrhages, the largest one located where the residual focal shear lesion is identified (arrow) in the T1 image (E). The FLAIR sequence (G) shows both PV and CS WM abnormalities, which can also be seen in the T2 image, although they are not always prominent there. The shear lesion has left a cavitation within the WM that has filled with CSF. The clinical rating in this patient is 1.0 for both PV and CS regions.

References

Adams JH, Graham DI, Jennett B: The neuropathology of the vegetative state after an acute brain insult. Brain 123:1327–1338, 2000

Anderson CV, Bigler ED: The role of caudate nucleus and corpus callosum atrophy in trauma-induced anterior horn dilation. Brain Inj 9:565–569, 1994

Anderson CV, Bigler ED: Ventricular dilation, cortical atrophy, and neuropsychological outcome following traumatic brain injury. J Neuropsychiatry Clin Neurosci 7:42–48, 1995

Anderson CV, Bigler ED, Blatter DD: Frontal lobe lesions, diffuse damage, and neuropsychological functioning in traumatic brain-injured patients. J Clin Exp Neuropsychol 17:900–908, 1995

Anderson CV, Wood DG, Bigler ED, et al: Lesion volume, injury severity, and thalamic integrity following head injury. J Neurotrauma 13:35–40, 1996

Arfanakis K, Haughton VM, Carew JD, et al: Diffusion tensor MR imaging in diffuse axonal injury. AJNR Am J Neuroradiol 23:794–802, 2002

Ariza M, Mataro M, Poca MA, et al: Influence of extraneurological insults on ventricular enlargement and neuropsychological functioning after moderate and severe traumatic brain injury. J Neurotrauma 21:864–876, 2004

Atlas S: Magnetic Resonance Imaging of the Brain and Spine, 3rd Edition. Hagerstown, MD, Lippincott Williams & Wilkins, 2001

Bain AC, Raghupathi R, Meaney DF: Dynamic stretch correlates to both morphological abnormalities and electrophysiological impairment in a model of traumatic axonal injury. J Neurotrauma 18:499–511, 2001

Barker LH, Bigler ED, Johnson SC, et al: Polysubstance abuse and traumatic brain injury: quantitative magnetic resonance imaging and neuropsychological outcome in older adolescents and young adults. J Int Neuropsychol Soc 5:593–608, 1999

Bergeson AG, Lundin R, Parkinson RB, et al: Clinical rating of cortical atrophy and cognitive correlates following traumatic brain injury. Clin Neuropsychol 18:1–12, 2004.

Bigler ED: Neuroimaging in pediatric traumatic head injury: diagnostic considerations and relationships to neurobehavioral outcome. J Head Trauma Rehabil 14:70–87, 1999

Bigler ED: Neuroimaging and rehabilitation outcome, in Handbook of Rehabilitation Psychology. Edited by Frank RG, Elliott TR. Washington, DC, American Psychological Association, 2000, pp 441–474

Bigler ED: The lesion(s) in traumatic brain injury: implications for clinical neuropsychology. Arch Clin Neuropsychol 16(2):95–131, 2001a

Bigler ED: Structural and functional neuroimaging of traumatic brain injury, in State of the Art Reviews in Physical Medicine and Rehabilitation: Traumatic Brain Injury. Edited by McDeavitt JT. Philadelphia, Hanley and Belfus, 2001b, pp 349–361

Bigler ED, Tate DF: Brain volume, intracranial volume and dementia. Invest Radiol 36:539–546, 2001

Bigler ED, Paver S, Cullum CM, et al: Ventricular enlargement, cortical atrophy and neuropsychological performance following head injury. Int J Neurosci 24:295–298, 1984

Bigler ED, Kurth S, Blatter D, et al: Degenerative changes in traumatic brain injury: post-injury magnetic resonance identified ventricular expansion compared to pre-injury levels. Brain Res Bull 28:651–653, 1992

Bigler ED, Blatter DD, Johnson SC, et al: Traumatic brain injury, alcohol and quantitative neuroimaging: preliminary findings. Brain Inj 10:197–206, 1996a

Bigler ED, Johnson SC, Anderson CV, et al: Traumatic brain injury and memory: the role of hippocampal atrophy. Neuropsychology 10:333–342, 1996b

Bigler ED, Anderson CV, Blatter DD: Temporal lobe morphology in normal aging and traumatic brain injury. AJNR Am J Neuroradiol 23:255–266, 2002a

Bigler ED, Kerr B, Victoroff J, Tate D, et al: White matter lesions, quantitative MRI and dementia. Alzheimer Dis Assoc Disord 16:161–170, 2002b

Bigler ED, Tate DF, Neeley ES, et al: Temporal lobe, autism and macrocephaly. AJNR Am J Neuroradiol 24:2066–2076, 2003

Bigler ED, Ryser DK, Gandhi P, et al: Day-of-injury computerised tomography, rehabilitation status, and long-term outcome as they relate to magnetic resonance imaging findings after traumatic brain injury. Brain Impairment 5:122–123, 2004

Blatter DD, Bigler ED, Gale SD, et al: MR-based brain and cerebrospinal fluid measurement after traumatic brain injury: correlation with neuropsychological outcome. AJNR Am J Neuroradiol 18:1–10, 1997

Blumbergs PC, Scott G, Manavis J, et al: Staining of amyloid precursor protein to study axonal damage in mild head injury. Lancet 344:1055–1056, 1994

Bowen JM, Clark E, Bigler ED, et al: Childhood traumatic brain injury: neuropsychological status at the time of hospital discharge. Dev Med Child Neurol 39:17–25, 1997

Bramlett HM, Dietrich WD: Quantitative structural changes in white and gray matter 1 year following traumatic brain injury in rats. Acta Neuropathologica 103:607–614, 2002

Cullum CM, Bigler ED: Ventricle size, cortical atrophy and the relationship with neuropsychological status in closed head injury: a quantitative analysis. J Clin Exp Neuropsychol 8:437–452, 1986

Derdeyn CP: Physiological neuroimaging: emerging clinical applications. JAMA 285:3065–3068, 2001

Diaz-Arrastia R, Agostini MA, Frol AB, et al: Neurophysiologic and neuroradiologic features of intractable epilepsy after traumatic brain injury in adults. Arch Neurol 57:1611–1616, 2000

Dikmen S, Machamer J, Miller B, et al: Functional status examination: a new instrument for assessing outcome in traumatic brain injury. J Neurotrauma 18:127–140, 2001

Ding Y, Yao B, Lai Q, et al: Impaired motor learning and diffuse axonal damage in motor and visual systems of the rat following traumatic brain injury. Neurol Res 23:193–202, 2001

Eisenberg RL: Radiology: An Illustrated History. St. Louis, Mosby Year Book, 1992

Filley CM: The Behavioral Neurology of White Matter. Oxford and NY, Oxford University Press, 2001

Gale SD, Burr RB, Bigler ED, et al: Fornix degeneration and memory in traumatic brain injury. Brain Res Bull 32:345–349, 1993

Gale SD, Johnson SC, Bigler ED, et al: Traumatic brain injury and temporal horn enlargement: correlates with tests of intelligence and memory. Neuropsychiatry Neuropsychol Behav Neurol 7:160–165, 1994

Gale SD, Johnson SC, Bigler ED, et al: Nonspecific white matter degeneration following traumatic brain injury. J Int Neuropsychol Soc 1:17–28, 1995a

Gale SD, Johnson SC, Bigler ED, et al: Trauma-induced degenerative changes in brain injury: a morphometric analysis of three patients with preinjury and postinjury MR scans. J Neurotrauma 12:151–158, 1995b

Garnett MR, Blamire AM, Rajagopalan B, et al: Evidence for cellular damage in normal-appearing white matter correlates with injury severity in patients following traumatic brain injury: a magnetic resonance spectroscopy study. Brain 123:1403–1409, 2000

Gean AD: Imaging of Head Trauma. New York, Raven Press, 1994

Goetz P, Blamire A, Rajagopalan B, et al: Increase in apparent diffusion coefficient in normal appearing white matter following human traumatic brain injury correlates with injury severity. J Neurotrauma 21:645–654, 2004

Gorrie C, Duflou J, Brown J, et al: Extent and distribution of vascular brain injury in pediatric road fatalities. J Neurotrauma 18:849–860, 2001

Govindaraju V, Gauger GE, Manley GT, et al: Volumetric proton spectroscopic imaging of mild traumatic brain injury. AJNR Am J Neuroradiol 25:730–737, 2004

Graham DI, Gennarelli TA, McIntosh TK: Trauma, in Greenfield's Neuropathology, 7th Edition, Vol. 2. Edited by Graham DI, Lantos PI. London, Arnold, 2002, pp 823–882

Groswasser Z, Reider G II, Schwab K, et al: Quantitative imaging in late TBI, part II: cognition and work after closed and penetrating head injury: a report of the Vietnam head injury study. Brain Inj 16:681–690, 2002

Guo Z, Cupples LA, Kurz A, et al: Head injury and the risk of AD in the MIRAGE study. Neurology 54:1316–1323, 2000

Hall KM, Hamilton BB, Gordon WA, et al: Characteristics and comparisons of functional assessment indices: disability rating scale, functional independence measure, and functional assessment measure. J Head Trauma Rehabil 8:60–74, 1993

Hamilton BB, Granger CV, Sherwin FS, et al: A uniform data system for medical rehabilitation, in Rehabilitation Outcomes: Analysis and Measurement. Edited by Fuhrer MJ. Baltimore, MD, Brooks, 1987

Haydel MJ, Preston CA, Mills TJ, et al: Indications for computed tomography in patients with minor head injury. N Engl J Med 343:100–105, 2000

Henry-Feugas MC, Azouvi P, Fontaine A, et al: MRI analysis of brain atrophy after severe closed-head injury: relation to clinical status. Brain Inj 14:597–604, 2000

Hofman PA, Stapert SZ, van Kroonenburgh MJ, et al: MR imaging, single-photon emission CT, and neurocognitive performance after mild traumatic brain injury. AJNR Am J Neuroradiol 22:441–449, 2001

Holsinger T, Steffens DC, Phillips C, et al: Head injury in early adulthood and the lifetime risk of depression. Arch Gen Psychiatry 59:17–22, 2002

Hopkins RO, McCourt A, Cleavinger HB, et al: White matter hyperintensities and neuropsychological outcome following traumatic brain injury. J Int Neuropsychol Soc 9:234, 2003

Jellison BJ, Field AS, Medow J, et al: Diffusion tensor imaging of cerebral white matter: a pictorial review of physics, fiber tract anatomy, and tumor imaging patterns. AJNR Am J Neuroradiol 25:356–369, 2004

Johnson SC, Bigler ED, Burr RB, et al: White matter atrophy, ventricular dilation, and intellectual functioning following traumatic brain injury. Neuropsychology 8:307–315, 1994

Johnson SC, Pinkston JB, Bigler ED, et al: Corpus callosum morphology in normal controls and TBI: sex differences, mechanisms of injury, and neuropsychological correlates. Neuropsychology 10:408–415, 1996

Jorge RE, Robinson RG, Moser D, et al: Major depression following traumatic brain injury. Arch Gen Psychiatry 61:42–50, 2004

Kurth SM, Bigler ED, Blatter DD: Neuropsychological outcome and quantitative image analysis of acute hemorrhage in traumatic brain injury: preliminary findings. Brain Inj 8:489–500, 1994

Laidlaw DH, Fleischer KW, Barr AH: Partial-volume Bayesian classification of material mixtures in MR volume data using voxel histograms. IEEE Trans Med Imaging 17:74–86, 1998

Lazar M, Weinstein DM, Tsuruda JS, et al: White matter tractography using diffusion tensor deflection. Human Brain Mapping, 18:306–321, 2003

Levin HS, Benavidez DA, Verger-Maestre K, et al: Reduction of corpus callosum growth after severe traumatic brain injury in children. Neurology 54:647–653, 2000

Levine B, Cabeza R, McIntosh AR, et al: Functional reorganisation of memory after traumatic brain injury: a study with H(2)(15)0 positron emission tomography. J Neurol Neurosurg Psychiatry 73:173–181, 2002

Litcher DG, Cummings JL: Frontal-subcortical circuits in psychiatric and neurologic disorders. New York, Guilford Press, 2001

Makris N, Worth AJ, Sorensen AG, et al: Morphometry of in vivo human white matter association pathways with diffusion-weighted magnetic resonance imaging. Ann Neurol 42:951–962, 1997

Marshall LF, Marshall SB, Klauber MR, et al: A new classification of head injury based on computerized tomography. J Neurosurg 75:S14–S20, 1991

Massman PJ, Bigler ED, Cullum CM, et al: The relationship between cortical atrophy and ventricular volume in Alzheimer's disease and closed head injury. Int J Neurosci 30:87–99, 1986

McGowan JC, Yang JH, Plotkin RC, et al: Magnetization transfer imaging in the detection of injury associated with mild head trauma. AJNR Am J Neuroradiol 21:875–880, 2000

Orrison WW: Neuroimaging. Philadelphia, PA, WB Saunders, 2000

Parkinson RB, Hopkins RO, Cleavinger HB, et al: White matter hyperintensities and neuropsychological outcome following carbon monoxide poisoning. Neurology 58:1525–1532, 2002

Plassman BL, Havlik RJ, Steffens DC, et al: Documented head injury in early adulthood and risk of Alzheimer's disease and other dementias. Neurology 55:1158–1166, 2000

Primus EA, Bigler ED, Anderson CV, et al: Corpus striatum and traumatic brain injury. Brain Inj 11:577–586, 1997

Rappaport M, Hall KM, Hopkins K, et al: Disability rating scale for severe head trauma: coma to community. Arch Phys Med Rehabil 63:118–123, 1982

Reider-Groswasser I, Groswasser Z, Ommaya AK, et al: Quantitative imaging in late traumatic brain injury, part I: late imaging parameters in closed and penetrating head injuries. Brain Inj 16:517–525, 2002

Scheid R, Preul C, Gruber O, et al: Diffuse axonal injury associated with chronic traumatic brain injury: evidence from T2*-weighted gradient-echo imaging at 3 T. Am J Neuroradiol 24:1049–1056, 2003

Shiozaki T, Akai H, Taneda M, et al: Delayed hemispheric neuronal loss in severely head-injured patients. J Neurotrauma 18:665–674, 2001

Sinson GP, Bagley LJ, Cecil KM, et al: Magnetization transfer imaging and proton MR spectroscopy in the evaluation of axonal injury: correlation with clinical outcome after traumatic brain injury. AJNR Am J Neuroradiol 22:143–151, 2001

State University of New York at Buffalo Department of Rehabilitation Medicine, School of Medicine and Biochemical Sciences Center for Functional Assessment Research. Guide for Use of the Uniform Data Set for Medical Rehabilitation Including the Functional Independence Measure (FIM), Version 3.1. New York, State University of New York, 1987, 1990 Research Foundation, 1990

Strich SJ: Diffuse degeneration of the cerebral white matter in severe dementia following head injury. J Neurol Neurosurg Psychiatry 19:163–185, 1956

Tate D, Bigler ED: Fornix and hippocampal atrophy in traumatic brain injury. Learn Mem 7:442–446, 2000

Thatcher R, Camacho M, Salazar A, et al: Quantitative MRI of the gray-white matter distribution in traumatic brain injury. J Neurotrauma 14:1–14, 1997

Toga AW, Thompson PM: Maps of the brain. Anat Rec 265:37–53, 2001

Tong KA, Ashwal S, Holshouser BA, et al: Diffuse axonal injury in children: clincial correlation with hemorrhagic lesions. Ann Neurol 56:36–50, 2004

Turkheimer E, Yeo RA, Bigler ED: Basic relations among lesion location, lesion volume and neuropsychological performance. Neuropsychologia 28:1011–1019, 1990

Umile EM, Sandel ME, Alavi A, et al: Dynamic imaging in mild traumatic brain injury: support for the theory of medial temporal vulnerability. Arch Phys Med Rehabil 83:1506–1513, 2002

van der Naalt J, Hew JM, van Zomeren AH, et al: Computed tomography and magnetic resonance imaging in mild to moderate head injury: early and late imaging related outcome. Ann Neurol 46:70–78, 1999

Vasa RA, Grados M, Slomine B, et al: Neuroimaging correlates of anxiety after pediatric traumatic brain injury. Biol Psychiatry 55:208–216, 2004

Victoroff J, Mack WJ, Grafton ST, et al: A method to improve interrater reliability of visual inspection of brain MRI scans in dementia. Neurology 44:2267–2276, 1994

Vos PE, Van Voskuilen AC, Beems T, et al: Evaluation of the traumatic coma data bank computed tomography classification for severe head injury. J Neurotrauma 18:649–655, 2001

Wakana S, Jiang H, Nagae-Poetscher LM, et al: Fiber tract-based atlas of human white matter anatomyq. Radiology 230:77–87, 2004

Wallesch C-W, Curio N, Galazky I, et al: The neuropsychology of blunt head injury in the early postacute stage: effects of focal lesions and diffuse axonal injury. J Neurotrauma 18:11–20, 2001

Wilson JTL, Wiedmann KD, Hadley DM, et al: Early and late magnetic resonance imaging and neuropsychological outcome after head injury. J Neurol Neurosurg Psychiatry 51:391–396, 1988

Wood DG, Bigler ED: Diencephalic changes in traumatic brain injury: relationship to sensory perceptual function. Brain Res Bull 38:545–549, 1995

Yount R, Raschke KA, Biru M, et al: Traumatic brain injury and atrophy of the cingulate gyrus. J Neuropsychiatry Clin Neurosci 14:416–423, 2002

Appendix 5–1

Summary of quantitative magnetic resonance studies of regions affected by traumatic brain injury

Brain structure or regions of interest	Atrophy	References
Total brain volume	***	6,8,11,19,26,27,29,32,35,38,39,42–44,54–56
Lobular volume		—
Frontal	***	3,11,31,32,41,46,51
Temporal	***	11,16,21,23,25,33,39,49,50
Ventricular system		19,27,41,51
Lateral ventricle	**	11,12,13,17,18,20,37,48
Anterior (frontal)	***	12,13,17
Body	***	12,13,17
Posterior (occipital)	***	12,13,17
Inferior (temporal)	***	12,13,17,41
III Ventricle	**	27,41
IV Ventricle	*	—
Basal ganglia	*	7,39,40
Caudate nucleus	*	1,9,40
Putamen	*	2,40
Globus pallidus		2,40
Diencephalon		—
Thalamus	*	2,4,34,52
Hypothalamus	*	2,4,10,36,47,52
Limbic system		—
Amygdala	**	11,29
Hippocampus	**	5,14–16
Fornix	*	22,24,25
Mammillary body	*	22,25
Anterior thalamus	*	—
Cingulate gyrus	*	53
Midbrain		
Cerebral peduncle	*	22,25
Hindbrain		—
Cerebellum	*	24
Tracts		—
Internal capsule	*	24,28
Corticospinal	*	24
Corpus callosum	***	24,28,30,31,39,51

Note. * = minimal; ** = moderate; *** = major.

References

1. Anderson CV, Bigler ED: The role of caudate nucleus and corpus callosum atrophy in trauma-induced anterior horn dilation. Brain Inj 9:565–569, 1994

2. Anderson CV, Bigler ED: Ventricular dilation, cortical atrophy, and neuropsychological outcome following traumatic brain injury. J Neuropsychiatry Clin Neurosci 7:42–48, 1995

3. Anderson CV, Bigler ED, Blatter DD: Frontal lobe lesions, diffuse damage, and neuropsychological functioning in traumatic brain-injured patients. J Clin Exp Neuropsychol 17:900–908, 1995

4. Anderson CV, Wood DG, Bigler ED, et al: Lesion volume, injury severity, and thalamic integrity following head injury. J Neurotrauma 13:35–40, 1996

5. Arciniegas DB, Topkoff JL, Rojas DC, et al: Reduced hippocampal volume in association with p50 nonsuppression following traumatic brain injury. J Neuropsychiatry Clin Neurosci 13:213–221, 2001

6. Arfanakis K, Haughton VM, Carew JD, et al: Diffusion tensor MR imaging in diffuse axonal injury. AJNR Am J Neuroradiol 23:794–802, 2002

7. Ariza M, Junque C, Mataro M, et al: Neuropsychological correlates of basal ganglia and medial temporal lobe NAA/Cho reductions in traumatic brain injury. Arch Neurol 61:541–544, 2004

8. Bagley LJ, Grossman RI, Galetta SL, et al: Characterization of white matter lesions in multiple sclerosis and traumatic brain injury as revealed by magnetization transfer contour plots. AJNR Am J Neuroradiol 20:977–981, 1999

9. Barker LH, Bigler ED, Johnson SC, et al: Polysubstance abuse and traumatic brain injury: quantitative magnetic resonance imaging and neuropsychological outcome in older adolescents and young adults. J Int Neuropsychol Soc 5:593–608, 1999

10. Beresford T, Arciniegas D, Rojas D, et al: Hippocampal to pituitary volume ratio: a specific measure of reciprocal neuroendocrine alterations in alcohol dependence. J Stud Alcohol 60:586–588, 1999

11. Bigler ED: Neuroimaging in pediatric traumatic head injury: diagnostic considerations and relationships to neurobehavioral outcome. J Head Trauma Rehabil 14:70–87, 1999

12. Bigler ED, Paver S, Cullum CM, et al: Ventricular enlargement, cortical atrophy and neuropsychological performance following head injury. Int J Neurosci 24:295–298, 1984

13. Bigler ED, Kurth S, Blatter D, et al: Degenerative changes in traumatic brain injury: post-injury magnetic resonance identified ventricular expansion compared to pre-injury levels. Brain Res Bull 28:651–653, 1992

14. Bigler ED, Blatter DD, Johnson SC, et al: Traumatic brain injury, alcohol and quantitative neuroimaging: preliminary findings. Brain Inj 10:197–206, 1996

15. Bigler ED, Johnson SC, Anderson CV, et al: Traumatic brain injury and memory: the role of hippocampal atrophy. Neuropsychology 10:333–342, 1996

16. Bigler ED, Anderson CV, Blatter DD: Temporal lobe morphology in normal aging and traumatic brain injury. AJNR Am J Neuroradiol 23:255–266, 2002

17. Blatter DD, Bigler ED, Gale SD, et al: MR-based brain and cerebrospinal fluid measurement after traumatic brain injury: correlation with neuropsychological outcome. AJNR Am J Neuroradiol 18:1–10, 1997

18. Bowen JM, Clark E, Bigler ED, et al: Childhood traumatic brain injury: neuropsychological status at the time of hospital discharge. Dev Med Child Neurol 39:17–25, 1997

19. Bramlett HM, Dietrich WD: Quantitative structural changes in white and gray matter 1 year following traumatic brain injury in rats. Acta Neuropathologica 103:607–614, 2002

20. Cullum CM, Bigler ED: Ventricle size, cortical atrophy and the relationship with neuropsychological status in closed head injury: a quantitative analysis. J Clin Exp Neuropsychol 8:437–452, 1986

21. Diaz-Arrastia R, Agostini MA, Frol AB, et al: Neurophysiologic and neuroradiologic features of intractable epilepsy after traumatic brain injury in adults. Arch Neurol 57:1611–1616, 2000

22. Gale SD, Burr RB, Bigler ED, et al: Fornix degeneration and memory in traumatic brain injury. Brain Res Bull 32:345–349, 1993

23. Gale SD, Johnson SC, Bigler ED, et al: Traumatic brain injury and temporal horn enlargement: correlates with tests of intelligence and memory. Neuropsychiatry Neuropsychol Behav Neurol 7:160–165, 1994

24. Gale SD, Johnson SC, Bigler ED, et al: Nonspecific white matter degeneration following traumatic brain injury. J Int Neuropsychol Soc 1:17–28, 1995

25. Gale SD, Johnson SJ, Bigler ED, et al: Trauma induced temporal horn dilation: neuropsychologic correlates. JINS 1:369–370, 1995

26. Govindaraju V, Gauger GE, Manley GT, et al: Volumetric proton spectroscopic imaging of mild traumatic brain injury. AJNR Am J Neuroradiol 25:730–737, 2004

27. Groswasser Z, Reider G II, Schwab K, et al: Quantitative imaging in late TBI, part II: cognition and work after closed and penetrating head injury: a report of the Vietnam head injury study. Brain Inj 16:681–690, 2002

28. Huisman TA, Schwamm LH, Schaefer PW, et al: Diffusion tensor imaging as potential biomarker of white matter injury in diffuse axonal injury. AJNR Am J Neuroradiol 25:370–376, 2004

29. Jantzen KJ, Anderson B, Steinberg FL, et al: A prospective functional MR imaging study of mild traumatic brain injury in college football players. AJNR Am J Neuroradiol 25:738–745, 2004

30. Johnson SC, Bigler ED, Burr RB, et al: White matter atrophy, ventricular dilation, and intellectual functioning following traumatic brain injury. Neuropsychology 8:307–315, 1994

31. Johnson SC, Pinkston JB, Bigler ED, et al: Corpus callosum morphology in normal controls and TBI: sex differences, mechanisms of injury, and neuropsychological correlates. Neuropsychology 10:408–415, 1996

32. Jorge RE, Robinson RG, Moser D, et al: Major depression following traumatic brain injury. Arch Gen Psychiatry 61:42–50, 2004

33. Kumar R, Gupta RK, Husain M, et al: Magnetization transfer MR imaging in patients with posttraumatic epilepsy. AJNR Am J Neuroradiol 24:218–224, 2003

34. Kurth SM, Bigler ED, Blatter DD: Neuropsychological outcome and quantitative image analysis of acute hemorrhage in traumatic brain injury: preliminary findings. Brain Inj 8:489–500, 1994

35. Levine B, Cabeza R, McIntosh AR, et al: Functional reorganisation of memory after traumatic brain injury: a study with H(2)(15)0 positron emission tomography. J Neurol Neurosurg Psychiatry 73:173–181, 2002

36. MacKenzie JD, Siddiqi F, Babb JS, et al: Brain atrophy in mild or moderate traumatic brain injury: a longitudinal quantitative analysis. AJNR Am J Neuroradiol 23:1509–1515, 2002

37. Masel BE: Rehabilitation and hypopituitarism after traumatic brain injury. Growth Horm IGF Res 14 (suppl A):108–113, 2004

38. Massman PJ, Bigler ED, Cullum CM, et al: The relationship between cortical atrophy and ventricular volume in Alzheimer's disease and closed head injury. Int J Neurosci 30:87–99, 1986

39. McGowan JC, Yang JH, Plotkin RC, et al: Magnetization transfer imaging in the detection of injury associated with mild head trauma. AJNR Am J Neuroradiol 21:875–880, 2000

40. Pierallini A, Pantano P, Fantozzi LM, et al: Correlation between MRI findings and long-term outcome in patients with severe brain trauma. Neuroradiology 42:860–867, 2002

41. Primus EA, Bigler ED, Anderson CV, et al: Corpus striatum and traumatic brain injury. Brain Inj 11:577–586, 1997

42. Reider-Groswasser I, Groswasser Z, Ommaya AK, et al: Quantitative imaging in late traumatic brain injury, part I: late imaging parameters in closed and penetrating head injuries. Brain Inj 16:517–525, 2002

43. Scheid R, Preul C, Gruber O, et al: Diffuse axonal injury associated with chronic traumatic brain injury: evidence from T2*-weighted gradient-echo imaging at 3 T. AJNR Am J Neuroradiol 24:1049–1056, 2003

44. Shanmuganathan K, Gullapalli RP, Mirvis SE, et al: Whole-brain apparent diffusion coefficient in traumatic brain injury: correlation with Glasgow Coma Scale score. AJNR Am J Neuroradiol 25:539–544, 2004

45. Sinson GP, Bagley LJ, Cecil KM, et al: Magnetization transfer imaging and proton MR spectroscopy in the evaluation of axonal injury: correlation with clinical outcome after traumatic brain injury. AJNR Am J Neuroradiol 22:143–151, 2001

46. Tate D, Bigler ED: Fornix and hippocampal atrophy in traumatic brain injury. Learn Mem 7:442–446, 2000

47. Tateno A, Jorge RE, Robinson RG: Clinical correlates of aggressive behavior after traumatic brain injury. J Neuropsychiatry Clin Neurosci 15:155–160, 2003

48. Thorley RR, Wertsch JJ, Klingbeil GE: Acute hypothalamic instability in traumatic brain injury: a case report. Arch Phys Med Rehab 82:246–249, 2001

49. Turkheimer E, Yeo RA, Bigler ED: Basic relations among lesion location, lesion volume and neuropsychological performance. Neuropsychologia 28:1011–1019, 1990

50. Umile EM, Sandel ME, Alavi A, et al: Dynamic imaging in mild traumatic brain injury: support for the theory of medial temporal vulnerability. Arch Phys Med Rehab 83:1506–1513, 2002

51. Vasa RA, Grados M, Slomine B, et al: Neuroimaging correlates of anxiety after pediatric traumatic brain injury. Biol Psychiatry 55:208–216, 2004

52. Verger K, Junque C, Levin HS, et al: Correlation of atrophy measures on MRI with neuropsychological sequelae in children and adolescents with traumatic brain injury. Brain Inj 15:211–221, 2001

53. Wood DG, Bigler ED: Diencephalic changes in traumatic brain injury: relationship to sensory perceptual function. Brain Res Bull 38:545–549, 1995

54. Yount R, Raschke KA, Biru M, et al: Traumatic brain injury and atrophy of the cingulate gyrus. J Neuropsychiatry Clin Neurosci 14:416–423, 2002

55. Zhang L, Ravdin LD, Relkin N, et al: Increased diffusion in the brain of professional boxers: a preclinical sign of traumatic brain injury? AJNR Am J Neuroradiol 24:52–57, 2003

56. Ariza M, Mataro M, Poca MA, et al: Influence of extraneurological insults on ventricular enlargement and neuropsychological functioning after moderate and severe traumatic brain injury. J Neurotrauma 21:864–876, 2004

6 Functional Imaging

Karen E. Anderson, M.D.

Katherine H. Taber, Ph.D.

Robin A. Hurley, M.D.

AS TECHNOLOGY RAPIDLY evolved in the last century, our ability to look into the brain and study its function increased exponentially. Structural imaging techniques such as skull X rays, computed tomography (CT), and magnetic resonance imaging (MRI), which provide information about the neuroanatomy of the skull, brain tissue, and blood vessels, have proved immensely helpful in assessment of extent of brain injury and in following the medical sequelae of traumatic brain injury (TBI), such as edema, intracranial bleeding, and degeneration. With improvements in technology, these tools provide increasing detail about bone and tissue injury sustained in TBI and many other medical conditions. However, these methods cannot assess "function," or underlying cerebral metabolic rate (CMR) and cerebral blood flow (CBF), in the brain. Subtle brain changes due to TBI that can affect a patient's ability to function at a normal level may not appear on structural imaging.

Functional brain imaging uses newer methods to capture brain activity as reflected by regional CMR (rCMR) or regional CBF (rCBF) (Table 6–1). Most clinical functional brain imaging in TBI is currently performed with single-photon emission CT (SPECT) or positron emission tomography (PET). In both techniques, a radioactive isotope is injected into the patient. Its uptake is measured to give an indication of brain metabolism or blood flow. Another technique, functional MRI (fMRI), makes use of the magnetic qualities of oxygenated blood to create rapid images of brain blood flow. Magnetic resonance spectroscopy (MRS) provides information on brain metabolites, which may indicate changes in tissue, such as cell death. An advantage of both fMRI and MRS is that neither of them requires injection of ionizing radiation. These four modalities represent the main functional imaging techniques

available at this time. The ultimate hope is that the use of these imaging methods, along with others not described here, will allow clinicians to more accurately assess damage to the brain's ability to function and predict potential for rehabilitation, as well as follow the brain's recovery of function with an objective measure. Use of functional imaging in the assessment of TBI has increased since the 1980s. The actual contribution of these modalities to improvement in clinical care and outcome, however, is not yet clear.

Despite limitations, functional imaging continues to hold promise as a tool for evaluation of neuropsychiatric sequelae of TBI. We begin this chapter with a discussion of how to evaluate the various types of studies available. We then review the literature for each modality, with an emphasis on controlled studies with clear outcome measures that address the use of functional imaging for clinical assessment of TBI. We also discuss studies that use functional imaging to examine possible neuropathological contributions to behavioral changes after TBI. SPECT and PET, which are the clinically relevant modalities, receive the most attention. Finally, we review recent work with fMRI and MRS, which may have promise for future clinical applications.

Understanding the Literature

As new techniques emerge, clinicians must be able to evaluate current research and critically review published studies. This section is a brief overview of the most critical factors in evaluation of research in functional brain imaging in TBI and in many other conditions. There are few controlled studies of the use of functional brain imaging for assessment and treatment of TBI patients. Many studies

TABLE 6–1.   Brain imaging techniques

Method	What is usually measured	Advantages	Approximate cost per study ($)	Time to complete study (minutes)	Limitations/issues
SPECT	Blood flow	Widely available; relatively inexpensive	800	≤30, depending on tracer	Requires ionizing radiation; resolution limited
PET	Metabolism or blood flow	Superior to SPECT for anatomical resolution; can measure metabolism	2,000	30–40 for FDG; 5 for ^{15}O	Requires ionizing radiation; not widely available
fMRI	Blood flow	No ionizing radiation; good anatomical resolution; repeat studies can be done quickly	Not applicable for TBI	Generally 45–60	Currently research-only for TBI; cognitive activation task must be used
MRS	Change in brain metabolites	No ionizing radiation; noninvasive neurochemical measurements	Not applicable for TBI	Generally 45–60	Currently research-only for TBI

Note.   FDG, fluorodeoxyglucose; fMRI, functional magnetic resonance imaging; MRS, magnetic resonance spectroscopy; PET, positron emission tomography; SPECT, single-photon emission computed tomography; TBI, traumatic brain injury.

use data from functional scans originally obtained for clinical purposes, meaning that imaging data were not collected in a systematic, uniform manner. In existing studies, standardized ratings of scans are the exception. Also, because the patients who are being studied must all be treated with the optimal therapies available at the time of the study, there are few opportunities for objective evaluations of treatment with functional imaging (because of the obvious ethical concerns). When TBI patient data are compared with those from noninjured control subjects, care must be taken to ensure that control subjects are matched to the patient groups with regard to important variables such as age, handedness, sex, and general health, all of which can affect brain blood flow and metabolism. As reviewed in the sections of this chapter that address abnormalities found by the use of functional brain imaging modalities in psychiatric conditions other than TBI, the presence of active psychiatric symptomatology, common in TBI, can also affect brain activity. Finally, many other factors seen in TBI such as bony injury, edema, changes in white matter integrity, and diffuse axonal injury may complicate interpretation of functional imaging findings acquired using any of the various modalities (see McAllister et al. 2001b for a review of these factors in mild TBI).

When reviewing the literature on functional imaging in TBI, the clinician must make important distinctions between the type of information acquired in resting scans—during which the patient lies motionless with eyes closed, sometimes in a darkened room—and the data acquired during performance of a cognitive activation task, such as memorization of words presented on a computer screen, which allows for assessment of function in a (relatively) isolated domain, such as language, spatial memory, or performance of a simple motor task. All functional imaging studies are limited in that other factors such as physiological changes unrelated to what is being assessed are also present. The use of an activation paradigm may help increase activity in a certain network of structures that are the focus of study. Activation studies are often limited to a single assessment at a point after TBI when recovery is believed to have occurred (sometimes measured by improvement on performance of neuropsychological tests). Fewer studies use pre- and postrecovery scans, which offer the benefit of allowing for comparison in the same patients. For activation studies, controlling for level of education, fluency in the language in which stimuli are presented, and other demographic variables may also be important because these factors may influence the subject's ability to perform the activation task and, ultimately, the functional imaging results.

Single-Photon Emission Computed Tomography

SPECT is a functional imaging modality that is used to determine brain blood flow based on the distribution of a radiopharmaceutical agent in the brain. A radiotracer is injected into a patient's vein. As the tracer decays, it emits a photon, which is detected and recorded by the SPECT gamma camera (Figure 6–1). The computer reconstructs these detections to produce a tomographic image of activity throughout the brain, similar to the "slices" produced by CT or MRI examination. Like MRI, coronal, sagittal, and axial SPECT views as well as three-dimensional reconstructions are available. This image can be visually interpreted by a nuclear medicine specialist and/or analyzed statistically using various software programs.

Older SPECT cameras, which were used for many of the studies discussed in the section below, Studies Using SPECT and Structural Imaging, had limited detectors and produced poor quality images (Figure 6–2). More credence should be given to studies performed with the newer "tri-

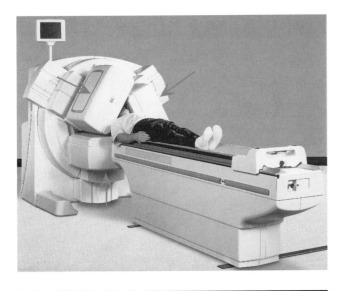

FIGURE 6–1.   Procedure for obtaining a SPECT scan.
The same scanner is used for imaging many body systems, including brain, heart, bone, and lung. Details of the procedure differ. Before brain imaging, the patient receives an intravenous injection of the radioactive tracer while lying in a darkened room. After a short period in the darkened room that allows the tracer to distribute through the brain, the patient is ready to be scanned. The tracer distribution is stable for several hours, thus allowing a considerable time window for scanning to occur. After the patient is positioned on the scanner table, the gamma camera head(s) are moved in as close to the patient's head as possible, as illustrated (IREX, Philips Medical Systems, Andover, MA). The three cameras of this multidetector system are indicated by arrows. The camera(s) rotate around the patient's head during the imaging examination. Data are collected from multiple positions as the camera(s) rotate around the patient's head. The data are transmitted to a computer that produces tomographic images in the desired plane(s) of section.
Source.   Picture courtesy of Philips Medical Systems.

ple head" cameras. These provide a resolution of approximately 1 cm, allowing assessment of much smaller structures than those assessed with older equipment (Figures 6–3 and 6–4). Use of companion structural imaging studies (CT or MRI) in the same patient can provide greater precision of anatomical location. This method is called "coregistration" of the structural and functional images.

Tracers

The most commonly used radiotracer for clinical SPECT is technetium-99m-hexamethylpropyleneamine oxime (^{99m}Tc-HMPAO), which accumulates in endothelial cell membranes a few minutes after injection. Concentrations of this tracer are thus highest in regions receiving the most plentiful blood flow shortly after the injection and remain so for up to 24 hours. Because of this long half-life, multiple scans can be performed after one injection, which can be helpful if the patient moves during a scan. However, because the tracer is taken up at a certain time, the location of tracer concentration in the brain does not change (e.g., for research purposes, one could not perform a vision activation study and then an auditory study on one patient using the same tracer injection).

Ligand studies, in which a radioactive ligand (marker) binds with a particular receptor, transporter, or protein, are becoming an important tool in both SPECT and PET and could contribute to future understanding of neurotransmitter change during cognitive processes. For example, if administration of a ligand that binds specifically to one neurotransmitter type is followed by a scan, and then an activation task is performed, a follow-up scan could potentially provide information on how much ligand was displaced by the endogenous neurotransmitter, suggesting involvement of that system in the task. Receptor studies (e.g., examining benzodiazepine receptor function in alcohol dependency [Lingford-Hughes et al. 1998] or dopamine transporter function in schizophrenia [Abi Dargham et al. 2000]) have also been conducted with SPECT but are not discussed in detail in this chapter (see Table 6–2 for a review of commonly used, U.S. Food and Drug Administration [FDA]-approved SPECT tracers). Similarly, these methods could be used in TBI to study disruption of neurotransmitter systems after brain injury. However, interpretation of these results is still in the preliminary stages (Laruelle 2000). We limit our discussion in this chapter to blood flow studies because they are the most clinically relevant at this time.

Practical Considerations

SPECT scans can be obtained in most large medical centers and are substantially more affordable than PET. For clinical

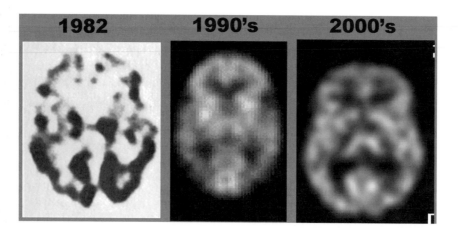

FIGURE 6–2.   SPECT imaging then and now.

Axial single-photon emission computed tomography images acquired in 1982, early 1990s, and early 2000s of brain. Note the significant improvement in resolution since the 1980s.

Source.   SPECT images (1982) reprinted by permission of the Society of Nuclear Medicine from Hill TC, et al: "Initial Experience With SPECT (Single Photon Computerized Tomography) of the Brain Using *N*-isopropyl I-123 *p*-iodoamphetamine: Concise Communication." *Journal of Nuclear Medicine* 23:193, 1982. SPECT images (early 1900s and 2000s) courtesy of Philips Medical Systems.

use, a resting SPECT scan of the whole brain is generally ordered. Intravenous radioactive tracer is injected into the patient a few minutes before scanning, preferably in a quiet, controlled environment to minimize blood flow changes due to anxiety and presence of loud noise. The patient should be able to lie still in a supine position in the scanner for the duration of the scan—up to half an hour. If the patient is too agitated to remain still, sedation may be given *after* tracer injection to minimize effects on the uptake and distribution of tracer. With the most commonly used SPECT tracer (i.e., ^{99m}Tc-HMPAO), the concentrations of tracer remain stable in the brain for up to a day, so the patient can be imaged several hours after the injection is given. Because the patient is exposed to ionizing radiation with this technique, consideration must be given to the number and recency of prior scans using radioactive tracers.

Indications

At this time, no clear guidelines exist for use of SPECT in evaluation and treatment of TBI. Clinicians generally order SPECT scans when brain injury is suspected but not seen on structural studies, or when structural studies do not indicate damage extensive enough to explain a patient's deficits.

Limitations

SPECT studies typically provide information only about relative CBF, not absolute CBF as can be evaluated with

PET. The xenon gas–inhalation technique produces quantitative CBF values, but the images are of relatively poor quality and low resolution compared with those obtained by PET, as discussed later in the section Positron Emission Tomography. There are no SPECT tracers for the study of cerebral metabolism. Interpretation is often performed by visual rating of scans for abnormalities rather than by use of statistical methods, which introduces problems inherent in the use of subjective, nonstandardized ratings. This circumstance introduces methodological difficulties, because interrater reliability cannot be standardized. Comparison of results from different studies becomes increasingly problematic because some groups may report only the presence of overall abnormality whereas others report the number of individual lesions seen in each scan (see Herscovitch 1996 for a detailed review of these issues).

Overview of Abnormal Findings in Other Psychiatric Disorders

There are some research applications of SPECT in psychiatry. It is sometimes useful in helping differentiate causes of dementia. It has also been used in small studies of headaches, pain, and sleep disorders. SPECT's use for psychiatric evaluation or prognosis in other conditions is still a matter of debate. Frontal lobe hypoperfusion is seen in most studies of depression, often in the lateral prefrontal cortex. Work with anxiety disorder patients has led to the discovery of abnormally increased flow in the anterior

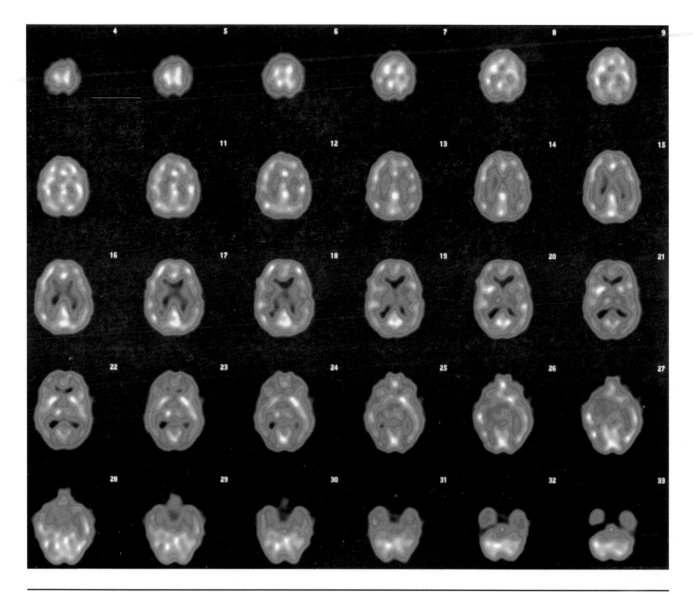

FIGURE 6–3. **Serial axial SPECT images of a normal adult brain.**

Reference numbers for brain slice order are shown next to each slice.

cingulate and orbitofrontal cortices in some patients with obsessive-compulsive disorder. Schizophrenic patients have been reported to have frontal cortex flow loss, along with basal ganglia and temporal lobe deficits. SPECT study abnormalities have also been seen in patients with substance abuse, sleep disorders, pain syndromes, and headaches. SPECT is more frequently used in neurological practice for assessment of patients with stroke, epilepsy, and ischemic attacks.

In evaluation of dementia, a pattern of bilateral posterior temporal and/or parietal decreases in blood flow (i.e., hypoperfusion) is suggestive of Alzheimer's disease (AD). However, a similar pattern of perfusion loss may be seen in Parkinson's disease patients who have dementia (Pizzolato et al. 1988). Reports of sensitivity and specificity of SPECT for detection of blood flow

changes related to AD vary. Bonte et al. (1997) correlated autopsy diagnosis, the gold standard for determining cause of dementia, with SPECT findings. They found that SPECT showed 86% sensitivity and 73% specificity for detection of AD. Jobst et al. (1998) found similar results with histological confirmation of diagnosis. Masterman et al. (1997) found SPECT to be less useful for differentiating probable AD from other dementias. In their study, sensitivity was 75% and specificity was 52% when comparing probable AD versus unlikely AD groups. Ishii et al. (1996) found a high sensitivity but low specificity for AD prediction with SPECT (95.2% and 56.9%, respectively). In some cases, SPECT may also be useful in distinguishing AD from vascular, frontotemporal, or Lewy body dementia (see Van Heertum et al. 2001 for a review).

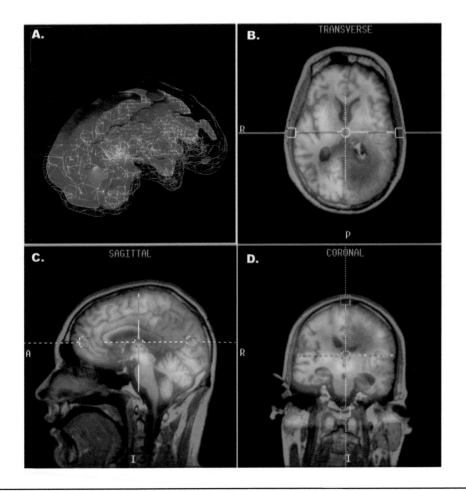

FIGURE 6–4.   Current SPECT imaging capabilities.

Three-dimensional reconstruction of SPECT results obtained 2 months post–traumatic brain injury (A). Areas of normal blood flow are red. Note the absence of flow in the right anterior temporal and frontal lobes (foreground), resulting in visualization of the left temporal and frontal lobes from the medial side. Seeing blood flow deficits in three dimensions improves appreciation of the extent of lesions. Merging blood flow data with anatomical imaging also improves identification of areas of abnormality. Sectional SPECT images overlaid on T1-weighted magnetic resonance images (B–D).

Source.   B–D, pictures courtesy of Philips Medical Systems.

Imaging work with migraine patients has shown variable results (see Cutrer et al. 2000 for a review). Interhemispheric asymmetry in superior frontal and occipital cortices of migraine patients has been reported (Mirza et al. 1998; see Aurora and Welch 2000 for a review of imaging in migraine). Cluster headache patients also show abnormalities on SPECT during experimental application of painful stimuli; the authors suggest that such ab-

TABLE 6–2.   U.S. Food and Drug Administration–approved, commonly used tracers for SPECT

Tracer	Parameter measured	Comments
^{99m}Tc-HMPAO	Blood flow	Most commonly used clinical tracer for SPECT. Slow washout, so scan can be done long after injection of tracer.
^{123}I-IMP	Blood flow	Distributes quickly in brain, so scan must be done within 1 hour of injection.
^{201}Tl	Blood flow	Used for cardiac studies and assessment of malignancies throughout the body.

Note. ^{99m}Tc-HMPAO=technetium-99m-hexamethylpropyleneamine oxime; ^{123}I-IMP=iodine-123 *N*-isopropyl-*p*-iodoamphetamine; ^{201}Tl= thallium-201.

normalities may reflect a modification of pain-detection systems (Di Piero et al. 1997). Studies of chronic pain and fibromyalgia have reported decreased thalamic flow (Mountz et al. 1995; Nakabeppu et al. 2001), which some groups suggest could be linked to low threshold for pain perception (Mountz et al. 1995). SPECT abnormalities have been reported in limited studies of primary insomnia (Smith et al. 2002), narcolepsy (Asenbaum et al. 1995), and rapid eye movement–sleep behavioral disorder (Shirakawa et al. 2002).

SPECT has been used for evaluation of other psychiatric conditions with varying results. Studies of depressed patients with SPECT have been inconclusive. There is some consensus that frontal lobe flow deficits are seen in patients with depression, usually affecting the lateral prefrontal cortex. SPECT studies have shown hypoperfusion of the prefrontal, temporal, and cingulate cortices and left caudate nucleus in depression (Devous 1992; Van Heertum and O'Connell 1991). The heterogeneous spectrum of patients seen with depression is probably a factor in the lack of consistency in these studies.

SPECT studies with obsessive-compulsive disorder patients have generally shown abnormally high blood flow (i.e., hyperperfusion) in the anterior cingulate and orbitofrontal cortices, with basal ganglia hyperperfusion also reported (Hoehn-Saric et al. 1991b; Machlin et al. 1991). A pre- and posttreatment SPECT study showed that perfusion normalized after successful treatment (Hoehn-Saric et al. 1991a). Hypoperfusion of the frontal lobes, caudate, and thalamus has also been found (Lucey et al. 1995).

In schizophrenia patients, SPECT most frequently shows frontal cortex hypoperfusion, especially during activation studies; basal ganglia and temporal lobe flow loss has also been reported (Woods 1992). However, medication status (whether the patient is taking or not taking medication) and presence of positive or negative symptoms may affect SPECT findings (Sabri et al. 1997).

Global, diffuse hypoperfusion has been shown in patients who abuse alcohol and those who abuse cocaine (Devous 1992; Holman et al. 1991). Blood flow abnormalities due to cocaine abuse may resolve after cessation of drug abuse (Holman et al. 1993). Abuse of other substances may produce similar blood flow deficits. Psychogenic disorders have been the subject of limited study with SPECT to date (Garcia-Campayo et al. 2001; Tiihonen et al. 1995; Yazici and Kostakoglu 1998), with heterogeneous results such as hyper- or hypoperfusion in sensorimotor, parietal, frontal, temporal, or cerebellar regions. In other work, Vuilleumier et al. (2001) found decreased flow to the basal ganglia and thalamus contralateral to the side of sensorimotor deficits in a study of seven patients with psychogenic symptoms that resolved after

recovery of function, suggesting failure to modulate voluntary motor function in psychogenic illness. The variability and range of psychiatric conditions that may cause blood flow changes provide a cautionary note in interpretation of SPECT and other imaging studies of TBI patients, who often have one or more comorbid psychiatric conditions.

Overview of Abnormal SPECT Findings in TBI

Despite the promise of SPECT as an accessible, low-cost method for the study of brain activity after TBI and during recovery from injury, there are relatively few methodologically sound studies in the literature. There are even fewer studies incorporating other methods of assessment, such as neuropsychological testing and standardized ratings for recovery, in conjunction with SPECT for evaluation of TBI.

Studies Using SPECT and Structural Imaging

SPECT has been used in combination with structural imaging in numerous studies (Abdel-Dayem et al. 1987; Audenaert et al. 2003; Gray et al. 1992; Ichise et al. 1994; Jacobs et al. 1994; Kesler et al. 2000; Newton et al. 1992; Oder et al. 1992; Prayer et al. 1993; Roper et al. 1991; Umile et al. 2002). It should be noted that in these studies, the SPECT scan was not coregistered with a structural image. Instead, the scans were interpreted separately, and functional results were compared with those from structural modalities.

In general, more abnormalities are seen on SPECT scans than on structural imaging scans such as CT and MRI in studies of patients with TBI over a wide range of recency and severity (Figures 6–5, 6–6, 6–7) (Abdel-Dayem et al. 1987; Audenaert et al. 2003; Gray et al. 1992; Ichise et al. 1994; Jacobs et al. 1994; Newton et al. 1992; Roper et al. 1991). MRI is generally superior to CT for visualization of anatomical regions, and thus more lesions are usually seen with MRI than CT. Factors such as bony artifact limit CT studies in areas of particular interest in TBI, such as the temporal lobes. Both MRI and SPECT results were found to be abnormal in a study of severe TBI patients with normal CT scans (Prayer et al. 1993). However, lesions seen with SPECT do not always correlate with abnormalities seen on MRI (Newton et al. 1992; Prayer et al. 1993). A large, recent study of patients with mild, moderate, or severe TBI (average of 3 years postinjury) found 67% agreement between SPECT and MRI on location of brain injury (Kesler et al. 2000). The very limited research in this area to date suggests that SPECT may be useful in cases of mild TBI in which there is no evidence of ab-

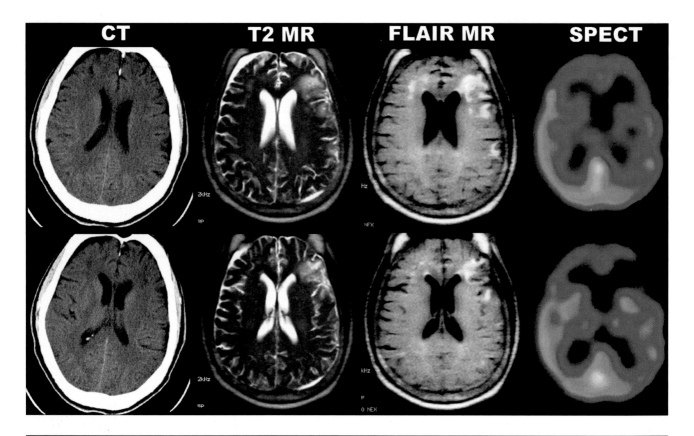

FIGURE 6–5.   Early subacute presentation of traumatic brain injury on SPECT.

A 61-year-old man had a single-motor-vehicle collision with a tree. This resulted in severe trauma with loss of consciousness requiring neurosurgical interventions. After several weeks of hospitalization, the patient was released. Within a few days, the patient's family brought him to a psychiatric emergency service with agitation, incoherence, cognitive impairment, and psychosis. Two different sectional levels in the brain are illustrated with companion axial CT, T2-weighted MR, FLAIR MR, and SPECT. Note that the injury is more apparent on the FLAIR images than on the T2-weighted MR and CT images. The true extent of the injury, however, can be appreciated only on the SPECT images. FLAIR=fluid attenuated inversion recovery.

normality on a structural scan. However, because structural scans and SPECT are both generally interpreted by subjective visual analyses, direct comparison of these differing modalities is difficult. It should be noted that few of the SPECT studies reviewed in this discussion used noninjured control comparison groups. One of the studies did have a control comparison group; Ichise et al. (1994) found neuroimaging abnormalities in a small number of noninjured control subjects, which the researchers attributed to possible underlying, unrecognized neurological abnormalities. This circumstance raises the issue of the importance of careful control selection in studies with any imaging modality.

The limited work that has been done at this time suggests that a normal SPECT scan after TBI is predictive of a good outcome (Abdel-Dayem et al. 1987; Jacobs et al. 1994; Oder et al. 1992). In one study, a negative initial SPECT, determined by expert visual rating, was 97% predictive of good clinical outcome for mild and

moderate TBI within 4 weeks of injury (Jacobs et al. 1994). Good clinical outcome in this study was judged according to neurological examination findings, questioning on postconcussive symptoms, and unspecified memory and concentration tests. Clinical evaluation for outcome was performed on all subjects, but only those with an initial abnormal scan received a follow-up SPECT scan. An initial SPECT rated as abnormal was a predictor of poor outcome only 59% of the time. At follow-up, 95% of patients with clinical evidence of TBI sequelae continued to show abnormal perfusion on SPECT. Abdel-Dayem et al. (1987) used SPECT to study comatose acute TBI patients and noninjured controls. They found that a bad outcome in patients (i.e., death) was related to size, multiplicity, and location of lesions, as rated by two experienced raters. In a study by Oder et al. (1992) of 12 patients in persistent vegetative states after TBI, SPECT global hypoperfusion had a 100% positive predictive value for poor outcome. However, evidence

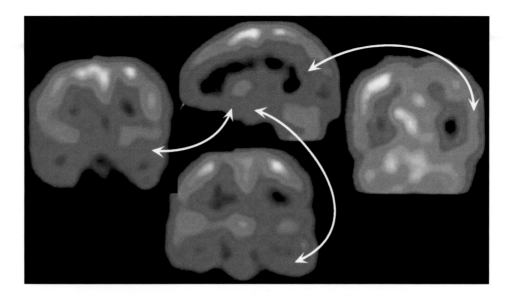

FIGURE 6–6.   Late subacute presentation of traumatic brain injury.

A 24-year-old man had a motor vehicle accident with no loss of consciousness 10 years after a mild head injury. Shortly thereafter, the patient presented with severe cognitive deficits, depression, agitation, aggression, and psychosis. Symptoms were sufficiently severe to require prolonged psychiatric hospitalization. MR examination during this time was normal. Numerous perfusion abnormalities were evident on SPECT scans acquired 2 years later (three coronal and a single sagittal section are illustrated). The most pronounced abnormality was moderately reduced perfusion in the left parietal lobe near the posterior Sylvian fissure and in both temporal lobes. Mildly reduced perfusion was noted in the occipital lobes (left greater than right) and basal ganglia (particularly near the caudate heads). Some of these abnormalities are visible on both the sagittal and coronal images, as indicated by arrows.

of focal flow deficits alone did not reliably predict good long-term outcome. All patients with poor outcome had MRI evidence of diffuse axonal injury, whereas none of those with good outcome showed such injury. Mazzini and others (2003) also found that degree of temporal lobe hypoperfusion on SPECT was one predictor of posttraumatic epilepsy in a series of 143 patients, approximately 19% of whom developed seizures.

Especially in cases of mild TBI, SPECT may show lesions where no abnormalities are seen on structural imaging, which may be helpful in explaining the cause of persistent behavioral changes. However, in some cases, lesions on structural scans are not detected with SPECT. An initial negative SPECT after TBI may be predictive of good clinical outcome; the use of an abnormal scan for prognosis is less clear. It should be noted that little work has been done to elucidate the true relationship between an abnormal scan and objective outcome measures, especially for cases of subtle hypoperfusion.

Studies Using Behavioral Measures

Only a few studies have tried to correlate abnormal cerebral perfusion patterns with behavioral changes after TBI. Behavioral problems are an important clinical confound, and accurate assessments of them are often missing. Use of SPECT for prediction of which patients may

be at risk to develop behavioral problems after TBI has not been explored to date.

Oder et al. (1992), in a study of severe TBI, found a significant correlation between frontal hypoperfusion and disinhibition, left hemisphere hyperperfusion and social isolation, and right hemisphere hypoperfusion and aggression. Varney et al. (1995) examined whether blood flow changes in mild TBI patients—relative to noninjured control subjects—were related to functional difficulties postinjury. Specifically, they studied employment difficulties in those patients who had been consistently employed before TBI and had normal postinjury structural scans. Both patient and control SPECT scans were rated by visual inspection, with the rater blind to whether the scan was from a patient or a control. All control SPECT scans were rated as normal. Two of the mild TBI scans were also rated as normal. The remaining 12 patient SPECT scans demonstrated flow changes, mainly in the anterior mesial temporal lobes and also, in some patients, in orbitofrontal regions. Quantitative analysis was also performed on the SPECT scans, showing hypoperfusion, mainly in the anterior mesial temporal regions, along with some indications of orbitofrontal flow loss in patients with employment difficulties. This study suggests that even mild TBI can have an impact on a patient's functional abilities. These preliminary studies indicate that

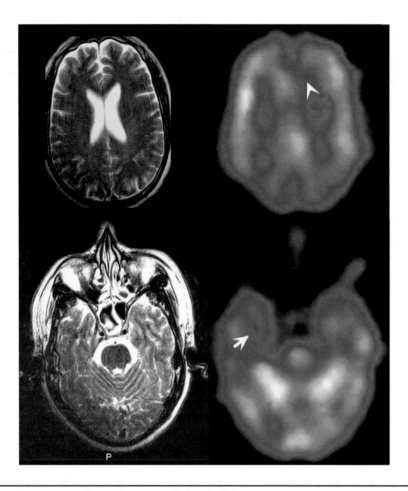

FIGURE 6–7.   Chronic presentation of traumatic brain injury.
A 52-year-old man had a high-impact closed head injury 30 years before scanning. He presented with a 30-year history of emotional incontinence and depression. Additionally, the patient reported a loss of singing ability after the accident. Two different sectional levels in the brain are illustrated with companion axial T2-weighted MR and SPECT. There are minimal white matter changes in the parietal region apparent on the MR. Mildly decreased perfusion is evident in the medial frontal lobes (left greater than right, arrowhead). Moderately decreased perfusion is evident in the right anterior temporal lobe adjacent to the Sylvian fissure (arrow).

SPECT may prove helpful in assessment of behavioral sequelae of TBI.

Studies Using Neuropsychological Assessments

There have been limited comparisons of blood flow changes and performance deficits on neuropsychological testing in TBI patients. SPECT results have not been consistently correlated with neuropsychological test results in most studies. In one study, a relationship was found between perfusion deficits and neuropsychological test performance in only 14 of 120 comparisons (Wiedmann et al. 1989). In a recent small study, Audenaert et al. (2003) found a relationship between location of focal frontal and temporal abnormalities on [57]Co SPECT and deficits in neuropsychological testing in six of eight mild TBI patients. Comparison of 28 mild TBI patients who had long-standing clinical complaints with 20 matched noninjured control subjects by another group found that

hypoperfusion of frontal, left posterior, and some subcortical regions on SPECT was predictive of performance deficits on neuropsychological evaluation. However, other brain regions did not show the same concordance with test results (Bonne et al. 2003). Umile and others (2002) also found that neuropsychological test performance deficits could not be consistently predicted by regional perfusion abnormalities using SPECT and PET in mild TBI patients with persistent postinjury symptoms. In another study, although neuropsychological tests predicted SPECT finding, the converse was not true (Umile et al. 1998). Thus, results have been less than encouraging. At the present time, SPECT cannot be used to predict neuropsychological/cognitive testing deficits.

Only preliminary work has been done to examine whether SPECT and neuropsychological test results can be used in conjunction to improve assessment of progress in rehabilitation. Laatsch et al. (1997, 1999) found flow increases in damaged regions after cognitive rehabilitation in two small studies of patients with varying levels of brain injury severity. However, in the first study (Laatsch et al. 1997) no prerehabilitation SPECT scan was performed; rather, the location of regions with suspected pathology was inferred from neuropsychological test results. If more studies confirm these results, SPECT may be helpful in assessing progress made through rehabilitation programs.

Activation Studies

As yet, no studies have been done using performance of an activation task to engage specific brain areas during SPECT studies of TBI.

Studies Using Comparisons With Other Patient Populations

Masdeu et al. (1994) compared 14 patients with mild TBI and normal brain CT scans with 15 noninjured control subjects and 12 patients with mild human immunodeficiency virus encephalopathy. Based on expert blind visual rating, 10 of the 14 TBI patients were differentiated from noninjured control subjects by both independent raters. No control subjects were misclassified as TBI patients via SPECT results. However, the raters could not reliably differentiate human immunodeficiency virus patients from those with TBI on the basis of SPECT data.

Recommendations

Clinically, SPECT scans may be helpful in assessment of brain function in TBI cases in which behavioral problems or cognitive change affects patient function but no lesion is found on structural imaging. However, a "normal" SPECT scan does not imply lack of pathology. When interpreting SPECT scan results for a particular patient, the clinician must take psychiatric comorbidity into account, because presence of symptoms such as depressed mood can affect SPECT results, as can substance abuse. SPECT abnormalities after TBI have not been shown to clearly correlate with behavioral change or neuropsychological test performance deficits; at this time, SPECT is not useful for evaluation of these problems, except possibly in cases of subtle TBI with behavioral and cognitive sequelae. SPECT research is limited, to date, by lack of standardized, objective measures of SPECT results. Finally, for both clinical purposes and in research studies, SPECT has limited resolution, especially with older cameras. Thus, discrimination of neuroanatomical detail is not possible. Coregistration with a companion structural image may partially correct this problem, but this technique requires sophisticated technology and is not widely used in clinical settings at this time.

Positron Emission Tomography

PET imaging uses a method similar to that used for SPECT but with different radioactive tracers and more sophisticated detection equipment, which has improved with new technologies (Figures 6–8 and 6–9). As with SPECT, the physics behind PET limit its resolution, which is approximately 4 mm on high-quality scanners. Thus, PET images are much clearer and show greater anatomical detail than SPECT images. As in the procedure used with SPECT, a radiotracer is injected into the patient intravenously. As it decays, a positron is released. After collision with an electron, two photons are produced that travel away from each other in a straight line at the speed of light. The photons are detected on opposite sides of the PET scanner simultaneously, and a computerized calculation is performed to pinpoint where in the brain the original positron was located. A record of these detections is made and can be transformed by a computer into a tomographic image (Figure 6–10). Because two photons must be detected at the same instant to be "counted," the technique reduces errors in detection. As with MRI and SPECT, coronal, sagittal, and axial views are available. The images can be visually interpreted but more commonly are analyzed statistically using various software programs.

Tracers

Like SPECT, PET requires the injection of a radioactive tracer but, because of differences in the tracers used, can image either CBF or metabolism. Fluoride 18 (^{18}F) fluorodeoxyglucose (FDG) is the most commonly used tracer for clinical PET scans. It is taken into cells via the glucose transport mechanism, after which it is phosphorylated into FDG-6-phosphate. Because it is not a substrate for the glycolytic process, the FDG-6-phosphate remains trapped in the cell. Thus, scans with FDG produce a measure of glucose metabolism rather than blood flow. A scan performed with FDG generally takes approximately 30–40 minutes. The oxygen 15 (^{15}O) tracer is more commonly used in research; Table 6–3 provides an overview of FDA-approved PET radiotracers. Because of the short half-life, ^{15}O scans are performed within a few minutes of when the patient is correctly positioned and in the scanner. The resolution obtained with ^{15}O tracer is inferior to that obtained with FDG. However, the use of short-acting

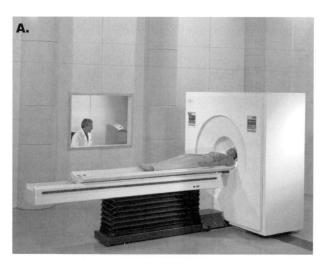
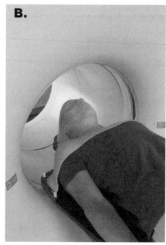

FIGURE 6–8. **Procedure for obtaining a PET scan.**

The patient receives an intravenous injection of the radioactive tracer while lying in a darkened room. After 20–30 minutes are spent in the darkened room to allow the tracer to distribute through the brain, the patient is ready to be scanned (A). Scanning usually begins within 1 hour of tracer injection and requires 30–45 minutes to complete. A headholder is often used to prevent head motion (B).

Source. Pictures courtesy of CTI Molecular Imaging, Inc.

isotopes permits repeat studies in the same subject in a short period. This circumstance is useful if a cognitive activation paradigm, such as performance of a verbal memory task, is to be compared with scans done in other states, such as motor activations (e.g., finger tapping) (Figure 6–11).

Practical Considerations

The method used for PET is similar to that used for SPECT, but the scan must take place within a few minutes or seconds of the injection because of the differing properties of the isotopes used in PET. As with SPECT, for most clinical purposes a resting whole-brain scan is ordered. Depending on the tracer used, the time of the scan is 2–40 minutes, during which time the patient must remain still in the scanner. FDG, the most commonly used PET tracer in clinical studies, requires a 30- to 40-minute scan. As with SPECT, sedation may be given after isotope injection if the patient is extremely anxious or unable to remain still while lying supine during the scan. In many centers, headholders are used during PET scanning to keep the patient's head in a stable position. Headholders can be constructed of thermoplastic and individually fitted to the patient's head. Alternatively, they may be made of foam rubber or other soft material placed around the head to prevent motion. The degree of stabilization gained must be weighed against the amount of discomfort caused to the patient, especially if he or she is claustrophobic or uncomfortable being somewhat restrained.

Indications

There are no clinical guidelines for use of PET in TBI at this time. As with SPECT, PET scans are often obtained when brain injury is suspected but not seen on structural studies or when structural studies do not indicate damage extensive enough to explain a patient's deficits.

Limitations

PET scans generally cost $2,000 for a clinical study. In comparison, SPECT scans are $800–$1,000 at most centers. The higher price of PET is due to several factors, including the advanced technology used in PET scanners compared with that used in SPECT scanners. For certain short-half-life isotopes, such as ^{15}O, the isotope must be made onsite, limiting its use to centers that have a cyclotron (another expense). Thus, PET is not available at many institutions.

Overview of Abnormal Findings in Other Psychiatric Disorders

As with SPECT, PET is used in the evaluation of many neurological disorders. The most common clinical uses are in the assessment of patients with epilepsy, central nervous system malignancies, and cerebrovascular accidents. However, in acute cerebrovascular accident, SPECT results have been shown to reflect abnormalities not seen with FDG-PET (Henkin 1996). PET is also use-

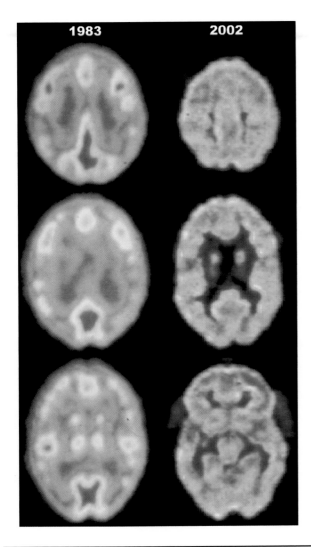

FIGURE 6–9.   PET imaging then and now.
Axial PET images of brain acquired in 1983 and 2002. Note the significant improvement in resolution since the 1980s.
Source.   Pictures courtesy of CTI Molecular Imaging, Inc.

ful, in some cases, in helping differentiate between different types of dementia. The ability of PET to detect perfusion changes consistent with AD may be superior to that of SPECT, with studies reporting sensitivity of 87%–94% and specificity of 85%–96% (Hoffman et al. 1996; Mielke and Heiss 1998; Van Heertum et al. 2000).

PET has also been used for research studies of headache. Flow reduction has been seen in migraine headache with and without auras (Bednarczyk et al. 1998; see Aurora and Welch 2000 for a review), although hyperperfusion of cortical regions and brainstem have also been reported in studies of migraine without aura (see Cutrer et al. 2000 for a review). Studies with PET suggest that cluster headaches may be associated with activation of the hypothalamus (May et al. 1999).

Research has been conducted in evaluation of pain with PET. According to studies primarily with nonpatient volunteers, the brain regions most consistently found to be associated with varying types of pain perception include the contralateral insula and anterior cingulate, bilateral thalamus and premotor cortex, and the vermis of the cerebellum, with magnitude of neuronal response increasing as level of pain is modulated upward (see Casey 1999 for a review). Hypothalamic and periaqueductal gray activation associated with pain perception has also been reported in other PET work with nonpatient volunteers (Hofbauer et al. 2001; Hsieh et al. 1996).

The use of PET in the evaluation of other psychiatric conditions has yet to be demonstrated. PET studies of patients with depression have shown prefrontal cortex flow and metabolic changes, which may resolve with treatment (Goodwin 1996). Some PET studies of patients with obsessive-compulsive disorder have shown increased metabolism in the caudate and/or orbitofrontal cortex (Baxter et al. 1987, 1988), although not all study results are consistent with these (Swedo et al. 1989). In schizophrenia, imaging studies suggest frontal metabolic and flow deficits (Andreasen et al. 1996; Liddle et al. 1992) and also have begun to demonstrate differences between patients with positive symptoms and those with more predominant negative symptoms (Lahti et al. 2001). Receptor ligand studies, similar to those described with SPECT, have also been conducted with PET for the study of psychiatric illnesses. In particular, work characterizing dopamine receptor change has been extremely important, especially in the study of schizophrenia (see Verhoeff 2001 for a review).

Limited PET investigations have been conducted in patients with psychogenic disorders. Hypometabolism in the caudate, putamen, and right precentral gyrus was found in one study of somatization disorder and somatoform disorder (Hakala et al. 2002). Reduced frontal activation was seen in three patients with limb weakness (Spence et al. 2000). In a single case study with PET, activations were produced during hypnotic paralysis similar to those observed with psychogenic paralysis (Halligen et al. 2000).

Overview of Abnormal PET Findings in TBI

PET has been used in several studies of TBI patients to assess many measures, including evidence of functional abnormalities in patients who have normal structural scans, prognosis, correlations between post-TBI behavioral disorders and brain injury, and correlations between neuroanatomical damage and neuropsychological test–

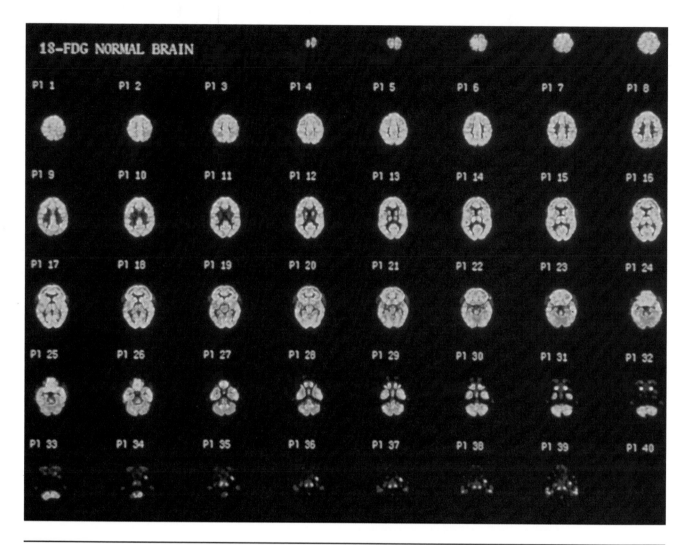

FIGURE 6–10.   Serial axial fluoride 18 fluorodeoxyglucose PET images of a normal adult brain.
Letter/number combinations below each image refer to brain slice order.
Source.   Picture courtesy of CTI Molecular Imaging, Inc.

performance deficits. Most of these studies involve small numbers of patients, making conclusions based on the data problematic. Use of PET for cognitive activation studies to look at neuroplasticity after TBI and for examination of neuropathological changes in these patients are two promising applications for PET. In general, the scope of the clinical studies with PET is smaller than those with SPECT, but research applications of PET may ultimately prove to be more fruitful.

Studies Using PET and Structural Imaging

In contrast to research with SPECT, little work has been done to assess whether PET is more accurate than structural imaging in assessment of lesions in TBI patients. Because PET can provide other data in addition to blood flow information, one might expect differing use of PET in prediction of outcome.

The limited work thus far suggests that, like SPECT, PET may be helpful in assessment of patients with TBI who have normal structural imaging but behavioral problems or cognitive deficits. Studies using FDG (glucose metabolism) or cobalt 55 (cell death) have indicated that PET provides additional information beyond that available from structural imaging (Fontaine et al. 1999; Jansen et al. 1996; Langfitt et al. 1986; Rao et al. 1984; Ruff et al. 1994; Umile et al. 2002). In all of these studies, more lesions were present on PET. In some of these studies, the authors suggest that these abnormalities correlated with behavioral and cognitive complaints. However, as with SPECT, a causal link between a specific lesion seen on functional imaging and behavioral changes seen in a patient is difficult to assess.

Other work has questioned whether the more extensive information obtained from PET is actually clinically

TABLE 6–3.   U.S. Food and Drug Administration–approved, commonly used tracers/ligands for PET

Tracer/radioligand	Parameter measured	Comments
[18]F	Glucose metabolism	Commonly used in clinical studies; longer half-life than [15]O means only one scan may be acquired in each scanning session.
[15]O	Blood flow	Short half-life means that multiple scans may be collected in one session with a subject; commonly used for cognitive research studies with cognitive activation paradigms.
[13]N	Blood flow	Used in cardiac assessment.
[55]Co	Calcium	Provides indications of areas where cell death is occurring.
[11]C	Dopaminergic system	Research use to study receptors.

useful in the management of TBI patients. Worley et al. (1995) examined PET results compared with CT or MRI data in 22 children and adolescents with severe TBI who were followed through a rehabilitation program. They concluded that PET was not more helpful than standard structural imaging in prediction of outcome after TBI in children. In a more recent study, Bergsneider et al. (2001) found that FDG-PET was not useful in following functional recovery from moderate and severe TBI, because the correlation between change in metabolism on follow-up PET and recovery from neurological damage was weak. Their PET findings did suggest that metabolic re-

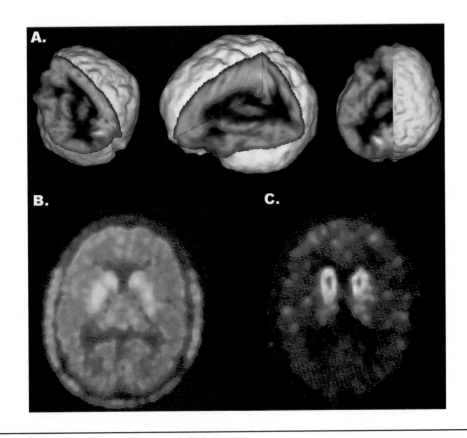

FIGURE 6–11.   **Current PET imaging capabilities.**

Three-dimensional (3D) reconstruction of PET results (A). 3D imaging improves appreciation of the extent of functional abnormalities. Neurotransmitter systems may also be imaged with PET. Presynaptic dopamine terminals can be labeled with [^{18}F]fluorodopa (B). Dopamine D_2 receptors can be labeled with [^{11}C]N-methylspiperone (C).

Source.   Pictures courtesy of CTI Molecular Imaging, Inc.

covery begins approximately 1 month after moderate or severe TBI, a concept that may have implications for the timing of pharmacological or rehabilitational interventions after TBI.

Some PET findings may indicate new directions for interventions post-TBI. Bergsneider et al. (1997) suggested that the apparent hyperglycolysis may be secondary to excitotoxicity or ischemia. Yamaki et al. (1996) studied CBF, oxygen ejection fraction, and cerebral metabolism for both oxygen and glucose in three patients with acute, severe, diffuse TBI. Their findings suggested that persistent anaerobic glycolysis (which may indicate excitotoxicity) is a predictor of poor outcome. PET findings suggest that hyperglycolysis (an influx of ions into cells that have not suffered irreversible damage) occurs after TBI (Bergsneider et al. 1997), possibly because more energy (i.e., glucose) is needed to pump out the ions and restore homeostasis (Hovda 1996). Coles and others (2004) also discuss the use of oxygen extraction fraction studies in TBI for evaluation of ischemic burden and newer methods for its determination. Other uses for PET in investigation of pathophysiology following TBI have also been proposed in recent work (Hattori et al. 2003; Hattori et al. 2004; Wu et al. 2004). These findings may encourage new interventions/treatment for severe acute TBI, such as diminution of persistent excitotoxicity.

PET consistently shows abnormalities not seen on structural imaging, especially in cases of mild TBI. However, the actual clinical usefulness of this information has not been proven. PET has not been found to be useful in assessment of recovery but has suggested new avenues for research into early interventions (Bergsneider et al. 1997; Yamaki et al. 1996).

Studies Using Behavioral Measures

Few studies have focused on the use of functional imaging to assess patients with behavioral symptoms after TBI. Given the changes seen on PET scans of patients with primary psychiatric illness, one might expect some correlation between PET data and post-TBI behavioral problems. Starkstein et al. (1990) used FDG-PET to evaluate patients with mania after TBI. Three patients who had only subcortical damage on structural imaging were scanned during mania; they showed right lateral basitemporal hypometabolism, implicating right-sided damage in the development of mania. Fontaine et al. (1999) also reported a relationship between behavioral disorders in severe TBI and mesial prefrontal and cingulate metabolic abnormalities. Further work with detailed behavioral information and psychiatric diagnosis is needed in this area before use can be assessed, although these prelimi-

nary studies suggest that PET studies in TBI may enhance research into neuroanatomical underpinnings of psychiatric symptoms.

Studies Using Neuropsychological Assessments

Several groups have compared PET results in TBI patients with results from their performance on neuropsychological tests, with varying results. Some studies found good correspondence between areas of abnormality on PET and neuropsychological test deficits (Fontaine et al. 1999; Langfitt et al. 1987; Rao et al. 1984; Ruff et al. 1994). On the other hand, the pattern of deficits on neuropsychological testing has not been shown to predict PET location of lesions (Jansen et al. 1996; Umile et al. 2002).

A single study has compared PET and SPECT directly for assessment of neuropsychological deficits in TBI (Abu-Judeh et al. 1998). SPECT scanning demonstrated frontal and parietal perfusion, concurring with neuropsychological test results, whereas FDG-PET results indicated normal glucose metabolism. The authors suggested that, at least in mild TBI, vascular compromise due to injury may cause SPECT findings of flow loss, although the normal glucose metabolism indicates that underlying tissue is still viable. Although this example illustrates the possibility that different information from the two modalities could be complementary, no work has been done to apply this finding clinically to date.

Activation Studies

Performance of a behavioral task during a scan, called a *cognitive activation paradigm*, may be helpful in studying the function of particular cognitive domains. In the largest PET activation study to date, Gross et al. (1996) compared FDG-PET results from 20 patients with mild TBI to those of noninjured control subjects. All subjects were scanned while performing a simple continuous performance task (i.e., press button when "zero" appears on screen). The authors concluded that even mild TBI may produce abnormalities both on neuropsychological test performance and behaviorally and that cerebral metabolism may be affected. They also noted that performance of an activation task during scanning may have affected brain activity, because patients with more damage may need to exert more effort to perform the task, which could be reflected in metabolic change. Similar results were seen in a study by Levine and others (2002), which examined brain activation differences in six moderate to severe TBI patients, with greater brain activation in the TBI patients relative to matched noninjured control subjects during performance of a cued recall task. The authors suggested this may be due to brain reorganization in response to diffuse axonal injury, possibly indicating compensation.

Studies Using Other PET Tracers

As with SPECT, PET ligand studies are becoming an important tool for research. Although these techniques have not yet been used to study TBI, they may well provide the most important future contributions from PET. Potentially, radioactive ligands (e.g., raclopride, which is used to study dopaminergic transmission) could provide information on disruption of receptor types, intracellular messengers, and proteins after TBI. Ligands are also available, but less widely so, for research use in investigations of serotonergic, acetylcholinergic, and other neurotransmitter systems.

Recommendations

As of this writing, PET does not have a large role in evaluation of TBI. In very select cases in which more exacting localization of lesions is important, PET may be helpful, although correlation of specific lesion location with function is often problematic. Otherwise, the lower cost and greater availability of SPECT make it the best functional assessment in those select cases in which functional imaging may enhance evaluation of TBI. As with SPECT, PET may sometimes be useful in detection of lesions in cases in which behavioral symptoms or cognitive deficits are present in the patient with no apparent structural injury. PET is generally superior to SPECT for use in research studies of cognitive function and brain injury because of its finer resolution. Use of ^{15}O as a PET tracer allows investigators to perform several studies on a patient in one session, which is important when studying cognition. PET may have a role in investigation of pathophysiology of TBI. Most important, it may be useful in determining whether pathophysiological events after TBI are dynamic in nature and, if so, when the optimum time for intervention is. In the future, PET scanning may also be a technique for the study of putative mechanisms of cellular damage after TBI, including excitotoxicity and changes in neurotransmitter systems.

Functional Magnetic Resonance Imaging

fMRI is a relatively new technique for the measurement of activity-related changes in CBF without the use of ionizing radiation. fMRI is based on the observation that the magnetic qualities of oxygenated and deoxygenated hemoglobin differ (Kwong et al. 1992; Ogawa et al. 1990). As brain activity increases in a certain region, metabolic demand also rises. Blood flow increases to meet the demand but increases slightly more than is required to sustain the activity. The resulting higher concentration of oxygenated hemoglobin in blood causes a slight increase in MRI signal intensity. This signal change is what is measured by fMRI. The computerized data are then reconstructed into images, with higher signal areas presumably reflecting regions of increased activation. These images are commonly coregistered with a companion structural MRI obtained in the same session, providing neuroanatomical detail. Some work has demonstrated the confirmation of fMRI findings with more established PET techniques during performance of cognitive activation tasks (Ojemann et al. 1998; Xiong et al. 1998).

Practical Considerations

Currently, fMRI is used only for research purposes. This technique holds great promise for future studies of normal brain function and for investigations of pathological change due to many conditions, including TBI. The advantages of fMRI include easy implementation on many existing scanners, lack of ionizing radiation exposure, ability to repeat multiple studies on one patient in a short time, and greatly improved anatomical resolution (1 mm) as compared to that possible with SPECT and PET.

Indications

fMRI is currently not used clinically in evaluation of TBI. The high resolution and the lack of ionizing radiation make it a promising technique for future investigations.

Limitations

Although fMRI can be performed on many standard MRI scanners after a few modifications, considerable technical expertise is needed to acquire reliable fMRI data. fMRI scans are generally not "read" as with PET or SPECT but rather are interpreted using statistical programs. Thus, knowledge of these programs and correct interpretation of the results generated by them are vital. Because there is presently no resting fMRI technique, subjects must be able to perform an activation task during scanning. This limits use to alert, cooperative subjects. Standardization of activation tasks before their performance would be needed before fMRI could be used widely for clinical purposes.

Overview of Abnormal Findings in Other Psychiatric Disorders

Most fMRI work to date has been with psychiatrically healthy volunteers in cognitive activation studies. However, interest in using fMRI clinically to assess neurological/neuropsychiatric illness is increasing. Evaluation of brain function, recovery, and reorganization after stroke is a promising potential area for its use (Cao et al. 1998; Marshall et al. 2000; Pineiro et al. 2002). It may also be of value in the presurgical evaluation of epilepsy patients for lateralization of language function, which is currently done with the Wada test (Binder et al. 1996; Detre et al. 1998). Preliminary studies have been conducted with psychiatric populations using fMRI. Sheline et al. (2001) found amygdala hyperactivity in depression, which normalized with antidepressant treatment. Menon et al. (2001) found prefrontal and parietal cortex function to be abnormal in patients with schizophrenia during performance of a working memory task. Studies have also been done in substance abuse populations (Garavan et al. 2000).

Overview of Abnormal fMRI Findings in TBI

Only a few studies have used fMRI in the TBI population. TBI patients may have significantly different and sometimes more extensive activation patterns from those seen in noninjured control subjects during performance of a cognitive activation task.

McAllister et al. (1999) imaged mild TBI patients during performance of a working memory task within 1 month of their injury. Although task performance did not differ between the two groups, the TBI patients showed significant activation changes, especially in the right parietal and right dorsolateral frontal regions, compared with noninjured control subjects. Further studies by the same group (McAllister et al. 2001a) found that mild TBI patients imaged a few weeks after injury showed increased activation relative to noninjured control subjects during a moderately difficult working memory–processing load. However, as task difficulty increased, the patients with mild TBI did not demonstrate the same increases in activation with higher processing demands, despite maintaining comparable performance. The authors of this study suggest that perhaps the TBI patients have already recruited all cognitive reserves at lower levels of task difficulty and do not have additional resources available to them because of injury-related pathology. As an alternative explanation, they propose that mild TBI patients do not have actual deficits in working memory ability, as evidenced by their task performance, but that the TBI pa-

tients have lost some ability to modulate the allocation of neural processing resources. They suggest that disruption of catecholaminergic systems, which are crucial to working memory function, may occur in many cases of TBI because of the frequency of frontal lobe damage (for reviews see Arnsten 1998; McIntosh 1994).

Christodoulou et al. (2001) also examined patterns of brain activation during performance of a working memory task in patients with moderate to severe TBI. TBI patients were able to perform the task but made significantly more errors than healthy controls. Cerebral activation in both groups was found in similar regions of the frontal, parietal, and temporal lobes. This resembles patterns of activation found in prior studies of working memory in healthy persons. However, the TBI group displayed a pattern of cerebral activation that was more regionally dispersed and more lateralized to the right hemisphere, especially in the frontal lobes. Both studies (Christodoulou et al. 2001; McAllister et al. 2001a) suggest that impairment in ability to modulate brain activation in response to task demands occurs in TBI.

Easdon and others (2004) compared brain activation during response inhibition on a "go-stop" task in five patients with variable degrees of TBI and five control subjects. A go-stop task is an executive task that relates to some of the behavioral changes seen in TBI patients, such as impulsivity. Despite similar performance on the task, TBI patients showed reduced activation in the dorsolateral prefrontal cortex when no response was to be made and in the cingulate when a response was indicated, brain areas implicated in decisions to withhold responses and monitor decision making, respectively. All three studies (Christodoulou et al. 2001; Easdon et al. 2004; McAllister et al. 2001a) suggest that regions modulating appropriate responses may be impaired in some cases of TBI. In other recent work (Scheibel et al. 2003), executive function in severe, diffuse TBI was evaluated in a single patient. Compared with noninjured control subjects, the severely affected patient showed more extensive frontal activation during working memory and response inhibition tasks. The authors suggest that recruitment of additional brain regions may occur to facilitate performance of these executive tasks in severe TBI. Thus, depending on the measures used and brain regions studied, TBI may be associated with reduced or increased activation during executive task performance.

Recommendations

fMRI is potentially a powerful tool for investigation of brain function, particularly cognition. As methods are standardized and comparisons to PET and SPECT results are conducted, application of this technique to studies of patient groups may be helpful clinically. The lack of ionizing radiation exposure makes fMRI ideal for extensive investigation of behavior and of cognitive processes—as well as their disruption—in TBI.

Magnetic Resonance Spectroscopy

MRS is another method for functional brain assessment. The basic principle is the same as for MRI, in which the signal comes from the protons in water and lipids, which are present in very high concentrations in the brain. In clinical MRS, either proton (^{1}H MRS)- or phosphorus (^{31}P MRS)-containing metabolites are measured. These are present in very low concentrations, so the signal is usually displayed as a spectrum rather than an image. The area under each peak represents the relative concentration of each metabolite. MRS studies provide information on intracellular function and, possibly, indications of microscopic tissue damage.

^{1}H MRS can provide quantification of neurochemicals, including N-acetylaspartate (NAA), choline (Cho), creatine (Cr), lactate, and several others (Table 6–4). NAA is thought to be a marker of neuronal integrity; loss of NAA is associated with neuron or axon loss. Cho is generally not visible to ^{1}H MRS because it is bound to cell membranes, lipids, and myelin. However, in pathological conditions, Cho is released and becomes visible on MRS. Thus, its presence suggests brain pathology. Cr is used as an internal reference, because it usually occurs in stable levels. Because levels of neurochemicals can vary depending on the exact ^{1}H MRS technique used, measures are often expressed as a ratio, relative to Cr (e.g., the NAA/Cr ratio, which reflects neuronal and axonal density and integrity). Lactate is also not usually seen with MRS; however, its presence is increased when abnormal states occur, leading to glycolysis or failed oxidative metabolism. The ^{31}P spectrum includes peaks for adenosine diphosphate, adenosine triphosphate, and phosphocreatine as well as phosphomono- and phosphodiesters (see Table 6–4). In addition, tissue pH can be calculated. Thus, MRS provides measures of both energy state and phospholipid metabolism.

Indications

As with fMRI, MRS holds great potential for study of brain function and change because of neuropathology. Because of its noninvasive nature, it has a promising future as a clinical tool. Because there is no ionizing radiation, multiple studies can be performed in a patient and can be repeated over time. Like fMRI, MRS can be performed on a standard MRI scanner with a few modifications, although higher magnet strength produces better resolution.

TABLE 6–4.   Compounds commonly studied with MRS

Nuclei measured	Compound studied	Parameter measured	Comments
^{1}H MRS	Creatine	Energy use	Provides reference point for measurement of other metabolites
	N-acetylaspartate	Decrease when neurons/axons damaged or lost	Measures neuronal integrity
	Choline	Neuropathology (suggestive)	Becomes "visible" to MRS when cell integrity is compromised
	Lactate	Glycolysis or failed oxidative metabolism (suggestive)	Only present in pathological states
^{31}P MRS	Phosphocreatine	Energy storage	Reference for chemical shift of other peaks in spectrum
	Adenosine triphosphate	High-energy phosphate metabolism	—
	Inorganic phosphate	Local tissue pH	Calculated based on the chemical shift of inorganic phosphate
	Phosphomonoesters	Membrane phospholipid metabolism	—
	Phosphodiesters	Membrane phospholipid metabolism	—

Limitations

As with fMRI, technical expertise is important to produce and interpret data from MRS. There is a need for standardized interpretation of the clinical relevance of MRS findings in TBI and in many other conditions.

Overview of Abnormal Findings in Other Psychiatric Disorders

MRS is rapidly becoming an important tool in many areas of behavioral research. It has been used to study carbon monoxide (CO) poisoning, particularly for assessment of CO-related white matter changes (Sakamoto et al. 1998; Sohn et al. 2000). In one report, MRS abnormalities after CO poisoning were seen before any changes in CBF or on structural imaging (Kamada et al. 1994). It has also been used successfully to image neurodegenerative disease, such as AD. Recent work indicates that MRS may prove useful for assessment of neuronal level effects of medications used for treatment of neurodegenerative disorders (Frederick et al. 2002). Auer et al. (2001) found reduction of thalamic NAA along with abnormal levels of other compounds in schizophrenia. The authors suggested that these abnormalities provide additional evidence for neuropathological change in schizophrenia. Bertolino et al. (2001) used MRS to detect cerebral changes in the brains of patients with schizophrenia posttreatment. They found increases in dorsolateral prefrontal cortex NAA levels after administration of antipsychotics.

Overview of Abnormal MRS Findings in TBI

There are promising preliminary results in the use of MRS to study TBI. MRS has been helpful in demonstrating persistent damage on a cellular level, even in remote mild TBI, and in assessment of the mechanisms by which cellular damage occurs after TBI. MRS has been useful in the detection of abnormalities in studies of patients with structurally normal scans but with persistent symptoms. It may have a role in prediction of outcome.

Son et al. (2000) examined metabolic changes in regions proximal to the area of injury seen on MRI after mild TBI using ^{1}H MRS. NAA/Cr was reduced at both early and late stages, suggesting persistent damage. Garnett et al. (2000) found reduced NAA/Cr and increased Cho/Cr in normal-appearing brain regions of TBI patients, which may help explain why TBI patients with normal-appearing structural scans can show cognitive and other deficits at follow-up. Friedman and others (1999) correlated ^{1}H MRS measures in normal-appearing occipitoparietal white and gray matter with neuropsychological testing. Early NAA concentrations in gray matter predicted overall neuropsychological test per-

formance, but other metabolite measures were not related to behavioral function at outcome. Garnett et al. (2001) assessed cellular metabolism with ^{31}P MRS. The alterations in metabolism seen in the TBI patients were suggestive of a loss of normal cellular homeostasis or a relative increase in glial cell density in damaged regions, providing evidence against simple ischemia as a cause of abnormalities.

Several studies have examined the correlation between functional measures and neurochemical state measured by MRS. Ariza et al. (2004) examined the correlation between neuropsychological test performance and neurochemical changes measured with MRS in 20 patients with moderate and severe TBI. Compared with 20 matched noninjured controls, NAA concentrations were decreased in TBI patients' basal ganglia and medial temporal cortical regions. Basal ganglia changes correlated with assessments measuring speed, motor scanning, and attention. Thus, neuronal death, as measured by decreases in NAA, was found in a focal region, which the authors hypothesize could help explain neuropsychological performance deficits due to frontal-striatal networks that figure prominently in some executive tasks. Other work has shown evidence of axonal recovery on MRS in a TBI patient who also made functional gains (Danielsen et al. 2003).

Recommendations

Many of the same challenges seen with fMRI currently arise with use of MRS in the clinical assessment of TBI patients. Methods must be standardized and validated. MRS may prove especially helpful in assessment of patients with mild TBI who have normal structural scans but persistent behavioral and cognitive impairment. As with many technologies used in psychiatry, MRS is rapidly evolving into a powerful research tool for use in studying effects of TBI on a cellular level.

Other Promising Modalities

There are two additional functional imaging techniques that deserve brief mention: magnetoencephalography (MEG) and xenon-enhanced CT (Xe/CT).

Magnetoencephalography

MEG is a noninvasive method that uses superconducting sensors to measure the neuromagnetic fields generated by neuronal activation. These fields pass through the skull and scalp without distortion. Thus, this method provides data similar to those provided by standard electroencephalogram (EEG) technology but with fewer arti-

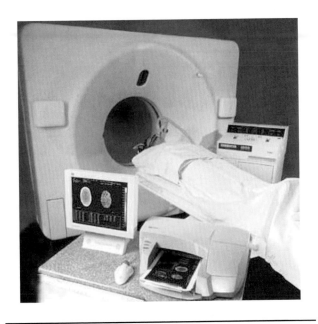

FIGURE 6–12. Procedure for obtaining a xenon-enhanced CT (Xe/CT) scan.

Normal clinical CT scans are acquired as the first stage in an Xe/CT study. The patient then inhales a mixture of xenon gas and oxygen via a face mask (as illustrated in this figure) for several minutes. Xe/CT images are acquired during inhalation. Generally, a solid headholder is used to minimize motion of the head. *Source.* Picture courtesy of Diversified Diagnostic Products, Inc.

facts. Using computerized models to generate activation maps, MEG can be used to localize patterns of brain activity. The spatial resolution that can be achieved from MEG data is greater than that from EEG data. Like EEG, MEG directly measures neuronal activity in milliseconds, unlike the other functional imaging techniques, all of which provide indirect measures of neuronal activity. The ability of MEG to monitor rapid changes in neuronal activity makes it possible to separate components of a cognitive task, such as word reading.

MEG has been used to study numerous neuropsychiatric conditions, including epilepsy and autism (Hurley et al. 2000; King et al. 2000; Lewine et al. 1999a). There have been small studies assessing use of MEG in TBI (Iwasaki et al. 2001; Lewine et al. 1999b). The preliminary work in TBI suggests that MEG may become a useful modality for evaluation of TBI patients, especially if combined with other imaging technologies. At present, MEG is available as a research tool only in a few large centers because of the high cost of the technology.

Xenon-Enhanced Computed Tomography

Xe/CT combines anatomical and CBF imaging. Stable xenon gas is both radiodense and lipid soluble. It dissolves in the blood and enters the brain parenchyma. Patients inhale a mixture of xenon gas and oxygen via a face mask (Figure 6–12). CT scans are acquired before, during, and sometimes after inhalation. The CBF calculation is based on the arrival of xenon at each standardized unit of brain measured (i.e., pixel) and the amount of xenon exhaled. In February of 2001, the historical FDA status of xenon as a "grandfathered" X-ray contrast agent was withdrawn, thus halting its clinical use. As of this writing, the pertinent FDA-required studies are in progress. It is hoped that xenon will be available again soon.

Xe/CT has several advantages over other functional imaging methods. Because of the rapid elimination of xenon from the body, Xe/CT can be repeated every 15 minutes as desired. It can provide functional imaging data for patients undergoing a standard structural CT scan at a relatively low cost (approximately $100 in addition to the cost of the standard CT). Xenon is nonradioactive, so the acquisition of the structural CT is the only radiation exposure required for the scan. The main drawback of Xe/CT is that patients may experience positive or negative changes in mood, either of which could be problematic, especially in neuropsychiatric populations. Nausea also occurs in some patients. Apnea is a rare and reversible side effect. Sedation may be needed for neuropsychiatric patients.

Xe/CT has been used primarily for the evaluation of cerebrovascular accidents, bleeds, and aneurysms (Kilpatrick et al. 2001; Latchaw 2004; Taber et al. 1999). Some work has been done with TBI patients, including assessment of ischemic regions after TBI and prediction of prognosis based on metabolic and blood flow changes in severe TBI (Kelly et al. 1996; Kushi et al. 1999; Marion and Bouma 1991; von Oettingen et al. 2002; Zurynski et al. 1995). Thus, Xe/CT may provide important research contributions to the understanding of the pathophysiology of TBI in the future (Figures 6–13, 6–14, and 6–15).

Summary

Despite the promise of functional brain imaging as a noninvasive means for evaluation of traumatic brain injury (TBI), clinical use has not been fully demonstrated at this time.

Single-photon emission computed tomography (SPECT) and positron emission tomography (PET) have each demonstrated lesions not seen on structural scans, especially in mild TBI, although the clinical significance of this finding for an individual patient with TBI has not been convincingly shown. SPECT and PET may have some role in prediction of outcome, which is presently their most common clinical use. Their use for assessment of brain changes correlating with findings on neuropsy-

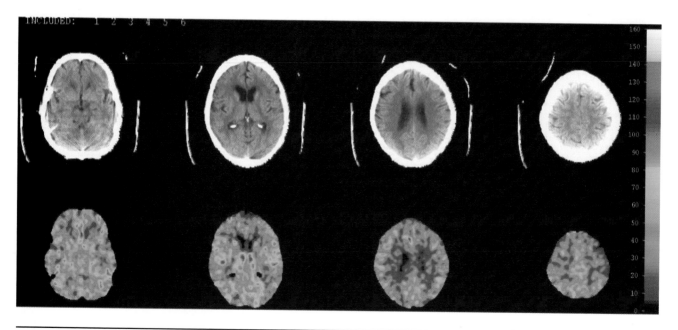

FIGURE 6–13.   Xenon-enhanced CT.

Axial CT (top row) and xenon-enhanced CT (bottom row) images of blood flow in normal brain. Blue areas indicate lower perfusion, and red areas indicate higher perfusion (see color key to the right of the figure).
Source.   Picture courtesy of Diversified Diagnostic Products, Inc.

chological testing, behavioral symptoms, and progress in rehabilitation is unclear. Despite the superior resolution of PET, its higher cost makes it difficult to justify over SPECT in evaluation of most TBI cases.

Functional magnetic resonance imaging (fMRI) and magnetic resonance spectroscopy (MRS) are promising methods for study of TBI. Activation paradigms are required for most fMRI work, so standardization of cogni-

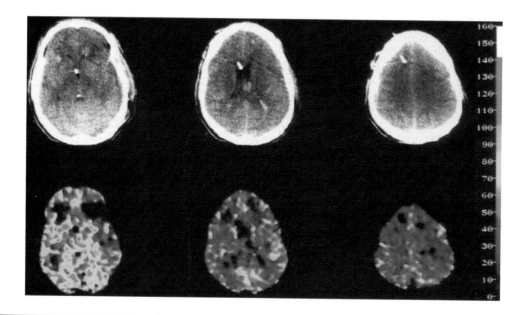

FIGURE 6–14.   Acute presentation of traumatic brain injury on xenon-enhanced CT.

Axial CT (top row) and xenon-enhanced CT (Xe/CT) (bottom row) images of blood flow after an acute brain injury. Blue areas indicate lower perfusion and red areas indicate higher perfusion (see color key to the right of the figure). Xe/CT was used in this case to adjust the ventilator settings to achieve optimal perfusion.
Source.   Picture courtesy of Diversified Diagnostic Products, Inc.

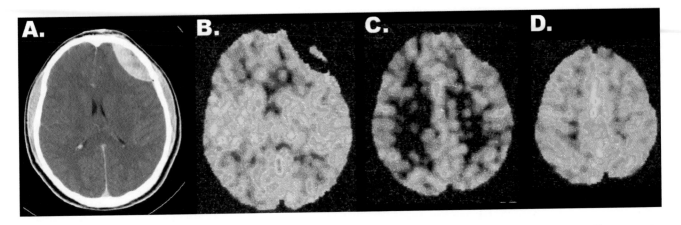

FIGURE 6–15. **Acute presentation of epidural hematoma on xenon-enhanced CT.**
Seventeen-year-old male patient status post–motor vehicle accident and seizure. CT (A) reveals an epidural hematoma in the left frontal region. Companion xenon-enhanced CT (B) shows a focal perfusion defect corresponding to the hematoma. Diffuse globally decreased perfusion is clearly present on the slice immediately above the hematoma (C). In the uppermost slice (D), blood flow is globally somewhat decreased with a more severe deficit on the side of the hematoma.
Source. Case contributed by Dr. Susan Weathers, Baylor College of Medicine.

tive tasks must occur if clinical studies are to become useful. MRS is emerging as an important tool for study of neuropathology at a cellular level. It may be capable of demonstrating pathological change after TBI even in patients with normal structural scans. As with PET and SPECT, the clinical applicability of this information has yet to be established in TBI.

With all functional imaging modalities, caution must be used in the interpretation of scans of TBI patients with concomitant (possibly preexisting) neurological or psychiatric conditions. Blood flow and metabolic changes are also seen on functional imaging studies of this population. In all functional imaging modalities used to study TBI, there is a need for more controlled studies using standardized methods to evaluate imaging data. Comparison of modalities in a single study is also important, because it will help establish how the modalities can be complementary to one another. Receptor studies may be important in future TBI work. As new ligands are developed, enabling studies of different neurotransmitter systems, it may be possible to image disruption of particular systems after TBI (e.g., dopamine transmission deficits) and to individualize treatment using these data.

It is probable that the most significant contribution of functional imaging to the study of TBI will be in understanding its pathophysiology. All of the modalities described in this chapter and many new ones still in development will contribute to knowledge of how cell injury and death occur in TBI. It is possible that this information could lead to new treatments, such as neuroprotective therapies that can be used immediately after TBI to minimize neuronal damage.

References

Abdel-Dayem H, Sadek SA, Kouris K, et al: Changes in cerebral perfusion after acute head injury: comparison of CT with Tc-99m HM-PAO SPECT. Radiology 165:221–226, 1987

Abi Darghum A, Rodenhiser J, Printz D, et al: Increased baseline occupancy of D_2 receptors by dopamine in schizophrenia. Proc Natl Acad Sci U S A 97:8104–8109, 2000

Abu-Judeh HH, Singh M, Masdeu JC, et al: Discordance between FDG uptake and technetium-99m-HMPAO brain perfusion in acute traumatic brain injury. J Nucl Med 39:1357–1359, 1998

Andreasen NC, O'Leary DS, Cizadlo T, et al: Schizophrenia and cognitive dysmetria: a positron-emission tomography study of dysfunctional prefrontal-thalamic-cerebellar circuitry. Proc Natl Acad Sci U S A 93:9985–9990, 1996

Ariza M, Junque C, Mataro M, et al: Neuropsychological correlates of basal ganglia and medial temporal lobe NAA/Cho reductions in traumatic brain injury. Arch Neurol 61:541–544, 2004

Arnsten AFT: Catecholamine modulation of prefrontal cortical cognitive function. Trends Cogn Sci 2:436–447, 1998

Asenbaum S, Zeithofer J, Saletu B, et al: Technetium-99-HMPAO SPECT imaging of cerebral blood flow during REM sleep in narcoleptics. J Nucl Med 36:1150–1155, 1995

Audenaert K, Jansen HM, Otte A, et al: Imaging of mild traumatic brain injury using ^{57}Co and ^{99m}Tc HMPAO SPECT as compared to other diagnostic procedures. Med Sci Monit 9:MT112–117, 2003.

Auer DP, Wilke M, Grabner A, et al: Reduced NAA in the thalamus and altered membrane and glial metabolism in schizophrenic patients detected by 1H-MRS and tissue segmentation. Schizophr Res 52:87–99, 2001

Aurora SK, Welch KM. Migraine: imaging the aura. Curr Opin Neurol 13:273–276, 2000

Baxter LR Jr, Phelps ME, Mazziotta JC, et al: Local cerebral glucose metabolic rates in obsessive-compulsive disorder: a comparison with rates in unipolar depression and in normal controls. Arch Gen Psychiatry 44:211–228, 1987

Baxter LR Jr, Schwartz JM. Massiotta JC, et al: Cerebral glucose metabolic rates in nondepressed patients with obsessive-compulsive disorder. Am J Psychiatry 145:1560–1563, 1988

Bednarczyk EM, Remier B, Weikart C, et al: Global cerebral blood flow volume and oxygen metabolism in patients with migraine headaches. Neurology 50:1736–1740, 1998

Bergsneider M, Hovda DA, Shalmon E, et al: Cerebral hyperglycolysis following severe traumatic brain injury in humans: a positron emission tomography study. J Neurosurg 86:241–251, 1997

Bergsneider M, Hovda DA, McArthur DL, et al: Metabolic recovery following human traumatic brain injury based on FDG-PET: time course and relationship to neurological disability. J Head Trauma Rehabil 16:135–148, 2001

Bertolino A, Callicott JH, Mattay VS, et al: The effect of treatment with antipsychotic drugs on brain N-acetylaspartate measures in patients with schizophrenia. Biol Psychiatry 49:39–46, 2001

Binder JR, Swanson SJ, Hammeke TA, et al: Determination of language dominance using functional MRI: a comparison with the Wada test. Neurology 46:978–984, 1996

Bonne O, Gilboa A, Louzoun Y, et al: Cerebral blood flow in chronic symptomatic mild traumatic brain injury. Psychiatry Res 124:141–152, 2003

Bonte FJ, Weiner MF, Bigio EH, et al: Brain blood flow in the dementias: SPECT with histopathologic correlation in 54 patients. Radiology 202:793–797, 1997

Cao Y, D'Olhaberriague L, Vikingstad EM, et al: Pilot study of functional MRI to assess cerebral activation of motor function after poststroke hemiparesis. Stroke 29:112–122, 1998

Casey KL: Forebrain mechanisms of nociception and pain: analysis through imaging. Proc Natl Acad Sci U S A 96:7668–7674, 1999

Christodoulou C, DeLuca J, Ricker JH, et al: Functional magnetic resonance imaging of working memory impairment after traumatic brain injury. J Neurol Neurosurg Psychiatry 71:161–168, 2001

Coles JP, Fryer TD, Smielewski P, et al: Defining ischemic burden after traumatic brain injury using 15O PET imaging of cerebral physiology. J Cereb Blood Flow Metab 24:191–201, 2004

Cutrer FM, O'Donnell A, Sanchez del Rio M: Functional neuroimaging: enhanced understanding of migraine pathology. Neurology 55 (suppl 2):S36–S45, 2000

Danielsen ER, Christensen PB, Arlien-Soborg P, Thomsen C: Axonal recovery after severe traumatic brain injury demonstrated in vivo by 1H MR spectroscopy. Neuroradiology 45 (10):722–724, 2003

Detre JA, Maccotta L, King D, et al: Functional MRI lateralization of memory in temporal lobe epilepsy. Neurology 50:926–932, 1998

Devous MD Sr: Comparison of SPECT applications in neurology and psychiatry. J Clin Psychiatry 53 (suppl):13–19, 1992

Di Piero V, Fiacco F, Tombari D, et al: Tonic pain: a SPET study in normal subjects and cluster headache patients. Pain 70:185–191, 1997

Easdon C, Levine B, O'Connor C, et al: Neural activity associated with response inhibition following traumatic brain injury: an event-related fMRI investigation. Brain Cogn 54:136–138, 2004

Fontaine A, Azouvi P, Remy P, et al: Functional anatomy of neuropsychological deficits after severe traumatic brain injury. Neurology 53:1963–1968, 1999

Frederick B, Satlin A, Wald LL, et al: Brain proton magnetic resonance spectroscopy in Alzheimer disease: changes after treatment with xanomeline. Am J Geriatr Psychiatry 10:81–88, 2002

Friedman SD, Brooks WM, Jung RE, et al: Quantitative proton MRS predicts outcome after traumatic brain injury. Neurology 52:1384–1391, 1999

Garcia-Campayo J, Sanz-Carrillo C, Baringo T, et al: SPECT scan in somatization disorder patients: an exploratory study of eleven cases. Aust N Z J Psychiatry 35:359–363, 2001

Garnett MR, Blamire AM, Corkill RG, et al: Early proton magnetic resonance spectroscopy in normal-appearing brain correlates with outcome in patients following traumatic brain injury. Brain 123 (Pt 10):2046–2054, 2000

Garnett MR, Corkill RG, Blamire AM, et al: Altered cellular metabolism following traumatic brain injury: a magnetic resonance spectroscopy study. J Neurotrauma 18:231–240, 2001

Garavan H, Pankiewicz J, Bloom A, et al: Cue-induced cocaine craving: neuroanatomical specificity for drug users and drug stimuli. Am J Psychiatry 157:1789–1798, 2000

Goodwin GM: Neuropsychological and neuroimaging evidence for the involvement of the frontal lobes in depression. J Psychopharmacol 11:115–122, 1997

Gray BG, Ichise M, Chung DG, et al: Technetium-99m-HMPAO SPECT in the evaluation of patients with a remote history of traumatic brain injury: a comparison with x-ray computed tomography. J Nucl Med 33:52–58, 1992

Gross H, Kling A, Henry G, et al: Local cerebral glucose metabolism in patients with long-term behavioral and cognitive deficits following mild traumatic brain injury. J Neuropsychiatry Clin Neurosci 8:324–334, 1996

Hakala M, Karlsson H, Ruotsalainen U, et al: Severe somatization in women is associated with altered cerebral glucose metabolism. Psychol Med 32:1379–1385, 2002

Halligen PW, Athwal BS, Oakley DA, et al: Imaging hypnotic paralysis: implications for conversion hysteria. Lancet 356:162–163, 2000

Hattori N, Huang SC, Wu HM, et al: PET investigation of post-traumatic cerebral blood volume and blood flow. Acta Neurochir Suppl 86:49–52, 2003

Hattori N, Huang SC, Wu HM, et al: Acute changes in regional cerebral (18)F-FDG kinetics in patients with traumatic brain injury. J Nucl Med 45:775–783, 2004

Henkin R. Nuclear medicine: the role of positron emission tomography in the investigation of neurological disorders. St. Louis, MO, Mosby, 1996, pp 1334–1346

Herscovitch P. Functional brain imaging—basic principles and application to head trauma, in Head Injury and Postconcussive Syndrome. Edited by Rizzo M, Tranel D. Churchill Livingstone, New York, 1996, pp 89–118

Hoehn-Saric R, Harris GJ, Pearlson GD, et al: A fluoxetine induced frontal lobe syndrome in an obsessive-compulsive patient. J Clin Psychiatry 52:131–133, 1991a

Hoehn-Saric R, Pearlson GD, Harris GJ, et al: Effects of fluoxetine on regional cerebral blood flow in obsessive-compulsive patients. Am J Psychiatry 148:1243–1245, 1991b

Hofbauer RK, Rainville P, Duncan GH, et al: Cortical representation of the sensory dimension of pain. J Neurophysiology 86:402–411, 2001

Hoffman JM, Hanson MW, Welsh KA, et al: Interpretation variability of [18]FDG positron emission tomography studies in dementia. Invest Radiol 31:316–322, 1996

Holman BL, Carvalho PA, Mendelson J, et al: Brain perfusion is abnormal in cocaine-dependent polydrug users: a study using technetium-99m-HMPAO and ASPECT. J Nucl Med 32:1206–1210, 1991

Holman BL, Mendelson J, Garada B, et al: Regional cerebral blood flow improves with treatment in chronic cocaine polydrug users. J Nucl Med 34:723–727, 1993

Hovda DA: Metabolic dysfunction, in Neurotrauma. Edited by Narayan RK, Wilberger JE, Povlishock JT. New York, McGraw-Hill, 1996, pp 1459–1478

Hsieh JC, Stahle-Baeckdahl M, Haeermark O, et al: Traumatic nociceptive pain activates the hypothalamus and the periaqueductal gray: a positron emission tomography study. Pain 64:303–314, 1996

Hurley RA, Lewine JD, Jones GM, et al: Application of magnetoencephalography to the study of autism. J Neuropsychiatry Clin Neurosci 12:1–3, 2000

Ichise M, Chung DG, Wang P, et al: Technetium-99m-HMPAO SPECT, CT and MRI in the evaluation of patients with chronic traumatic brain injury: a correlation with neuropsychological performance. J Nucl Med 35:217–226, 1994

Ishii K, Mori E, Kitagaki H, et al: The clinical utility of visual evaluation of scintigraphic perfusion patterns for Alzheimer's disease using I-123 IMP SPECT. Clin Nucl Med 21:106–110, 1996

Iwasaki M, Nakasato N, Kanno A, et al: Somatosensory evoked fields in comatose survivors after severe traumatic brain injury. Clin Neurophysiol 112:205–211, 2001

Jacobs A, Put E, Ingels M, et al: Prospective evaluation of technetium-99m-HMPAO SPECT in mild and moderate traumatic brain injury. J Nucl Med 35:942–947, 1994

Jansen HML, van der Naalt J, van Zomeron AH, et al: Cobalt-55 positron emission tomography in traumatic brain injury: a pilot study. J Neurol Neurosurg Psychiatry 60:221–224, 1996

Jobst KA, Barnetson LP, Shepstone BJ: Accurate prediction of histologically confirmed Alzheimer's disease and the differential diagnosis of dementia: the use of NINCDS-ADRDA and DSM-III-R criteria, SPECT, X-ray CT, and Apo E4 in medial temporal lobe dementias. Int Psychogeriatr 10:271–302, 1998

Kamada K, Houkin K, Aoki T, et al: Cerebral metabolic changes in delayed carbon monoxide sequelae studied by proton MR spectroscopy. Neuroradiology 36:104–106, 1994

Kelly DF, Kordestani RK, Martin NA, et al: Hyperemia following traumatic brain injury: relationship to intracranial hypertension and outcome. J Neurosurg 85:762–771, 1996

Kesler SR, Adams HF, Bigler ED: SPECT, MR, and quantitative MR imaging: correlates with neuropsychological and psychological outcome in traumatic brain injury. Brain Inj 14:851–857, 2000

Kilpatrick MM, Yonas H, Goldstein S, et al: CT-based assessment of acute stroke: CT, CT angiography, and xenon-enhanced CT cerebral blood flow. Stroke 32:2543–2549, 2001

King DW, Park YD, Smith JR, et al: Magnetoencephalography in neocortical epilepsy. Adv Neurol 84:415–423, 2000

Kushi H, Moriya T, Saito T, et al: Importance of metabolic monitoring systems as an early prognostic indicator in severe head injured patients. Acta Neurochir Suppl (Wien) 75:67–68, 1999

Kwong KK, Belliveau JW, Chesler DA, et al: Dynamic magnetic resonance imaging of human brain activity during primary sensory stimulation. Proc Natl Acad Sci U S A 89:5675–5679, 1992

Laatsch L, Jobe T, Sychra J, et al: Impact of cognitive rehabilitation therapy on neuropsychological impairments as measured by brain perfusion SPECT: a longitudinal study. Brain Inj 11:851–863, 1997

Laatsch L, Pavel D, Jobe T, et al: Incorporation of SPECT imaging in a longitudinal cognitive rehabilitation therapy programme. Brain Inj 13:555–570, 1999

Lahti AC, Holcomb HH, Medoff DR, et al: Abnormal patterns of regional cerebral blood flow in schizophrenia with primary negative symptoms during an effortful auditory recognition task. Am J Psychiatry 158:1797–1808, 2001

Langfitt TW, Obrist WD, Alavi A, et al: Computerized tomography, magnetic resonance imaging, and positron emission tomography in the study of brain trauma: preliminary observations. J Neurosurg 64:760–767, 1986

Langfitt TW, Obrist WD, Alavi A, et al: Regional structure and function in head-injured patients: correlation of CT, MRI, PET, CBF, and neuropsychological assessment, in Neurobehavioral Recovery from Head Injury. Edited by Levin HS, Grafman J, Eisenberg HM. New York, Oxford University Press, 1987, pp 30–42

Laruelle M: Imaging synaptic neurotransmission with in vivo binding competition techniques: a critical review. J Cereb Blood Flow Metab 20:423–451, 2000

Latchaw RE: Cerebral perfusion imaging in acute stroke. J Vasc Interv Radiol 15 (1 pt 2):S29–S46, 2004

Levine B, Cabeza R, McIntosh AR, et al: Functional reorganisation of memory after traumatic brain injury: a study with H(2)(15)O positron emission tomography. J Neurol Neurosurg Psychiatry. 73:173–181, 2002

Lewine JD, Andrews R, Chez M, et al: Magnetoencephalographic patterns of epileptiform activity in children with regressive autism spectrum disorders. Pediatrics 104 (3 pt 1):405–418, 1999a

Lewine JD, Davis JT, Sloan JH, et al: Neuromagnetic assessment of pathophysiologic brain activity induced by minor head trauma. AJNR Am J Neuroradiol 20:857–866, 1999b

Liddle PF, Friston KJ, Frith CD, et al: Patterns of cerebral blood flow in schizophrenia. Br J Psychiatry 160:179–186, 1992

Lingford-Hughes AR, Acton PD, Gacinovic S, et al: Reduced levels of GABA-benzodiazepine receptor in alcohol dependency in the absence of grey matter atrophy. Br J Psychiatry 173:116–122, 1998

Lucey JV, Costa DC, Blanes T, et al: Regional cerebral blood flow in obsessive-compulsive disordered patients at rest: differential correlates with obsessive-compulsive and anxious-avoidant dimensions. Br J Psychiatry 167:629–663, 1995

Machlin SR, Pearlson GD, Hoehn-Saric R, et al: Elevated frontal cerebral blood flow in obsessive-compulsive patients: a SPECT study. Am J Psychiatry 148:1240–1242, 1991

Marshall RS, Perera GM, Lazar RM, et al: Evolution of cortical activation during recovery from corticospinal tract infarction. Stroke 31:656–661, 2000

Masdeu JC, Van Heertum RL, Kleiman A, et al: Early single photon emission computed tomography in mild head trauma: a controlled study. J Neuroimaging 4:177–181, 1994

Masterman DL, Mendez MF, Fairbanks LA, et al: Sensitivity, specificity, and positive predictive value of technetium 99-HMPAO SPECT in discriminating Alzheimer's disease from other dementias. J Geriatr Psychiatry Neurol 10:15–21, 1997

Marion DW, Bouma GJ: The use of stable xenon-enhanced computed tomographic studies of cerebral blood flow to define changes in cerebral carbon dioxide vasoresponsivity caused by a severe head injury. Neurosurgery 29:869–873, 1991

May A, Ashburner J, Buchel C, et al: Correlation between structural and functional changes in brain in an idiopathic headache syndrome. Nat Med 5:836–838, 1999

Mazzini L, Cossa FM, Angelino E, et al: Posttraumatic epilepsy: neuroradiologic and neuropsychological assessment of long-term outcome. Epilepsia 44 (4):569–574, 2003

McAllister TW, Saykin AJ, Flashman LA, et al: Brain activation during working memory 1 month after mild traumatic brain injury: a functional MRI study. Neurology 53:1300–1308, 1999

McAllister TW, Sparling MB, Flashman LA, et al: Differential working memory load effects after mild traumatic brain injury. Neuroimage 14:1004–1012, 2001a

McAllister TW, Sparling MB, Flashman LA, et al: Neuroimaging findings in mild traumatic brain injury. J Clin Exp Neuropsychol 23:775–791, 2001b

McIntosh TK: Neurochemical sequelae of traumatic brain injury: therapeutic implications. Cerebrovasc Brain Metab Rev 6:109–162, 1994

Menon V, Anagnoson RT, Mathalon DH, et al: Functional neuroanatomy of auditory working memory in schizophrenia: relation to positive and negative symptoms. Neuroimage 13:433–446, 2001

Mielke R, Heiss WD: Positron emission tomography for diagnosis of Alzheimer's disease and vascular dementia. J Neural Transm Suppl 53:237–250, 1998

Mirza M, Tutus A, Erdogan F, et al: Interictal SPECT with Tc-99m HMPAO studies in migraine patients. Acta Neurol Belg 98:190–194, 1998

Mountz JM, Bradley LA, Modell JG, et al: Fibromyalgia in women: abnormalities of regional cerebral blood flow in the thalamus and the caudate nucleus are associated with low pain threshold levels. Arthritis Rheum 38:926–938, 1995

Nakabeppu Y, Nakajo M, Gushiken T, et al: Decreased perfusion of the bilateral thalami inpatients with chronic pain by Tc-99m-ECD SPECT with statistical parametric mapping. Ann Nucl Med 15:459–463, 2001

Newton MR, Greenwood RJ, Britton KE, et al: A study comparing SPECT with CT and MRI after closed head injury. J Neurol Neurosurg Psychiatry 55:92–94, 1992

Obrist WD, Langfitt TW, Jaggi JL, et al: Cerebral blood flow and metabolism in comatose patients with acute head injury: relationship to intracranial hypertension. J Neurosurg 61:241–253, 1984

Oder W, Goldenberg G, Spatt J, et al: Behavioural and psychological sequelae of severe closed head injury and regional cerebral blood flow: a SPECT study. J Neurol Neurosurg Psychiatry 55:475–480, 1992

Ogawa S, Lee TM, Kay AR, et al: Brain magnetic resonance imaging with contrast dependent on blood oxygenation. Proc Natl Acad Sci U S A 87:9868–9872, 1990

Ojemann JG, Buckner RL, Akbudak E, et al: Functional MRI studies of word-stem completion: reliability across laboratories and comparison to blood flow imaging with PET. Hum Brain Map 6:203–215, 1998

Pineiro R, Pendlebury S, Johansen-Berg H, et al: Altered hemodynamic responses in patients after subcortical stroke measured by functional MRI. Stroke 33:103–109, 2002

Pizzolato G, Dam M, Borsato N, et al: [99mTc]-HM-PAO SPECT in Parkinson's disease. J Cereb Blood Flow Metab 8:S101–S108, 1988

Prayer L, Wimberger D, Oder W, et al: Cranial MR imaging and cerebral 99mTc HM-PAO-SPECT in patients with subacute or chronic severe closed head injury and normal CT examinations. Acta Radiologica 34:593–599, 1993

Rao N, Turski PA, Polcyn RE, et al: 18F positron emission computed tomography in closed head injury. Arch Phys Med Rehabil 65:780–785, 1984

Roper SN, Mena I, King WA, et al: An analysis of cerebral blood flow in acute closed-head injury using technetium-99m-HMPAO SPECT and computed tomography. J Nucl Med 32:1684–1687, 1991

Ruff RM, Crouch A, Troster AI, et al: Selected cases of poor outcome following a minor brain trauma: comparing neuropsychological and positron emission tomography assessment. Brain Inj 8:297–308, 1994

Sabri O, Erkwoh R, Schreckenberger M, et al: Correlation of positive symptoms exclusively to hyperperfusion or hypoperfusion of cerebral cortex in never-treated schizophrenics. Lancet 349:1735–1739, 1997

Sakamoto K, Murata T, Omori M, et al: Clinical studies on three cases of the interval form of carbon monoxide poisoning: serial proton magnetic resonance spectroscopy as a prognostic predictor. Psychiatry Res 83:179–192, 1998

Scheibel RS, Pearson DA, Faria LP, et al: An fMRI study of executive functioning after severe diffuse TBI. Brain Inj 17:919–930, 2003

Sheline YI, Barch DM, Donnelly JM, et al: Increased amygdala response to masked emotional faces in depressed subjects resolves with antidepressant treatment: an fMRI study. Biol Psychiatry 50:651–658, 2001

Shirakawa SI, Takeuchi N, Uchimura N, et al: Study of image findings in rapid eye movement sleep behavioural disorder. Psychiatry Clin Neurosci 56:291–292, 2002

Smith MT, Perlis ML, Chengazi VU, et al: Neuroimaging of NREM sleep in primary insomnia: a Tc-99-HMPAO single proton emission computed tomography study. Sleep 25:325–335, 2002

Sohn YH, Jeong Y, Kim HS, et al: The brain lesion responsible for parkinsonism after carbon monoxide poisoning. Arch Neurol 57:1214–1218, 2000

Son BC, Park CK, Choi BG, et al: Metabolic changes in pericontusional oedematous areas in mild head injury evaluated by 1H MRS. Acta Neurochir Suppl 76:13–16, 2000

Spence SA, Crimlisk HL, Cope H, et al: Discrete neurophysiological correlates in prefrontal cortex during hysterical and feigned disorder of movement. Lancet 355:1243–1244, 2000

Starkstein SE, Mayberg HS, Berthier ML, et al: Mania after brain injury: neuroradiological and metabolic findings. Ann Neurol 27:652–659, 1990

Swedo SE, Schapiro MB, Grady CL, et al: Cerebral glucose metabolism in childhood onset obsessive compulsive disorder. Arch Gen Psychiatry 46:518–523, 1989

Taber KH, Zimmerman JG, Yonas H, et al: Applications of xenon CT in clinical practice: detection of hidden lesions. J Neuropsychiatry Clin Neurosci 11:423–425, 1999

Tiihonen J, Kuikka J, Viinamaki H, et al: Altered cerebral blood flow during hysterical paresthesia. Biol Psychiatry 37:134–135, 1995

Umile EM, Plotkin RC, Sandel ME: Functional assessment of mild traumatic brain injury using SPECT and neuropsychological testing. Brain Inj 12:577–594, 1998

Umile EM, Sandel ME, Alavi A, et al: Dynamic imaging in mild traumatic brain injury: support for the theory of medial temporal vulnerability. Arch Phys Med Rehabil 83:1506–1513, 2002

Van Heertum RL, O'Connell RA: Functional brain imaging in the evaluation of psychiatric illness. Semin Nucl Med 21:24–39, 1991

Van Heertum RL, Tikofsky RS, Rubens AB: Dementia, in Functional Cerebral SPECT and PET Imaging, 3rd Edition. Edited by Van Heertum RL, Tikovsky RS. New York, Lippincott Williams & Wilkins, 2000, pp 127–188

Van Heertum RL, Drocea C, Ichise M, et al: Single photon emission CT and positron emission tomography in the evaluation of neurologic disease. Radiol Clin North Am 39:1007–1033, 2001

Varney NR, Bushnell DL, Nathan M, et al: NeuroSPECT correlates of disabling mild head injury: preliminary findings. J Head Trauma Rehabil 10:18–28, 1995

Verhoeff PLG: Imaging of dopaminergic transmission in neuropsychiatric disorders. Curr Opin Psychiatry 4:227–239, 2001

von Oettingen G, Bergholt B, Gyldensted C, et al: Blood flow and ischemia within traumatic cerebral contusions. Neurosurgery 50:781–788, 2002

Vuilleumier P, Chicherio C, Assal F, et al: Functional neuroanatomical correlates of hysterical sensorimotor loss. Brain 124:1077–1090, 2001

Wiedmann KD, Wilson JT, Wyper D, et al: SPECT cerebral blood flow, MR imaging, and neuropsychological findings in traumatic head injury. Neuropsychology 3:267–281, 1989

Woods SW: Regional cerebral blood flow imaging with SPECT in psychiatric disease: focus on schizophrenia, anxiety disorders and substance abuse. J Clin Psychiatry 53 (suppl):20–25, 1992

Worley G, Hoffman JM, Paine SS, et al: 18-Fluorodeoxyglucose positron emission tomography in children and adolescents with traumatic brain injury. Dev Med Child Neurol 37:213–220, 1995

Wu HM, Huang SC, Hattori N, et al: Selective metabolic reduction in gray matter acutely following human traumatic brain injury. J Neurotrauma 21:149–161, 2004

Xiong J, Rao S, Gao JH, et al: Evaluation of hemispheric dominance for language using functional MRI: a comparison with positron emission tomography. Hum Brain Mapp 6:42–58, 1998

Yamaki T, Imahori Y, Ohmori Y, et al: Cerebral hemodynamics and metabolism of severe diffuse brain injury measured by PET. J Nucl Med 37:1166–1170, 1996

Yazici KM, Kostakoglu L: Cerebral blood flow changes in patients with conversion disorder. Psychiatry Res 83:163–168, 1998

Zurynski YA, Dorsch NW, Pearson I: Incidence and effects of increased cerebral blood flow velocity after severe head injury: a transcranial Doppler ultrasound study, I: prediction of post-traumatic vasospasm and hyperemia. J Neurol Sci 134:33–40, 1995

7

Electrophysiological Techniques

David B. Arciniegas, M.D.

C. Alan Anderson, M.D.

Donald C. Rojas, Ph.D.

CLINICAL ELECTROPHYSIOLOGY OFFERS a variety of powerful and informative methods for studying cerebral function and dysfunction after traumatic brain injury (TBI). Electroencephalography (EEG) was the first clinical diagnostic tool to provide evidence of abnormal brain function due to TBI (Glaser and Sjaardema 1940; Jasper et al. 1940). Such early observations led to the development of more sophisticated electrophysiological techniques, including quantitative EEG (QEEG), topographic QEEG (also known as *brain electrical activity mapping*, or BEAM), evoked potentials (EPs), event-related potentials (ERPs), and magnetoencephalography (MEG) and magnetic source imaging (MSI). Each of these techniques provides a means of measuring brain activity noninvasively and with temporal resolution vastly superior to that achieved with any of the several presently available functional neuroimaging methods (e.g., positron emission tomography, single-photon emission computed tomography, and functional magnetic resonance imaging [MRI]) (Neylan et al. 1997).

Although conventional (i.e., visually inspected) EEG is commonly used in clinical neuropsychiatry and neurology, it is the least technologically sophisticated of currently available techniques and has only limited utility in the evaluation of the traumatically brain-injured patient (Cantor 1999). Computer-assisted and quantitative methods of electrophysiological data acquisition and analysis, including complementary data acquisition methods (e.g., EP/ERP, MEG/MSI), offer more informative and potentially more useful tools for the evaluation and study of individuals with brain injury than conventional EEG.

These techniques may provide information about the mechanisms of impaired perception, selective and sustained attention, memory, and executive function produced by TBI that is not accessible through conventional electroencephalographic recording and visual inspection (John et al. 1977; Lewine et al. 1999; Thatcher et al. 1989, 2001b). Some of these methods may index disturbances in specific neuronal networks and neurotransmitter systems underlying cognitive impairments produced by TBI (Arciniegas et al. 1999, 2000, 2001), the subtle nature of which precludes their identification with conventional EEG. Other electrophysiological techniques afford sensitivity and specificity to the types of neurophysiological changes produced by TBI that far exceed conventional EEG or even structural MRI (Lewine et al. 1999; Thatcher et al. 1999, 2001b).

Clinical and research application of electrophysiological techniques requires substantial knowledge of human electrophysiology, familiarity and experience with the principles of electrophysiological recording, and the ability to analyze and interpret the complex data sets that these tools produce. Clinicians working with traumatically brain-injured patients should, at a minimum, be familiar with electrophysiological techniques, their strengths and limitations, and their role in the evaluation, treatment, and study of these patients.

This chapter is intended to provide a broad overview of the principles of clinical electrophysiology and a brief discussion of some of the more interesting and potentially important findings from studies of electrodiagnostic techniques in traumatically brain-injured individuals. The basic principles of electrophysiological recording are presented first, followed by a brief discussion of each of the electrophysiological recording techniques noted above. Because a complete review of all findings of relevance to the neuropsychiatry of TBI is beyond the scope of the present work, the remainder of this chapter focuses on the applications and limitations of recently developed electrophysiological techniques to the evaluation, treatment, or study of this population.

Basic Principles of Clinical Electrophysiology

Neurons of the cortical mantle are organized into columns in which electrical activity occurs at the cortical surface and is transmitted inward to the neurons and axons. Such activity within the cortical columns establishes an electrical dipole whose orientation is parallel to that of the cortical column. The charge of that dipole at the cortical surface is a function of the neurotransmitter-receptor interactions occurring at the apical dendrites on cortical neurons, which can be either of an excitatory or inhibitory nature. Excitatory and inhibitory amino acids (e.g., glutamate and γ-aminobutyric acid, respectively) appear to regulate the thalamocortical circuits involved in immediate information processing, whereas the major neurotransmitters (e.g., acetylcholine, norepinephrine, dopamine, serotonin, and histamine) modulate the overall state of cerebral activity and establish the context within which more immediate information processing occurs (Coull 1998; McCormick 1992a, 1992b). The electrical activity generated by a single excitatory or inhibitory postsynaptic potential at a single dendrite does not generate an electrical field potential of sufficient strength to be detected by a surface electrode; instead, the summation of many millions, or more, of these potentials at the apical dendrites of superficial cortical neurons is required to generate a positively or negatively charged electrical field potential amenable to surface recording using presently available recording techniques.

Normal Electrophysiological Rhythms

The activity of cortical columnar neurons is influenced by amino acid and other neurotransmitter afferents from deeper structures, particularly the thalamus and the reticular activating system (Hughes 1982). The interaction of these deeper structures with the cortex creates a complex system within which cortical rhythms are regulated (Hughes and John 1999). Under conditions of modestly increased neuronal excitability and cortical activation,

neurons within these information-processing circuits fire asynchronously (or, relatively independently of other neurons) and rapidly as they perform their respective tasks. Relatively rapid neuronal firing of neurons within these information-processing circuits produces an oscillatory rhythm of relatively high frequency (>12.5 Hz). Oscillatory rhythms in this range of 12.5–25.0 Hz are designated as "beta activity."

Some elements of this complex electrochemical system also display an intrinsic rhythmicity when freed from reticular-activating influences. "Pacemaker" neurons distributed throughout the thalamus oscillate at a frequency of approximately 8.0–12.5 Hz (the alpha range); when the cortex is not engaged in information processing ("idling"), cortical neurons are driven by the thalamic pacemaker neurons to oscillate at these frequencies, producing oscillatory activity that is referred to as the "alpha rhythm" (Misulis 1997). In principle, all neocortical areas will develop an alpha rhythm when not actively processing information. However, the prominence of this easily evoked rhythm over the posterior (occipital) in the awake, eyes-closed state has led to its description by electroencephalographers as the "posterior dominant rhythm" (Hughes 1982; Misulis 1997).

The oscillating frequency of the thalamic pacemaker neurons is modulated by the nucleus reticularis of the thalamus, a thin layer of cells between the posterior limb of the internal capsule and the external medullary lamina that receives projections from brainstem reticular formation and cortical neurons and that sends inhibitory afferents into the thalamus (Mesulam 2000). The effect of the reticular nucleus of the thalamus on thalamic pacemaker neurons is to slow their oscillatory activity to 3.5–8.0 Hz (theta range), thereby inhibiting transmission of ascending, descending, and corticothalamocortical information. Cortical areas "at rest" and connected to these inhibited thalamic pacemaker neurons consequently oscillate at theta frequencies, such as may occur during drowsiness and light sleep.

When the thalamic neurons are insufficiently activated by the reticular formation/cortex or are markedly inhibited by the reticular nucleus of the thalamus, or both, they become unable to either drive cortical activity or transmit corticocortical and ascending sensory information effectively. Freed of both brainstem reticular and thalamic influences, as may occur in deep sleep and a variety of pathological states, these neurons oscillate at a frequency of approximately 1.5–3.5 Hz (delta range) (Hughes 1982; Hughes and John 1999).

The frequency and degree of synchrony of cortical rhythms may be understood most simply as reflecting the state of cortical activation: faster and relatively more

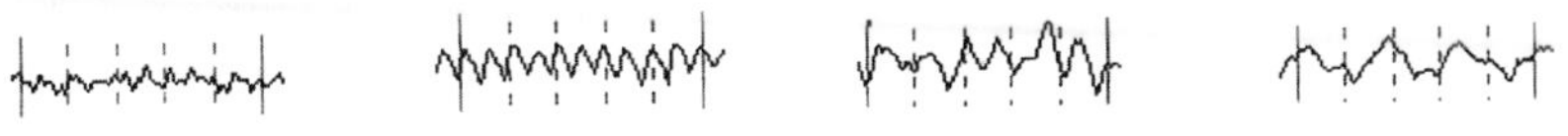

Beta activity   Alpha rhythm   Theta activity   Delta activity

FIGURE 7–1. Examples of electroencephalography tracings illustrating activity in each of the four major frequency domains (1 second per block, sensitivity = 7 μV/mm).

asynchronous (beta) activity reflects heightened arousal, cortical activation, and/or active information processing; activity in the alpha range reflects cortex at rest ("idling"); activity in the theta range reflects modestly diminished arousal and reduced information flow to and from the cortex; and activity in the delta range reflects substantially diminished arousal and a reduced cortical activity (Figure 7–1 and Table 7–1).

Abnormal Electrophysiological Events and Rhythms

Abnormal events and patterns of cortical electrical activity generally fall into two major categories, paroxysmal spikes (and sharp waves) and slow waves. Spikes are relatively high-voltage paroxysmal electrical events with a duration of 70 milliseconds or less. Sharp waves are similar events lasting 70–200 milliseconds. Spikes and sharp waves indicate abnormal paroxysms of cortical activity. *Slow waves* refers to waveforms with a frequency of less than 8 Hz in a waking record and are usually considered abnormal in such records. In some cases, spikes and slow waves occur together, forming spike-and-wave complexes, such as may be seen in a variety of epilepsies.

Both slow and fast activity may be observed in some EEG recordings; for example, the background rhythm may slow into the theta range while some fast (beta) activity continues. This admixture of abnormally slow background rhythm with superimposed fast activity in a waking record is referred to as *intermixed slowing*. Such slowing may be diffuse (generally indicating an encephalopathy) or focal (generally indicating a structural lesion).

The capacity for making transitions between slower, synchronous rhythms and faster, asynchronous rhythms in response to stimulation, referred to as *reactivity*, requires that the reticular activating system, thalamus, and relevant sensory cortices are capable of being engaged in different information processing states. Diminished reactivity is indicative of cerebral dysfunction of the sort that may be produced by TBI (Gütling et al. 1995).

Neurophysiological Recording

The neurophysiological activity of cortical neurons may be recorded using either surface electrodes or magnetometers (a magnetic recording device). The selection of one method of recording over another depends, at least in

TABLE 7–1. Major electroencephalography (EEG) bands, their respective frequencies, probable neural generators, and most characteristic location in a normal surface EEG recording

Band	Frequency range (Hz)	Principal neural generators	Characteristic surface electrode location
β (beta)	>12.5	Corticocortical and thalamocortical networks involved in information processing	Maximal over frontal and central regions
α (alpha)	8.0–12.5	Thalamic pacemaker neurons	Occipital and perhaps central when eyes are closed
θ (theta)	3.5–8.0	Thalamic pacemaker neurons under the influence of inhibitory input from the reticular nucleus of the thalamus	If present in the waking record at all, amplitude is low and content is small; may be most obvious in central regions; becomes more obvious with drowsiness and sleep
δ (delta)	<3.5	Oscillatory neurons in the deep cortical layers and within the thalamus	Not typically seen in the awake record of healthy adults; diffusely present in deeper sleep stages; may be focally located over cortical lesions; may become prominent in frontal/central regions due to disruption of corticothalamocortical circuits

part, on the areas of cortex to be recorded. Because the cerebral cortex contains both gyral and sulcal surfaces, the columnar organization of cortex results in the production of both radially and tangentially oriented electrical dipoles (Figure 7–2). Radially oriented dipoles are generated by gyral cortex; the dipole at the gyral surface would, if extended, form a radial line from the center of the head to the surface of the scalp (Figure 7–2, left). Tangentially oriented currents are generated by sulcal cortex, the orientation of which is tangential to the scalp surface that overlies them (Figure 7–2, right). Although both radially and tangentially oriented dipoles contribute to the electrical fields on the scalp, radially oriented currents are the predominant contributor to scalp surface electrical fields. Tangentially oriented electrical fields generated by sulcal cortex are not as readily amenable to recording by a scalp electrode because they do not generate as substantial an electrical potential difference at the scalp surface as radially oriented dipoles. However, tangentially oriented electrical dipoles produce a magnetic field that is radially oriented with respect to the scalp that is detectable through magnetoencephalographic recordings using an appropriately positioned magnetometer (Figure 7–3).

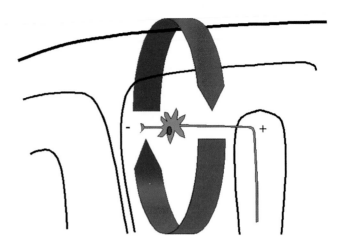

FIGURE 7–3. Illustration of the magnetic field generated by a tangentially oriented electrical dipole.
At the top of the diagram is the scalp surface. Below, a coronal cross section through two gyri is depicted. On the sulcal surface of the gyrus on the right, a single neuron in a cortical column is illustrated. When this neuron produces an electrical current, the magnetic field it generates is oriented perpendicular to that current. Many adjacent and simultaneously active tangentially oriented cortical neuronal columns produce magnetic fields whose flux lines are radially oriented with respect to the scalp and may be recorded by a magnetic recording device overlying this area.

Basic Methods of Electroencephalographic Recording

Electroencephalographic methods are standardized to facilitate improved reliability of both recording and interpretation, particularly with respect to the detection and approximate localization of abnormal electrical activity. In most clinical settings, electrodes are placed on the patient's scalp according to the 10–20 International System of Electrode Placement (Figure 7–4); higher density electrode arrays are sometimes used, particularly in neuropsychiatric research. Once electrodes are placed, they are connected to one another to create recording channels. Multiple electroencephalographic channels are arranged in a variety of ways to create electroencephalographic montages (see Figure 7–5 for a few examples). Through these different arrangements, several different views of cortical electrical activity can be established that facilitate both identification and approximate localization of abnormal cortical activity (e.g., seizure focus, contusion, infarction, subdural hematoma).

Once recorded, the electroencephalographic record is visually inspected for normal and abnormal findings. Although this remains the most common and generally accepted method of electroencephalographic interpreta-

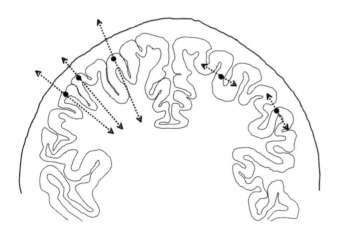

FIGURE 7–2.   Illustration of the cortical mantle in the coronal plane.
The radial orientation of electrical dipoles generated by gyral cortical columns is illustrated on the left, including their projection to the scalp surface. On the right, the tangential orientation of electrical dipoles generated by sulcal cortical columns is illustrated. Note that the tangentially oriented dipoles do not project to the scalp surface directly overlying them. Instead, the electrical fields associated with tangentially oriented dipoles eventually project to more distant (far-field) scalp areas. As a result of the longer distance and greater amounts of tissue traversed before emerging at the scalp, the electrical fields of tangentially oriented dipoles are relatively more attenuated and diffused before emerging at the scalp surface than are those of radially oriented electrical dipoles.

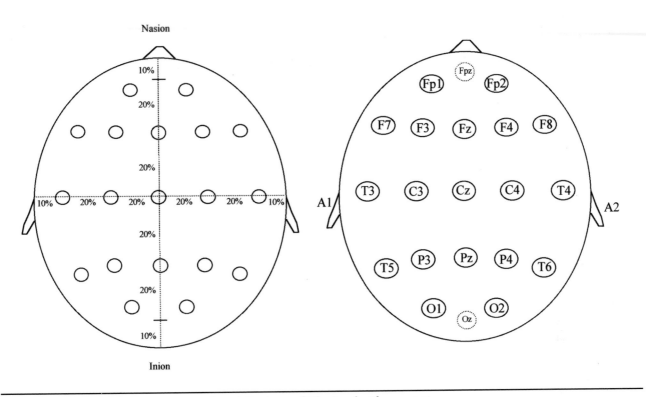

FIGURE 7–4.   The 10-20 International System of Electrode Placement.
Electrodes are labeled according to their approximate locations over the hemispheres (F = frontal, T = temporal, C = central, P = parietal, and O = occipital; z designates midline); left is indicated by odd numbers and right by even numbers. A parasagittal line running between the nasion and inion and a coronal line between the preauricular points is measured. Electrode placements occur along these lines at distances of 10% and 20% of their lengths, as illustrated. In most clinical laboratories, the Fpz and Oz electrodes are not placed, but are instead used only as reference points. Fp1 is placed posterior to Fpz at a distance equal to 10% of the length of the line between Fpz-T3-Oz; F7 is placed behind Fp1 by 20% of the length of that line. O1 is placed anterior to Oz at a distance equal to 10% of the length of the line between Oz-T3-Fpz; T5 is placed anterior to O1 by 20% of the length of that line. F3 is placed halfway between Fp1 and C3 along the line created between Fp1-C3-O1; P3 is placed halfway between O1 and C3 along that same line. Right hemisphere electrodes are placed in similar fashion. Reference electrodes, in this case placed on the ears, are labeled A1 and A2.

tion, digitization and computer-assisted methods permit quantitative electroencephalographic analyses that are not possible through visual inspection alone (Hughes and John 1999). These methods include quantified analysis of the frequency composition of the EEG over a given period (spectral analysis), analysis of absolute and relative amplitude (µV/cycle/second) and power (µV²/cycle/second) within a frequency range or at each channel, coherence (correlation between activity in two channels), phase (relationships in the timing of activity between two channels), or symmetry between homologous pairs of electrodes (Hughes and John 1999; Neylan et al. 1997; Nuwer 1990; Thatcher 1999). Values derived from quantitative electroencephalographic analyses can be mapped onto a representation of the entire scalp surface, a procedure known as *brain electrical activity mapping* (BEAM). Statistical probability mapping of BEAM data can be used to construct topographic maps of the results

of such analyses (Duffy et al. 1981), which offers a visual and potentially more intuitive method of inspecting these complex data sets (Figure 7–6).

There are reasonable concerns about the potential for misinterpretation and distortion of data subjected to quantitative electroencephalographic analyses without concurrent visual inspection by a qualified electroencephalographer (Jerrett and Corsak 1988; Nuwer 1997). For example, spike detection using presently available QEEG software packages is poor, thereby limiting the application of quantitative electroencephalographic procedures in the inspection of records for epileptiform activity. Although these issues remain the subject of ongoing debate in the literature (Hughes and John 1999; Neylan et al. 1997; Nuwer 1997; Thatcher 1999), quantitative electroencephalographic interpretation and analysis continue to hold promise for the investigation of neuropsychiatric disorders in general and the neuropsychiatric consequences of TBI in particular.

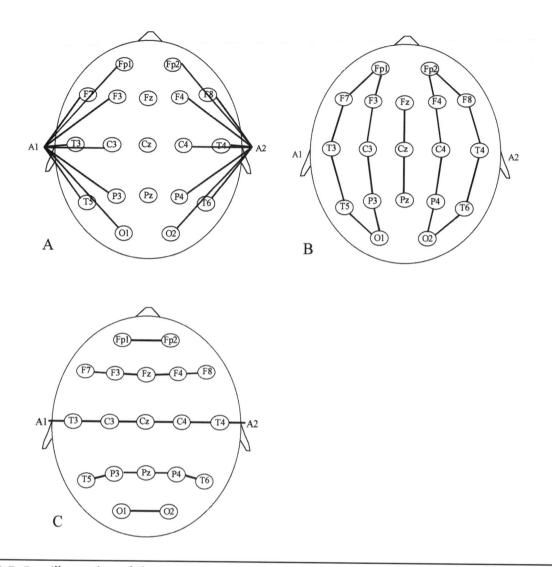

FIGURE 7–5. Illustration of three common electroencephalographic montages, including referential **(A)**, parasagittal bipolar **(B;** sometimes referred to as the *double-banana* montage**),** and transverse bipolar **(C).**

Regardless of the method of electroencephalographic data analysis, the limitations of electroencephalographic recordings are important to acknowledge. Cerebrospinal fluid, meningeal tissue, bone, connective tissue, muscle, and skin attenuate the amplitude of high-frequency signals, leaving at least part of the frequency spectrum (beta and higher) less than optimally represented on scalp surface recordings. These tissues, as well as sweat and skin oils, diffuse the electrical signal (now an electrical field) across the scalp surface. Hence, deeper sources of electrical signals within the brain are subject to greater attenuation and diffusion before arrival at the scalp surface. Consequently, surface electrodes tend to be relatively insensitive to signals of low strength or those generated by deep (e.g., subcortical, orbitofrontal, medial temporal, inferotemporal, and inferior occipitotemporal) structures. Signal diffusion across the scalp presents serious

challenges to precise signal source localization using electrophysiological recording techniques, particularly with respect to localizing relatively deep signal sources. Placement of special (e.g., nasopharyngeal and sphenoidal) electrodes may modestly improve signal detection from the cortex to which they are most proximate, but in general these areas are relatively inaccessible to conventional EEG recording.

Basic Methods of Magnetoencephalographic Recording

Magnetoencephalographic systems use superconducting quantum interference devices (SQUIDs) to record cortically generated magnetic fields. Because fluctuating magnetic fields (such as are produced by the cortex) induce electrical currents in conducting wires oriented

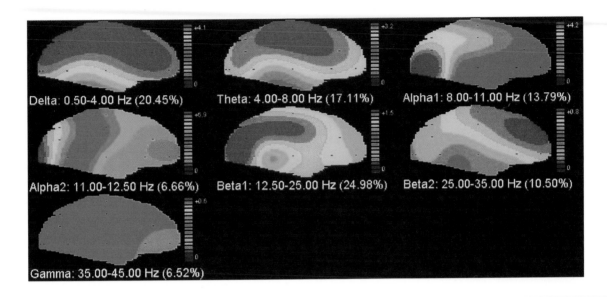

FIGURE 7–6.   An example of spectral mapping.

This map describes relative power (percentage of total power) in the right hemisphere across several frequency ranges in a 25-year-old man with diffuse intermixed slowing on visual inspection of the electroencephalography record.

perpendicular to the direction of flow of the magnetic field, current is induced in the wire coil when it is placed over an area of active cortex (Reite et al. 1999). The wire detector is itself inductively coupled to the SQUID and its electronics, which together comprise a sensitive magnetic field measuring device. Because the magnetic fields produced by cortical activity are closer to the magnetic field detector than are most environmental sources, this device is reasonably sensitive to the fluctuating gradients produced by cortical activity and less affected by the more stable field gradients of distant environmental magnetic sources (Rojas et al. 1999). A variety of MEG detection coils are available, each differing in their signal sensitivity and capacity for noise reduction. Modern magnetoencephalographic systems may have as many as 300 individual magnetic detectors (which are analogous to electroencephalographic electrodes). Pairing magnetic field detectors creates channels for signal recording; these channels can be arranged to create recording montages. Arrays of multiple magnetoencephalographic channels may also be used for these purposes or arranged in a variety of ways to create magnetoencephalographic counterparts to electroencephalographic montages. Smaller arrays offer more limited and/or focused areas of signal detection, as might be used in magnetoencephalographic evoked field or MSI recordings.

Magnetic field strength is not significantly attenuated by the tissue interposed between the source of the signal and the magnetometer positioned to detect it (Cuffin

1993). As such, MEG may be better able to detect both very high-frequency (up to 400–700 Hz) and ultra-low frequency (<1 Hz) signals that are not amenable to electroencephalographic recording (Lewine et al. 1999; Reite et al. 1999). However, there remain substantial technical challenges to recording cortically generated magnetic fields that offset this theoretical advantage (see Rojas et al. 1999 for a review). Although many of these technological challenges are manageable by presently available recording devices, the equipment, the magnetically shielded environment in which it must be operated, and the routine operation of such recording systems are cost, expertise, and labor intensive. These challenges may be reasons for the limited availability and application of MEG in TBI research to date.

Electrophysiological Techniques and TBI

The neurophysiological recording methods introduced in the preceding sections offer a variety of powerful and informative methods for studying cerebral function and dysfunction after TBI. In this section, results of studies using each of these electrophysiological techniques of particular relevance to the neuropsychiatry of TBI are reviewed. Because neuropsychiatrists are generally involved in the evaluation and treatment of patients in the postacute and late periods after TBI, greater emphasis is given to the review of studies examining electro-

TABLE 7–2.   Normal and trauma-related electroencephalographic findings

Condition	Typical electroencephalographic findings
Healthy adult	Low-voltage beta frequencies predominate with eyes open, posterior dominant (alpha) rhythm emerges with eyes closed; central alpha may be present, but is of lower amplitude than posterior alpha; theta and delta are not prominent, although a small amount of bihemispheric theta may be detectable with digital frequency (spectral) analysis
Normal aging	Diminished amplitude of beta activity; decreased amplitude of the posterior dominant rhythm, possible shift of the posterior dominant rhythm to the low alpha range; possible increase in temporal theta; possible diffuse increase in delta and theta in advanced aging
Focal cortical contusion, hemorrhage, infarction, or abscess	Focal slowing at the borders of infarction and decrease in beta activity over the area of contusion or infarction; focal slowing may be superimposed on a relatively normal-appearing background if there is only a small, discrete contusion or infarction; rhythms overlying such lesions consist of intermittent or continuous polymorphic delta and superimposed theta; sharp waves or spikes
White matter injury (relatively severe)	Continuous polymorphic delta activity that is not reactive to stimuli; deeper lesions causing a disconnection of subcortical nuclei and cortex may also produce FIRDA
Anterior brainstem/diencephalic injury	Bilateral FIRDA that is reactive to stimuli and not apparent during sleep; bifrontal theta may be seen with slow-growing deep midline tumors
Encephalopathy (delirium)	Diffuse slowing with irregular high-voltage delta activity
Acute agitated delirium	Low-voltage fast activity
Acute confusional state	Diffuse intermixed slowing
Seizure disorders	Focal or generalized spikes, sharp waves, and spike-and-wave complexes
Complex partial seizures	Focal spike-and-wave or sharp-wave discharges
Skull defect	Markedly asymmetrical, high-amplitude, focal beta activity recorded from the scalp overlying the defect (breach rhythm)
Subdural hematoma	Asymmetrical suppression of normal rhythms recorded from the scalp overlying the subdural hematoma; slower rhythms may eventually develop
Medications	Increased beta activity (sedative-hypnotics, anticonvulsants); diffuse intermixed slowing

Note.   FIRDA = frontal intermittent rhythmic delta activity.

physiological disturbances in these periods when such are available.

Electroencephalography

EEG was the first clinical diagnostic tool to provide evidence of transient abnormal brain function due to TBI (Glaser and Sjaardema 1940; Jasper et al. 1940). Williams and Denny-Brown (1941) experimentally demonstrated similar electroencephalographic abnormalities after TBI, including electroencephalographic attenuation and slowing in the acute injury period followed by resolution of these abnormalities over time. Consistent with these observations, there is general agreement among electroencephalographers that in the acute injury period the EEG often demonstrates a variety of abnormalities consistent with the severity of injury, the type and location of injury, and the patient's age (Table 7–2).

Immediately after mild TBI, the EEG is typically normal or only mildly abnormal, but may demonstrate slowing of the background rhythm into the theta range, attenuation of alpha, and increase in delta activity. More severe TBIs, particularly those affecting cortical, subcortical, and mesencephalic areas, may result in more severe electroencephalographic abnormalities such as prominent and diffuse delta with minimal or no alpha and theta activity, lack of reactivity, a burst suppression pattern, or frank electrocerebral silence (Gütling et al. 1995; Theilen et al. 2000; Tippin and Yamada 1996). In general, there is a relatively robust correlation between depth of coma and the degree of electroencephalographic abnormality, and clinically apparent focal neurological deficits tend to be associated with electroencephalographic abnormalities referable to the cortical injuries responsible for such deficits (Rumpl et al. 1979). Electroencephalographic abnormalities of this sort may include focal and asymmetrical slowing, generalized slowing of the background rhythm, focal spikes or spike-and-wave discharges, focal loss or asymmetry of reactivity, or some combination of these (Gütling et al. 1995; Rumpl et al. 1979; Tippin and Yamada 1996). In the acute injury period, and particularly in children, electroencephalographic abnormalities may be present even in the absence of frank neuroimaging (computed tomography) abnormalities (Liguori et al. 1989); when present, such abnormalities should raise clinical concern for the possibility of a traumatically induced structural abnormality.

Several studies suggest that EEG may be a useful tool for monitoring cerebral function after TBI (Jordan 1993), including the identification of focal ischemia, diffuse hypoxia, nonconvulsive seizures, the efficacy of pentobarbital treatment of increased intracerebral pressure (Winter et al. 1991), and the effect of hyperventilation on cerebral function (Bricolo et al. 1972). Prognosis after TBI may also be predicted using EEG, other complementary electrophysiological techniques, or combinations of these (Evans and Bartlett 1995; Gütling et al. 1995; Rae-Grant et al. 1991).

For example, Rae-Grant et al. (1996) studied EEG, somatosensory and brainstem auditory EPs (SSEPs and BAEPs, respectively), ocular plethysmography, transcranial Doppler sonography, and computed tomographic assessments in 69 acutely injured patients for the purpose of determining the techniques' ability to predict long-term outcome after TBI. Among these several assessments, only EEG (based on ratings of background activity, symmetry, reactivity, variability, and additional abnormal patterns) independently predicted the Glasgow Outcome Scale score at 6 months. However, electroencephalographic assessment in the acute injury period offered no advantage in outcome prediction over the Glasgow Coma Scale (GCS) score determined at day 7 postinjury.

Synek (1990a, 1990b) suggests that the pattern of EEGs obtained during acute posttraumatic coma may yet be of prognostic value. He reports that benign patterns (e.g., alpha or theta background, reactivity) predict survival and relatively good outcome, whereas malignant patterns (e.g., burst suppression, low-output or isoelectric EEG, nonreactive alpha or theta coma patterns) are highly associated with death. Hutchinson et al. (1991) demonstrated similar but less striking findings, including the association of either isoelectric EEG and lack of electroencephalographic reactivity with poor outcome and benign patterns with relatively good outcome after TBI. This study also demonstrated that modestly abnormal electroencephalographic patterns did not consistently predict outcome after TBI.

Among patients with mild TBI, the value of EEG in the acute setting is less clear. Although generalized slow-ing may occur in the first several hours after injury (Geets and De Zegher 1985), these and other abnormalities are seen in less than 20% of mildly injured individuals and tend to abate with time after injury (Tippin and Yamada 1996). Voller et al. (1999) compared MRI, EEG, and neuropsychological testing results of 12 patients with very mild TBI (no or only brief loss of consciousness [LOC], posttraumatic amnesia of less than 1 hour, GCS = 15, no disorientation, and normal neurological examination) within 24 hours of injury and at 6 weeks to those of comparably aged and educated control subjects. Significant differences in neuropsychological performance between these groups were demonstrated. MRI abnormalities were observed in 25% of the subjects with TBI. However, none of the subjects with very mild TBI had electroencephalographic abnormalities of any kind, including those with mild structural abnormalities, suggesting that routine EEG is not sensitive to subtle electroencephalographic abnormalities even in patients with mild TBI with structural abnormalities on MRI.

Early studies suggested that as many as 44%–50% of patients with persistent postconcussive symptoms have electroencephalographic abnormalities in the late postinjury period, including generalized or focal slowing and occasional epileptiform discharges (Denker and Perry 1954; Torres and Shapiro 1961). More recent studies using rigidly defined conventional electroencephalographic rating criteria do not support these earlier observations (Haglund and Persson 1990; Jacome and Risko 1984), leaving uncertain the relationship between postconcussive symptoms and conventional electroencephalographic findings.

It is possible for patients to have electroencephalographic abnormalities on a post-TBI recording that are unrelated to their symptoms or that may have antedated their injuries. Conversely, patients may have postconcussive symptoms, including posttraumatic epilepsy, without readily apparent abnormalities on conventional EEG. Nonetheless, abnormal electroencephalographic findings whose location, type, and severity correlate well with clinical problems occurring after TBI should be regarded as strongly suggestive of injury-induced electrophysiological abnormalities. It is important to note that epileptiform electroencephalographic abnormalities are relatively uncommon findings in the immediate postinjury period, and, even when present, they do not robustly predict the development of posttraumatic epilepsy (Tippin and Yamada 1996). Nonetheless, persistence of epileptiform abnormalities in a patient with paroxysmal clinical events consistent with seizures after TBI strongly suggests posttraumatic epilepsy. Additionally, a markedly abnormal background rhythm, mildly abnormal rhythms not better accounted for by medications or concurrent medical conditions, focal slowing, or focal epileptiform discharges in the late postinjury period should raise concern for the possibility of underlying structural abnormalities.

In summary, conventional EEG may contribute to the evaluation of severely brain-injured patients in the days to weeks after injury. Severe electroencephalographic abnormalities, as well as combinations of less severe but still abnormal findings, may be of value when making prognoses about survival and functional outcome after severe TBI. Less severe electroencephalographic abnormalities tend to improve significantly or resolve over time in patients who survive their TBI. However, persistent electroencephalographic abnormalities whose type and location are clinically correlated with certain neurological or neuropsychiatric disturbances in the late period after TBI indicate the presence of functionally important physiological and, possibly structural, brain abnormalities. Conventional electroencephalographic evaluations may be particularly useful in the evaluation of patients with events suggestive of posttraumatic epilepsy in either the acute or late postinjury periods. However, the absence of epileptiform abnormalities on EEG does not necessarily suggest that such events are of a nonepileptic nature (e.g., psychogenic or cardiogenic). Put another way, an absence of evidence of electrophysiological abnormalities on conventional EEG does not constitute evidence of absence of such. Because routine EEG is relatively insensitive to many of the subtleties of cerebral electrophysiology and to deeper sources of electrophysiological activity, it should be regarded as having only limited utility in the neuropsychiatric evaluation of patients with TBIs.

Quantitative Electroencephalography

Quantification of the EEG provides methods of data analysis that may be more sensitive to electrophysiological subtleties than conventional visual inspection of the electroencephalographic record (Hughes and John 1999). Although there has been considerable debate about the validity, reliability, sensitivity, and specificity of quantitative electroencephalographic findings associated with TBI (Hughes and John 1999; Nuwer 1997; Thatcher et al. 1999), these methods of electroencephalographic interpretation and analysis continue to hold promise for the investigation of neuropsychiatric disorders in general and the neuropsychiatric consequences of TBI in particular (Gevins et al. 1992).

Several early studies of acutely brain-injured patients suggested that spectral analysis of frequency data demonstrated abnormalities that predicted outcome (Bricolo et al. 1979; Steudel and Kruger 1979; Strnad and Strnadova

1987). In these studies, slower monotonous rhythms and limited or poor reactivity after TBI were associated with death in as many as 86% of subjects, whereas relatively greater amounts of alpha and theta activity portended better survival rates. More recently, Theilen et al. (2000) applied spectral analysis to frontally acquired electroencephalographic data in acutely severely injured patients to determine the predictive value of the electroencephalogram silence ratio (ESR). The ESR was defined as intervals of suppression of electroencephalographic activity lasting more than 240 milliseconds in which the electroencephalographic amplitude did not exceed 5 μV (also known as the *burst-suppression ratio*). This measure was inversely correlated with outcome at 6 months as assessed using Glasgow Outcome Scale scores and Rappaport Disability Rating Scale scores. In other words, increased electrical silence in the EEG in the acute injury period was highly correlated with poor functional outcome and/or death at 6 months. Although this finding echoes early reports of poor outcome in association with electrocerebral silence assessed by visual inspection of conventional electroencephalographic recordings (Hockaday et al. 1965), the ESR offers an easily measured and quantified variable for inclusion in postinjury prognostications. When used in the fashion described by Theilen et al. (2000), the ESR predicted outcome with an accuracy of 90%, exceeding that offered by somatosensory evoked potentials (84%), GCS at 6 hours postinjury (75%), or age (68%).

Kane et al. (1998) demonstrated the potential value of topographic analysis of relative electroencephalographic power in the prediction of 6-month and 1-year outcome after severe TBI. In particular, they demonstrated significant correlations between left frontocentral beta and alpha; left centrotemporal beta, alpha, theta, and delta; right frontocentral beta; and right centrotemporal beta and alpha power and outcome from posttraumatic coma. In particular, loss of left frontocentral beta and centrotemporal beta and alpha power was associated with poor outcome after TBI.

Thatcher et al. (1991) applied a topographic analysis of electroencephalographic power, coherence, phase, and symmetry to outcome predictions in a group of 162 patients with TBI at various levels of severity. They demonstrated highly significant correlations between Rappaport Disability Rating Scale scores and measures of electroencephalographic coherence and phase between multiple frontal and frontocentral electrodes. In this study, the combined GCS scores obtained at the time of electroencephalographic recording (on average, 7.5 days after TBI) and the measures of electroencephalographic coherence and phase provided 95.8% discriminant accuracy between good outcome and death. Unlike the more recent study by Kane et al. (1998), Thatcher and colleagues did not find electroencephalographic power values of similar significance in prognostic predictions. It is possible that the inclusion of a relatively more mildly injured group of subjects may have reduced the likelihood of significant power reductions, as mild injuries are less likely to produce the types and severities of cortical, diencephalic, and brainstem injuries likely to produce coma (as in the Kane et al. study) and related reductions in beta and alpha power. Instead, the inclusion of relatively more mildly injured patients may have increased the likelihood of finding significant changes in more subtle measures of brain network function (i.e., coherence and phase) in these subjects. Despite their methodological differences, both studies demonstrate that topographic quantitative electroencephalographic analyses offer information not available with conventional EEG that may be useful in predicting outcome after TBI.

QEEG may also be useful for the evaluation of patients in the postacute and late periods after TBI. Montgomery et al. (1991) evaluated bilateral temporoparietal electroencephalographic spectra in 26 patients with mild TBI and postconcussive symptoms acutely and at 6 weeks after TBI and demonstrated a relative excess of theta power bilaterally immediately after TBI that significantly improved by the time of subsequent assessment. This study did not report correlations between relative normalization of theta power and resolution of postconcussive symptoms, leaving unanswered the strength of this relationship, if any. Additionally, more comprehensive assessment of other measures (coherence, phase, and symmetry) were not undertaken by Montgomery and colleagues. Nonetheless, this study suggests that QEEG may be useful for tracking the recovery of electrophysiological function after TBI.

Other neuropsychiatric consequences of TBI, including hostility (Demaree and Harrison 1996), postconcussive syndrome (Fenton 1996), and treatment-resistant depression (Mas et al. 1993), have been studied using QEEG. In these conditions, the principal application of QEEG has been to define electrophysiological abnormalities (typical changes in power in one or more frequency bands) that might improve understanding of the neurobiology of these sequelae of TBI.

Comparatively greater efforts have been put toward the development of QEEG-based discriminant functions (a statistically derived set of measures that permit pattern recognition in complex data sets) capable of accurately identifying electrophysiological changes that discriminate robustly those individuals with TBI from those without TBI (Thatcher et al. 1989, 2001b). QEEG-based dis-

criminant functions that index injury severity might improve predictions of clinical outcome and assist in the development of rehabilitation strategies for patients with known TBI. Additionally, such discriminant functions might improve diagnostic accuracy if capable of robustly distinguishing between individuals with and without TBI. Such functions might also be of benefit in the medicolegal evaluation of patients with mild TBI whose clinical symptoms and neuropsychological impairments are not corroborated by abnormalities on conventional EEG or structural neuroimaging.

In an early study of the potential usefulness of discriminant functions comprised of multiple quantitative electroencephalographic variables, Randolph and Miller (1988) studied 10 patients with neuropsychologically significant TBI in the late (2-to 4-year) postinjury period and 10 matched controls. Spectral analysis demonstrated increased amplitudes in the beta, theta, and delta ranges; increased amplitude variance; and reduced correlation coefficients between homologous electrode sites. Among these findings, increased amplitude variance in temporal areas correlated with poorer neuropsychological performance. The authors note that these findings suggest the persistence of clinical significant electrophysiological dysfunction after TBI that is not amenable to detection with conventional electroencephalographic analysis, and that several quantitative electroencephalographic variables appear to offer some discriminant validity for the detection of symptomatic TBI survivors.

In an effort to develop a QEEG-based discriminant function capable of accurately distinguishing between individuals with and without mild TBI, Thatcher et al. (1989) studied 608 individuals with documented uncomplicated mild TBI (GCS = 13–15) producing either no LOC or LOC less than 20 minutes and 108 noninjured comparison subjects. The initial phases of the study included the assessment of 243 patients with mild TBI and 83 noninjured comparison subjects, the results of which were used to build sets of variables to be entered into the discriminant function. After defining the relevant electroencephalographic variables, their use in the proposed discriminant function was independently cross-validated in three additional series of patients. Data from one of these series demonstrated that the discriminant function offered a high level of test-retest reliability. From these studies, three classes of neurophysiological variables provided the basis for the discriminant function: increased coherence and decreased phase in frontal and frontotemporal regions, decreased power differences between anterior and posterior cortical regions, and reduced alpha power in posterior cortical regions. Using these variables, the discriminant function affords 96.6% sensitivity and

89.2% specificity for mild TBI versus no injury, and also offers a positive predictive value of 93.6% and a negative predictive value of 97.4% (Thatcher et al. 1999).

Increased coherence and decreased phase in frontal and frontotemporal regions may suggest a loss of functional differentiation between frontal and frontotemporal areas that would not be expected in a noninjured brain (Thatcher et al. 1989). A similar interpretation of reduced anteroposterior power differences was also offered. Reduced posterior alpha was taken to suggest reduced cortical excitability, consistent with previous observations of postinjury alpha reductions described in the conventional EEG literature. Thus, each of three classes of neurophysiological variables comprising the discriminant function were understood as modifications of brain function attributable to the effects of mechanical brain injury.

Thatcher and colleagues subsequently demonstrated correlations between electroencephalographic coherence (1998b), amplitude (1998a), and power (2001a) and increases in T2 relaxation times in cortical gray matter and white matter in patients with TBI. These findings suggest that subtle alterations in the composition of these tissues are associated with abnormalities of electrophysiological function and provide support for the hypothesis that the variables in the TBI discriminant function reflect reduced functional differentiation of the brain areas whose function they index.

Thornton (1999) reported a similar study of a mild TBI discriminant function predicated on the work of Thatcher et al. (1989) but extending the frequency spectrum of interest to include higher ranges (32–64 Hz) than those included previously. Quantitative electroencephalographic variables were collected from 91 adult and adolescent subjects, including 32 TBI subjects with LOC less than 20 minutes ("mild TBI"), seven TBI subjects with LOC greater than 20 minutes, and 52 noninjured comparison subjects. Thornton reported that the mild TBI discriminant function correctly identified 79% of subjects, even 43 years postinjury. His additional high-frequency discriminant correctly identified 87% of the mild TBI subjects across all time periods after injury and 100% of subjects within 1 year of accident. The combination of the original mild TBI discriminant function and the additional high-frequency discriminant variables correctly classified 100% of the TBI subjects.

In the most recent study of this sort, Thatcher et al. (2001b) extended the discriminant function to patients with moderate and severe TBI and noted similar alterations in coherence, phase, and amplitude to those described in the mild TBI discriminant function. Additionally, more severe QEEG discriminant function scores were correlated with more severe neuropsychological im-

pairments, even when such assessments were performed months to years after TBI. Taken together, these studies suggest that quantitative electroencephalographic variables may usefully index the presence, severity, and neuropsychological effects of TBI at all levels of severity.

Although the quantitative electroencephalographic discriminant functions described by Thatcher and colleagues (1989, 2001b) appear to distinguish robustly between patients with TBI at various levels of initial injury severity and also between TBI and noninjured comparison subjects, they are not intended to provide a method for distinguishing patients with TBI and those presenting with similar cognitive impairments due to other causes such as depression, attention deficit hyperactivity disorder, substance abuse, and so forth. Although these other neuropsychiatric conditions have been characterized using QEEG (see Evans and Abarbanel 1999 for a review), direct comparisons of the discriminant validity of these patterns when compared not against controls subjects but against other clinical conditions are not available at present. Therefore, it is not appropriate to compare an individual patient's quantitative electroencephalographic data with one or another of these databases in the hope of identifying the "correct diagnosis." It is entirely likely that the set of quantitative electroencephalographic variables that discriminate between patients with mild TBI and controls will not be the same as those that discriminate between mild TBI and other neuropsychiatric conditions. With this in mind, Thatcher et al. (1999) and Duffy et al. (1994) stated quite clearly that clinical diagnoses should not be made solely by virtue of fitting electroencephalographic data with one or another quantitative electroencephalographic discriminant score. Until studies designed to ascertain the accuracy with which the TBI discriminant function distinguishes TBI from these other conditions are completed, the routine clinical use of discriminant function databases claiming to offer diagnoses across a range of neuropsychiatric conditions is not advisable.

It is also important for clinicians working with traumatically brain-injured patients in either clinical or medicolegal contexts to be aware that the use of QEEG and the mild TBI discriminant function are subjects of substantial, and at times acrimonious, debate. Shortly after the mild TBI discriminant function was described (Thatcher et al. 1989), a position paper offered by the American Academy of Neurology (AAN) (1989) characterized QEEG as experimental and therefore without clear indication for use in routine clinical practice. Almost a decade later, Nuwer (1997), writing on behalf of the AAN and American Clinical Neurophysiology Society (ACNS), offered a review of the evidence supporting the usefulness of QEEG and, in particular, the mild TBI discriminant function described by Thatcher et al. (1989). He concluded that "evidence of clinical usefulness or consistency or results are not considered sufficient for us to support its [QEEG] use in diagnosis of patients with postconcussion syndrome, or minor or moderate head injury." Additionally, this position paper rejected the use of QEEG in medicolegal contexts. This paper was followed by two rebuttals by Thatcher et al. (1999) and Hoffman et al. (1999). These rebuttal papers described problems in the AAN and AAN/ACNS reports, including factual misrepresentations, omissions, and biases, and their authors suggested that these problems are of a severity sufficient to merit reconsideration and/or frank dismissal of the official AAN/ACNS position on QEEG in TBI. It is not our intention here to offer an opinion with respect to the merits of the AAN/ACNS position paper or the rebuttal papers it prompted. Instead, we strongly suggest that clinicians involved in the care and medicolegal evaluation of individuals with mild TBI review these papers independently before forming either a clinical or a medicolegal opinion about these issues.

Evoked Potentials and Event-Related Potentials

EPs reflect neurophysiological processing along the pathways from sensation to primary sensory cortex (Misulis and Fakhoury 2001). EPs develop 1–150 milliseconds after presentation of the stimulus used to evoke them, with the exact timing (latency) of the EP after stimulus delivery dependent on the location of its neural generators along the processing pathway in which it is evoked. In general, EPs reflect automatic sensory information processes occurring before conscious recognition and intentional processing of the stimulus. ERPs reflect the neurophysiological processes associated with cognitive, sensory, or motor events (Pfefferbaum et al. 1995). ERPs develop 70–500 milliseconds after the event that evokes them. The speed with which these neurophysiological processes occur makes them relatively inaccessible to study using self-report, neuropsychological assessment, behavioral assessments, or functional neuroimaging methods (Pfefferbaum et al. 1995; Reeve 1996). The exquisite temporal resolution of EPs and ERPs offers a method of investigating the earliest components of sensory and cognitive function and dysfunction that would otherwise be difficult, if not impossible, to study in living human subjects.

EPs and ERPs are generally named according to their polarity and latency; the names of EPs are often also qualified by indicating the sensory modality in which they are evoked. The polarity of an EP or ERP is defined by the

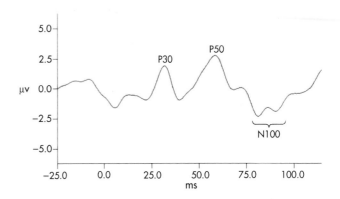

FIGURE 7–7. **P30 and P50 evoked potentials (EPs).** P30 and P50 EPs to a short-duration, moderate intensity, broad-frequency binaural stimulus in a 34-year-old male control subject. The actual latencies of these EPs vary from their stated latency by approximately 10 milliseconds (ms); this degree of variability is normal and is expected in most recordings. The low-amplitude N100 in this tracing is "split," meaning that two definable but partially overlapping waveforms contribute to the EP observed in this tracing.

positive or negative deflection of its waveform in the electroencephalographic tracing. The *latency* of an EP refers to the time after stimulus delivery at which the EP or ERP develops. For example, the positive waveforms evoked approximately 30 and 50 milliseconds after the delivery of an auditory stimulus are referred to as the *P30* and *P50*, respectively; the largest auditory evoked negative waveform between 70–100 milliseconds is designated the *N100* (Figure 7–7).

The amplitude of EPs and ERPs is quite small (0.1–10 μV) compared with that of the background EEG (10–100 μV). Consequently, computer-assisted signal averaging of many stimulus-evoked response sets is used to improve detection of these small signals. The signal-averaging process assumes that the amplitude of EP or ERP is stable (signal) and that the waveforms in the background EEG are random (noise). Averaging the results of many stimulus-EP trials results in reduction of the amplitude of the background electroencephalographic waveforms because the mathematical average of random noise approximates zero. This process improves the signal-to-noise ratio within EP and ERP data sets, enhances signal detection, and facilitates recognition of subtle differences in the effects of stimuli or events on the waveforms they evoke (Cudmore and Segalowitz 2000).

Short-Latency Evoked Potentials

A number of studies have used short-latency somatosensory, auditory, or visual EPs to characterize brain function in deeply comatose, sedated, or pharmacologically paralyzed, uncooperative patients after severe TBI in the acute and postacute injury periods (Guerit 2000). Short-latency EPs have been of particular interest in the study of EP predictions of outcome after traumatically induced coma. Given that coma may result from injury to the reticular or diencephalic areas, EPs that reflect function in these areas may usefully index the extent of injury to them. Short-latency EPs are relatively less susceptible to artifacts related to medications, and they appear to reflect more elemental reticular-diencephalic-cortical connections than either long-latency EPs or ERPs (Newlon 1983; Tippin and Yamada 1996). Because short-latency EPs assess the integrity of elemental brain areas and because there is a reasonable correlation between the integrity of these areas and short-term outcome after TBI (Wedekind et al. 2002), short-latency EPs may be useful for prediction of outcome after severe TBI (Jordan 1993).

A pattern of absent cortical but preserved brainstem activities suggests ischemic-anoxic encephalopathy, whereas major abnormalities of somatosensory conductions at the midbrain and cortical level, with variable additional involvement of auditory pontine and cortical and visual cortical pathways, is more consistent with severe TBI (Guerit 1994; Guerit et al. 1993). Because severe TBI often entails both mechanical and hypoxic-ischemic injury (Halliday 1999; McIntosh et al. 1999), both patterns may be observed after such injuries. The outcome is worse in the absence of improving multimodal EP patterns (i.e., patterns that do not normalize in the acute injury period) and better when these EPs suggest both nonfixed mesencephalic dysfunction and a relative preservation of cortical function (Guerit 1994).

Several studies suggest that somatosensory EPs (SEPs) alone are sensitive predictors of outcome after severe TBI (Goldberg and Karazim 1998; Guerit 1994; Jabbari et al. 1987; Kane et al. 1996). Anderson et al. (1984) observed that SEPs were more accurate predictors of clinical outcome after severe TBI than intracranial pressure, pupillary light reaction, or motor findings on clinical examination. SEPs also accurately identify impending clinical deterioration in the postacute injury period (Dauch 1991; Ganes and Lundar 1988; Newlon et al. 1982). Dauch (1991) demonstrated that diminution in amplitude or disappearance of the primary cortical SEP predicted clinical deterioration 4–144 hours earlier than deterioration of pupillary findings on clinical examination. Ganes and Lundar (1988) similarly observed that the first neurophysiological parameter indicating a grave prognosis was the disappearance of the cortical SEPs bilaterally, which often occurred hours to days before cessation of the spontaneous electroencephalographic activity. These observations suggest that ongoing EP assessments in the acute and postacute injury period

may improve early recognition of worsening cerebral dysfunction, thereby facilitating the delivery of timely therapeutic interventions.

Many studies have demonstrated that multimodal EPs are useful in identification of severe cerebral, diencephalic, and brainstem dysfunction after TBI and may facilitate accurate prognostication of outcome after TBI (Tippin and Yamada 1996). For example, Narayan et al. (1981) demonstrated outcome prediction accuracy of 91% using multimodal EPs, and their use yielded no falsely pessimistic outcome predictions. In their study, multimodal EPs offered better outcome prediction than clinical examination, computed tomography findings, or intracranial pressure. Although a few studies suggest that outcome prediction is improved with the combined use of SEPs and brainstem auditory evoked responses (Mahapatra 1990) or SEPs and QEEG-based assessments (Montgomery et al. 1991; Tsubokawa et al. 1990), no single or combination electrophysiological method of outcome prediction is superior to any other. Instead, it appears that in the hands of a skilled clinical electrophysiologist each of these tools usefully contribute to outcome prediction after severe TBI.

Short-latency auditory EPs have been used to investigate whether mild TBI is associated with changes similar to those observed in more severely injured patients and whether EP abnormalities are correlated with the development and persistence of postconcussive symptoms. Brainstem auditory EPs are abnormal in 10%–30% of mild TBI patients, including delayed latencies (Benna et al. 1982; McClelland et al. 1994; Rizzo et al. 1983; Rowe and Carlson 1980; Schoenhuber and Gentilini 1986; Schoenhuber et al. 1987, 1988) and reduced amplitudes (Haglund and Persson 1990). These findings suggest that mild TBI produces pathophysiologic changes similar to severe TBI, although perhaps less often. However, the relationship between abnormal short-latency EPs and persistent postconcussive symptoms is not robust (Gaetz and Weinberg 2000; Schoenhuber and Gentilini 1986; Schoenhuber et al. 1988; Werner and Vanderzant 1991) and are not useful for distinguishing between mildly brain-injured individuals with and without "true" postconcussive symptoms.

A major methodological flaw of such studies is their lack of an a priori hypothesis regarding the relationship between a particular EP abnormality and a specific postconcussive symptom. Most attempt correlations between short-latency EP abnormalities and any of several postconcussive symptoms without clearly articulating the nature of the proposed relationship between them. One exception is the study by Rowe and Carlson (1980), which found a predicted relationship between short-latency brainstem auditory EPs (which index the function of cranial nerve VIII) and postconcussive dizziness. This finding suggests that some abnormal EPs in patients with mild TBI may bear a relationship to postconcussive symptoms when both are predicated on dysfunction of the same neural pathways and systems. Pairing postconcussive symptoms and EPs and EPRs may yield more useful information about the physiology of such symptoms, particularly when the neural bases of both the symptoms and the EPs or ERPs are well understood. Although the short-latency EPs do not appear to facilitate such pairings, middle- and long-latency EPs and ERPs appear better suited to such investigations.

Middle-Latency Evoked and Event-Related Potentials

Using EPs and ERPs to investigate specific symptoms produced by TBI is characteristic of more recent investigations in this area, although only a few studies investigating middle-latency EPs in TBI are available for review. Among these are several recent studies of the P50 evoked response to paired auditory stimuli after TBI performed in our laboratories.

We have suggested that impairment of the hippocampally mediated, cholinergically dependent, preattentive process of sensory gating may, at least in part, underlie persistent attention and memory impairments after TBI (Arciniegas et al. 1999) and might be reflected by abnormal P50 evoked responses to paired auditory stimuli. The auditory P50 is a middle-latency EP that reflects cortical processing of auditory stimuli (Freedman et al. 1994). Although there are several neural systems that generate a P50 EP to auditory stimuli (Reite et al. 1988), the manner in which P50 responses are evoked by closely paired stimuli differ between these systems (Clementz et al. 1998). The hippocampus is a principal generator of the P50 (Bickford-Wimer et al. 1990), and it responds to closely paired auditory stimuli by inhibiting (or "gating") its evoked responses to the second of these pairs (Figure 7–8). This response is dependent on adequate cholinergic input to the hippocampus (Adler et al. 1999; Freedman et al. 1994; Luntz-Leybman et al. 1992). Failures in P50 gating are associated with symptoms of impaired auditory gating in patients with schizophrenia (Adler et al. 1998, 1999; Boutros et al. 1991, 1995; Freedman et al. 1994, 1996; Nagamoto et al. 1989, 1991) and in patients with several other psychiatric diagnoses (Baker et al. 1987) in which either or both cholinergic dysfunction and hippocampal abnormalities occur.

Multiple animal (Ciallella et al. 1998; DeAngelis et al. 1994; Dixon et al. 1994a, 1994b, 1997a, 1997b; Saija et al.

1988) and human (Dewar and Graham 1996; Murdoch et al. 1998) studies suggest that TBI results in dysfunction of hippocampal cholinergic systems. We hypothesized that hippocampal cholinergic dysfunction contributes to persistent sensory gating impairments after TBI and that impaired sensory gating contributes, at least in part, to TBI-induced attention and memory dysfunction (Arciniegas et al. 1999, 2000). We further suggested that abnormal P50 physiology among patients with chronic impairments in auditory sensory gating, attention, and memory after TBI might serve as a putative marker of cholinergic dysfunction in these patients.

We demonstrated impaired P50 suppression among TBI survivors with persistent symptoms of impaired auditory gating in the late (>1 year) postinjury period in two reports. The first described abnormal P50 suppression in a case series of three individuals with traumatically induced persistent impairments in auditory gating (Arciniegas et al. 1999). The second described a study comparing 20 subjects with TBI of varying levels of initial injury severity and persistently impaired auditory sensory gating in the late postinjury period to a group of age- and gender-matched noninjured comparison subjects (Arciniegas et al. 2000). Importantly, this study matched patients for clinical outcome (not initial injury) severity and the presence of symptoms of impaired auditory sensory gating. Comparable degrees of P50 nonsuppression were observed among subjects with symptoms of impaired auditory gating after TBI irrespective of initial TBI severity. In a subsequent study, we demonstrated marked bilateral hippocampal volume reductions in subjects with TBI and persistent P50 nonsuppression (Arciniegas et al. 2001). We suggested that these findings provide convergent evidence of functional and structural hippocampal abnormalities in these affected individuals. More recently, we used donepezil HCl (a cholinesterase inhibitor) as a pharmacologic probe of the hippocampal cholinergic system in these subjects. Ten subjects with remote (>1 year) TBI of at least mild severity and persistent symptoms of impaired auditory gating, attention, and memory received treatment with donepezil HCl in a randomized, double-blind, placebo-controlled, crossover design. One-half of the subjects received donepezil HCl, 5 mg daily for 6 weeks, followed by donepezil HCl, 10 mg daily for 6 weeks, and two 6-week periods of treatment with matching placebos. The other half of the subjects received two 6-week periods of placebo followed by 6 weeks of donepezil HCl, 5 mg daily, and then donepezil HCl, 10 mg daily. The group P50 ratio was significantly reduced during treatment with low-dose donepezil HCl but not during treatment with high-dose donepezil HCl or placebo (Arciniegas et al. 2002).

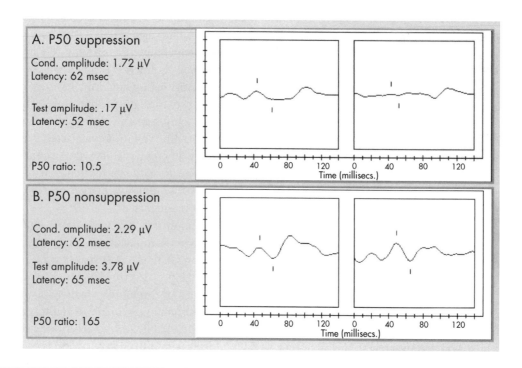

FIGURE 7–8.   P50 suppression (A) and nonsuppression (B).

Part A illustrates normal P50 response in a noninjured control subject. Part B illustrates abnormal P50 response in a 19-year-old patient approximately 1 year after mild traumatic brain injury. In both parts, the P50 response to the conditioning click is on the left, and the P50 response to the test click is on the right.

Source.   Adapted from Arciniegas D, Olincy A, Topkoff J, et al: "Impaired Auditory Gating and P50 Nonsuppression Following Traumatic Brain Injury." *Journal of Neuropsychiatry and Clinical Neurosciences* 12:77–85, 2000.

These studies suggest that at least some individuals who experience a TBI will develop impairments in auditory sensory gating and P50 nonsuppression that persist well into the late postinjury period. The observation that neurophysiological abnormalities normalized in response to low-dose cholinergic augmentation in these subjects is consistent with the suggestion that P50 nonsuppression in this population reflects cholinergic dysfunction. As such, the quality of P50 physiology may serve as a marker of cholinergic function in the late postinjury period after TBI, and both this marker and the clinical symptoms with which it is associated may index patients whose cognitive impairments might respond to treatment with medications that augment cholinergic functioning.

Similar pairings of postconcussive symptoms and EPs have been performed in the visual system. Rizzo et al. (1983) reported that approximately 10% of subjects with postconcussive syndrome demonstrated abnormal visual EP latencies. However, Freed and Hellerstein (1997) reported cortical visual EP abnormalities in 39 of 50 (78%) patients with mild TBI presenting for optometric rehabilitation in the postacute and late period after injury. In other words, the frequency of visual EP abnormalities is appreciably higher among patients who do not simply have "postconcussive symptoms," but whose postconcussive symptoms specifically include visual disturbances. Eighteen of these patients underwent optometric rehabilitation, and the remainder received no specific visual therapy. When visual EP testing was performed 12–18 months later, only 38% of the treated patients with mild TBI demonstrated persistent visual EP abnormalities, whereas 78% of the untreated patients continued to demonstrate abnormal visual EPs. Although the nature of the interaction between optometric rehabilitation and improvement in visual EPs is not clear, these findings suggest that pairing the EP of interest to specific postconcussive symptoms (in this case, visual disturbances) may offer information substantiating the presence of neurobiological dysfunction related to the symptom and thereby provide a method of monitoring neurobiological changes during treatment.

Long-Latency Evoked and Event-Related Potentials

Long-latency EPs and ERPs appear to be particularly useful markers of novel stimulus detection (Näätänen 1986, 1992), of attention and related aspects of cognition

(Gaetz et al. 2000), and of the allocation of cerebral resources for the performance of cognitive tasks (Kramer et al. 1985). Because patients with persistent cognitive impairments after TBI frequently report difficulty performing cognitive tasks that are related to these functions, long-latency EPs and ERPs have been used extensively in the study of TBI-related cognitive impairments and the postconcussive syndrome (Tippin and Yamada 1996).

The most frequently studied long-latency EPs and ERPs in the TBI population include the auditory mismatch negativity (MMN), auditory N200 (N2), P300 (P3), and contingent negative variation (CNV) (Gaetz et al. 2000). The MMN is an anteriorly distributed negative response occurring approximately 100 milliseconds after stimulus delivery and reflects stimulus change detection at the level of the cortex (Pfefferbaum et al. 1995). The N2 is a negative ERP that occurs approximately 200–250 milliseconds after stimulus delivery and is maximally distributed in the frontal regions. The N2 is generally regarded as the earliest ERP reflection of target categorization (N2 latency) and the attentional effort associated with that categorization (N2 amplitude) (Fitzgerald and Picton 1983).

The P3 is a positive ERP that occurs approximately 250–500 milliseconds after stimulus delivery and involves two major components: the quickly evoked P3a and more slowly developing late positivity, referred to by some authors as the *P3b* (Näätänen 1986). The P3a describes a positive EP occurring 250–300 milliseconds after stimulus delivery that is maximally represented over the frontocentral scalp areas. It appears P3a reflects transient allocation of attentional resources to novel stimuli, particularly task-irrelevant stimuli that automatically (and involuntarily) capture attention. The most common task used to evoke the P3a is an "oddball" paradigm. Most versions of this task consist of infrequently occurring target tones in a much larger set of frequently occurring nontarget tones, during the delivery of which the subject is instructed to count silently the number of target tones, to respond quickly to the target tones, or to perform some other operation verifying the subject's recognition of the target tones. The amplitude of the P3a may be most simply understood as the magnitude of the resources captured by irrelevant stimuli.

The P3b denotes a more slowly developing positive peak that occurs approximately 300–500 milliseconds after stimulus delivery, with more specific latencies related to the stimulus and task parameters of the experimental paradigm in which it is evoked. The P3b is evoked in response to attended targets and appears to be influenced by the time required to categorize or "evaluate" the stimulus, and its amplitude appears to be proportional to the attentional effort associated with that categorization (Näätänen 1986; Rugg et al. 1993). Both the P3a and P3b are included under the more general heading of P300, and both may be abnormal after even mild TBI (Solbakk et al. 1999).

The CNV is a sustained negative evoked response that develops over the vertex approximately 400 milliseconds after delivery of a stimulus warning the patient of an upcoming and required response. The CNV reaches a maximum approximately 800 milliseconds after the warning stimulus is delivered and may have an amplitude as high as 50 μV. The CNV is sometimes referred to as the *readiness potential* because it seems to reflect the preparation of the cortex to facilitate a response to an expected stimulus (Misulus and Fakhoury 2001; Neylan et al. 1997).

There are many reports of long-latency EPs and ERPs abnormalities after TBI, only a small subset of which is described herein. There are descriptions of the relationship between these measures and the severity of cognitive dysfunction in the acute injury period after severe (Papanicolaou et al. 1984) and mild (Pratap-Chand et al. 1988) TBI, as well as reports indicating the prognostic value of ERP abnormalities after severe (Kane et al. 1996) and mild (Lew et al. 1999) TBI. More commonly, long-latency EPs and ERPs have been used to investigate the nature of persistent cognitive impairments in the late injury period after severe (Kaipio et al. 2000; Keren et al. 1998; Rizzo et al. 1978; Rugg et al. 1993) and mild (Solbakk et al. 1999, 2000) TBI. Although the results of these studies vary depending on injury severity, the timing of recording with respect to initial injury, the specific experimental paradigm used, and the question asked by the investigators, a few consistent themes arise from this literature. Significantly reduced amplitudes or delayed latencies N2, P3b, and CNV suggest reduced and inefficient allocation of attentional processing resources after TBI, including mild TBI (Solbakk et al. 2000). Delayed development of the P3a suggests slowed detection of stimulus novelty, reduced P3a amplitude suggests inadequate allocation of novelty detection systems to incoming stimuli (e.g., inattention), and exaggerated P3a amplitude suggests excessive direction of resources to novelty (e.g., distractibility). In general, more severe long-latency EP and ERP abnormalities are associated with more severe and more recent injuries, are often associated with demonstrable neuropsychological dysfunction, and tend to improve to some degree with time after injury and as neuropsychological performance improves (Solbakk et al. 1999).

Several recent studies are particularly noteworthy in the context of the neuropsychiatry of TBI. Reinvang et al.

(2000) compared cognitive ERPs (N100, P200, N200, P300) in a modified oddball paradigm requiring both novelty detection and stimulus categorization and found evidence of deficits in early processing of neutral and nontarget stimuli in TBI subjects. As suggested above, their findings suggest that persistently cognitively impaired TBI patients are less efficient in terminating processing of irrelevant stimuli and tend to misallocate attentional resources as a whole.

The possibility that long-latency ERPs reflect subtle but physiologically important abnormalities in attention and processing resource allocation has been pursued in several recent studies of the postconcussive syndrome. Gaetz and Weinberg (2000) observed abnormally long (>2.5 standard deviations above normal) visual P3 latencies in 40% of patients with a remote (>1 year) TBI and persistent postconcussive symptoms and no comparable abnormalities in a noninjured control group. Sangal and Sangal (1996) observed increased visual P3 latencies in 75% of mild TBI subjects with postconcussive symptoms, including impaired alertness and mild cognitive complaints in the absence of overt neurological or psychiatric problems. Gaetz et al. (2000) also observed significantly delayed visual P3 latencies among persons with multiple (three or more) TBIs and demonstrated a significant correlation between the severity of memory complaints and P3 latency and slowness/difficulty in thinking and N2 and P3 latencies. These findings also support the theory that postconcussive symptoms are associated with subtle but definable neurophysiological abnormalities consistent with TBI and are not solely attributable to symptom exaggeration or malingering.

It does appear that recovery of function after concussion is associated with normalization of P3 latency (Pratap-Chand 1988; von Bierbrauer and Weissenborn 1998), although P3 amplitudes may remain abnormal (Dupuis et al. 2000). Segalowitz et al. (2001) studied a group of highly functional college students with a remote history of mild TBI and demonstrated substantially and significantly reduced P3 amplitudes and subsequent attenuation on all of the oddball tasks in their paradigm, whether those tasks were easy or difficult. They suggested that despite excellent behavioral recovery, subtle attentional and information processing deficits persist long after TBI even though such deficits may be well compensated for behaviorally and therefore not apparent on standard neuropsychological tests.

Finally, it is worth noting that P3 amplitude is reduced and P3 latency is prolonged under conditions of relative cholinergic depletion, and that these abnormalities may be normalized during administration of cholinesterase inhibitors (Frodl-Bauch et al. 1999; Hammond et al. 1987; Meador et al. 1987). Pratap-Chand et al. (1988) noted the links between cholinergic dysfunction after TBI, cholin-

ergic dysfunction and P3 abnormalities, and P3 abnormalities and postconcussive cognitive dysfunction. They suggested that recognition of these links afford an opportunity for investigation of cholinergic pharmacotherapies for cognitive dysfunction after TBI using the P3 as a metric of cholinergic function. Although this avenue of research has not, at the time of this writing, been pursued in this population, the hypothesis suggested by these authors and that described using the P50 paradigm reflect common formulations with respect to the usefulness of EPs and ERPs as neurophysiological markers of cholinergic dysfunction and attentional impairments after TBI. Additional investigations clarifying these electrophysiological-neurochemical relationships are needed, and their results may suggest a role for EPs and ERPs in the identification of neurochemical dysfunction and the selection of treatments for cognitive impairment due to TBI.

Magnetoencephalography

At the time of this writing, MEG remains an underused technology in the study of TBI. Lewine et al. (1999) investigated the usefulness of MEG and MSI for demonstrating neurophysiological abnormalities associated with mild TBI in comparison to more conventional EEG and MRI measures. Based on quantitative electroencephalographic observations of a relative shift of the power spectrum to lower frequencies, they hypothesized that MEG might reveal similar abnormal low-frequency magnetic activity (ALFMA) and that MSI would more sensitively detect areas of dysfunctional cortex than either conventional MRI or EEG.

They characterized three subject groups with these measures: group A included 20 noninjured comparison subjects; group B included 10 fully recovered subjects with mild TBI at least 2 months postinjury; group C included 20 subjects with mild TBI at least 2 months postinjury with persistent postconcussive symptoms. All noninjured comparison and asymptomatic TBI subjects had normal MRI examinations, whereas 20% of the persistently symptomatic mild TBI patients had abnormal MRI examinations. One noninjured comparison subject (5%) and one asymptomatic TBI subject (10%) had abnormal EEGs, whereas five of the symptomatic mild TBI subjects (20%) had abnormal EEGs. The MSI of all noninjured comparison and asymptomatic TBI subjects was normal. However, 13 (65%) of the symptomatic mild TBI subjects had abnormal MSI confirmed by both computer-assisted analysis and visual inspection. In this group, clusters of ALFMA localized to either the coup or contrecoup location known from the patient's injury history.

The authors noted that in the symptomatic TBI group, the MSI findings made "clinical sense" with respect to the relationship between symptom type and ALFMA location. Nine of the 13 subjects reported problems with short-term memory, and all had ALFMA localized to either the left or right temporal lobe. Four of these 13 had ALFMA localized to parietal cortices in the context of attentional impairments.

The authors also reexamined 15 subjects (10 noninjured comparison and 5 symptomatic TBI) using these procedures approximately 2–4 months after the initial assessments. None of the noninjured comparison subjects had MSI abnormalities. Two of the TBI patients experienced resolution of their symptoms in the interval between examination and were without MSI abnormalities at their second assessment. One TBI subject had partial alleviation of symptoms and partial resolution of MSI abnormalities, and the two persistently symptomatic TBI subjects had stable and still abnormal MSI findings at the time of reassessment.

These findings suggest that excessive AFLMA may index postconcussive symptoms more effectively than either conventional MRI or EEG and that the degree of MSI abnormality relates to the degree of symptomatic recovery. Preliminary analysis from this small group of subjects suggests that MSI had a sensitivity of 0.81 for detection of abnormalities in patients with cognitive dysfunction and that the MSI findings, interpreted conservatively, offered a specificity of 0.95 for this group and 0.90 for the asymptomatic TBI group. Although a single study provides no foundation for conclusions about the clinical utility of MEG in the evaluation of TBI patients, it seems reasonable to suggest that additional investigation of the application of this technique is worth undertaking.

Summary

Clinical electrophysiology offers a variety of powerful and informative methods for studying cerebral function and dysfunction after traumatic brain injury (TBI). Electroencephalography (EEG), quantitative EEG (QEEG) and topographic QEEG, evoked potentials (EPs) and event-related potentials (ERPs), and magnetoencephalography (MEG)/magnetic source imaging (MSI) measure different aspects of brain activity noninvasively and with temporal resolution vastly superior to that achieved with any of the several presently available functional neuroimaging methods. Although conventional EEG is commonly used in clinical neuropsychiatry and neurology, it has limited utility in the evaluation of the traumatically brain-injured patient. QEEG, EPs and ERPs, and MEG/MSI offer more informative and potentially more useful tools for the evaluation and study of individuals with brain injury than conventional EEG, but they also entail a much greater level of technical and analytical complexity that limits their application to clinical practice. Additionally, there remain substantial controversies about the use, clinical interpretation, and medicolegal application of these technologies, about which clinicians working with this population should be aware.

Each of the presently available electrophysiological techniques provides information about cerebral function after TBI, and some have the capacity to provide both diagnostic and predictive information. Among these, EP-, ERP-, and QEEG-based analyses offer the best hope for advancing the understanding of the neurophysiological mechanisms underlying cognitive impairments caused by TBI. MEG and MSI may be of similar use, but more research into MEG-based analyses in this population is needed before any evaluation of the merits of this technology is warranted.

Clinical and research applications of electrophysiological techniques requires substantial knowledge of human electrophysiology, familiarity and experience with the principles of electrophysiological recording, and the ability to analyze and interpret the complex data sets that these tools produce. Clinicians wishing to make routine use of electrophysiological techniques in clinical and research settings are well advised to pursue specialized training in the selection of these techniques and interpretation of the data they yield. Other clinicians working with TBI patients should, at a minimum, be familiar with the electrophysiological techniques presented in this chapter, their strengths and limitations, and their role in the evaluation, treatment, and study of these patients.

References

Adler LE, Olincy A, Waldo M, et al: Schizophrenia, sensory gating, and nicotinic receptors. Schizophr Bull 24:189–202, 1998

Adler LE, Freedman R, Ross RG, et al: Elementary phenotypes in the neurobiological and genetic study of schizophrenia. Biol Psychiatry 46:8–18, 1999

American Academy of Neurology: Assessment: EEG brain mapping. Report of the American Academy of Neurology, Therapeutics and Technology Assessment Subcommittee. Neurology 39:1100–1101, 1989

Anderson DC, Bundlie S, Rockswold GL: Multimodality evoked potentials in closed head trauma. Arch Neurol 41:369–374, 1984

Arciniegas D, Adler L, Topkoff J, et al: Attention and memory dysfunction after traumatic brain injury: cholinergic mechanisms, sensory gating, and a hypothesis for further investigation. Brain Inj 13:1–13, 1999

Arciniegas D, Olincy A, Topkoff J, et al: Impaired auditory gating and P50 nonsuppression following traumatic brain injury. J Neuropsychiatry Clin Neurosci 12:77–85, 2000

Arciniegas DB, Topkoff J, Rojas DC, et al: Reduced hippocampal volume in association with P50 nonsuppression following traumatic brain injury. J Neuropsychiatry Clin Neurosci 13:213–221, 2001

Arciniegas DB, Topkoff JL, Anderson CA, et al: Low-dose donepezil normalizes P50 physiology in traumatic brain injury patients. J Neuropsychiatry Clin Neurosci 14:115, 2002

Baker N, Adler LE, Franks RD, et al: Neurophysiological assessment of sensory gating in psychiatric inpatients: comparison between schizophrenia and other diagnoses. Biol Psychiatry 22:603–617, 1987

Benna P, Bergamasco B, Bianco C, et al: Brainstem auditory evoked potentials in postconcussion syndrome. Ital J Neurol Sci 3:281–287, 1982

Bickford-Wimer PC, Nagamoto H, Johnson R, et al: Auditory sensory gating in hippocampal systems: a model system in the rat. Biol Psychiatry 27:183–192, 1990

Boutros NN, Zouridakis G, Overall J: Replication and extension of P50 findings in schizophrenia. Clin Electroencephalogr 22:40–45, 1991

Boutros N, Torello MW, Burns EM, et al: Evoked potentials in subjects at risk for Alzheimer's disease. Psychol Res 57:57–63, 1995

Bricolo A, Formenton A, Turella G, et al: Clinical and EEG effects of mechanical hyperventilation in acute traumatic coma. Eur Neurol 8:219–224, 1972

Bricolo A, Turazzi S, Faccioli F: Combined clinical and EEG examinations for assessment of severity of acute head injuries. Acta Neurochir Suppl (Wien) 28:35–39, 1979

Cantor DS: An overview of quantitative EEG and its applications to neurofeedback, in Introduction to Quantitative EEG and Neurofeedback. Edited by Evans JR, Abarbanel A. San Diego, CA, Academic Press, 1999, pp 3–28

Ciallella JR, Yan HQ, Ma X, et al: Chronic effects of traumatic brain injury on hippocampal vesicular acetylcholine transporter and M2 muscarinic receptor protein in rats. Exp Neurol 152:11–19, 1998

Clementz BA, Geyer MA, Braff DL: Multiple site evaluation of P50 suppression among schizophrenia and normal comparison subjects. Schizophr Res 30:71–80, 1998

Coull JT: Neural correlates of attention and arousal: insights from electrophysiology, functional neuroimaging and psychopharmacology. Prog Neurobiol 55:343–361, 1998

Cudmore LJ, Segalowitz SJ: Signal-to-noise ratio sensitivity in ERPs to stimulus and task complexity: different effects for early and late components. Brain Cogn 43:130–134, 2000

Cuffin BN: Effects of local variations in skull and scalp thickness on EEGs and MEGs. IEEE Trans Biomed Eng 40:42–48, 1993

Dauch WA: Prediction of secondary deterioration in comatose neurosurgical patients by serial recording of multimodality evoked potentials. Acta Neurochirurgica 111:84–91, 1991

DeAngelis MM, Hayes RL, Lyeth BG: Traumatic brain injury causes a decrease in M2 muscarinic cholinergic receptor binding in the rat brain. Brain Res 653:39–44, 1994

Demaree HA, Harrison DW: Case study: topographical brain mapping in hostility following mild closed head injury. Int J Neurosci 87:97–101, 1996

Denker PG, Perry GF: Postconcussion syndrome in compensation and litigation: analysis of 95 cases with electroencephalographic correlations. Neurology 4:912–918, 1954

Dewar D, Graham DI: Depletion of choline acetyltransferase but preservation of Ml and M2 muscarinic receptor binding sites in temporal cortex following head injury: a preliminary human postmortem study. J Neurotrauma 13:181–187, 1996

Dixon CE, Bao J, Bergmann JS, Johnson KM: Traumatic brain injury reduces hippocampal high-affinity [^{3}H]choline uptake but not extracellular choline levels in rats. Neurosci Lett 180:127–130, 1994a

Dixon CE, Hamm RJ, Taft WC, et al: Increased anticholinergic sensitivity following closed skull impact and controlled cortical impact traumatic brain injury in the rat. J Neurotrauma 11:275–287, 1994b

Dixon CE, Ma X, Marion DW: Effects of CDP-choline treatment on neurobehavioral deficits after TBI and on hippocampal and neocortical acetylcholine release. J Neurotrauma 14:161–169, 1997a

Dixon CE, Ma X, Marion DW: Reduced evoked release of acetylcholine in the rodent neocortex following traumatic brain injury. Brain Res 749:127–130, 1997b

Duffy FH, Bartels PH, Burchfiel JL: Significance probability mapping: an aid in the topographical analysis of brain electrical activity. Electroencephalogr Clin Neurophysiol 51:455–462, 1981

Duffy FH, Hughes JR, Miranda F, et al: Status of quantitative EEG (QEEG) in clinical practice. Clin Electroencephalogr 25:VI–XXII, 1994

Dupuis F, Johnston KM, Lavoie M, et al: Concussions in athletes produce brain dysfunction as revealed by event-related potentials. Neuroreport 11:4087–4092, 2000

Evans BM, Bartlett JR: Prediction of outcome in severe head injury based on recognition of sleep reactivity in the polygraphic electroencephalogram. J Neurol Neurosurg Psychiatry 59:17–25, 1995

Evans JR, Abarbanel A: Introduction to Quantitative EEG and Neurofeedback. San Diego, CA, Academic Press, 1999

Fenton GW: The postconcussional syndrome reappraised. Clin Electroencephalogr 27:174–182, 1996

Fitzgerald PG, Picton TW: Event-related potentials recorded during the discrimination of improbable stimuli. Biol Psychiatry 17:241–276, 1983

Freed S, Hellerstein LF: Visual electrodiagnostic findings in mild traumatic brain injury. Brain Inj 11:25–36, 1997

Freedman R, Adler LE, Bickford P, et al: Schizophrenia and nicotinic receptors. Harv Rev Psychiatry 2:179–192, 1994

Freedman R, Adler LE, Myles-Worsley M, et al: Inhibitory gating of an evoked response to repeated auditory stimuli in schizophrenic and normal subjects: human recordings, computer simulation, and an animal model. Arch Gen Psychiatry 53:1114–1121, 1996

Frodl-Bauch T, Bottlender R, Hegerl U: Neurochemical substrates and neuroanatomical generators of the event-related P300. Neuropsychobiology 40:86–94, 1999

Gaetz M, Weinberg H: Electrophysiological indices of persistent post-concussion symptoms. Brain Inj 14:815–832, 2000

Gaetz M, Goodman D, Weinberg H: Electrophysiological evidence for the cumulative effects of concussion. Brain Inj 14:1077–1088, 2000

Ganes T, Lundar T: EEG and evoked potentials in comatose patients with severe brain damage. Electroencephalogr Clin Neurophysiol 69:6–13, 1988

Geets W, De Zegher F: EEG and brainstem abnormalities after cerebral concussion: short term observations. Acta Neurologica Belgica 85:277–283, 1985

Gevins A, Le J, Brickett P, et al: The future of high-resolution EEGs in assessing neurocognitive effects of mild head injury. J Head Trauma Rehabil 7:78–90, 1992

Glaser MA, Sjaardema H: The value of electroencephalogram in craniocerebral injuries. West J Surg Obstet Gynecol 48:689–695, 1940

Goldberg G, Karazim E: Application of evoked potentials to the prediction of discharge status in minimally responsive patients: a pilot study. J Head Trauma Rehabil 13:51–68, 1998

Guerit JM: The interest of multimodality evoked potentials in the evaluation of chronic coma. Acta Neurol Belg 94:174–182, 1994

Guerit JM: The usefulness of EEG, exogenous evoked potentials, and cognitive evoked potentials in the acute stage of post-anoxic and post-traumatic coma. Acta Neurol Belg 100:229–236, 2000

Guerit JM, de Tourtchaninoff M, Soveges L, et al: The prognostic value of three-modality evoked potentials (TMEPs) in anoxic and traumatic comas. Neurophysiologie Clinique 23:209–226, 1993

Gütling E, Gonser A, Imhof H-G, Landis T: EEG reactivity in the prognosis of severe head injury. Neurology 45:915–918, 1995

Haglund Y, Persson HE: Does Swedish amateur boxing lead to chronic brain damage? 3: a retrospective clinical neurophysiology study. Acta Neurol Scand 82:353–360, 1990

Halliday AL: Pathophysiology, in Traumatic Brain Injury. Edited by Marion DW. New York, Thieme Medical, 1999, pp 29–38

Hammond EJ, Meador KJ, Aung-Din R, et al: Cholinergic modulation of human P3 event-related potentials. Neurology 37:346–350, 1987

Hockaday JM, Potts F, Bonazzi A, et al: Electroencephalographic changes in acute cerebral anoxia from cardiac or respiratory arrest. Electroencephalogr Clin Neurophysiol 18:575–586, 1965

Hoffman DA, Lubar JF, Thatcher RW, et al: Limitations of the American Academy of Neurology and American Clinical Neurophysiology Society paper on QEEG. J Neuropsychiatry Clin Neurosci 11:401–407, 1999

Hughes JR: EEG in Clinical Practice. New York, Butterworth Publishers, Inc., 1982

Hughes JR, John ER: Conventional and quantitative electroencephalography in psychiatry. J Neuropsychiatry Clin Neurosci 11:190–208, 1999

Hutchinson DO, Frith NA, Shaw NA, et al: A comparison between electroencephalography and somatosensory evoked potentials for outcome prediction following severe head injury. Electroencephalogr Clin Neurophysiol 78:228–233, 1991

Jabbari B, Vance SC, Harper MG, et al: Clinical and radiological correlates of somatosensory evoked potentials in the late phase of head injury: a study of 500 Vietnam veterans. Electroencephalogr Clin Neurophysiol 67:289–297, 1987

Jacome DE, Risko M: EEG features in post-traumatic syndrome. Clin Electroencephalogr 15:214–221, 1984

Jasper HH, Kershman J, Elvidge A: Electroencephalographic studies of injury to the head. Arch Neurol 44:328–348, 1940

Jerrett SA, Corsak J: Clinical utility of topographic EEG brain mapping. Clin Electroencephalogr 19:134–143, 1988

John ER, Karmel BZ, Corning WC, et al: Neurometrics: numerical taxonomy identifies different profiles of brain functions within groups of behaviorally similar people. Science 210:1255–1258, 1977

Jordan KG: Continuous EEG and evoked potential monitoring in the neuroscience intensive care unit. J Clin Neurophysiol 10:445–475, 1993

Kaipio ML, Cheour M, Ceponiene R, et al: Increased distractibility in closed head injury as revealed by event-related potentials. Neuroreport 11:1463–1468, 2000

Kane NM, Curry SH, Rowlands CA, et al: Event-related potentials—neurophysiological tools for predicting emergence and early outcome from traumatic coma. Intensive Care Med 22:39–46, 1996

Kane NM, Moss TH, Curry SH, et al: Quantitative electroencephalographic evaluation of non-fatal and fatal traumatic coma. Electroencephalogr Clin Neurophysiol 106:244–250, 1998

Keren O, Ben Dror S, Stern MJ, et al: Event-related potentials as an index of cognitive function during recovery from severe closed head injury. J Head Trauma Rehabil 13:15–30, 1998

Kramer AF, Wickens CD, Donchin E: Processing of stimulus properties: evidence for dual-task integrality. J Exp Psychol Hum Percept Perform 11:393–408, 1985

Lew HL, Slimp J, Price R, et al: Comparison of speech-evoked v tone-evoked P300 response: implications for predicting outcomes in patients with traumatic brain injury. Am J Phys Med Rehabil 78:367–371, 1999

Lewine JD, Davis JT, Sloan JH, et al: Neuromagnetic assessment of pathophysiologic brain activity induced by minor head trauma. AJNR Am J Neuroradiol 20:857–866, 1999

Liguori G, Foggia L, Buonaguro A, et al: EEG findings in minor head trauma as a clue for indication to CT scan. Childs Nerv Syst 5:160–162, 1989

Luntz-Leybman V, Bickford P, Freedman R: Cholinergic gating of response to auditory stimuli in rat hippocampus. Brain Res 587:130–136, 1992

Mahapatra AK: Evoked potentials in severe head injuries: a prospective study of 40 cases. J Indian Med Assoc 88:217–220, 1990

Mas F, Prichep LS, Alper K: Treatment resistant depression in a case of minor head injury: an electrophysiological hypothesis. Clin Electroencephalogr 24:118–122, 1993

McClelland RJ, Fenton GW, Rutherford W: The postconcussional syndrome revisited. J R Soc Med 87:508–510, 1994

McCormick DA: Neurotransmitter actions in the thalamus and cerebral cortex. J Clin Neurophysiol 9:212–223, 1992a

McCormick DA: Neurotransmitter actions in the thalamus and cerebral cortex and their role in neuromodulation of thalamocortical activity. Prog Neurobiol 39:337–388, 1992b

McIntosh TK, Juhler M, Raghupathi R, et al: Secondary brain injury: neurochemical and cellular mediators, in Traumatic Brain Injury. Edited by Marion DW. New York, Thieme Medical, 1999, pp 39–54

Meador KJ, Loring DW, Adams RJ, et al: Central cholinergic systems and the P3 evoked potential. Int J Neurosci 33:199–205, 1987

Mesulam M-M: Principles of Behavioral and Cognitive Neurology, 2nd Edition. Philadelphia, PA, FA Davis, 2000

Misulis KE: Essentials of Clinical Neurophysiology, 2nd Edition. Boston, MA, Butterworth–Heinemann, 1997

Misulis KE, Fakhoury T: Spehlmann's Evoked Potential Primer, 3rd Edition. Boston, MA, Butterworth–Heinemann, 2001

Montgomery EA, Fenton GW, McClelland RJ, et al: The psychobiology of minor head injury. Psychol Med 21:375–384, 1991

Murdoch I, Perry EK, Court JA, et al: Cortical cholinergic dysfunction after human head injury. J Neurotrauma 15:295–305, 1998

Näätänen R: The orienting response theory: an integration of informational and energetical aspects of brain function, in Adaptation to Stress and Task Demands: Energetical Aspects of Human Information Processing. Edited by Hockey RGJ, Gaillard AWK, Coles M. Dordrecht, The Netherlands, Martinus Nijhoff, 1986, pp 91–111

Näätänen R: Attention and Brain Function. Hillsdale, NJ, Lawrence Erlbaum, 1992

Nagamoto HT, Adler LE, Waldo MC, et al: Sensory gating in schizophrenics and normal controls: effects of changing stimulation intervals. Biol Psychiatry 25:549–561, 1989

Nagamoto HT, Adler LE, Waldo MC, et al: Gating of auditory response in schizophrenics and normal controls: effects of recording site and stimulation interval on the P50 wave. Schizophr Res 4:31–40, 1991

Narayan RK, Greenberg RP, Miller JD, et al: Improved confidence of outcome prediction in severe head injury: a comparative analysis of the clinical examination, multimodality evoked potentials, CT scanning, and intracranial pressure. J Neurosurg 54:751–762, 1981

Newlon PG, Greenberg RP, Hyatt MS, et al: The dynamics of neuronal dysfunction and recovery following severe head injury assessed with serial multimodality evoked potentials. J Neurosurg 57:168–177, 1982

Newlon PG, Greenberg RP, Enas GG, et al: Effects of therapeutic pentobarbital coma on multimodality evoked potentials recorded from severely head-injured patients. Neurosurgery 12:613–619, 1983

Neylan TC, Reynolds CF, Kupfer DJ: Electrodiagnostic techniques in neuropsychiatry, in Textbook of Neuropsychiatry. Edited by Yudofsky SC, Hales RE. Washington, DC, American Psychiatric Press, 1997, pp 165–180

Nuwer MR: The development of EEG brain mapping. J Clin Neurophysiol 7:459–471, 1990

Nuwer MR: Assessment of digital EEG, quantitative EEG and EEG brain mapping: report of the American Academy of Neurology and the American Clinical Neurophysiology Society. Neurology 49:292, 1997

Papanicolaou AC, Levin HS, Eisenberg HM, et al: Evoked potential correlates of posttraumatic amnesia after closed head injury. Neurosurgery 14:676–678, 1984

Pfefferbaum A, Roth WT, Ford JM: Event-related potentials in the study of psychiatric disorders. Arch Gen Psychiatry 52:559–563, 1995

Pratap-Chand R, Sinniah M, Salem FA: Cognitive evoked potential (P300): a metric for cerebral concussion. Acta Neurol Scand 78:185–189, 1988

Rae-Grant AD, Barbour PJ, Reed J: Development of a new EEG rating scale for head injury using dichotomous variables. Electroencephalogr Clin Neurophysiol 79:349–357, 1991

Rae-Grant AD, Eckert N, Barbour PJ, et al: Outcome of severe brain injury: a multimodality neurophysiologic study. J Trauma 40:401–407, 1996

Randolph C, Miller MH: EEG and cognitive performance following closed head injury. Neuropsychobiology 20:46–50, 1988

Reeve A: Clinical neurophysiology in neuropsychiatry, in Neuropsychiatry. Edited by Fogel BS, Schiffer RB, Rao SM. Baltimore, MD, Williams & Wilkins, 1996, pp 65–92

Reinvang I, Nordby H, Nielsen CS: Information processing deficits in head injury assessed with ERPs reflecting early and late processing stages. Neuropsychologia 38:995–1005, 2000

Reite M, Teale P, Zimmerman J, et al: Source origin of a 50-msec latency auditory evoked field component in young schizophrenic men. Biol Psychiatry 24:495–506, 1988

Reite M, Teale P, Rojas DC: Magnetoencephalography: applications in psychiatry. Biol Psychiatry 45:1553–1563, 1999

Rizzo PA, Amabile G, Caporali M, et al: A CNV study in a group of patients with traumatic head injuries. Electroencephalogr Clin Neurophysiol 45:281–285, 1978

Rizzo PA, Pierelli F, Pozzessere G, et al: Subjective posttraumatic syndrome: a comparison of visual and brain stem auditory evoked responses. Neuropsychobiology 9:78–82, 1983

Rojas DC, Arciniegas DB, Teale PD, et al: Magnetoencephalography and magnetic source imaging: technology overview and applications in psychiatric neuroimaging. CNS Spectrums 4:37–43, 1999

Rowe MJ III, Carlson C: Brainstem auditory evoked potentials in postconcussion dizziness. Arch Neurol 37:679–683, 1980

Rugg MD, Pickles CD, Potter DD, et al: Cognitive brain potentials in a three-stimulus auditory "oddball" task after closed head injury. Neuropsychologia 31:373–393, 1993

Rumpl E, Lorenzi E, Hackl JM, et al: The EEG at different stages of acute secondary traumatic midbrain and bulbar brain syndromes. Electroencephalogr Clin Neurophysiol 46:487–497, 1979

Saija A, Robinson SE, Lyeth BG, et al: The effects of scopolamine and traumatic brain injury on central cholinergic neurons. J Neurotrauma 5:161–170, 1988

Sangal RB, Sangal JM: Closed head injury patients with mild cognitive complaints without neurological or psychiatric findings have abnormal visual P300 latencies. Biol Psychiatry 39:305–307, 1996

Schoenhuber R, Gentilini M: Auditory brain stem responses in the prognosis of late postconcussional symptoms and neuropsychological dysfunction after minor head injury. Neurosurgery 19:532–534, 1986

Schoenhuber R, Gentilini M, Scarano M, et al: Longitudinal study of auditory brain-stem response in patients with minor head injuries. Arch Neurol 44:1181–1182, 1987

Schoenhuber R, Gentilini M, Orlando A: Prognostic value of auditory brain-stem responses for late postconcussion symptoms following minor head injury. J Neurosurg 68:742–744, 1988

Segalowitz SJ, Bernstein DM, Lawson S: P300 event-related potential decrements in well-functioning university students with mild head injury. Brain Cogn 45:342–356, 2001

Solbakk AK, Reinvang I, Nielsen C, et al: ERP indicators of disturbed attention in mild closed head injury: a frontal lobe syndrome? Psychophysiology 36:802–817, 1999

Solbakk AK, Reinvang I, Neilsen CS: ERP indices of resource allocation difficulties in mild head injury. J Clin Exp Neuropsychol 22:743–760, 2000

Steudel WI, Kruger J: Using the spectral analysis of the EEG for prognosis of severe brain injuries in the first post-traumatic week. Acta Neurochir Suppl (Wien) 28:40–42, 1979

Strnad P, Strnadova V: Long-term follow-up EEG studies in patients with traumatic apallic syndrome. Eur Neurol 26:84–89, 1987

Synek VM: Revised EEG coma scale in diffuse acute head injuries in adults. Clin Exp Neurol 27:99–111, 1990a

Synek VM: Value of a revised EEG coma scale for prognosis after cerebral anoxia and diffuse head injury. Clin Electroencephalogr 21:25–30, 1990b

Thatcher RW: EEG database-guided neurotherapy, in Introduction to Quantitative EEG and Neurofeedback. Edited by Evans JR, Abarbanel A. San Diego, CA, Academic Press, 1999, pp 29–65

Thatcher RW, Walker RA, Gerson I, et al: EEG discriminant analyses of mild head trauma. Electroencephalogr Clin Neurophysiol 73:93–106, 1989

Thatcher RW, Cantor DS, McAlaster R, et al: Comprehensive predictions of outcome in closed head-injured patients: the development of prognostic equations. Ann N Y Acad Sci 620:82–101, 1991

Thatcher RW, Biver C, McAlaster R, et al: Biophysical linkage between MRI and EEG amplitude in closed head injury. Neuroimage 7:352–367, 1998a

Thatcher RW, Biver C, McAlaster R, et al: Biophysical linkage between MRI and EEG coherence in closed head injury. Neuroimage 8:307–326, 1998b

Thatcher RW, Moore N, John ER, et al: QEEG and traumatic brain injury: rebuttal of the American Academy of Neurology 1997 Report by the EEG and Clinical Neuroscience Society. Clin Electroencephalogr 30:94–98, 1999

Thatcher RW, Biver C, Gomez JF, et al: Estimation of the EEG power spectrum using MRI T(2) relaxation time in traumatic brain injury. Clin Neurophysiol 112:1729–1745, 2001a

Thatcher RW, North DM, Curtin RT, et al: An EEG severity index of traumatic brain injury. J Neuropsychiatry Clin Neurosci 13:77–87, 2001b

Theilen HJ, Ragaller M, Tscho U, et al: Electroencephalogram silence ratio for early outcome prognosis in severe head trauma. Crit Care Med 28:3522–3529, 2000

Thornton KE: Exploratory investigation into mild brain injury and discriminant analysis with high frequency bands (32–64 Hz). Brain Inj 13:477–488, 1999

Tippin J, Yamada T: The electrophysiologic evaluation of head-injured patients: value and limitations, in Head Injury and Postconcussive Syndrome. Edited by Rizzo M, Tranel D. New York, Churchill Livingstone, 1996, pp 119–138

Torres F, Shapiro SK: Electroencephalograms in whiplash injury. Arch Neurol 5:28–35, 1961

Tsubokawa T, Yamamoto T, Katayama Y: Prediction of outcome of prolonged coma caused by brain damage. Brain Inj 4:329–337, 1990

Voller B, Benke T, Benedetto K, et al: Neuropsychological, MRI and EEG findings after very mild traumatic brain injury. Brain Inj 13:821–827, 1999

von Bierbrauer A, Weissenborn K: P300 after minor head injury (a follow-up examination). Acta Neurol Belg 98:21–26, 1998

Wedekind C, Hesselmann V, Lippert-Gruner M, et al: Trauma to the pontomesencephalic brainstem—a major clue to the prognosis of severe traumatic brain injury. Br J Neurosurg 16:256–260, 2002

Werner RA, Vanderzant CW: Multimodality evoked potential testing in acute mild closed head injury. Arch Phys Med Rehabil 72:31–34, 1991

Williams SD, Denny-Brown D: Cerebral electrical changes in experimental concussion. Brain 64:223–238, 1941

Winter JW, Rosenwasser RJ, Jimenez F: Electroencephalographic activity and serum and cerebrospinal fluid pentobarbital levels in determining the therapeutic end point during barbiturate coma. Neurosurgery 29:739–742, 1991

8 Issues in Neuropsychological Assessment

Mary F. Pelham, Psy.D.

Mark R. Lovell, Ph.D.

NEUROPSYCHOLOGICAL ASSESSMENT HAS become a useful tool in neuropsychiatry and provides specific information regarding neurobehavioral functioning. The neuropsychological evaluation is focused on the formal assessment of brain–behavior relationships, using psychometric methods. This evaluation provides important information regarding type and severity of brain injury and course and process of recovery, and is particularly useful in structuring rehabilitation. This chapter reviews the use of neuropsychological assessment, with particular reference to the neuropsychiatric evaluation and treatment of the patient with traumatic brain injury (TBI).

Role of the Neuropsychologist

In the traumatically brain-injured population, the neuropsychologist most often works as part of a multidisciplinary team and contributes to treatment by determining the extent of cognitive, behavioral, and emotional deficits produced by damage to the central nervous system. In addition to identifying deficits, one of the primary purposes of neuropsychological assessment is the quantification of the individual's relative strengths and weaknesses. The data gathered from psychometric testing are integrated with nonpsychometric information acquired during the clinical interview and review of records. This multifaceted approach incorporates premorbid functioning, type of injury, patient history (med-

ical, psychiatric, social), cultural variables, behavioral observations, and the circumstances surrounding the examination (e.g., referral question) and enables the clinician to develop a comprehensive picture of the patient's overall functioning. Additionally, this collaboration greatly enhances the diagnostic accuracy of the evaluation and leads to the development of more effective treatment recommendations for the rehabilitation team, the patient, and his or her family. Neuropsychology's emphasis on the measurement of the behavioral expression of brain injury within the context of the patient's interpersonal, social, and familial environment enables the treatment team to better address both pharmacological and psychosocial needs.

Although modern anatomical and functional neuroimaging procedures have become increasingly helpful in localizing the site of brain injury after TBI, contemporary neuropsychological assessment focuses on understanding the relationship between the patient's neurocognitive deficits and the behavioral expression of these deficits within his or her environment.

Approaches to Neuropsychological Assessment of Patients With TBI

Traditionally, three approaches to neuropsychological assessment have been popular: a fixed battery of neuropsychological tests, a flexible battery approach, and a combination of fixed and flexible approaches.

Fixed Battery Approach

The fixed battery is a preset selection of tests that are given to every patient in a standard manner regardless of the referral question or the patient's symptoms. The advantages of the fixed battery are its comprehensive assessment of multiple cognitive domains and the usefulness of its standardized format for research purposes. However, the battery's lengthy administration time and lack of flexibility in different clinical situations pose a disadvantage. The Halstead-Reitan Neuropsychological Test Battery (HRNB; Reitan and Wolfson 1993) is no doubt the most frequently used fixed test battery within neuropsychology (Lovell and Nussbaum 1994).

The HRNB is a comprehensive battery comprised of five tests that measure cognitive functioning across multiple domains. Additionally, the battery is frequently supplemented with measures of general intelligence (Wechsler Adult Intelligence Scale—III [WAIS-III; Wechsler 1997a]), memory (Wechsler Memory Scale—III [WMS-III; Wechsler 1997b]), aphasia, sensory-perceptual skills, and grip strength (Franzen 2000). The five HRNB test results are used to calculate the Impairment Index, which represents the proportion of scores that fall within the impaired range. Although the Impairment Index was intended for making gross diagnostic discriminations, research indicates that conclusions regarding the simple presence or absence of brain damage based on this index have been found to be less accurate than those obtained by clinical judgment based on tests, interviews, and medical history (Tsushima and Wedding 1979). Other criticisms of the HRNB are its lengthy time of administration (6–8 hours), inappropriateness for elderly or demented patients and those with sensory or motor handicaps, and cumbersome testing materials. Nonetheless, it is a widely researched battery that is effective in discriminating a variety of neurological conditions (Franzen 2000). The well-established reliability and validity of the HRNB as well as normative data for comparisons of psychiatric populations likely contributes to its extensive use in forensic settings. Additionally, some of the subtests demonstrate ecological validity in their correlation with occupational, social, and independent living criteria (Heaton and Pendleton 1981).

Flexible Battery Approach

The flexible battery is a battery of tests that are selected by the neuropsychologist based on the patient's presenting illness or referral question. Thus, the battery is tailored to each individual based on the specific diagnostic question. The advantages of using a flexible approach include a possible shorter administration time, lower economic costs, and the ability to adapt to varying patient situations and needs. Disadvantages include the potential for examiner bias or omission of deficits through a lack of comprehensiveness, a lack of standardized administration rules for some of the tests, and a limited ability to develop a research database (Lovell and Nussbaum 1994). A more common approach is for the examiner to use a core set of tests that assess the major cognitive domains and to supplement the battery with additional tests as needed. This approach is increasing in popularity as health maintenance organizations continue to restrict reimbursement for lengthy neuropsychological evaluations.

Neuropsychological Assessment Process

There are several major cognitive domains that should be assessed in a comprehensive neuropsychological examination for TBI. These include attention, memory, executive functioning, speech and language, visuospatial and visuoconstructional skills, intelligence, and psychomotor speed, strength, and coordination (Vanderploeg 1994b). Measures of psychological functioning are also frequently administered and are an important aspect of the evaluation given that mild, moderate, and severe TBI are associated with increased risk of onset of psychiatric illness after injury (Fann et al. 2004). There are numerous neuropsychological tests that purport to measure specific aspects of neurocognitive functioning, and some of the more popular test instruments are listed in Table 8–1. This table provides a list of the major cognitive domains and examples of neuropsychological tests that are used to assess those domains.

Alertness and Orientation

Impairment in alertness and orientation is common in patients with TBI, particularly in the immediate hours and days after their injury. A neuropsychological evaluation during this period would be difficult and most likely invalid. Traumatically brain-injured patients have a high probability of developing a disorder of alertness in the presence of certain etiological factors that further compromise brain function (brainstem reticular activating system damage, supratentorial and subtentorial lesions, reduction in brain metabolism, organ failure, increased or decreased body temperature, seizure) as well as from sedating medications and lack of sleep (Stringer 1996).

TABLE 8–1. Cognitive domains and representative neuropsychological tests

Attention and concentration

Digit Span (WAIS-III, WMS-III; Wechsler 1997a, 1997b)

Spatial Span (WMS-III; Wechsler 1997b)

Digit Symbol (WAIS-III; Wechsler 1997a)

Continuous Performance Test (Rosvold et al. 1956)

Paced Auditory Serial Addition Task (Gronwall 1977)

Stroop Color and Word Test (Golden 1978)

Consonant Trigrams (Peterson and Peterson 1959)

Memory and learning

Wechsler Memory Scale—III (WMS; Wechsler 1997b)

California Verbal Learning Test (Delis et al. 1987, 2001)

Rey-Osterrieth Complex Figure Test (Osterrieth 1944)

Hopkins Verbal Learning Test (Brandt 1991)

Rey Auditory-Verbal Learning Test (Rey 1964)

Benton Visual Retention Test (Benton et al. 1983)

Brief Visuospatial Memory Test—Revised (Benedict 1997)

Executive functioning, concept formation, and planning

Booklet Category Test (DeFilippis and McCampbell 1997)

Wisconsin Card Sorting Test (Heaton 1981)

Design Fluency (Jones-Gotman and Milner 1977)

Controlled Oral Word Association Test (Benton and Hamsher 1978)

Trail Making Test—Part B (Reitan 1958)

Matrix Reasoning (WAIS-III; Wechsler 1997a)

Language

Boston Diagnostic Aphasia Examination (Goodglass and Kaplan 1972)

Multilingual Aphasia Examination (Benton and Hamsher 1978)

Western Aphasia Battery (Kertesz 1979)

Aphasia Examination (Russel et al. 1970)

Boston Naming Test (Kaplan et al. 1983)

Visuospatial and visuoconstructional skills

Visual Form Discrimination Test (Benton et al. 1983)

Judgment of Line Orientation Test (Benton et al. 1983)

Hooper Visual Organization Test (Hooper 1958)

Rey-Osterrieth Complex Figure (Copy Condition) (Osterrieth 1944)

Block Design (WAIS-III; Wechsler 1997a)

Intelligence

Wechsler Adult Intelligence Scale (WAIS-III; Wechsler 1997a)

TABLE 8–1. Cognitive domains and representative neuropsychological tests *(continued)*

Motor processes

Finger Tapping Test (Reitan and Wolfson 1993)

Grooved Pegboard Test (Matthew and Klove 1964)

Note. WAIS=Wechsler Adult Intelligence Scale; WMS=Wechsler Memory Scale.

Patients with psychiatric disorders such as depression, schizophrenia, factitious disorder, and conversion disorder can appear sleepy, apathetic, or unresponsive, and psychiatric disorders should be ruled out when determining if the patient has impaired alertness. However, misattributing a patient's impaired alertness to psychiatric causes can have life-threatening consequences for the patient if the cause is actually physiological.

The Galveston Orientation and Amnesia Test (GOAT; Levin et al. 1979) is a brief test that is often administered at bedside to assess the patient's current level of orientation and recall of events that occurred before and after the accident (Figure 8–1). The GOAT is particularly useful for determining posttraumatic amnesia within the acute hospital setting. During posttraumatic amnesia, the patient is disoriented and confused, and his or her ability to learn and remember new information is disrupted. Posttraumatic amnesia is acute and time-limited, and its duration can be an important prognostic indicator of recovery from brain injury, with a longer period of posttraumatic amnesia (> 1 or 2 weeks) predictive of poor recovery (Lovell and Franzen 1994).

Attentional Processes

Disorders of attention are a common consequence of TBI and frequently occur with rapid deceleration injuries such as in traffic accidents. Attentional impairments can interfere with rehabilitation, especially if the deficit is severe. Patients with severe attentional impairments may be too distractible and unable to focus their attention long enough to learn compensatory strategies or to benefit from retraining (Lezak 1995).

Assessment of attention is necessary because it is a prerequisite for successful performance in other cognitive domains. Additionally, deficits in attention can mimic other cognitive deficits. For example, a patient who is unable to fully attend to the stimuli on a memory test will not adequately encode the information. This patient's test scores may indicate memory impairment when in fact the deficit is in attention, rather than in memory. Patients

Name: _____   Date of test: _____

Age: _____   Sex: M   F   Day of the week: S   M   T   W   Th   F   S

Date of birth:_____ /_____ /_____   Time: _____ A.M. _____ P.M.

Diagnosis: _____   Date of injury: _____ /_____ /_____

Instructions: Error Points (shown in parentheses after each question) are scored for *incorrect* answers and are entered in the two columns on the extreme right side of the test form. Enter the total error points accrued for the 10 items in the lower right hand corner of the test form. The GOAT score equals 100 minus the total error points. Recovery of orientation is depicted by plotting serial GOAT scores on at least a daily basis.

	Error	Points

1. What is your name? (2)
   When were you born? (4)
   Where do you live? (4)		

2. Where are you now? (5) city (5) hospital (unnecessary to state name of hospital)		
3. On what date were you admitted to this hospital? (5) How did you get here? (5)		
4. What is the first event you can remember *after* the injury? (5) Can you describe in detail (e.g., date, time, companions) the first event you can recall *after* the injury? (5)		
5. Can you describe the last event you recall *before* the accident? (5) Can you describe in detail (e.g., date, time, companions) the first event you can recall *before* the injury? (5)		
6. What time is it now? (1) for each 1/2 hour *removed* from correct time to maximum of 5		
7. What day of the week is it? (1) for each day *removed* from correct one to a maximum of 5		
8. What day of the month is it? (1) for each day *removed* from correct date to a maximum of 5		
9. What is the month? (5) for each month *removed* from correct one to a maximum of 15		
10. What is the year? (10) for each year *removed* from correct one to a maximum of 30		
Total		

FIGURE 8–1.   The Galveston Orientation and Amnesia Test (GOAT).

Source.   Reprinted from Levin HS, O'Donnell VM, Grossman RG: "The Galveston Orientation and Amnesia Test: A Practical Scale to Assess Cognition After Head Injury." *Journal of Nervous and Mental Disease* 167:675–684, 1979. Copyright © Williams & Wilkins, 1979. Used with permission.

with attentional deficits can also appear to have problem-solving deficits even though these cognitive processes are intact (Fisher and Beckly 1999). For example, a patient with an attentional deficit may respond impulsively or have difficulty maintaining his or her attention on the task long enough to correctly solve it. Behaviorally, a patient with an attentional impairment may start many new tasks or projects but is unable to complete them. Socially, his or her conversation may shift from topic to topic without

any issue being dealt with thoroughly (Stern and Prohaska 1996).

There are multiple components of attention, and specific tests are used to evaluate the different aspects of attention. An individual's attention to the task at hand requires him or her to focus on some aspect of the environment (focused and/or selective attention), to sustain that focus for as long as necessary (sustained attention and/or vigilance), and to shift the focus when required (cognitive flexibility and/or divided attention) (Anderson 1994; Campbell 1996).

When assessing attention, it is first important to assess general level of arousal. Next, the attention span, or density of information the person can hold in attention at one time, is assessed. Tests such as Digit Span and Spatial Span (WMS-III; Wechsler 1997b) are often used to assess auditory and visual attention span. Divided attention (e.g., being able to maintain a conversation while ignoring environmental distractions) is often assessed with the Stroop Color and Word Test (Golden 1978) or the Paced Auditory Serial Addition Task (PASAT; Gronwall 1977). The Stroop test is commonly used because it addresses multiple aspects of attention such as focused and divided attention as well as executive functioning abilities. The Interference score on the Stroop test has been particularly useful in looking at the ability to inhibit an over-learned response and cognitive flexibility (Groth-Marnat 2000). The PASAT, a challenging test of sustained and divided attention, is particularly useful as a measure of recovery from mild brain injury and is sensitive to the subtle but meaningful deficits that may occur after multiple head injuries. The PASAT is also useful for assessing information processing deficits in patients with brain injury (Gronwall 1977).

The third component of attention that should be assessed is sustained attention, or vigilance. This area is frequently referred to as *distractibility* and is the ability to sustain concentration on a set of stimuli that falls within the person's span of concentration while ignoring extraneous stimuli (Stringer 1996). Thus, vigilance is the ability to maintain attention over time. The Continuous Performance Test (Rosvold et al. 1956) is commonly used to measure vigilance, as are the Digit Symbol Test from the WAIS-III (Wechsler 1997a) and letter and number cancellation tests.

Memory

Memory impairment is one of the most common complaints after TBI. Memory represents a multifaceted process that can generally be described as the ability, process, or act of remembering or recalling, and the ability to reproduce what has been learned or experienced (Campbell 1996). Memory deficits can be temporary, as occurs with posttraumatic amnesia, or more permanent. In general, memory impairment can be classified as either retrograde amnesia or anterograde amnesia. Retrograde amnesia involves memory loss for events in a time period before the injury. Anterograde amnesia involves memory loss for events after the injury. Similar to attentional processes, memory is a multidi-

mensional cognitive process that involves multiple underlying brain structures. In neuropsychological assessment, memory for verbal and visual information is formally measured. Memory for material immediately after the material has been presented is referred to as *immediate memory*. Memory for information after a delay of minutes to hours is referred to as *delayed recall* or *recent memory* (Anderson 1994). Additionally, the patient's acquisition, retention, and retrieval of newly learned information should be assessed.

Although patients with mild brain injury frequently complain of memory problems, their perceived problems may often be the result of impairment in the ability to attend to or acquire the material rather than to a memory disorder per se. Patients with more focal damage, as can occur in penetrating injuries, are likely to demonstrate material-specific deficits in learning and remembering as a result of selective damage to the language-dominant (usually left) or nondominant hemisphere (usually right). Specifically, patients with dominant hemisphere damage are more likely to have impaired recall of verbal material but preserved recall of nonverbal material, although this is not always the case. The California Verbal Learning Test (CVLT; Delis et al. 1987), Hopkins Verbal Learning Test (Brandt 1991), and Rey Auditory-Verbal Learning Test (Rey 1964) are commonly used to assess verbal memory.

Visual memory is typically assessed through tests that require the patient to learn and reproduce spatial designs. The Rey-Osterrieth Complex Figure (Osterrieth 1944) assesses visual memory by having the patient reproduce a drawing of a geometric design at different time intervals after the initial presentation (which involves copying the figure) (Lovell and Franzen 1994). The Benton Visual Retention Test (Benton et al. 1983) is another commonly used test of visual memory that requires the patient to draw a series of simple designs. The WMS-III (Wechsler 1997b) is a battery of tests specifically designed to measure various aspects of memory functioning. Clinicians often supplement their evaluations with one or more of the subtests (e.g., Logical Memory and Visual Reproduction) from the Weschler Memory Scale batteries. More recently, the Brief Visuospatial Memory Test—Revised (Benedict 1997) has become a popular visual memory assessment tool. The patient is asked to draw a series of six designs over three 10-second exposures to the test stimuli. Delayed memory is evaluated by having the patient draw the designs after a 25-minute delay.

One aspect of memory that is frequently compromised after TBI is working memory. Working memory is a form of short-term memory that encompasses the ability to hold or retain information in a temporary storage system while simultaneously concentrating on another task (Stringer 1996). The Auditory Consonant Trigrams (ACT) test, also known as the *Brown-Peterson test of memory* (Peterson and Peterson 1959), assesses short-term (working) memory, divided attention, and information-processing capacity. It is a 10-minute test that was originally designed for adults but currently has versions appropriate for children ages 9–15 years. The ACT is useful for a variety of populations but is particularly sensitive to mild head injury (Spreen and Strauss 1998). The ACT requires the patient to hold information in mind (three letters) while simultaneously performing another task (counting backward by threes).

Executive Functioning

Executive functioning encompasses the abilities necessary for an individual to perform a problem-solving task from beginning to end. The major areas of executive functioning include judgment, reasoning, concept formation, and abstraction; initiation and fluency; planning and organizing; set maintenance and mental flexibility; and disinhibition and impulse control. These skills enable a person to engage with others effectively, plan activities, solve problems, and interact with the environment to have his or her needs met (Sbordone 2000). A deficit of executive functioning can be the most crippling impairment that afflicts the TBI patient and can intensify deficits seen in other cognitive processes such as memory (Lezak 1995). Research suggests that executive functioning is often impaired when a frontal-subcortical circuit or loop is damaged (Cummings and Trimble 1995). This damage can occur from lesions in the frontal-subcortical circuits or from alterations in metabolic activity of the neural structures that form the circuit. Cummings and Trimble (1995) described five frontal-subcortical circuits. Three of these circuits (dorsolateral prefrontal, lateral orbitofrontal, and medial frontal/anterior cingulate) play an important role in executive function, and damage in these areas produces a neurobehavioral syndrome with executive functioning impairments. Thus, instead of one global "frontal lobe syndrome" there are three distinct "frontal syndromes" that display executive impairments. Damage to the dorsolateral prefrontal area results in a syndrome characterized by an inability to maintain set, disassociation between verbal and motor behavior, deficits in motor programming and concrete thinking, poor mental control, and stimulus-bound behavior (Sbordone 2000). Orbitofrontal lesions produce a syndrome characterized by tactlessness, disinhibition, emotional lability, insensitivity to the needs and welfare of others, and antisocial acts. Damage to the medial frontal/anterior cingulate area produces a syndrome characterized by apathy, diminished motivation and interest, psychomotor retardation, diminished social involvement, and reduced communication (Cummings and Trimble 1995). The cluster of executive deficits that accompany the previously mentioned neurobehavioral syndromes can be misinterpreted as emotional problems or personality aberrations (Lezak 1997). For example, the apathy, diminished initiative, reduced motor and verbal output, and impaired motivation that are typical of medial frontal/anterior cingulate injuries mimic depression.

Executive functioning deficits can severely impact a patient's adaptive functioning. Problems with planning, impulsivity, and disinhibition can adversely affect everyday skills such as preparing a meal, handling finances, and social appropriateness (Sbordone 2000). Additionally, impaired executive functioning has been found to be one of four of the most reliable correlates of unemployment (Crepeau and Scherzer 1993). The Wisconsin Card Sorting Test (WCST; Heaton 1981) and the Category Test (Reitan and Wolfson 1993) are two measures typically used to assess different aspects of executive functioning. The Category Test and its more portable and efficient format the Booklet Category Test (DeFilippis and McCampbell 1997) are considered tests of abstract concept formation, reasoning, and logical analysis abilities. Successful performance requires mental flexibility, attention and concentration, learning and memory, and visuospatial skills (Mitrushina et al. 1999). The WCST (Heaton 1981) is an abstract problem-solving test that is particularly useful because there has been substantial research on its ability to measure perseveration (Flashman et al. 1991). In general, the WCST provides information across multiple behavioral domains, including ability to form concepts, problem-solving ability, ability to learn from experience, and capacity to shift conceptual sets.

Speech and Language

Language processes are often disrupted after TBI and vary greatly depending on the nature, localization, and severity of brain injury. TBI patients who do sustain damage to the language centers tend to have minimal to no deficits on verbal tests of overlearned material, culturally common information, and reading, writing, and speech. However, they may demonstrate difficulties with verbal retrieval of names of objects, places, and persons. TBI patients' dysnomias, or word-finding problems, tend to present as slow recall of the word, paraphasias, and semantically related misnamings (Lezak 1995).

Injuries that are focal or penetrating and involve the language-dominant hemisphere are more likely to cause language impairments. Aphasia is a disorder of oral language and can include compromised verbal expression and comprehension. In addition, written communication (alexia and agraphia) is also frequently impaired in patients with aphasia. There are specific lesion locations that are likely to produce certain types of aphasia. For example, Broca's aphasia often results from lesions in the frontal operculum that extend to subjacent white matter, the anterior parietal lobe, the insula, and both banks of the rolandic fissure. Conduction aphasia often results from lesions in the arcuate fasciculus (Stringer 1996). The major types of aphasia are differentiated by assessing three language domains: fluency, comprehension, and repetition. Although other aspects of language may be compromised, these three areas are typically considered the "cardinal" symptoms. For example, a patient with Broca's aphasia will have deficits in fluency and repetition, but relatively adequate comprehension. Those with Wernicke's aphasia are fluent (although their verbalizations may be incomprehensible) but have poor repetition and comprehension.

Evaluation of speech and language usually involves assessing spontaneous speech; repetition of words, phrases, and sentences; speech comprehension; naming; reading; and writing (Lezak 1995). During the evaluation, it is important to attend to fluency, prosody, articulatory errors, grammar and syntax, and the presence of paraphasias (Goodglass 1986). The Aphasia Examination (Russel et al. 1970) is a useful screening instrument for uncovering language deficits that may need further assessment. The Boston Diagnostic Aphasia Examination (Goodglass and Kaplan 1972) is a comprehensive and sensitive battery that is excellent for the description of aphasic disorders and for treatment planning (Lezak 1995). Rather than using the entire battery, many clinicians selectively use portions of the battery in combination with other neuropsychological tests.

Assessment of Motivation and Malingering

Although the majority of traumatically brain-injured patients have bona fide deficits, the issue of secondary gain should always be considered. In addition to assessing the major cognitive domains detailed above, the neuropsychologist should also include formal tests of motivation and malingering within the evaluation. This is particularly true in cases in which litigation may be pursued to assign blame and/or financial responsibility for the resulting disability. In these cases, a patient may attempt to fake or exaggerate a brain injury. Similarly, some patients who have legitimate deficits after their TBI may not put forth their full effort in an attempt to

receive needed treatments (rehabilitation), services (home care), and compensation (disability benefits) (Lovell and Franzen 1994). This can create difficulty in determining the patient's actual strengths and weaknesses and hinders the evaluation process. Addressing the issues of effort and motivation early in the evaluation can help prevent unnecessary testing and an invalid evaluation. Tests that are commonly used to assess for motivation and malingering are

- Test of Memory Malingering (Tombaugh 1996)
- 21-Item Test (Iverson et al. 1991)
- Rey 15-Item Memory Test (Rey 1964)
- Portland Digit Recognition Test (Binder 1990)
- Victoria Symptom Validity Test (Slick et al. 1997)

The 21-Item Test (Iverson et al. 1991) can be used to initially screen for exaggerated deficits in verbal memory. The Rey 15-Item Memory Test (Rey 1964) was specifically designed to detect attempts at faking memory deficits. The patient is told the difficulty of remembering the 15 items before their presentation. However, the stimuli are overlearned sequences and redundant, which makes the items relatively simple to remember (Stringer 1996). Symptom validity testing is a method in which 100 trials of forced-choice stimuli that are relevant to the patient's presenting complaint are presented. Malingering is suggested if the patient performs below 50% correct (suggesting a performance that is worse than chance) (Crosson 1994). Although some measures are specifically constructed for malingering and motivation, other tests of cognitive functioning (e.g., memory) attempt to include subtests that are useful for assessing motivation. The most common method is the use of a forced-choice format. Many instruments, such as the WMS-III (Wechsler 1997b) and CVLT-II (Delis et al. 2001), include these subtests in their measures. The premise of forced-choice tests is that the patient has a 50% chance of answering approximately one-half of the items correctly without even trying. Thus, a patient who incorrectly answers 90% of the items is likely demonstrating poor effort. Recent research (Bender and Rogers 2004) has focused on the use of multiple measures and strategies to detect feigning. These researchers found Magnitude of Error to be a useful detection strategy: "The Magnitude of Error assumes that feigners will not be especially concerned about which incorrect responses they select" (p. 50). In other words, the malingerer may focus on what item to fail rather than how the item should be failed (e.g., the plausibility of the error).

In addition to administering tests designed to assess for malingering and biased responding, the clinician should compare the patient's performance on neuropsychological measures to his or her ability to function in everyday activities. For example, a patient who performs in the severely impaired range on neuropsychological testing yet continues to perform well in graduate-level coursework is demonstrating an inconsistency between his test performance and academic functioning. Obviously, this disparity suggests suboptimal effort on testing. Last, when assessing for malingering it is important to keep in mind that some patients may appear to be malingering but are not. A variety of factors can influence neuropsychological test performance (e.g., psychiatric disorders such as depression, poor rapport with the evaluator, uncooperativeness, and the context in which the evaluation is conducted) (Franzen and Iverson 1997). Franzen and Iverson (1997) stated that when assessing for malingering "It is important to remember that these test instruments evaluate the likelihood of nonoptimal performance, not malingering itself. As such, the specific assessment instruments provide information about biased responding, that is, information about the probability that variables other than skill level have adversely affected the level of effort" (p. 396).

Neuropsychological Screening Instruments

Time constraints, patient fatigue or noncompliance, and lack of health insurance and financial restrictions may necessitate the administration of a screening battery rather than a full neuropsychological evaluation. However, although the advantages of neuropsychological screening are cost-effectiveness and short administration time, this approach has limited value in making differential diagnoses. For example, the Mini-Mental State Examination (MMSE) is useful in determining the presence or absence of dementia, but it is not useful for differentiating Alzheimer's disease from other types of dementia. Additionally, screening devices are limited in their ability to discriminate mild head injury, and they do not provide specific information about rehabilitation needs (e.g., memory retraining) and individual strengths and weaknesses (e.g., impaired auditory memory but intact visual memory). Some examples of screening instruments are

- Mini-Mental State Examination (Folstein et al. 1975)
- Repeatable Battery for the Assessment of Neuropsychological Status (Randolph 1998)
- Neurobehavioral Cognitive Status Examination (Kiernan et al. 2001)
- Shipley Institute of Living Scale (Revised Manual) (Zachary 1986)

- BNI Screen for Higher Cerebral Functions (Prigatano 1991)

The MMSE is a well-known screening instrument that is brief and easy to administer. The MMSE is most useful for moderate to severe impairment in dementia patients. However, its sensitivity and specificity decline with other patient populations, particularly those with mild cognitive impairment, focal neurological deficits, and psychiatric disorders (Spreen and Strauss 1998).

The Repeatable Battery for the Assessment of Neuropsychological Status (Randolph 1998) is a relatively new cognitive screening instrument that takes less than 30 minutes to administer and provides a total scale score and five specific cognitive ability index scores. It was designed for the dual purpose of identifying and characterizing abnormal cognitive decline in the older adult and as a neuropsychological screening battery for younger patients (Randolph et al. 1998). It has also been found to be particularly useful in evaluating neuropsychological change in patients with schizophrenia (Wilk et al. 2002).

Differential Diagnosis of TBI From Other Neuropsychiatric Conditions

Determining Premorbid Level of Functioning

TBI occurs within many different contexts, and one of the primary challenges to the neuropsychologist working with these patients is the separation of TBI-related sequelae from preexisting conditions. In addition, the neurocognitive affects of psychiatric disorders and TBI may be synergistic.

The initial task of the neuropsychologist is to assess the patient's probable level of preinjury functioning. This provides the basis for assumptions about post-TBI level of functioning and is an important aspect of the evaluation process. This is necessary because only rarely has the TBI patient undergone preinjury neuropsychological testing that would allow a direct comparison to his or her postinjury level of functioning. Although preinjury neuropsychological test results are not often available, intellectual and achievement testing is becoming increasingly popular in the school system, and these data can be useful in estimating premorbid functioning. Collateral information provided by spouses, co-workers, and employers; school performance; educational level; and work history all contribute to the determination of premorbid functioning.

An additional method of estimating the patient's level of premorbid functioning involves the analysis of the pattern of neuropsychological test scores. This method is based on the assumption that cognitive processes such as basic reading skills and vocabulary tend to be less affected by TBI than other skill areas. A few tests that are considered to be relatively resistant to neurological impairment are the Vocabulary, Information, Picture Completion, and Object Assembly subtests from the WAIS—Revised (Vanderploeg 1994a; Wechsler 1981) and WAIS-III (Wechsler 1997a). These have traditionally been known as "hold" tests and have been considered to be relatively unaffected by TBI. However, caution is advised when implementing this method because the traditional "hold" tests can indeed be influenced by different types of brain injury, particularly if it is of a focal nature. For example, patients with aphasia would obviously perform poorly on the Vocabulary and Information subtests. Reading skill, as mentioned previously, is also considered to be resistant to TBI, and, as a result, basic word reading tests, such as the North American Adult Reading Test, are frequently used for premorbid estimates. Another common method for estimating premorbid functioning is the use of demographic variable methods. This is based on the premise that certain demographic variables such as social class and education are correlated with scores on intelligence tests (Franzen 2000). In general, most clinicians use a combination of methods and measures to predict premorbid functioning.

Depression

Depression can interfere with the normal expression of cognitive abilities and can also cloud the diagnostic picture in an individual who has had a TBI. Depressed patients who have not had a TBI may demonstrate cognitive difficulties such as slowed mental processing, psychomotor retardation, mild attentional deficits, decreased drive and initiation, and impairments in short-term recall and learning for verbal and visuospatial material. Cognitive impairment is most frequently encountered in the areas of attention, specific aspects of memory, and psychomotor speed. Impairment in language, perception, and spatial abilities tends to be secondary to poor attention, motivation, or organizational abilities (Mayberg et al. 1997).

A large body of research on depressed patients has focused on memory processes. In attempting to differentiate the neurocognitive effects of depression from TBI, there are certain key factors that should be considered. Neuropsychological testing of patients diagnosed with depression reveals that the "memory deficit" is often expressed in free-recall retrieval errors rather than as a deficit in actually learning the information. As a result, the patient requires a cue or recognition stimulus for the memory to become available for recall (Lezak 1995). This can be evaluated by tests such as the CVLT (Delis et al. 1987) that assess the ability to learn across trials as well as the patient's ability to benefit from semantic cues and recognition.

Differential diagnosis of the cognitive consequences of depression versus TBI is often clouded by the comorbidity of depressed mood with TBI. A review by Busch and Alpern (1998) suggests that the prevalence of depression after mild TBI is at least 35%. A careful and thorough history addressing the patient's premorbid cognitive and emotional functioning is essential in attempting to understand the contribution of both disorders. Examining the pattern of the patient's performance on neuropsychological testing (e.g., learning vs. retrieval) is helpful, as well as qualitatively looking at individual subtest scores and performance. For example, if given extra time and encouragement, many depressed patients perform adequately. Memory disturbances in depressed patients are likely the result of attention and concentration difficulties typically associated with depression, whereas patients with TBI may have a more consistent pattern across the tests designed to assess memory. Assessing the rate of forgetting of information from immediate recall to a delayed recall is one method that can contribute to the differential diagnosis.

Anxiety

Anxiety can interfere with the patient's ability to attend to, learn, and remember new information and therefore can be similar to the pattern of deficits seen after mild TBI. The experience of anxiety is also common during the neuropsychological evaluation process and may relate to performance anxiety or general frustration on the part of the patient. It is therefore important for the clinician to create an atmosphere that reduces the normal anxiety that a patient might feel when undergoing the evaluation process. Patients with a history of anxiety disorders can have particular difficulty in participating in formal neuropsychological assessment and may manifest mental efficiency problems such as slowing, scrambled or blocked thoughts and words, memory failure, and increased distractibility (Lezak 1995). Additionally, patients who are anxious about appearing "stupid" may respond with "I don't know" rather than providing their best response to a particular question. Encouraging patients to make their best guess and trying to optimize their effort is essential to obtaining a valid neuropsychological profile. In addition to performance-related anxieties that can occur during the evaluation, there are specific anxiety disorders that are likely to be more prevalent among the TBI population.

Posttraumatic Stress Disorder

Posttraumatic stress disorder (PTSD) is common after TBI, and many patients with mild TBI vividly recall and are distressed by the details of their injury. Additionally, there is symptom overlap between postconcussion syndrome and PTSD (Cummings et al. 1995). In general, postconcussive symptoms tend to decrease or remit within 3–6 months, whereas the course and duration of PTSD may be much longer (Evans 2000; Silver et al. 1997). Similar symptoms include, but are not limited to, amnesia for certain aspects of the traumatic event, difficulty concentrating, somatic complaints (headache, dizziness, fatigue, insomnia), perceptual symptoms (sensitivity to noise and light), and irritability (American Psychiatric Association 2000; Silver et al. 1997). Although much of the research on TBI and PTSD focuses on mild head injury, there is evidence to suggest that PTSD can develop after severe TBI even with impaired consciousness during the trauma and a relative absence of traumatic memories of the event (Bryant et al. 2000; Harvey et al. 2003).

Turnbull et al. (2001) investigated whether memory loss of the injury event and whether the type of memory (e.g., traumatic or nontraumatic) influence the development of PTSD symptoms. Subjects were divided into three groups on the basis of memory of the injury event: those with no memory of the injury event, those who remembered the injury but had nontraumatic memory of the event, and those who had a traumatic memory of the injury event. The results of this research indicated that patients with no memory of the injury and patients with memories that are traumatic reported higher levels of psychological distress than the group without traumatic memories. However, ratings of PTSD symptoms were less severe in the "no memory" group as compared to those with traumatic memories of the event. Thus, they found that amnesia did not protect against PTSD but does protect against the severity and presence of specific intrusive symptoms. Feinstein et al. (2002) addressed the relationship between the length of posttraumatic amnesia and symptoms of PTSD after TBI. They found that patients with brief posttraumatic amnesia (<1 hour) are more likely to experience a PTSD reaction than those with longer posttraumatic amnesia (>1 hour). Mayou et al. (2000) examined the relationship between unconsciousness, amnesia, and psychiatric symptoms after road traffic accidents. In general, their results suggested that PTSD, anxiety, and depression were more common at 3 months in those patients who had documented unconsciousness than in patients who had no loss of consciousness. However, at 1-year follow-up there were no differences between the two groups. They found clear evidence that PTSD is at least as common in those who experience brief unconsciousness as in those who were not unconscious. Explanations for the onset of PTSD in patients with posttraumatic amnesia are that the intrusive memories may relate to events before or after the period of amnesia, and there may be islands of preserved memory (Parker 1996). It has also been suggested that there are implicit memories that result in "intensive psychological distress on exposure to internal or external cues that symbolize or resemble an aspect of the traumatic event" (Bryant et al. 2000).

In terms of treatment for PTSD symptoms, Bryant et al. (2003) found that brief cognitive behavioral therapy provided early (2 weeks postinjury) to patients with mild brain injury was more effective than supportive counseling for treatment of acute stress disorder as well as for prevention of PTSD symptoms at 6-month follow-up.

Obsessive-Compulsive Disorder

Obsessive-compulsive–like behaviors can occur after TBI. These behaviors frequently evolve when mental inefficiency, such as the attentional deficits that are typically associated with slowed processing and diffuse damage, is the prominent feature (Lezak et al. 1990). Rigidity in thinking and perseverative tendencies can be evidenced on some of the tests typically used to assess executive functioning such as the WCST. Perseveration can also be detected across different subtests (e.g., carrying aspects of one subtest into the next subtest). Socially, these patients may act inappropriately and be disruptive due to failing to respond to social cues (Stringer 1996). Patients who are perseverative may repeat a task in a stereotyped manner or may have difficulty switching topics during a conversation and appear to repeat themselves. They can also appear hypervigilant (Stern and Prohaska 1996).

Schizophrenia

Using neuropsychological testing to differentiate the cognitive sequelae of schizophrenia from TBI is difficult, given that patients with schizophrenia often demonstrate impairment on formal neuropsychological testing (Crosson 1994). It has been suggested that at least in some cases of schizophrenia the disorder may be the result of earlier cerebral insult rather than being merely an expression of the disease entity. This hypothesis is based on the high incidence of premorbid neurological disorders such as head injury, perinatal complications, and childhood illnesses in patients with schizophrenia (Lezak 1995; McAllister 1998).

Neuropsychological studies indicate that persons with schizophrenia demonstrate difficulties in attention, motor behavior, speed of processing, abstraction, learning, and memory (Sackeim and Stern 1997). However, reviews of the research suggest that the deficits seen in schizophrenia can be broad, and no cognitive domain is entirely spared. It has also been suggested that cognitive deficits are not present in every individual at all times, and the pattern of deficits can change over time within an individual (Tamminga 1997). Malloy and Duffy (1994) reviewed literature on the frontal lobes in neuropsychiatric disorders and found that frontal dysfunction has been linked to the negative subtype of schizophrenia on the basis of neuropsychological, structural and functional imaging, and electrophysiological studies. However, they state that there is controversy as to whether the results indicate distinct subtypes of schizophrenic patients or predominant symptoms that occur at different stages of the schizophrenic process in the same patient. A study by Sachdev et al. (2001) compared patients with TBI who developed schizophrenia-like psychosis (SLP) after their injury and patients with TBI who did not develop SLP. Their results indicated that the patients with TBI who developed SLP had a mean age at onset of 26.3 years, a mean latency of 54.7 months after the head injury, and usually a gradual onset and a subacute or chronic course. They also found that prodromal symptoms were common as well as the presence of depression at the onset of SLP. The predominant features were paranoid delusions and auditory hallucinations. However, formal thought disorder, catatonic features, and negative symptoms were uncommon. Additionally, the SLP group had more widespread brain damage on neuroimaging, particularly in the left temporal and right parietal regions, and was more cognitively impaired than the TBI group without SLP. Last, they found that a positive family history of psychosis and duration of loss of consciousness were the best predictors of SLP. The results from the Sachdev et al. study (2001) are inconsistent with past studies (Bond 1984; Kwentus et al. 1985), which indicate that schizophrenia-like symptoms after TBI are more likely to be of the negative subtype, with flat affect, suspiciousness, and social withdrawal as opposed to positive symptoms of delusions and hallucinations. The variability in research findings points to the need for further research into possible subtypes of schizophrenia and course of cognitive deficits.

Attention-Deficit/Hyperactivity Disorder

Attention-deficit/hyperactivity disorder (ADHD) is a disorder involving disturbances in attention span (e.g., poor attention to task), self-regulation (e.g., inability to consider consequences of behavior), activity level (e.g., motoric overactivity), and impulse control (e.g., impulsive behaviors) (Teeter and Semrud-Clikeman 1997).

As mentioned throughout this chapter, deficits in attention are common after TBI. The diagnosis ADHD not otherwise specified can technically be used to diagnose adults with attentional deficits resulting from brain damage. However, this diagnosis is misleading given that ADHD is considered a developmental disorder, and some of the symptoms must be present before age 7 (Stringer 1996). During the clinical interview, it is important to assess for premorbid diagnosed and undiagnosed ADHD symptoms. It is useful to ask developmentally oriented questions and to seek information collaterally. This is particularly important because there are commonalities in behavioral and cognitive sequelae of TBI and ADHD, particularly in response inhibition (Konrad et al. 2000). Konrad et al. (2000) compared children with TBI and children with developmental ADHD during two inhibition tasks. Additionally, they divided the children with TBI, according to Actigraph data, into hypo-, hyper-, and normokinetic subgroups. They concluded that slowing of information processing speed is a general consequence of TBI in childhood and that inhibitory deficits are associated with postinjury hypo- and hyperactivity. Specifically, hyperactive children with TBI had the same inhibitory deficit patterns as children with developmental ADHD.

Neuropsychological testing can contribute to the diagnosis of persons with ADHD without TBI and TBI patients with a history of ADHD that predates their injury by highlighting the cognitive strengths and weaknesses and helping to distinguish attentional disturbances from an underlying memory disorder. Because there is a high comorbidity of ADHD with learning disorders, neuropsychological testing can also diagnose the presence of learning disabilities or other deficits that may be contributing to the clinical presentation of the patient (Cohen and Salloway 1997).

Learning Disorders

A learning disorder involves a deficit in the acquisition and performance of certain academic skills (Popper and Steingard 1996). DSM-IV-TR (American Psychiatric Association 2000) addresses four classifications of learning disorders: reading disorder, mathematics disorder, disorder of written expression, and learning disorders not otherwise specified. Although learning disorders are usually first evident in childhood, they can have major consequences for lifetime functioning. The cognitive effects of learning disorders can be mistaken for those of head injury (Crosson 1994), and a careful neuropsychological evaluation can assist in differentiating these two conditions. This process should involve a careful education and social history as well as the review of school transcripts.

Summary

This chapter provides a summary of the role of neuropsychological assessment strategies in the evaluation of traumatically brain-injured individuals. Neuropsychological testing can be a useful adjunctive tool within the neuropsychiatric context and can help to separate TBI from other disorders, thus guiding the treatment planning and rehabilitation process. Neuropsychological assessment is helpful in identifying psychosocial and neurological components of TBI and is particularly helpful with regard to differential diagnosis.

References

American Psychiatric Association: Diagnostic and Statistical Manual of Mental Disorders, 4th Edition, Text Revision. Washington, DC, American Psychiatric Association, 2000

Anderson RM Jr: Practitioner's Guide to Clinical Neuropsychology. New York, Plenum, 1994

Bender SD, Rogers R: Detection of neurocognitive feigning: development of a multi-strategy assessment. Arch Clin Neuropsychol 19:49–60, 2004

Benedict R: Revision of the Brief Visuospatial Memory Test: studies of normal performance, reliability, and validity. Psychol Assess 8:145–153, 1997

Benton AL, Hamsher K: Multilingual Aphasia Examination. Iowa City, IA, The University of Iowa Press, 1978

Benton AL, Hamsher K, Varney NR, et al: Contributions to Neuropsychological Assessment: A Clinical Manual. New York, Oxford University Press, 1983

Binder LM: Malingering following minor head trauma. Clin Neuropsychol 4:25–36, 1990

Bond MR: The psychiatry of closed head injury, in Closed Head Injury: Psychological, Social and Family Consequences. Edited by Brooks N. Oxford, UK, Oxford University Press, 1984, pp 148–178

Brandt J: The Hopkins Verbal Learning Test: development of a new memory test with six equivalent forms. Clin Neuropsychol 5:125–142, 1991

Bryant RA, Marosszeky JE, Crooks J, Gurka JA: Post-traumatic stress disorder after severe traumatic brain injury. Am J Psychiatry 157:629–631, 2000

Bryant RA, Moulds M, Guthrie R, et al: Treating acute stress disorder following mild traumatic brain injury. Am J Psychiatry 160:585–587, 2003

Busch CR, Alpern HP: Depression after mild traumatic brain injury: a review of current research. Neuropsychol Rev 8:95–108, 1998

Campbell RJ: Psychiatric Dictionary, 7th Edition. New York, Oxford University Press, 1996

Cohen RA, Salloway S: Neuropsychiatric aspects of disorders of attention, in The American Psychiatric Press Textbook of Neuropsychiatry, 3rd Edition. Edited by Yudofsky SC, Hales RE. Washington, DC, American Psychiatric Press, 1997, pp 413–446

Crepeau F, Scherzer P: Predictors and indicators of work status after traumatic brain injury: a meta-analysis. Neuropsychological Rehabilitation 3:5–35, 1993

Crosson B: Application of neuropsychological assessment results, in Clinician's Guide to Neuropsychological Assessment. Edited by Vanderploeg RD. Hillsdale, NJ, Lawrence Erlbaum, 1994, pp 113–163

Cummings JL, Trimble MD: Concise Guide to Neuropsychiatry and Behavioral Neurology. Washington, DC, American Psychiatric Press, 1995

DeFilippis NA, McCampbell E: The Booklet Category Test Professional Manual, 2nd Edition. Odessa, FL, Psychological Assessment Resources, 1997

Delis DC, Kramer JH, Kaplan E, et al: The California Verbal Learning Test—Adult Version. San Antonio, TX, The Psychological Corporation/Harcourt Brace Jovanovich, 1987

Delis DC, Kaplan E, Kramer JH, Ober RA: The California Verbal Learning Test—2nd Edition, Adult Version: A Comprehensive Assessment of Verbal Learning and Memory. San Antonio, TX, The Psychological Corporation, 2001

Evans RW: Postconcussion syndrome, in Prognosis of Neurological Disorders, 2nd Edition. Edited by Evans RW, Baskin DS, Yatsu FM. New York, Oxford University Press, 2000, pp 366–380

Fann JR, Burington B, Leonetti A, et al: Psychiatric illness following traumatic brain injury in an adult health maintenance organization population. Arch Gen Psychiatry 61:54–61, 2004

Feinstein A, Hershkop S, Ouchterlony D, et al: Posttraumatic amnesia and recall of a traumatic event following traumatic brain injury. J Neuropsychiatry Clin Neurosci 14:25–30, 2002

Fisher BC, Beckley RA: Attention Deficit Disorder: Practical Coping Methods. Boca Raton, FL, CRC Press, 1999

Flashman LA, Horner MD, Freides D: Note on scoring perseveration on the Wisconsin Card Sorting Test. Clin Neuropsychol 5:190–194, 1991

Folstein MF, Folstein SE, McHugh PR: "Mini-Mental State": a practical method for grading the cognitive state of patients for the clinician. J Psychiatr Res 12:189–198, 1975

Franzen MD: Critical Issues in Neuropsychology: Reliability and Validity in Neuropsychological Assessment, 2nd Edition. New York, Kluwer Academic/Plenum, 2000

Franzen MD, Iverson GL: The detection of biased responding in neuropsychological assessment, in The Neuropsychology Handbook: Foundations and Assessment, Vol. 1. Edited by Webster J, MacNeill-Horton A, Wedding D. New York, Springer, 1997, pp 393–421

Golden CJ: Stroop Color and Word Test. Chicago, IL, Stoelting Co, 1978

Goodglass H: The assessment of language after brain damage, in Handbook of Clinical Neuropsychology, Vol. 2. Edited by Filskov SB, Boll TJ. New York, Wiley, 1986

Goodglass H, Kaplan E: Assessment of Aphasia and Related Disorders. Philadelphia, PA, Lea and Febiger, 1972

Gronwall D: Paced Auditory Serial Addition Task: a measure of recovery from concussion. Percept Mot Skills 44: 367–373, 1977

Groth-Marnat G: Neuropsychological Assessment in Clinical Practice: A Guide to Test Interpretation and Integration. New York, Wiley, 2000

Harvey AG, Brewin CR, Jones C, et al: Coexistence of posttraumatic stress disorder and traumatic brain injury: towards a resolution of the paradox. J Int Neuropsychol Soc 9:633–676, 2003

Heaton RK: Wisconsin Card Sorting Test Manual. Odessa, FL, Psychological Assessment Resources, 1981

Heaton RK, Pendleton MG: Use of neuropsychological tests to predict adult patients' everyday functioning. J Consult Clin Psychol 49:807–821, 1981

Hooper HE: The Hooper Visual Organization Test Manual. Los Angeles, CA, Western Psychological Services, 1958

Iverson GL, Franzen MD, McCracken LM: Evaluation of an objective assessment technique for the detection of malingered memory deficits. Law Hum Behav 15:667–676, 1991

Jones-Gotman M, Milner B: Design fluency: the invention of nonsense drawings after focal cortical lesions. Neuropsychologia 15:653–674, 1977

Kaplan EF, Goodglass H, Weintraub S: The Boston Naming Test, 2nd Edition. Philadelphia, PA, Lea and Febiger, 1983

Kertesz A: Aphasia and Associated Disorders. New York, Grune & Stratton, 1979

Kiernan RJ, Mueller J, Langston JW: Cognistat (Neurobehavioral Cognitive Status Examination). Lutz, FL, Psychological Assessment Resources, Inc., 2001

Konrad K, Gauggel S, Manz A, Scholl M: Inhibitory control in children with traumatic brain injury (TBI) and children with attention deficit/hyperactivity disorder (ADHD). Brain Inj 14:859–875, 2000

Kwentus JA, Hart RP, Peck ET, Kornstein S: Psychiatric complications of closed head trauma. Psychosomatics 26:8–17, 1985

Levin HS, O'Donnell VM, Grossman RG: The Galveston Orientation and Amnesia Test: a practical scale to assess cognition after head injury. J Nerv Ment Dis 167:675–684, 1979

Lezak MD: Neuropsychological Assessment, 3rd Edition. New York, Oxford University Press, 1995

Lezak MD: Principles of neuropsychological assessment, in Behavioral Neurology and Neuropsychology. Edited by Feinberg TE, Farah MJ. New York, McGraw–Hill, 1997, pp 43–54

Lezak MD, Whitham R, Bourdette D: Emotional impact of cognitive inefficiencies in multiple sclerosis (MS). J Clin Exp Neuropsychol 12:50, 1990

Lovell MR, Franzen MD: Neuropsychological assessment, in Neuropsychiatry of Traumatic Brain Injury. Edited by Silver JM, Yudofsky SC, Hales RE. Washington, DC, American Psychiatric Press, 1994, pp 133–160

Lovell MR, Nussbaum PD: Neuropsychological assessment, in Textbook of Geriatric Neuropsychiatry. Edited by Coffey CE, Cummings JL. Washington, DC, American Psychiatric Press, 1994, pp 129–144

Malloy PF, Duffy J: The frontal lobes in neuropsychiatric disorders, in Handbook of Neuropsychology, Vol. 9. Edited by Boller F, Grafman J. Amsterdam, Elsevier North-Holland, 1994, pp 203–232

Matthew CG, Klove H: Instruction Manual for the Adult Neuropsychology Test Battery. Madison, WI, University of Wisconsin Medical School, 1964

Mayberg HS, Mahurin RK, Brannan SK: Neuropsychiatric aspects of mood and affective disorders, in The American Psychiatric Press Textbook of Neuropsychiatry, 3rd Edition. Edited by Yudofsky SC, Hales RE. Washington, DC, American Psychiatric Press, 1997, pp 883–902

Mayou RA, Black J, Bryant B: Unconsciousness, amnesia and psychiatric symptoms following road traffic accident injury. Br J Psychiatry 177:540–545, 2000

McAllister TW: Traumatic brain injury and psychosis: what is the connection? Semin Clin Neuropsychiatry 3:211–223, 1998

Mitrushina MN, Boone KB, D'Elia LF: Handbook of Normative Data for Neuropsychological Assessment. New York, Oxford University Press, 1999

Osterrieth PA: Le test de copie d'une figure complexe. Archives de Psychologie 30:206–356, 1944

Parker RS: The spectrum of emotional distress and personality changes after minor head injury incurred in a motor vehicle accident. Brain Inj 10:287–302, 1996

Peterson LR, Peterson MJ: Short-term retention of individual verbal items. J Exp Psychol 58:193–198, 1959

Popper CW, Steingard RJ: Disorders usually first diagnosed in infancy, childhood, or adolescence, in The American Psychiatric Press Synopsis of Psychiatry. Edited by Hales RE, Yudofsky SC. Washington, DC, American Psychiatric Press, 1996, pp 681–774

Prigatano GP: BNI Screen for higher cerebral functions: rationale and initial validation. BNI Q 7:2–9, 1991

Randolph C: Repeatable Battery for the Assessment of Neuropsychological Status. San Antonio, TX, Psychological Corporation, 1998

Randolph C, Tierney MC, Mohr E, Chase TN: The Repeatable Battery for the Assessment of Neuropsychological Status (RBANS): preliminary clinical validity. J Clin Exp Neuropsychol 20:310–319, 1998

Reitan RM: Validity of the Trail Making Test as an indicator of organic brain damage. Perceptual Motor Skills 8:271–276, 1958

Reitan RM, Wolfson D: The Halstead-Reitan Neuropsychological Test Battery: Theory and Clinical Interpretation, 2nd Edition. Tucson, AZ, Neuropsychology Press, 1993

Rey A: L'examen clinique en psychologie. Paris, Presses Universitaires de France, 1964

Rosvold HE, Mirsky AF, Sarason EF, et al: A continuous performance test of brain damage. J Consult Clin Psychol 20:343–350, 1956

Russel EW, Neuringer C, Goldstein G: Assessment of Brain Damage: A Neuropsychological Key Approach. New York, Wiley-Interscience, 1970

Sachdev P, Smith JS, Cathcart S: Schizophrenia-like psychosis following traumatic brain injury: a chart-based descriptive and case control study. Psychol Med 31:231–239, 2001

Sackeim HA, Stern Y: Neuropsychiatric aspects of memory and amnesia, in The American Psychiatric Press Textbook of Neuropsychiatry, 3rd Edition. Edited by Yudofsky SC, Hales RE. Washington, DC, American Psychiatric Press, 1997, pp 499–501

Sbordone RJ: The executive functions of the brain, in Neuropsychological Assessment in Clinical Practice: A Guide to Test Interpretation and Integration. Edited by Groth-Marnat G, New York, Wiley, 2000, pp 437–456

Silver JM, Hales RE, Yudofsky SC: Neuropsychiatric aspects of traumatic brain injury, in The American Psychiatric Press Textbook of Neuropsychiatry, 3rd Edition. Edited by Yudofsky SC, Hales RE. Washington, DC, American Psychiatric Press, 1997, pp 521–560

Slick DJ, Hopp G, Strauss E, Thompson GB: Victoria Symptom Validity Test Professional Manual. Odessa, FL, Psychological Assessment Resources, 1997

Spreen O, Strauss E: A Compendium of Neuropsychological Tests, 2nd Edition: Administration, Norms, and Commentary. New York, Oxford University Press, 1998

Stern RA, Prohaska ML: Neuropsychological evaluation of executive functioning. American Psychiatric Press Review of Psychiatry 15:243–266, 1996

Stringer AY: A Guide to Adult Neuropsychological Diagnosis. Philadelphia, PA, FA Davis Company, 1996

Tamminga CA: Neuropsychiatric aspects of schizophrenia, in The American Psychiatric Press Textbook of Neuropsychiatry, 3rd Edition. Edited by Yudofsky SC, Hales RE. Washington, DC, American Psychiatric Press, 1997, pp 855–882

Teeter PA, Semrud-Clikeman, M: Child Neuropsychology: Assessment and Interventions for Neurodevelopmental Disorders. Needham Heights, MA, Allyn and Bacon, 1997

Tombaugh TN: Test of Memory Malingering. New York, Multi Health Systems, 1996

Tsushima WT, Wedding D: A comparison of the Halstead-Reitan Neuropsychological Battery and computerized tomography in the identification of brain disorder. J Nerv Ment Dis 167:704–707, 1979

Turnbull SJ, Campbell EA, Swann IJ: Post-traumatic stress disorder symptoms following a head injury: does amnesia for the event influence the development of symptoms? Brain Inj 15:775–785, 2001

Vanderploeg RD: Estimating premorbid level of functioning, in Clinician's Guide to Neuropsychological Assessment. Edited by Vanderploeg RD. Hillsdale, NJ, Lawrence Erlbaum, 1994a, pp 43–68

Vanderploeg RD: Interview and testing: The data collection phase of neuropsychological evaluations, in Clinician's Guide to Neuropsychological Assessment. Edited by Vanderploeg RD. Hillsdale, NJ, Lawrence Erlbaum, 1994b, pp 1–41

Wechsler D: Wechsler Adult Intelligence Scale—Revised Manual. New York, Psychological Corporation, 1981

Wechsler D: Wechsler Memory Scale—Revised Manual. New York, Psychological Corporation, 1987

Wechsler D: Wechsler Adult Intelligence Scale—III. San Antonio, TX, Psychological Corporation, 1997a

Wechsler D: Wechsler Memory Scale—III. San Antonio, TX, Psychological Corporation, 1997b

Wilk CM, Gold JM, Bartko JJ, et al: Test-retest stability of the Repeatable Battery for the Assessment of Neuropsychological Status in schizophrenia. Am J Psychiatry 159:838–844, 2002

Zachary RA: Shipley Institute of Living Scale. Revised Manual. Los Angeles, CA, Western Psychological Services, 1986

PART II

Neuropsychiatric Disorders

9 Delirium and Posttraumatic Amnesia

Paula T. Trzepacz, M.D.

Richard E. Kennedy, M.D.

What Is Delirium?

Defining Delirium in Traumatic Brain Injury

Delirium is a neuropsychiatric disorder composed of diffuse cognitive deficits, language and thought abnormalities, psychomotor and affective changes, and sleep-wake cycle disturbances. It is caused by a wide variety of medical, pharmacological, and postoperative conditions. Approximately 18% of general hospital patients are delirious (Trzepacz et al. 2002), and delirium point prevalence ranges from 10%–30% in general hospital patients (Fann 2000). Some surgical populations have an even higher incidence of delirium—approximately 30% in postcardiotomy patients (Smith and Dimsdale 1989) and as much as 50% in elderly hip surgery patients (Williams et al. 1985). The incidence of delirium after traumatic brain injury (TBI) is uncertain because of classification issues in the TBI literature, but appears to be high, especially with severe injuries and loss of consciousness (LOC). However, brief confusional periods occur after minor concussions (Lipowski 1990; Teasdale and Jennett 1974) and "disturbed consciousness is a feature found in most cases of head injury" (Russell and Smith 1961).

The term *delirium* is not commonly used in TBI literature, although there is a growing appreciation that a confusional state occurs and includes more than just memory and orientation deficits (Sandel et al. 1995; Yuen and Benzing 1996). Terms such as *states of impaired consciousness, posttraumatic amnesia* (PTA), *posttraumatic agitation, posttraumatic disorientation, posttraumatic confusional state,*

altered consciousness, and *loss of consciousness* (coma) are used, often without clear definitions of signs and symptoms or, when defined, without a clear consensus regarding usage or practical assessment (Fortuny et al. 1980; Gronwall and Wrightson 1980; Sandel et al. 1995; Stuss et al. 1999; Tate et al. 2000). The varying definitions and criteria make a review of delirium after TBI difficult and interpretation of research on PTA confusing. In psychiatric nosology, delirium and amnesia are not the same, the former being made up of impairment of attention, memory, orientation, and visuoconstructional ability in addition to many other noncognitive symptoms, whereas the latter involves only memory impairment. However, the term *posttraumatic amnesia* is not used by nonpsychiatrists solely to denote memory impairment after a TBI event.

The closest term to *delirium* that is widely used in the TBI literature is *posttraumatic amnesia;* however, this is loosely used and may encompass coma at one extreme or only focal memory deficits at the other and overlaps with a number of neuropsychiatric terms applied to those different clinical stages (Figure 9–1). However, definitions of PTA found in most of the TBI literature overlap significantly with what psychiatrists would call *delirium followed by an amnestic disorder. Posttraumatic amnesia* was defined as the "time elapsed from injury until recovery of full consciousness and the return of ongoing memory" (Grant and Alves 1987). *Posttraumatic amnesia* also has been defined as "a period of clouded consciousness which precedes the attainment of full orientation and continuous awareness in persons recovering from head injuries" and as "characterized primarily by a failure of amnestic processes" (Mandleberg 1975). Thus, PTA overlaps with

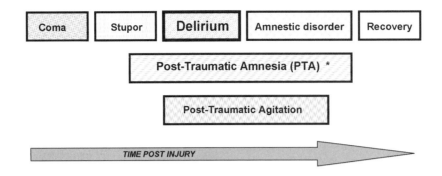

FIGURE 9–1.   Comparing physiatric and neuropsychiatric terminology for post–traumatic brain injury (TBI) changes in level of consciousness and cognition.

Posttraumatic amnesia (PTA) is a term used in the TBI literature. PTA overlaps with many of the symptoms of delirium, although the term also is used to denote the phase after the resolution of delirium (confusion) when more isolated cognitive impairment (usually memory deficits) persists without other behavioral symptoms. At times, stupor is included in the definition of PTA, whereas stupor is distinct from delirium in neuropsychiatric terminology. When agitation is accompanied by other neuropsychiatric symptoms, posttraumatic agitation overlaps with the hyperactive variant of delirium, but agitation can also occur as an isolated symptom.
*Some older studies included coma and stupor in PTA.

coma, stupor, delirium, and amnestic syndrome. However, Ommaya and Gennarelli (1974) defined delirium ("confusion") as a separate state from either coma or amnesia in patients with TBI and specified the expected temporal relationship between them (Figure 9–2). This paradigm has not been well integrated into the TBI literature, however. Katz (1992) also recognized the confusional state embedded in PTA. Thus, *posttraumatic confusional state* would be a more accurate term to denote delirium (Stuss et al. 1999).

Delirium resulting from any cause is an abnormal state of consciousness that exists on a continuum between stupor or coma and normal consciousness (Figure 9–3). However, patients often progress directly from coma into delirium without a clearly defined stupor stage. The placement of a particular delirious episode along this continuum depends on the severity of that delirium. *Subclinical delirium* describes a phase before or during the resolution of an episode of diagnosable delirium that is less severe and detectable only by more subtle examination of

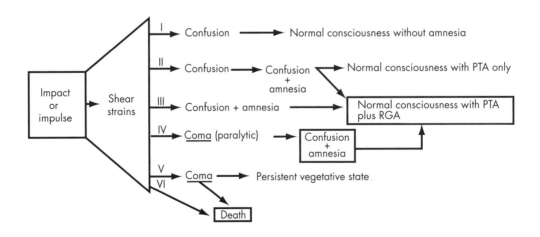

FIGURE 9–2.   Temporal relationships of coma, confusion, and posttraumatic amnesia (PTA) after traumatic brain injury.

Coma and levels of confusion (delirium) after traumatic brain injury, with PTA occurring after resolution of delirium and in the context of normal consciousness, according to Ommaya and Gennarelli (1974). This model differentiates PTA from delirium states.
Source.   Reprinted from Ommaya AK, Gennarelli TA: "Cerebral Concussion and Traumatic Unconsciousness." *Brain* 97:633–654, 1974. Used with permission of Oxford University Press.

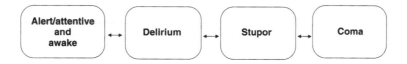

FIGURE 9–3. **Delirium and continuum of levels of consciousness.**

Delirium occurs on a continuum between normal consciousness and stupor and/or coma. Delirium often has a prodrome of milder symptoms, called *subclinical delirium,* as an intermediate state between full-blown delirium and normal consciousness; subclinical delirium also occurs during the resolution of an episode of delirium.

the patient. This is an important concept in TBI because of the need to distinguish lingering amnestic deficits after a resolved delirium from a subclinical delirium that involves more diffuse cognitive deficits accompanied by other behavioral symptoms. Often, these other psychiatric symptoms are not evaluated in patients with TBI in whom clinicians and researchers focus more on cognition—especially orientation, attention, and memory (see the section Rating Scales).

Additionally, delirium can have hypoactive, hyperactive, or mixed motoric presentations that may be subtypes of delirium (Meagher and Trzepacz 2000). These differing motor presentations are often accompanied by other behavioral symptoms, such as yelling, punching, and mood lability in hyperactive delirious patients. The term *posttraumatic agitation* overlaps with the hyperactive subtype of delirium, but because agitation can be either an isolated symptom or associated with other psychiatric and medical conditions besides delirium, delirium and agitation are not synonymous in patients with TBI. Fugate et al. (1997a, 1997b) surveyed by telephone 157 United States physiatrists for their understanding of symptoms of agitation and delirium during the acute recovery phase after TBI. Although there was some overlap in symptoms, they did not appreciate use of the term *delirium* from DSM-III-R symptoms (American Psychiatric Association 1987), although they did associate disorientation, amnesia, and memory impairment with agitation during acute recovery. Symptoms of disorganized thinking, perceptual disturbance, disorientation and disturbed sleep-wake cycle were associated with "delirium."

There are few studies of the relationships between various signs and symptoms common to delirium and other posttraumatic sequelae. Tate et al. (2000), in a study of severely brain-injured patients, found that disorientation resolved before amnesia in 94% of TBI cases, which supports the idea that a confusional (delirium) phase precedes an amnestic phase. Both disorientation and amnesia occur in delirium, so as TBI delirium resolves, disorientation would be expected to improve, whereas some form of memory impairment could persist depending on the

trauma-related lesion locations (often frontotemporal). Similar results can occur after mild injury; one study showed only 38% of patients to be well oriented during PTA (Gronwall and Wrightson 1980). A study of behavioral disturbances after TBI showed that restlessness and agitation resolved in all patients before the resolution of PTA (van der Naalt et al. 2000), which suggests that the delirium phase includes motoric disturbance. Corrigan et al. (1992) reported that agitation and cognition showed 50% shared variance, with most of this shared variance accounted for by attention. Attentional disturbance is the cardinal feature of delirium and a required criterion for diagnosis. However, all of the variance explained by cognition could not be accounted for by agitation, or vice versa, suggesting that not all delirium patients are hyperactive and not all agitated TBI patients have confusional states. Ewert et al. (1989) studied types of memory impairment during PTA and found that during the confusional phase both procedural and declarative memory were impaired, but as confusion resolved the procedural memory deficits resolved before the declarative ones.

Our own findings from our prospective TBI delirium study at the Traumatic Brain Injury Model Systems in Mississippi are consistent with previous studies (Nakase-Thompson et al. 2004). Forty consecutive patients rated as Rancho Los Amigos Cognitive Scale level IV or better during inpatient rehabilitation hospitalization were prospectively evaluated using both neuropsychiatric and rehabilitation rating instruments. All subjects were rated on the Delirium Rating Scale (DRS) and independently using the Agitated Behavior Scale (ABS) and Galveston Orientation and Amnesia Test (GOAT). Twenty-four subjects met DSM-IV delirium diagnostic criteria (American Psychiatric Association 1994), whereas 26 did not. Using GOAT and ABS in a logistic regression model, the two groups were classified with 77.5% accuracy. Inspection of individual scores revealed that some subjects in the delirium group had scores meeting the cutoff for "normal" on the ABS (22.5%) and GOAT (7.5%), whereas some subjects in the nondelirious group had scores in the impaired range on the ABS (7.5%) and GOAT (27.5%). This sug-

TABLE 9–1.   Delirium symptoms and characteristics

Disorientation (time, place, person)

Attentional deficits

Memory impairment (short and long term)

Deficits in higher-order thinking

Visuoconstructional dysfunction

Change in mood/affective lability

Disorganized thinking

Delusions (distinguish from confabulation)

Perceptual disturbances

Language impairments

Psychomotor behavior changes

Sleep-wake cycle disturbances

Abrupt onset

Fluctuating course

Usually reversible

gests that there is significant but incomplete overlap between these clinical syndromes.

Signs and Symptoms of Delirium

Delirium involves a range of cognitive deficits, differentiating it from other psychiatric disorders, except for advanced dementias. Attentional deficits are a hallmark to diagnose delirium in contrast to memory impairment being cardinal in dementia. Delirium cognitive impairments include disorientation to time, place, and person (usually impaired in that order); deficits in attention and concentration; impaired short-term memory with an inability to learn and retain new information; long-term memory impairment; impaired executive functions (e.g., abstraction, conceptualization, temporal ordering, sequencing, and mental flexibility); and impaired visuoconstructional ability (including wandering and getting lost). Such a breadth of cognitive impairment can occur after TBI depending on the severity of injury. Concussion seems to be a brief, transient mild delirium.

In addition to these cognitive deficits, delirium involves many other neuropsychiatric symptoms (Table 9–1). These include an alteration in mood (anxious, depressed, irritable, hostile), affective lability (sometimes to the proportions of pseudobulbar palsy), and mood incongruency. Thinking is disorganized and may be rambling, tangential, circumstantial, or even loosely associated. Language abnormalities are variable, but can include

word-finding difficulty, paraphasias, dysnomia, dysgraphia, impaired repetition, impaired articulation, impaired comprehension, and perseveration of words or phrases. In the most severe cases, speech resembles a fluent or a global aphasia. However, deficits in semantics of communication are the most characteristic language disturbance of delirium and serve to distinguish it from the language abnormalities associated with other psychiatric disorders. Psychomotor behavior may evidence retardation or agitation, often mixed together (related concepts are the motor subtypes of delirium, called *hypoactive* or *hyperactive*); patients may appear depressed and withdrawn, or may be agitated and remove intravenous lines, or may wander or pace around. Hypoactive delirium is commonly misdiagnosed as depression. Perceptual disturbances are common and may take the form of either illusions or hallucinations; visual (and occasionally tactile) hallucinations strongly suggest delirium, though auditory hallucinations or illusions also occur in delirium. Suspiciousness and persecutory delusions are common, but the latter usually are poorly formed and not well systematized, often incorporating many of the caregivers into the delusional ideation. Patients may refuse tests because of suspiciousness, thus interfering with their own medical care. The sleep-wake cycle is disrupted and fragmented throughout the 24-hour period, with napping and nocturnal arousals that are often accompanied by nocturnal confusion and an inability to distinguish nightmares or dreams from reality. In the extreme, delirious patients may have severe sleeplessness.

These symptoms of delirium typically wax and wane in severity to some degree during a 24-hour period, with phases of increased lucidity alternating with more severe impairment. This waxing and waning makes it more difficult to assess the severity of delirium for short time frames and complicates determining exactly when the episode has ended. DSM-IV-TR criteria (American Psychiatric Association 2000) for diagnosing delirium require disturbance of consciousness and/or attentional deficits, as well as a change in memory, language, orientation, or perceptual disturbances with a fairly abrupt onset and a fluctuating course, and physical factors that can be implicated as causative (Table 9–2).

Descriptions of the clinical symptoms of PTA covering the period after emergence from coma until the later phase of focal memory deficits are essentially descriptions of delirium. This is a period of "confusion, restlessness, perplexity, irritability, aggression, withdrawal, and frank psychosis" (Grant and Alves 1987) and of "restlessness, agitation, combativeness, confusion, hallucinations and other disturbed perceptions, disorientation, depression, paranoid ideation, hypomania, and confabulation" (Fisher 1985).

TABLE 9-2.   DSM-IV-TR diagnostic criteria for delirium due to a general medical condition

A. Disturbance of consciousness (i.e., reduced clarity of awareness of the environment) with reduced ability to focus, sustain, or shift attention.

B. A change in cognition (e.g., memory deficit, disorientation, language disturbance) or the development of a perceptual disturbance that is not better accounted for by a preexisting, established, or evolving dementia.

C. The disturbance develops over a short period of time (usually hours to days) and tends to fluctuate during the course of the day.

D. There is evidence from the history, physical examination, or laboratory findings that the disturbance is caused by the direct physiological consequences of a general medical condition.

Source. Reprinted from American Psychiatric Association: *Diagnostic and Statistical Manual of Mental Disorders*, 4th Edition, Text Revision. Washington, DC, American Psychiatric Association, 2000. Used with permission.

These clinical descriptions highlight the hyperactive variant of delirium, which may be more common in TBI or may be more easily recognized by staff. Ewert et al. (1989) described PTA as the "initial stage of recovery from TBI after emergence from coma and characterized by anterograde and retrograde amnesia, disorientation, and rapid forgetting," but not necessarily accompanied by attentional deficits, confusion, and changes in behavior. This latter description focuses on impaired memory and downplays other cognitive and behavioral symptoms of delirium. Wechsler Adult Intelligence Scale test results have revealed diffuse cognitive deficits in PTA (abstraction, comprehension, attention, general information, visuomotor skill, and vocabulary) and performance scores that were somewhat worse than verbal scores; scores improved after resolution of the PTA (Mandleberg 1975).

Rao and Lyketsos (2000) describe four groups of cognitive deficits according to when they occur in relation to the phases of TBI (Figure 9–4). The first period is LOC or coma soon after injury. The second phase, which lasts from a few days to a month, is characterized by a mixture of cognitive and behavioral abnormalities, including agitation, confusion, disorientation, and alteration in psychomotor activity with inability to recall events, sequence time, and learn new information, called *posttraumatic delirium*. The third phase is a rapid cognitive recovery period lasting from 6 to 12 months and plateauing 12–24 months after injury. Phase four is permanent cognitive sequelae.

Motoric agitation is common after acute brain injury and includes combativeness, truncal rocking, and arm thrashing (Levin and Grossman 1978). In this study, such agitation was more common in younger patients, although the duration of coma was shorter (less than 24 hours) in those who were agitated than in those who were not (Levin and Grossman 1978). Also, agitation was not related to focal neurological signs, focal frontotemporal injury, or (inferred) mesencephalic injury, but was associated with visual and auditory hallucinations and delusions. This parallels descriptions of hyperactive delirium from other causes when hyperactivity is more associated with psychosis than hypoactivity (Meagher and Trzepacz 2000). Reyes et al. (1981) showed that patients with restlessness and agitation at the time of hospital discharge eventually had better recovery of premorbid physical and cognitive functions, but with a greater need for psychological intervention. van der Naalt et al. (2000) found that agitation and restlessness resolved before PTA did and that approximately one-half of patients with TBI had agitation during PTA.

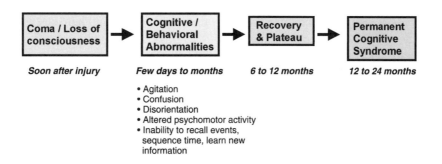

FIGURE 9-4.   Cognitive deficits in posttraumatic brain injury: four phases.

There are four phases of cognitive deficits during recovery from posttraumatic brain injury. Delirium occurs after emergence from stupor or coma and persists until either full neuropsychiatric recovery or a plateau phase of persisting cognitive and behavioral symptoms that do not meet criteria for a delirium diagnosis.

Source. Adapted from Rao V, Lyketsos C: "Neuropsychiatric Sequelae of Traumatic Brain Injury." *Psychosomatics* 41:95–103, 2000.

Memory studies have been performed in PTA, although the complexity of the tests suggests that these patients were not severely delirious. Both declarative and procedural long-term memory have been studied in TBI (Ewert et al. 1989; Levin et al. 1985). Disoriented PTA patients had poorer recall of autobiographical information as compared with their recall after PTA resolution (Levin et al. 1985). In this same study, both retrograde and anterograde memory deficits occurred in PTA patients. In a test of visual memory, PTA patients had more difficulty in acquisition of material and forgot at a faster rate than did recovered PTA patients (Levin et al. 1988a). In a group of patients with frontal lobe lesions, procedural memory improved over the course of PTA, whereas declarative memory deficits remained stable (Ewert et al. 1989). Thus, delirium in TBI involves an alteration of both declarative and procedural memory. This is interesting because procedural memory remains relatively intact in amnestic patients, is implicit, and is not affected by the temporal lobe–diencephalon areas of the brain (Squire 1986). In contrast, declarative memory is impaired in amnestic syndrome; is "explicit" (conscious); is subserved by the medial temporal lobe, hippocampus, diencephalon, and ventromedial frontal lobe; and consolidates over time (Squire 1986). This suggests a possible difference in the neuroanatomical substrates of amnestic syndrome and delirium.

Distinguishing the type of memory impairment may help distinguish between delirium and residual memory deficits that persist (i.e., amnestic syndrome) (Tate et al. 2000). Using daily ratings of memory and orientation in 31 patients with severe TBI diagnosed with PTA, Tate et al. (2000) found that disorientation recovered first—person, then place, and then time—replicating a prior study (High et al. 1990). This paralleled the pattern of cognitive recovery after electroconvulsive therapy–induced delirium (Daniel et al. 1987). In 94% of these patients, memory deficits resolved before disorientation; however, orientation to person preceded improvement in visual recognition memory, followed by orientation to place, then to time, and, finally, free recall (Tate et al. 2000). Thus, their most sensitive memory measure was actually last to improve, and there was much individual variation. Geffen et al. (1991) studied PTA and found that orientation returned first, followed by recognition and cued recall, and free recall was last. Schwartz et al. (1998) compared 91 patients with TBI (mild to severe) to 27 trauma center control subjects using serial GOAT ratings and ability to learn/retain new information (three words and three pictures). For the TBI group, the time sequence was later for recovering recall memory than for either recognition memory or obtaining a normal GOAT score, irrespective of TBI severity level, although recovery occurred sooner in subjects with milder

injury. Picture memory recovered before verbal memory. Stuss et al. (1999) studied patterns of cognitive recovery in 108 patients with TBI and found that recognition memory improved before verbal recall memory (which was last), and attentional deficits were the first to recover. Ability to perform simpler tests preceded more effortful or strategic ones. An auditory continuous performance task was used to measure attention.

Attentional deficits and disorientation are hallmarks of delirium, further supporting the premise that PTA patients were likely delirious. Improvement of attentional deficits and disorientation may be critical in determining the end of delirium. Sisler and Penner (1975) studied 28 patients with severe TBI in whom the temporal course of orientation and memory improvement was highly variable, with both resolving simultaneously in 50% of cases.

To examine the extent to which posttraumatic stress disorder (PTSD) symptoms require memory for the traumatic event, the relationship between PTSD and PTA was explored in 282 outpatients a mean of 53 days after TBI (Feinstein et al. 2002). The investigators found that patients whose PTA lasted longer than a week could still have PTSD symptoms, though such symptoms were more likely if PTA was briefer (i.e., lasted less than 1 hour).

Baker (2001) played taped and live music to 22 patients with TBI and found that 77% recalled the music program while in PTA (scoring <9 on the Westmead PTA scale). Music was recalled better than pictures—on average, at least one song was recalled by day 3 and one picture by day 5; by day 6, recall was similar for both.

Based on a compilation of findings from these various studies, Figure 9–5 shows the progression of recovery of cognitive abilities as posttraumatic delirium resolves. Because not all of the abilities were simultaneously measured in each study, these are not definitive in their relationship to each other. In addition, there is probably individual variation for order of recovery, and some functions can recover simultaneously as well.

Causes of Delirium

Delirium is caused by physiological, structural, and/or pharmacological etiologies that affect the brain directly or indirectly. Often, more than one etiology exists in a given patient. Table 9–3 summarizes categories and common etiologies for delirium. The most common causes include drug intoxication and withdrawal (polypharmacy is common) and metabolic, cardiovascular, infectious, and traumatic causes. The first step in the management of delirium is the diagnosis and treatment of these underlying etiologic factors.

Table 9–4 lists etiologies of delirium that are more specific to the TBI population, although any of the prob-

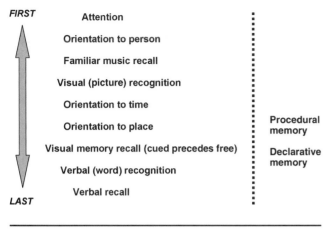

FIRST
Attention
Orientation to person
Familiar music recall
Visual (picture) recognition
Orientation to time
Orientation to place — Procedural memory
Visual memory recall (cued precedes free) — Declarative memory
Verbal (word) recognition
Verbal recall
LAST

FIGURE 9–5. Time course of recovery of cognitive abilities during resolution of posttraumatic delirium. Delirium involves impairment of many cognitive functions, in addition to other neuropsychiatric disturbances. The time course of recovery of these, on the basis of a compilation of results from separate studies (in which only several of these functions were compared), suggests that certain functions (e.g., attention and orientation) recover before others (e.g., music recall before verbal recall; procedural memory before declarative memory).

lems listed in Table 9–3 also need to be considered in patients with TBI. In addition to TBI itself, patients are at increased risk of morbidity and mortality from a variety of other causes, with seizures, circulatory diseases, and respiratory diseases being particularly common (Kalisky et al. 1985; Shavelle et al. 2001). Delirium in TBI can be caused by both direct effects on the brain (e.g., coup-contrecoup, concussion, subdural hematoma, intraparenchymal hemorrhage, and contusion) and by extracranial injuries such as multiple trauma, hypoxemia from chest trauma or a compromised airway, and shock. TBI patients with systemic hypoxia or hypertension have an increased mortality (Gentleman and Jennett 1990). Increased intracranial pressure has been associated with a greatly increased mortality in TBI, and strategies such as hyperventilation and barbiturate coma have been used to reduce acute brain swelling and metabolic rate (Lobato et al. 1988). These treatments, however, as well as these TBI complications, may cause delirium (see the section Functional Neuroimaging in this chapter as well as Chapter 6, Functional Imaging, for a discussion of cerebral blood flow [CBF]).

Risk Factors

Factors that increase the risk of delirium are listed in Table 9–5. Low serum albumin is an important risk factor

TABLE 9–3. Etiologies for delirium in any population

Category	Causes
Drug intoxication	Anticholinergics, digoxin, histamine antagonists, antiarrhythmics, phenytoin, opioids, and others
Drug withdrawal	Alcohol, benzodiazepine, barbiturate
Metabolic	Hepatic or renal insufficiency, change in pH, hyper- or hypoglycemia, hypothermia, hyponatremia, hypercalcemia, vitamin deficiency, dehydration
Infection	Any systemic type, encephalitis, meningitis, abscess, tertiary syphilis
Endocrine	Hypothyroidism, hypo- or hypercortisolism, hyperparathyroidism
Seizures	Ictal and postictal states
Cancer	Metastases, brain tumor, carcinomatous meningitis, remote effects
Vascular	Stroke, transient ischemic attack, hypoperfusion, hypoxemia, subdural hematoma, shock, increased intracranial pressure, acute hypertension, pulmonary embolus, cardiac arrhythmia, myocardial infarction, vasculitis
Environmental/ physical	Heat stroke, radiation, toxins, heavy metals (lead, mercury), industrial solvents, pesticides, electrocution, burns, carbon monoxide

that has been elucidated in a number of different patient samples (Levkoff et al. 1988; Trzepacz and Francis 1990). It can indicate poor nutrition or change in pharmacokinetics with increased free (unbound) serum levels of drugs and consequent increased potential for central nervous system (CNS) toxicity. Elderly patients are more vulnerable to delirium (Francis et al. 1990) and are a sometimes forgotten population susceptible to head trauma (Galbraith 1987). Ellenberg et al. (1996) found older age, low initial Glasgow Coma Scale (GCS) score, nonreactive pupils, coma duration, and use of phenytoin to be associated with more prolonged PTA. Wilson et al. (1994) found a correlation between PTA duration and number of hemispheric lesions on magnetic resonance imaging (MRI) ($r=0.37$) and number of central brain areas with lesions ($r=0.57$). However, patients who are traditionally considered to have a higher risk for delirium are nearly

TABLE 9–4. Causes of delirium in patients with traumatic brain injury

Mechanical effects (acceleration or deceleration, contusion, and others)

Cerebral edema

Hemorrhage

Infection

Subdural hematoma

Seizure

Hypoxia (cardiopulmonary or local ischemia)

Increased intracranial pressure

Alcohol intoxication or withdrawal; Wernicke's encephalopathy

Illicit drug intoxication or withdrawal

Reduced hemoperfusion related to multiple trauma

Fat embolism

Change in pH

Electrolyte imbalance

Medications (barbiturates, steroids, opioids, and anticholinergics)

TABLE 9–5. Risk factors predisposing toward delirium

Low serum albumin

Geriatric age, with or without dementia

Brain damage or central nervous system disease

Prior episode of delirium

Serious medical disease

Polypharmacy

Basal ganglia lesions on magnetic resonance imaging

Cerebral atrophy with right-hemisphere focal lesions

always excluded from PTA studies—especially alcoholic patients, elderly patients, those with prior psychiatric and neurological histories, and those with prior brain injury.

Rating Scales

PTA assessment tools include those that diagnose or measure severity of symptoms. Many tools are from the rehabilitation literature, whereas delirium scales are from the psychiatry literature. All of the scales assess cognitive elements or level of consciousness of PTA, agitation, or a full range of delirium symptoms (Table 9–6). Although the rehabilitation scales have been used to characterize, follow the clinical course of, or assess the outcome of PTA, each scale has drawbacks, and none of them adequately assesses delirium. There is a growing appreciation for the inadequacies of scales that focus only on cognition or agitation and do not include a fuller range of symptoms (Sandel et al. 1995; Tate et al. 2000). In addition, without measuring a wider range of symptoms, it can be difficult to determine when the confusional state ends and a more persistent focal cognitively impaired state begins. It is unusual for these scales to be compared with one another in research.

The GCS (Teasdale and Jennett 1974) (see Chapter 1, Epidemiology; Table 1–2) was devised to assess the depth and duration of impaired consciousness and coma by measuring three axes (consisting of motor responsiveness, verbal performance, and eye opening), each on a separately scored subscale. Although this scale has some utility in quantifying some clinical symptoms of coma, it does not assess delirium. The GCS has been used to rate patients with TBI on admission to the hospital and then to compare various outcome measures; it has also been used to select study samples of patients with TBI, depending on certain cutoff scores, to indicate initial severity of TBI (Changaris et al. 1987). Its simplicity makes it ideal for nonresearchers (e.g., ward nurses) to perform ratings.

The GOAT (Levin et al. 1979b) (see Chapter 8, Issues in Neuropsychological Assessment; Figure 8–1) was developed for serial use in assessing cognitive status after TBI, and it specifically focuses on orientation and ability to remember events preceding and the earliest valid memory after the injury. It does not address the other cognitive deficits present in delirium, nor does it rate behavioral symptoms of delirium (e.g., mood, sleep, psychomotor, psychotic, perceptual, and others). Delirious patients can become oriented on this scale before amnesia has resolved (Gronwall and Wrightson 1980). A cutoff score of 75 out of 100 points has been used as an indicator that PTA has resolved (Ewert et al. 1989); however, given the nature of the questions, 75 is probably too low, and too many false-negative deliria may occur using this criterion. The GOAT identifies a stage in recovery most consistent with recovery of recognition memory after simple attention recovers (Stuss et al. 1999).

The Rancho Los Amigos Cognitive Scale (Hagen et al. 1972; see Table 4–6 in Chapter 4, Neuropsychiatric Assessment) is an 8-point scale describing the patient's behavior along a continuum from coma to a state close to normal, but often with persistent cognitive deficits (level VIII). It is often used for rating individuals who are in long-term rehabilitation settings and who have chronic sequelae of TBI. Levels IV and V include delirium symp-

TABLE 9–6. Instruments that can be used to rate posttraumatic amnesia (PTA), agitation, and/or delirium in traumatic brain injury

PTA scales (references)	Agitation scales (reference)	Delirium scales (references)
Galveston Orientation and Memory Test: Orientation and retrograde memory (Levin et al. 1979b)	Agitation Behavior Scale: Agitation (Corrigan et al. 1989)	Delirium Rating Scale: Cognition, psychosis, psychomotor behavior, perception, sleep-wake cycle, temporal course (Trzepacz et al. 1988a)
Oxford PTA scale: Anterograde memory and orientation (Fortuny et al. 1980)	Overt Agitation Severity Scale (Yudofsky et al. 1997)	Delirium Rating Scale-Revised-98: Orientation, attention, short-term memory, long-term memory, visuospatial ability, sleep-wake cycle, language, thought processes, delusions, psychomotor behavior, perception, temporal course (Trzepacz et al. 2001)
Westmead PTA scale: Orientation and anterograde memory (Shores et al. 1986)		
Orientation Group Monitoring System: Orientation (Corrigan and Mysiw 1984; Corrigan et al. 1985)		
Julia Farr Centre PTA scale: Orientation, recognition and recall memory (Geffen et al. 1991)		Confusion Assessment Method: Temporal course, inattention, disorganized thinking, altered level of consciousness (Inouye et al. 1990)
Rivermead PTA Protocol: Return of continuous memory (King et al. 1997)		Confusion Assessment Method for the Intensive Care Unit: Temporal course, inattention, disorganized thinking, altered level of consciousness (Ely et al. 2001a, 2001b)
Neurobehavioral Rating Scale: Wide variety of psychiatric symptoms that are not specific to delirium (Levin et al. 1987)		
Rancho Los Amigos Cognitive Scale: Cognition in broad categories, overlapping with levels of consciousness (Hagen et al. 1972)		Cognitive Test for Delirium: Attention span, orientation, memory, vigilance, comprehension (Hart et al. 1996)
Glasgow Coma Scale: Coma to normal consciousness (Teasdale and Jennett 1974)		

toms, whereas level III corresponds more closely to stupor, and levels I and II correspond to coma.

Early attempts were made to address broader psychiatric symptoms of PTA (Levin and Grossman 1978; Levin et al. 1979a) using the Brief Psychiatric Rating Scale (Overall and Gorham 1962), which is usually used to rate psychotic patients, in particular patients with schizophrenia. This was an important step in recognizing other psychiatric symptoms of TBI delirium. The Neurobehavioral Rating Scale (Levin et al. 1987) was developed by incorporating parts of the Brief Psychiatric Rating Scale and adding a number of other psychiatric symptoms considered to be relevant to the evaluation of TBI patients. The Neurobehavioral Rating Scale is more comprehensive than the GOAT or the GCS, with 27 clinician-rated items, each scored on a 7-point severity scale. Items include disorientation, inattention, anxiety, disinhibition, guilt, agitation, poor insight, depressed mood, fatigability, hallucinations, blunted affect, and speech articulation deficit. The problem with its use for delirium is its great breadth and lack of focus on delirium—it mentions most symptoms seen in nearly any psychiatric disorder. Its main utility might be as

a screening tool to increase clinical detection of various psychiatric disorders occurring after TBI.

The Oxford scale for PTA (Fortuny et al. 1980) is a simple questionnaire composed of demographic information, orientation, and visual memory. It involves presentation of three pictures and the examiner's face and name, all to be recalled the following day, with a recognition component to assist free recall, including distractor items and enough different items for 21 days of daily assessment.

The Westmead scale for PTA adapted the Oxford memory procedure with personal information plus memory and orientation. It has only one set of distractor pictures for recognition memory testing, and target pictures can change, with already used ones becoming distractors, so it is a more demanding test (Tate et al. 2000). It measures new learning (anterograde memory). A perfect score means resolution of PTA.

The Julia Farr Centre PTA scale (Geffen et al. 1991) separately assesses word recognition and free recall, in addition to orientation.

The Rivermead PTA Protocol (King et al. 1997) is a retrospective clinical interview for patients' free recall of memories after TBI, in chronological order, to determine the point of return of normal continuous memory. It was tested in 12 patients with severe TBI who were within 2 years of injury, 40 TBI patients within 6 months of injury, and 22 TBI patients 7–10 days after injury and in 116 TBI patients with both early and 6-month assessments. This method is more geared to amnestic syndrome than to delirium.

Wilson et al. (1999) recommended tests of orientation, memory, attention, and visuospatial function for patients with PTA on the basis of their serial neuropsychological testing of patients with severe TBI in PTA ($n=9$), patients with severe TBI without PTA ($n=10$) and healthy control subjects ($n=13$). Specifically, they suggested measures of orientation, reaction time, visual recognition memory, and speed of information processing because patients with PTA show a much wider range of deficits than people with chronic memory impairment or amnestic syndrome. PTA does not appear to be solely a disorder of memory or orientation as suggested by the GOAT or Westmead.

The DRS (Trzepacz et al. 1988a) specifically rates the severity of many symptoms of delirium and differentiates patients with delirium from patients with psychosis and dementia. Each of its 10 items, which are rated by trained clinicians, is scored on the basis of descriptive ratings for severity, and total scores above 10 or 12 points have been used to indicate delirium of varying severity. One of the items rates the degree of cognitive dysfunction and depends on specific testing of cognition. Detection of subclinical delirium (a score between 8 and 12 points) is enhanced by concurrent use of bedside cognitive screening tests. Its sensitivity and specificity are high and range from 82% to 94% and 82% to 94%, respectively, across studies (Trzepacz 1999a). The DRS has recently been used in acute recovery phase TBI patients, in whom it detects delirium (Thompson et al. 2001). The DRS has been translated into 12 languages.

The DRS-Revised-98 (DRS-R-98; Trzepacz et al. 2001) is a substantially revised version of the DRS, with 13 severity and 3 diagnostic items rated on the basis of descriptions. These items are sleep-wake cycle disturbance, perceptual disturbances and hallucinations, delusions, lability of affect, language, thought process abnormalities, motor agitation, motor retardation, orientation, attention, short-term memory, long-term memory, visuospatial ability, temporal onset of symptoms, fluctuation of symptom severity, and physical disorder. On the basis of receiver operating characteristic analyses, scores 15 or higher on the severity scale and 18 or higher on the total scale indicate delirium. The DRS-R-98 differentiated delirium patients (including some patients with TBI) from patients with schizophrenia, depression, and dementia

($P<0.001$) during blind ratings, and it correlated highly with the DRS ($r=0.81$) and the Cognitive Test for Delirium (CTD) ($r=-0.62$). Internal consistency is high, whereas sensitivity ranges from 91% to 100% and specificity from 85% to 100%, depending on the cutoff score used. The DRS-R-98 is being or has been translated into 11 languages. It has been administered to patients with TBI in acute recovery phase, though these data are not yet published.

The Confusion Assessment Method (CAM; Inouye et al. 1990) is a commonly used screening test for delirium especially in nonpsychiatric settings such as medical-surgical wards or emergency departments. The four-item algorithm version is easily used by nonpsychiatrists for screening possible cases of delirium. The CAM for the Intensive Care Unit (ICU) is an adaptation of the CAM algorithm for use by ICU nurses, but unlike the original CAM it includes standardized examples of how to administer each of the four items (i.e., cognitive items from the CTD, described in the following paragraph). It was validated in two different samples and has high sensitivity (95% to 100%) and specificity (93% to 100%) as compared with an independent DSM-IV diagnosis (Ely et al. 2001a, 2001b).

A commonly used 30-point cognitive screening test is the Mini-Mental State Examination (MMSE; Folstein et al. 1975), which assesses orientation, concentration, short-term verbal memory, visuoconstructional ability, comprehension, naming, repetition, and writing. Scores below 24 indicate cognitive dysfunction but do not specifically indicate delirium. The CTD (Hart et al. 1996) correlates highly with the MMSE in delirium patients but has advantages of measuring broader cognitive functions than the MMSE and does not require the patient to speak or write responses. The CTD has been used in acutely recovering TBI patients (Kennedy et al. 2002). Receiver operating characteristic analysis with delirious and nondelirious patients shows an optimum cutoff value of 22; at this level, sensitivity was 72% and specificity 71%. Although these levels are generally acceptable for clinical use, there are clear limitations in using purely cognitive measures such as the CTD for the detection of delirium. Measures such as the CAM-ICU, which incorporate both cognitive and noncognitive aspects of delirium, may have advantages for this purpose.

Other Features of TBI Delirium

Severity and Location of Injury

It is believed that more severe brain injuries result in more prolonged coma and PTA (Williams et al. 1990). PTA may persist for weeks or months, although it is not known whether this indicates a continuing delirium, a subclinical delirium, a dementia, or another process. A variety of brain lesions, especially those in the brainstem, have been associated with protracted coma and PTA (Jellinger and Seitelberger 1970). Deeper brain lesions were associated with more severe brain injury (Ommaya and Gennarelli 1974), and resulted in longer duration and degree of coma and/or PTA (Katz et al. 1989; Levin et al. 1988b; Ommaya and Gennarelli 1974). The degree of mechanical shearing caused by acceleration/deceleration forces may determine the depth of lesion along a continuum from the surface of the cortex to the brainstem (Ommaya and Gennarelli 1974). Basal ganglia (Katz et al. 1989) and basal forebrain lesions (Salazar et al. 1986) were more associated with unconsciousness than more superficial lesions. The severity of impaired consciousness did not differ among lesions located in frontal and temporal lobes, however (Levin et al. 1988b). Hemispheric lateralization of lesions was not related to behavioral sequelae (Levin and Grossman 1978), but left-sided lesions were associated with longer duration of PTA than right-sided lesions (Levin et al. 1989). Patients with severe TBI had more symptoms consistent with delirium (conceptual disorganization, unusual thought content, excitement, and disorientation) even though patients were studied after the most severe confusional symptoms had resolved (Levin and Grossman 1978).

Posttraumatic Amnesia and Outcome

Several features of PTA are related to outcome after TBI (Levin et al. 1979a; Katz et al. 1989). Residual medical, cognitive, behavioral, linguistic, and psychosocial problems all may impede recovery to premorbid levels (Levin 1995). The relationship between duration of coma or duration of PTA to outcome varies in different studies (Smith 1961). Although increased duration of coma correlates with poorer outcome and duration of PTA increases with longer coma, duration of PTA may or may not correlate with outcome. A study of 314 patients with severe TBI found that PTA duration was predicted by coma duration and initial GCS score, suggesting a relationship between coma and delirium (Ellenberg et al. 1996). Smith (1961) found that after excluding patients with focal injuries, duration of PTA correlated better with outcome; also, longer duration of PTA was associated with a higher incidence of seizures.

Ellenberg et al. (1996) found that duration of PTA, nonreactive pupils, time in coma, and use of phenytoin were predictive of the 6-month outcome after severe TBI in their retrospective study of 314 patients. Wilson et al. (1994) found that TBI coma survivors whose PTA was disproportionately long compared with coma duration (i.e., brief coma) had more numerous hemispheric lesions on MRI than patients whose LOC was more proportional to PTA duration. In a study of 65 TBI acute-care or rehabilitation inpatients, 45 of whom met DSM-IV criteria for delirium, Nakase-Thompson et al. (2002) found that those whose delirium was not resolved by discharge had higher levels of disability and lower cognitive function ratings than those whose delirium resolved before discharge, even after controlling for severity of injury and initial admission ratings for these variables.

Reyes et al. (1981) reported a better outcome from TBI in those patients who had hyperactive delirium as compared with hypoactive. Nakase-Thompson et al. (2002) studied the relationship between DSM-IV–diagnosed delirium and disability status in 65 consecutive TBI rehabilitation inpatients who scored IV or above on the Rancho Los Amigos Cognitive Scale. They diagnosed delirium in 45 patients on initial ratings, which resolved by discharge in all but 14 patients who also were found to have significantly greater levels of disability and cognitive impairment at discharge, even after controlling for severity of injury and admission ratings. This suggests that persistent delirium affects recovery from TBI.

There is a debate about the reversibility of delirium after an index admission to a medical-surgical ward, especially in the elderly. Some consider persistent cognitive impairments to be permanent damage related to the delirium, whereas others consider these symptoms to have been present though not yet diagnosed at the index hospitalization. The latter would explain the increased risk for delirium as well as the etiology of so-called persistent cognitive deficits during follow-up. Thus, many geriatric delirious patients are considered to have had an underlying dementia that keeps progressing over time. Rockwood et al. (1999) found an 18% annual incidence of dementia in delirium patients—more than three times higher than the incidence in nondelirious patients, after adjusting for age and comorbid illness severity. Camus et al.'s (2000) cross-sectional study of consecutive psychogeriatric admissions found that preexisting cognitive impairment was the only factor linked to incomplete symptom resolution after a delirium episode. If we draw an analogy between these dementia data and TBI, CNS trauma/lesions increase the risk for a delirium episode and also explain persistent cognitive deficits long after the delirium episode has resolved. A more specific definition for PTA would then be focused only on the memory (amnestic) impairments that persist long after the delirium has resolved. Supporting this are the data from Ewert et al. (1989) that show that the type of long-term memory impairment during the confusional phase (procedural and declarative) evolves toward just declarative memory deficits as the confusion resolves.

Early studies by Russell (1932) found that older, more severely injured patients had longer PTA duration such that advanced age itself may be a risk factor independent of injury severity. Ellenberg et al. (1996) found that the proportion of 16- or 25-year-olds still in PTA was lower than that of 40-year-olds (Cox proportional hazards survival curves) when determined by a GOAT score 75 points or higher after emergence from coma. Salazar et al. (1986) found that coma was more associated with left hemisphere penetrating head injury (in 26% of patients) versus right-sided wounds (in 9% of patients). Levin et al. (1989) found longer median duration of coma in patients with TBI with left-sided lesions (32.8 days) versus right-sided lesions (8.8 days) on the basis of the time from injury until they were able to obey commands.

Among 30 patients with severe TBI, those who overestimated their actual behavioral competencies several months after injury had significantly longer duration of PTA ($r=0.41$, $P<0.05$) and lower admission GCS scores ($r=-0.39$, $P=0.05$) (Prigatano et al. 1998). This suggests that more severe delirium may result in worse self-awareness, thereby affecting level of disability during recovery from TBI.

Duration of PTA was predictive of functional outcome in 276 TBI patients admitted to a level 1 trauma center (Zafonte et al. 1997). Duration of PTA was even more predictive of Disability Rating Scale and Functional Independence Measures scores, with PTA accounting for 20%–45% of the variance.

Duration of delirium associated with TBI, as measured by traditional PTA scales, seems to be longer than for the average duration of other causes of delirium. For example, at 30 days after coma emergence, 65% of patients with TBI remained in PTA (GOAT cutoff of 75), and at 65 days 35% were still in PTA (Ellenberg et al. 1996). Patients with severe TBI with reactive pupils whose PTA lasted 10 days had an 80% probability of a satisfactory outcome, whereas the worst prognosis was PTA longer than 40 days and nonreactive pupils. Tate et al. (2001) used the modified Oxford PTA scale and the GOAT for daily ratings of early PTA duration from measurements during the first week after injury. However, they excluded patients with important and common delirium risk factors from their study, including prior neurological events, psychiatric problems, developmental disability, and drug/alcohol dependency.

Neuropathophysiology of Delirium in TBI

Delirium is considered to be a syndrome—that is, a constellation of signs and symptoms that result from a variety of different causes and culminate in a common presentation. At what point these various etiologies converge neurophysiologically to form this syndrome is unknown, but a final common neural pathway has been proposed (Trzepacz et al. 2002) that emphasizes a perturbation of acetylcholine and dopamine balance and involvement of certain neural pathways (Figure 9–6). On the basis of structural and functional neuroimaging studies, certain brain regions may be more implicated in delirium—in particular, prefrontal cortex, thalamus, right posterior parietal cortex, and fusiform cortex (Trzepacz 1999b). Most of these brain regions also play a role in various components of attention. A plethora of evidence supports a role for a deficiency of acetylcholine in delirium (Trzepacz 1996; Trzepacz et al. 2002) in conjunction with an excess activity of dopamine. Although a number of different neurotransmitters may be involved or affected from the various etiologies of delirium, these two neurotransmitters may play a particular role in a final neural common pathway that produces the constellation of symptoms of delirium (Trzepacz 2000). Of interest is that in an experimental rat model of TBI (Dixon et al. 1994), acetylcholine initially rises immediately after the injury (along with the excitatory neurotransmitter glutamate) but then sharply declines followed by a prolonged period of continued cholinergic hypofunction (Figure 9–7). Using this model for humans with TBI, delirium would occur during the acute phase of severe decline in cholinergic neurotransmission and then amnestic or other more circumscribed

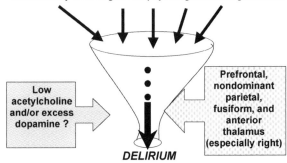

FIGURE 9–6.   Delirium final common pathway.
Certain brain regions and neurotransmitters may be responsible for the neuropathogenesis of delirium. Therefore, diverse physiological or structural perturbations affecting the brain caused by a wide variety of etiologies can result in a common set of symptoms that make up delirium.
Source.   Reprinted with permission from Trzepacz PT, Meagher DJ, Wise M: "Neuropsychiatry of Delirium," in *Textbook of Neuropsychiatry*. Edited by Yudofsky SC, Hales RE. Washington, DC, American Psychiatric Publishing, 2002, pp 525–564.

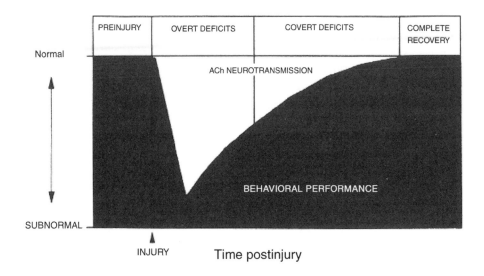

FIGURE 9–7.   Brain cholinergic hypoactivity after traumatic brain injury (TBI).
Initially, acetylcholine (ACh) release is increased, followed by a hypocholinergic state that may coincide with delirium (and posttraumatic amnesia) that gradually lessens over time but underlies more isolated cognitive deficits and increases susceptibility to anticholinergic medication effects.
Source. Reprinted from Dixon CE, Hamm RJ, Taft WC, Hayes RL: "Increased Anticholinergic Sensitivity Following Closed Skull Impact and Controlled Cortical Impact Traumatic Brain Injury in the Rat." *Journal of Neurotrauma* 1:275–287, 1994. Used with permission.

cognitive disorders would occur/persist after the delirium clears when cholinergic activity is still suppressed but less so than during the delirium phase. TBI patients are sensitive to cognitive impairment due to use of anticholinergic drugs during their recovery, consistent with the rat data. Medications to treat posttraumatic delirium may need to have different characteristics from those to treat postdelirium cognitive problems, on the basis of an evolving neurochemical and clinical picture.

Electroencephalography

Since the seminal research in the 1950s by Engel and Romano, it has been recognized that a diagnosis of delirium is supported by an objective finding of generalized slowing on electroencephalography (EEG; see Chapter 7, Electrophysiological Techniques), particularly of the dominant posterior rhythm (Engel and Romano 1959; Trzepacz et al. 1988b). Most cases of delirium are associated with electroencephalographic slowing, except for some cases of alcohol or sedative-hypnotic withdrawal (superimposed increased fast-wave activity), partial complex status epilepticus (epileptiform complexes), or superimposed focal brain lesions (focal abnormalities). Most studies of PTA are consistent with the usual finding of diffuse slowing in delirium (Levin and Grossman 1978). Focal findings are appropriately indicative of a focal lesion, such as contusion, ischemic injury, hemorrhage, or

hematoma. Diffuse slowing occurs during "psychosis with amnesia" in TBI and may not resolve for weeks; focal lesions are also common and tend to normalize within several months, persisting longer in patients with traumatic epilepsy (Koufen and Hagel 1987). These abnormal foci have been associated with focal neurological signs and skull fractures. Abnormal sleep EEG with sleep spindles preceded the more classical generalized slowing phase (Koufen and Hagel 1987). Computed tomography (CT) scans showed evidence of cerebral edema associated with electroencephalographic slowing (Koufen and Hagel 1987). However, interpretation of EEGs in patients with TBI may be affected by barbiturates and other medications. The degree and type of electroencephalographic abnormality are correlated with prognosis during traumatic coma, showing reactivity (i.e., changes in the electroencephalographic pattern in response to various maneuvers such as eye opening, alerting, or hyperventilation) to be as important as the background activity (Synek 1988, 1990).

Somatosensory evoked potentials show delayed conduction in traumatic coma and PTA; conduction times improve as the PTA clears (Houlden et al. 1990; Hume and Cant 1981). The degree of abnormality correlates with outcome when performed within the first 3.5 days after injury (Hume and Cant 1981). Damage to subcortical areas, including the medial lemniscus, has been hypothesized in TBI in addition to cortical factors (Hume and Cant 1981; Lindsay et al. 1981). These findings are consistent with the slowed conduction of somatosensory evoked potentials in delirious patients with hepatic insufficiency, wherein a subcortical, as well as a cortical, pathophysiology was considered (Trzepacz et al. 1989b).

More recently, quantitative electroencephalographic techniques have been used in delirium and TBI. Quantitative EEG (QEEG) is a family of related technologies and techniques based on digital EEG, a paperless acquisition of the EEG using computerized instrumentation that allows post hoc changes in filters, adjustment of horizontal and vertical scales, and montage reformatting that is not possible with paper recordings (Nuwer 1997). QEEG involves mathematical processing of the digital electroencephalographic signal to better identify certain waveform components, transform the EEG into another format, or associate numerical data with electroencephalographic data for subsequent comparison. Frequency or spectral analysis converts the original electroencephalographic signal into frequency components, with the magnitude of each component corresponding to the amount of energy that the original EEG possesses at each frequency (Nuwer 1997). Electroencephalographic data may then be mapped onto a stylized or actual brain image, called *topographic EEG display* or *EEG brain mapping*. However, data are gathered from relatively few reference points on the scalp; thus, these maps lack the detail of neuroimaging studies, despite the pictorial representation of the entire brain (Wallace et al. 2001).

QEEG offers several potential advantages over conventional EEG, particularly for delirium (Jacobson and Jerrier 2000; Leuchter and Jacobson 1991). Quantitative electroencephalographic processing improves signal detection in the delta and beta bands, which are particularly important in the diagnosis of delirium. QEEG may reduce data acquisition time because a single recording can be reformatted to an entire series of montages, which is essential in studying the agitated delirious patient. Finally, quantitative electroencephalographic numerical data are more easily compared than traditional electroencephalographic waveforms, making serial studies easier. However, disadvantages include not recognizing traditional electroencephalographic artifacts, such as eye movements, that may be recorded as quantitative electroencephalographic abnormalities. Brief abnormalities, such as epileptiform spikes or transient slowing, may be overlooked or misinterpreted. Finally, quantitative electroencephalographic techniques vary considerably between laboratories, which makes generalization difficult.

The American Academy of Neurology (Nuwer 1997) states that QEEG allows the detection of diminished alpha activity and increased slowing in delirium, similar to the EEG, and frequency analysis may detect excess slowing more readily than routine EEG. The degree of slowing on quantitative electroencephalographic frequency analysis has been correlated with the severity of hepatic encephalopathy.

Koponen et al. (1989) used QEEG in elderly delirious patients (most of whom had comorbid dementia) and found reduced alpha percentage, increased theta and delta power, and slowing of the peak and mean frequencies. Reduced alpha percentage and mean frequency correlated with declining cognitive function, whereas increases in delta percentage were correlated with longer duration of delirium and hospitalization. Patients with delirium and dementia had the most abnormal QEEG. Also, patients with "hyperactive" and "hypoactive" delirium showed no differences in mean electroencephalographic frequency. Jacobson et al. (1993) compared elderly delirious patients with dementia and control subjects using QEEG. They found an increase in slow-wave power and decrease in alpha power that were correlated with worsening delirium and MMSE scores.

The literature regarding QEEG in TBI is small, with most focusing on coma (Ricker and Zafonte 2000). Similar to electroencephalographic monitoring in coma due to severe head injury, QEEG has been useful for predicting prognosis and in detecting nonconvulsive seizures (Nuwer 1997; Wallace et al. 2001).

Several QEEG studies have shown increased focal or diffuse theta activity, decreased alpha activity, decreased coherence, and increased asymmetry in patients with severe TBI. These are also found in mild to moderate TBI (Hughes and John 1999). One study of patients with mild TBI found three quantitative electroencephalographic features not present in control subjects: 1) increased coherence and decreased phase in frontal and fronto-temporal regions, 2) reduced alpha band amplitudes in the parieto-occipital regions, and 3) decreased power differences between anterior and posterior cortical regions (Thatcher et al. 1989). These changes may relate to symptoms of postconcussive syndrome. They may also be related to similar symptoms in delirium, although such studies have yet to be performed. The frontal changes are consistent with axonal injuries and localized contusions, which would be associated with attentional deficits, emotional instability, and difficulty with planning and sequencing. The parieto-occipital changes are consistent with coup-contrecoup injuries, and the anterior-posterior differences are consistent with changes in long axonal systems. These injuries may result in diminished information processing and ability to perform concurrent mental tasks (Wallace et al. 2001). However, these results may not be generalizable because the study did not exclude comorbidities that may affect the QEEG.

Thatcher et al. (2001) did not find a correlation between QEEG discriminant scores (coherence, phase, and amplitude) and PTA duration in 108 TBI patients, but did find a correlation between QEEG and GCS score ($r=-0.85$, $P=0.001$) and hours of LOC ($r=0.56$, $P=0.001$).

A pilot study correlated quantitative electroencephalographic techniques with MRI imaging in the TBI postacute to chronic period (Thatcher et al. 1998). Gray matter lesions were related to decreased QEEG alpha and beta amplitudes, and white matter lesions to increased QEEG delta amplitudes. White matter lesions could disrupt neural circuits important in causing delirium. Cognitive deficits were correlated with increased delta amplitude and decreased alpha and beta amplitudes, as also would be expected in delirium.

Structural Neuroimaging

CT scans are useful in evaluating TBI delirium to diagnose structural lesions such as hemorrhage, subdural hematoma, stroke, and contusions (Feuerman et al. 1988; see Chapter 5, Structural Imaging). Cerebral atrophy (at times preexisting) usually suggests a brain that is more vulnerable to delirium. In addition, evidence of cerebral edema from compression of the third ventricle and basal cisterns correlates closely with increased intracranial pressure (Teasdale et al. 1984), which is a known cause of delirium and coma in TBI. Overall, reports suggest a relationship between more intracranial lesions and a higher incidence of longer duration of delirium.

One study focused on the relationship between early behavioral disturbances and admission CT scans in 43 patients with mild TBI and 24 patients with moderate TBI (van der Naalt et al. 2000). Initial CT scans were available from 55 patients. Behavioral disturbances—agitation, inappropriate behavior, and restlessness—were seen in 52% of patients and occurred more commonly in moderate injury. In all patients, restlessness and agitation disappeared before PTA resolved, and PTA was significantly increased among patients with agitation and restlessness. Early behavioral disturbances were correlated with the number of lesions on CT, with affected patients having more than twice as many lesions as those who were unaffected. Patients with behavioral disturbances had significantly more lesions on CT (81% vs. 39%), which were mostly located in the frontotemporal region. Feinstein et al. (2002) divided 282 TBI outpatients into four groups according to PTA duration (<1 hour, <24 hours, <1 week, and >1 week). The percentage in each group who had an abnormal CT scan was significantly different ($P=0.001$), with higher percentages for groups with more prolonged PTA

(lowest=28% to highest=63.2%). Livingston et al. (2000) found that even grade 3 concussions (brief LOC or PTA) seen in a emergency department (GCS=14 or 15) had intracranial abnormalities on unenhanced CT scan in 217 of 1,788 prospectively studied TBI cases (13% positive rate).

Several studies have shown MRI to be more sensitive than CT in detecting intracranial abnormalities after TBI (Levin et al. 1992). However, initial neuropsychological deficits after TBI tend to be pervasive in nature and poorly associated with focal abnormalities (Levin et al. 1992; Wilson et al. 1988). Correlation with injury location and neuropsychological deficits were more consistent after several months of recovery, at which time many lesions had improved or resolved (Levin et al. 1992; Wilson et al. 1988). This suggests that diffuse lesions, edema, subtle damage not detected on structural neuroimaging, focal lesions with widespread downstream effects (e.g., diaschisis), or neurochemical abnormalities may underlie the acute confusional phase.

Using the MRI pulse sequence FLAIR (fluid-attenuated inversion recovery) in 45 patients with mild TBI during PTA, Wakamoto et al. (1998) detected changes not evident on MRI or CT. These changes were apparent only if PTA lasted >2 hours and consisted of periventricular lesions in the anterior horn of the lateral ventricle (60%), basal frontal lobe (16%), and/or deep cerebral white matter (24%). Etiology was presumed to be consistent with either brain edema or contusion with hemorrhage. Increased duration of PTA was associated with increased frequency of these lesions: 19% in PTA less than 30 minutes, 63% in PTA greater than 30 minutes and less than 2 hours, and 88% in PTA greater than 2 hours. Lesions had resolved by 1-month follow-up. This may be evidence of reversible microstructural damage causing delirium, affecting brain regions that could disrupt neural circuits connecting thalamus, prefrontal cortex, and basal ganglia.

Proton magnetic resonance spectroscopy studies in hepatic encephalopathy have shown decreased levels of myoinositol and choline and increased levels of glutamate. These abnormalities resolved after liver transplantation, suggesting that these were markers reflecting the reversible nature of the disorder (Lerner and Rosenstein 2000). In contrast, magnetic resonance spectroscopy studies in TBI have generally shown elevations in myoinositol and choline and reductions in N-acetylaspartate, which are thought to indicate neuronal loss or metabolic depression (Brooks et al. 2001). Such changes tend to normalize over a period of several months, indicating potential neuronal recovery. Patients with persistent abnormalities tend to have poorer outcomes (Brooks et al. 2001). Other studies have shown substantial correlations between neurometabolite ratios with PTA (Garnett et al.

2001) and general cognitive function (Friedman et al. 1998).

Functional Neuroimaging

CBF studies using xenon single-photon emission CT (SPECT) scans have been performed in TBI patients who are in coma or emerging from coma in an effort to better understand the underlying physiology of brain damage (Deutsch and Eisenberg 1987; Jaggi et al. 1990; Obrist et al. 1984; see Chapter 6, Functional Imaging). Under most circumstances, CBF is coupled to metabolism in essentially a 1:1 relationship (Raichle et al. 1976), except for acute vascular events such as stroke when luxury perfusion of an ischemic area is much higher than the actual metabolic demand and CBF does not accurately reflect physiological needs (Lassen 1966). A reduction of frontal CBF as compared with the normal resting pattern (i.e., a reversal of the normal anteroposterior gradient) was noted in comatose patients after TBI (Deutsch and Eisenberg 1987); with increased global blood flow (hyperemia), this pattern was more exaggerated, but on regaining consciousness, this frontal defect normalized.

Acute brain trauma is another condition in which metabolism and CBF are not tightly coupled (Obrist et al. 1984). Xenon-SPECT scan quantitative CBF measures were compared with arteriojugular venous oxygen differences in two groups of TBI coma patients (hyperemic patients and patients with reduced CBF), and cerebral metabolism for oxygen was estimated (Obrist et al. 1984). Metabolism was reduced in all TBI coma patients as a consequence of normal metabolic coupling between CBF and metabolism; uncoupling occurred only in the hyperemic cases. Hyperemia was often associated with intracranial hypertension and was believed to result in luxury perfusion, perhaps related to cerebrospinal fluid lactic acidosis or failure of CBF autoregulation (Obrist et al. 1984). Hyperventilation of patients with reduced CBF was cautioned against as risking ischemia from vasoconstriction (Obrist et al. 1984), which would increase susceptibility to delirium. Lower levels of cerebral oxygen metabolism are related to poorer outcome, and when hyperemic patients are excluded, lower CBF also predicts a poorer outcome (Jaggi et al. 1990). On recovery, CBF and, presumably, metabolism increase. Although not yet directly studied, it may be hypothesized that CBF progresses toward normal during delirium.

SPECT studies in hepatic encephalopathy have demonstrated decreased levels of CBF (Lerner and Rosenstein 2000). Specific deficits have been noted in the right anterior cingulate gyrus (O'Carroll et al. 1991) and frontal and anterior cortices (Trzepacz 1994). SPECT studies

in systemic lupus erythematosus with neuropsychiatric symptoms have also shown decreased cortical perfusion (Lerner and Rosenstein 2000). These studies have typically shown lesions in the left parietal cortex (Rubbert et al. 1993), in the left parietal and occipital lobe (Sabbadini et al. 1999), and in the territory of the middle cerebral artery (Colamussi et al. 1995).

In TBI, SPECT studies detect lesions not apparent on CT and MRI, particularly in mild to moderate head injury (van Heertum et al. 2001). These functional lesions also correlate better with neurological clinical findings than with anatomical studies (Camargo 2001). The pattern of abnormalities differs depending on the severity and type of injury (i.e., motor vehicle, blunt trauma, or fall) (Abdel-Dayem et al. 1998). A rather specific pattern for TBI consists of focal, well-circumscribed areas of decreased perfusion at one or more sites, although other less specific patterns can also be seen. It remains to be seen if delirium resulting from TBI shows similar focal deficits on SPECT as do other disorders. The correlation between SPECT abnormalities and neuropsychological deficits is more complicated. Preliminary studies indicate that neuropsychological deficits have correlates on SPECT scans, but SPECT abnormalities may not have neuropsychological correlates (Umile et al. 1998). Most improvement on neuropsychological testing correlates with improved perfusion on SPECT (Laatsch et al. 1999).

Positron emission tomography (PET) studies in TBI typically show a triphasic pattern of cerebral metabolic glucose utilization (Bergsneider et al. 2001). After a brief period of hyperglycolysis, the brain enters into a second period of metabolic depression, followed by a third phase of metabolic recovery. In animal studies, persistent neurologic deficits remain during the period of metabolic depression, and the rate of recovery of behavioral function parallels that of recovery of metabolic function. Similarly, decreases in cortical blood flow occurred in a recent PET study of hepatic encephalopathy (Lerner and Rosenstein 2000). Deficits in flow to the anterior cingulate gyrus were correlated with attentional deficits on neuropsychological testing. Simultaneously, there were increases in blood flow to subcortical structures. Making an exact association between delirium and PET changes in TBI is difficult—though one might speculate that a cortical metabolic depression phase would occur during delirium. Human studies have shown that metabolic reductions on PET do not correlate with level of consciousness at the time of scanning (Bergsneider et al. 2000). Another study found no apparent association between injury severity and the time course or magnitude of metabolic depression (Bergsneider et al. 2001), although delirium is believed to be more common with more severe injuries.

Correlations between PET and neuropsychological studies in TBI have also shown that PET scans may show regional abnormalities that have no clear clinical correlation (Ruff et al. 1994).

Treatment

Treatment of delirium after TBI is not standardized and differs among different specialists. Many psychiatrists treat TBI delirium in essentially the same way as delirium from other causes (Lipowski 1990). The principles of treatment involve a workup for etiologies, treatment of the underlying etiology when possible, manipulation of the environment, and medication.

Search for Underlying Causes

The search for underlying causes can be guided by considering the many possible etiologies as outlined above and as listed in Tables 9–4 and 9–5, individualized according to each patient's needs. The clinician must reduce polypharmacy, discontinuing or replacing medications that produce delirium. Laboratory tests, cerebrospinal fluid examination, CT or MRI brain scans, arterial blood gases, intracranial pressure monitoring, electrocardiogram, blood cultures, and so on can all be performed as needed to investigate various potential causes. If the diagnosis of delirium is uncertain, use of a specific delirium symptom rating scale can be used along with EEG and bedside cognitive tests. The EEG shows the usual pattern of diffuse background slowing (Engel and Romano 1959; Koufen and Hagel 1987), sometimes with the presence of sleep spindles (Koufen and Hagel 1987). Bedside cognitive tests such as the MMSE; Trail Making Tests (Trzepacz et al. 1988b); CTD; and specific attentional, visuoconstructional, and executive function tasks (see Chapter 8, Issues in Neuropsychological Assessment) are useful in determining the degree of diffuse cognitive dysfunction and can be followed over time. In addition, physiatrists use other cognitive tests such as the GOAT and Rancho Los Amigos scales.

Environmental Manipulations

Traditionally, efforts are made to help familiarize and structure the delirious patient's environment (Table 9–7). The delirious patient requires external structure to compensate for a disorganized and cognitively impaired internal mental state. When the patient is so confused or frightened that physical harm might inadvertently happen or uncooperativeness with medical treatment occurs,

TABLE 9–7. Environmental manipulations in the treatment of delirium

Familiarize the environment	Put family pictures nearby
	Play familiar music
Structure the environment	Have a clock in full view
	Put large calendar on wall, with days marked off
	Use night-light
	Reorient patient frequently
	Have natural window light to assist day-night biorhythms
Adjust sensory stimulation level	Minimize loud noises
	Do not remove all stimulation
	Use soft-walled portable room for severe agitation
Assure safety	Use a sitter
	Minimize use of restraints whenever possible

then physical restraints may be appropriate. Restraints must never be used to replace good nursing observation but rather should be used only to supplement other treatment efforts. However, some have expressed opinions about the negative aspects of using restraints in patients with TBI (Berrol 1988; DeChancie et al. 1987). The increased use of restraints in patients with TBI has been associated with a patient's alcohol use but not with a lower level of consciousness (Edlund et al. 1991); these restrained patients also had longer lengths of stay, more combativeness and aggression, and more alcohol withdrawal symptoms, but few were seen in consultation by a psychiatrist. The use of sitters can often reduce the need for restraints while assisting with observations and reassurance of the confused patient.

One view is that instead of medication ("too sedating") and restraints ("increases agitation") for agitated delirious TBI patients, a portable, Naugahyde padded room enclosure should be used to allow freer movement (DeChancie et al. 1987). This is essentially a seclusion room, a comfortable room with a mattress and devoid of objects, which is well known to psychiatrists and has been used for decades to reduce distracting sensory stimulation and provide safety. Although this may be a useful adjunct, it should not preclude appropriate use of medication, because changing the environment will not by itself alter the pathophysiology of delirium. In addition, a balance must be struck between minimizing excessive or confusing sounds and providing enough environmental structure (e.g., family photos) to reduce anxiety from disorientation and cognitive deficits that contribute to agitation. Deafness, blindness, and other causes of sensory deprivation actually increase the risk for delirium (Lipowski 1990).

In one study, playing music increased calmness and enhanced orientation to year and place in agitated PTA patients, significantly decreasing scores on the ABS ($P<0.001$) (Baker 2001). Both taped and live music, chosen on the basis of the patient's preference in style, were effective.

Medication

Appropriately chosen and monitored medication for reducing the cognitive, behavioral, and psychotic symptoms of delirium is the clinical standard of care. Neuroleptic medication is the treatment of choice for TBI delirium (Cassidy 1990; Gualtieri 1991; Lipowski 1985). Of the conventional neuroleptics, haloperidol is most often used. Its sedating side effect can be used to the patient's benefit initially to enhance and consolidate nocturnal sleep by dosing at bedtime. This sedating effect is minimized by using lower doses than conventionally used for mania or schizophrenia and diminishes after several days. Furthermore, haloperidol is not sedating to all patients. In addition, delirium itself involves napping and drowsy periods.

Haloperidol is generally given in 0.5- to 1-mg doses at night or twice a day initially, titrated upward according to the patient's response (up to 5-mg total daily dose or even to 20 mg in severe cases). It can be given orally, intramuscularly, or intravenously, although the latter route has not been approved by the U.S. Food and Drug Administration. At low doses, extrapyramidal side effects are uncommon, especially when given intravenously (Menza et al. 1987). Haloperidol can be given intravenously (Sos and Cassem 1980) without respiratory depression, but is associated with idiopathic torsades de pointes tachyarrhythmia. The risk of torsades is generally thought to be low, though most data are from patients with schizophrenia (Glassman and Bigger 2001). In one study of 223 critically ill patients who received haloperidol for agitation, the incidence of torsades was 3.6% (Sharma et al. 1998). A more recent, growing literature suggests this potentially lethal tachyarrhythmia is indeed a concern for intravenous haloperidol, being associated with prolongation of the QTc interval (Trzepacz et al. 2002). American Psychiatric Association treatment guidelines for delirium (American Psychiatric Association 1999) recommend monitoring of serum magnesium and potassium and also if QTc is prolonged, cardiac monitoring and/or consultation, or medication discontinuation. Dystonic reactions

tend to occur at the initiation of treatment, and akathisia may increase restlessness. These are uncommon complications when haloperidol is used in low doses for brief periods. Neuroleptic malignant syndrome is even less common but must be considered in the differential diagnosis of fever, increased confusion, and lead-pipe muscle rigidity (Guze and Baxter 1985). The response to haloperidol in delirium is often remarkable. By promptly reducing the symptoms of delirium, the patient becomes more aware and able to begin rehabilitation.

Neuroleptics should be tapered and discontinued after the TBI delirium clears (Gualtieri 1991) and continued only if a psychotic disorder persists (or preexisted, such as mania or schizophrenia) into the rehabilitation phase. Some speculate that the dopamine blocking effects of neuroleptics may delay or interfere with the TBI patient's cognitive rehabilitation (Feeney et al. 1982; Gualtieri 1991) because dopaminergic medications have been shown to enhance memory (Gualtieri 1991) and even to arouse chronically comatose TBI patients (Cope 1990). The danger is in overstating these caveats, because assumptions have been made from motor cortex animal models about human cognition in TBI (Feeney et al. 1982) and from one phase of TBI recovery (coma or amnestic syndrome) about another phase's (delirium's) neurochemical mechanisms. The brief duration of antidelirium treatment and the morbidity and mortality associated with delirium argue for careful use of neuroleptics in TBI delirium.

Animal studies in both rats and cats have shown that doses of haloperidol can reinstate motor deficits after frontal cortex injuries, although only certain behaviors are affected (Feeney and Sutton 1987). Haloperidol has also been shown to block the acceleration of motor recovery produced by amphetamine in animal models and to block the acceleration of depth perception recovery produced by amphetamine in cats (Feeney and Sutton 1987). However, whether the findings from these animal studies have relevance to CNS injuries in humans remains to be seen.

One retrospective review of patients with severe TBI showed no statistical difference in the rehabilitation outcomes of patients who were treated with haloperidol versus those not receiving haloperidol (Rao et al. 1995). There were trends toward poorer outcome in the haloperidol-treated group; however, individuals treated with haloperidol also had significantly longer PTA. Because PTA is widely used as a marker for injury severity, it would not be surprising that the more severely injured group would also have poorer outcome. Although no controlled trials have been conducted for supporting evidence, many physiatrists have reported individual cases in which haloperidol was effective when other drugs failed (Fugate et al. 1997b). Droperidol, a butyrophenone like haloperidol, has been used for agitation in TBI (Stanislaw 1997). Intramuscular droperidol in 1.25- to 10-mg single doses was compared retrospectively to other intramuscular drugs in 27 inpatients with acute TBI. Time to achieve calming with one dose was shorter with droperidol (mean=27 minutes) than with intramuscular haloperidol, lorazepam, or diphenhydramine (mean=36.2 minutes). However, droperidol has been withdrawn from the market in Europe in relation to cardiac risks.

Atypical antipsychotics may offer new alternatives in the treatment of delirium after TBI. Their side-effect profiles tend to be more tolerable than typical neuroleptics, making their use more acceptable to patients. Furthermore, the atypical antipsychotic drugs act more specifically in the neuroanatomical areas thought to be responsible for the symptoms of delirium (Morton et al. 2000). In addition to their antipsychotic effects, clozapine (Ratey et al. 1993), olanzapine (Edell and Tunis 2001; Kinon et al. 2001; Meehan et al. 2001, 2002; Wright et al. 2001), and risperidone (Czobor et al. 1995) have been efficacious in reducing aggression, which may be related to their effects on serotonin receptors (Bell and Cardenas 1995). Case reports on the use of risperidone, olanzapine, and clozapine have demonstrated a more benign side-effect profile and improved patient participation in social activities compared with typical neuroleptics. These case studies have also demonstrated a substantial reduction in delusions, aggression, and agitation (Jeanblanc and Davis 1995; Madhusoodanan et al. 1995). Cognition-enhancing effects have been found for risperidone administered to dementia patients (Owens and Risch 1998) and olanzapine in Lewy body dementia (Cummings et al. 2002). There is rat in vivo microdialysis evidence that olanzapine has procholinergic effects in the prefrontal cortex and hippocampus (Kennedy et al. 2001), and these effects were not apparent to the same degree with the other atypicals studied. Procholinergic effects would be expected to be helpful in treating delirium.

There have been few investigations of atypical antipsychotics for the TBI population. One series of case reports noted that clozapine was effective in treating patients with post-TBI psychosis, agitation, and aggression (Michals et al. 1993). However, the incidence of side effects (including seizures) was reportedly high for clozapine. Zimnitsky et al. (1996) described the successful use of risperidone to treat a 19-year-old man with ischemic brain damage–related psychosis after failed trials of typical antipsychotics and valproate. No trials using atypical antipsychotic treatment for TBI-associated delirium were found in the literature.

The atypical antipsychotics are increasingly being used to treat delirium from a variety of causes. Case reports suggest possible efficacy for risperidone (Furmaga et al. 1997; Mittal et al. 2001; Sipahimalani and Masand 1997; Sipahimalani et al. 1997), quetiapine (Schwartz and Masand 2000; Torres et al. 2001), and ziprasidone (Leso and Schwartz 2002). Case series as well as open-label trials suggest possible efficacy for olanzapine (Breitbart et al. 2002; Khouzam and Gazula 2001; Kim et al. 2001; Passik and Cooper 1999; Sipahimalani and Masand 1998). A few of these reports have included some patients with posttraumatic delirium. However, there are also reports of some patients developing delirium associated with risperidone (Ravona-Springer et al. 1998; Tavcar and Dernovsek 1998) and quetiapine (Sim et al. 2000). Because of its side-effect profile, the antipsychotic clozapine is not generally used in delirium, and there are no reports in the literature. Additionally, there have been several reports of delirium induced by clozapine, in part due to its strong anticholinergic activity (Banki and Vojnik 1978; Jackson et al. 1995; Schuster et al. 1977; Szymanski et al. 1991; Wilkins-Ho and Hollander 1997). Ziprasidone use in a patient with delirium was associated with prolonged QTc (8.4% increase in QTc) that necessitated its discontinuation (Leso and Schwartz 2002).

As with haloperidol, low doses of the atypical antipsychotics are generally thought to be effective in treating delirium, though this is off-label use (Schwartz and Masand 2002). Recommendations are the initiation of risperidone at 0.25 to 0.5 mg twice daily; olanzapine, 2.5 to 5 mg at nighttime; and quetiapine, 25 to 50 mg twice daily. Doses may be increased further if needed, and occasionally doses in the full antipsychotic range are necessary (up to 4 mg/day for risperidone, 20 mg/day for olanzapine, and 600 mg/day for quetiapine). As-needed doses may also be given for increased symptoms.

Wilson et al. (2003) compared effects of haloperidol and olanzapine on recovery from lateral fluid-percussion–induced TBI in rats. Treatment for 15 days postinjury with haloperidol caused further impairment of cognition as compared with injured control subjects and a trend toward impairment in motor functions at higher doses, whereas treatment with olanzapine did not impair cognitive or motor recovery as compared with injured control subjects.

The risk/benefit ratio of prescribing antipsychotic drugs for the short-term treatment of agitated delirium remains unclear. Antipsychotic medications may cause cognitive and motor impairment in healthy individuals (Killian et al. 1984). However, for patients who are severely agitated, the potential side effects of antipsychotic medications may be less harmful than the long-term disruptive effects of agitation on cognitive recovery. When a comorbid psychotic disorder is present, antipsychotics are the treatment of choice to treat psychosis and agitation (Rowland and DePalma 1995).

The uncertainty related to the risk/benefit ratio of antipsychotic drug treatment is reflected in the prescribing practices of many physiatrists. The physiatric field as a whole infrequently prescribes antipsychotic medication. In a recent survey, haloperidol was the antipsychotic medication most likely to be prescribed. However, it was ranked only the fourth most frequently used drug to treat TBI-related agitation among physicians classified as "nonexperts" (less than 70% of practice devoted to TBI). Among "experts," haloperidol was ranked as only the eighth most frequently prescribed drug for TBI-related agitation (Fugate et al. 1997b). Target symptoms for haloperidol use were typically aggression or disinhibition. Frequently cited reasons for haloperidol use included sedating effects, rapid onset, availability of multiple modes of administration, and effectiveness when other treatments failed (Fugate et al. 1997b). Despite less severe side-effect profiles, atypical antipsychotics were seldom administered.

Three TBI patients in rehabilitation were administered serial neuropsychological tests over a 3-week period during taper and discontinuation of an antipsychotic drug each had been taking (Stanislav 1997). Thioridazine-discontinued patients showed more improvement when not taking the drug than did patients who discontinued haloperidol on certain cognitive tests (e.g., Trail Making A). This was attributed to greater anticholinergic effects of thioridazine. However, these patients were tested years after their TBI and apparently were not still in delirium.

Intramuscular haloperidol and ziprasidone are available for patients who cannot take oral administration. More uniquely, a rapidly dissolving oral formulation of olanzapine (administered on the tongue) offers advantages for uncooperative or agitated patients, though it has not been systematically evaluated in TBI patients. An intramuscular form of olanzapine has been approved by the U.S. Food and Drug Administration for treatment of agitation in mania and schizophrenia.

The selection of an antipsychotic drug to treat TBI-related agitation should be based on minimizing adverse side effects because there have been no studies demonstrating a consistent advantage of one drug over another in this population. As noted, atypical antipsychotics have the most favorable side-effect profiles. When administering antipsychotic drugs to treat agitation, the common practice is to start with low doses and slowly titrate upward, monitoring responsiveness to treatment with a standardized scale (e.g., the ABS [Corrigan et al. 1989] or Overt Agitation Scale [Yudofsky et al. 1997]). To avoid dose-related side effects, scheduled low dosing, with provisions for treating "breakthrough" symptoms on an as-needed basis, is the most beneficial course of treatment. Once the agitated behavior has been controlled, medication administration should be tapered.

Benzodiazepines can worsen delirium and further impair cognition and therefore are usually avoided unless specifically indicated. Most clinicians reserve benzodiazepines as an adjunct to haloperidol only for complicating conditions of alcohol (or other sedative-hypnotic drug) withdrawal (Edlund et al. 1991). Benzodiazepines are the safest of the sedative class of drugs and can be used if the sleep-wake cycle disturbance does not normalize after adjusting the dose of haloperidol, or if extreme agitation is not responsive to haloperidol, although this is usually not necessary. The choice depends on the need—lorazepam has a shorter half-life than diazepam. Unlike most benzodiazepines, lorazepam can be effectively administered intramuscularly because it is well absorbed by that route. Longer-acting agents may be helpful in treating alcohol withdrawal. The use of barbiturates during TBI suggests more caution when subsequently using benzodiazepines; also, the use of barbiturates may delay the onset of alcohol withdrawal symptoms, which generally peak 3–5 days after cessation of drinking.

Agents that enhance acetylcholine, such as physostigmine and donepezil, theoretically should treat delirium by restoring the balance between dopamine and acetylcholine (Trzepacz 1994, 1996, 2000; Trzepacz et al. 2001). This has been shown in a few uncontrolled reports (Fischer 2001; Stern 1983; Wengel et al. 1999). Cholinomimetic agents have been used for treatment of long-term cognitive deficits after TBI, though with mixed results (Blount et al. 2002). Such agents have not been tested in the acute phase of recovery in human TBI.

Agitation in 21 patients with severe TBI improved more on propranolol LA, 60–240 mg, than placebo in a double-blind randomized trial (Brooke et al. 1992), as measured by the Overt Aggression Scale. Agitation intensity and need for restraints decreased for patients taking propranolol, whereas episode frequency did not differ; these patients may not have been delirious, however.

Electroconvulsive therapy has been reported to treat cases of both prolonged "organic stupor" and agitated delirium after TBI (Kant et al. 1995; Silverman 1964). Carbamazepine, 400 mg/day, plus buspirone, 30 mg/day, reduced delirium in four TBI patients within 36 hours (Pourcher et al. 1994).

Conclusion

There is a need for nomenclature clarification in the TBI literature for research on the phenomenological features, risk factors, duration, treatment, neuropathophysiology, prognosis, and outcome of delirium after TBI to proceed in a meaningful way. The broad adoption by rehabilitation clinicians and researchers of diagnostic criteria for delirium and the use of rating scales and cognitive tests that assess the whole range of behavioral symptoms of delirium are necessary. Delirium after TBI must be more clearly differentiated from agitation and amnestic syndrome, implying that the term *posttraumatic amnesia* (PTA) should be replaced by more specific terminology for the individual phases of recovery than the term *PTA* covers. More uniform use of the term *delirium* or even *posttraumatic confusional state* would be helpful.

The exclusion of certain patients from most TBI PTA studies has excluded some of the patients at greatest risk for TBI, namely those who abuse alcohol (Honkanen and Smith 1991; Yates et al. 1987) and other substances, and those with antisocial personality disorder, mania, schizophrenia, suicidal depression, and so on. Whether these psychiatrically impaired persons have a higher risk for delirium is unknown but could be hypothesized for at least some of them (alcoholic and bipolar patients). Neurologically impaired persons are also excluded from TBI PTA studies, yet they are at higher risk for delirium. A person with impaired cognition or prior brain injury that alters personality (e.g., aggressive) or frontal lobe executive functions (e.g., judgment and abstraction) may be at increased risk for recurrent TBI from fighting or falling, for example, and would likely have an increased risk for delirium after TBI. Elderly patients, with or without dementia, have diminished brain reserve and reduced ability to withstand the effects of TBI (Galbraith 1987), probably also with increased TBI delirium. In fact, the TBI literature has mounting evidence that the more brain damage, the more delirium and the longer the delirium lasts.

A methodological problem in many studies is not accounting for effects of medications in study outcomes; for example, in research on the duration of PTA. Naturalistic studies without treatment or carefully controlling medications in a randomized, blinded fashion are needed to more accurately determine relationships between outcomes and other variables.

The neuropathophysiology of TBI delirium probably involves deficiency of cholinergic neurotransmission that may include an imbalance with dopamine. This excess of dopamine may not persist in later phases of recovery, when dopaminergic agents can be helpful for cognitive functioning. Randomized, double-blind, placebo-controlled trials are needed in TBI delirium to determine whether any of the agents currently being used is truly effective; otherwise the natural course of episode duration and variability among individuals might explain so-called treatment responses.

References

Abdel-Dayem HM, Abu-Judeh H, Kumar M, et al: SPECT brain perfusion abnormalities in mild or moderate traumatic brain injury. Clin Nucl Med 23:309–317, 1998

American Psychiatric Association: Diagnostic and Statistical Manual of Mental Disorders, 3rd Edition, Revised. Washington, DC, American Psychiatric Association, 1987

American Psychiatric Association: Diagnostic and Statistical Manual of Mental Disorders, 4th Edition. Washington, DC, American Psychiatric Association, 1994

American Psychiatric Association: Practice guideline for the treatment of patients with delirium: American Psychiatric Association. Am J Psychiatry 156 (5 suppl):1–20, 1999

American Psychiatric Association: Diagnostic and Statistical Manual of Mental Disorders, 4th Edition, Text Revision. Washington, DC, American Psychiatric Association, 2000

Baker F: The effects of live, taped, and no music on people experiencing posttraumatic amnesia. J Music Ther 38:170–92, 2001

Banki CM, Vojnik M: Comparative simultaneous measurement of cerebrospinal fluid 5-hydroxyindoleacetic acid and brain serotonin levels in delirium tremens and clozapine-induced delirious reaction. J Neurol Neurosurg Psychiatry 41:420–4, 1978

Bell KR, Cardenas DC: New frontiers of neuropharmacologic treatment of brain injury agitation. Neurorehabilitation 5:233–244, 1995

Bergsneider M, Hovda DA, Lee SM, et al: Dissociation of cerebral glucose metabolism and level of consciousness during the period of metabolic depression following human traumatic brain injury. J Neurotrauma 17:389–401, 2000

Bergsneider M, Hovda DA, McArthur DL, et al: Metabolic recovery following human traumatic brain injury based on FDG-PET: time course and relationship to neurological disability. J Head Trauma Rehabil 16:135–148, 2001

Berrol S: Risks of restraints in head injury. Arch Phys Med Rehabil 69:537–538, 1988

Blount PJ, Nguyen CD, McDeavitt JT: Clinical use of cholinomimetic agents: a review. J Head Trauma Rehabil 17:314–321, 2002

Breitbart W, Tremblay A, Gibson C: An open trial of olanzapine for the treatment of delirium in hospitalized cancer patients. Psychosomatics 43:175–183, 2002

Brooke MM, Patterson DR, Questad KA, et al: The treatment of agitation during initial hospitalization after traumatic brain injury. Arch Phys Med Rehabil 73:917–921, 1992

Brooks WM, Friedman SD, Gasparovic C: Magnetic resonance spectroscopy in traumatic brain injury. J Head Trauma Rehabil 16:149–164, 2001

Camus V, Gonthier R, Dubos G, et al: Etiologic and outcome profiles in hypoactive and hyperactive subtypes of delirium. J Geriatr Psychiatry Neurol 13:38–42, 2000

Carmago EE: Brain SPECT in neurology and psychiatry. J Nucl Med 42:611–623, 2001

Cassidy JW: Pharmacological treatment of post-traumatic behavioral disorders: aggression and disorders of mood, in Neurobehavioural Sequelae of Traumatic Brain Injury. Edited by Wood RL. New York, Taylor and Francis, 1990, pp 227–229

Changaris DG, McGraw CP, Richardson JD, et al: Correlation of cerebral perfusion pressure and Glasgow Coma Scale. J Trauma 27:1007–1013, 1987

Colamussi P, Giganti M, Cittanti C, et al: Brain single-photon emission tomography with 99mTc-HMPAO in neuropsychiatric systemic lupus erythematosus: relations with EEG and MRI findings and clinical manifestations. Eur J Nucl Med 22:17–24, 1995

Cope DN: Pharmacology for behavioral deficits: disorders of cognition and affect, in Neurobehavioural Sequelae of Traumatic Brain Injury. Edited by Wood RL. Taylor and Francis, New York, 1990, p 255

Corrigan JD, Mysiw WJ: Prospective system for monitoring length of post-traumatic amnesia. Arch Phys Med Rehabil 65:652, 1984

Corrigan JD, Arnett JA, Houck LJ, et al: Reality orientation for brain injured patients: group treatment and monitoring of recovery. Arch Phys Med Rehabil 66:675–689, 1985

Corrigan JD, Mysiw WJ, Gribble MW, et al: Agitation, cognition and attention during post-traumatic amnesia. Brain Inj 6:155–160, 1992

Cummings JL, Street J, Masterman D, et al: Efficacy of olanzapine in the treatment of psychosis in dementia with Lewy bodies. Dement Geriatr Cogn Disord 13:67–73, 2002

Czobor P, Volavka J, Meibach RC: Effect of risperidone on hostility in schizophrenia. J Clin Psychopharmacol 15:243–249, 1995

Daniel WF, Crovitz HF, Weiner RD: Neuropsychological aspects of disorientation. Cortex 23:169–187, 1987

DeChancie H, Walsh JM, Kessler LA: An enclosure for the disoriented head-injured patient. J Neurosci Nurs 19:341, 1987

Deutsch G, Eisenberg HM: Frontal blood flow changes in recovery from coma. J Cereb Blood Flow Metab 7:29–34, 1987

Dixon CE, Hamm RJ, Taft WC, et al: Increased anticholinergic sensitivity following closed skull impact and controlled cortical impact traumatic brain injury in the rat. J Neurotrauma 1:275–287, 1994

Edell WS, Tunis SL: Antipsychotic treatment of behavioral and psychological symptoms of dementia in geropsychiatric inpatients. Am J Geriatr Psychiatry 9:289–297, 2001

Edlund MJ, Goldberg RJ, Morris PLP: The use of physical restraint in patients with cerebral contusion. Int J Psychiatry Med 21:173–182, 1991

Ellenberg JH, Levin HS, Saydjari C: Posttraumatic amnesia as a predictor of outcome after severe closed head injury. Arch Neurol 53:782–91, 1996

Ely EW, Inouye SK, Bernard GR, et al: Delirium in mechanically ventilated patients: validity and reliability of the Confusion Assessment Method for the Intensive Care Unit (CAM-ICU). JAMA 286:2703–2710, 2001a

Ely EW, Margolin R, Francis J, et al: Evaluation of delirium in critically ill patients: validation of the Confusion Assessment Method for the Intensive Care Unit (CAM-ICU). Crit Care Med 29:1370–1379, 2001b

Engel G, Romano J: Delirium: a syndrome of cerebral insufficiency. J Chron Dis 9:260–277, 1959

Ewert J, Levin HS, Watson MG, et al: Procedural memory during posttraumatic amnesia in survivors of severe closed head injury: implications for rehabilitation. Arch Neurol 46:911–916, 1989

Fann JR: The epidemiology of delirium: a review of studies and methodological issues. Semin Clin Neuropsychiatry 5:64–75, 2000

Feeney DM, Sutton RL: Pharmacotherapy for recovery of function after brain injury. Crit Rev Neurobiol 3:135–197, 1987

Feeney DM, Gonzalez A, Law WA: Amphetamine, haloperidol, and experience interact to affect rate of recovery after motor cortex injury. Science 217:855–857, 1982

Feinstein A, Hershkop S, Ouchterlony D, et al: Posttraumatic amnesia and recall of a traumatic event following traumatic brain injury. J Neuropsychiatry Clin Neurosci 14:25–30, 2002

Feuerman T, Wackym PA, Gade GF, et al: Value of skull radiography, head computed tomographic scanning, and admission for observation in cases of minor head injury. Neurosurgery 22:449–453, 1988

Fischer P: Successful treatment of nonanticholinergic delirium with a cholinesterase inhibitor. J Clin Psychopharmacol 21:118, 2001

Fisher JM: Cognitive and behavioral consequences of closed head injury. Semin Neurol 5:197–204, 1985

Folstein MF, Folstein SE, McHugh PR: "Mini-Mental State": a practical method for grading the cognitive state of patients for the clinician. J Psychiatr Res 12:189–198, 1975

Fortuny LA, Briggs M, Newcombe F, et al: Measuring the duration of post-traumatic amnesia. J Neurol Neurosurg Psychiatry 40:377–379, 1980

Francis J, Martin D, Kapoor W: A prospective study of delirium in hospitalized elderly. JAMA 263:1097–1101, 1990

Friedman SD, Brooks WM, Jung RE, et al: Proton MR spectroscopic findings correspond to neuropsychological function in traumatic brain injury. AJNR Am J Neuroradiol 19:1879–1885, 1998

Fugate LP, Spacek LA, Kresty LA, et al: Definition of agitation following traumatic brain injury, I: a survey of the brain injury special interest group of the American Academy of Physical Medicine and Rehabilitation. Arch Phys Med Rehabil 78:917–923, 1997a

Fugate LP, Spacek LA, Kresty LA, et al: Measurement and treatment of agitation following traumatic brain injury, II: a survey of the Brain Injury Special Interest Group of the American Academy of Physical Medicine and Rehabilitation. Arch Phys Med Rehabil 78:924–928, 1997b

Furmaga KM, DeLeon OA, Sinha SB, et al: Psychosis in medical conditions: response to risperidone. Gen Hosp Psychiatry 19:223–228, 1997

Galbraith S: Head injuries in the elderly. Br Med J (Clin Res Ed) 294:325, 1987

Garnett MR, Corkill RG, Blamire AM, et al: Altered cellular metabolism following traumatic brain injuryL a magnetic resonance spectroscopy study. J Nuerotrauma 18:231–240, 2001

Geffen GM, Encel JS, Forrester GM: Stages of recovery during post-traumatic amnesia and subsequent everyday memory deficits. Neuroreport 2:105–108, 1991

Gentleman D, Jennett B: Audit of transfer of unconscious head-injured patients to a neurosurgical unit. Lancet 1:330–334, 1990

Glassman AH, Bigger JT Jr: Antipsychotic drugs: prolonged QTc interval, torsades de pointes, and sudden death. Am J Psychiatry 158:1774–1782, 2001

Grant I, Alves W: Psychiatric and psychosocial disturbances in head injury, in Neurobehavioral Recovery From Head Injury. Edited by Levin HS, Grafman J, Eisenberg HM. New York, Oxford University Press, 1987, pp 234–235

Gronwall D, Wrightson P: Duration of post-traumatic amnesia after mild head injury. J Clin Neuropsychol 2:51–60, 1980

Gualtieri CT: Neuropsychiatry and Behavioral Pharmacology. New York, Springer-Verlag, 1991

Guze BH, Baxter LR: Neuroleptic malignant syndrome. N Engl J Med 313:463–466, 1985

Hagen C, Malkmus D, Durham P: Rancho Los Amigos levels of cognitive functioning scale. Downey, CA, Professional Staff Association, 1972

Hart RP, Levenson JL, Sessler CN, et al: Validation of a cognitive test for delirium in medical ICU patients. Psychosomatics 37:533–546, 1996

High WM, Levin HS, Gary HE: Recovery of orientation following closed head injury. J Clin Exp Neuropsychol 12:703–714, 1990

Honkanen R, Smith G: Impact of acute alcohol intoxication on patterns of non-fatal trauma: cause-specific analysis of head injury effect. Injury 22:225–229, 1991

Houlden DA, Li C, Schwartz ML, et al: Median nerve somatosensory evoked potentials and the Glasgow Coma Scale as predictors of outcome in comatose patients with head injuries. Neurosurgery 27:701–708, 1990

Hughes JR, John ER: Conventional and quantitative electroencephalography in psychiatry. J Neuropsychiatry Clin Neurosci 11:190–208, 1999

Hume AL, Cant BR: Central somatosensory conduction after head injury. Ann Neurol 10:411–419, 1981

Inouye SK, van Dyck CH, Alessi CA, et al: Clarifying confusion: the Confusion Assessment Method. Ann Intern Med 113:941–948, 1990

Jackson CW, Markowitz JS, Brewerton TD: Delirium associated with clozapine and benzodiazepine combinations. Ann Clin Psychiatry 7:139–141, 1995

Jacobson S, Jerrier H: EEG in delirium. Semin Clin Neuropsychiatry 5:86–92, 2000

Jacobson SA, Leuchter AF, Walter DO, et al: Serial quantitative EEG among elderly subjects with delirium. Biol Psychiatry 34:135–140, 1993

Jaggi JL, Obrist WD, Gennarelli TA, et al: Relationship of early cerebral blood flow and metabolism to outcome in acute head injury. J Neurosurg 72:176–182, 1990

Jeanblanc W, Davis YB: Risperidone for treating dementia-related aggression. Am J Psychiatry 152:1239, 1995

Jellinger K, Seitelberger F: Protracted post-traumatic encephalopathy: pathology, pathogenesis and clinical implications. J Neurol Sci 10:51–94, 1970

Kalisky Z, Morrison DP, Meyers CA, et al: Medical problems encountered during rehabilitation of patients with head injury. Arch Phys Med Rehabil 66:25–29, 1985

Kant R, Bogyi AM, Carosella NW, et al: ECT as a therapeutic option in severe brain injury. Convuls Ther 11:45–50, 1995

Katz DI: Neuropathology and neurobehavioral recovery from closed head injury. J Head Trauma Rehabil 7:1–15, 1992

Katz DI, Alexander MP, Seliger GM, et al: Traumatic basal ganglia hemorrhage: clinicopathologic features and outcome. Neurology 39:897–904, 1989

Kennedy JS, Zagar MS, Bymaster F, et al: The central cholinergic system profile of olanzapine compared with placebo in Alzheimer's disease. Int J Geriatr Psychiatry 16:S24–S32, 2001

Kennedy RE, Thompson RN, Nick TG, et al: Use of the Cognitive Test for Delirium in TBI patients (abstract). J Neuropsychiatry Clin Neurosci 14:116, 2002

Khouzam HR, Gazula K: Clinical experience with olanzapine in the course of post-operative delirium associated with psychosis in geriatric patients: a report of three cases. Int J Psych Clin Pract 5:63–66, 2001

Killian GA, Holzman PS, Davis JM, et al: Effects of psychotropic medication on selected cognitive and perceptual measures. J Abnorm Psychol 93:58–70, 1984

Kim KS, Pae CU, Chae JH, et al: An open pilot trial of olanzapine for delirium in the Korean population. Psychiatry Clin Neurosci 55:515–519, 2001

King NS, Crawford S, Wenden FJ, et al: Measurement of post-traumatic amnesia: how reliable is it? J Neurol Neurosurg Psychiatry 62:38–42, 1997

Kinon BJ, Roychowdhury SM, Milton DR, et al: Effective resolution with olanzapine of acute presentation of behavioral agitation and positive symptoms in schizophrenia. J Clin Psychiatry 62:17–21, 2001

Koponen H, Partanen J, Paakkonen A, et al: EEG spectral analysis in delirium. J Neurol Neurosurg Psychiatry 52:980–985, 1989

Koufen H, Hagel K-H: Systematic EEG follow-up study of traumatic psychosis. Eur Arch Psychiatry Neurol Sci 237:2–7, 1987

Laatsch L, Pavel D, Jobe T, et al: Incorporation of SPECT imaging in a longitudinal cognitive rehabilitation therapy programme. Brain Inj 13:555–570, 1999

Lassen NA: The luxury-perfusion syndrome and its possible relation to acute metabolic acidosis localized within the brain. Lancet 2:1113–1115, 1966

Lerner DM, Rosenstein DL: Neuroimaging in delirium and related conditions. Semin Clin Neuropsychiatry 5:98–112, 2000

Leso L, Schwatrz TL: Ziprasidone treatment of delirium. Psychosomatics 43:61–63, 2002

Levin HS: Prediction of recovery from traumatic brain injury. J Neurotrauma 12:913–922, 1995

Levin HS, Grossman RG: Behavioral sequelae of closed head injury: a quantitative study. Arch Neurol 35:720–727, 1978

Levin HS, Grossman RG, Rose JE, et al: Long-term neuropsychological outcome of closed head injury. J Neurosurg 50:412–422, 1979a

Levin HS, O'Donnell VM, Grossman RG: The Galveston Orientation and Amnesia Test: a practical scale to assess cognition after head injury. J Nerv Ment Dis 167:675–684, 1979b

Levin HS, High WM, Meyers CA, et al: Impairment of remote memory after closed head injury. J Neurol Neurosurg Psychiatry 48:556–563, 1985

Levin HS, High WM, Goethe KE, et al: The Neurobehavioral Rating Scale: assessment of the behavioral sequelae of head injury by the clinician. J Neurol Neurosurg Psychiatry 50:183–193, 1987

Levin HS, High WM, Eisenberg HM: Learning and forgetting during posttraumatic amnesia in head-injured patients. J Neurol Neurosurg Psychiatry 51:14–20, 1988a

Levin HS, Williams D, Crofford MJ, et al: Relationship of depth of brain lesions to consciousness and outcome after closed head injury. J Neurosurg 69:861–866, 1988b

Levin HS, Gary HE, Eisenberg HM: Duration of impaired consciousness in relation to side of lesion after severe head injury. Lancet 1:1001–1003, 1989

Levin HS, Williams DH, Eisenberg HM, et al: Serial MRI and neurobehavioral findings after mild to moderate closed head injury. J Neurol Neurosurg Psychiatry 55:255–262, 1992

Levkoff SE, Safran C, Cleary PD, et al: Identification of factors associated with the diagnosis of delirium in elderly hospitalized patients. J Am Geriatr Soc 36:1099–1104, 1988

Lindsay KW, Carlin J, Kennedy I, et al: Evoked potentials in severe head injury—analysis and relation to outcome. J Neurol Neurosurg Psychiatry 44:796–802, 1981

Lipowski ZJ: Delirium (acute confusional state), in Handbook of Clinical Neurology. Edited by Vinken PJ, Bruyn GW, Klawans HL. New York, Elsevier, 1985, pp 523–559

Lipowski ZJ: Delirium, in Head Injury, Epilepsy and Brain Tumor. New York, Oxford University Press, 1990, pp 399–401

Livingston DH, Lavery RF, Passannante MR, et al: Emergency department discharge of patients with a negative cranial computed tomography scan after minimal head injury. Ann Surg 232:126–132, 2000

Lobato RD, Sarabia R, Cordobes F, et al: Posttraumatic cerebral hemispheric swelling: analysis of 55 cases studied with computerized tomography. J Neurosurg 68:417–423, 1988

Madhusoodanan S, Brenner R, Araujo L, et al: Efficacy of risperidone treatment of psychoses associated with schizophrenia, schizoaffective disorder, bipolar disorder, or senile dementia in 11 geriatric patients: a case series. J Clin Psychiatry 56:514–518, 1995

Mandleberg IA: Cognitive recovery after severe head injury: WAIS during post-traumatic amnesia. J Neurol Neurosurg Psychiatry 38:1127–1132, 1975

Meagher DJ, Trzepacz PT: Motoric subtypes of delirium. Semin Clin Neuropsychiatry 5:76–85, 2000

Meehan K, Zhang F, Dabid S, et al: A double-blind randomized comparison of the efficacy and safety of intramuscular injections of olanzapine, lorazepam, or placebo in treating acutely agitated patients diagnosed with bipolar mania. J Clin Psychopharmacol 21:389–397, 2001

Meehan KM, Wang H, David SR, et al: Comparison of rapidly acting intramuscular olanzapine, lorazepam, and placebo: a double-blind, randomized study in acutely agitated patients with dementia. Neuropsychopharmacology 26:494–504, 2002

Menza MA, Murray GB, Holmes VF, et al: Decreased extrapyramidal symptoms with intravenous haloperidol. J Clin Psychiatry 48:278–280, 1987

Michals ML, Crismon ML, Roberts S, Childs A: Clozapine response and adverse effects in nine brain-injured patients. J Clin Psychopharmacol 13:198–203, 1993

Mittal D, Jimerson N, Peoples E, et al: Successful treatment of delirium with risperidone: a case series (abstract). Presented to the International College of Geriatric Psychoneuropharmacology, Honolulu, HI, December 14–15, 2001

Morton RO, Gleason OC, Yates WR: Delirium: multiple neural system dysregulation—implications for therapy. Med Psychiatry 3:23–34, 2000

Nakase-Thompson RN, Sherer M, Yablon SA, et al: Persistent delirium and outcome following TBI. J Int Neuropsychol Soc 8:219, 2002

Nakase-Thompson R, Sherer M, Yablon SA, et al: Acute confusion following traumatic brain injury. Brain Inj 18:131–142, 2004

Nuwer M: Assessment of digital EEG, quantitative EEG, and EEG brain mapping: report of the American Academy of Neurology and the American Clinical Neurophysiology Society. Neurology 49:277–292, 1997

Obrist WD, Langfitt TW, Jaggi JL, et al: Cerebral blood flow and metabolism in comatose patients with acute head injury: relationship to intracranial hypertension. J Neurosurg 61:241–253, 1984

O'Carroll RE, Hayes PC, Ebmeier KP, et al: Regional cerebral blood flow and cognitive function in patients with chronic liver disease. Lancet 337:1250–1253, 1991

Ommaya AK, Gennarelli TA: Cerebral concussion and traumatic unconsciousness. Brain 97:633–654, 1974

Overall JE, Gorham DR: The Brief Psychiatric Rating Scale. Psychol Rep 10:799, 1962

Owens MJ, Risch SC: Atypical antipsychotics, in Textbook of Psychopharmacology, 2nd Edition. Edited by Schatzberg AF, Nemeroff CB. Washington, DC, American Psychiatric Press, 1998, pp 323–348

Passik SD, Cooper M: Complicated delirium in a cancer patient successfully treated with olanzapine. J Pain Symptom Manage 17:219–223, 1999

Pourcher E, Filteau MJ, Bouchard RH, et al: Efficacy of the combination of buspirone and carbamazepine in early post-traumatic delirium. Am J Psychiatry 151:150–151, 1994

Prigatano GP, Bruna O, Mataro M, et al: Initial disturbances of consciousness and resultant impaired awareness in Spanish patients with traumatic brain injury. J Head Trauma Rehabil 13:29–38, 1998

Raichle ME, Grubb RL Jr, Gado MH, et al: Correlation between regional cerebral blood flow and oxidative metabolism: in vivo studies in man. Arch Neurol 33:523–526, 1976

Rao N, Jellinek HM, Woolston DC: Agitation in closed head injury: haloperidol effects on rehabilitation outcome. Arch Phys Med Rehabil 66:30–34, 1995

Rao V, Lyketsos C: Neuropsychiatric sequelae of traumatic brain injury. Psychosomatics 41:95–103, 2000

Ratey JJ, Leveroni C, Kilmer D, et al: The effects of clozapine on severely aggressive psychiatric inpatients in a state hospital. J Clin Psychiatry 54:219–223, 1993

Ravona-Springer R, Dolberg OT, Hirschmann S, et al: Delirium in elderly patients treated with risperidone: a report of three cases. J Clin Psychopharmacol 18:171–172, 1998

Reyes RL, Bhattacharyya AK, Heller D: Traumatic head injury: restlessness and agitation as prognosticators of physical and psychological improvement in patients. Arch Phys Med Rehabil 62:20–23, 1981

Ricker JH, Zafonte RD: Functional neuroimaging and quantitative electroencephalography in adult traumatic head injury: clinical applications and interpretive cautions. J Head Trauma Rehabil 15:859–868, 2000

Rockwood K, Cosway S, Carver D, et al: The risk of dementia and death after delirium. Age Ageing 28:551–556, 1999

Rowland T, DePalma L: Current neuropharmacologic interventions for the management of brain injury agitation. Neurorehabilitation 5:219–232, 1995

Rubbert A, Marienhagen J, Pirner K, et al: Single-photon-emission computed tomography analysis of cerebral blood flow in the evaluation of central nervous system involvement in patients with systemic lupus erythematosus. Arthritis Rheum 36:1253–1262, 1993

Ruff RM, Crouch JA, Troster AI, et al: Selected cases of poor outcome following a minor brain trauma: comparing neuropsychological and positron emission tomography assessment. Brain Inj 8:297–308, 1994

Russell WR: Cerebral involvement in head injury. Brain 55:549–603, 1932

Russell WR, Smith A: Post-traumatic amnesia in closed head injury. Arch Neurol 5:4–17, 1961

Sabbadini MG, Manfredi AA, Bozzolo E, et al: Central nervous system involvement in systemic lupus erythematosus patients without overt neuropsychiatric manifestations. Lupus 8:11–19; 1999

Salazar AM, Grafman JH, Vance SC, et al: Consciousness and amnesia after penetrating head injury: neurology and anatomy. Neurology 36:178–187, 1986

Sandel ME, Zwil AS, Fugate LP: An interdisciplinary perspective on the agitated brain injured patient. Neurorehabilitation 5:299–308, 1995

Schuster P, Gabriel E, Kufferle B, et al: Reversal by physostigmine of clozapine-induced delirium. Clin Toxicol 10:437–441, 1977

Schwartz ML, Carruth F, Binns MA, et al: The course of posttraumatic amnesia: three little words. Can J Neurol Sci 25:108–116, 1998

Schwartz TL, Masand PS: Treatment of delirium with quetiapine. Prim Care Companion J Clin Psychiatry 2:10–12, 2000

Schwartz TL, Masand PS: The role of atypical antipsychotics in the treatment of delirium. Psychosomatics 43:171–174, 2002

Sharma ND, Rosman HS, Padhi ID, et al: Torsades de pointes associated with intravenous haloperidol in critically ill patients. Am J Cardiol 81:238–240, 1998

Shavelle RM, Strauss D, Whyte J, et al: Long-term causes of death after traumatic brain injury. Am J Phys Med Rehabil 80:510–516, 2001

Shores EA, Marosszeky JE, Sandanam J, et al: Preliminary validation of a clinical scale for measuring the duration of posttraumatic amnesia. Med J Aust 144:569–572, 1986

Silverman M: Organic stupor subsequent to a severe head injury treated with ECT. Br J Psychiatry 119:648–650, 1964

Sim FH, Brunet DG, Conacher GW: Quetiapine associated with acute mental status changes. Can J Psychiatry 45:299, 2000

Sipahimalani A, Masand PS: Use of risperidone in delirium: case reports. Ann Clin Psychiatry 9:105–107, 1997

Sipahimalani A, Masand PS: Olanzapine in the treatment of delirium. Psychosomatics 39:422–429, 1998

Sipahimalani A, Sime RA, Masand PS: Treatment of delirium with risperidone. Int J Geriatr Psychopharmacol 1:24–26, 1997

Sisler G, Penner H: Amnesia following severe head injury. Can Psychiatr Assoc J 20:333–336, 1975

Smith A: Duration of impaired consciousness as an index of severity in closed head injuries: a review. Dis Nerv Syst 22:70–74, 1961

Smith LW, Dimsdale J: Postcardiotomy delirium: conclusions after 25 years. Am J Psychiatry 146:452–458, 1989

Sos J, Cassem NH: Intravenous use of haloperidol for acute delirium in intensive care settings, in Psychic and Neurological Dysfunctions After Open Heart Surgery. Edited by Speidel H, Rodewald G. Stuttgart, Georg Thieme Verlag, 1980, pp 196–199

Squire LR: Mechanisms of memory. Science 232:1612–1619, 1986

Stanislav SW: Cognitive effects of antipsychotic agents in persons with traumatic brain injury. Brain Inj 11:335–341, 1997

Stern TA: Continuous infusion of physostigmine in anticholinergic delirium: case report. J Clin Psychiatry 44:463–464, 1983

Stuss DT, Binns MA, Carruth FG, et al: The acute period of recovery from traumatic brain injury: posttraumatic amnesia. J Neurosurg 90:635–643, 1999

Synek VM: EEG abnormality grades and subdivisions of prognostic importance in traumatic and anoxic coma in adults. Clin Electroencephalogr 19:160–166, 1988

Synek VM: Value of a revised EEG coma scale for prognosis after cerebral anoxia and diffuse head injury. Clin Electroencephalogr 21:25–30, 1990

Szymanski S, Jody D, Leipzig R, et al: Anticholinergic delirium caused by retreatment with clozapine. Am J Psychiatry 148:1752, 1991

Tate RL, Pfaff A, Jurjevic L: Resolution of disorientation and amnesia during post-traumatic amnesia. J Neurol Neurosurg Psychiatry 68:178–185, 2000

Tate RL, Perdices M, Pfaff A, et al: Predicting duration of post-traumatic amnesia (PTA) from early PTA measurements. J Head Trauma Rehabil 16:525–542, 2001

Tavcar R, Dernovsek MZ: Risperidone-induced delirium. Can J Psychiatry 43:194, 1998

Teasdale E, Cardoso E, Galbraith S, et al: CT scan in severe diffuse head injury: physiological and clinical correlations. J Neurol Neurosurg Psychiatry 47:600–603, 1984

Teasdale G, Jennett B: Assessment of coma and impaired consciousness: a practical scale. Lancet 2:81–84, 1974

Thatcher RW, Walker RA, Gerson I, et al: EEG discriminant analyses of mild head trauma. Electroencephalogr Clin Neurophysiol 73:94–106, 1989

Thatcher RW, Biver C, McAlaster R, et al: Biophysical linkage between MRI and EEG amplitude in closed head injury. Neuroimage 7:352–367, 1998

Thatcher RW, North DM, Curtin RT, et al: An EEG severity index of traumatic brain injury. J Neuropsychiatry Clin Neurosci 13:77–87, 2001

Torres R, Mittal D, Kennedy R: Use of quetiapine in delirium: case reports. Psychosomatics 42:347–349, 2001

Trzepacz PT: The neuropathogenesis of delirium: a need to focus our research. Psychosomatics 35:374–391, 1994

Trzepacz PT: Anticholinergic model for delirium. Semin Clin Neuropsychiatry 1:294–303, 1996

Trzepacz PT: The Delirium Rating Scale: its use in C/L psychiatry research. Psychosomatics 40:193–204, 1999a

Trzepacz PT: Update in neuropathogenesis of delirium. Dement Geriatr Cogn Disord 10:330–334, 1999b

Trzepacz PT: Is there a final common neural pathway in delirium? focus on acetylcholine and dopamine. Semin Clin Neuropsychiatry 5:132–148, 2000

Trzepacz PT, Baker RW, Greenhouse JB: A symptom rating scale for delirium. Psychiatry Res 23:89–97, 1988a

Trzepacz PT, Brenner RP, Coffman G, et al: Delirium in liver transplantation candidates: discriminant analysis of multiple test variables. Biol Psychiatry 24:3–14, 1988b

Trzepacz PT, Sclabassi RJ, Van Thiel DH: Delirium: a subcortical phenomenon? J Neuropsychiatry Clin Neurosci 1:283–290, 1989b

Trzepacz PT, Francis J: Low serum albumin and risk of delirium. Am J Psychiatry 147:675, 1990

Trzepacz PT, Mittal D, Torres R, et al: Validation of the Delirium Rating Scale-Revised-98: comparison with the Delirium Rating Scale and cognitive test for delirium. J Neuropsychiatry Clin Neurosci 13:229–242, 2001

Trzepacz PT, Meagher DJ, Wise M: Neuropsychiatry of delirium, in Textbook of Neuropsychiatry, 4th Edition. Edited by Yudofsky SC, Hales RE. Washington. DC, American Psychiatric Publishing, 2002, pp 525–564

Umile EM, Plotkin RC, Sandel ME: Functional assessment of mild traumatic brain injury using SPECT and neuropsychologic testing. Brain Inj 12:577–594, 1998

van der Naalt J, van Zomeren AH, Sluiter WJ, et al: Acute behavioral disturbances related to imaging studies and outcome in mild-to-moderate head injury. Brain Inj 14:781–788, 2000

van Heertum RL, Drocea C, Ichise M, et al: Single photon emission CT and positron emission tomography in the evaluation of neurologic disease. Radiol Clin North Am 39:1007–1033, 2001

Wakamoto H, Miyazaki H, Inaba M, et al: FLAIR images of mild head trauma with transient amnesia. No Shinkei Geka 11:985–990, 1998

Wallace BA, Wagner AK, Wagner EP, et al: A history and review of quantitative electroencephalography in traumatic brain injury. J Head Trauma Rehabil 16:165–190, 2001

Wengel SP, Burke WJ, Roccaforte WH: Donepezil for postoperative delirium associated with Alzheimer's disease. J Am Geriatr Soc 47: 379–380, 1999

Wilkins-Ho M, Hollander Y: Toxic delirium with low-dose clozapine. Can J Psychiatry 42:429–430, 1997

Williams MA, Campbell EB, Raynor WJ, et al: Reducing acute confusional states in elderly patients with hip fractures. Res Nurs Health 8:329–337, 1985

Williams MA, Levin HS, Eisenberg HM: Mild head injury classification. Neurosurgery 27:422–428, 1990

Wilson BA, Evans JJ, Emslie H, et al: Measuring recovery from post traumatic amnesia. Brain Inj 13:505–520, 1999

Wilson JT, Wiedmann KD, Hadley DM, et al: Early and late magnetic resonance imaging and neuropsychological outcome after head injury. J Neurol Neurosurg Psychiatry 51:391–396, 1988

Wilson JT, Teasdale GM, Hadley DM, et al: Posttraumatic amnesia: still a valuable yardstick. J Neurol Neurosurg Psychiatry 57:198–201, 1994

Wilson MS, Gibson CJ, Hamm RJ: Haloperidol, but not olanzapine, impairs cognitive performance after traumatic brain injury in rats. Am J Phys Med Rehabil 82:871–879, 2003

Wright P, Birkett M, David SR, et al: Double-blind placebo-controlled comparison of intramuscular olanzapine and intramuscular haloperidol in the treatment of acute agitation in schizophrenia. Am J Psychiatry 158:1149–1151, 2001

Yates DW, Hadfield JM, Peters K: Alcohol consumption of patients attending two accident and emergency departments in north-west England. J R Soc Med 80:486–489, 1987

Yudofsky SC, Kopecky HJ, Kunik M, et al: The Overt Agitation Severity Scale for the objective rating of agitation. J Neuropsychiatry Clin Neurosci 9:541–548, 1997

Yuen HK, Benzing P: Treatment methodology: guiding of behavior through redirection in brain injury. Brain Inj 10:229–238, 1996

Zafonte RD, Mann NR, Mullis SR, et al: Posttraumatic amnesia: its relation to functional outcome. Arch Phys Med Rehabil 78:1103–1106, 1997

Zimnitzky BM, DeMaso DR, Steingard RJ: Use of risperidone in psychotic disorder following ischemic brain damage. J Child Adolesc Psychopharmacol 6:75–78, 1996

10 Mood Disorders

Robert G. Robinson, M.D.

Ricardo E. Jorge, M.D.

ASSOCIATIONS BETWEEN TRAUMATIC brain injury (TBI) and a variety of neuropsychiatric disorders have been reported in the medical literature for many years. Lishman (1986), in his classic study on the Oxford collection of head injury records, analyzed potential etiological factors involved in the development of psychiatric disturbances after TBI. These studies stressed the importance of biological variables such as the extent of brain damage, lesion location, and presence of posttraumatic epilepsy in determining the type and duration of psychiatric disorder.

There have been relatively few studies, however, that have examined the prevalence of mood disorders associated with TBI and their effect on outcome variables. Issues such as the prevalence of major depressive disorder after TBI, clinical variables that predict the development of major depression, the natural course of post-TBI major depression, and the influence of mood disorders on the longitudinal evolution of post-TBI physical and intellectual impairments are relatively unexplored and deserve further investigation.

Prevalence of Depressive Disorders

Mood and anxiety disorders appear to be frequent psychiatric complications among patients with TBI. The presence of such neuropsychiatric disorders may play an important role in shaping long-term outcome.

The reported frequency of depressive disorders after TBI has varied from 6% to 77% (Levin and Grossman 1978; Rutherford et al. 1997; Varney et al. 1987). McKinlay et al. (1981) reported indirect evidence of a depressed mood in approximately half of their patients at 3, 6, or 12 months after severe brain injury. Kinsella et al. (1988) reported in a series of 39 patients within 2 years of severe brain injury that 33% were classified as depressed and 26%

as having anxiety. Schoenhuber and Gentilini (1988) found depressive symptoms in 39% of 103 patients with mild head injury interviewed at 1-year follow-up and concluded that these patients had an increased risk of developing depression compared with an appropriate control group. More recently, Gualtieri and Cox (1991) estimated that the frequency of major depression in TBI patients lies between 25% and 50%. The variability in the reported frequency of depressive disorders, particularly major depression, may be due to the lack of uniformity in the psychiatric diagnosis. Most of the studies relied on rating scales or relatives' reports rather than on structured interviews of the patient and established diagnostic criteria (e.g., DSM-IV-TR [American Psychiatric Association 2000]).

Hibbard et al. (1998) used a structured interview and DSM-IV (American Psychiatric Association 1994) criteria to identify Axis I psychopathology in 100 adults with TBI who were evaluated 8 years (on average) after trauma. The prevalence of major depression in this series was 61%. More recently, Kreutzer et al. (2001) studied the prevalence of major depressive disorder among a sample of 722 outpatients with TBI who were evaluated an average of 2.5 years after brain injury. Major depression, defined using DSM-IV criteria, was diagnosed in 303 patients (42%).

In addition, Koponen et al. (2002) reported that major depression had a lifetime prevalence of 26.7% in a group of 60 TBI patients followed for an average of 30 years. These findings emphasize the need for careful psychiatric follow-up of patients who have experienced TBI.

The authors of this chapter studied the prevalence, duration, and clinical correlates of mood and anxiety disorders in a group of 66 patients admitted with TBI to the Shock Trauma Center of the Maryland Institute of Emergency Medical Services System (Fedoroff et al. 1992). The patients in our sample were mostly white men of

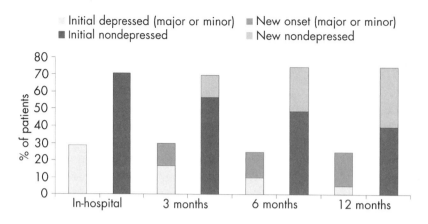

FIGURE 10–1. **The frequency of depressed and nondepressed patients over 12 months after traumatic brain injury.**

The overall frequency of major depression was 26% in-hospital, 22% at 3 months, 23% at 6 months, and 19% at 12 months. The remainder of the patients with depression had minor depression.

Source. Data from Jorge RE, Robinson RG, Arndt SV, et al: "Depression Following Traumatic Brain Injury: A 1 year Longitudinal Study." *Journal of Affective Disorders* 27:233–243, 1993.

lower socioeconomic classes in their 30s. The principal cause of brain injury was motor vehicle accidents. The majority of patients (68%) had moderate brain injuries, 11 patients (17%) had severe brain injuries, and 10 patients (15%) had mild head injuries. Almost one-third of the patients (30%) had a history of alcohol/drug abuse, and 11 patients (17%) had a personal history of psychiatric disorder (excluding alcoholism and/or drug abuse).

In the acute stage of TBI (i.e., approximately 1 month after brain injury), 17 of 66 patients (26%) developed major depression, and 2 patients (3%) developed minor (dysthymic) depression (Fedoroff et al. 1992). The prevalence of major depression during the year after TBI remained stable at 25%, with some patients recovering from major depression and other patients developing delayed-onset depressions (Jorge et al. 1993c) (Figure 10–1). Minor depression was diagnosed in 8 patients during the course of the year. Of the 17 acutely depressed patients, 7 patients (41%) also met DSM-III-R (American Psychiatric Association 1987) criteria for the presence of generalized anxiety disorder, whereas none of the 47 nondepressed patients met criteria for this disorder (Jorge et al. 1993d). There were 11 patients who developed delayed-onset major depression at some point during the follow-up period (i.e., 4 patients at 3 months, 4 patients at 6 months, and 3 patients at 12 months after brain injury). Thus, 28 of the 58 patients (47%) for whom we have follow-up data met DSM-III-R criteria for major depression during the first year after the traumatic episode (Jorge et al. 1993b).

In this series, patients who developed major depression during the acute period had an estimated mean duration

depression of 4.7 months, with a minimum of 1.5 months and a maximum of 12 months. In addition, we identified two patients with recurrent depressions who had major depression in hospital but were not depressed at the 3- or 6-month evaluation, only to become depressed again at 1-year follow-up (Jorge et al. 1993c). Anxious depression (median duration of 7.5 months) had a significantly longer duration than nonanxious depression (median duration of 1.5 months) (Jorge et al. 1993c). Delayed-onset major depression, in turn, had an estimated duration of 4.0 months (Jorge et al. 1993b).

The authors of this chapter are currently analyzing the findings observed in a different group of 89 consecutive patients with closed-head injury admitted to the University of Iowa Hospitals and Clinics in Iowa City (*n*=58) and the Iowa Methodist Medical Center in Des Moines, Iowa (*n*=31) who enrolled in a 2-year prospective observational study (Jorge et al. 2004). Twenty-six patients with multiple traumas but without clinical or radiological evidence of central nervous system involvement (i.e., without primary or secondary brain damage or spinal cord injury) consecutively admitted to the University of Iowa Hospital and Clinics constituted our control group. Sixty-seven of the 89 patients with TBI (75.3%) and 19 of the 26 patients in the control group (73.1%) were injured in a motor vehicle accident. Severity of TBI was classified as mild in 31 patients (35%), moderate in 36 patients (40%), and severe in 22 patients (25%).

Of the 89 TBI patients enrolled in the study, 44 (49%) developed mood disorders during the first year after TBI, compared with 7 out of 26 patients (27%) in the control group. Thus, the frequency of mood disorders was significantly higher in brain-injured patients compared with patients who had a similar severity of physical impairment but without brain damage ($P=0.04$).

Of the 44 patients with post-TBI mood disorders, major depressive disorder occurred in 30 of 75 patients (40%) followed up for 1 year after TBI. Major depression occurred in 15 patients at the initial evaluation, 9 patients at 3 months, and 6 patients at 6 months. The average duration of major depression among this group was 6.1 months, spanning from 8 weeks to 12 months.

Major depressive disorder was associated with prominent anxiety symptoms. Of the 30 patients with major depression, 23 (76.7%) met DSM-IV criteria for anxiety disorder, compared with 10 of 45 patients (22.2%) who did not develop a mood disorder during the course of the 1-year follow-up but met criteria for anxiety disorder. In addition, major depressive disorder was significantly associated with aggression. Aggressive behavior was found in 33.7% of TBI patients during the first 6 months after injury. A major depression diagnosis was significantly more frequent among the aggressive group than the nonaggressive group ($P=0.01$).

Diagnosis of Depression

Diagnostic Criteria

To characterize the affective disturbances occurring after TBI, we have adopted a disease perspective (McHugh and Slavney 1998), assuming that mood disorders, although diagnosed through a recognized constellation of symptoms, have an identifiable biological substrate, a distinct clinical prognosis, and a predictable treatment response. Using DSM-IV-TR diagnostic criteria, depressive disorders associated with TBI are categorized as mood disorder due to a general medical condition with the predominant symptom type indicated by one of the following subtypes: with depressive features, with major depressive-like episode, with manic features, or with mixed features.

One of the basic issues in the diagnosis of post-TBI depression is the specificity of symptoms on which these diagnostic criteria are based. For example, symptoms of major depression such as changes in sleep, appetite, or libido may occur in patients with TBI as a consequence of brain injury or as a nonspecific consequence of an acute medical illness. Thus, symptoms used to diagnose depressive disorders could be independent of the associated mood disturbance. Consequently, major depressive disorder could be systematically overdiagnosed. On the other hand, patients may deny the presence of a depressed mood as part of a general unawareness of deficit or a denial syndrome. This situation would result in underdiagnosis of depression.

Specificity of Diagnostic Criteria

We longitudinally examined the specificity of symptoms of depression after TBI (Jorge et al. 1993a). Depressive symptoms were divided into "autonomic" and "psychological" subtypes using the distinctions proposed by Davidson and Turnbull (1986). We then analyzed their frequency among patients who presented with a depressed mood (no other depressive symptoms were required) compared with those who presented without a depressed mood. We found that among patients who acknowledged a depressed mood, the mean frequency of autonomic symptoms was 2.7 (SD=1.4), and the mean frequency of psychological symptoms was 3.1 (SD=1.9). These frequencies were more than three times higher than the frequency of autonomic (0.8 [SD=0.8]) and psychological (0.9 [SD=0.9]) symptoms found in patients who denied having a depressed mood.

Because there were depressive symptoms that were not specific to depression, one might question whether existing DSM criteria for depression due to TBI with major depressive–like episode should be modified to account for this finding. If we required the presence of at least three specific symptoms (including depressed mood) as a criterion for diagnosing major depression, standard DSM-IV-TR criteria would have a 100% sensitivity and 94% specificity at the initial evaluation, 88% sensitivity and 94% specificity at 3 months, 91% sensitivity and 96% specificity at 6 months, and 80% sensitivity and 100% specificity at 1-year follow-up. Thus, the standard diagnostic criteria (DSM-based) have a high sensitivity and specificity for identifying depressed patients when compared with alternative specific symptom diagnostic criteria. We have concluded, therefore, that standard DSM-IV-TR criteria are the most logical criteria to use for the diagnosis of major depression in the TBI population.

On the other hand, other authors (Rosenthal et al. 1998) argue that the use of categorical variables (e.g., depressed vs. nondepressed) might ignore important dimensional information that characterize the complex affective response of a patient recovering from TBI. The combination of structured diagnostic interviews, self-report, and caregiver-based measures may represent a comprehensive approach to the assessment of depression after TBI.

Differential Diagnosis of Post-TBI Depression

The differential diagnosis of post-TBI major depression includes adjustment disorder with depressed mood, apathy, emotional lability, and posttraumatic stress disorder. Patients with adjustment disorders develop short-lived and relatively mild emotional disturbances within 3 months of a stressful life event. Although they may present with depressive symptoms, they do not meet DSM-IV-TR criteria for major depressive–like episode. Posttraumatic stress disorder is another differential diagnosis. It occurs after an unusually severe distressing event and it is characterized by symptoms of reexperiencing the trauma ranging from transient flashbacks or vivid nightmares to severe dissociative states in which the patient behaves as if he or she is actually living the traumatic event. In addition, patients typically avoid all the circumstances related to the trauma and become withdrawn and emotionally blunted.

Pathological laughing and crying (PLC) is another differential diagnosis of major depression. It is characterized by the presence of sudden and uncontrollable affective outbursts (i.e., crying or laughing) that may be congruent or incongruent with the patient's mood. These emotional displays are recognized by the patient as being excessive to the underlying mood and can occur spontaneously or may be triggered by minor stimuli. This condition lacks the pervasive alteration of mood as well as the specific vegetative symptoms associated with a major depressive episode. In our new series of TBI patients, the prevalence of PLC during the first year after TBI was 10.9%. Compared with patients without PLC, patients with PLC were significantly more anxious and aggressive and had poorer social functioning. Furthermore, PLC was associated with the occurrence of focal prefrontal lesions (Tateno et al., in press).

Finally, TBI patients may present with apathetic syndromes that interfere with the rehabilitation process (Marin et al. 1995). A study of 83 consecutive TBI patients referred to a neuropsychiatric clinic because of behavioral disturbance showed that 59 patients (71.1%) were apathetic. However, 50 of these 59 patients were also depressed (Kant et al. 1998). In our experience, apathy is frequently associated with psychomotor retardation and emotional blunting. Among patients with stroke, we reported that half of the patients with apathy also met diagnostic criteria for major or minor depression (Starkstein et al. 2003). Thus, apathy is often comorbid with depression but can be distinguished from it by failure to meet appropriate diagnostic criteria. Although apathy is frequently associated with frontal lobe damage, the relationship between apathy and the type, extent, and location of TBI has not been systematically studied (see Chapter 18, Disorders of Diminished Motivation).

Relationship to Background and Impairment Variables

In our first group of patients examined for acute-onset post-TBI major depression (n=17), nondepressed patients (n=47)

TABLE 10–1. Demographic data and history of psychiatric disorders in 64 patients with acute traumatic brain injury, for depressed and nondepressed groups

Variable	Major depression (n=17)	Nondepressed (n=47)
Age, mean (SD)	26.8 (5.8)	29.5 (10.7)
Sex, % male	82.4	87.2
Race, % black	29.4	23.4
Handedness, % left	5.9	8.5
Mean education in years (SD)	12.4 (2.0)	12.3 (2.1)
Hollingshead socioeconomic status, % class IV or V	75	72
Family history of psychiatric disorder, %	47.0 (8/17)	48.9 (23/47)
Personal history of psychiatric disorder, including substance abuse, %[a]	70.6 (12/17)	37.0 (17/46)

[a]$P<0.05$.

did not differ from the depressed patients with respect to demographic variables, type or severity of brain injury, family history of psychiatric disorder, or degree of physical or cognitive impairment. There was, however, a significantly greater frequency of personal history of psychiatric disorder (including substance abuse) in the group with major depression (Table 10–1). Patients with major depression also had significantly poorer premorbid social functioning (as measured by initial Social Functioning Examination [SFE] scores) than the nondepressed group (Fedoroff et al. 1992). In addition, cross-sectional analysis at 3-, 6-, and 12-month follow-up evaluations showed that poor social functioning was the strongest and most consistent clinical correlate of major depression (Jorge et al. 1993c).

Findings from our most recent series of TBI patients are generally consistent with our previous findings (Jorge et al. 2004). A personal history of mood disorders or anxiety disorders was significantly more frequent in those patients who developed post-TBI major depressive disorder compared with those who did not ($P=0.03$) (Table 10–2). However, depressed patients and nondepressed patients were not significantly different with regard to the frequency of personal history of substance abuse. We did, however, confirm our previous finding that impaired so-

TABLE 10–2. History of psychiatric illness

Variable present in history	Major depression (*n*=30)	Nondepressed, (*n*=45)
Mood disorders[a] (%)	36.7	11.1
Anxiety disorders[a] (%)	20	4.4
Alcohol abuse (%)	21.4	17.8
Drug abuse (%)	20	6.7

[a]$P = 0.03$.

cial functioning was the only impairment significantly associated with major depression (Jorge et al. 2004) (Table 10–3).

Secondary Mania

Secondary manic and hypomanic states have been reported in a number of organic disorders such as thyroid disease (Corn and Checkley 1983), uremia (Thomas and Neale 1991), and vitamin B_{12} deficiency (Goggan 1984) as well as after open heart surgery (Isles and Orrell 1991). Mania has also been associated with brain tumors (Robinson et al. 1988), central nervous system infection (Thienhaus and Kosla 1984), stroke (Cummings and Mendez 1984), and TBI (Bamrah and Johnson 1980). Shukla et al. (1987) reported on 20 patients who developed manic syndromes after closed head trauma. They found a significant association between mania and the presence of posttraumatic seizures, predominantly of the partial complex type (e.g., temporal lobe epilepsy). However, these authors found no association with a family history of bipolar disorder among 85 first-degree relatives.

We have studied the prevalence of manic syndromes among a sample of 66 TBI patients (Jorge et al. 1993e). There were 6 patients (9%) who developed secondary mania at some point during the follow-up period (i.e., 5 patients at 3 months and 1 patient at 6 months after brain injury).

Although manic episodes only lasted approximately 2 months, elevated or expansive mood had a mean duration of 5.7 months. Secondary mania was not related to the type or severity of brain injury, degree of physical or intellectual impairment, level of social functioning, or the presence of family or personal history of psychiatric disorder. In addition, it was not associated with the development of posttraumatic epilepsy. Secondary mania, however, was associated with the presence of basopolar temporal lesions.

TABLE 10–3. Baseline impairment variables

Variable	Major depression (*n*=30)	Nondepressed (*n*=45)
Glasgow Coma Scale	12.3 (2.2)	11.5 (3.1)
Abbreviated Injury Scale	16.7 (6.7)	17.8 (7.9)
Functional Independence Measure	62.6 (10.7)	62.5 (9.9)
Mini-Mental State Examination	27.7 (1.5)	27.4 (2.8)
Social Functioning Examination[b]	0.215 (0.140)	0.128 (0.114)
Social Ties Checklist	3.8 (1.8)	3.4 (1.9)

[a]All values are mean (standard deviation).
[b]$P = 0.01$.

The development of abnormal activation patterns in limbic networks, functional changes in aminergic inhibitory systems, and the presence of aberrant regeneration pathways may play a role in the genesis of manic syndromes.

Diagnosis

DSM-IV-TR defines secondary manic syndromes as an Axis I disorder: mood disorder due to a general medical condition, with manic or with mixed features. As with depressive disorders due to TBI, the presence of TBI should be noted on Axis III.

This diagnosis should not be made if the mood disturbance occurs only during the course of a delirium characterized by sudden onset, fluctuating level of consciousness, disorientation, and prominent attentional deficits. In addition, the diagnosis of delirium requires clinical evidence of the presence of a medical or metabolic derangement (e.g., urinary tract infection, hyponatremia, and medication toxicity).

Differential Diagnosis

The differential diagnosis of mania after TBI includes the following:

1. *Substance-induced mood disorder*, which may occur as a result of intoxication or withdrawal from different drugs. This is a particularly important consideration with regard to patients with TBI, who show an increased frequency of substance abuse and who are often medicated with psychotropic drugs for their medi-

cal condition. Substance-induced mood disorder is usually identified by a careful clinical interview and/or toxicological screening.

2. *Psychosis associated with epilepsy* is frequently observed among patients with epileptic foci located in limbic or paralimbic cortices. Psychotic episodes may be temporally linked to seizures or may have a more prolonged interictal course. In the latter case, the clinical picture is characterized by the presence of partial and/or complex-partial seizures and of a schizoaffective syndrome. Electroencephalographic and functional neuroimaging studies (e.g., single-photon emission computed tomography and positron emission tomography) usually define ictal and interictal disturbances.

3. *Personality change* due to TBI may include mood instability, paranoid ideation, and poor control over aggression, as well as disinhibited behavior and hypersexuality. However, these patients lack the pervasive alteration of mood that characterizes secondary manic syndromes.

Physiological Correlations

Numerous studies have identified the complex pathological processes that occur after brain trauma with the hope of designing effective specific interventions to prevent neuronal death and foster restorative change. These processes include an array of neurochemical and structural changes, including the release of neurotransmitters and neuropeptides, the expression of several transcription factors, and the activation of the molecular cascades associated with necrotic cell death and neuronal apoptosis (Raghupathi et al. 2000). Other complex delayed processes include microglial activation and release of inflammatory cytokines, as well as mechanisms of repair and regeneration that include reactive synaptogenesis and axonal sprouting (Graham et al. 2000).

The role that these changes play in mediating the behavioral outcome of TBI patients, particularly in relation to the onset and course of psychiatric disorders, has not been elucidated and represents a fertile area of research.

Perhaps the most compelling hypothesis linking a pathological change characterized at a biological molecular level and a behavioral outcome is the one relating the expression of amyloid precursor protein and the increased deposition of β-amyloid peptides post-TBI, which ultimately leads to the onset of dementia (Nakagawa et al. 1999). This appears to be the likely mechanism for the association observed in epidemiological studies between a

history of TBI and the development of Alzheimer's disease (Luukinen et al. 1999).

A recent community study suggested an association between a history of TBI and an increased lifetime prevalence of major depression. The physiopathological basis of such an association remains to be explained (Holsinger et al. 2002). There have also been numerous recent examinations of posttraumatic changes in the major neurotransmitter systems in the brain. Glutamate has been extensively studied because of its role in excitotoxic injury. Excitotoxic injury has a sequential mechanism, including sodium and chloride influx with resultant cytotoxic edema, followed by calcium influx leading to increased expression of early transcription factors and other acute phase proteins, followed by activation of different cellular kinases as well as activation of caspases, proteolytic enzymes that mediate neuronal apoptosis (Clark et al. 2000). Clinical studies have reported that glutamate concentrations are significantly elevated for several days in the cerebrospinal fluid of TBI patients (Palmer et al. 1994). Thus, it is conceivable that excitotoxic injury could be prevented through pharmacological intervention. Glutamate antagonists have shown a beneficial effect in experimental models of TBI (McIntosh et al. 1998). In addition, the use of inhibitors of glutamate release such as riluzole (Stutzmann and Doble 1995) or lubeluzole (Ashton et al. 1997) or the use of mild to moderate hypothermia may be an alternative to postsynaptic glutamatergic blockade, which is known to be associated with severe psychiatric side effects (McIntosh et al. 1998). There is also evidence that magnesium chloride administered early after TBI attenuates cortical histological damage and improves behavioral outcome (Bareyre et al. 2000).

Cholinergic neuronal activity appears to be increased immediately after TBI. Blockade of massive acetylcholine release resulting from pathological excitation of basal forebrain nuclei at the time of injury may prevent neuronal cell loss and associated behavioral deficits (Lyeth and Hayes 1992; Schmidt and Grady 1995). There is also evidence of a hypofunctional cholinergic state occurring later in the course after TBI. A reduction of cholinergic transmission in hippocampal and neocortical areas has been observed after cortical contusion brain injury (Dixon et al. 1996). In addition, experimental models in rats have demonstrated dysfunction of the septohippocampal cholinergic pathway, which might play a significant role in the development of posttraumatic cognitive and behavioral deficits (Leonard et al. 1997). Although cholinergic systems have not been systematically studied in clinical populations of TBI patients, cholinergic deficits observed in patients with Alzheimer's disease have been associated with behavioral changes, including apathy, anhedonia, and disinhibited behavior (Cummings and Kaufer 1996).

Ascending biogenic amine pathways have also been implicated in the pathophysiological processes determining the clinical presentation and even the long-term outcome of TBI patients. Circulating levels of catecholamines have been shown to significantly correlate with TBI severity as measured by the Glasgow Coma Scale (Hamill et al. 1987). Markianos et al. (1992) found that TBI patients showed an increase in both serotonergic and noradrenergic metabolites in the cerebrospinal fluid. They also hypothesized that prolonged increase of the synaptic concentration of these neurotransmitters would result in subacute or chronic downregulation of aminergic transmission and, eventually, depressive symptoms. In addition, aminergic neurotransmitters may be implicated in the restorative processes that occur in the chronic phase of TBI, an effect that may be mediated by neurotrophic factors.

An extensive body of research associates both primary and brain injury–related mood disorders with the disruption of neural circuits involving the prefrontal cortex, amygdala, hippocampus, basal ganglia, and thalamus. It is not surprising that TBI, a pathological condition that selectively affects prefrontal and anterior temporal structures and produces widespread axonal injury, is associated with an increased prevalence of mood disorders.

Lishman (1988) reported that several years after penetrating brain injury, depressive symptoms were more common among patients with right hemisphere lesions. Depressive symptoms were also more frequent among patients with frontal and parietal lesions than among patients with other lesion locations. Grafman et al. (1986) also reported that several years after head injury, depressive symptoms were more frequently associated with penetrating injuries involving the right hemisphere (i.e., right orbitofrontal lesions) than with any other lesion location.

In our first series of 66 TBI patients (Fedoroff et al. 1992), there were no significant differences between the major depressed and the nondepressed groups in the frequency of diffuse or focal patterns of injury. In addition, there were no significant between-group differences in the frequency of extraparenchymal hemorrhages, contusions, or intracerebral or intraventricular hemorrhages. A logistical regression model taking all of the sites of brain injury into account, however, showed that major depression after acute TBI was associated with the presence of left lateral frontal and/or left basal ganglia lesions and, to a lesser extent, with right hemisphere and parietooccipital lesions. Left lateral frontal and left basal ganglia lesions were strongly associated with major depression during the initial

in-hospital evaluation; these may have been strategic lesion locations that elicited neurochemical and metabolic responses that ultimately led to the clinical manifestation of depression. By 3-month follow-up, however, the major correlates of depression were history of psychiatric disorder and impaired social functioning, a fact that underscores the role of psychosocial factors in the causation of prolonged and delayed-onset depressions.

It is clear that the biological variables contributing to the pathophysiology of mood disorders must be studied with more specific hypotheses than the ones previously cited using both physiological and neuroimaging techniques, including functional magnetic resonance imaging, mapping of neurotransmitter receptors, and magnetic resonance spectroscopy.

Effect of Mood Disorders on the Outcome of TBI Patients

TBI has been associated with a host of physical, cognitive, and behavioral deficits that influence the community reintegration of these patients (Fann et al. 1995). Although there has been significant progress in determining the factors associated with poor outcome, we are still uncertain about what are the most successful restorative interventions. For instance, estimates of the number of patients with TBI that will return to competitive employment are still alarmingly low, varying from 10% to 70% (Yasuda et al. 2001).

We examined the factors that contributed to deterioration in either social functioning, activities of daily living (ADL), or intellectual function during the first year after TBI (Jorge et al. 1994). Change was estimated for each patient using a simple linear regression of time (months postinjury) on each of three impairment scales—Mini-Mental State Examination (MMSE), Johns Hopkins Functional Inventory (JHFI), and SFE. The slope (B) was taken as the degree of change that individuals showed on that scale. Negative slopes for JHFI and SFE and a positive slope for MMSE reflected recovery. The poor-outcome groups were defined by identifying those patients who 1) had a deteriorating slope in the linear regression of time on SFE, JHFI, or MMSE scores and 2) fell outside the interquartile range (i.e., 25%–75%). There were 11 patients (21%) who fulfilled these criteria for SFE, 7 (13%) for JHFI, and 11 (21%) for MMSE. The rest of the patients (e.g., 52–11=41 for SFE) constituted the control group.

Age, sex, education, socioeconomic status, premorbid levels of social functioning, personal history of psychiatric disorder, or previous history of alcohol and drug abuse did not appear to be significant predictors of poor psychosocial, cognitive, or ADL outcome. Logistic regression analysis identified race (i.e., black) as the only background variable significantly associated with a poor psychosocial outcome. Patients with poor outcome in recovery of ADL had a significantly higher frequency of focal (mass) injuries when compared with the control group. Logistic regression analysis disclosed a significant association between the presence of right hemisphere lesions and a poor psychosocial outcome.

We assumed that an effect of depression on long-term outcome would only be identifiable in those depressive disorders with a longer course. Thus, patients with prolonged major depression (i.e., ≥6 months) constitute the major depression group. There was a significant association between poor psychosocial outcome and the presence of major depression. Patients with short-term depression (i.e., <3 months) recovered like nondepressed patients. Half of the patients with major depression and initial ADL impairment had poor outcomes, whereas none of the nondepressed patients had a poor ADL outcome. Thus, major depression had a deleterious effect on both psychosocial and ADL outcome. The negative impact of depression on recovery from brain injury has been observed in other groups of patients. For example, Gillen et al. (2001) reported that stroke patients with higher levels of depressive symptoms used rehabilitation services less efficiently than those with lower levels. In addition, a history of depression was associated with longer hospital stays. Rappaport et al. (2003) found that 22 patients with major depression after mild TBI had poorer outcome on the Neurobehavioral Rating Scale and Glasgow Outcome Scale than 130 mild TBI patients without depression. It is conceivable that depression negatively influences patients' participation in rehabilitation efforts and social interaction early during their course of recovery and that depressed patients are unable to recover these early losses, even when the depression is over.

Finally, assessment of negative outcome after TBI must include suicide. Suicidal ideation, suicide attempts, and completed suicides have all been shown to occur more frequently in patients with TBI compared with non-brain-injured control subjects (Oquendo et al. 2004; Silver et al. 2001; Teasdale and Engberg 2001). Teasdale et al. (2001) found that patients with concussion (N=126,114), cranial fracture (N=7,650), or cerebral contusion or traumatic hemorrhage (N=11,766) had mortality ratios from suicide that were, respectively, 3.0, 2.7, and 4.1 times the general population rate. Similarly, Silver et al. (2001) found that among 5,034 individuals in a community sample from New Haven, 361 patients had a significantly higher lifetime risk of suicide attempts compared to those without head injury. Finally, Oquendo et al. (2004) found that among 325 patients hospitalized

for unipolar or bipolar depression, those with mild TBI (N=109) were more likely to have attempted suicide (60% vs. 47%) than patients without a history of TBI. The strongest predictors of suicide attempts among the TBI survivors were strong feelings of hostility and aggression.

Treatment of Mood Disorders

Treatment of psychiatric disorders occurring after TBI involves different pharmacological and nonpharmacological strategies. Therapeutic interventions may be implemented at different points in the pathophysiological process initiated by brain trauma. One would assume that treatment of the neurobehavioral consequences of TBI should begin early in the acute phase after injury. If it is possible to modify the processes associated with neuronal damage, the intervention should be started as early as possible. Doing so would presumably lead to the greatest amount of recovery in cognition, motivation, activity levels, and emotional disorder. For instance, if one prevents the occurrence of excitotoxic injury to the hippocampus, one attenuates memory deficits and emotional dysregulation associated with hippocampal damage.

Despite the progress observed in elucidating neuronal pathologic mechanisms at a biomolecular level, however, therapeutic interventions based on experimental models have been disappointing. For instance, although calcium kinetics and the production of reactive oxygen species have been consistently implicated in cellular injury, controlled trials have shown no clinical benefit from calcium channel blockers or reactive oxygen species scavenger agents. Further interventions at different points in the pathological cascades (e.g., inhibition of caspases) might be more successful (McIntosh et al. 1998).

Although progress in basic research allows us to envision a promising future for therapeutic intervention after TBI, there is a lack of adequately controlled clinical studies, which are needed to provide a solid scientific basis for neuropsychiatric treatment. Currently, only anecdotal cases and clinical experience support many of our daily treatment decisions.

Patients with brain injury are more sensitive to the side effects of medications, especially psychotropics. Silver et al. (1991) proposed several general guidelines for their use in this population. Doses of psychotropics must be prudently increased, minimizing side effects (i.e., "start low, go slow"). However, the patient must receive an adequate therapeutic trial with regard to dosage and duration of treatment. Brain-injured patients must be frequently reassessed to determine changes in treatment schedules. Special care must be taken in monitoring drug interactions. Finally, if there is evidence of a partial response to a specific medication, augmentation therapy may be warranted, depending on the augmenting drug's mechanism of action and potential side effects.

To our knowledge, there have been no double-blind, placebo-controlled studies of the efficacy of pharmacological treatments of depression in patients with acute TBI.

There is some preliminary evidence that desipramine may be effective for treating depression in patients with severe TBI (Wroblewski et al. 1996). An 8-week, nonrandomized, placebo run-in trial of sertraline in 15 patients with mild TBI showed statistically significant improvement in psychological distress, anger, and aggression as well as in the severity of postconcussive symptoms (Fann et al. 2001). Sertraline may also lead to a beneficial effect on cognitive functioning (Fann et al. 2000).

Selection among competing antidepressants is usually guided by their side-effect profiles. Mild anticholinergic activity, minimal lowering of seizure threshold, and low sedative effects are the most important factors to be considered in the choice of an antidepressant drug in this population (Silver et al. 1990). Tricyclic antidepressants have important anticholinergic effects that may interfere with cognitive and memory functions. In addition, they may lower the seizure threshold. If, however, a decision is made to administer tricyclic antidepressants, nortriptyline (starting at 10 mg/day) constitutes a reasonable alternative, provided that blood levels and toxic effects are carefully monitored (Silver et al. 1990). Selective serotonin reuptake inhibitors are antidepressants that appear to have a less adverse side-effect profile. The most common side effects include headache, gastrointestinal complaints, insomnia, diminished libido, and sexual dysfunction. S-citalopram (starting at 5 mg/day), sertraline (starting at 25 mg/day), or paroxetine (starting at 5–10 mg/day) are among the most useful drugs in this group. Trazodone and nefazodone are alternative antidepressants that block 5-HT_2 receptors and also inhibit serotonin reuptake. These can be useful for the treatment of patients with prominent anxiety symptoms and sleep disturbance. Nefazodone dosage should be gradually increased from 100 mg/day to 500 mg/day. Trazodone is also started at low doses (50–100 mg) at bedtime after a snack. The dose may be gradually increased every 3–4 days up to 400 mg. The most troublesome side effects are sedation and orthostatic hypotension (Silver et al. 1990).

There are case reports of successful treatments of post-TBI depression with psychostimulants (Zasler 1992), including dextroamphetamine (8–60 mg/day) and methylphenidate (10–60 mg/day). Stimulants might also be useful to treat deficits in attention and apathetic symptoms that are frequently seen in patients with TBI. How-ever, the magnitude and temporal course of their therapeutic effect is still a matter of controversy. Stimulants are usually given twice a day, with the last dose given at least 6 hours before sleep to prevent initial insomnia. Treatment is begun at lower doses that are later gradually increased. Patients taking stimulants need close medical observation to prevent abuse or toxic effects. The most common side effects are anxiety, dysphoria, headaches, irritability, anorexia, insomnia, cardiovascular symptoms, dyskinesias, and even psychotic symptoms (Zasler 1992).

Amantadine, a drug with complex pharmacologic effects on dopaminergic, cholinergic, and N-methyl-D-aspartate receptors, might be of some use for the treatment of motivational deficits. It is usually started at low dosages (50 mg bid) and gradually increased to 200 mg bid. There is also some empirical evidence of the beneficial effects of cholinesterase inhibitors such as donepezil on cognitive functioning, motivation, and general well-being. The dosage range is 5–10 mg/day, and the more common side effects are insomnia, diarrhea, and dizziness. These side effects are usually transient and may be minimized by a gradual increase in dosage (Masanic et al. 2001).

Electroconvulsant therapy is not contraindicated in TBI patients and may be considered if other methods of treatment prove to be unsuccessful. Electroconvulsant therapy should be administered with the lowest possible effective energy, using pulsatile, nondominant, unilateral currents, with an interval of 2–5 days between treatments and four to six treatments for a complete course.

Buspirone, a drug that has an agonist effect on 5-HT_1 receptors and an antagonist effect on D_2 dopaminergic receptors, has proved to be a safe and efficacious anxiolytic. Initial dosing is 15 mg/day given in three divided doses, and the dosage may gradually be increased (5 mg every 4 days) to 60 mg/day. The most common side effects are dizziness and headaches (Gualtieri 1991).

Finally, we have already mentioned the role that social intervention and adequate psychotherapeutic support may play in the treatment of depression after TBI (Prigatano 1991; Sbordone 1990). There have been no systematic studies of the treatment of secondary mania. There are, however, several reports of potentially useful treatment modalities. Bakchine et al. (1989) conducted a double-blind, placebo-controlled study in a single patient with secondary mania after TBI. Clonidine (600 μg/day) was effective in reverting manic symptoms, carbamazepine (CBZ; 1,200 mg/day) did not elicit mood changes, and levodopa/benserazide (375 mg/day) resulted in an increase of manic symptoms.

Lithium (Starkstein et al. 1987), CBZ (Bouvy et al. 1988), and valproate (Kim and Humaran 2002; Pope et al. 1988) therapies have also been reported to be efficacious in individual cases. Lithium has been reported to impair cognitive performance in traumatic-brain-injured patients (Hornstein and Seliger 1989). In addition, it may lower the seizure threshold. Some authors limit its use to patients in whom bipolar disorder preceded the onset of TBI (Silver et al. 1990). The mood stabilizer and anticonvulsant CBZ should be gradually increased to obtain therapeutic blood levels (8–12 μg/mL). Complete blood counts should be obtained every 2 weeks for the first 2 months of therapy and every 3 months thereafter. Liver function tests should be obtained every 3 months. Frequent side effects include sedation, dry mouth, gastrointestinal upset, drowsiness, impaired concentration, ataxia, nystagmus, and rash. Severe complications include pancytopenia, aplastic anemia, and cholestatic jaundice. Valproic acid may be progressively increased from 500 mg/day to the dose necessary to obtain plasma levels between 50 and 100 μg/mL. The maximum recommended dosage is 60 mg/kg/day divided into two to four doses. Valproic acid may have potentially serious side effects, including hepatotoxicity that ranges from a discrete elevation of transaminases and serum ammonia levels to irreversible liver failure. Hemorrhagic pancreatitis has also been reported. The most common side effects are drowsiness, tremor, gastritis, and increased weight. Liver function tests and serum amylase levels should be monitored. The role of other anticonvulsants such as lamotrigine and topiramate as mood stabilizers has not been tested in TBI populations.

Finally, pathological emotions may respond to treatment with antidepressants (Robinson et al. 1993; Schiffer et al. 1985; Seliger et al. 1991). There is, however, a great variability in treatment response among brain-injured patients, with some showing a rapid response at relatively low dosages and others requiring more time and higher dosages.

From this discussion of therapeutic interventions, it is obvious that treatment options are based on logic and current standards of practice rather than empirically based controlled treatment trials. There is a great need for randomized, double-blind, placebo-controlled trials to establish the most effective treatments for the variety of mood disorders that occurs in TBI patients.

References

American Psychiatric Association: Diagnostic and Statistical Manual of Mental Disorders, 3rd Edition, Revised. Washington, DC, American Psychiatric Association, 1987

American Psychiatric Association: Diagnostic and Statistical Manual of Mental Disorders, 4th Edition. Washington, DC, American Psychiatric Association, 1994

American Psychiatric Association: Diagnostic and Statistical Manual of Mental Disorders, 4th Edition, Text Revision. Washington, DC, American Psychiatric Association, 2000

Ashton D, Willems R, Wynants J, et al: Altered sodium channel function as an in vitro model of the ischemic penumbra: action of lubeluzole and other neuroprotective drugs. Brain Res 745:210–221, 1997

Bakchine S, Lacomblez L, Benoit N, et al: Manic-like state after orbitofrontal and right temporoparietal injury: efficacy of clonidine. Neurology 39:777–781, 1989

Bamrah JS, Johnson J: Bipolar affective disorder following head injury. Br J Psychiatry 258:117–119, 1980

Bareyre FM, Saatman KE, Raghupathi R, et al: Postinjury treatment with magnesium chloride attenuates cortical damage after traumatic brain injury in rats. J Neurotrauma 17:1029–1039, 2000

Bouvy PF, Van de Wetering BJM, Meerwaldt JD, et al: A case of organic brain syndrome following head injury successfully treated with carbamazepine. Acta Psychiatr Scand 77:361–363, 1988

Clark RS, Kochanek PM, Watkins SC, et al: Caspase-3 mediated neuronal death after traumatic brain injury in rats. J Neurochem 74:740–753, 2000

Corn TH, Checkley SA: A case of recurrent mania with recurrent hyperthyroidism. Br J Psychiatry 143:74–76, 1983

Cummings JL, Kaufer D: Neuropsychiatric aspects of Alzheimer's disease: the cholinergic hypothesis revisited. Neurology 47:876–883, 1996

Cummings JL, Mendez MF: Secondary mania with focal cerebrovascular lesions. Am J Psychiatry 141:1084–1087, 1984

Davidson J, Turnbull CD: Diagnostic significance of vegetative symptoms in depression. Br J Psychiatry 148:442–446, 1986

Dixon CE, Bao J, Long DA, et al: Reduced evoked release of acetylcholine in the rodent hippocampus following traumatic brain injury. Pharmacol Biochem Behav 53:679–686, 1996

Fann JR, Katon WJ, Uomoto JM, et al: Psychiatric disorders and functional disability in outpatients with traumatic brain injuries. Am J Psychiatry 152:1493–1499, 1995

Fann JR, Uomoto JM, Katon WJ: Sertraline in the treatment of major depression following mild traumatic brain injury. J Neuropsychiatry Clin Neurosci 12:226–232, 2000

Fann JR, Uomoto JM, Katon WJ: Cognitive improvement with treatment of depression following mild traumatic brain injury. Psychosomatics 42:48–54, 2001

Fedoroff JP, Starkstein SE, Forrester AW, et al: Depression in patients with acute traumatic brain injury. Am J Psychiatry 149:918–923, 1992

Gillen R, Tennen H, McKee TE, et al: Depressive symptoms and history of depression predict rehabilitation efficiency in stroke patients. Arch Phys Med Rehabil 82:1645–1649, 2001

Goggan FC: A case of mania secondary to vitamin B-12 deficiency. Am J Psychiatry 141:300–301, 1984

Grafman J, Vance SC, Swingartner H: The effects of lateralized frontal lesions on mood regulation. Brain 109:1127–1148, 1986

Graham DI, McIntosh TK, Maxwell WL, et al: Recent advances in neurotrauma. J Neuropathol Exp Neurol 59:641–651, 2000

Gualtieri CT: Buspirone: neuropsychiatric effects. J Head Trauma Rehabil 6:90–92, 1991

Gualtieri CT, Cox DR: The delayed neurobehavioral sequelae of traumatic brain injury. Brain Inj 5:219–232, 1991

Hamill RW, Woolf PD, McDonald JV, et al: Catecholamines predict outcome in traumatic brain injury. Ann Neurol 21:438–443, 1987

Hibbard MR, Uysal S, Kepler K, et al: Axis I psychopathology in individuals with traumatic brain injury. J Head Trauma Rehabil 13:24–39, 1998

Holsinger T, Steffens DC, Phillips C, et al: Head injury in early adulthood and the lifetime risk of depression. Arch Gen Psychiatry 59:17–22, 2002

Hornstein A, Seliger G: Cognitive side effects of lithium in closed head injury. J Neuropsychiatry Clin Neurosci 1:446–447, 1989

Isles LJ, Orrell MW: Secondary mania after open-heart surgery. Br J Psychiatry 159:280–282, 1991

Jorge RE, Robinson RG, Arndt SV: Are depressive symptoms specific for a depressed mood in traumatic brain injury? J Nerv Ment Dis 181:91–99, 1993a

Jorge RE, Robinson RG, Arndt SV, et al: Comparison between acute- and delayed-onset depression following traumatic brain injury. J Neuropsychiatry Clin Neurosci 5:43–49, 1993b

Jorge RE, Robinson RG, Arndt SV, et al: Depression following traumatic brain injury: a 1 year longitudinal study. J Affect Disord 27:233–243, 1993c

Jorge RE, Robinson RG, Starkstein SE, et al: Depression and anxiety following traumatic brain injury. J Neuropsychiatry Clin Neurosci 5:369–374, 1993d

Jorge RE, Robinson RG, Starkstein SE, et al: Secondary mania following traumatic brain injury. Am J Psychiatry 150:916–921, 1993e

Jorge RE, Robinson RG, Starkstein SE, et al: Influence of major depression on 1 year outcome in patients with traumatic brain injury. J Neurosurg 81:726–733, 1994

Jorge RE, Robinson RG, Moser D, et al: Major depression following traumatic brain injury. Arch Gen Psychiatry 61:42–50, 2004

Kant R, Duffy JD, Pivovarnik A: Prevalence of apathy following head injury. Brain Inj 12:87–92, 1998

Kim E, Humaran TJ: Divalproex in the management of neuropsychiatric complications of remote acquired brain injury. J Neuropsychiatry Clin Neurosci 14:202–205, 2002

Kinsella G, Moran C, Ford B: Emotional disorders and its assessment within the severe head injured population. Psychol Med 18:57–63, 1988

Koponen S, Taiminen T, Portin R, et al: Axis I and II psychiatric disorders after traumatic brain injury: a 30 year follow-up study. Am J Psychiatry 159:1315–1321, 2002

Kreutzer JS, Seel RT, Gourley E: The prevalence and symptom rates of depression after traumatic brain injury: a comprehensive examination. Brain Inj 15:563–576, 2001

Leonard JR, Grady MS, Lee ME, et al: Fluid percussion injury cause disruption of the septohippocampal pathway in the rat. Exp Neurol 143:177–187, 1997

Levin HS, Grossman RG: Behavioral sequelae of closed head injury: a quantitative study. Arch Neurol 35:720–727, 1978

Lishman WA: Brain damage in relation to psychiatric disability after head injury. Br J Psychiatry 114:373–410, 1968

Lishman WA: Physiogenesis and psychogenesis in the post-concussional syndrome. Br J Psychiatry 153:460–469, 1988

Luukinen H, Viramo P, Koski K, et al: Head injuries and cognitive decline among older adults: a population-based study. Neurology 52:557–562, 1999

Lyeth BG, Hayes RL: Cholinergic and opioid mediation of traumatic brain injury. J Neurotrauma 9:S463–S474, 1992

Marin RS, Fogel BS, Hawkins J, et al: Apathy: a treatable syndrome. J Neuropsychiatry Clin Neurosci 7:23–30, 1995

Markianos M, Seretis A, Kotsou S, et al: CSF transmitter metabolites and short term outcome of patients in coma after head injury. Acta Neurol Scand 86:190–193, 1992

Masanic CA, Bayley MT, VanReekum R, et al: Open-label study of donepezil in traumatic brain injury. Arch Phys Med Rehabil 82:896–901, 2001

McHugh PR, Slavney PR: The Perspectives of Psychiatry. Baltimore, MD, Johns Hopkins University Press, 1998

McIntosh TK, Juhler M, Wieloch T: Novel pharmacologic strategies in the treatment of experimental traumatic brain injury: 1998. J Neurotrauma 15:731–769, 1998

McKinlay WW, Brooks DN, Bond MR, et al: The short-term outcome of severe blunt head injury as reported by the relatives of the head injury person. J Neurol Neurosurg Psychiatry 44:527–533, 1981

Nakagawa Y, Nakamura M, McIntosh TK, et al: Traumatic brain injury in young, amyloid-beta peptide overexpressing transgenic mice induces marked ipsilateral hippocampal atrophy and diminished Abeta deposition during aging. J Comp Neurol 411:390–398, 1999

Oquendo MA, Friedman JH, Grunebaum MF, et al: Suicidal behavior and mild traumatic brain injury in major depression. J Nerv Ment Dis 192:430–434, 2004

Palmer AM, Marion DW, Botscheller ML, et al: Increased transmitter amino acid concentration in human ventricular CSF after brain trauma. Neuroreport 6:153–156, 1994

Pope HG, McElroy SL, Satlin A, et al: Head injury, bipolar disorder and response to valproate. Compr Psychiatry 29:34–38, 1988

Prigatano GP: Disordered mind, wounded soul: the emerging role of psychotherapy in rehabilitation after brain injury. J Head Trauma Rehabil 6:1–10, 1991

Raghupathi R, Graham DI, McIntosh TK: Apoptosis after traumatic brain injury. J Neurotrauma 17:927–38, 2000

Rappaport MJ, McCullagh S, Streiner D, et al: The clinical significance of major depression following mild traumatic brain injury. Psychosomatics 44:31–37, 2003

Robinson RG, Boston JD, Starkstein SE, et al: Comparison of mania with depression following brain injury: casual factors. Am J Psychiatry 145:172–178, 1988

Robinson RG, Parikh RM, Lipsey JR, et al: Pathological laughing and crying following stroke: validation of measurement scale and double-blind treatment study. Am J Psychiatry 150:286–293, 1993

Rosenthal M, Christensen BK, Ross TP: Depression following traumatic brain injury. Arch Phys Med Rehabil 79:90–103, 1998

Rutherford WH, Merrett JD, McDonald JR: Sequelae of concussion caused by minor head injuries. Lancet 1:1–4, 1977

Sbordone RJ: Psychotherapeutic treatment of the client with traumatic brain injury: a conceptual model, in Community Integration Following Traumatic Brain Injury. Edited by Kreutzer JS, Wehman P. Paul H. Baltimore, MD, Brookes Publishing, 1990

Schiffer RB, Herndon RM, Rudick RA: Treatment of pathological laughing and weeping with amitriptyline. N Engl J Med 312:1480–1482, 1985

Schmidt RH, Grady MS: Loss of forebrain cholinergic neurons following fluid-percussion injury: implications for cognitive impairment in closed head injury. J Neurosurg 83:496–502, 1995

Schoenhuber R, Gentilini M: Anxiety and depression after mild head injury: a case control study. J Neurol Neurosurg Psychiatry 51:722–724, 1988

Seliger GM, Hornstein A, Flax J, et al: Fluoxetine improves emotional incontinence. Brain Inj 6:267–270, 1991

Shukla S, Cook BL, Mukherjee S, et al: Mania following head trauma. Am J Psychiatry 144:93–96, 1987

Silver JM, Hales RE, Yudofsky SC: Psychopharmacology of depression in neurologic disorders. J Clin Psychiatry 51:33–39, 1990

Silver JM, Yudofsky SC, Hales RE: Depression in traumatic brain injury. Neuropsychiatry Neuropsychol Behav Neurol 4:12–23, 1991

Silver JM, Kramer R, Greenwald S, et al: The association between head injuries and psychiatric disorders: findings from the New Haven NIMH Epidemiologic Catchment Area Study. Brain Inj 15 (11):935–945, 2001

Starkstein SE, Pearlson GD, Boston J, et al: Mania after brain injury: a controlled study of causative factors. Arch Neurol 44:1069–1073, 1987

Starkstein SE, Federoff JP, Price TR, et al: Apathy following cerebrovascular lesions. Stroke 24:1625–1630, 1993

Stutzmann JM, Doble A: Blockade of glutaminergic transmission and neuroprotection: the strange case of riluzole, in Neurodegenerative Disease. Edited by Jolles G, Stutzmann JM. New York, Academic Press, 1995, pp 205–214

Tateno A, Jorge RE, Robinson RG: Clinical correlates of aggressive behavior after traumatic brain injury. J Neuropsychiatry Clin Neurosci 15:155–160, 2003

Tateno A, Jorge RE, Robinson RG: Pathological laughing and crying following traumatic brain injury. J Neuropsychiatry Clin Neurosci (in press)

Teasdale TW, Engberg AW: Suicide after traumatic brain injury: a population study. J Neurol Neurosurg Psychiatry 71 (4):436–440, 2001

Thienhaus OJ, Kosla N: Meningeal cryptococcosis misdiagnosed as a manic episode. Am J Psychiatry 141:1459–1460, 1984

Thomas CS, Neale TJ: Organic manic syndrome associated with advanced uraemia due to polycystic kidney disease. Br J Psychiatry 158:119–121, 1991

Varney NR, Martzke JS, Roberts RJ: Major depression in patients with closed head injury. Neuropsychology 1:7–9, 1987

Wroblewski BA, Joseph AB, Cornblatt RR: Antidepressant pharmacotherapy and the treatment of depression in patients with severe traumatic brain injury: a controlled, prospective study. J Clin Psychiatry 57:582–587, 1996

Yasuda S, Wehman P, Targett P, et al: Return to work for persons with traumatic brain injury Am J Phys Med Rehabil 80:852–864, 2001

Zasler ND: Advances in neuropharmacological rehabilitation for brain dysfunction. Brain Inj 6:1–14, 1992

11 Psychotic Disorders

Cheryl Corcoran, M.D.

Thomas W. McAllister, M.D.

Dolores Malaspina, M.D.

AN ASSOCIATION BETWEEN traumatic brain injuries (TBIs) and later serious psychopathology, including psychosis, has been observed since the nineteenth century (von Krafft-Ebing 1868). Early in the twentieth century, Adolf Meyer's 1904 paper on what he termed "traumatic insanity" (Meyer 1904) gave credence to the idea that trauma to the brain could result in significant psychopathology, including psychosis. He also emphasized that many of his patients had preexisting psychiatric disturbances or family histories of psychiatric illness, or both. Shortly thereafter, Emil Kraepelin hypothesized that head injuries in childhood might either cause or release predisposition to schizophrenia, implicating a causative role for TBI in psychotic illness (Kraepelin 1919).

The establishment of an association between TBI and psychosis is important because it has implications for the prevention of psychotic disorders, and it may shed light on the pathophysiology of both psychosis and TBI. In fact, there is extensive evidence of such an association between TBI and psychosis, as psychotic symptoms are consistently found to occur more frequently in individuals who have had a TBI, and patients with psychotic disorders are consistently more likely to have had a prior TBI than the general population. Although psychosis is not among the most common psychiatric sequelae of TBI, it

is a disturbing and disabling outcome with great morbidity and cost. One to two million people incur a TBI in the United States each year: these individuals have a two- to fivefold greater risk of developing psychosis than does the general population (Ahmed and Fujii 1998).

Psychosis is a plausible outcome of severe brain injury. Individuals are at greatest risk for a TBI between their mid-teens and mid-20s, before the onset of most psychotic disorders, with males having a several-fold higher risk for TBI than females (Jager et al. 2000). Also, key brain regions implicated in the etiology of psychosis (and schizophrenia), such as the prefrontal cortex, temporal lobes, and hippocampus, are particularly vulnerable to TBI. The bony protrusions adjacent to the orbitofrontal and anterior temporal lobes render these areas vulnerable to damage from the differential motion of the brain within the fixed skull. Axons are stretched and sheared from the rotation of the brain, which may injure important corticocortical pathways. Secondary damage to the hippocampus remote from the point of impact in TBI is particularly evident from both human and animal studies.

In this chapter, we review 1) diagnostic issues in relation to TBI and psychotic illness, 2) follow-up studies of psychosis in individuals who have incurred TBI (with an examination of factors that may predict later psychosis af-

This work was supported in part by the National Alliance for Research on Schizophrenia and Depression (Dr. Corcoran); by National Institute on Disability and Rehabilitation Research grants H133G70031 and H133000136, National Institutes of Health grant R01 NS40472–01, the Ira DeCamp Foundation, and New Hampshire Hospital (Dr. McAllister); and by the G. Harold and Leila Y. Mathers Charitable Foundation and National Institute of Mental Health grants R01 MH50727, U01 MH46289, and K24 MH01699 (Dr. Malaspina).

ter TBI), 3) assessments of rates of premorbid TBI in patients with psychosis (with a look at how these patient groups may differ), 4) similarities between psychotic disorders and TBI, 5) the neurobiology of TBI and how it might lead to psychosis, 6) vulnerable populations, and 7) assessment, treatment, and prevention strategies.

Diagnosis

According to DSM-IV-TR (Andreasen et al. 2000), the term *psychosis* has historically meant different things, and as yet there is no universal acceptance for any one definition. Different definitions have included "loss of ego boundaries," "gross impairment in reality testing," and even "impairment that grossly interferes with the capacity to meet ordinary demands of life." Over time, the concept of psychosis has been operationalized and more strictly defined, as reflected in DSM-IV-TR (American Psychiatric Association 2000). In its narrowest sense, psychosis is presently defined as the presence of delusions or hallucinations, without insight that the hallucinations are pathological in nature. This definition of psychosis is used for "psychosis due to a general medical condition." A broader sense of psychosis is drawn from the positive symptoms of schizophrenia, which extend beyond delusions and hallucinations to encompass disorganized speech and grossly disorganized or catatonic behavior.

Posttraumatic psychosis is a generic term for psychotic illness in a person who has experienced brain trauma. It is an empirical description that denotes a temporal rather than a causal relationship. Posttraumatic psychosis is not itself a DSM-IV-TR diagnosis, so in any given individual, this phenomenon falls either under the rubric of "psychotic disorder due to a medical condition" or a primary psychotic disorder. The boundaries between these choices are blurred, and the diagnosis can be ambiguous, as it is often not easy to ascertain that the psychotic disorder is caused by the TBI.

The DSM-IV-TR criteria for psychotic disorder due to a general medical condition are shown in Table 11–1. To meet the criteria, the psychotic disturbance must be etiologically related to the general medical condition through a physiological mechanism. According to DSM-IV-TR:

> A careful and comprehensive assessment of multiple factors is necessary to make this judgment. Although there are no infallible guidelines for determining whether the relationship between the psychotic disturbance and the general medical condition is etiological, several considerations provide some guidance in this area. One con-

TABLE 11–1.   DSM-IV-TR criteria for psychotic disorder due to a general medical condition

A. Prominent hallucinations or delusions.

B. There is evidence from the history, physical examination, or laboratory findings that the disturbance is the direct physiological consequence of a general medical condition.

C. The disturbance is not better accounted for by another mental disorder.

D. The disturbance does not occur exclusively during the course of a delirium.

Code on the basis of predominant symptom:

With Delusions: if delusions are the predominant symptom

With Hallucinations: if hallucinations are the predominant symptom

Source.   Reprinted from *Diagnostic and Statistical Manual of Mental Disorders*, 4th Edition, Text Revision. Washington, DC, American Psychiatric Association, 2000. Copyright 2000, American Psychiatric Association. Used with permission.

sideration is the presence of a temporal association between the onset, exacerbation, or remission of the general medical condition and that of the psychotic disturbance. A second consideration is the presence of features that are atypical for a primary psychotic disorder (e.g., atypical age at onset or presence of visual or olfactory hallucinations). Evidence from the literature that suggests that there can be a direct association between the general medical condition in question and the development of psychotic symptoms can provide a useful context in the assessment of a particular situation. In addition, the clinician must also judge that the disturbance is not better accounted for by a primary Psychotic Disorder, a Substance-Induced Psychotic Disorder, or another primary mental disorder. (American Psychiatric Association 2000, p. 335)

Establishing a diagnosis of psychotic disorder due to a general medical condition (TBI) can be uncertain for a number of reasons. First, the temporal association may not be entirely clear. DSM-IV-TR does not specify an appropriate time delay between the general medical condition and psychosis. Existing literature suggests that psychosis may follow a TBI months to years later. For example, in a series of case reports of patients with schizophrenia and premorbid TBI, the onset of psychosis occurred, respectively, 1, 9, 7, 16, and 11 years after TBI was incurred (Buckley et al. 1993). A retrospective case-control study of 45 patients with posttraumatic psychosis showed a mean latency of 54.7 months from time of injury to onset of psychosis. A follow-up study of brain-injured World

War II veterans found that psychosis occurred from 2 days to 48 years later, with 42% of those studied experiencing their first psychotic episode more than 10 years after the brain injury (Achte et al. 1969). Other latency periods from brain injury to psychosis include a mean of 5.9 years (range, 3 months to 19 years) (Fujii and Ahmed 1996), 4.6 years (range, 0 to 15 years) (Fujii and Ahmed 2001), and 4.6 years (range, 2 weeks to 17 years) (Sachdev et al. 2001).

Second, although atypical psychotic features may suggest an etiological role for TBI in the psychosis of some individuals, the absence of these features does not rule out TBI as a causative factor. That is, atypical psychotic features have specificity but not sensitivity for determining posttraumatic psychosis. There is evidence to suggest that atypical features of psychosis such as olfactory and tactile hallucinations, and misidentification syndromes such as Capgras syndrome may follow a TBI. However, there is also evidence, as described below, that posttraumatic psychoses may be phenomenologically indistinguishable from a primary mental disorder, such as schizophrenia, and may be better accounted for by a primary psychotic disorder. According to DSM-IV-TR, in those cases, primary mental disorder, and not psychotic disorder due to a medical condition, should be diagnosed (American Psychiatric Association 2000). It is important to keep in mind, however, that TBI may contribute to the etiology of primary mental disorders, which are complex disorders that result from interactions of genes and environment.

Third, evidence of a correlation between TBI and subsequent psychosis in the existing literature is strong, though not definitive. Schizophrenia and other primary psychotic disorders are complex heterogeneous illnesses that arise from the interaction of multiple etiologies, including genes, obstetric complications, and other exposures. TBI may be an etiological factor with small or large effects, depending on inherent genetic vulnerability and other exposures.

Therefore, it is difficult to discern that any case of posttraumatic psychosis is directly caused by TBI, and the diagnosis of primary psychotic disorder versus psychotic disorder due to a general medical condition is a difficult diagnosis to make. In any given individual, TBI and later psychosis may be 1) etiologically related (i.e., TBI contributes to the psychosis), 2) independent and unrelated phenomena, or 3) two conditions that result from a separate third factor (i.e., the neuromotor incoordination inherent in vulnerability to schizophrenia could predispose an individual both to incurring TBI and psychosis). Having relatives with schizophrenia increases one's risk for both incurring TBI and for developing schizophrenia, but then exposure to TBI further

elevates the risk for schizophrenia in individuals with a family history (Malaspina et al. 2001). In such a complex disorder, it is difficult, if not impossible, to determine that psychosis is the direct physiological consequence of TBI.

Efforts to Validate the Diagnosis of Psychosis Due to a General Medical Condition

Feinstein and Ron (1998) followed a cohort of 44 patients over 4 years in an effort to determine the predictive and construct validity of the diagnosis of psychosis due to a general medical condition. Participants had 1) a neurological disorder known to involve the brain, 2) delusions and/or hallucinations, 3) an absence of delirium, and 4) an absence of prominent and persistent mood symptoms. Epilepsy was the most common neurological condition. Subjects were recruited from psychiatry departments in urban hospitals and were approximately 50% male, with a mean age of 39.3 ± 13.3 years. There was no control group of either neurological patients without psychosis or individuals with psychosis without neurological disorder. However, the authors argued that the disorder of psychosis due to a general medical condition was differentiated from schizophrenia by 1) later mean age at onset of psychosis (approximately age 35 years), 2) fewer premorbid schizoid and paranoid personality traits, 3) lower incidence of having a first-degree relative with schizophrenia (7%), 4) briefer duration of psychosis, 5) more rapid response to low-dose neuroleptics, 6) less need for maintenance neuroleptics, and 7) better outcome with greater return to premorbid work levels. In sum, there may be group differences between this patient group and psychotic patients without a diagnosis of neurological disorder, but there is substantial overlap in characteristics of these two groups.

Follow-Up Studies of Psychosis After TBI

Many studies have attempted to explore the link between brain injury and psychosis since Kraepelin (1919) first proposed that such injury might cause dementia praecox. Together, these studies offer substantial evidence of increased rates of psychosis among those exposed to TBI. However, the reported rates vary greatly, and many of these studies have methodological problems, such as the absence of clear diagnostic criteria. Kornilov (1980) followed 340 patients with brain injury and found "psychotic symptoms" and a "personality transformation" consistent with negative symptoms in 26.5% of these patients. In a 10- to 15-year follow-up study of 40 patients who incurred severe TBI, 20% were found to develop posttraumatic psychosis (Thomsen 1984). However, the criteria for psychosis were not defined; rather, patients were described as having regression, impulsivity, and aggression. Of note, hallucinations and delusions were not mentioned. However, many patients had features characteristic of the deficit symptoms of schizophrenia, including loss of social contact (68%), lack of interest (55%), aspontaneity (53%), slowness (53%), and speech abnormalities (Thomsen 1984). In an earlier study of Finnish veterans that also did not use standardized criteria, 7.95% of 415 soldiers with a brain injury went on to develop posttraumatic psychosis (Hillbom 1960). Approximately one-third of the posttraumatic psychosis group had a clinical picture resembling schizophrenia, with paranoia and hallucinations. A significant percentage (40%) of the group had sustained temporal lobe injuries.

A much lower rate of posttraumatic psychosis is found when using more contemporary diagnostic criteria. In a retrospective chart review study of 670 World War II British soldiers with penetrating head injuries (Lishman 1968) only 5 of the veterans (0.7%) developed psychosis during the 4 years of follow-up. This study was among the first to use contemporary diagnostic criteria, and, notably, mood disorders, dementias, and amnestic disorders were counted separately. The patients were all evaluated and treated at the same head injury unit, and vigorous efforts were made to follow up the patients, with annual questionnaires sent to patients, relatives, employers, general practitioners, and social service agencies. However, patients with psychosis were not contrasted with other groups, and the follow-up period was only 4 years. Furthermore, the focus on penetrating brain injuries may limit the generalizability of the results to those with more diffuse injuries.

An analysis of consolidated data from eight long-term follow-up studies published between 1917 and 1964 yielded an overall rate of psychosis after brain trauma of 0.7%–9.8%, with a median of 1.35% (Davison and Bagley 1969). The subjects of these reports ranged from civilians who incurred concussions to soldiers who experienced combat injury. Different diagnostic criteria were used, and follow-ups ranged from as little as 3 months to more than 20 years. The two lowest rates of posttraumatic psychosis resulted from two studies with follow-ups of only 3 months and 2 years. Davison and Bagley (1969) noted that the incidence of psychosis increased over time and that many individuals did not become psychotic until years after the injury. In comparing this range of 0.7%–9.8% (with a median of 1.35%) to the 0.8% lifetime incidence of psychosis in the general population over a period of 25 years, Davison and Bagley concluded that brain

trauma increased the observed incidence of psychosis by two- to threefold over a period of 10–20 years.

More recent studies report rates of posttraumatic psychosis that are in the range found by Davison and Bagley in their survey. For example, post-TBI psychosis was found in 7.6% of 10,000 veterans in a national Finnish cohort (Achte et al. 1991). Record review found posttraumatic delusional states in 3.4% of 530 patients on a neurosurgical unit in a Belgian hospital over a 1- to 10-year follow-up period (Violon and De Mol 1987). One-third of these posttraumatic delusional patients were reported to have a chronic course similar to schizophrenia, although none of the cases was fully described. Posttraumatic delusions were defined as "regressive or chronic acquired delusional states appearing after a head injury in non-demented patients."

As mentioned, the lower rates of posttraumatic psychosis in some of these studies may be due to a limited duration of follow-up, because the onset of psychosis can be remote from the injury, occurring months and even years later. Frequently, confounding variables, such as age, gender, and even exposure to war, were not controlled for. Furthermore, many studies had low statistical power and contained imprecise data on TBI exposure and diagnosis of subsequent psychiatric disorders. Investigators have only rarely been blind to proband status. Other likely sources of variance in these studies include case ascertainment strategies, retrospective versus prospective designs, inclusion of various categories of psychosis, and different methods of case evaluation.

Childhood TBI and Psychosis

Although Kraepelin (1919) suggested that brain injury during childhood may predispose an individual to psychosis, this has not been borne out by prospective studies of children incurring TBI, though it must be noted that only a few studies have been done and the time of follow-up in these studies was brief, on the order of 1–2 years. For example, in a prospective study of 32 children who had severe TBI (characterized by 7 days of posttraumatic amnesia [PTA]), only one child (3.2%) was observed to develop psychosis over a 2-year follow-up (Brown et al. 1981). No specific psychiatric diagnosis was given, though the patient was described as having agitation, flight of ideas, ideas of reference, silly giggling, grimacing, changed intonation of speech, and expression of odd ideas. Black et al. (1981) followed children with mild TBI for 1 year and found that 80% had no posttraumatic sequelae. However, this study did not use standardized psychiatric instruments. In 50 children ages 6–14 years who incurred TBI requiring hospitalization, Max et al.

(1997) found that after 2 years, predictors of a new psychiatric diagnosis included severity of brain injury, preinjury family function, and preinjury psychiatric history. Although their study was prospective and used standardized criteria, the follow-up was short. None of the children in this study became psychotic.

Comparisons Among Brain-Injured Patients With and Without Posttraumatic Psychosis

The follow-up studies of brain-injured adults described in the preceding sections suggest a posttraumatic incidence of psychosis that is greater than the incidence of psychosis in the general population. Newer studies have endeavored to characterize predictors of posttraumatic psychosis through the comparison of brain-injured individuals who go on to develop psychosis with those who do not.

Fujii and Ahmed (2001) performed a retrospective chart review of 25 state hospital inpatients with "psychosis secondary to TBI" compared with a control group of 21 outpatients with TBI but no psychosis, all of whom were selected through referral to a tertiary care center for neuropsychological evaluation. The diagnosis of "psychosis secondary to TBI" was made using criteria both from DSM-IV-TR (Andreasen et al. 2000) and additional criteria described by Cummings (1988). The criteria included: 1) hallucinations or delusions, 2) historical or laboratory evidence indicating the psychosis is the direct physiological consequence of the medical condition, 3) psychotic symptoms not better accounted for by another mental disorder, 4) psychotic symptoms not occurring exclusively within the course of delirium, 5) no family history of psychosis, 6) no prior history of psychosis, 7) a history of TBI, 8) onset of symptoms after TBI, and 9) the existence of cognitive deficits. Therefore, the authors endeavored to identify patients with clear psychosis due to a general medical condition, as described by DSM-IV-TR. It should be noted that 17 of these 25 patients had previously been diagnosed as having schizophrenia.

The study by Fujii and Ahmed (2001) did not identify any clear predictors of psychosis among brain-injured patients, as there was no difference between the groups with respect to handedness, IQ, socioeconomic status, average age for sustaining TBI, and type or severity of TBI. The study could not determine whether family history of psychosis was a predictor of posttraumatic psychosis, because this was an exclusion criterion. This study had a number of strengths, including its use of operationalized criteria for establishing posttraumatic psychosis and for determining severity of TBI. Furthermore, the time from TBI to assessment for the nonpsychotic group was long enough at a mean of 9.2 years (range, 1–23 years) to ensure that most of these individuals were truly control subjects and not brain-injured individuals who were yet to develop psychosis. However, patients and control subjects were not matched on age, gender, or ethnicity, so it is difficult to discern whether these may be confounding factors. For example, the patient group was comprised of 24 men and 1 woman, whereas the control subjects were 9 men and 12 women.

Sachdev et al. (2001) recently reported the results of a case-control study of 45 patients with "schizophrenia-like psychosis following TBI" and 45 brain-injured subjects without psychosis who were matched on gender, age at injury (± 1 year), current age (± 2 years), and time since injury (± 2 years). Participants were drawn from those referred to a tertiary care neuropsychiatry unit or from a medico-legal evaluation. "Schizophrenia-like psychosis following TBI" in this study was defined as 1) meeting DSM-IV-TR criteria A, B, C, and E for schizophreniform disorder or schizophrenia; 2) no past dementia, mania, major depression, or alcohol or drug dependence and no current delirium; and 3) history of TBI preceding psychosis that led to medical treatment and either loss of consciousness for more than 5 minutes or anterograde amnesia for more than 1 hour, as documented by an emergency medical technician or emergency department staff. Control subjects had experienced a TBI but had no history of psychosis, major depression, or drug or alcohol dependence.

The authors performed an extensive review of records pertaining to the TBI, psychotic phenomenology, birth and developmental history, psychiatric history, drug and alcohol use history, sociodemographics, family history of schizophrenia and other psychiatric disorders, and serial physical examinations. All participants had 1) a computed tomography (CT) scan that was reviewed for focal lesions and atrophy, diffuse atrophy, and ventricular dilatation and 2) neuropsychological testing that included assessments of IQ, verbal and nonverbal memory, frontal executive functioning, parietal functioning (constructional ability, agnosia, and apraxia), and language.

Type of injury, prior alcohol and drug use, and posttraumatic behavioral and personality changes did not differ between cases and control subjects (Sachdev et al. 2001). The major predictors of posttraumatic psychosis were a positive family history of schizophrenia and duration of loss of consciousness after the TBI. Compared with nonpsychotic brain-injured individuals, patients with posttraumatic psychosis were found to have 1) more evidence of left temporal damage on CT scan and 2) greater neuropsychological deficits, with lower IQ, worse verbal and visual memory, and language impairment. It could not be determined, of course, whether these factors preceded or resulted from the TBI. Strengths of this study include matching of age and gender in control subjects, use of operationalized criteria for TBI and "schizophrenia-like psychosis following TBI," consistent ascertainment of cases and control subjects, direct patient interviews and use of informants, and collection of both structural imaging and neuropsychological data (although neuroimaging data were qualitative and read by different radiologists and a standard neuropsychological battery was not used).

What Predicts Psychosis in Brain-Injured Individuals?

The preceding studies are the most recent and perhaps most methodologically sound attempts at clarifying the characteristics of injury that place someone at risk for developing psychosis after brain injury. A variety of other studies have looked at other specific factors that may contribute to the development of posttraumatic psychosis, including location and extent of injury, and genetic vulnerability.

Location of Injury

Accumulated evidence suggests that injuries to the left hemisphere and to the temporal lobes may be most closely associated with risk of posttraumatic psychosis (Davison and Bagley 1969). As noted, Sachdev et al. (2001) found that those with a TBI who developed psychosis had more CT scan evidence of brain damage, especially in the left temporal and parietal regions, than those who did not develop a psychosis, though this did not survive Bonferroni correction. In a logistic regression model, only left temporal damage significantly predicted the occurrence of psychosis after TBI. In an earlier study, Hillbom (1960) found that 40% of individuals with posttraumatic psychosis had temporal lobe injuries, a significantly higher occurrence than in those with nonpsychotic psychiatric disturbance. Of the group with psychosis, 63% had left-hemisphere injuries (a higher value than for nonpsychotic psychiatric disturbance), 26% had right-hemisphere lesions, and 11% had bilateral injuries. The individuals with schizophrenia-like syndromes had more severe injuries and were more likely to have left hemispheric injury.

Koufen and Hagel (1987) evaluated electroencephalographic abnormalities in a cohort of 100 patients with psychosis on a brain injury hospital ward and found that posttraumatic psychosis was associated with abnormal foci in the temporal lobes bilaterally in the majority of cases. However, in this study, psychosis was not well defined, and criteria for the diagnosis of posttraumatic psychosis were not well described.

The suggestion of a link between left-hemisphere injury, particularly of the temporal lobe, and psychosis is consistent with findings in other neurological disorders. Davison and Bagley (1969) found that in a series of 150 cases of schizophrenia-like psychoses related to diverse neurological disorders, the lesions were usually in the left hemisphere and temporal lobes.

Severity of Injury

Many studies have found that severity of TBI is related to risk of posttraumatic psychosis. As early as the 1960s, Davison and Bagley (1969) found in their review of eight studies that increased severity of injury with more diffuse brain damage and coma longer than 24 hours were risk factors for the development of posttraumatic psychosis. Thomsen (1984) also found a link between severity of brain injury and subsequent psychosis. Hillbom (1960) found that the rate of psychosis increased with the severity of the injury: 2.8% of those with mild injuries, 7.2% of those with medium-severity injuries, and 14.8% of those with severe injuries had become psychotic. Furthermore, in Hillbom's study, the patients who appeared to have schizophrenia had more severe injuries than the other patients with psychosis. These findings are corroborated by the more rigorous case-control study of Sachdev et al. (2001), who found that measures of injury severity, including duration of unconsciousness, evidence of brain damage on CT scan, and cognitive deficits on neuropsychological testing, predicted posttraumatic schizophrenia-like psychosis.

However, the link between injury severity and psychosis is not a universal finding. Violon and De Mol (1987) found that severity of injury did not predict psychosis after TBI. In the Fujii and Ahmed (2001) study noted earlier, there was a trend for the control group to have had more severe injuries. In the posttraumatic psychosis group, 16 of 22 patients had only had a mild brain injury. Also, for members of families with a history of bipolar disorder and schizophrenia, the risk of developing schizophrenia associated with having had a TBI was found to be unrelated to the severity of the TBI (Malaspina et al. 2001).

Other Features of Injury

The type of brain injury may also be related to psychosis risk. Davison and Bagley (1969) found that closed-head injury was related to risk of posttraumatic psychosis, and Lishman (1968) found a low rate of psychosis after penetrating head injury in veterans (though follow-up was only 4 years). However, newer studies have not found a link between psychosis risk and type of injury (closed vs. open) (Fujii and Ahmed 2001; Sachdev et al. 2001). Age at injury has not been found to determine psychosis risk (Fujii and Ahmed 2001); nor have behavioral and personality changes after TBI (Sachdev et al. 2001).

Inherent Vulnerability to Psychosis

Risk of posttraumatic psychosis has been linked to pretraumatic psychological characteristics and vulnerability to psychosis. Previous psychopathological disturbances have been reported for 83% of individuals who develop psychosis after TBI (Violon and De Mol 1987). Lishman (1987) found that psychosis is more likely to follow TBI in individuals who are predisposed to schizophrenia. In the recent study by Sachdev et al. (2001) genetic vulnerability to psychosis, as indicated by having a first-degree relative with a psychotic disorder, was found to be among the strongest predictors of who would develop psychosis after a TBI.

Gender

There are no studies that clearly evaluate the role of gender in risk for posttraumatic psychosis. Many of the earlier studies focused on veterans, who were invariably men. Although Fujii and Ahmed (2001) reported a preponderance of males in a sample of state hospital inpatients who developed posttraumatic psychosis (as compared with brain-injured outpatient control subjects), this may simply be an artifact of the selection process. Also, Sachdev et al.'s (2001) sample of patients with posttraumatic psychosis had more men than women, but this may simply be due to the greater prevalence of TBI in men.

IQ/Cognition

Although one recent study found no differences in IQ between brain-injured persons who went on to develop psychosis and those who did not (Fujii and Ahmed 2001), another recent study (Sachdev et al. 2001) found that the group that developed a schizophrenia-like psychosis had more neurological deficits than brain-injured control subjects, with lower IQ, significantly worse verbal and nonverbal memory, and greater impairments in language and frontal and parietal lobe functioning, consistent with a diffuse impairment in neuropsychological functioning. However, the authors acknowledge that it cannot be determined to what extent psychosis itself may have contributed to these deficits.

Socioeconomic Status

There are few data on the role of socioeconomic status in risk for posttraumatic psychosis. In one recent study, no differences in level of education attained was found between the group with psychosis secondary to TBI and a control group with TBI only (Fujii and Ahmed 2001).

Substance Abuse

There are few data on substance use or dependence as a risk factor for psychosis after TBI. In the newer case-control studies, there was more general previous substance use among those who developed posttraumatic psychosis (Fujii and Ahmed 2001) but no difference in use of psychosis-inducing substances such as lysergic acid diethylamide, amphetamines, and cocaine (Fujii and Ahmed 2001) and no difference in history of alcohol or drug dependence (Sachdev et al. 2001).

Prior Neurological Disorder

Fujii and Ahmed (2001) found that patients who went on to develop psychosis after a TBI had significantly more premorbid neurological pathology than did the brain-injured control subjects (80% vs. 40%; $\chi^2 = 7.99$; $P < 0.01$), including prior brain injury (14/25), seizures (3/25), learning disability (3/25), birth complications (2/25), attention deficit hyperactivity disorder (1/25), and congenital syphilis (1/25). This supports their hypothesis that psychosis may be more likely to follow TBI if the brain was already vulnerable before the injury. However, Sachdev et al. (2001) did not find differences in perinatal or developmental abnormalities between the group that developed psychosis after TBI as compared with the brain-injured control subjects.

Posttraumatic Epilepsy

Delusions and hallucinations are known to be prevalent in temporal lobe epilepsy, which can result from brain injury (Flor-Henry 1969; Garyfallos et al. 1988; Lishman 1987; McKenna et al. 1985). A prospective study of patients with temporal lobe epilepsy found that 10% developed psychotic symptoms (Lindsay et al. 1979). A rigorous study in Iceland that involved clinical interviews found that 7% of epilepsy patients had psychotic symptoms (Gudmundsson 1966). Furthermore, patients with psychosis are 3–7 times more likely than the general population to have features of epilepsy, and interictal psychoses frequently resemble chronic schizophrenia. Hillbom (1960) found that the incidence of posttraumatic epilepsy in brain-injured Finnish veterans who developed psychosis was 57.5%, compared with only 31.8% in those with no psychiatric sequelae; however, the relationship between posttraumatic psychosis and epilepsy was not specific, because the incidence of posttraumatic epilepsy was 55.6% in the group of brain-injured veterans who had any significant psychiatric sequelae (psychotic and nonpsychotic).

The more recent studies by Fujii and Ahmed (2001) and Sachdev et al. (2001) did not find a link between epilepsy and posttraumatic psychosis; in fact, Sachdev et al. found a trend toward less epilepsy in patients compared with control subjects. These findings appear paradoxical given that schizophrenia-like psychosis is 6–12 times more likely to occur in the context of epilepsy than in the general population (Sachdev 1998), and TBI is clearly known to be associated with the onset of seizures. It is reasonable to hypothesize that seizures could be a mediating phenomenon between TBI and psychosis, but the newer data do not support this theory. It may be that a longer time of follow-up after TBI might be needed to detect a relationship, because Davison and Bagley (1969) found that posttraumatic epilepsy was associated with delayed onset of psychosis, as opposed to immediate onset of psychosis; the mean interval between onset of seizures and onset of psychosis was noted to be approximately 14 years.

History of TBI in Patients With Schizophrenia

A connection between TBI and subsequent psychosis is also supported by retrospective studies of premorbid brain injury in patients with schizophrenia, which reveal elevated rates of prior TBI compared with other groups. In a review of five studies published between 1932 and 1961, Davison and Bagley (1969) found the frequency of premorbid TBI in hospitalized patients with schizophrenia to range from 1% to 15%. This wide range of values likely derives from differences in definitions of brain injury and schizophrenia. Wilcox and Nasrallah (1987) reviewed the records for a history of TBI in 659 patients admitted to a large tertiary care center. Psychiatric diagnoses were made according to research diagnostic criteria, and TBI was defined as brain trauma occurring before age 10 years and resulting in either loss of consciousness for at least 1 hour or medical complica-

tions (vomiting, confusion, visual changes). They found a premorbid history of TBI in 11% of patients with schizophrenia, compared with 4.9% of patients with mania, 1.5% of patients with depression, and 0.7% of surgical control subjects. Likewise, in a sample of Nigerian patients diagnosed with research diagnostic criteria, patients with schizophrenia were found to have significantly more premorbid TBI than did patients with mania (Gureje et al. 1994). Malaspina et al. (2001) found a threefold greater rate of reported TBI for individuals with schizophrenia compared with their never mentally ill family members in a combined pedigree sample of families with bipolar disorder and schizophrenia, for a total of 1,832 members. (However, patients with schizophrenia were not significantly more likely to have incurred TBI than were patients with bipolar or depressive disorder.) In a replication, AbdelMalik et al. (2003) also found more childhood TBI among schizophrenia patients than in their unaffected siblings (OR=2.35; CI=1.03–5.36).

Does Posttraumatic Psychosis Differ From Psychosis That Occurs Without Premorbid TBI?

Atypical Versus Typical Symptoms

One criterion listed in DSM-IV-TR for distinguishing psychosis secondary to a general medical condition from a primary psychotic disorder is the presence of atypical features such as visual and olfactory hallucinations (i.e., burning rubber or unpleasant smells). For example, there are case reports of Lilliputian hallucinations occurring in individuals with previous brain trauma (Cohen et al. 1994). Furthermore, there appears to be a link between right hemispheric injury and content-specific misidentification delusions such as Capgras' syndrome (loved ones replaced by identical-appearing impostors), Fregoli's syndrome (persecutor able to change appearances and appear as different people), and reduplicative paramnesia (familiar place exists in two different places at the same time) (reviewed in Edelstyn and Oyebode 1999; Forstl et al. 1991; McKenna et al. 1985) However, only between 25% and 40% of cases of Capgras' syndrome are associated with neurological disorders, so such atypical symptoms are not pathognomonic for psychosis due to a general medical condition. Additionally, posttraumatic psychosis frequently occurs without these atypical symptoms. For example, in a study of 45 individuals with schizophrenia-like psychosis after TBI, none of the sample demonstrated misidentification syndromes, only 15% had religious delusions, 20% had visual hallucinations, and 4% had tactile hallucinations (Sachdev et al. 2001). In contrast, 55% of these patients with posttraumatic schizophrenia-like psychosis had persecutory delusions and 84% had auditory hallucinations, which are common symptoms in schizophrenia. The low rates of atypical psychotic symptoms and high rates of typical symptoms in the Sachdev et al. (2001) study may be related to the study design, because individuals had to meet DSM-IV-TR Criteria A, B, C, and E for schizophrenia or schizophreniform disorder to be included. A more inclusive sample of any posttraumatic psychosis might demonstrate more atypical and fewer typical psychotic symptoms. However, others have also reported that paranoia and delusions are common symptoms in post-TBI psychosis (Cutting 1987).

In contrast to the overlap of positive symptoms of psychosis, only 22% of Sachdev et al.'s (2001) sample displayed negative symptoms (such as flattening of affect, avolition, or asociality), and only 4% had derailment or thought disorder. This is consistent with previous reports of relative absence of formal thought disorder and of blunting of affect in schizophrenia after TBI (McKenna 1994). However, the finding of low rates of negative symptoms is not consistent with the study by Thomsen (1984), which found that patients who developed psychoses after severe blunt brain trauma often developed deficit types of symptoms, including anhedonia, aspontaneity, and loss of social contact, probably related to the high rate of frontal injuries.

The course of psychotic illness among the brain-injured individuals with psychosis in the Sachdev et al. (2001) study was similar to that of schizophrenia not associated with TBI, because the patients had prodromal symptoms such as scholastic or work deterioration and social withdrawal, with a gradual onset of psychotic symptoms at a similar age accompanied frequently by depression (50%) and a subsequent subacute or chronic course.

Cognition

As with positive and negative symptoms, there is no clear consensus as to whether posttraumatic psychosis can be differentiated from primary psychotic disorders by the extent of cognitive impairment. In a Nigerian sample of patients with schizophrenia, those with a history of childhood brain trauma that required hospitalization had poorer scholastic performance as children (Gureje et al. 1994). They were also found to have mixed laterality as adults, possibly due to left hemi-spheric damage. However, we have found (Corcoran et al. 2000) that among patients with schizophrenia, those with a history of TBI actually had better cognition than those who did not.

Family History/Genetic Vulnerability

An early study suggested that brain trauma could contribute to schizophrenia either 1) directly or 2) through an interaction with latent vulnerability, and that these two pathways yielded different symptom patterns (Shapiro 1939). Shapiro (1939) evaluated 2,000 cases of dementia praecox (schizophrenia) in residents of a large public hospital and found that "a large number . . . showed some relationship to a severe head injury." To establish a sample in which there was less doubt that the brain injury and psychosis were linked, he selected 21 cases in which the schizophrenia-like psychosis quickly ensued after the brain injury, beginning within a few hours to 3 months afterward. Ten of the 21 patients had no grossly obvious signs suggestive of the sequelae of the trauma; all 10 of these patients demonstrated a predisposition to schizophrenia such as positive family history or "introverted" premorbid personality. Shapiro concluded that in these 10 patients, the brain trauma acted as a precipitating factor. The other 11 patients showed symptoms not only typical of schizophrenia but other "neurological" features as well, such as headache, seizures, confusion, dizziness, disorientation, and memory impairment. In this group, only 2 of the 11 showed "hereditary tainting," and 7 of the 11 had "well-integrated" premorbid personalities. Shapiro concluded that in this group, brain trauma not only precipitated but directly contributed to the etiology of the psychosis.

Other studies have suggested that TBI can contribute to schizophrenia risk, because among schizophrenia patients, those without premorbid TBI have more genetic vulnerability for psychotic disorders than do those with prior TBI, who have no greater rates of family members with psychosis than do the general population (Davison and Bagley 1969). In a reexamination of a database of 722 probands with schizophrenia (originally studied by Rudin), the diagnosis of schizophrenia was confirmed in a subsample of 660, and the prevalence of schizophrenia in the parents and siblings of these 660 probands was examined (Kendler and Zerbin-Rudin 1996). It was found that the risk for schizophrenia was particularly low in siblings of probands whose onset of illness occurred within a year of major brain trauma. Malaspina et al. (2001) found that TBI may interact with schizophrenia genetic vulnerability to increase the risk for schizophrenia.

What Are Common Cognitive Features of TBI and Schizophrenia?

The presence of similar features in TBI and schizophrenia may shed light on the pathophysiological mechanisms by which these phenomena may be associated. Key similarities between TBI and schizophrenia include deficits in insight, executive function, and memory, which indicate pathology in similar neuroanatomical sites, such as, respectively, the orbitofrontal regions, dorsolateral prefrontal cortex, and hippocampi. Common deficits in sensory gating may implicate abnormal connectivity between various parts of the brain in both conditions.

Poor Insight

Up to one-half of individuals with moderate to severe TBI have reduced awareness of their deficits (Flashman et al. 1998; see Chapter 19, Awareness of Deficits). Poor insight is highly prevalent in schizophrenia patients and is characterized by deficits in awareness of having a mental disorder, of response to medication, of the social consequences of the mental disorder, and of specific symptoms of the illness (Amador et al. 1994; Pini et al. 2001). Poor insight complicates compliance with treatment recommendations in both those with brain injury and those with psychotic disorders.

Neuropsychological Function

Cognitive deficits are common in both brain-injured individuals and those with schizophrenia. Impairments in executive functions occur frequently in both groups, such as planning and problem solving needed for activities such as balancing bank accounts, writing letters, planning one's week, and driving or taking public transportation (Mazaux et al. 1997). Formal neurocognitive tests of executive function include the Trail Making Test B, Wisconsin Card Sorting Test, and Tower of Hanoi. Poor performance on these tests is a common finding both in individuals with a TBI (Brooks et al. 1999; Callahan and Hinkebein 1999; Leon-Carrion et al. 1998; Wiegner and Donders 1999) and in individuals with schizophrenia (reviewed in Johnson-Selfridge and Zalewski 2001). Individuals with both schizophrenia and brain injury also show deficits in explicit memory, which is the deliberate recall of facts such as dates and phone numbers, as well as decrements in volume of the hippocampus, the part of the brain thought to be responsible for explicit memory. In both groups of patients, the extent of memory deficit is associated with the degree of volume reduction of the hippocampus (Gur et al. 2000; Tate and Bigler 2000).

Neuroanatomical Effects of TBI and Implications for Psychosis Pathophysiology

Perhaps accounting for the overlap in cognitive deficits seen in both groups, there is significant overlap between the brain regions implicated in schizophrenia and those regions that are vulnerable to TBI, including the frontal and temporal cortices and the hippocampus.

Primary Sites of Lesion

Brain injury frequently results in damage to the frontal and temporal cortices. Similar regions are often involved in individuals who develop psychosis from other neurological conditions such as metachromatic leukodystrophy and cerebrovascular disease (Buckley et al. 1993; Hyde et al. 1992; Levine and Grek 1984; Miller et al. 1991; Rabins et al. 1991; Richardson 1992). In epilepsy, visual hallucinations have been found to result from seizure foci in the temporal lobes or orbitofrontal regions (Fornazzari et al. 1992) and delusions of passivity ("forces are acting upon me," "I am being controlled") have been linked to left temporal lobe seizure foci (Perez and Trimble 1980; Trimble and Thompson 1981). Of interest, in early experiments of stimulation of the brains of awake patients undergoing neurosurgery, stimulation of the temporal lobes elicited auditory hallucinations (Mullan and Penfield 1959). Abnormalities in the prefrontal cortex are common in schizophrenia, and it has been hypothesized that the attendant working memory deficits (holding information online while attending to other tasks) may be the key pathophysiological feature of schizophrenia.

Secondary Sites of Lesion

Brain injury also results in damage to regions far from the primary site of impact (diaschisis) (Joashi et al. 1999). Animal studies of TBI, including weight-drop and fluid percussion models, show that the hippocampus is particularly vulnerable to TBI, even injuries that have a primary impact far from the hippocampus (Bramlett et al. 1997; Chen et al. 1996; Colicos et al. 1996; Lowenstein et al. 1992; Qian et al. 1996; Tang et al. 1997b; Yamaki et al. 1998). Furthermore, hippocampal injury in animals leads to memory impairments (Chen et al. 1996; Tang et al.

1997a). Of note, the cell loss in the hippocampus is progressive longer than 1 year after TBI in rats, suggesting a possible explanation for what is observed in humans: ongoing changes in the brain months to years after the initial injury (i.e., a chronically progressive degenerative process initiated by brain trauma) (Smith et al. 1997a).

This special vulnerability of the hippocampus to trauma may be due to axon stretching and diffuse axonal injury, which are common features of brain trauma in animals and humans. When diffuse axonal injury was replicated in pigs through nonimpact inertial loading, there was widespread multifocal injury observed of axons and neurons, especially in regions of the hippocampus (Smith et al. 1997b). In nonhuman primates with acceleration-induced experimental brain injury, 59% developed hippocampal lesions: 46% of animals with mild injury (brief unconsciousness and no residual neurologic deficit) and 94% of animals with severe injuries. Cell death in the hippocampus occurred without a drop in cerebral perfusion pressure or increase in intracranial pressure and did not seem to be a consequence of low oxygen, because other regions of the brain vulnerable to hypoxia did not have cell death (Kotapka et al. 1991). Traumatic injury to the hippocampus also occurs in humans in the absence of elevated intracranial pressure (Kotapka et al. 1994).

Abnormalities in hippocampal structure and function are common in schizophrenia. A meta-analysis of 18 studies showed a bilateral reduction of volume in the hippocampus in schizophrenia of 4% (Nelson et al. 1998). Magnetic resonance spectroscopy studies suggest that neuronal integrity is compromised in the hippocampus in schizophrenia, because low *N*-acetylaspartate has been found across several studies (reviewed in Poland et al. 1999 and Soares and Innis 1999). Silbersweig et al. (1995) found increased blood flow in the hippocampus during hallucinations. Postmortem studies provide evidence that there is synaptic and, hence, circuitry abnormality in both the hippocampus and the prefrontal cortex (Harrison 1999). Intriguingly, cognitive and magnetic resonance imaging volumetric assessments of twins discordant for schizophrenia suggest that hippocampal abnormality is more prevalent in the affected twin, suggesting nongenetic influences operating on the hippocampus in schizophrenia (Baare et al. 2001; Cannon et al. 2000; Suddath et al. 1990).

Disturbances in connectivity among different regions of the brain are a common result of TBI and have been hypothesized to play a role in the genesis of some symptoms of schizophrenia. For example, Frith (1996) suggested hallucinations result from disruption in connectivity among parts of the brain responsible for intentional speech and observation/interpretation of speech, so that auditory sensory phenomena are misattributed to external sources. Furthermore, TBI can impair the ability to filter incoming sensory information; deficits in the gating/filtering of sensory information are also characteristic of schizophrenia. It has been hypothesized that these abnormalities result from disruptions in connections between different parts of the brain, and that the inability to filter out stimuli can lead to sensory "flooding" by irrelevant information.

Populations Who Are Vulnerable to Posttraumatic Psychosis

Homeless Individuals

Homeless people have high rates of schizophrenia-like psychosis and TBI history (Silver and Felix 1999). Studies have shown that homeless persons have an elevated prevalence of schizophrenia that ranges between 13.7% (Koegel et al. 1988) and 25% (Susser et al. 1989). More than 40% of homeless individuals with a schizophrenia-like psychosis who were treated at a university hospital in New York had a history of premorbid TBI (Silver and McKinnon 1993).

Death Row Prisoners

An interesting study of 15 death row inmates showed that all 15 had histories of severe brain injury and 9 had recurrent psychoses (with hallucinations, delusions, thought disorder, and bizarre behavior) that antedated incarceration (Lewis et al. 1986). Remarkably, these subjects were not selected for clinical evaluation because of any evident psychopathology but rather were chosen for neuropsychological testing in the hope of appealing for clemency when their executions were imminent. That is, these were individuals who had not been identified as mentally ill but who were at the final stages of their appeals process. All had repetitive episodes of brain trauma beginning in childhood that were quite dramatic—severe physical abuse, falling from heights, being hit by and run over by cars, being hit with baseball bats. The episodes of brain trauma were corroborated by scars, indentations of the cranium, hospital records, and CT scans. They had comprehensive evaluations by a board-certified psychiatrist lasting from 4 to 16 hours that involved detailed birth, development, neurological, psychiatric, medical, educational, family, and social histories; interviews of family members; physical examinations; CT scans; and electroencephalography. The inmates largely tried to conceal their psychotic symptoms. Of note, all but one had a normal IQ.

Children and Teens

The National Institutes of Health Consensus Development Panel on Rehabilitation of Persons With Traumatic Brain Injury (Consensus conference 1999) reports the highest incidence of brain trauma is among individuals 15–24 years old (and the elderly), with another peak in children younger than 5 years. Motor vehicle accidents are the major cause of TBIs in the 15- to 24-year-old group, and alcohol is frequently involved. Sports injuries and violence also are a major cause of brain injury in teens. Child abuse and assault is also a significant cause of TBI in children. Of note, reported rates of prior child abuse are 20/38, or 52%, of patients with first-episode psychosis (Greenfield et al. 1994) and 27/61, or 44%, of patients with chronic psychosis (Goff et al. 1991).

Evaluation of Posttraumatic Psychosis

A thorough assessment of the patient with posttraumatic psychosis is an essential prerequisite to the prescription of any treatment (Arciniegas et al. 2000). A comprehensive evaluation must include detailed histories of birth, development, neurological features, psychiatric symptoms, medical status, education, substance use, social functioning, and any family illnesses, as well as physical and neurological examinations, detailed mental status examination, neuropsychological testing using a standardized battery, structural imaging (CT or magnetic resonance imaging), and electroencephalography. Premorbid history and current medication treatment are important because they can influence neuropsychiatric symptoms (Arciniegas et al. 2000). Family members and other corroborating sources should be included in the examination because individuals may not recall details of brain injury if it occurred either when they were children or when they were intoxicated, and the neuropsychological correlates of both psychosis and TBI can interfere with the ability to recall one's history in detail (McAllister 1998).

Posttraumatic Amnesia

In the initial period after injury, during the period of PTA, numerous features of delirium are likely to occur (see Chapter 9, Delirium and Posttraumatic Amnesia), including restlessness, fluctuating level of consciousness, agitation, combativeness, emotional lability, emotional withdrawal or excessive dependency, confusion, distractibility, disorientation, and amnesia (Trzepacz 1994). Hallucinations and delusions may also occur during this period, although delusions are seldom well organized (Goethe and Levin 1984; McAllister and Ferrell 2002; Trzepacz 1994). Expressive and receptive speech and language disturbances, including perseveration, are frequently present during this period and can produce a clinical picture similar to the disorder of thought and language found in schizophrenia (Goethe and Levin 1984). Many of these symptoms are likely to improve as the period of PTA improves.

Posttraumatic Epilepsy

Psychotic syndromes associated with posttraumatic epilepsy occur in the peri-ictal period (either during seizures or in the immediate postictal period) or interictally, in which case the psychotic symptoms are more commonly chronic rather than episodic (McAllister and Ferrell 2002; Trimble 1991). The most common of these entities is the postictal acute confusional state characterized by generalized confusion, fluctuating sensorium, agitation, hallucinations, and delusions, which is similar to the posttraumatic delirium described in the preceding section. This condition generally resolves within a few hours after the seizure, although it may rarely persist for several days. It is important to detect whether the patient has a seizure disorder, because this can be treated with anticonvulsants and also because so many psychiatric medications can lower the seizure threshold.

Mood Disorders

Mood disorders are a common occurrence after TBI, and both depression and mania can present with psychotic symptoms. Manic syndromes with associated psychosis and schizoaffective syndromes after TBI have been described largely in single case reports or small series. Shukla et al. (1987), for example, reported on 20 patients with manic or schizoaffective symptoms and a history of TBI. In this series, psychotic symptoms occurred in a high percentage of patients. Grandiosity occurred in 90%, pressured speech in 80%, and flight of ideas in 75%. No one in this series had a positive family history for bipolar disorder, indicating that genetic loading is not a necessary prerequisite for development of mania after brain injury. Psychotic symptoms are prominent in many of the cases of mania subsequent to TBI reported in the literature (Bracken 1987; Clark and Davison 1987; Nizamie et al. 1988; Pope et al. 1988; Reiss et al. 1987). Depression is more common than mania after TBI and can also be associated with psychotic symptoms in approximately 25% of individuals (Hibbard et al. 1998; McAllister and Ferrell 2002). Obviously, it is important to recognize mood disorders as the cause of psychotic symptoms, because the treatment follows logically from this diagnosis.

Treatment of Posttraumatic Psychosis

Any existing delirium, seizure disorder, mood disorder, or substance abuse or dependence must be diagnosed and attended to in the treatment of posttraumatic psychosis. If these disorders are not present, if psychotic symptoms are life-threatening, or if psychotic symptoms persist beyond the treatment of these disorders, then an antipsychotic medication may be warranted. Care should be taken in administering neuroleptics, as animal studies suggest that dopamine antagonists (antipsychotic medications) can impede recovery after brain injury (Feeney et al. 1982). Problems with motor function, gait, arousal, and speed of information processing are common in brain-injured patients and may be exacerbated by the sedation, psychomotor slowing, parkinsonism, and anticholinergic side effects of neuroleptics. Of note, there are no controlled studies of treatments for psychosis in patients with premorbid TBI. Information comes from case reports and extrapolation from studies in other populations of patients with brain damage. Given these caveats, most clinicians advise that neuroleptics should be used specifically for psychotic symptoms and not for agitation only.

Medication dosing should be "low and slow." Many experts suggest starting with one-third to one-half of the usual dose (McAllister 1998). The clinician must be wary of medications with significant sedative and anticholinergic properties. Therefore, among typical neuroleptics, high-potency antipsychotic medications such as haloperidol (Haldol) may produce fewer of these side effects than low-potency antipsychotics such as chlorpromazine (Thorazine). However, it should be noted that TBI may also make patients more vulnerable to developing tardive dyskinesia (Kane and Smith 1982).

Atypical antipsychotic drugs have emerged as first-line drugs for treatment of psychotic disorders. These drugs offer two main advantages over conventional neuroleptic drugs. They have greater efficacy, especially in decreasing negative as well as positive symptoms of schizophrenia and in decreasing agitation and aggression. The latter effect can be of particular benefit in some individuals with TBI. Most important, the atypical antipsychotics carry significantly less risk of causing extrapyramidal symptoms (EPSs) and tardive dyskinesia. Like all drugs with antipsychotic activity, the atypicals have some blocking effect on dopamine-2 receptors but proportionally less so than conventional drugs. The atypical class also shows a preference for limbic dopamine-2 receptors

with minimal nigrostriatal effects, and thus less risk of EPSs.

Clozapine is a candidate for the treatment of posttraumatic psychosis in that it yields a low incidence of EPSs and tardive dyskinesia. Case reports of clozapine suggest efficacy in patients with posttraumatic psychosis. For example, 400 mg of clozapine daily was effective for a 34-year-old man who had a 10-year history of refractory and persistent voices and delusions after a brain injury at age 12 years (Burke et al. 1999). However, a less clear picture was observed in an open trial of clozapine in a series of nine brain-injured patients with either refractory psychotic symptoms or treatment-resistant outbursts of rage and aggression (Michals et al. 1993). In this series, one-third of patients had, respectively, marked improvement, mild improvement, and indeterminate improvement. However, seizures occurred in two of the nine patients, including new onset of seizures in one patient who was taking 600 mg/day of clozapine, along with pimozide and amoxapine. The other patient had a preexisting seizure disorder and developed a recurrence while taking low doses of clozapine (75–100 mg/day) despite also taking an anticonvulsant (valproate, 4,000 mg/day) and a benzodiazepine (lorazepam, 3 mg/day.)

These data suggest that clozapine should be given primarily to individuals with posttraumatic psychosis without a history of seizures, and that prophylactic anticonvulsants such as valproate may be indicated to prevent the onset of new seizures. Clozapine can also cause sedation and dizziness, for which brain-injured patients may have greater vulnerability. Additionally, there are risks of agranulocytosis (minimized with weekly blood draws), tachycardia, orthostatic hypotension, hypersalivation, and weight gain. Because of this side-effect profile, clozapine is not usually the first of the atypical antipsychotics to try. We suggest trying at least two of the other atypical antipsychotic drugs before beginning a clozapine trial. Among the other atypical antipsychotics, none shows clearly superior efficacy. A particular patient's history of previous response, minimizing certain side effects, and the clinician's familiarity with one drug or another all affect choice of drug. In some instances, one might wish to use a side effect such as sedation or tendency to cause weight gain to advantage. One should strive to make one change at a time to prevent confusion about the cause of subsequent clinical changes. Ineffective drugs should be discontinued. When adding a drug to the regimen, consider stopping the current drug to avoid polypharmacy.

A variety of case reports and small case series suggest that most of the atypical antipsychotics, including olanzapine, risperidone, and quetiapine, can be used to effectively treat psychosis resulting from TBI, although there are no randomized controlled trials to date (Ferrell 2000; McAllister and Ferrell 2002).

Benzodiazepines should be used sparingly, if at all. Augmenting the effects of one medication by using a second low-dose agent with a different method of action is a way to address the problem of sensitivity to specific side effects in certain patients.

Prevention of Posttraumatic Psychosis

Although psychosis is not among the most common psychiatric sequelae of TBI, it is a disturbing and disabling outcome with great morbidity and cost. We have estimated previously that TBI accounts for 1%–17% of all cases of schizophrenia, the most debilitating of all psychotic disorders (Corcoran and Malaspina 2001). The National Advisory Mental Health Council reported that in 1993 the total cost of schizophrenia (both direct and indirect costs) in the United States was $33 billion. If 50% of all TBI-induced schizophrenia could be prevented, this would mean a savings of $16.5–$280.5 million each year in the United States alone.

Individuals with a family history of psychosis may be most vulnerable to developing psychosis after incurring a TBI. Therefore, the prevention of TBI or the modification of the brain response to the trauma could plausibly decrease the incidence of posttraumatic psychosis. There are important public health implications if immediate medical approaches to brain injury can minimize resultant neurotoxicity in individuals who are vulnerable or at risk for developing major mental illness. New medications now given immediately after brain trauma may stop oxidative damage from evolving. Promising neuroprotective strategies implemented in the immediate aftermath of a TBI include the use of hypothermia, glutamate receptor antagonists, calcium channel antagonists, free radical scavengers, and cyclosporin A. Also promising may be the reduction of increased intracranial pressure, which is a common complication of severe TBI and is frequently associated with the development of secondary brain damage (Clausen and Bullock 2001).

Conclusion

The relationship between traumatic brain injury and psychosis is complex. It seems clear on the basis of the available evidence that TBI increases the risk of developing a psychotic syndrome and increases the risk of developing schizophrenia (among other disorders) if one already has a genetic vulnerability to this disorder. It may be the case

that having certain psychiatric disorders also increases the risk of sustaining a TBI. The overlap between the brain regions commonly affected by TBI and those implicated in the genesis of schizophrenia and its prominent symptoms (e.g., hallucinations and delusions) may account for this interaction. Psychotic syndromes also can be seen as part of the period of posttraumatic amnesia, posttraumatic epilepsy, and posttraumatic mood disorders. Treatment involves making the appropriate distinction between these different contexts in which psychosis can be seen and then the judicious use of medications appropriate to the context.

References

AbdelMalik P, Husted J, Chow EW, et al: Childhood head injury and expression of schizophrenia in multiply affected families. Arch Gen Psychiatry 60:231–236, 2003

Achte KA, Hillbom E, Aalberg V: Psychoses following war brain injuries. Acta Psychiatr Scand 45:1–18, 1969

Achte K, Jarho L, Kyykka T, et al: Paranoid disorders following war brain damage: preliminary report. Psychopathology 24:309–315, 1991

Ahmed I, Fujii D: Posttraumatic psychosis. Semin Clin Neuropsychiatry 3:23–33, 1998

Amador XF, Flaum M, Andreasen NC, et al: Awareness of illness in schizophrenia and schizoaffective and mood disorders. Arch Gen Psychiatry 51:826–836, 1994

American Psychiatric Association: Diagnostic and Statistical Manual of Mental Disorders, 4th Edition, Text Revision. Washington, DC, American Psychiatric Association, 2000

Arciniegas DB, Topkoff J, Silver JM: Neuropsychiatric aspects of traumatic brain injury. Curr Treat Options Neurol 2:169–186, 2000

Baare WF, van Oel CJ, Hulshoff Pol HE, et al: Volumes of brain structures in twins discordant for schizophrenia. Arch Gen Psychiatry 58:33–40, 2001

Black P, Blumer D, Wellner AM, et al: Head trauma in children: neurological, behavioral and intellectual sequelae, in Brain Dysfunction in Children: Etiology, Diagnosis and Management. Edited by Black P. New York, Raven, 1981, pp 171–180

Bracken P: Mania following head injury. Br J Psychiatry 150:690–692, 1987

Bramlett HM, Dietrich WD, Green EJ, et al: Chronic histopathological consequences of fluid-percussion brain injury in rats: effects of post-traumatic hypothermia. Acta Neuropathol (Berl) 93:190–199, 1997

Brooks J, Fos LA, Greve KW, et al: Assessment of executive function in patients with mild traumatic brain injury. J Trauma 46:159–163, 1999

Brown G, Chadwick O, Shaffer D, et al: A prospective study of children with head injuries, III: psychiatric sequelae. Psychol Med 11:63–78, 1981

Buckley P, Stack JP, Madigan C, et al: Magnetic resonance imaging of schizophrenia-like psychoses associated with cerebral trauma: clinicopathological correlates. Am J Psychiatry 150:146–148, 1993

Burke JG, Dursun SM, Reveley MA: Refractory symptomatic schizophrenia resulting from frontal lobe lesion: response to clozapine. J Psychiatry Neurosci 24:456–461, 1999

Callahan CD, Hinkebein J: Neuropsychological significance of anosmia following traumatic brain injury. J Head Trauma Rehabil 14:581–587, 1999

Cannon TD, Huttunen MO, Lonnqvist J, et al: The inheritance of neuropsychological dysfunction in twins discordant for schizophrenia. Am J Hum Genet 67:369–382, 2000

Chen Y, Constantini S, Trembovler V, et al: An experimental model of closed head injury in mice: pathophysiology, histopathology, and cognitive deficits. J Neurotrauma 13:557–568, 1996

Clark AF, Davison K: A report of two cases and a review of the literature. Br J Psychiatry 150:841–844, 1987

Clausen T, Bullock R: Medical treatment and neuroprotection in traumatic brain injury. Curr Pharm Des 7:1517–1532, 2001.

Cohen MA, Alfonso CA, Haque MM: Lilliputian hallucinations and medical illness. Gen Hosp Psychiatry 16:141–143, 1994

Colicos MA, Dixon CE, Dash PK: Delayed, selective neuronal death following experimental cortical impact injury in rats: possible role in memory deficits. Brain Res 739:111–119, 1996

Consensus conference. Rehabilitation of persons with traumatic brain injury. NIH Consensus Development Panel on Rehabilitation of Persons With Traumatic Brain Injury. JAMA 282:974–983, 1999

Corcoran CM, Malaspina D: Traumatic brain injury and schizophrenia risk. Int J Ment Health 30:17–32, 2001

Corcoran CM, Goetz R, Amador X, et al: Depression and higher IQ associated with premorbid traumatic brain injury in schizophrenia. Biol Psychiatry 47:1S-17S, 2000

Cummings JL: Organic psychosis. Psychosomatics 29:16–26, 1988

Cutting J: The phenomenology of acute organic psychosis: comparison with acute schizophrenia. Br J Psychiatry 151:324–332, 1987

Davison K, Bagley CR: Schizophrenia-like psychoses associated with organic disorders of the central nervous system: a review of the literature. Br J Psychiatry 4:113–184, 1969

Edelstyn NM, Oyebode F: A review of the phenomenology and cognitive neuropsychological origins of the Capgras syndrome. Int J Geriatr Psychiatry 14:48–59, 1999

Feeney DM, Gonzalez A, Law WA: Amphetamine, haloperidol, and experience interact to affect rate of recovery after motor cortex injury. Science 217:855–857, 1982

Feinstein A, Ron M: A longitudinal study of psychosis due to a general medical (neurological) condition: establishing predictive and construct validity. J Neuropsychiatry Clin Neurosci 10:448–452, 1998

Ferrell R: Pharmacotherapy of disruptive behaviors associated with brain disease. Semin Clin Neuropsychiatry 5:283–289, 2000

Flashman LA, Amador X, McAllister TW: Lack of awareness of deficits in traumatic brain injury. Semin Clin Neuropsychiatry 3:201–210, 1998

Flor-Henry P: Psychosis and temporal lobe epilepsy: a controlled investigation. Epilepsia 10:363–395, 1969

Fornazzari L, Farcnik K, Smith I, et al: Violent visual hallucinations and aggression in frontal lobe dysfunction: clinical manifestations of deep orbitofrontal foci. J Neuropsychiatry Clin Neurosci 4:42–44, 1992

Forstl H, Almeida OP, Owen AM, et al: Psychiatric, neurological and medical aspects of misidentification syndromes: a review of 260 cases. Psychol Med 21:905–910, 1991

Frith C: The role of the prefrontal cortex in self-consciousness: the case of auditory hallucinations. Philos Trans R Soc Lond B Biol Sci 351:1505–1512, 1996

Fujii D, Ahmed I: Psychosis secondary to traumatic brain injury. Neuropsychiatry Neuropsychol Behav Neurol 9:133–138, 1996

Fujii DE, Ahmed I: Risk factors in psychosis secondary to traumatic brain injury. J Neuropsychiatry Clin Neurosci 13:61–69, 2001

Garyfallos G, Manos N, Adamopoulou A: Psychopathology and personality characteristics of epileptic patients: epilepsy, psychopathology and personality. Acta Psychiatr Scand 78:87–95, 1988

Goethe KE, Levin HS: Behavioral manifestation during the early and long-term stages of recovery after closed head injury. Psychiatr Ann 14:540–546, 1984

Goff DC, Brotman AW, Kindlon D, et al: Self-reports of childhood abuse in chronically psychotic patients. Psychiatry Res 37:73–80, 1991

Greenfield SF, Strakowski SM, Tohen M, et al: Childhood abuse in first-episode psychosis. Br J Psychiatry 164:831–834, 1994

Gudmundsson G: Epilepsy in Iceland: a clinical and epidemiological investigation. Acta Neurol Scand 43 (suppl 25):1–124, 1966

Gur RE, Turetsky BI, Cowell PE, et al: Temporolimbic volume reductions in schizophrenia. Arch Gen Psychiatry 57:769–775, 2000

Gureje O, Bamidele R, Raji O: Early brain trauma and schizophrenia in Nigerian patients. Am J Psychiatry 151:368–371, 1994

Harrison PJ: The neuropathology of schizophrenia: a critical review of the data and their interpretation. Brain 122 (pt 4):593–624, 1999

Hibbard MR, Uysal S, Kepler K, et al: Axis I psychopathology in individuals with traumatic brain injury. J Head Trauma Rehabil 13:24–39, 1998

Hillbom E: After-effects of brain injuries: research on the symptoms causing invalidism of persons in Finland having sustained brain-injuries during the wars of 1939–1940 and 1941–1944. Acta Psychiatr Scand 35 (suppl 142):1–195, 1960

Hyde TM, Ziegler JC, Weinberger DR: Psychiatric disturbances in metachromatic leukodystrophy: insights into the
neurobiology of psychosis. Arch Neurol 49:401–406, 1992

Jager TE, Weiss HB, Coben JH, et al: Traumatic brain injuries
evaluated in U.S. emergency departments, 1992–1994.
Acad Emerg Med 7:134–140, 2000

Joashi UC, Greenwood K, Taylor DL, et al: Poly(ADP ribose)
polymerase cleavage precedes neuronal death in the hippocampus and cerebellum following injury to the developing
rat forebrain. Eur J Neurosci 11:91–100, 1999

Johnson-Selfridge M, Zalewski C: Moderator variables of executive functioning in schizophrenia: meta-analytic findings.
Schizophr Bull 27:305–316, 2001

Kane JM, Smith JM: Tardive dyskinesia: prevalence and risk factors, 1959 to 1979. Arch Gen Psychiatry 39:473–481, 1982

Kendler KS, Zerbin-Rudin E: Abstract and review of "Zur Erb-
pathologie der Schizophrenie" (Contribution to the genetics of schizophrenia): 1916. Am J Med Genet 67:343–346,
1996

Koegel P, Burnam MA, Farr RK: The prevalence of specific psychiatric disorders among homeless individuals in the inner
city of Los Angeles. Arch Gen Psychiatry 45:1085–1092,
1988

Kornilov AA: Clinical features and course of schizophrenia developing in patients during remote periods following
cranio-cerebral injuries. Zh Nevropatol Psikhiatr Im S S
Korsakova 80:1687–1692, 1980

Kotapka MJ, Gennarelli TA, Graham DI, et al: Selective vulnerability of hippocampal neurons in acceleration-induced experimental head injury. J Neurotrauma 8:247–258, 1991

Kotapka MJ, Graham DI, Adams JH, et al: Hippocampal pathology in fatal human head injury without high intracranial
pressure. J Neurotrauma 11:317–324, 1994

Koufen H, Hagel KH: Systematic EEG follow-up study of traumatic psychosis. Eur Arch Psychiatry Neurol Sci 237:2–7,
1987

Kraepelin E: Dementia Praecox and Paraphrenia. Edinburgh,
Livingston, 1919

Leon-Carrion J, Alarcon JC, Revuelta M, et al: Executive functioning as outcome in patients after traumatic brain injury.
Int J Neurosci 94:75–83, 1998

Levine DN, Grek A: The anatomic basis of delusions after right
cerebral infarction. Neurology 34:577–582, 1984

Lewis DO, Pincus JH, Feldman M, et al: Psychiatric, neurological, and psychoeducational characteristics of 15 death row
inmates in the United States. Am J Psychiatry 143:838–
845, 1986

Lindsay J, Ounsted C, Richards P: Long-term outcome in children with temporal lobe seizures, III: psychiatric aspects in
childhood and adult life. Dev Med Child Neurol 21:630–
636, 1979

Lishman WA: Brain damage in relation to psychiatric disability
after head injury. Br J Psychiatry 114:373–410, 1968

Lishman WA: Organic Psychiatry: The Psychological Consequences of Cerebral Disorder, 2nd Edition. Oxford, UK,
Blackwell Scientific, 1987

Lowenstein DH, Thomas MJ, Smith DH, et al: Selective vulnerability of dentate hilar neurons following traumatic
brain injury: a potential mechanistic link between head
trauma and disorders of the hippocampus. J Neurosci
12:4846–4853, 1992

Malaspina D, Goetz RR, Friedman JH, et al: Traumatic brain
injury and schizophrenia in members of schizophrenia and
bipolar disorder pedigrees. Am J Psychiatry 158:440–446,
2001

Max JE, Robin DA, Lindgren SD, et al: Traumatic brain injury
in children and adolescents: psychiatric disorders at two
years. J Am Acad Child Adolesc Psychiatry 36:1278–1285,
1997

Mazaux JM, Masson F, Levin HS, et al: Long-term neuropsychological outcome and loss of social autonomy after traumatic
brain injury. Arch Phys Med Rehabil 78:1316–1320, 1997

McAllister TW: Traumatic brain injury and psychosis: what is the
connection? Semin Clin Neuropsychiatry 3:211–223, 1998

McAllister TW, Ferrell R: Evaluation and treatment of psychosis
after traumatic brain injury. Neurorehabilitation 17:357–
368, 2002

McKenna PJ, Kane JM, Parrish K: Psychotic syndromes in epilepsy: Am J Psychiatry 142:895–904, 1985

McKenna PJ: Schizophrenia and Related Syndromes. New
York, Oxford University Press, 1994

Meyer A: The anatomical facts and clinical varieties of traumatic
insanity. American Anthropological Association 17:373–
442, 1904.

Michals ML, Crismon ML, Roberts S, et al: Clozapine response
and adverse effects in nine brain-injured patients. J Clin
Psychopharmacol 13:198–203, 1993

Miller BL, Lesser IM, Boone KB, et al: Brain lesions and cognitive function in late-life psychosis. Br J Psychiatry 158:76–
82, 1991

Mullan S, Penfield W: Illusions of comparative interpretation
and emotion: production of epileptic discharge and by electrical stimulation in the temporal cortex. AMA Arch Neurol Psychiatry 81:269–284, 1959

Nelson MD, Saykin AJ, Flashman LA, et al: Hippocampal volume reduction in schizophrenia as assessed by magnetic
resonance imaging: a meta-analytic study. Arch Gen Psychiatry 55:433–440, 1998

Nizamie SH, Nizamie A, Borde M, et al: Mania following head
injury: case reports and neuropsychological findings. Acta
Psychiatr Scand 77:637–639, 1988

Perez MM, Trimble MR: Epileptic psychosis: diagnostic comparison with process schizophrenia. Br J Psychiatry
137:245–249, 1980

Pini S, Cassano GB, Dell'Osso L, et al: Insight into illness in
schizophrenia, schizoaffective disorder, and mood disorders
with psychotic features. Am J Psychiatry 158:122–125, 2001

Poland RE, Cloak C, Lutchmansingh PJ, et al: Brain N-acetyl
aspartate concentrations measured by H MRS are reduced
in adult male rats subjected to perinatal stress: preliminary
observations and hypothetical implications for neurodevelopmental disorders. J Psychiatr Res 33:41–51, 1999

Pope HG, McElroy SL, Satlin A, et al: Head injury, bipolar disorder, and response to valproate. Compr Psychiatry 29:34–38, 1988

Qian L, Nagaoka T, Ohno K, et al: Magnetic resonance imaging and pathologic studies on lateral fluid percussion injury as a model of focal brain injury in rats. Bull Tokyo Med Dent Univ 43:53–66, 1996

Rabins PV, Starkstein SE, Robinson RG: Risk factors for developing atypical (schizophreniform) psychosis following stroke. J Neuropsychiatry Clin Neurosci 3:6–9, 1991

Reiss H, Schwartz CE, Klerman GL: Manic syndrome following head injury: another form of secondary mania. J Clin Psychiatry 48:29–30, 1987

Richardson JK: Psychotic behavior after right hemispheric cerebrovascular accident: a case report. Arch Phys Med Rehabil 73:381–384, 1992

Sachdev P: Schizophrenia-like psychosis and epilepsy: the status of the association. Am J Psychiatry 155:325–336, 1998

Sachdev P, Smith JS, Cathcart S: Schizophrenia-like psychosis following traumatic brain injury: a chart-based descriptive and case-control study. Psychol Med 31:231–239, 2001

Shapiro LB: Schizophrenic-like psychosis following head injuries. Ill Med J 76:250–254, 1939

Shukla S, Cook BL, Mukherjee S, et al: Mania following head trauma. Am J Psychiatry 144:93–96, 1987

Silbersweig DA, Stern E, Frith C, et al: A functional neuroanatomy of hallucinations in schizophrenia. Nature 378:176–179, 1995

Silver JM, Felix A: Neuropsychiatry and the homeless, in Neuropsychiatry and Mental Health Services. Edited by Ovsiew F. Washington, DC, American Psychiatric Press, 1999, pp 319–333

Silver MA, McKinnon K: Characteristics of homeless patients discharged from an intensive placement unit. Hosp Community Psychiatry 44:576–578, 1993

Smith DH, Chen XH, Pierce JE, et al: Progressive atrophy and neuron death for one year following brain trauma in the rat. J Neurotrauma 14:715–727, 1997a

Smith DH, Chen XH, Xu BN, et al: Characterization of diffuse axonal pathology and selective hippocampal damage following initial brain trauma in the pig. J Neuropathol Exp Neurol 56:822–834, 1997b

Soares JC, Innis RB: Neurochemical brain imaging investigations of schizophrenia. Biol Psychiatry 46:600–615, 1999

Suddath RL, Christison GW, Torrey EF, et al: Anatomical abnormalities in the brains of monozygotic twins discordant for schizophrenia. N Engl J Med 322:789–794, 1990

Susser E, Struening EL, Conover S: Psychiatric problems in homeless men: lifetime psychosis, substance use, and current distress in new arrivals at New York City shelters. Arch Gen Psychiatry 46:845–850, 1989

Tang YP, Noda Y, Hasegawa T, et al: A concussive-like brain injury model in mice, I: impairment in learning and memory. J Neurotrauma 14:851–862, 1997a

Tang YP, Noda Y, Hasegawa T, et al: A concussive-like brain injury model in mice, II: selective neuronal loss in the cortex and hippocampus. J Neurotrauma 14:863–873, 1997b

Tate DF, Bigler ED: Fornix and hippocampal atrophy in traumatic brain injury. Learn Mem 7:442–446, 2000

Thomsen IV: Late outcome of very severe blunt head trauma: a 10–15 year second follow-up. J Neurol Neurosurg Psychiatry 47:260–268, 1984

Trimble MR: Interictal psychoses of epilepsy. Adv Neurol 55:143–152, 1991

Trimble MR, Thompson PJ: Memory, anticonvulsant drugs and seizures. Acta Neurol Scand Suppl 89:31–41, 1981

Trzepacz PT: Delirium, in Neuropsychiatry of Traumatic Brain Injury. Edited by Silver J, Yudofsky SC, Hales RE. Washington, DC, American Psychiatric Press, 1994, pp 189–218

Violon A, De Mol J: Psychological sequelae after head traumas in adults. Acta Neurochir (Wein) 85:96–102, 1987

von Krafft-Ebing R: [Ueber die durch Gehirnerschutterung und Kopfverletzung hervorgerufenen psychischen Krankheiten. Eine klinisch-forensische Studie (German)]. Erlangen, Germany, Verlag von Ferdinand Enke, 1868

Wiegner S, Donders J: Performance on the Wisconsin Card Sorting Test after traumatic brain injury. Assessment 6:179–187, 1999

Wilcox JA, Nasrallah HA: Childhood head trauma and psychosis. Psychiatry Res 21:303–306, 1987

Yamaki T, Murakami N, Iwamoto Y, et al: Cognitive dysfunction and histological findings in rats with chronic-stage contusion and diffuse axonal injury. Brain Res Brain Res Protoc 3:100–106, 1998

12 Posttraumatic Stress Disorder and Other Anxiety Disorders

Deborah L. Warden, M.D.

Lawrence A. Labbate, M.D.

ANXIETY OCCURS COMMONLY after traumatic brain injury (TBI). Patients may have anxiety in the immediate wake of the accident, in the postacute period, and sometimes chronically. Many problems may contribute to anxiety, including worry about physical injuries and possible cognitive decline as well as disruption of neural circuits implicated in the development of anxiety. Anxiety may have cognitive, behavioral, and somatic presentations that become disabling and interfere with patients' recovery and adaptation to life after brain injury. Although lack of awareness of one's cognitive and behavioral injuries may occur in moderate to severe TBI (see Chapter 19, Awareness of Deficits), individuals may still worry about their injuries and exhibit components of anxiety syndromes (e.g., irritability) that may respond to treatment. Hence, the clinician must be aware of how these anxiety problems present and the potential need for treatment. Although any of the anxiety states may develop, there are few longitudinal studies of consecutive brain-injured patients that examine the frequency and outcome of these states. Strong evidence regarding treatment for anxiety states related to TBI is currently lacking.

Cognitive and Behavioral Consequences of Anxiety

After TBI, individuals may worry about their capacity to do what were once simple tasks. Especially in the first few months after TBI when recovery may not yet be complete, frustration and anxiety regarding the performance of tasks that were once simple and automatic may occur. This difficulty may lead to additional distress and free-floating anxiety. Patients may abandon their attempts to complete tasks because of fear of failure or misperception about their abilities, especially if they are aware that tasks take longer to complete than they did before the brain injury. Patients may develop a cognitive distortion causing the belief that they are unable to do such tasks, even though these patients are simply slower and less facile than they once were.

After TBI, patients may respond to their decreased abilities by avoidance. For example, people who are physically disfigured may lose self-esteem and feel uncomfortable around others with whom they once felt at ease and then may avoid social contact. Difficulty processing mul-

The opinion or assertions contained herein are the private views of the author(s) and are not to be construed as official or as reflecting the views of the Department of the Army or the Department of the Defense.

tiple stimuli in a social setting may cause feelings of discomfort and anxiety in the patient in this setting and lead to avoidance of future social gatherings because of the anxiety they produce. Individuals with mild brain injury may also become self-conscious about cognitive deficits and therefore wish to avoid the anxiety and humiliation of those deficits being revealed to others. This self-consciousness may lead to worsened anxiety and further avoidance of situations that could reveal deficits, as demonstrated in the following case example:

> Mr. A was a 29-year-old plumber who experienced a mild TBI (MTBI) and a broken leg when his car crashed on the highway during a rainstorm. He lost consciousness for less than 30 minutes and experienced 1 day of posttraumatic amnesia (PTA) while in the hospital. Brain magnetic resonance imaging (MRI) findings were unremarkable. After the accident, he had no neurological deficits and had mild headaches that were relieved by ibuprofen. On return to work, he found that he was unable to concentrate on his job and that it took him twice as long to complete simple plumbing tasks. He became worried about "losing his mind" and would ruminate about the loss of his livelihood and about not being able to support his family; he thought that he had "become retarded." He had trouble sleeping, felt his heart racing all the time, and felt very uncomfortable when visiting with friends because he felt humiliated that he was not his former self. He quit playing softball with his friends because he didn't want to "make a fool of himself." Six months after the accident, the patient was enrolled in an occupational therapy program and ultimately was able to reconcile his relatively modest cognitive decline and return to work, doing simpler tasks initially. His anxiety was then greatly reduced.

Somatic Consequences of Anxiety

As in patients with idiopathic anxiety disorders, patients with brain injury may complain of many somatic symptoms of anxiety, especially cardiopulmonary, gastrointestinal, and neurological symptoms. These symptoms may be difficult to tease out from injury to other body systems in cases of multiple traumas, or there may be considerable overlap with the neurological symptoms of the postconcussive syndrome (PCS). That is, some patients may experience vertigo, headache, or even complex partial seizures that may be mistaken as anxiety. On the other hand, patients with multiple bodily injuries may develop anxiety that worsens these bodily symptoms. Sorting out the contributions of bodily injury, neurological disorders, and anxiety is not an easy task. However, treating identifiable problems associated with trauma such as pain, headache, and epilepsy is paramount before ascribing the symptoms to anxiety.

Young people, in particular, those who have never been medically ill, may report many somatic symptoms in response to their loss of function. They may have trouble sleeping or concentrating or may develop panic attacks or free-floating anxiety. In an effort to quell anxiety and improve sleep, patients may drink alcohol. Moreover, many patients involved in motor vehicle accidents (MVAs) have premorbid alcohol abuse or dependence, and the return to alcohol use may only precipitate more somatic symptoms, especially disrupted sleep and gastrointestinal symptoms. In heavier alcohol users, mild alcohol withdrawal symptoms may be mistaken for primary anxiety. Only after other causes of somatic symptoms are excluded should somatic symptoms be ascribed to anxiety associated with TBI. Clues that anxiety is the culprit include specific phobias, panic attacks in association with specific behaviors, and somatic anxiety symptoms combined with rituals to reduce symptoms. The following case example illustrates somatic consequences of anxiety related to brain injury:

> Mr. B was a 26-year-old motorcycle enthusiast who lost control of his motorcycle while racing with a friend after drinking in a bar. He experienced a mild brain injury as well as a ruptured spleen, fractured femur, and orbital fracture and remained in the intensive care unit for 2 weeks due to pneumonia. Medical and surgical treatments were considered successes. However, the patient had a slow recovery of walking ability and complained continually of fears of falling and constant feelings of dizziness and blurred vision associated with walking. He felt that he was unable to stand without a cane, even though his physical therapists believed that he should be able to walk. One month after the accident, he developed panic attacks with prominent vertigo and dyspnea. He then surreptitiously resumed drinking alcohol, up to 10 beers per evening. His girlfriend reported that he walked *better* after drinking a few beers. The patient's anxiety symptoms worsened with continued drinking, and he was unable to walk without feeling dizzy or experiencing panic. He felt that he needed his girlfriend with him to walk for fear of fainting. Eventually, through discussing his fears about his inability to be his former, fearless self and with the addition of

sertraline, 75 mg/day, his somatic symptoms and panic attacks subsided.

Relationship of TBI to Development of Anxiety Disorders

It is often difficult to assign causality of an anxiety disorder after TBI. The anxiety disorder may be due to the brain injury directly or to the accumulation of severe life experiences that immediately follow the brain injury or to the combination of both events. Because the pathophysiology of anxiety disorders remains unknown, only inferences can be made about the contribution of the brain injury to the development of posttraumatic anxiety. The temporal association of the TBI with the development of anxiety disorders is helpful although not definitive in assigning causation of the TBI to the anxiety disorder. Current understanding suggests that the sooner a new anxiety disorder follows a TBI, the more likely that the anxiety disorder is related to the TBI. Similarly, an exacerbation of anxiety symptoms after TBI in persons with preexisting anxiety disorders may be due to the direct effects of the brain trauma.

It is reasonable to think that injuries affecting systems known to be relevant to anxiety disorders may be the cause of a newly acquired anxiety disorder. For example, a finding on brain MRI of a contusion in the frontal lobe pathways connecting with the caudate nucleus would be reasonable evidence of the role of the TBI in a new case of obsessive-compulsive disorder (OCD). In many cases, however, the imaging is not so clear-cut, and a patient's injuries may be diffuse. Moreover, anxiety disorders starting a considerable time after the injury—perhaps 1 year after the TBI—are less likely to be caused by the TBI, although anxiety may develop in response to ongoing cognitive or other persisting sequelae and the individual's possibly diminished functioning because of these sequelae. In many cases, a combination of biological, interpersonal, and social factors likely contribute to the development of anxiety disorders after TBI.

Incidence Studies of Anxiety Disorders After TBI

A number of studies in the past 10 years have evaluated the frequency and types of anxiety disorders that follow TBI. However, few case series have evaluated consecutive brain-injured patients soon after the brain injury to establish the natural history and frequency of anxiety disorders after TBI. Some studies have evaluated patients who were referred for psychiatric evaluation after brain injury some time after the injury. Clearly, the referral studies may be biased toward reporting higher rates of psychiatric disorders than in unselected samples. In addition, it is still not clear whether the development of anxiety after TBI exhibits different characteristics or occurs at different frequencies in patients with mild compared with moderate to severe brain injury.

Few studies have evaluated the presence of all of the anxiety disorders post-TBI. That is, investigators have examined the development of generalized anxiety disorder (GAD) but not OCD or other anxiety disorders after brain injury (Salazar et al. 2000). There are few comprehensive studies that have followed the natural history of anxiety disorders after brain injury. Moreover, without the benefit of knowing the neuroanatomic correlates of brain injury and anxiety disorders, researchers remain uncertain about whether anxiety disorders are due to specific or multiple neuropathologic lesions and/or the psychosocial consequences of disability in an individual with a given biologic vulnerability for developing anxiety disorders. Likely, a combination of these factors contributes to the development of post-TBI anxiety disorders, but this connection has not been established.

The medical literature is dotted with case reports and case series of individual anxiety disorders after brain injury, although without the benefit of control groups, it remains unknown whether these are chance findings or whether the anxiety disorder is truly secondary to the brain injury. Although most clinical investigators support the causal association between brain injury and the development of anxiety disorders, the hypothesis has not been proved. This review focuses on the larger prospective studies but mentions the case reports of anxiety after brain injury.

Fann et al. (2000) evaluated 50 consecutive patients who were referred to a university brain rehabilitation clinic. Patients were evaluated, on average, 3 years after their brain injury. Most patients had mild brain injury. Patients were evaluated using structured clinical interviews, and DSM-III-R (American Psychiatric Association 1987) criteria were applied for making diagnoses. This sample, on average, did not demonstrate gross cognitive impairment as evidenced by a screening neuropsychological evaluation. Patients were evaluated only for the following anxiety disorders: panic disorder, agoraphobia, and GAD. Patients were not assessed for other phobias, posttraumatic stress disorder (PTSD), or OCD.

The authors of the aforementioned study found that 24% of patients had GAD at the time of interview. Some of these patients also had concurrent major depression. The authors noted, however, that 34% of the patients had a history of GAD, thus making it somewhat difficult to interpret whether the GAD was because of the brain injury. These high rates could represent a selection bias of patients presenting for brain injury rehabilitation. Anxiety disorder patients also had greater medical and social disability rates than patients without anxiety. The authors found, perhaps surprisingly, that 2% of the patients had panic disorder, a rate no different from that of the general population. Hence, this study suggests that anxiety is common and contributes to disability, but the link between anxiety and TBI is far from clear.

In a well-designed study by Deb et al. (1998), investigators evaluated 148 patients in Wales whose conditions were diagnosed as TBI during a visit to a hospital. Patients were contacted by mail and questionnaire, and some were then interviewed in person approximately 1 year after the brain injury. Diagnoses of anxiety disorders were made by a structured interview—the Schedule for Clinical Assessment in Neuropsychiatry—which corresponds with diagnoses in the *International Statistical Classification of Diseases and Related Health Problems*, 10th Revision. It is unclear which anxiety disorders were queried, although the frequency of GAD, panic disorder, phobic disorder, and OCD were reported. Most patients had mild brain injury.

The authors found that panic disorder in this sample occurred in 7% of patients. Hence, the rate of panic was several times higher than that in the general population. Unlike the high rates of anxiety disorders seen in the referral patients in other studies (Fann et al. 1995, 2000; Hibbard et al. 1998), GAD (1.8%) and OCD (1.2%) occurred at approximately the same rate as that in the general population. "Nightmare" was diagnosed in 4.2% of the sample, but no mention is made of the frequency of PTSD. Hence, this study, which represented an unselected series of patients evaluated after brain injury, found that anxiety disorders occurred but were somewhat less frequent than might be expected. It may have been the case that patients experienced anxiety but that these anxiety symptoms were subsyndromal. Perhaps many patients do not experience significant anxiety by 1 year.

In a prospective study evaluating the benefits of cognitive rehabilitation, Salazar et al. (2000) evaluated 120 consecutive active-duty military members after a moderate to severe brain injury. Nearly all patients were men (95%). Patients were generally evaluated by 1 month after the brain injury and then systematically evaluated during a 1-year follow-up. Structured clinical interviews were used to make DSM-IV-TR diagnoses (American Psychiatric Association 2000). The only anxiety disorder reported in this study was GAD. The authors found that 10% of patients had generalized anxiety at baseline, and at 1 year after enrollment, 15% of patients met criteria for generalized anxiety. This study, similar to the study by Deb et al. (1998), is important because patients were not selected just because they had psychological problems. This study represents a naturalistic longitudinal history of a consecutive group of mostly young

men who experienced brain injury. However, the report did not address the frequency of other anxiety disorders.

Mayou and Bryant (1994) and Mayou et al. (1993) evaluated 188 people soon after a motor vehicle accident, then 3 months later, and then 1 year later. Patients were interviewed in person with structured clinical interviews and several rating scales. Only some of these patients (n=51) had mild brain injuries, and severe brain injuries were excluded. Forty-four of the patients with head injury had no memory of the accident. The investigators were interested in determining the frequency and time course of psychiatric disorders, especially PTSD and travel anxiety, after an MVA. One hundred seventy-one patients were evaluated at the 1-year point. The authors found that soon after the accident, many subjects experienced high levels of anxiety and depression. Moreover, many patients avoided car travel or were anxious in their everyday life events. Anxiety disorders other than PTSD were not systematically recorded.

In a similar and more recent study, Mayou et al. (2000) evaluated psychiatric symptoms after motor vehicle accidents in 1,441 patients. Patient diagnoses and psychiatric problems were identified via a questionnaire sent through the mail rather than by direct interview. The findings of this study may be limited by the questionable validity of the method used. From this larger sample, a subset of 60 patients who had evidence of mild brain injury (i.e., definite or probable unconsciousness) was analyzed. The authors found that at 3 months and at 1 year after the accident, approximately 20% of the patients with TBI were experiencing travel anxiety. Travel anxiety was considered a specific phobia by the authors.

In a small sample of patients (n=18), Van Reekum et al. (1996) examined patients after TBI for the presence of DSM-III-R mental disorders using a structured interview. The sample was nearly split in severity, with 8 patients experiencing mild or moderate TBI and 10 experiencing severe TBI. Patients were recruited using a letter that described the study as one examining "emotional and cognitive well-being" after brain injury. This patient selection may have biased the sample toward patients with higher rates of emotional distress. The authors found that 7 patients (39%) met criteria for an anxiety disorder, although only 4 of these developed the disorder after the TBI. GAD was the most common diagnosis among the patients with anxiety disorders. Because of the small sample size and methodological limitations, these findings may not be as readily generalized.

Using a very different study design, Hibbard et al. (1998), evaluated 100 patients with a mean of 8 years between TBI and structured clinical interview. Patients were recruited by advertisements in brain injury newsletters in New York. Severity of brain injury ranged widely, with 40% of patients having severe TBI by self-report. The authors found that

TABLE 12–1.   Rates of anxiety disorders after traumatic brain injury, from case series

Anxiety disorder	Rate (%)
Generalized anxiety disorder	8–24
Panic disorder	2–7
Obsessive-compulsive disorder	1–9
Specific phobia (especially driving)	≤25
Social phobia	Not known
Posttraumatic stress disorder	0–42

80% of patients met the criteria for a DSM-IV-TR mental disorder on the basis of patients' reports after their brain injury. The validity of these retrospective diagnoses, however, may be questioned because of the long duration between injury and interview. Moreover, patients' cognitive limitations may potentially exaggerate or minimize past events. Additionally, many of the mental disorders that reportedly followed TBI had already resolved at the time of the interview. At the time of the interview, however, a number of patients had anxiety disorders, including PTSD (10%), OCD (9%), GAD (8%), and panic disorder (4%). These rates of anxiety disorders (Table 12–1) are consistent with other reports, although the high incidence of OCD stands apart from results of other reports. One of the problems with this sample, however, is that many of the patients reported preexisting mental disorders, including 40% with substance abuse disorders. At a minimum, this study suggests that for some patients, especially those with preexisting mental disorders, anxiety disorders may persist long after TBI.

In an analysis of the New Haven National Institute of Mental Health Epidemiologic Catchment Area Study data, Silver et al. (2001) demonstrated a significantly higher rate of panic disorder, phobic disorder, and OCD in persons who said yes to the question "Have you ever had a severe head injury that was associated with a loss of consciousness or confusion?" In a clinical sample, a greater proportion of TBI patients with anxiety disorders and comorbid major depressive disorder were identified than patients with anxiety disorder alone (Jorge et al. 2004).

Posttraumatic Stress Disorder in TBI

Required for the diagnosis of PTSD is the experience of a traumatic event that later evokes physiological reactivity, emotional distress upon reminders of the event, and reexperiencing phenomena (e.g., flashbacks, nightmares, and intrusive thoughts of the traumatic event). Although anxiety after TBI has been described for some time, more controversial has been the issue of PTSD occurring after brain injury with neurogenic amnesia for the event, specifically because amnesia due to the brain injury might protect the individual from developing such memories and future PTSD symptoms of flashbacks and nightmares. The incidence studies discussed in the following section focus on the topic of PTSD after TBI with amnesia.

Incidence Studies

Evidence That PTSD Does Not Follow TBI With Amnesia

According to research about the Coconut Grove disaster, a devastating fire in a busy Boston nightclub, survivors who sustained loss of consciousness (LOC) longer than 1 hour were less likely to develop psychiatric complications (Adler 1943). In a later report of MVA patients, Mayou et al. (1993) reported that 19 of 188 individuals developed PTSD within the first year after injury. This study included only individuals with LOC less than 15 minutes. PTSD did not develop in patients with brief unconsciousness; the development of PTSD was strongly associated with the presence of "horrific memories" and was not associated with prior psychological problems, baseline depression, or neuroticism. In a brief report, McCarthy et al. (1998) investigated 196 hospitalized patients with TBI who were followed for 1 year. Five individuals developed PTSD; 4 still had PTSD at the 1-year interview. All 5 who developed PTSD recalled their injury and had experienced brief or no LOC.

In a consecutive series of military subjects with moderate to severe TBI, Warden et al. (1997) reported that 0 of 47 patients met full DSM-III-R criteria for PTSD; 6 of 47 (13%) met all criteria for PTSD except for the reexperiencing phenomena, which included intrusive memories. Significant comorbidity was reported, with 5 of 6 individuals meeting criteria for either DSM-III-R organic anxiety or mood disorder. In a study of individuals who had received diagnoses previously, Sbordone and Liter (1995) compared individuals with PTSD to another group with PCS. None of the 42 individuals with PTSD had lost consciousness, and all could give a detailed history of the trauma, whereas 24 of 28 individuals with PCS had lost consciousness, and none could give a detailed account of the trauma. No individual had both PTSD and PCS, leading Sbordone and Liter to suggest that the two did not occur simultaneously.

Evidence That PTSD May Follow TBI With Amnesia

Contrary to the results discussed in the preceding section, individual case reports (Bryant 1996; King 1997;

McMillan 1991) suggest that PTSD may follow TBI with amnesia for the event. A case series by McMillan (1996) reported that 10 individuals out of 312 evaluated met criteria for PTSD, although vivid reexperiencing was uncommon. Women were overrepresented in the PTSD sample (60% with PTSD, vs. 25% of the sample), and 6 of 10 individuals with PTSD also experienced chronic pain and/or depression. McMillan's patients were drawn from admissions for rehabilitation or for forensic evaluation; all individuals with PTSD were at least 9 months postinjury. McMillan suggested that PTSD is relatively rare after TBI and that other researchers had not found it in consecutive series reports for that reason.

Overrepresentation of women developing PTSD after TBI was also reported in a mixed sample of 60 mild- and 9 moderate-TBI patients (Levin et al. 2001). Feinstein et al. (2002) investigated the frequency of intrusive symptoms in a group of 282 mixed-severity-TBI outpatients who averaged 53 days postinjury when evaluated. Patients with the less severe TBI (PTA <1 hour) had significantly higher intrusion and avoidance scores than patients with more severe brain injury. The authors note that because this was not their a priori hypothesis, the finding must be replicated. Hickling et al. (1998) reported equivalent frequencies of PTSD in MVA patients with MTBI and in MVA patients without TBI in a sample referred to a private psychology practice. In this group, individuals with PTSD and no TBI did not perform worse on a neuropsychological battery of attention and memory items when compared with individuals without PTSD. In another series, 33% of a mixed sample of patients with TBI and stroke developed DSM-III-R PTSD (Ohry et al. 1996). On self-report instruments, reexperiencing phenomena were the least common symptoms noted, and women were overrepresented in the PTSD group. In a small series of emergency department patients, 3 of 9 MVA patients with head injury developed PTSD (Epstein and Ursano 1994), although additional information was not available.

Silver et al. (1997) reported on a series of seven referred patients who experienced PTSD after mild to moderate TBI. Most patients experienced no or very brief LOC. Several patients developed PTSD related to events that they recalled either before LOC or on regaining consciousness, suggesting the existence of mechanisms for establishing traumatic memories for PTSD even if no memories are encoded at the time of the accident and LOC.

In a report on community dwellers recruited from brain injury organization newsletters, PTSD was the most common anxiety disorder reported (Hibbard et al.

1998). Of the 17% of the subjects who reported PTSD developing after injury, 41% of them had experienced resolution of their symptoms by the time of the interview. Subjects in this study were approximately 7.6 years postinjury. Approximately one-half of the individuals had experienced an Axis I disorder before the TBI, although equivalent rates of patients with and without prior Axis I diagnoses developed PTSD after TBI.

In a series of papers, Bryant and others reported an incidence of PTSD of 24% in patients with mild TBI (Bryant and Harvey 1998) and 27% in patients with severe TBI (Bryant et al. 2000). PTSD was diagnosed by the PTSD Interview on the basis of DSM-III-R criteria. Patients with severe TBI uncommonly reported intrusive memories, and the reexperiencing criterion was met in these patients largely by emotional reactivity. When intrusive memories did occur, however, they were highly predictive of PTSD. Patients with chronic pain were more likely to develop PTSD (Bryant et al. 1999); patients with PTSD also had higher Beck Depression Inventory scores (Bryant et al. 2001) and Overt Aggression Scale scores. At least one of the patients described having nightmares on the basis of photographs of his car that he viewed after the accident. PTSD negatively affected outcome: a diagnosis of PTSD was associated with greater functional disability as measured by the Functional Assessment Measure and Community Integration Questionnaire—Productivity. Individuals with PTSD also reported lower satisfaction with life, as measured by the Community Integration Questionnaire.

Finally, a recent prospective study of admissions to a rehabilitation unit reported that PTSD is much less likely to develop in TBI patients with more prolonged loss of consciousness (Glaesser et al. 2004).

Characteristics of Posttraumatic Stress Disorder After TBI

Relationship to Acute Stress Disorder

The development of acute stress disorder was predictive of PTSD in MTBI patients at 6 months (Bryant and Harvey 1998) and 2 years (Bryant et al. 2000). Compared with MTBI patients without PTSD, MTBI patients with PTSD experienced more headache, dizziness, fatigue, and visual disturbances. Possible comorbidity with depression or other anxiety disorders was not discussed. In an earlier study of patients seen within 1 month of injury, Bryant and Harvey (1995) noted less acute stress disorder in patients who had experienced an MVA and an MTBI (27% PTSD) than in control patients who had experienced an MVA and no TBI (42%). Patients with acute stress disorder and MTBI reported significantly fewer intrusive reexperiencing phenomena and less fear and helplessness than those without brain injury. At 6 months, both groups reported comparable amounts of intrusive symptoms. Intrusive symptoms and acute stress symptoms were not correlated with anxiety in TBI patients, unlike in non-TBI patients. The authors state that "the lack of a positive correlation between anxiety and intrusive symptoms in the head injured patients points to different processes mediating the experience of anxiety in head injured and non-head injured patients" (Bryant and Harvey 1995, p. 872).

Comorbidity of Posttraumatic Stress Disorder and Depression in TBI

Increased symptom severity of depression and a trend toward more frequent diagnosis of depression was noted in a TBI sample compared with a general trauma control group in a study of patients with mild and moderate TBI (Levin et al. 2001). In a study of individuals presenting to the Veterans Administration with psychiatric disability claims, Vasterling et al. (2000) studied comorbidity of PTSD (using the Structured Clinical Interview for DSM-IV) and depression. Approximately one-half of claimants gave a self-report of TBI. Approximately the same percentage of individuals with TBI reported depression and PTSD, but the severity of depression was greater in the TBI group. Using regression analysis, the researchers concluded that depression is related to TBI, but PTSD is not. This study, however, is limited by its retrospective design and self-report of head injury without verification of the occurrence or severity of TBI.

Cognition and Posttraumatic Stress Disorder in TBI

The presence of PTSD did not affect measures of attention and memory in a TBI population studied by Hickling et al. (1998). However, increased severity of TBI was associated with decreased performance in measures of memory and attention. Future reports on this topic are welcome, because PTSD patients without TBI may demonstrate decreased performance on memory and attention testing (Bremner et al. 1993; Vasterling et al. 2002); these cognitive changes are also observed after TBI.

Summary

Taken together, these studies suggest that PTSD after TBI does occur but may be modified by the brain injury. Specifically, intrusive memories are less common than in non-TBI individuals and in less severely injured individuals with TBI. It is possible that some patients develop PTSD related to memories of events that follow the brain injury. Specifically, patients may respond to the story of the event, photographs of the accident, or seeing injuries that they sustained from the accident, all of which may lead them to create a version of the trauma. It is also possible that patients do not encode the events as explicit memory but have an emotional memory that leads to the development of anxiety symptoms. The rate of PTSD appears to increase over time, although few studies offer longitudinal follow-up. PTSD has been described for a range of traumatic memories, including events immediately before LOC, events experienced after regaining consciousness, information learned on regaining consciousness (e.g., from photographs), and traumas reactivated from earlier life events.

Neurobiology of Anxiety and Anxiety Disorders

Recent developments in neurobiology offer insights into the pathophysiology of PTSD and other anxiety disorders. TBI involves diffuse brain injury as well as frequent focal injuries to frontal and temporal structures (Levin and Kraus 1994), including the hippocampus and amygdala (Bigler 2001), areas implicated in the neurobiology of anxiety.

The physiological response to acute stress involves multiple neuroendocrine and neurotransmitter responses, including increased levels of circulating cortisol and catecholamines. As catecholamines ready the organism for "fight or flight," cortisol facilitates negative feedback on the hypothalamus and pituitary to shut down the stress response. The amygdala participates in the stress/fear response, sending projections to brain areas involved in the autonomic nervous system (sympathetic and parasympathetic) and the hypothalamic-pituitary-adrenal axis. The amygdala and hippocampus are located in close proximity in the temporal lobes. Work by LeDoux (1992) demonstrates the existence of amygdala circuits for emotional memory that are separate from hippocampal circuits involved in explicit memory. Thus, a fear response to an injury (e.g., a burn) would be encoded at an amygdala/"emotional" level, which is separate from the pathway for processing explicit information that could include a lexical encoding of the details of the experience. The amygdala circuit is phylogenetically older than the hippocampal circuit. If consciousness is lost during the traumatic event, it seems consistent that the organism could subsequently respond in an avoidant, fearful manner to subsequent exposure without a full recall of previous exposures.

The inverted, U-shaped curve describes well how increasing levels of anxiety/arousal may enhance performance, but beyond a certain threshold, anxiety/arousal is detrimental to performance. The relationship of chronic stress and elevated cortisol levels to neurotoxicity to hippocampal neurons is a subject of active research (Gilbertson et al. 2002; Sapolsky 1994, 2000). The effects of chronic elevation of cortisol have been postulated to damage hippocampal neurons; neuroimaging findings of reduced hippocampal size in individuals with PTSD are discussed in the next section. Other researchers suggest a cortisol-independent mechanism of neurotoxicity of hippocampal neurons in PTSD (see Sapolsky 2000 for review).

Although Yehuda (2001) suggested that high levels of cortisol contribute to the development of PTSD, other recent studies suggest that basal cortisol levels are low in individuals with PTSD (Yehuda and McFarlane 1995) and in those at risk for PTSD (Yehuda 1999) and that lower cortisol levels in MVA patients in the emergency department are predictive of later PTSD (Yehuda et al. 1998). Moreover, increased number and sensitivity of glucocorticoid receptors have also been reported in the hippocampus in individuals with PTSD (Yehuda 2001).

Other work has investigated the potential genetic contributions to vulnerability to the development of anxiety disorders (True et al. 1993). A genetic contribution to the development of PTSD in non-TBI cohorts has been reported; this biological diathesis could also influence the development of PTSD after TBI but must be confirmed. New molecular genetic techniques permit the investigation of stress at the molecular level. For example, a recent study suggests that glucocorticoid-mediated stress is associated with a change in the ratio of two splice products of a rat acetylcholinesterase gene (Meshorer et al. 2002), which may be associated with hypersensitivity to acetylcholinesterases. Understanding how gene products are formed in response to stress may offer opportunities for future treatment interventions.

Because the frontal poles of the temporal lobes are often affected by trauma, it is not unreasonable to believe that the amygdala is often involved in TBI-related anxiety disorders. Hence, direct trauma or secondary effects of trauma from stress may affect amygdala functioning after TBI and lead to the start of anxiety symptoms. Although the exact neuroanatomic disruption leading to anxiety disorders after TBI remains unknown, limbic structures in the temporal lobes, especially the amygdala and hippocampus, remain the best hypothetical sites for the confluence of anatomical and physiological evidence related to anxiety.

Insight From Neuroimaging

Neuroimaging of Posttraumatic Stress Disorder in Non-TBI patients

Structural imaging studies have identified decreased volume of hippocampal structures (right—Bremner et al. 1995; left—Bremner et al. 1997; bilateral—Gurvits et al. 1996) in cross-sectional studies of individuals with PTSD.

A prospective longitudinal study of hippocampal volume in patients with new onset of PTSD failed to demonstrate a difference between hippocampal volumes in PTSD patients and control subjects studied at 1 week and 6 months after diagnosis (Bonne et al. 2001), suggesting that changes in hippocampal volume do not underlie the development of the PTSD in this population. Decreased volume of the hippocampus has been suggested to relate to glutamate-mediated neurotoxicity in hippocampal neurons through a glucocorticoid or non-glucocorticoid-mediated mechanism (Sapolsky 2000).

A recent study of monozygotic twins in which one twin was a Vietnam combat veteran explored the contributions of genetics and combat exposure/PTSD in hippocampal volume. Hippocampal volumes were smaller in both twins (the twin who was combat-exposed and developed more severe PTSD as well as the twin who was not combat-exposed and did not have PTSD) compared with twins who had not been combat-exposed and who did not have PTSD. Also, by demonstrating no significant difference in hippocampal volumes between the combat-exposed/PTSD twin and the nonexposed/non-PTSD twin, the authors suggested that smaller hippocampi in PTSD represent a preexisting, familial vulnerability factor (Gilbertson et al. 2002). An emerging literature on the neuroimaging of children with PTSD may prove useful to understanding the pathophysiology of PTSD (Vasa et al. 2004).

Finally, functional imaging has the ability to use symptom provocation and cognitive activation to study structures involved in PTSD. Symptom-provocation studies have demonstrated activation of amygdala (Liberzon et al. 1999; Rauch et al. 1996) and decreased activity of the anterior cingulated gyrus (functional MRI—Lanius et al. 2001; positron emission tomography—Bremner et al. 1999; Shin et al. 1999).

Relevance for TBI Patients

Taken together, imaging studies demonstrate involvement of amygdala, hippocampus, and other limbic/paralimbic structures in PTSD. The vulnerability of frontal and temporal lobes to structural damage from TBI was documented in early computed tomography studies (Levin and Kraus 1994). MRI studies have additionally identified decreased volume of the hippocampus and cingulate gyrus after TBI (Bigler 2001). On the basis of the finding of decreased hippocampal volume in subjects after TBI (Bigler 2001), a common substrate/pathway may exist for the development of PTSD after TBI. Injury to these structures during TBI may predispose patients to the development of anxiety symptoms and/or alter the expression/manifestations of PTSD. By inference from animal studies of acquisition and extinction of conditioned fear, injury to prefrontal areas may also predispose individuals with TBI to increased anxiety and fear (Morgan and LeDoux 1995). Future studies are needed to pursue these findings as well as findings of the relative resilience of many individuals who do not develop anxiety symptoms after TBI.

Possible Implications for the Neuroanatomy/Physiology of Anxiety Disorders

The observation that patients with PTSD after TBI are less likely to report intrusive memories or nightmares is compatible with studies of fear conditioning. A traumatic injury with amnesia could potentially result in one's responding with a fear response to certain stimuli, yet one may not have the memory of specifics of the event that would presumably be needed to produce reexperiencing phenomena of nightmares, flashbacks, or the sense that one was reliving the trauma. Still, physiological reactivity and avoidant responses after the trauma could in themselves be quite distressing.

Similarly, an individual who is told details and shown photographs of a horrific accident may begin to recall that learned information and relate it to the event that elicits the fear response. In this way, individuals may have reexperiencing symptoms for the events of the injury or even for events leading to the trauma. It also follows that mem-

ories that were not initially available to the person may be regained, especially in cases of brief LOC in which the PTA resolves over time.

With a better understanding of why certain individuals develop anxiety disorders, researchers will have better interventions for prevention and treatment. These understandings must then be linked to knowledge regarding the pathophysiology of TBI to relate more fully to TBI patients with anxiety disorders.

Treatment of Anxiety Associated With TBI

Psychotherapy

Even though anxiety commonly complicates the clinical status and rehabilitation of patients experiencing TBI, there is no clear evidence about how to best treat this phenomenon. There are no controlled trials of psychotherapy for anxiety disorders after TBI.

Whether anxiety is readily apparent during a patient interview depends on the severity of the patient's deficits, the extent of the anxiety, and the situation in which the anxiety occurs. Other cognitive or somatic complaints may mask the anxiety symptoms. Therefore, collateral information from family members and others involved with the patient's care is crucial to uncovering the extent and contribution of anxiety in the clinical picture. Without family input, the clinician may not learn about how the patient's anxiety led to avoidance of feared situations or activities.

Education—for both the patient and family—is critically important. Educating the patient and his or her family about the natural course of the illness and the expected level of disability over time is crucial for the development of realistic expectations regarding what capacities may reasonably improve and what capacities are less likely to improve. Even though the patient may lack insight or be unable to appreciate this information, at least the family can be supportive during rehabilitation and allow the patient to cope with the attendant frustration and anxiety. Because patients are frequently frustrated and anxious about loss of past skills, helping patients accept the new reality is crucial in controlling anxiety.

Many patients will be anxious about the loss of what they once were and have concerns about whether they will ever regain that sense of self. They may also fear that they will "lose their mind" if they are aware of their deficits and persisting anxiety. Patients require calm reassurance and the steady presence of a therapist to validate their experience.

Supportive psychotherapy appears intuitively important to patients during the acute and subacute recovery periods to help allay unrealistic fears and help patients adjust to their deficits. There are, however, no controlled studies to establish whether supportive therapy or any other form of psychotherapy is beneficial for treating anxiety symptoms associated with TBI. There are anecdotal reports that cognitive, behavioral, or psychodynamic therapies may benefit patients with TBI, but there are no controlled studies to substantiate any of these claims for the efficacy of psychotherapy. For example, exposure therapy for avoidance of feared activities makes sense, but the efficacy of this approach in patients with TBI has not been established.

For mildly brain-injured patients with anxiety, behavioral therapy may be a reasonable option. Because cognitive abilities and sensory filtering may be impaired, exposure to feared objects should be done very slowly and with realistically graded expectations to allow for incremental success. Patients need frequent reassurance that anxiety may be slightly worsened with initial treatment and that difficulty with mastering avoided behaviors is expected. Initial behavioral changes must be simple and clearly understood. Patients may have difficulty comprehending the sequence of events that the entire therapy might encompass and are probably best served by being introduced to small pieces of the therapy at a time. Behavioral treatments frequently need to include family members and other therapists, such as occupational or physical therapists, to maximize benefits and aid in the in vivo experience that is frequently required at the beginning of treatment.

A recent randomized trial of a series of individual cognitive behavior therapy or supportive counseling in 24 civilian MTBI survivors with acute stress disorder demonstrated superiority of the cognitive behavior therapy in reducing the development of PTSD at the end of treatment and at 6-month follow-up. These results are very encouraging (Bryant et al. 2003).

Psychopharmacology

Some patients require treatment with medication in combination with supportive psychotherapy or other psychotherapy. Again, the data regarding treatment of anxiety or anxiety syndromes associated with TBI are anecdotal and not well established. The usual pharmacological treatments for anxiety, including benzodiazepines, buspirone, and antidepressants, are often used, although benefits may be complicated by sensitivity to drug-associated adverse effects. The anticonvulsants also may have anxiolytic benefits, although these too are unstudied in anxiety syndromes related to TBI.

Benzodiazepines

The benzodiazepines may be useful in the setting of acute brain injury to reduce anxiety. Short-half-life drugs such as lorazepam are probably best used. For long-term use, the benzodiazepines may be problematic because of their adverse effects on concentration, motor coordination, and memory. In cases of severe anxiety, however, the benzodiazepines may actually help patients focus and improve sleep, thus improving cognition. For patients with a history of alcohol or drug dependence before their brain injury, the benzodiazepines should generally be avoided outside of supervised environments. These patients are at risk for misuse and behavior problems with benzodiazepines. For many patients, other pharmacological agents or nonpharmacological treatments can reduce anxiety. In most cases, benzodiazepine treatment of anxiety in brain-injured patients should be short-term, and efforts should be made to reduce or discontinue the medication after a reasonable period of symptom control. Because brain-injured patients are also at greater risk for behavioral disinhibition, use of this class of drug outside of controlled environments should be done cautiously and should begin with the lowest possible doses.

Serotonin Reuptake Inhibitor Antidepressants

The serotonin reuptake inhibitor (SRI) antidepressants have become the mainstay of the treatment of anxiety disorders because of limited adverse effects, minimal abuse potential, and effectiveness in the treatment of a wide range of anxiety symptoms. Although there are anecdotal reports of the benefits of SRIs in the treatment of anxiety in association with TBI, there are no controlled trials to establish SRI efficacy in patients whose anxiety is considered secondary to brain injury. Hence, although the SRIs frequently improve PTSD, panic attacks, social anxiety, obsessional symptoms, and free-floating anxiety, rigorous study of SRIs in TBI patients is missing. An open-label study of sertraline in the treatment of 15 patients with major depression after TBI found that 13 of the patients had at least a 50% improvement in depressive symptoms (Fann et al. 2000). Randomized, controlled trials are needed to determine whether the benefits are drug- or placebo-mediated. There is no compelling reason to believe that these drugs would not be beneficial for the treatment of anxiety; however, side effects may be problematic in brains compromised by cerebral injury, and the etiology underpinning anxiety related to brain injury may be different from the etiology in idiopathic cases.

In general, injured brains are less plastic and more vulnerable to pharmacological toxicity. Although the SRIs are largely free of cardiovascular and anticholinergic toxicity, they may still have central nervous system (CNS) and other systemic adverse effects. Although many CNS adverse effects are possible, including sedation, insomnia, worsened anxiety, and tremor, two clinically relevant CNS adverse effects of the SRIs should be carefully monitored when SRIs are used in brain-injured patients. These two common SRI-related adverse effects are drug-induced apathy and sexual dysfunction.

The SRIs appear to have both beneficial and problematic effects on executive function. In the case of obsessions or worry, diminished frontal overactivity may be beneficial, although if these effects are excessive then it is possible that apathy or indifference may result. Apathy or indifference may occur as a side effect of SRIs in the treatment of idiopathic anxiety disorders, especially at higher doses. In brain-injured patients, this side effect of SRIs could worsen preexisting apathy related to frontal injury or introduce a side effect that is potentially more problematic than the targeted anxiety. Hence, SRI treatment should begin at the lowest possible dose.

Sexual dysfunction (e.g., decreased libido, delayed orgasm) may also occur with SRI treatment, which may be more troublesome for younger brain-injured patients. Assessment of pretreatment sexual functioning (whether in a relationship or masturbation) is important before patients begin taking SRIs, and patients should be made aware of the potential for drug-induced sexual problems. Young males frequently do not tolerate an unforeseen side effect and discontinue the medication because of sexual side effects. Again, gradual dose titration is key in limiting sexual side effects. Sometimes, dose reduction or tolerance results in improved sexual functioning, although other times treatment with sildenafil or change to a non-SRI is required. Among agents potentially beneficial for treating anxiety, mirtazapine, nefazodone, buspirone, and the benzodiazepines have limited sexual dysfunction associated with their use.

Buspirone

Anecdotal reports of buspirone use with brain-injured patients suggest therapeutic effects, particularly with aggression and agitation. Buspirone may have a role as an add-on medication in the treatment of OCD, PTSD, and panic disorder. No controlled trials address the efficacy of buspirone in anxiety syndromes with brain injury.

Antipsychotics

The antipsychotics reduce anxiety associated with psychosis. Brain-injured patients, however, may be particu-

larly sensitive to extrapyramidal adverse effects, especially akathisia and dystonia. Hence, older, high-potency agents, such as haloperidol or fluphenazine, may be particularly problem prone in a young person with a brain injury. Outside of acute use in post-TBI delirium, the older, high-potency antipsychotics should be avoided in most cases. The antipsychotics, in general, should not be used as first-line agents for anxiety and should be reserved for patients with psychotic symptoms.

The newer antipsychotic agents, however, are better tolerated and may be beneficial for patients with psychosis and associated anxiety. With the exception of clozapine and quetiapine, these agents may still cause extrapyramidal adverse effects, and they must be used judiciously. Patients may also be sensitive to the orthostatic effects of the newer antipsychotics, particularly clozapine, quetiapine, and risperidone. Olanzapine may be particularly useful for sleep and anxiety, although sedation and weight gain are often problematic.

Anticonvulsants

The anticonvulsants may be helpful for anxiety associated with manic symptoms or agitation associated with brain injury. There is anecdotal evidence of benefits from the use of valproic acid in patients with idiopathic panic disorder (Woodman and Noyes 1994); however, these benefits are not established in placebo-controlled trials, and valproic acid has not been tested for the treatment of anxiety associated with TBI. There is limited evidence that gabapentin may be useful for the treatment of idiopathic PTSD (Hamner et al. 2001) and that lamotrigine may benefit patients with PTSD (Hertzberg et al. 1999), although the benefits for treating anxiety have not been studied in anxiety disorders after brain injury. The anticonvulsants may be a reasonable treatment alternative for patients with anxiety associated with aggressiveness. The anticonvulsants are intuitively appealing for treating anxiety after brain injury, especially when partial seizures contribute to the anxiety, although further work is needed to establish the benefit of anticonvulsants for the treatment of TBI-associated anxiety. Neurotoxic side effects may be amplified in patients with TBI, and using these agents requires slow titration.

References

Adler A: Neuropsychiatric complications in victims of Boston's Coconut Grove Disaster. JAMA 123:1098–1101, 1943

American Psychiatric Association: Diagnostic and Statistical Manual of Mental Disorders, 3rd Edition, Revised. Washington, DC, American Psychiatric Association, 1987

American Psychiatric Association: Diagnostic and Statistical Manual of Mental Disorders, 4th Edition, Text Revision. Washington, DC, American Psychiatric Association, 2000

Bigler ED: The lesion(s) in traumatic brain injury: implications for clinical neuropsychology. Arch Clin Neuropsychol 16:95–131, 2001

Bonne O, Brandes D, Gilboa A, et al: Longitudinal MRI study of hippocampal volume in trauma survivors with PTSD. Am J Psychiatry 158:1248–1251, 2001

Bremner JD, Scott TM, Delaney RC, et al: Deficits in short-term memory in posttraumatic stress disorder. Am J Psychiatry 150:1015–1019, 1993

Bremner J, Randall P, Scott T, et al: MRI-based measurement of hippocampal volume in patients with combat-related posttraumatic stress disorder. Am J Psychiatry 152:973–981, 1995

Bremner J, Randall P, Vermetten E, et al: Magnetic resonance imaging-based measurement of hippocampal volume in posttraumatic stress disorder related to childhood physical and sexual abuse—a preliminary report. Biol Psychiatry 41:23–32, 1997

Bremner JD, Staib LH, Kaloupek D, et al: Neural correlates of exposure to traumatic pictures and sound in Vietnam combat veterans with and without posttraumatic stress disorder: a positron emission tomography study. Biol Psychiatry 45:806–816, 1999

Bryant R: Posttraumatic stress disorder, flashbacks, and pseudomemories in closed head injury. J Trauma Stress 9:621–629, 1996

Bryant RA, Harvey AG: Acute stress response: a comparison of head injured and non-head injured patients. Psychol Med 25:869–873, 1995

Bryant R, Harvey A: Relationship between acute stress disorder and posttraumatic stress disorder following mild traumatic brain injury. Am J Psychiatry 155:625–629, 1998

Bryant R, Marosszeky J, Crooks J, et al: Interaction of posttraumatic stress disorder and chronic pain following traumatic brain injury. J Head Trauma Rehabil 14:588–594, 1999

Bryant RA, Marosszeky JE, Crooks J, et al: Posttraumatic stress disorder after severe traumatic brain injury. Am J Psychiatry 157:629–631, 2000

Bryant R, Marosszeky J, Crooks J, et al: Posttraumatic stress disorder and psychosocial functioning after severe traumatic brain injury. J Nerv Ment Dis 189:109–113, 2001

Bryant RA, Moulds M, Guthrie R, et al: Treating acute stress disorder following traumatic brain injury. Am J Psychiatry 160:585–587, 2003

Deb S, Lyons I, Koutzoukis C: Neuropsychiatric sequelae one year after a minor head injury. J Neurol Neurosurg Psychiatry 65:899–902, 1998

Epstein RS, Ursano RJ: Anxiety disorders, in Neuropsychiatry of Traumatic Brain Injury. Edited by Silver JM, Yudofsky SC, Hales RE. Washington, DC, American Psychiatric Press, 1994, pp 285–311

Fann J, Katon WJ, Uomoto JM, et al: Psychiatric disorders and functional disability in outpatients with traumatic brain injuries. Am J Psychiatry 152:1493–1499, 1995

Fann J, Uomoto JM, Katon WJ: Sertraline in the treatment of major depression following mild traumatic brain injury. Brain Inj 12:226–232, 2000

Feinstein A, Hershkop S, Ouchterlony D, et al: Posttraumatic amnesia and recall of a traumatic event following traumatic brain injury. J Neuropsychiatry Clin Neurosci 14:25–30, 2002

Gilbertson MW, Shenton ME, Ciszewski A, et al: Smaller hippocampal volume predicts pathologic vulnerability to psychological trauma. Nat Neurosci 5:1242–1247, 2002

Glaesser J, Neuner F, Lutgehetmann R, et al: Posttraumatic stress disorder in patients with traumatic brain injury. BMC Psychiatry 4:5, 2004

Gurvits TV, Shenton ME, Hokama H, et al: Magnetic resonance imaging study of hippocampal volume in chronic, combat-related posttraumatic stress disorder. Biol Psychiatry 40:1091–1099, 1996

Hamner MB, Brodrick PS, Labbate LA: Gabapentin in PTSD: a retrospective, clinical series of adjunctive therapy. Ann Clin Psychiatry 13:141–146, 2001

Hertzberg MA, Butterfield MI, Feldman ME, et al: A preliminary study of lamotrigine for the treatment of posttraumatic stress disorder. Biol Psychiatry 45:1226–1229, 1999

Hibbard M, Uysal S, Kepler K, et al: Axis I psychopathology in individuals with traumatic brain injury. J Head Trauma Rehabil 13:24–39, 1998

Hickling EJ, Gillen R, Blanchard EB, et al: Traumatic brain injury and posttraumatic stress disorder: a preliminary investigation of neuropsychological test results in PTSD secondary to motor vehicle accidents. Brain Inj 12:265–274, 1998

Jorge RE, Robinson RG, Moser D, et al: Major depression following traumatic brain injury. Arch Gen Psychiatry 61:42–50, 2004

King NS: Post-traumatic stress disorder and head injury as a dual diagnosis: "islands" of memory as a mechanism. J Neurol Neurosurg Psychiatry 62:82–84, 1997

Lanius RA, Williamson PC, Densmore M, et al: Neural correlates of traumatic memories in posttraumatic stress disorder: a functional MRI investigation. Am J Psychiatry 158:1920–1922, 2001

LeDoux J: Emotional memories in the brain, in Neuropsychology of Memory. Edited by Squire LR, Butters N. New York, Guilford Press, 1992, pp 463–469

Levin H, Kraus MF: The frontal lobes and traumatic brain injury. J Neuropsychiatry Clin Neurosci 6:443–454, 1994

Levin HS, Brown SA, Song JX, et al: Depression and posttraumatic stress disorder at three months after mild to moderate traumatic brain injury. J Clin Exp Neuropsychol 23:754–769, 2001

Liberzon I, Taylor SF, Amdur R, et al: Brain activation in PTSD in response to trauma-related stimuli. Biol Psychiatry 45:817–826, 1999

Mayou R, Black J, Bryant B: Unconsciousness, amnesia and psychiatric symptoms following road traffic accident injury. Br J Psychiatry 177:540–545, 2000

Mayou R, Bryant B: Effects of road traffic accidents on travel. Injury 25:457–460, 1994

Mayou R, Bryant B, Duthie R: Psychiatric consequences of road traffic accidents. BMJ 307:647–651, 1993

McCarthy G, Lyons I, Koutzoukis C, et al: Loss of consciousness and post-traumatic stress disorder. Br J Psychiatry 173:537, 1998

McMillan T: Post-traumatic stress disorder and severe head injury. Br J Psychiatry 159:431–433, 1991

McMillan T: Post-traumatic stress disorder following minor and severe closed head injury: 10 single cases. Brain Inj 10:749–758, 1996

Meshorer E, Erb C, Gazit R, et al: Alternative splicing and neuritic mRNA translocation under long-term neuronal hypersensitivity. Science 295:508–512, 2002

Morgan MA, LeDoux JE: Differential contribution of dorsal and ventral medial prefrontal cortex to the acquisition and extinction of conditioned fear in rats. Behav Neurosci 109:681–688, 1995

Ohry A, Rattok J, Solomon Z: Post-traumatic stress disorder in brain injury patients. Brain Inj 10:687–695, 1996

Rauch SL, van der Kolk BA, Fisler RE, et al: A symptom provocation study of posttraumatic stress disorder using positron emission tomography and script-driven imagery. Arch Gen Psychiatry 53:380–387, 1996

Salazar A, Warden D, Schwab K, et al: Cognitive rehabilitation for traumatic brain injury: a randomized trial. Defense and Veterans Head Injury Program (DVHIP) Study Group. JAMA 283:3075–3081, 2000

Sapolsky R: Glucocorticoids, stress and exacerbation of excitotoxic neuron death. Semin Neurosci 6:323–331, 1994

Sapolsky R: Glucocorticoids and hippocampal atrophy in neuropsychiatric disorders. Arch Gen Psychiatry 57:925–935, 2000

Sbordone RJ, Liter JC: Mild traumatic brain injury does not produce post-traumatic stress disorder. Brain Inj 9:405–412, 1995

Shin LM, McNally RJ, Kosslyn SM, et al: Regional cerebral blood flow during script-driven imagery in childhood sexual abuse-related PTSD: a PET investigation. Am J Psychiatry 156:575–584, 1999

Silver JM, Rattok J, Anderson K: Posttraumatic stress disorder and traumatic brain injury. Neurocase 3:151–157, 1997

Silver JM, Kramer R, Greenwald S, et al: The association between head injuries and psychiatric disorders: findings from the New Haven NIMH Epidemiologic Catchment Area Study. Brain Inj 15:935–945, 2001

True W, Rice J, Eisen S, et al: A twin study of genetic and environmental contributions to liability for posttraumatic stress symptoms. Arch Gen Psychiatry 50:257–264, 1993

Van Reekum R, Bolago I, Finlayson MA, et al: Psychiatric disorders after traumatic brain injury. Brain Inj 10:319–327, 1996

Vasa RA, Grados M, Slomine B, et al: Neuroimaging correlates of anxiety after pediatric traumatic brain injury. Biol Psychiaty 55:208–216, 2004

Vasterling J, Constans J, Hanna-Pladdy B: Head injury as a predictor of psychological outcome in combat veterans. J Trauma Stress 13:441–451, 2000

Vasterling JJ, Duke LM, Brailey K, et al: Attention, learning, and memory performances and intellectual resources in Vietnam veterans: PTSD and no disorder comparisons. Neuropsychology 16:5–14, 2002

Warden D, Labbate L, Salazar A, et al: Posttraumatic stress disorder in patients with traumatic brain injury and amnesia for the event. J Neuropsychiatry Clin Neurosci 9:18–22, 1997

Woodman CL, Noyes R Jr: Panic disorder: treatment with valproate. J Clin Psychiatry 55:134–136, 1994

World Health Organization: International Statistical Classification of Diseases and Related Health Problems, 10th Revision, Vol 1. Geneva, World Health Organization, 1992

Yehuda R: Biological factors associated with susceptibility to posttraumatic stress disorder. Can J Psychiatry 44:34–39, 1999

Yehuda R: Biology of posttraumatic stress disorder. J Clin Psychiatry 62:41–46, 2001

Yehuda R, McFarlane A: Conflict between current knowledge about posttraumatic stress disorder and its original conceptual basis. Am J Psychiatry 152:1705–1713, 1995

Yehuda R, McFarlane AC, Shalev AY: Predicting the development of posttraumatic stress disorder from the acute response to a traumatic event. Biol Psychiatry 44:1305–1313, 1998

13 Personality Disorders

Gregory J. O'Shanick, M.D.
Alison Moon O'Shanick, M.S., C.C.C.-S.L.P.

NEUROSCIENCE RESEARCH HAS intensified in the pursuit of the neuroanatomical and neurophysiological bases for personality traits and dysfunction. Development and application of functional neuroimaging methods such as positron emission tomography and functional magnetic resonance imaging provide in vivo measures of cortical processing, allowing real-time mapping of the neuroanatomical localization of behavior. These techniques provide a more comprehensive understanding of the complex interaction between nature and experience in the development of coping mechanisms and personality style.

Although no significant gains have been realized in reducing the mortality rates associated with severe traumatic brain injury (TBI) in the past decade, morbidity reduction has been a major focus in both neuromedical and neurobehavioral domains. Changes in discharge planning and resource availability now result in a reduced length of hospitalization and rehabilitation, with a proportionate increase and shift of care and supervision to the family and community at large. Interactional patterns in this setting of reduced environmental structure and core knowledge underscore the personality-altering aspects of TBIs.

Studies of individuals with TBI find that personality changes are the most significant problems at 1, 5, and 15 years postinjury (Livingston et al. 1985; Thomsen 1984; Weddell et al. 1980). At one extreme, there may be subtle awareness on the part of the person and his or her most intimate friends of an attitudinal shift or interpersonal "clumsiness," whereas at the other extreme, there may be dramatic departures from socially acceptable norms of behavior. Such idiosyncratic changes in personality create substantial problems in quantifying these changes after TBI.

On the whole, these changes have been believed to represent exaggerations of premorbid traits in the face of the overwhelming anxiety of illness (Strain and Grossman 1975), although no definitive study exists. Focal cerebral contusions may elicit a pattern of behaviors that initially suggest a personality change. In the course of longitudinal contact with the individual, it is often observed that these discrete areas exist in the context of the person's overall premorbid personality style. The manifestations of these personality changes vary as a function of fatigue, anxiety, styles of the other individuals involved, and environmental cues. Development of chameleon-like or "as if" attributes can create diagnostic confusion with patients who have disorders due to early disturbances of separation-individuation (Gunderson and Singer 1975; Mahler et al. 1975; Munro 1969). Patients may be diagnosed as having borderline personality disorder when they display the impulsivity, lack of empathy, lack of sense of self, and inability to self-monitor that are typical of frontal lobe dysfunction.

Developmental milestones during the life cycle mediate certain elements of personality change subsequent to TBI. An Eriksonian model provides a functional yardstick against which to measure such traits (Erikson 1950). The maturational arrests that are observed after TBI may, in part, be a function of a critical insult that stalls further developmental sequences. Actions that are acceptable from a 15-year-old adolescent are not congruent with those of a 35-year-old. Yet those who sustained their TBI in adolescence are caught in precisely this "time warp" that adversely affects their relationships.

Dissection of these issues requires a relationship between the physician and the individual that allows coping strategies to be observed and assessed in multiple settings and under varying conditions. By their very nature, personality changes show modest response to a crisis intervention approach to treatment. In this chapter, we review the complexities of these personality alterations.

Definition of Personality Alteration After TBI

In 1978, Lezak described alterations in personality after TBI as 1) impaired social perceptiveness, 2) impaired self-control and regulation, 3) stimulus-bound behavior, 4) emotional change, and 5) inability to learn from social experience (Lezak 1978). These deficits, either singly or collectively, impair the ability of the individual to engage in an acceptable social interaction and create a high potential for alienation from others. Frequently, the loss of self-monitoring is overtly manifest as the externalization of responsibility for failed social interactions. As a result, this behavior can appear similar to a narcissistic disorder. Whether this lack of interpersonal awareness or insight represents an organically based agnosia (failure to recognize one's behavior) or is a result of a defensive use of denial is unclear (Sandifer 1946). The term *organic denial* has been proposed to describe this phenomenon.

The search for correlates between brain lesions and behavior after TBI resulted in a reworking and refinement of Lezak's work. Describing a population of individuals with frontal lobe injuries, Lezak (1982) defined the following attributes: 1) problems with initiation, 2) inability to shift responses, 3) difficulty stopping ongoing behavior, 4) inability to monitor oneself, and 5) profound concreteness. The clinician often observes the apathetic, abulic patient who lacks sufficient "motivation" to get going (similar to bradykinesia) after experiencing a TBI.

Neuroanatomical and Neurophysiological Substrates of Personality

Harlow (1868) described a nineteenth-century railroad worker, Phineas Gage, who experienced a penetrating brain injury with a tamping rod and had personality alterations described as apathy, disinhibition, lability, and loss of appropriate social behavior. Hibbard et al. (2000), using a more sophisticated tool, the Structured Clinical Interview for DSM-IV Axis II Personality Disorders (First 1997), found that two-thirds of their cohort of individuals with brain injury met criteria for a DSM-IV (American Psychiatric Association 1994) personality disorder diagnosis after injury that was independent of injury severity, age at injury, or time since injury occurred. Such alterations are illustrative of the effects of both focal and diffuse changes that accompany TBI. Focal trauma to the tips of the temporal lobes, inferior orbital frontal

regions, or frontal convexities may occur without neuroradiographical evidence of injury and yet may have devastating clinical ramifications for the patient and the family (Jenkins et al. 1986; Langfitt et al. 1986; Wilson and Wyper 1992). Diffuse axonal injury is the underlying pathophysiological change that accompanies TBI regardless of its severity (Meythaler et al. 2001; Strich 1956, 1961). Diffuse axonal injury results in the "unplugging" of neural networks from one another, with a decrease or loss of the associational matrix within the central nervous system (CNS). These changes create "networking" lapses for the individual during functional activities. Lapses may vary from transient problems with initiation that affect one's ability to appropriately begin a pattern, such as a conversation or a problem-solving sequence, to more overt problems with stopping ongoing behaviors.

Researchers, past and present, have attempted to define the location of personality in the human brain. From the efforts of Wolford et al. (2000) in identifying the left hemisphere as the locus of searching for patterns in events to Gazzaniga's (1998) postulated "hypothesis generator" in the left hemisphere, research into the brain–behavior substrate for personality and judgment has continued to find hemispheric differentiation. Alternatively, functional magnetic resonance imaging studies have demonstrated activation of the frontopolar cortex and medial frontal gyrus in judgment settings without emotional significance, whereas moral judgment activated regions in the right anterior temporal cortex, lenticular nucleus, and cerebellum as well (Moll et al. 2001).

Localization of personality to any one structure or set of structures in the CNS is a difficult task. The set of characteristic reactions and psychological defenses to an anxiety-inducing stimulus results from a complex interaction among limbic-mediated drive states, paralimbic cortical inhibition of certain of those states, contextual elements relating to pattern recognition of similar past events, and selection of a response pattern predicated on a cost/benefit analysis for the event in question. All of these cognitive events must occur subsequent to the sensory recognition of the provocative event. Diffuse injury that occurs in TBI can affect any of these events. Pathway reduplication and parallel systems in the CNS may contribute to the behavioral variability over time. This creates the potential for an irregularly irregular syndrome. Nondominant parietal structures and frontal executive structures may define awareness of body in space and integration of sensory signals. Indeed, damage to these regions can result in a syndrome of guarded hypervigilance similar to a paranoid style. Damage the temporal lobe in the region of the amygdala may affect the "coloration," or affective intensity, of an event. Rage and fear responses associated with these lesions are discussed in Chapter 14, Aggressive Disorders.

Basic science research provides insights into the regional localization of temperament, inhibition, and impulsivity in animal models and infants. Right frontal hemispheric influences are implicated in most of these processes. Intense defensiveness in rhesus monkeys manifested by elevations in cortisol concentration (viewed as traitlike fear-related behaviors) occurs in those animals with extreme right frontal asymmetry (Kalin et al. 1998). Similarly, 4-month-old human infants also demonstrated greater right frontal electroencephalographic activity in direct proportion to level of inhibited behavior (Calkins et al. 1996). Conversely, impulsivity in a rat model has been correlated with selective lesions in the nucleus accumbens, but not with lesions in the anterior cingulate or medial prefrontal cortices (Cardinal et al. 2001). Frontal reactivity as measured by event-related potentials (ERPs) are linked to sensation-seeking behavior. In this research, frontal P3 ERP amplitudes in a cohort of high-sensation seekers (i.e., skydivers) were larger than in control subjects. The implication that such large amplitudes reflect the capacity to improve automatic attentional processes has been suggested (Pierson et al. 1999).

The definition of frontal lobe syndromes has been the subject of multiple articles and a comprehensive work by Stuss and Benson (1986). Functional correlates of regional changes in these lobes are important, with focal lesions such as arteriovenous malformations, neoplastic disease, and focal hemorrhagic events. However, caution is advised when ascribing definitive importance to frontal lesions in TBI when the critical neuropathological change is diffuse axonal injury. Nonetheless, some elements of frontal lobe localization may be evident after TBI. Orbital frontal lesions resulting from contusions of neural tissue against the floor of the anterior cranial vault can occur when an individual falls backward, striking the occiput against a firm surface. A subtle dysfunction in olfaction (cranial nerve I) may be detected as a result of either complete avulsion from the cribriform plate or stretching of fibers on the inferior surface of the frontal lobes (Costanzo and Zasler 1992). Such a finding is often accompanied by neurobehavioral alterations, including impulsivity, euphoria, and manic symptoms. These individuals also have been described as "pseudosociopathic" because they have diminished capacity for introspection and self-awareness. Damage to the medial surfaces or the frontal convexities defines a syndrome of apathy, abulia, and indifference, as described above. These individuals present a "lobotomized" image, much as Jack Nicholson portrayed in the closing scenes of *One Flew Over the Cuckoo's Nest*. The term *pseudodepressed* has been applied to this population.

Reasoning and creativity have been localized as frontal lobe functions. Measurements of regional cerebral blood flow in anterior prefrontal, frontotemporal, and superior frontal regions define increases bilaterally on a divergent thinking task assessing creativity (Carlsson et al. 2000). The predictability of a task has implications as to the activation of frontal regions. An expected sequential task engaged the medial anterior prefrontal cortex and ventral striatum, whereas unpredictable tasks involved the polar prefrontal and dorsolateral striatum (Koechlin et al. 2000). Functional neuroimaging studies reveal the frontal lobe as the site of accessing information previously encoded and required for problem solving. Fletcher and Henson (2001) noted ventrolateral frontal cortex activation, with successful encoding and initial stage of retrieval of data from long-term stores into working memory. Data selection, manipulation, and monitoring activate the dorsolateral frontal cortex for complex encoding and analysis of relevance of information retrieved for use. Cortical activation anterior to the anterior edge of the inferior frontal gyrus (anterior frontal cortex [AFC]) occurs with goal selection and data coordination function between the ventrolateral and dorsolateral frontal cortex. Online monitoring of goal-directed behavior and shifting cognitive sets also activate the AFC. A recent analysis of right hemispheric function by Devinsky (2000) found that awareness of physical and emotional self-constructs (e.g., body image, relationship of body to environmental space, and social function) reside in the AFC.

Frontal activation on functional imaging studies is demonstrated in localization studies of empathy, emotional distress, forgiveness, self-monitoring, and constructs of "the self." Imaging studies assessing social reasoning define activation of the left superior frontal gyrus, orbitofrontal gyrus, and precuneus in both empathy and forgiveness. Empathy-related activation is also found in the left anterior middle temporal and left inferior frontal gyri. Forgiveness activates the posterior cingulate gyrus (Farrow et al. 2001). Frontal ERP measurement during an error-monitoring task defines amplitude variability inversely correlated to negative affect and emotionality in study subjects (Luu et al. 2000). Basal ganglia–thalamocortical circuits modulate generation, switching, and blending in executive functions (Saint-Cyr et al. 1995). Self-monitoring during a verbal inhibitory exercise activates the left dorsolateral prefrontal cortex (and, to a lesser degree, the anterior cingulate) (Chee et al. 2000). Nondominant frontal lobe dysfunction as measured by single-photon emission computed tomography has a strong correlation with loss of "self" (Miller et al. 2001).

Implicit gender stereotyping and overlearned social knowledge link to ventromedial cortex function (Milne and Grafman 2001).

The neurochemical basis of personality attributes is an emerging area of interest. Whereas models of dopamine receptor activity relating to vigilance, expectation, and reward have been proffered (Gershanik et al. 1983; McEntee et al. 1987), serotonin has recently been implicated in large-scale studies of hostility in those with type A personality (Tyrer and Seivewright 1988; Williams 1991). Of great clinical interest is the correlation between high circulating levels of catecholamines and their metabolites and a good outcome post-TBI (Clifton et al. 1981; Woolf et al. 1987). This laboratory finding supports the long-held clinical wisdom that the patient who is agitated and "hits the ground running" has a much better prognosis than his or her lethargic, apathetic counterpart.

Preinjury Factors and Personality

Controversy exists regarding the importance of premorbid personality in predicting the occurrence of TBI. "Clinical wisdom" initially suggested that TBI was not strictly a random event and tended to affect those with a proclivity for "living on the edge." Studies, however, find that there is no overrepresentation of risk takers or substance abusers in adolescents with TBI (Lehr 1990). Ruff et al. (1996) noted that those with significant dependency issues, grandiosity, overachievement, perfectionism, and borderline personality have a compromised outcome. Bigler (2001) noted no demonstrable effect of antisocial traits with frontal lobe injury. Studies by Cantu (1997) suggest an increasing risk of concussion in football-related injuries as the number of events increase: the first event creates a threefold increase in vulnerability to a second event, whereas a second event increases this to an eightfold statistical probability.

Recent work on the neural basis of personality disorders suggests frontal lobe regional influences in impulsive personality disorders and aggressive personality disorders (Siever et al. 1999). A reduction in metabolic function for serotonergic modulation in orbitofrontal, ventral medial, and cingulate cortices is implicated in this study. Studies of borderline personality disorder define reduced frontal cortex glucose metabolism on positron emission tomography in those meeting DSM III-R criteria (Goyer et al. 1994). These populations "at risk" for frontal abnormalities at baseline might exhibit enhanced vulnerability for personality dysfunction post–brain injury.

Premorbid personality factors affect the defense mechanisms used to cope with the stresses of TBI. The schema developed by Strain and Grossman (1975) for stresses of

hospitalization, as shown in Table 13–1, can be adapted to focus on the stresses specific to the experience of TBI. The loss of self is a primary focus of individual psychotherapy, as discussed in Chapter 35, Psychotherapy. The loss of sense of self pervades every aspect of life for those with TBI, resulting in significant anxiety. In an attempt to contain this anxiety, the patient uses the defenses that have provided the greatest past success in stress reduction. This exaggeration of premorbid style is identical to that described in a study of personality types in acutely ill medical patients (Kahana and Bibring 1964). The authors observed that these styles became exaggerated under stress. Because stress is reduced by the correction of Axis I or Axis III disturbances, the individual gradually returns to the preillness level of homeostasis. In the case of TBI, the level of stress becomes chronic because there is a seemingly permanent exaggeration of personality style.

Assessment of Personality

Personality changes after TBI have been assessed in many ways since the 1930s. Projective tests such as the Rorschach were believed to have predictive validity regarding post-TBI personality disturbance (Perline 1979). A more neurologically based approach was offered by Bender (1938) in the development of the test of visual motor gestalt. Although this instrument tapped integrative deficits, it lacked an objective scoring strategy or a high degree of interrater reliability. Attempts to use large population-based measures such as the Minnesota Multiphasic Personality Inventory (MMPI) in individuals with TBI have created potential for misdiagnosis of response profiles for a variety of reasons (Levin et al. 1976). Foremost among these is the length of this instrument even in the shortened 168-item version published in 1974 (Vincent et al. 1984). In clinical use, the slowed rate of information processing that occurs in TBI results in an inordinate time for proper administration of the MMPI. Patient impulsivity results in invalid scores or inaccurate data. Language-mediated problems, which affect up to 85% of individuals post-TBI, may preclude adequate reading, comprehension, or analytic skills, resulting in an inability to honestly answer the items (Groher 1977). At least one study (Kaimann 1983) has correlated elevations in MMPI scores with neuropathological findings on computed tomography scans. In this study, a high degree of correlation was noted between elevations of the depression scale and nondominant temporal lobe lesions, elevations of the psychoticism scale and periventricular lesions, and elevations of the psychopathic deviance scale and lesions of the frontal lobes. The exclusive use of the MMPI in lieu of a comprehensive clinical

TABLE 13-1. Manifestations of stress in hospitalized patients with traumatic brain injury

Threat to one's sense of self

Change in self-identity

Short-term memory impairment

Disorientation

Stranger anxiety

Short-term memory impairment

Loss of anticipatory capacity

Impaired visual memory or recognition

Visual field cuts

Inattention syndromes (anosognosia)

Separation anxiety

Disorientation

Loss of anticipatory capacity

Short-term memory impairment

Fear of losing love or approval

Social role disruption

Interpersonal intrusiveness

Loss of intimacy and approval

Impaired self-observational skills

Fear of losing control of developmentally mastered milestones

Loss of impulse control

Bowel or bladder incontinence

Motor dysfunction (apraxia)

Functional independence changes in activities of daily living

Language disturbances (aphasia, aprosodia, and alexia)

Fear of loss of or injury to body parts

Craniotomy scars

Percutaneous endoscopic gastrostomy tube sites

Tracheostomy scars

Urinary catheters

Fears of retribution, guilt, or shame

Retribution or expiation themes

Survivor guilt

Source. Adapted from Strain J, Grossman S: "Psychological Reactions to Medical Illness and Hospitalization," in *Psychological Care of the Medically Ill: A Primer in Liaison Psychiatry.* Edited by Strain J, Grossman S. New York, Appleton-Century-Crofts, 1975, pp 23–36.

interview conducted by a skilled professional is to be absolutely avoided in the evaluation of individuals with TBI. Face-to-face interaction between the examiner and the patient is always indicated to allow the assessment of non-

TABLE 13-2. Subtypes of personality change due to a general medical condition (DSM-IV-TR)

Labile

Disinhibited

Aggressive

Apathetic

Paranoid

Other (e.g., associated with a seizure disorder)

Combined

Unspecified

Source. Reprinted from *Diagnostic and Statistical Manual of Mental Disorders,* 4th Edition, Text Revision. Washington, DC, American Psychiatric Association, 2000. Copyright 2000, American Psychiatric Association. Used with permission.

verbal elements. Because of the multiple problems with written and symbolic language that are found after TBI, a pencil-and-paper analysis alone neglects intact communication pathways that may enable the patient to better communicate his or her strengths and weaknesses.

Efforts to objectively quantify personality changes after TBI have relied on factor analysis of multicenter studies such as the National Traumatic Coma Databank (Levin et al. 1990). One such instrument is the Neurobehavioral Rating Scale (see Fig. 4-2) (Levin et al. 1987; Vanier et al. 2000). This 27-item, observer-rated scale incorporates elements of the Brief Psychiatric Rating Scale (Overall and Gorham 1962) and provides a profile of personality and behavioral change that can demonstrate recovery over time. An assessment has been developed for the pediatric population that incorporates a more age-appropriate profile of memory changes (Ewing-Cobbs et al. 1990).

Diagnostic categories for these changes in DSM-IV-TR (American Psychiatric Association 2000) are included in the section "Personality Change Due to a General Medical Condition." The elements are that a persistent disturbance in previous personality characteristics exists that is due to a nonpsychiatric medical condition. Marked impairment in social or occupational functioning or marked distress occurs. Subtypes are also proposed (Table 13–2).

Clinical Manifestations of Personality Disorders in TBI

Loss of "Sense of Self"

The "innate sense of self" or the individuality of a person rests with his or her idiosyncratic analytic capacities that are developed throughout life and represents an amalgamation of experience, genetic endowment, defensive structure, and social reinforcers at any point in time. Changes in the environment play a major role in the regression observed in hospitalized patients without TBI (see Table 13–1, adapted from Strain and Grossman 1975). These same factors may influence individuals with a chronic medical disability such as TBI. Pressures to conform to an external set of behaviors in addition to the "chameleon-like" effect of TBI on personality further serve to confound the individual's sense of self. This "chameleon" quality relates to the patient's assuming the behavioral characteristics of individuals in the immediate environment. A patient with brain injury may well act like one with a severe psychotic disorder when hospitalized on an acute admission unit or chronic care facility. This issue has been the basis for class action suits that endeavor to eliminate such commingling in state mental health facilities. When in the presence of more functional individuals, the patient shows a higher level of competence. Subtle deficits in executive functions that accompany frontal lobe injuries in mild TBI or concussive injuries may affect those individuals who rely primarily on these skills for vocational or interpersonal success, such as lawyers, health care professionals, and entrepreneurs. Integrative deficits in sensory areas may undermine the confidence and skills of craftsmen whose jobs rely on these functions, such as welders, electricians, and artists. The chronic and enduring nature of these deficits requires a reworking of the internal representation of oneself, which may be hindered by the impairment in self-appraisal.

Childish Behavior

Childish behavior results from a combination of changes after TBI that include language deficits, cognitive deficits, and egocentricity. Pragmatic language deficits (Table 13–3) are implicated most frequently in the childish behavior observed after TBI (Szekeres et al. 1987). From a developmental perspective, the same conversational or behavioral response is not expected from a 6-year-old as from a 30-year-old. Developmentally acquired skills such as taking turns, sharing, not interrupting, and inviting expansion on a conversational topic all require awareness of others and ongoing appraisal of the environment during social discourse. A childish style emerges when these elements are absent or diminished. Developmental arrests that result from hospitalization, as observed in infatuations with therapy staff or nurses, also may be perceived as childish.

One component of this type of childish behavior relates to the Eriksonian stage (Table 13–4) that is present at the highest risk period for the occurrence of TBI (15 to 24 years old). At that age, the stage of identity versus dif-

TABLE 13–3. Pragmatic language dysfunction after traumatic brain injury

Decreased intelligibility

Choppy rhythm

Impaired prosody

Limited gesturing with avoidant posturing

Limited affect and eye gaze

Constricted operational vocabulary

Use of ungrammatical syntax

Random, diffuse, and disjointed verbal style

Limited use of language with reliance on stereotypical uses

Abrupt shift of topic

Perseveration

Inability to alter message when communication failure occurs

Frequent interruptions of others

Limited initiation and/or listening

Source.   Adapted from Ehrlich J, Sipesk A: "Group Treatment of Communication Skills for Head Trauma Patients." *Cognitive Rehabilitation* 3:32–37, 1985. Used with permission.

fusion precedes the stage of intimacy versus isolation. A task of adolescence is to define oneself independent of one's parents, and then to share that self with another in an intimate relationship. In the setting of a rehabilitation hospital, the need for a strong therapeutic alliance between patient and therapist is critical, and similar to that required for successful psychotherapy. The patient needs to relinquish control to the therapist for a period of time and to suspend defensive barriers to permit the reeducation of a dysfunctional process. Similarly, both activities require delaying gratification and assuming a more vulnerable position relative to the therapist. The therapist, in both settings, must carefully avoid the creation of potentially damaging scenarios and misperceptions of the motivation behind the therapist's actions. Infatuations may arise out of a misguided enthusiasm for helping the pa-

TABLE 13–4. Eriksonian stages

Trust vs. mistrust

Autonomy vs. shame and doubt

Industry vs. inferiority

Identity vs. diffusion

Intimacy vs. isolation

Generativity vs. stagnation

Integrity vs. despair

tient, which is misinterpreted by the patient as a process that is more intimate than professional. Further complicating this set of interactions is the fact that most TBIs occur in young males, whereas the staff caring for these patients are typically younger female professionals. The avoidance of such childish responses rests in large measure on the concurrent supervision of therapeutic staff by seasoned senior supervisors and the establishment of therapeutic limits early in the treatment process. Mental health professionals who have received psychotherapy supervision at some point in their training are often more aware of these elements in the therapeutic process. Use of this unique expertise by the rehabilitation team can minimize staff and patient conflicts.

Judgment/Social Unawareness/ Inappropriate Behavior

Judgment may be impaired due to difficulty in accurately assessing a current situation on the basis of previously acquired information from past situations. This requires the correct and efficient retrieval of information from long-term databanks and an active comparative process to assess similar and dissimilar elements of the setting. Difficulties in accurate scanning of the situation, assessing the relevant components of the situation, and impulsivity also may be manifested as impairments in judgment. Inappropriate reactions to social cues may also result from impaired prosodic language and failure to appreciate the gestalt of a situation. This demonstrates deficiencies with multitasking and nonverbal task analysis. These difficulties constitute neurolinguistic deficits associated with the pragmatics of language (see Table 13–3, adapted from Ehrlich and Sipesk 1985; see also Prutting and Kirchner 1983). A patient may accurately appraise a situation, effectively review past strategies for interaction, and still execute an inappropriate response due to a failure to coordinate propositional language with the intended prosodic component. This can occur when the patient misreads a sarcastic remark as one that is sincere.

Aggression/Irritability

Irritability and aggressive behavior reflect an inability to filter environmental "noise" combined with defective inhibitory capacity. Arousal or vigilance may range from heightened to impaired. Low-vigilance states are associated with a poorer prognosis for functional independence (Clifton et al. 1981; Woolf et al. 1987). These problems most frequently are correlated with reduction in dopaminergic activity (Feeney and Sutton 1988; Lal et al. 1988; Neppe 1988) or increases in cholinergic activity in the CNS (Nissen et al. 1987; Rusted and Warburton 1989). Hypervigilant states

may portend a better clinical prognosis; however, the heightened arousal may predispose the patient to aggressive behavior (Eichelman 1987). Serotonergic and noradrenergic mechanisms have been implicated in aggressive states. These behaviors may be observed to increase in frequency in response to fatigue, pain (both acute and chronic), autonomic arousal (such as seen in posttraumatic stress disorder), and confrontation with affectively critical settings.

Affective Lability/Instability

One's inability to modulate and control emotional expression is a result of impaired capacity to monitor volume combined with failure or inefficiency of inhibiting behavior. This inability may escalate in the context of either affectively charged or neutral subject matter or setting. Loss of affective resonance with subject content is found in prosodic dysfunction and "pseudobulbar" states. Frequently associated with fatigue and complex social settings, these alterations may be mistakenly ascribed to depressive disorder or Cluster B personality disorders. The use of tricyclic antidepressants and selective serotonin reuptake inhibitors has reduced such episodes.

Attention

Disorders of attention are a common consequence of TBI and may be overlooked by the casual observer (Stuss et al. 1985, 1989; Van Zomeren 1981). The inability to attend to one distinct stimulus may be manifest in any sensory domain, including visual, auditory, and tactile. Whereas the neural substrate for the perception of the event may be intact, the capacity to "lock on" to the target is reduced. This reduction has been termed a *loss of phasic attention* by Van Zomeren (1981). This is in contrast to the phenomenon of an increased scanning attention, whereby the person is seeking meaningful stimuli from the environment. The loss of filtering capacity is presumably mediated by descending pathways that suppress simultaneous reception of competing sensory stimuli. Clinically, this is displayed in the reduced capacity to converse in noisy settings (e.g., parties, malls), impaired ability to read maps and blueprints, and problems interpreting simultaneous sensory events.

Concentration is the capacity to maintain attention on a fixed stimulus for a given period. Although in certain frontal lobe syndromes concentration appears to be present, this actually represents the loss of capacity to stop ongoing behavior such as watching television. The deficits are believed to be due to damage to pathways that inhibit transmission of afferent impulses (Gualtieri and Evans 1988; Gualtieri et al. 1989).

Memory

The classically described memory change subsequent to TBI is a loss of short-term memory for events that transpire in the individual's immediate life, such as misplacing objects and the inability to recall lists of items. These occasions of memory loss arise from an impairment in the capacity for encoding incoming data, which presumably resides in the region of the hippocampus. The high frequency of this occurrence in TBI may be explained by the vulnerable location of the hippocampus. The hippocampus resides in the anterior temporal lobe where force vectors may propel neuronal tissue into the sphenoidal ridge. The translation of information from storage to active memory also requires manipulation by hippocampal structures. Again, after TBI retrieval of data also may be faulty.

These changes in memory may be reflected in verbal or nonverbal functions, or both. Attempts to define variations in memory capacity may lead to more efficient retraining strategies; however, from a clinical perspective such differences have not proven useful. Memory dysfunction also might be dichotomized as effortful versus incidental in nature. Effortful memory would involve those processes needed to respond accurately to a "fill-in-the-blank" question. In this situation, the patient's recall process must conform to the external structure imposed by the examiner. Incidental memory, conversely, is demonstrated in the capacity to answer essay questions by using one's own idiosyncratic neural association pathways to arrive at the correct response. After TBI, incidental memory is more intact than effortful memory. Therefore, the examiner may obtain more information using an open-ended design than a structured interview format, such as is required by the MMPI, Structured Clinical Interview for DSM-III-R (Spitzer et al. 1986), and Beck Depression Inventory (Beck and Steer 1984), which may therefore produce inaccurate results. However, the open-ended design involves more investment of time for the examiner.

Cognition may be defined as the sum total of all processes involved in the analysis and management of data-based activity. This includes data acquisition through sensory inputs, discernment of a hierarchy of choice and nonchoice options on the basis of a predefined set of comparisons, and execution of the option chosen. A further element of follow-up analysis also occurs that expands the predefined set of comparisons. These steps have been labeled "executive functions" (Table 13–5). Disturbances in these functions occur after TBI with a frequency that approaches 100% (Szekeres et al. 1987).

TABLE 13–5.   Executive functions

Setting goals

Assessing strengths and weaknesses

Planning and/or directing activity

Initiating and/or inhibiting behavior

Monitoring current activity

Evaluating results

Source.   Adapted from Szekeres SF, Ylvisaker M, Cohen SB: "A Framework for Cognitive Rehabilitation Therapy," in *Community Reentry for Head Injured Adults.* Edited by Ylvisaker M, Gobble EMR. Boston, MA, College-Hill Press, 1987, pp 87–136.

Abstraction

The capacity for abstract thought may be reduced after TBI with injury to structures in the frontal lobes. This ability requires a multistep sequencing process that analyzes both face content and metaphoric elements. Because abstract reasoning is a high level of cognitive development, this process is keenly vulnerable to attack. Loss of abstract reasoning also involves an impaired capacity to move from a linear analysis to one based on a systems analytic approach. For example, an individual may appreciate that an employer expects punctuality when he or she is present, but may not demonstrate the same time skills when the boss is on vacation. Levin et al. (1991) provided the most useful discussion of this subject.

Problems in understanding abstract concepts, or concreteness, that occur in frontal lobe dysfunction result from the inability to maintain one set of information and to perform a simultaneous comparison with another set of data. The inability to perform divergent rather than linear analyses results in a "loss of the abstract attitude" and a decrease in sense of humor. Those individuals who have maintained their humor after TBI may, in fact, have a better clinical prognosis. Premorbid capacity for humor and the social modeling of those with whom the individual resides are other important factors in recovery.

Language/Pragmatic Deficits

Language disturbance is observed in 8%–85% of individuals after TBI (Groher 1977). Observed changes may include problems with verbal memory, auditory processing, integration and synthesis of linguistic information, word retrieval, and spelling. These problems most commonly arise from the combined effects of diffuse injury and focal cortical contusions. Loss of spontaneity of speech may occur in even the most trivial of injuries. Disturbances in the intonation of language (prosodic dysfunction) can influence both the ability to convey affect in speech (motor aprosodia) and to perceive affect in speech (sensory aprosodia). Cortical regions in analogous position to Broca's and Wernicke's areas in the nondominant hemisphere are believed to subserve expressive and receptive prosodic speech, respectively. In motor aprosodia, the patient may be misdiagnosed as depressed with blunted affect or thought disordered with flattened affect. The inability to impart tonal color to one's language often requires the use of either physical mannerisms (shaking fists or pounding the table) or invective to punctuate one's intended message clearly.

Pure sensory prosodic dysfunction is rarely observed. Substantial regions of the nondominant hemisphere and the inferior surfaces of both temporal lobes are involved in sensory prosody, possibly due to the adaptive evolutionary advantage that exists in the capacity to visually recognize affect in others. More commonly after TBI, dysfunction of auditory sensory prosody is seen and is manifest as the inability to correctly interpret affect in situations in which visual cuing is absent. This typically would be encountered in telephone conversations and crowd settings where the capacity to lock on to one individual's face may be compromised. In such situations, the individual may respond out of context to another's conversation predicated on his or her own mood state.

Evaluation of post-TBI neurolinguistic problems mandates a comprehensive speech-language assessment performed by a speech-language pathologist with experience in TBI. Attention to developmental language issues is required to adequately define the context in which the TBI changes occur. Audiometric evaluation may also be needed to diagnose occult peripheral hearing and processing deficits that may further worsen language capability.

Perception

Perceptual problems arise post-TBI due to diffuse damage to subcortical pathways responsible for interpretation of visual, auditory, kinesthetic, olfactory, and gustatory stimuli. Although end-organ damage may coexist to further compromise perception, deficient central processing occurs in most levels of TBI. Visual processing problems may be manifested by defects in visual organization, visual figure–ground awareness, three-dimensional perception, and visual tracking. These changes are often so subtle that the individual fails to recognize the existence of any problem. Rather, the presenting complaint is often one of anxiety that is situation specific. For example, an interior designer decreased the complexity of wallpaper hung after the disastrous event of hanging an entire room upside down. In another sit-

uation, a seamstress pieced a pattern in such a manner that the sleeves were inside out.

Auditory perceptual problems include auditory figure–ground, vigilance, and attention disturbances. Although the individual may possess intact afferent pathways for hearing, central integrative deficits may render the person functionally deaf (i.e., auditory agnosia or pure word deafness). Figure–ground deficits render the individual unable to accurately perceive one voice amidst a crowd of many, as may occur at a party or mall. The inability to lock on to one stimulus source, again, is the underlying problem.

Olfactory disturbances may involve not only disruption of the olfactory nerve, but also perceptual changes due to injury to the rhinencephalic cortex. Some association with sexual dysfunction exists in the literature, although no controlled study exists. These deficits have significant survival ramifications, as seen in the inability to smell smoke, food spoilage, or leaking natural gas. Adaptations to olfactory disturbances might include the use of smoke detectors, visually inspecting the contents of a container before ingestion, and gas alarms to warn of leakage.

Treatment

Changes of intellect have received vast interest as the development of more rigorously standardized assessment instruments have been introduced. As shown in Chapter 4, Neuropsychiatric Assessment, and Chapter 8, Issues in Neurological Assessment, comprehensive neuropsychological evaluation has been the mainstay of TBI intellectual assessment since the 1980s. The ability to perform these evaluations over many points in time with minimal test–retest effect has aided in quantification of recovery curves. These quantification studies have been primarily authored by neuropsychologists, with little recognition of the contributions of other rehabilitation professionals in the evaluation and treatment of neurocognitive and neurolinguistic deficits after brain injury (Levin et al. 1982, 1991; Prigatano 1986). Although neurolinguistic experts and those with neurosensory integration backgrounds have been consulted in the area of treatment of TBI in children, the developmental approach has been neglected in the current evaluation and treatment of adults. In individuals who have sustained either classic concussive or mild TBI injuries, the sensitivity of standardized neuropsychological testing batteries may miss the "higher" cognitive problems that require more facile manipulation of symbolic language. A comprehensive evaluation includes assessments by the psychiatrist, neuropsychologist, occupational therapist, physical therapist, and speech-language pathologist.

The clinical use of an Eriksonian model to identify the psychosocial stage of the patient in the rehabilitation setting provides a method of understanding the emotional recovery from the traumatic event. Development of basic trust in the form of a therapeutic alliance with the treatment team is the core necessity for successful outcome. Becoming increasingly independent in activities of daily living prepares the patient for the increasing complexity of group-based therapeutic activities. Competitive issues arise at this stage, which require caution on the therapist's part to avoid unduly delaying a successful treatment outcome. The individual gradually regains a sense of new identity, which incorporates elements of the preaccident style with the residua of the neurological damage. Attempts to seek intimacy with peers from the preinjury period may result in rejection due to antipathy for changes resulting from TBI or normal developmental maturation of those peers beyond the patient's current level. Creation of a productive, enriching environment allows for continued growth and productivity, with the resulting personal satisfaction.

Therapeutic interventions in TBI combine the use of pharmacological manipulation with a series of structured exercises of graded difficulty. The use of splints and adaptive equipment supports the maximal physical independence of the individual when total return to premorbid functional levels would otherwise be impossible. Just as TBI rarely results in an improved physical state, the patient's behavior is seldom improved after TBI. The goal of treatment is to return the person to his or her premorbid level of function. For the adult, the goal is to rehabilitate rather than habilitate.

Pharmacotherapy

Pharmacotherapy serves as a mechanism to provide a "splint" or "adaptive device" on the neurochemical milieu while the intrinsic healing of the CNS occurs. Selection of the agent is predicated on a cost–benefit analysis of desired therapeutic effects countered against the known side effects. This includes an awareness of the idiosyncratic responses observed in individuals after TBI (O'Shanick 1991).

Indications and contraindications relate to those agents that can adversely affect the recovery of the CNS. These might include dopamine antagonists, which may inhibit recovery curves in the acute phase postinjury (Feeney et al. 1982). Anticholinergic agents may in high concentrations induce delirium or worsen cognitive performance (Nissen et al. 1987; O'Shanick 1991; Rusted and Warburton 1989). Agents that lower seizure threshold require careful monitoring to prevent seizure induc-

TABLE 13–6. Target symptoms for stimulant therapy

Depression

Excessive daytime drowsiness

Fatigue

Impaired concentration

Decreased arousal

Decreased initiation

tion (O'Shanick and Zasler 1990). Any medication that shares metabolic degradation pathways with an anticonvulsant in use requires scrutiny of levels early in the course of therapy and regularly thereafter (O'Shanick 1987).

Several agents are useful in increasing arousal, decreasing fatigue, and improving affective continence (Gualtieri et al. 1989; Lal et al. 1988; Neppe 1988; O'Shanick 1991) (Tables 13–6 and 13–7). Stimulants exert their therapeutic effect primarily through augmenting the release of catecholamines into the synapse (Gualtieri and Evans 1988). Serotonergic actions have been described at higher concentrations. Dextroamphetamine is the prototype, although methylphenidate is a more potent releaser of dopamine from storage vesicles. Numerous stimulant formulations (e.g., dextroamphetamine [Adderall XR] and methylphenidate [Concerta, Metadate]) have been developed that provide an extended-release mechanism lasting 6–12 hours after ingestion to allow for once-a-day dosing convenience. Such dosing minimizes potential noncompliance due to memory deficits. Although pemoline has a longer half-life, it is seldom used because of the need to rapidly clear medication effects in the event of an adverse action. An alternative intervention for arousal and abulia is the use of agents that directly affect the synthesis of dopamine (Table 13–8). By increasing the precursor (as with L-dopa/carbidopa [Sinemet]), reducing degradation through inhibition of monoamine oxidase (as with L-deprenyl [Eldepryl]), or disrupting feedback inhibition

TABLE 13–7. Doses of stimulants in traumatic brain injury

Drug	Dosage
Methylphenidate	5–15 mg qd–qid
Dextroamphetamine	15–20 mg qd–bid
Modafinil	100–800 mg/day

TABLE 13–8. Dopamine agonist doses in traumatic brain injury

Drug	Dosage
Amantadine (Symmetrel)	100 mg qd–tid
L-Deprenyl (Eldepryl)	5–10 mg/day
Levodopa/carbidopa (Sinemet)	Up to a total daily dose of 100 mg levodopa
Bromocriptine (Parlodel)	2.5–30.0 mg qd–tid
Pergolide (Permax)	0.05–1.5 mg qd–tid
Ropinirole (Requip)	0.125–0.5 mg qd–tid
Pramipexole (Mirapex)	0.125–1.0 mg qd–tid

of dopamine production (as with amantadine [Symmetrel]), a net gain can be attained. These strategies require an intact neuron for successful treatment. If substantial cell death has occurred, a limited response is observed. The use of direct agents with a predominant agonist action provides benefit. These include ropinirole, pramipexole, bromocriptine, and pergolide (Berg et al. 1987; Crismon et al. 1988).

Opiate antagonists have been shown to be of benefit in situations involving hypothalamic dysregulation. Disorders of satiety that have been described as "organic bulimia" have shown response to naltrexone (Childs 1987). Self-injurious behaviors also respond to naltrexone, much as has been described in the developmental disability literature (Herman et al. 1986) (Table 13–9).

Psychotherapy Treatment

Verbal therapies with individuals with TBI require careful monitoring to ensure that auditory processing problems do not interfere with the therapeutic process. Ylvisaker and Feeney (1996) described a model of supported cognition and self-advocacy to improve real-world executive functioning.

TABLE 13–9. Opiate antagonists

Indications

Organic bulimia

Self-injurious behavior

Prader-Willi syndrome

? Other hypothalamic dysregulation

Dosage

Naltrexone, 25–50 mg bid–qid

Short-term memory problems also may be mistaken for resistance in the setting of a traditional psychotherapeutic relationship. The use of a notebook or audiotape for the patient's benefit remedies this problem. A flexible treatment schedule that also includes a period with an involved outside observer is advantageous in providing corroborating data unavailable to the patient because of frontal lobe injuries. Care with issues of a confidential nature that could compromise the trust in the therapist is essential. A close alliance with healthy family members can provide the therapist with a base of understanding of system needs and tolerances. Additional information concerning individual, behavioral, cognitive, and family therapies appears in Chapters 34–38.

Summary

Personality and cognitive changes after TBI result from a complex array of forces that affect biological, psychological, and social spheres of the individual's life. Comprehensive evaluation based on an understanding of the myriad subtle changes in information processing is a mandatory prerequisite for therapeutic success. The astute clinician considers these parameters not only in clearly identified situations of TBI, but also in those patients previously labeled as "functionally" disordered whose symptoms have become "treatment refractory." In these cases, either misdiagnosis or insufficient diagnosis may subject an individual to inadequate if not harmful interventions.

References

American Psychiatric Association: Diagnostic and Statistical Manual of Mental Disorders, 4th Edition. Washington, DC, American Psychiatric Association, 1994

American Psychiatric Association: Diagnostic and Statistical Manual of Mental Disorders, 4th Edition, Text Revision. Washington, DC, American Psychiatric Association, 2000

Beck AT, Steer RA: Internal consistencies of the original and revised Beck Depression Inventory. J Clin Psychol 40 (6):1365–1367, 1984

Bender L: A visual motor gestalt test and its clinical use. American Orthopsychiatric Association Research Monographs No 3, 1938

Berg MJ, Ebert B, Willis DK, et al: Parkinsonism—drug treatment, I. Drug Intell Clin Pharm 21:10–21, 1987

Bigler ED: Frontal lobe pathology and antisocial personality disorder (letter). Arch Gen Psychiatry 58:601–603, 2001

Calkins SD, Fox NA, Marshall TR: Behavioral and physiological antecedents of inhibited and uninhibited behavior. Child Dev 67:523–540, 1996

Cantu R: Reflection on head injuries in sport and the concussion controversy. Clin J Sports Med 7:83–84, 1997

Cardinal RN, Pennicott DR, Sugathapala CL, et al: Impulsive choice induced in rats by lesions of the accumbens core. Science 292:2499–2501, 2001

Carlsson I, Wendt PE, Risberg J: On the neurobiology of creativity: differences in frontal activity between high and low creative subjects. Neuropsychologia 38:873–885, 2000

Chee MW, Sriram N, Soon CS, et al: Dorsolateral prefrontal cortex and the implicit association of concepts attributes. Neuroreport 11:135–140, 2000

Childs A: Naltrexone in organic bulimia: a preliminary report. Brain Inj 1:49–55, 1987

Clifton GL, Ziegler MG, Grossman RG: Circulating catecholamines and sympathetic activity after head injury. Neurosurgery 8:10–14, 1981

Costanzo RM, Zasler ND: Epidemiology and pathophysiology of olfactory and gustatory dysfunction in head trauma. J Head Trauma Rehabil 7:15–24, 1992

Crismon ML, Childs A, Wilcox RE, et al: The effect of bromocriptine on speech dysfunction in patients with diffuse brain injury (akinetic mutism). Clin Neuropharmacol 11:462–466, 1988

Ehrlich J, Sipesk A: Group treatment of communication skills for head trauma patients. Cognitive Rehabilitation 13:32–37, 1985

Eichelman B: Neurochemical and psychopharmacologic aspects of aggressive behavior, in Psychopharmacology: The Third Generation of Progress. Edited by Meltzer HY. New York, Raven, 1987, pp 697–704

Erikson E: Childhood and Society. New York, WW Norton, 1950

Ewing-Cobbs L, Levin HS, Fletcher JM, et al: The children's orientation and amnesia test: relationship to severity of acute head injury and to recovery of memory. Neurosurgery 27:683–691, 1990

Farrow TF, Zheng Y, Wilkinson ID, et al: Investigating the functional anatomy of empathy and forgiveness. Neuroreport 12:2433–2438, 2001

Feeney DM, Sutton RL: Catecholamines and recovery of function after brain damage, in Pharmacological Approaches to the Treatment of Brain and Spinal Cord Injury. Edited by Stein DG, Sabel BA. New York, Plenum, 1988, pp 121–142

Feeney DM, Gonzalez A, Law WA: Amphetamine, haloperidol and experience interact to affect rate of recovery after motor cortex injury. Science 217:855–857, 1982

First MB, Gibbon M, Spitzer RL, et al: Structured Clinical Interview for DSM-IV Axis II Personality Disorders. Washington, DC, American Psychiatric Association, 1997

Fletcher PC, Henson RN: Frontal lobes and human memory: insights from functional neuroimaging. Brain 124:849–881, 2001

Gazzaniga MS: The Minds Past. Berkeley and Los Angeles, CA, University of California Press, 1998, pp 123–148

Gershanik O, Heikkila RE, Duvoisin RC: Behavioral correlations of dopamine receptor activation. Neurology 33:1489–1492, 1983

Goyer PF, Andreason PJ, Semple WE, et al: Positron-emission tomography and personality disorders. Neuropsychopharmacology 10:21–28, 1994

Groher M: Language and memory disorders following closed head trauma. J Speech Hearing Res 20:212–223, 1977

Gualtieri CT, Evans RW: Stimulant treatment for the neurobehavioural sequelae of traumatic brain injury. Brain Inj 2:273–290, 1988

Gualtieri CT, Chandler M, Coons TB, et al: Amantadine: a new clinical profile for traumatic brain injury. Clin Neuropharmacol 12:258–270, 1989

Gunderson JG, Singer MT: Defining borderline patients: an overview. Am J Psychiatry 132:1–10, 1975

Harlow JM: Recovery from the passage of an iron bar through the head. Publications of the Massachusetts Medical Society 2:327–346, 1868

Herman BH, Hammock MK, Arthur-Smith A, et al: A biochemical role for opioid peptides in self-injurious behavior. Paper presented at the annual meeting of the American Academy of Child and Adolescent Psychiatry, Los Angeles, CA, October 1986

Hibbard MR, Bogdany J, Uysal S, et al: Axis II psychopathology in individuals with traumatic brain injury. Brain Inj 14:45–61, 2000

Jenkins A, Teasdale G, Hadley MDM, et al: Brain lesions detected by magnetic resonance imaging in mild and severe head injuries. Lancet 2:445–446, 1986

Kahana R, Bibring G: Personality types in medical management, in Psychiatry and Medical Practice in a General Hospital. Edited by Zimberg NE. New York, International Universities Press, 1964, pp 108–123

Kaimann CR: A neuropsychological investigation of multiple sclerosis. Unpublished doctoral dissertation, University of Nebraska, Lincoln, Nebraska, 1983

Kalin NH, Larson C, Shelton, SE, et al: Asymmetric frontal brain activity, cortisol, and behavior associated with fearful temperament in rhesus monkeys. Behav Neurosci 112:286–292, 1998

Koechlin E, Corrado G, Pietrini P, et al: Dissociating the role of the medial and lateral anterior prefrontal cortex in human planning. Proc Natl Acad Sci 97:7651–7656, 2000

Lal S, Merbitz CP, Grip JC: Modification of function in head-injured patients with Sinemet. Brain Inj 2:225–233, 1988

Langfitt TW, Obrist WD, Alavi A, et al: Computerized tomography, magnetic resonance imaging, and positron emission tomography in the study of brain trauma. J Neurosurg 64:760–767, 1986

Lehr E: Incidence and etiology, in Psychological Management of Traumatic Brain Injuries in Children and Adolescents. Edited by Lehr E. Rockville, MD, Aspen Publishers, 1990, pp 1–13

Levin HS, Grossman RG, Kelley PJ: Aphasic disorders in patients with closed head injury. J Neurol Neurosurg Psychiatry 39:1062–1070, 1976

Levin HS, Benton AL, Grossman RG: Neurobehavioral Consequences of Closed Head Injury. New York, Oxford University Press, 1982

Levin HS, High WM, Goethe KE, et al: The Neurobehavioral Rating Scale: assessment of the behavioral sequelae of head injury by the clinician. J Neurol Neurosurg Psychiatry 50:183–193, 1987

Levin HS, Gary HE, Eisenberg HM: Neurobehavioral outcome one year after severe head injury: experience of the traumatic coma databank. J Neurosurg 73:699–709, 1990

Levin HS, Eisenberg HM, Benton AL: Frontal Lobe Function and Dysfunction. New York, Oxford University Press, 1991

Lezak MD: Living with the characterologically altered brain injured patient. J Clin Psychiatry 39:592–598, 1978

Lezak MD: The problem of assessing executive functions. Int J Psychol 17:281–297, 1982

Livingston M, Brooks N, Bond M: Patient outcome in the year following severe head injury and relatives' psychiatric and social functioning. J Neurol Neurosurg Psychiatry 48:876–881, 1985

Luu P, Collins P, Tucker DM: Mood, personality, and self-monitoring: negative affect and emotionality in relation to frontal lobe mechanisms of error monitoring. J Exp Psychol Gen 129:43–60, 2000

Mahler MS, Pine F, Bergman A: The Psychological Birth of the Human Infant. New York, Basic Books, 1975

McEntee WJ, Mair RG, Langlais PJ: Neurochemical specificity of learning: dopamine and motor learning. Yale J Biol Med 60:187–193, 1987

Meythaler JM, Peduzzi-Nelson J, Eleftheriou E, et al: Current concepts: diffuse axonal injury associated traumatic brain injury. Arch Phys Med Rehabil 82:1461–1471, 2001

Miller BL, Seeley WW, Mychack P, et al: Neuroanatomy of the self: evidence from patients with frontotemporal dementia. Neurology 57:817–821, 2001

Milne E, Grafman J: Ventromedial prefrontal cortex lesions in humans eliminate implicit gender stereotyping. J Neurosci 21:RC150, 2001

Moll J, Eslinger PJ, Oliveira-Souza R: Frontopolar and anterior temporal cortex activation in a moral judgment task: preliminary functional MRI results in normal subjects. Arq Neuropsiquiatr 59:657–664, 2001

Munro A: Parent-child separation—is it really the cause of psychiatric illness in adult life? Arch Gen Psychiatry 20:598–604, 1969

Neppe VM: Management of catatonic stupor with L-DOPA. Clin Neuropharmacol 11:90–91, 1988

Nissen MJ, Knopman DS, Schacter DL: Neurochemical dissociation of memory systems. Neurology 37:789–794, 1987

O'Shanick GJ: Clinical aspects of psychopharmacologic treatment in head-injured patients. J Head Trauma Rehabil 2:59–67, 1987

O'Shanick GJ: Cognitive function after brain injury: pharmacologic interference and facilitation. Neurorehabilitation 1:44–49, 1991

O'Shanick GJ, Zasler ND: Neuropsychopharmacological approaches to traumatic brain injury, in Community Integration Following Traumatic Brain Injury. Edited by Kreutzer JS, Wehman P. Baltimore, MD, Brooks Publishing, 1990, pp 15–27

Overall JE, Gorham DR: The Brief Psychiatric Rating Scale. Psychol Rep 10:799–812, 1962

Perline IH: Computer Interpreted Rorschach. Tempe, AZ, Century Diagnostics, 1979

Pierson A, Le Houezec J, Fossaert A, et al: Frontal reactivity and sensation seeking an ERP study in skydivers. Prog Neuropsychopharmacol Biol Psychiatry 23:447–463, 1999

Prigatano GP: Neuropsychological Rehabilitation After Brain Injury. Baltimore, MD, Johns Hopkins University Press, 1986

Prutting C, Kirchner D: Applied pragmatics, in Pragmatic Assessment and Intervention Issues in Language. Edited by Gallagher T, Prutting L. San Diego, CA, College-Hill Press, 1983, pp 32–41

Ruff RM, Camenzuli L, Mueller J: Miserable minority: emotional risk factors that influence the outcome of a mild traumatic brain injury. Brain Inj 10:551–565, 1996

Rusted JM, Warburton DM: Cognitive models and cholinergic drugs. Neuropsychobiology 21:31–36, 1989

Saint-Cyr JA, Taylor AE, Nicholson K: Behavior and the basal ganglia. Adv Neurol 65:1–28, 1995

Sandifer P: Anosognosia and disorders of body scheme. Brain 69:122–137, 1946

Siever LJ, Buchsbaum MS, New AS, et al: D,L-fenfluramine response in impulsive personality disorder assessed with [^{18}F]fluorodeoxyglucose positron emission tomography. Neuropsychopharmacology 20:413–423, 1999

Spitzer R, William JB, Gibbon M: Structured Clinical Interview for DSM-III-R. New York, Biometrics Research Department, New York State Psychiatric Institute, 1986

Strain J, Grossman S: Psychological reactions to medical illness and hospitalization, in Psychological Care of the Medically Ill: A Primer in Liaison Psychiatry. Edited by Strain J, Grossman S. New York, Appleton-Century-Crofts, 1975, pp 23–36

Strich SJ: Diffuse degeneration of the cerebral white matter in severe dementia following head injury. J Neurol Neurosurg Psychiatry 19:163–185, 1956

Strich SJ: Shearing of nerve fibers as a cause of brain damage due to head injury, a pathological study of twenty cases. Lancet 2:443–448, 1961

Stuss DT, Benson DF: The Frontal Lobes. New York, Raven, 1986

Stuss DT, Ely P, Hugenholtz H, et al: Subtle neuropsychological deficits in patients with good recovery after closed head injury. Neurosurgery 17:41–47, 1985

Stuss DT, Stethem LL, Hugenholtz H, et al: Reaction time after head injury: fatigue, divided and focused attention, and consistency of performance. J Neurol Neurosurg Psychiatry 52:742–748, 1989

Szekeres SF, Ylvisaker M, Cohen SB: A framework for cognitive rehabilitation therapy, in Community Reentry for Head Injured Adults. Edited by Ylvisaker M, Gobble EMR. Boston, MA, College-Hill Press, 1987, pp 87–136

Thomsen I: Late outcome of very severe blunt head trauma: a 10–15 year second follow-up. J Neurol Neurosurg Psychiatry 47:260–268, 1984

Tyrer P, Seivewright N: Pharmacological treatment of personality disorders. Clin Neuropharmacol 11:493–499, 1988

Van Zomeren AH: Reaction Time and Attention After Closed Head Injury. Lisse, The Netherlands, Swets & Zeitlinger, 1981

Vanier M, Mazaux JM, Lambert J, et al: Assessment of neuropsychological impairments after head injury: interrater reliability and factorial and criterion validity of the Neurobehavioral Rating Scale–Revised. Arch Phys Med Rehabil 81:796–806, 2000

Vincent KR, Castillo IM, Hauser RI, et al: MMPI-168: Codebook. Norwood, NJ, Ablex Publishing, 1984

Weddell R, Oddy M, Jenkins D: Social adjustment after rehabilitation: a two year follow-up of patients with severe head injury. Psychol Med 10:257–263, 1980

Williams R: A relook at personality type and coronary heart disease. Progress in Cardiology 4:91–97, 1991

Wilson JTL, Wyper D: Neuroimaging and neuropsychological functioning following closed head injury: CT, MRI, and SPECT. J Head Trauma Rehabil 7:29–39, 1992

Wolford G, Miller MB, Gazzaniga M: The left hemisphere's role in hypothesis formation. J Neurosci 20:RC64, 2000

Woolf PD, Hamill RW, Lee LA, et al: The predictive value of catecholamines in assessing outcome in traumatic brain injury. J Neurosurg 66:875–882, 1987

Ylvisaker M, Feeney T: Executive functions after traumatic brain injury: supported cognition and self-advocacy. Semin Speech Lang 17:217–232, 1996

14 Aggressive Disorders

Jonathan M. Silver, M.D.

Stuart C. Yudofsky, M.D.

Karen E. Anderson, M.D.

EXPLOSIVE AND VIOLENT behavior has long been associated with focal brain lesions, as well as with diffuse damage to the central nervous system (CNS) (Elliott 1992). Irritability and/or aggressiveness are major sources of disability to individuals with brain injury and sources of stress to their families. Agitation that occurs during the acute stages of recovery from brain injury can endanger the safety of the patients and their caregivers. Agitation may be predictive of longer length of hospital stay and decreased cognition (Bogner et al. 2001). Subsequently, low frustration tolerance and explosive behavior may develop that can be set off by minimal provocation or occur without warning. These episodes range in severity from irritability to outbursts that result in damage to property or assaults on others. In severe cases, it may be unsafe for affected individuals to remain in the community or with their families, and they often are referred to long-term psychiatric or neurobehavioral facilities. Therefore, it is essential that all psychiatrists be aware of neurologically induced aggression and its assessment and treatment so that they can provide effective care to patients with this condition and to their families.

Prevalence

It has been reported that during the acute recovery period, 35%–96% of individuals with brain injury exhibit agitated behavior (Levin and Grossman 1978; Rao et al. 1985) (Table 14–1). After the acute recovery phase, irritability or bad temper is common. There have been two prospective studies of the occurrence of aggression, agitation, or restlessness that has been monitored by an objective rating instrument: the Overt Aggression Scale (OAS) (Brooke et al. 1992, Tateno et al. 2003). Brooke and colleagues found that of 100 patients with severe traumatic brain injury (TBI) (Glasgow Coma Scale score <8, >1 hour of coma, and >1 week of hospitalization), only 11 patients exhibited agitated behavior. Only 3 patients manifested these behaviors for more than 1 week. However, 35 individuals were observed to be restless but not agitated. In a study of 89 patients assessed during the first 6 months after TBI, Tateno et al. (2003) found aggressive behavior in 33.7% of individuals with TBI, compared with 11.5% of patients with multiple trauma but without TBI. In a study of psychiatric disorders in 100 self-referred individuals who had TBI several years earlier, Hibbard et al. (1998) found that 34% admitted to symptoms of irritability (i.e., increase in number of arguments/fights, making quick impulsive decisions, complaining, cursing at self, feeling impatient, or threatening to hurt self), and 14% admitted to aggressive behavior (i.e., cursing at others, screaming/yelling, breaking/throwing things, being arrested, hitting/pushing others, threatening to hurt others). In follow-up periods ranging from 1 to 15 years after injury, these behaviors occurred in 31%–71% of patients who experienced severe TBI. In a survey of all skilled nursing facilities in Connecticut, 45% of facilities had individuals with a primary diagnosis of TBI who met the definition of agitation (Wolf et al. 1996). In a series of 67 patients admitted with mild to moderate TBI and rated prospectively, restlessness occurred in 40% and agitation occurred in 19% (van der Naalt et al. 2000). Studies of mild TBI have evaluated individuals for much briefer periods of time: 1-year estimates of irritability, temper, or agitation from these studies range from 5% to 70%. A small study of death row inmates found that 75% had a history of TBI (Freedman and Hemenway 2000). Carlsson et al. (1987) examined the relationship between the number of TBIs associated with loss of consciousness and various symptoms and demonstrated that irritability increased with subsequent injuries. Of men who did not have head injuries with loss of consciousness, 21% reported irritability, whereas 31% of men with one injury with loss of consciousness and 33% of men with two or more injuries with loss of consciousness admitted to this symptom (P=0.0001). Prediction of who will develop aggres-sive behaviors after brain injury is challenging. Risk factors may include irritability, impulsivity, and a preinjury history of aggression; neuropsychological test performance does not consistently predict propensity toward violence in those who have experienced brain injury (Greve et al. 2001). In a study of patients in the first 6 months after TBI, aggressive behavior was significantly associated with the presence of major depression, frontal lobe lesions, poor premorbid social functioning, and a history of alcohol and substance abuse (Tateno et al. 2003). In a group of 30 patients who developed major depression in the first year after TBI, 17 patients (56.7%) exhibited aggressive behavior (Jorge et al. 2004).

TABLE 14–1.   **Prevalence of aggression after traumatic brain injury**

Studies (by type of occurrence)	Severity	N	Follow-up	Irritability or temper (%)	Agitation (%)
Acute					
Levin and Grossman 1978	All	62	Acute	—	35.0
Rao et al. 1985	Severe	26	Acute	—	96.0
Brooke et al. 1992	Severe	100	Acute	35 (restless)	11.0
Tateno et al. 2003	All	89	6 months		33.7 (aggression)
Van der Naalt et al. 2000	Mild–moderate	67		40 (restless)	19.0
Chronic					
Rao et al. 1985	Severe	—	Rehabilitation	—	42.0
McKinlay et al. 1981	Severe	55	1 year	71	67.0
Brooks et al. 1986[a]	Severe	42	5 years	64	64.0
Oddy et al. 1985	Severe	44	7 years	43	31.0
Thomsen 1984	Severe	40	2–5 years	38	—
Thomsen 1984	Severe	—	10–15 years	48	—
Van Zomeren and Van Den Berg 1985	Severe	57	2 years	39	—
Levin et al. 1979	Severe	27	1 year	37	—
McMillan and Glucksman 1987[b]	Moderate	24	—	64	—
Schoenhuber and Gentili 1988	Mild	—	1 year	54	—
Dikmen et al. 1986[c]	Mild	20	1 month/1 year	70	40.0
Rutherford et al. 1977	Mild	131	1 year	5	—

[a]Same patients as McKinlay et al. 1981; only 42 participated in the 5-year follow-up evaluation.
[b]16% were orthopedic control subjects.
[c]Control subjects: 45% irritability, 30% temper; not significant.

Characteristics of Aggression After Brain Injury

In the acute phase after brain injury, patients often experience a period of agitation and confusion that may last from days to months. In rehabilitation facilities, these patients are described as "confused, agitated" (a Rancho Los Amigos Scale score of 4 [Hagen et al. 1972; see Table 4–6]) and have characteristics similar to those associated with delirium (see Chapter 9, Delirium and Posttraumatic Amnesia). Brooke et al. (1992) suggest that agitation usually appears in the first 2 weeks of hospitalization and resolves within 2 weeks. Restlessness may appear after 2 months and may persist for 4–6 weeks. In our clinical experience, after the acute recovery phase has resolved, continuing aggressive outbursts have typical characteristics (Table 14–2). These episodes may occur in the presence of other emotional changes or neurological disorders that occur secondary to brain injury, such as mood lability or seizures.

Certain behavioral syndromes have been related to damage to specific areas of the frontal lobe. The orbitofrontal syndrome is associated with behavioral excesses (e.g., impulsivity, disinhibition, hyperactivity, distractibility, and mood lability). Outbursts of rage and violent behavior occur after damage to the inferior orbital surface of the frontal lobe and anterior temporal lobes. The diagnostic category in DSM-IV-TR is "personality change due to a general medical condition" (American Psychiatric Association 2000) (Table 14–3). Patients with aggressive behavior would be specified as "aggressive type," whereas those with mood lability would be specified as "labile type."

TABLE 14–2. Characteristic features of aggression after brain injury

Type	Features
Reactive	Triggered by modest or trivial stimuli
Nonreflective	Usually does not involve premeditation or planning
Nonpurposeful	Aggression serves no obvious long-term aims or goals
Explosive	Buildup is NOT gradual
Periodic	Brief outbursts of rage and aggression punctuated by long periods of relative calm
Ego-dystonic	After outbursts, patients are upset, concerned, and/or embarrassed, as opposed to blaming others or justifying behavior

TABLE 14–3. DSM-IV-TR criteria for personality change due to a general medical condition

Diagnostic criteria for personality change due to a general medical condition

A. A persistent personality disturbance that represents a change from the individual's previous characteristic personality pattern. (In children, the disturbance involves a marked deviation from normal development or a significant change in the child's usual behavior patterns lasting at least 1 year).

B. There is evidence from the history, physical examination, or laboratory findings that the disturbance is the direct physiological consequence of a general medical condition.

C. The disturbance is not better accounted for by another mental disorder (including other mental disorders due to a general medical condition).

D. The disturbance does not occur exclusively during the course of a delirium.

E. The disturbance causes clinically significant distress or impairment in social, occupational, or other important areas of functioning.

Specify type:

Labile Type: if the predominant feature is affective lability

Disinhibited Type: if the predominant feature is poor impulse control as evidenced by sexual indiscretions, etc.

Aggressive Type: if the predominant feature is aggressive behavior

Apathetic Type: if the predominant feature is marked apathy and indifference

Paranoid Type: if the predominant feature is suspiciousness or paranoid ideation

Other Type: if the presentation is not characterized by any of the above subtypes

Combined Type: if more than one feature predominates in the clinical picture

Unspecified Type

Source. Reprinted from American Psychiatric Association: *Diagnostic and Statistical Manual of Mental Disorders*, 4th Edition, Text Revision. Washington, DC, American Psychiatric Association, 2000. Used with permission.

Pathophysiology of Aggression

Neuroanatomy of Aggression

Many areas of the brain are involved in the production and mediation of aggressive behavior, and lesions at dif-

TABLE 14–4. Neuropathology of aggression

Locus	Activity
Hypothalamus	Orchestrates neuroendocrine response via sympathetic arousal, monitors internal status
Limbic system	
Amygdala	Activates and/or suppresses hypothalmus, input from neocortex
Temporal cortex	Associated with aggression in both ictal and interictal status
Frontal neocortex	Modulates limbic and hypothalamic activity, associated with social and judgment aspects of aggression

Source. Reprinted from Silver JM, Hales RE, Yudofsky SC: "Neuropsychiatric Aspects of Traumatic Brain Injury," in *The American Psychiatric Press Textbook of Neuropsychiatry*, 2nd Edition. Edited by Yudofsky SC, Hales RE. Washington, DC, American Psychiatric Press, 1992, pp 363–395. Used with permission.

ferent levels of neuronal organization can elicit specific types of aggressive behaviors. van der Naalt (2000) found that more lesions, mainly localized in the frontotemporal region, were found in those patients manifesting restlessness and agitation (81% vs. 39%). Several anatomic areas of the brain are important in the production (or lack of suppression) of "irritative aggression," that is, feelings of irritability with occasional explosions. Table 14–4 summarizes the roles of key regions of the brain in mediating aggression.

Hypothalamus

Many areas of the brain are involved in the production and mediation of aggressive behavior, and lesions at different levels of neuronal organization can elicit specific types of aggressive behaviors. The regulation of the neuroendocrine and autonomic responses is controlled by the hypothalamus, which is involved in "flight or fight" reactions. Investigations have shown that lesions in the hypothalamus in animals who have undergone cortical ablation result in nondirected rage with stereotypic behavior (e.g., scratching, biting) (Valzelli 1981). Stimulation of only the posterior lateral hypothalamus in decorticate animals induced sham-rage episodes of fierce behavior with no external provocation (Bard 1928). Stimulation of the ventromedial hypothalamus may lead to inhibition of aggression, although some animals may assume defensive posturing (Roberts 1958). Similarly, humans with hypothalamic tumors can exhibit aggressive behavior (Malamud 1967).

Limbic System

The limbic system, especially the amygdala, is responsible for mediating impulses from the prefrontal cortex and hypothalamus, and it adds emotional content to cognition and to associating biological drives to specific stimuli (e.g., searching for food when hungry) (Halgren 1992). Activation of the amygdala, which can occur in seizurelike states or in kindling, may result in enhanced emotional reactions, such as outrage at personal slights. Damage to the amygdaloid area has resulted in violent behavior (Tonkonogy 1991). Injury to the anterior temporal lobe, which is a common site for contusions, has been associated with the "dyscontrol syndrome." Some patients with temporal lobe epilepsy exhibit emotional lability, impairment of impulse control, and suspiciousness (Garyfallos et al. 1988).

Neocortex

The most recent region of the brain to evolve, the neocortex, coordinates timing and observation of social cues, often before the expression of associated emotions. Because of the location of prominent bony protuberances in the base of the skull, this area of the brain is highly vulnerable to traumatic injury. Lesions in this area give rise to disinhibited anger after minimal provocation characterized by an individual showing little regard for the consequences of the affect or behavior. Patients with violent behavior have been found to have a high frequency of frontal lobe lesions (Heinrichs 1989). A recent review of the literature concluded that injury to the orbitofrontal region may put an individual at a particularly high risk for commission of violent acts (Brower and Price 2001). New et al. (2002) used positron emission tomography to assess regional metabolic activity in response to a serotonergic stimulus in patients (without TBI) who manifested impulsive aggression. They found that the patients did not activate the left anteromedial orbital cortex (as did nonaggressive control subjects), and the anterior cingulate was deactivated. The posterior cingulate was activitated in patients and deactivated in control subjects. Tateno et al. (2003) found that the frequency of frontal lobe lesions was significantly higher among aggressive patients, and those with focal frontal lesions exhibited higher aggressive scores as measured by the OAS. Those individuals with TBI who were nonaggressive had a greater frequency of diffuse injury. Frontal lesions may result in the sudden discharge of limbic- and/or amygdala-generated affects—affects that are no longer modulated, processed, or inhibited by the frontal lobe. In this condition, the patient overreacts with rage and/or aggression on thoughts or feelings that would have ordinarily been modulated, inhibited, or suppressed. In healthy volunteers, imagined aggressive behaviors were associated with significant emotional reactivity and cerebral blood flow reductions in the ventromedial prefrontal cortex, suggesting that a functional deactivation occurs (Pietrini et al. 2000). We hypothesize that injury to this area causes a structural deactivation, which "deinhibits" limbic structures.

Neurotransmitters in Aggression

Many neurotransmitters are involved in the mediation of aggression, and this area has been reviewed in detail by Eichelman (1987). Among the neurotransmitter systems, serotonin, norepinephrine (NE), dopamine, acetylcholine, and the γ-aminobutyric acid (GABA) systems have prominent roles in influencing aggressive behavior. It is often difficult to translate studies of aggression in various species of animals to a complex human behavior. Multiple neurotransmitter systems may be altered simultaneously by an injury that affects diffuse areas of the brain, and it may not be possible to relate any one neurotransmitter change to a specific behavior, such as aggression. In addition, different transmitters affect one another, and frequently the critical factor is the relationship among the neurotransmitters. However, in reviewing the available research data, we can advance certain generalizations that have merit in helping researchers understand the neurobiology of aggression and provide treatment.

The major NE tracts in the brain start in the locus coeruleus and the lateral tegmental system and course to the forebrain, and are thus vulnerable to traumatic injury (Cooper et al. 1991). β_1-adrenergic receptors are located in the limbic forebrain and cerebral cortex, areas known to be involved in the mediation of aggressive behavior (Alexander et al. 1979). In patients who have sustained TBI, elevations of plasma NE have been documented (Clifton et al. 1981; Hamill et al. 1987). Animal studies suggest that NE enhances aggressive behavior, including sham rage, affective aggression, and shock-induced fighting (Eichelman 1987). Higley et al. (1992) found an association between aggression in free-ranging Rhesus monkeys and NE in cerebrospinal fluid (CSF). Humans who exhibit aggressive or impulsive behavior have been shown to have increased levels of the NE metabolite 3-methoxy-4-hydroxyphenylglycol (MHPG) (G. L. Brown et al. 1979). Stimulation of the amygdala produces sham rage and is associated with a decrease in brainstem levels of NE (indicative of NE release) (Reis 1972).

Serotonergic neurons originate in the raphe located in the pons and upper brainstem and project to the frontal cortex. Olivier et al. (1990) suggested that serotonin-specific drugs with putative antiaggressive properties bind to the 5-hydroxytryptamine type 1B (5-HT_{1B}) serotonin receptor, which can be found in the neocortex and hypothalamus among other brain regions. Changes in serotonin activity have been found in patients who have sustained TBI, although these findings have been inconsistent (Bareggi et al. 1975; Van Woerkom et al. 1977; Vecht et al. 1975). Concentrations of CSF 5-hydroxyindoleacetic acid (5-HIAA) are correlated with the concentration of 5-HIAA in the frontal lobe (Knott et al. 1989; Stanley et al. 1985). Lowered levels of serotonergic activity have been associated with increased aggression in a number of studies, including studies of predatory aggression and shock-induced fighting in rats (Eichelman 1987) and in a study of free-ranging Rhesus monkeys (Higley et al. 1992). Clinical studies have confirmed the role of decreased serotonin in the expression of aggressiveness and impulsivity in humans (Kruesi et al. 1992; Linnoila and Virkkunen 1992), particularly as it applies to self-destructive acts.

Some studies have shown an increase in 5-HT_2 receptor binding in the frontal cortex of suicide victims (Arango et al. 1990), although not all results are consistent with these findings (Cheetham et al. 1988). A link between the gene for tryptophan hydroxylase and levels of CSF 5-HIAA in impulsive-aggressive individuals has been reported (Nielsen et al. 1994). 5-HT_2 receptor antagonists, including antipsychotic drugs, have antiaggressive properties (Mann 1995). Other work looking at receptor subtypes in rats found multifaceted relationships between serotonin receptor type and aggression. Only 5-HT_2 agonists decreased defensive aggression, but agonists 5-HT_{1A}, 5-HT_{1B} and 5-HT_2 all reduced offensive aggression (Muehlencamp et al. 1995). It has been reported that deleting the 5-HT_{1B} gene increases aggression (Hen et al. 1993).

Dopamine systems are prominent in both mesolimbic and mesocortical regions. Although some investigators have found decreased levels of lumbar CSF homovanillic acid levels, the metabolite of brain dopamine, in patients after severe TBI (Bareggi et al. 1975; Vecht et al. 1975), Porta et al. (1975) reported that ventricular CSF homovanillic acid was elevated. Hamill et al. (1987) reported elevated serum dopamine levels that correlated with the severity of the injury and with poorer outcome. Increases in dopamine may lead to aggression in several animal models (Eichelman 1987), and agitation is a common symptom in schizophrenia, often treated with antidopaminergic medications. Levodopa has been shown to cause aggression in animals, and personality changes in Parkinson's disease patients treated with this medication have also been reported (Lammers and van Rossum 1968; Saint-Cyr et al. 1993). Some work has also shown a reduction in the dopaminergic metabolites of patients who have attempted suicide (Roy et al. 1986; Traskman et al. 1981).

A cholinergic complex is found in the basal forebrain and the pontomesencephalotegmental area (Cooper et al. 1991). Elevated acetylcholine levels have been found in fluid obtained from intraventricular catheters or lumbar puncture in patients after TBI (Grossman et al. 1975). Acetylcholine has been reported to increase aggressive behaviors (Eichelman 1987). However, use of acetylcholinesterase inhibitors has been suggested as a treatment for disruptive patients with Alzheimer's disease (Kaufer et al. 1998).

GABA is an inhibitory neurotransmitter found throughout the brain. Although no studies have examined GABA levels after brain injury, it would be expected that injured neurons would produce less GABA. Increasing GABA via benzodiazepines results in reduced aggressive behavior in animals (Eichelman 1987), and GABA agonists such as the benzodiazepines have been reported to be associated with paradoxical rage attacks (Salzman et al. 1974).

Physiology of Aggression

Aggressive behavior may result from neuronal excitability of limbic system structures. For example, subconvulsive stimulation (i.e., kindling) of the amygdala leads to permanent changes in neuronal excitability (Post et al. 1982). Epileptogenic lesions in the hippocampus in cats, induced by the injection of the excitotoxic substance kainic acid, result in interictal defensive rage reactions (Engel et al. 1991). During periods when the cat experiences partial seizures, the animal exhibits heightened emotional reactivity and lability. In addition, defensive reactions can be elicited by excitatory injections to the midbrain periaqueductal gray region. Hypothalamus-induced rage reactions can be modulated by amygdaloid kindling.

Assessment

Differential Diagnosis

Individuals who exhibit aggressive behavior after sustaining TBI require a thorough assessment. Multiple factors may play a significant role in the production of aggressive behaviors in these patients. During the time period of emergence from coma, agitated behaviors can occur as the result of delirium. The usual clinical picture is one of restlessness, confusion, and disorientation. (The assessment and treatment of delirium are discussed in Chapter 9, Delirium and Posttraumatic Amnesia.) For patients who become aggressive after TBI, it is important to systematically assess the presence of concurrent neuropsychiatric

TABLE 14–5. Irritability and Axis I disorders post–traumatic brain injury

Disorder	Irritability (%) Yes	Irritability (%) No
Major mood disorder	46	23[a]
Anxiety disorder	47	25[a]
Major depression and anxiety disorder	52	28[a]
Aggression and Axis I disorders		
Major mood disorder	21	8[b]
Anxiety disorder	18	11
Major depression and anxiety disorder	24	11[b]

Source. Adapted from Hibbard MR, Uysal S, Kepler K, et al: "Axis I Psychopharmacology in Individuals With Traumatic Brain Injury." *The Journal of Head Trauma Rehabilitation* 13:24–39, 1998.
[a]$P < 0.05$.
[b]$P < 0.10$.

disorders, because such assessment may guide subsequent treatment. Thus, the clinician must diagnose psychosis, depression, mania, mood lability, anxiety, seizure disorders, and other concurrent neurological conditions.

When aggressive behavior occurs during later stages of recovery, after confusion and posttraumatic amnesia (PTA) have resolved, it must be determined whether the aggressivity and impulsivity of the individual antedated, was caused by, or was aggravated by the brain injury. Those who have experienced a TBI may have a history of neuropsychiatric problems including learning disabilities, attentional deficits, behavioral problems, or personality disorders. A preinjury history of drug and substance abuse is associated with aggressive behavior in the first 6 months after TBI (Tateno et al. 2003). Coexistent anxiety and depressive disorders are associated with increased aggression and irritability (Hibbard et al. 1998; Tateno et al. 2003). In a self-report of symptoms, individuals with anxiety and/or depression had a greater frequency of irritability and aggression (Table 14–5).

Because previous impulse dyscontrol and lability are exacerbated by brain injury, traits intensify after damage to the prefrontal areas and other brain regions that inhibit preexisting aggressive impulses. Many patients are able to differentiate between the aggressivity exhibited before brain injury and their current dyscontrol. One patient stated, "Before the accident, I engaged in hostile behavior when I wanted to and when it served my purpose; now I have no control over when I explode."

Drug effects and side effects commonly result in disinhibition or irritability (Table 14–6). By far, the drug

TABLE 14–6. Medications and drugs associated with aggression

Alcohol: intoxication and withdrawal states

Hypnotic and antianxiety agents (barbiturates and benzodiazepines): intoxication and withdrawal states

Analgesics (opiates and other narcotics): intoxication and withdrawal states

Steroids (prednisone, cortisone, and anabolic steroids)

Antidepressants: especially in initial phases of treatment

Amphetamines and cocaine: aggression associated with manic excitement in early stages of abuse and secondary to paranoid ideation in later stages of use

Antipsychotics: high potency agents that lead to akathisia

Anticholinergic drugs (including over-the-counter sedatives) associated with delirium and central anticholinergic syndrome

TABLE 14–7. Common etiologies of aggression in individuals with traumatic brain injury

Medications, alcohol and other abused substances, and over-the-counter drugs

Delirium (hypoxia, electrolyte imbalance, anesthesia and surgery, uremia, and so on)

Alzheimer's disease

Infectious diseases (encephalitis, meningitis, pneumonia, urinary tract infections)

Epilepsy (ictal, postictal, and interictal)

Metabolic disorders: hyperthyroidism or hypothyroidism, hypoglycemia, vitamin deficiencies

most commonly associated with aggression is alcohol, during both intoxication and withdrawal. Patients who were using alcohol when they incurred a brain injury exhibit longer durations of agitation compared to those of patients with TBI with no detectable blood alcohol level at the time of hospitalization (Sparadeo and Gill 1989). Stimulating drugs, such as cocaine and amphetamines, as well as the stimulating antidepressants may produce severe anxiety and agitation in patients with or without brain lesions. Because patients with TBI have an increased occurrence of concomitant alcohol or substance abuse, the clinician must consider the effects of illicit substances in all TBI patients with irritability. Antipsychotic medications often increase agitation through anticholinergic side effects, and agitation and irritability usually accompany severe akathisia. Many other drugs may produce confusional states, especially anticholinergic medications that cause agitated delirium (Beresin 1988). Drugs such as the tricyclic antidepressants (e.g., amitriptyline, imipramine, and doxepin) and the aliphatic phenothiazine antipsychotic drugs (e.g., chlorpromazine and thioridazine) are well known to have potent anticholinergic effects. However, other drugs have anticholinergic properties that are usually not considered to have these effects. These drugs include digoxin, ranitidine, cimetidine, theophylline, nifedipine, codeine, and furosemide (Tune et al. 1992).

Patients with TBI are susceptible to developing other medical disorders that may increase aggressive behaviors (Table 14–7), and comorbidity must always be considered in the individual who exhibits agitation after TBI. The clinician should not, a priori, assume that the brain injury

per se is the cause of the aggressivity but rather should assess the patient for the presence of other common etiologies of aggression. Because patients with neurological disorders are more susceptible to accidents, falls, and other sources of brain disorders, a neurological disorder may be the "underlying condition" that leads to the traumatic injury. In addition, when there are exacerbations or recurrences of aggressive behavior in a patient who has been in good control, an investigation must be completed to search for other etiologies, such as medication effects, infections, pain, or changes in social circumstances.

Studies of the emotional and psychiatric syndromes associated with epilepsy have documented an increase in hostility, irritability, and aggression interictally (Mendez et al. 1986; Robertson et al. 1987). Weiger and Bear (1988) describe interictal aggression in patients with temporal lobe epilepsy. They have observed that interictal aggression is characterized by behavior that is justified on moral or ethical grounds and may develop over protracted periods of time. This aggressive behavior is distinguished from the violent behavior that occurs during the ictal or postictal period, which is characterized by its nondirected quality and the presence of an altered level of consciousness. Even in patients with temporal lobe epilepsy, there are many factors that influence aggression. In a retrospective survey of aggressive and nonaggressive patients with temporal lobe epilepsy, Herzberg and Fenwick (1988) found that aggressive behavior was associated with early onset of seizures, a long duration of behavioral problems, and the male gender. There was no significant correlation of aggression with electroencephalogram or computed tomography scan abnormalities or a history of psychosis. These findings are consistent with those of Stevens and Hermann (1981), who critically examined the scientific literature on the association between temporal lobe epilepsy and violent behavior. They concluded that the significant factor predisposing to violence is the site of the lesion, particularly damage or dysfunction in the limbic areas of the brain.

Psychosocial factors are important in the expression of aggressive behavior. Those who have experienced a TBI may be acutely sensitive to changes in their environment or to variations in emotional support. Social conditions and support networks that existed before the injury affect the symptoms and course of recovery (G. Brown et al. 1981). Factors such as higher levels of education, income, and socioeconomic status positively affect a person's ability to return to work after mild brain injury (Rimel et al. 1981). Certain patients become aggressive only in specific circumstances, such as in the presence of particular family members. This suggests that there is some maintained level of control over aggressive behaviors and that the level of control may be modified by behavioral therapeutic techniques. Most families require professional support to adjust to the impulsive behavior of a violent relative with organic dyscontrol of aggression. Frequently, efforts to avoid triggering a rageful or violent episode lead families to withdraw from a patient. This can result in a paradox: the patient learns to gain attention by being aggressive. Thus, the unwanted behavior is unwittingly reinforced by familial withdrawal.

Documentation of Aggressive Behavior

Before therapeutic intervention is initiated to treat violent behavior, the clinician should document the baseline frequency of these behaviors. There are spontaneous day-to-day and week-to-week fluctuations in aggression that cannot be validly interpreted without prospective documentation. In our study of over 4,000 aggressive episodes in chronically hospitalized patients, hospital records failed to document 50%–75% of episodes (Silver and Yudofsky 1987, 1991). This study and others also indicated that aggression—like certain mood disorders—may have cyclic exacerbations. It is essential that the clinician establish a treatment plan, using objective documentation of aggressive episodes to monitor the efficacy of interventions and to designate specific time frames for the initiation and discontinuation of pharmacotherapy for acute episodes and for the initiation of pharmacotherapy for chronic aggressive behavior.

The OAS is an operationalized instrument of proven reliability and validity that can be used to easily and effectively rate aggressive behavior in patients with a wide range of disorders (Silver and Yudofsky 1987, 1991; Yudofsky et al. 1986) (Figure 14–1). The scale includes items that assess verbal aggression, physical aggression against objects, physical aggression against self, and physical ag-

gression against others. Each category of aggression has four levels of severity that are defined by objective criteria. An aggression score can be derived by obtaining the sum of the most severe ratings of each type of aggressive behavior over a particular time course. Aggressive behavior can be monitored by staff or family members using the OAS. Documentation of agitation can be objectively rated with the Overt Agitation Severity Scale (Yudofsky et al. 1997) (Figure 14–2). The Agitated Behavior Scale (Bogner et al. 1999), which rates 14 problematic behaviors, has been used in acute and long-term rehabilitation settings (Figure 14–3).

Treatment

Aggressive and agitated behaviors may be treated in a variety of settings, ranging from the acute brain injury unit in a general hospital, to a "neurobehavioral" unit in a rehabilitation facility, to outpatient environments including the home setting. A multifactorial, multidisciplinary, collaborative approach to treatment is necessary in most cases. The continuation of family treatments, psychopharmacologic interventions, and insight-oriented psychotherapeutic approaches is often required. In establishing a treatment plan for patients with agitation or aggression, the overarching principle is that diagnosis comes before treatment. The history of the development of symptoms in a biopsychosocial context is usually the most critical part of the evaluation. It is essential to determine the mental status of the patient before the agitated or aggressive event, the nature of the precipitant, the physical and social environment in which the behavior occurs, the ways in which the event is mitigated, and the primary and secondary gains related to agitation and aggression (Corrigan et al. 1993; Yudofsky et al. 1998).

Although there is no medication that is approved by the U.S. Food and Drug Administration specifically for the treatment of aggression, medications are widely used (and commonly misused) in the management of patients with acute or chronic aggression. The reported effectiveness of these medications is highly variable, as are the reported rationales for their prescription. Some of these medications are offered to inhibit excessive activity in temporolimbic areas (e.g., anticonvulsants), to reduce "hyperactive" limbic monoaminergic neurotransmission (e.g., noradrenergic blockade with propranolol, dopaminergic blockade with haloperidol), or to augment orbitofrontal and/or dorsolateral prefrontal cortical activity with monoaminergic agonists (e.g., amantadine, methylphenidate, perhaps buspirone), or increase serotonergic input (i.e., selective serotonin reuptake inhibitors). There

OVERT AGGRESSION SCALE (OAS)

Stuart Yudofsky, M.D., Jonathan Silver, M.D., Wynn Jackson, M.D., and Jean Endicott, Ph.D.

IDENTIFYING DATA

Name of Patient	Name of Rater
Sex of Patient: 1 Male 2 Female	Date / / (mo/da/yr) Shift: 1 Night 2 Day 3 Evening

☐ No aggressive incident(s) (verbal or physical) against self, others, or objects during the shift. (check here)

AGGRESSIVE BEHAVIOR (Check all that apply)

VERBAL AGGRESSION

☐ Makes loud noises, shouts angrily
☐ Yells mild personal insults, e.g., "You're stupid!"
☐ Curses viciously, uses foul language in anger, makes moderate threats to others or self
☐ Makes clear threats of violence toward others or self (I'm going to kill you.) or requests to help to control self

PHYSICAL AGGRESSION AGAINST SELF

☐ Picks or scratches skin, hits self, pulls hair, (with no or minor injury only)
☐ Bangs head, hits fist into objects, throws self onto floor or into objects (hurts self without serious injury)
☐ Small cuts or bruises, minor burns
☐ Mutilates self, makes deep cuts, bites that bleed, internal injury fracture, loss of consciousness, loss of teeth

PHYSICAL AGGRESSION AGAINST OBJECTS

☐ Slams door, scatters clothing, makes a mess
☐ Throws objects down, kicks furniture without breaking it, marks the wall
☐ Break objects, smashes windows
☐ Sets fires, throws objects dangerously

PHYSICAL AGGRESSION AGAINST OTHER PEOPLE

☐ Makes threatening gesture, swings at people, grabs at clothes
☐ Strikes, kicks, pushes, pulls hair (without injury to them)
☐ Attacks others causing mild–moderate physical injury (bruises, sprain, welts)
☐ Attacks others causing severe physical injury (broken bones, deep lacerations, internal injury)

Time incident began: _ _ : _ _ AM/PM	Duration of incident: _ _ : _ _ (hours/minutes)

INTERVENTION (check all that apply)

☐ None
☐ Talking to patient
☐ Closer observation
☐ Holding patient

☐ Immediate medication given by mouth
☐ Immediate medication given by injection
☐ Isolation without seclusion (time out)
☐ Seclusion

☐ Use of restraints
☐ Injury requires immediate medical treatment for patient
☐ Injury requires immediate treatment for other person

COMMENTS

FIGURE 14–1. The Overt Aggression Scale.

Source. Reprinted from Yudofsky SC, Silver JM, Jackson W, et al: "The Overt Aggression Scale for the Objective Rating of Verbal and Physical Aggression." *American Journal of Psychiatry* 143:35–39, 1986. Used with permission.

is a paucity of rigorous, double-blind, placebo-controlled studies (i.e., "Level I" studies) and even prospective cohort studies (i.e., "Level II") to guide clinicians in the use of pharmacologic interventions. The International Brain Injury Association has assembled a task force to review the literature pertaining to the neurobehavioral consequences of TBI (in progress). At this time, we suggest us-

ing the Consensus Guidelines for the Treatment of Agitation in the Elderly with Dementia as a framework for the assessment and management of agitation and aggression after TBI (Alexopolous et al. 1998). After appropriate assessment of possible etiologies of these behaviors, treatment is focused on the occurrence of comorbid neuropsychiatric conditions (e.g., depression, psychosis, in-

OVERT AGITATION SEVERITY SCALE (OASS)
Yudofsky SC, Kopecky HJ, Kunik M, Silver JM, Endicott J

INTENSITY (I)	BEHAVIOR	FREQUENCY (F)					SEVERITY SCORE (SS) (IxF=SS)
A.	**Vocalizations & Oral/Facial Movements**	NOT PRESENT	RARELY	SOME OF THE TIME	MOST OF THE TIME	ALWAYS PRESENT	
1	Whimpering, whining, moaning, grunting, crying	0	1	2	3	4	=
2	Smacking or licking of lips, chewing, clenching jaw; licking, grimacing, spitting	0	1	2	3	4	=
3	Rocking, twisting, banging of head	0	1	2	3	4	=
4	Vocal perseverating, screaming, cursing, threatening, wailing	0	1	2	3	4	=
B.	**Upper Torso & Upper Extremity Movements**						
1	Tapping fingers, fidgeting, or wringing of hands, swinging or flailing arms	0	1	2	3	4	=
2	Task perseverating (e.g., opening and closing drawers, folding and unfolding clothes, picking at objects, clothes, or self, pulling at own hair)	0	1	2	3	4	=
3	Rocking (back & forth), bobbing (up and down), twisting, writhing of torso; rubbing or masturbating self	0	1	2	3	4	=
4	Slapping, swatting, hitting at objects or others	0	1	2	3	4	=
C.	**Lower Extremity Movements**						
1	Tapping toes, clenching toes, tapping heel, extending, flexing or twisting foot	0	1	2	3	4	=
2	Shaking legs, tapping knees and/or thighs, thrusting pelvis, stomping	0	1	2	3	4	=
3	Pacing, wandering	0	1	2	3	4	=
4	Thrashing legs, kicking at objects or others	0	1	2	3	4	=

Instructions for Completing Form

Step One: For each behavior, circle the corresponding frequency after 15 minutes of observation.

Step Two: For every behavior _exhibited_, multiply the Intensity score (I) by the Frequency (F) and record as the Severity Score (SS).

Step Three: For the OVERT AGITATION SEVERITY SCORE (OASS), total all severity scores and record as Total OASS.

Step Four: Does this patient have a Neuromuscular Disorder (i.e., Parkinson's Disease, tardive dyskinesia), affecting Total OASS?   Yes   No

Step Five: If yes, please establish a baseline OASS in non-agitated state and subtract from above Total OASS for Revised OASS.

Total OASS [ ]

Subtract Baseline OASS [ ]

Revised OASS [ ]

COMMENTS:

DIAGNOSIS:_____   NAME OF RATER:_____
SEX OF PATIENT: MALE(1); FEMALE(2)   TIME OF OBSERVATION:_____
AGE:_____   DATE:_____

CURRENT MEDICATION:		
Name:	Dose:	Frequency:
Name:	Dose:	Frequency:
Name:	Dose:	Frequency:
Name:	Dose:	Frequency:
Name:	Dose:	Frequency:

FIGURE 14–2.   The Overt Agitation Severity Scale.

Source.   Reprinted from Yudofsky SC, Kopecky HJ, Kunik ME, et al: "The Overt Agitation Severity Scale for the Objective Rating of Agitation." *The Journal of Neuropsychiatry and Clinical Neurosciences* 9:541–548, 1997. Used with permission.

Patient _____   Period of Observation:
Observ. Environ._____ .   From:_____am/pm___/___/___
Rater/Disc. _____   To:_____am/pm___/___/___

At the end of the observation period, indicate whether the behavior described in each item was present and, if so, to what degree: slight, moderate, or extreme. Use the following numerical values and criteria for your ratings.

1 = Absent: the behavior is not present.
2 = Present to a slight degree: the behavior is present but does not prevent the conduct of other contextually appropriate behavior. (The individual may redirect spontaneously, or the continuation of the agitated behavior does not disrupt appropriate behavior.)
3 = Present to a moderate degree: the individual needs to be redirected from an agitated to an appropriate behavior but benefits from such cueing.
4 = Present to an extreme degree: the individual is not able to engage in appropriate behavior because of the interference of the agitated behavior, even when external cueing or redirection is provided.

DO NOT LEAVE BLANKS.

_____ 1. Short attention span, easy distractibility, inability to concentrate.
_____ 2. Impulsive, impatient, low tolerance for pain or frustration.
_____ 3. Uncooperative, resistant to care, demanding.
_____ 4. Violent and/or threatening violence toward people or property.
_____ 5. Explosive and/or unpredictable anger.
_____ 6. Rocking, rubbing, moaning or other self-stimulating behavior.
_____ 7. Pulling at tubes, restraints, etc.
_____ 8. Wandering from treatment areas.
_____ 9. Restlessness, pacing, excessive movement.
_____10. Repetitive behaviors, motor and/or verbal.
_____11. Rapid, loud or excessive talking.
_____12. Sudden changes of mood.
_____13. Easily initiated or excessive crying and/or laughter.
_____14. Self-abusiveness, physical and/or verbal.
_____ Total Score

FIGURE 14–3. Agitated Behavior Scale.

Source.   Adapted from Bogner JA, Corrigan JD, Stange M, et al: "Reliability of the Agitated Behavior Scale." *The Journal of Head Trauma Rehabilitation* 14:91–96, 1999.

somnia, anxiety, delirium) (Figure 14–4), whether the treatment is in the acute (hours to days) or chronic (weeks to months) phase, and the severity of the behavior (mild to severe). The clinician must be aware that patients may not respond to just one medication but instead may require combination treatment, similar to the pharmacotherapeutic treatment for refractory depression.

Acute Aggression

Antipsychotic Drugs

Antipsychotics are the most commonly used medications in the treatment of aggression. Although these agents are appropriate and effective when aggression is derivative of active psychosis, the use of neuroleptic agents to treat chronic aggression, especially chronic aggression secondary to TBI, is often ineffective, and the patient may develop serious complications. Usually, it is the sedative side effects rather than the antipsychotic properties of antipsychotics that are used (i.e., misused) to "treat" (i.e., mask) the aggression. Often, patients develop tolerance to the sedative effects of the neuroleptics and therefore require increasing doses. As a result, extrapyramidal side effects (EPS) and anticholinergic-related side effects occur. Paradoxically (and frequently), because of the development

of akathisia, the patient may become more agitated and restless as the dose of neuroleptic is increased, especially when a high-potency antipsychotic such as haloperidol (Haldol) is administered. The akathisia is often mistaken for increased irritability and agitation, and a vicious cycle of increasing neuroleptics and worsening akathisias occurs.

There is some evidence from studies of injury to motor neurons in animals that have found that haloperidol decreases recovery. This effect was only seen when ani-

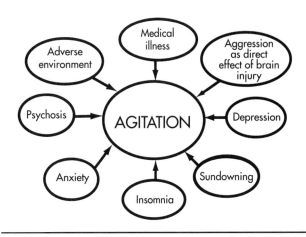

FIGURE 14–4. Neuropsychiatric factors associated with agitation and aggression.

mals actively participated in a behavioral task and not when the animals were restrained after drug administration (Feeney et al. 1982). It is possible that the effect on decreasing dopamine and inhibiting neuronal function, which may be the mechanism of action to treat aggression, may have other detrimental effects on recovery. Rao et al. (1985) found that patients treated with haloperidol in the acute period after TBI experienced significantly longer periods of PTA, although the acute rehabilitation outcome did not differ from that of those not treated with this medication. Whether this finding is generalizable to recovery in brain injury and with the "atypical antipsychotics" remains unclear. However, the finding raises important potential risk/benefit issues that must be considered before antipsychotic drugs are used to treat aggressive behavior in patients with neuronal damage.

In patients with brain injury and acute aggression, we recommend starting an atypical antipsychotic medication such as risperidone at low doses of 0.5 mg po with repeated administration every hour until control of aggression is achieved. If after several administrations of risperidone the patient's aggressive behavior does not improve, the hourly dose may be increased until the patient is so sedated that he or she no longer exhibits agitation or violence. Once the patient is not aggressive for 48 hours, the daily dosage should be decreased gradually (i.e., by 25%/ day) to ascertain whether aggressive behavior reemerges. In this case, consideration should then be given to whether it is best to increase the dose of risperidone and/ or to initiate treatment with a more specific antiaggressive drug. Other atypical antipsychotic medications such as olanzapine, quetiapine (which has few EPS), or ziprasidone may be used, although there is no published experience with the use of these medications to treat aggression in TBI patients.

Sedatives and Hypnotics

There is an inconsistent literature on the effects of the benzodiazepines in the treatment of aggression. The sedative properties of benzodiazepines are especially helpful in the management of acute agitation and aggression. Most likely, this is because of the amplifying effect of benzodiazepines on the inhibitory neurotransmitter GABA. Paradoxically, several studies report increased hostility and aggression and the induction of rage in patients treated with benzodiazepines. However, these reports are balanced by the observation that this phenomenon is rare (Dietch and Jennings 1988). Benzodiazepines can produce amnesia, and preexisting memory dysfunction can be exacerbated by the use of benzodiazepines. Brain-injured patients may also experience increased problems with coordination and balance with benzodiazepine use. For this reason, we prefer not to use benzodiazepines in the treatment of acute aggression in patients with TBI.

Chronic Aggression

If a patient continues to exhibit periods of agitation or aggression beyond several weeks, the use of specific anti-aggressive medications should be initiated to prevent these episodes from occurring. Because no medication has been approved by the Food and Drug Administration for treatment of aggression, the clinician must use medications that may be antiaggressive but that have been approved for other uses (e.g., seizure disorders, depression, hypertension) (Yudofsky et al. 1998). Although the pathophysiology of aggression may not be similar in different neuropsychiatric disorders (e.g., dementia, mental retardation), we often have to extrapolate from data obtained in non-TBI studies.

Antipsychotic Medications

If, after thorough clinical evaluation, it is determined that the aggressive episodes result from psychosis, such as paranoid delusions or command hallucinations, then antipsychotic medications are the treatment of choice. There have been double-blind, placebo-controlled studies of risperidone showing efficacy in the treatment of agitation in elderly patients with dementia (De Deyn et al. 1999; Katz et al. 1999) as well as in the treatment of children with autism and serious behavioral problems (McCracken et al. 2002). Olanzapine appears to be more sedating, and quetiapine may have fewer EPS than does risperidone. Quetiapine appears to be the antipsychotic medication (except for clozapine) least likely to produce EPS in vulnerable populations, such as those with Parkinson's disease (Fernandez et al. 2002). Clozapine may have greater antiaggressive effects than other antipsychotic medications (Michals et al. 1993; Ratey et al. 1993). However, the increased risk of seizures must be carefully assessed. Anticholinergic properties of the older aliphatic phenothiazines have been related to impairments in cognition (Stanislav 1997) and new-onset delusions (Sandel et al. 1993).

Antianxiety Medications

Serotonin appears to be a key neurotransmitter in the modulation of aggressive behavior. In preliminary open case studies, buspirone, a 5-HT$_{1A}$ agonist, has been reported to be effective in the management of aggression and agitation for patients with brain injury (Gualtieri 1991a, 1991b; Levine 1988) as well as dementia, developmental disabilities, and autism (Yudofsky et al. 1998). In rare instances, we have found that some patients become more aggressive when treated with buspirone. We recommend that buspirone be initiated at low dosages (i.e., 7.5 mg bid) and increased to 15 mg bid after 1 week. Dosages of 45–60 mg/day may be required before there is improvement in aggressive behavior, although we have noted dramatic improvement within 1 week.

Clonazepam may be effective in the long-term management of aggression, although evidence is restricted to case reports. Freinhar and Alvarez (1986) found that clonazepam decreased agitation in three elderly patients with organic brain syndromes. Keats and Mukherjee (1988) reported antiaggressive effects of clonazepam in a patient with schizophrenia and seizures. We use clonazepam when pronounced aggression and anxiety occur together, or when aggression occurs in association with neurologically induced tics and similarly disinhibited motor behaviors. Doses should be initiated at 0.5 mg bid and may be increased to as high as 2–4 mg bid, as tolerated. Sedation and ataxia are frequent side effects.

Anticonvulsant Medications

The anticonvulsant carbamazepine has been shown to be effective for the treatment of bipolar disorders and has also been advocated for the control of aggression in both epileptic and nonepileptic populations. Open studies have indicated that carbamazepine may be effective in decreasing aggressive behavior associated with developmental disabilities and schizophrenia and in patients with a variety of other organic brain disorders (Yudofsky et al. 1998). There have been several studies that have included individuals with TBI. Chatham-Showalter (1996) observed improvement after 4 days of treatment in seven multiple-trauma TBI patients treated openly with carbamazepine. One open study by Patterson (1987) on assaultive behavior in eight patients (only two had brain injury from gunshot wounds) reported that the number of aggressive episodes decreased by over 50% as documented by nursing staff. In a study by Azouvi et al. (1999) of 10 patients presenting with agitation and anger outbursts after severe TBI, the researchers describe a significant reduction in such behaviors as assessed using six relevant items on the Neurobehavioral Rating Scale—Revised (Vanier et al. 2000) during 8 weeks of treatment with carbamazepine (mean dose, 9.47±2.9 mg/kg/day). However, 4 of the 10 patients experienced significant drowsiness during the course of the study, necessitating the use of lower doses than had been initially planned and which may have reduced the effectiveness of this treatment. One patient developed a significant allergic cutaneous reaction necessitating discontinuation of carbamazepine. Although the authors report no significant changes in cognition during the course of this trial, their primary measure of cognition was the Mini-Mental State Examination—a measure that is widely regarded as a poor instrument for the assessment of cognition after TBI because of its insensitivity to executive dysfunction and to speed and efficiency of information processing. Hence, a failure to find no change in cognition in this study must be regarded with some caution because the measure used is unlikely to be sensitive to other functionally important aspects of cognitive performance after TBI.

In our experience and that of others, the anticonvulsant valproic acid may also be helpful to some patients with organically induced aggression (Geracioti 1994; Giakas et al. 1990; Mattes 1992). There have been a limited number of open case reports published on patients with TBI. Horne and Lindley (1995) reported on a 70-year-old woman whose emotional lability and irritability improved with use of valproate. Wroblewski et al. (1997) reported on five individuals whose aggression improved within 1–2 weeks.

Gabapentin may be beneficial for the treatment of agitation in patients with dementia (Herrmann et al. 2000; Roane et al. 2000). Doses have ranged from 200 to 2,400 mg/day. However, Childers and Holland (1997) reported an increase in anxiety and restlessness (i.e., agitation) in two cognitively impaired TBI patients for whom gabapentin was prescribed to reduce chronic pain.

For patients with aggression and epilepsy whose seizures are being treated with anticonvulsant drugs such as phenytoin and phenobarbital, switching to carbamazepine or to valproic acid may treat both conditions. Oxcarbazepine may be an alternative to carbamazepine, although there are no published reports on this use of oxcarbazepine at this time.

Antimanic Drugs

Although lithium is known to be effective in controlling aggression related to manic excitement, many studies suggest that it may also have a role in the treatment of aggression in selected, nonbipolar patient populations, including individuals with mental retardation who exhibit self-injurious or aggressive behavior, children and adolescents with behavioral disorders, prison inmates, and those with other organic brain syndromes (Yudofsky et al. 1998). Two individuals in state psychiatric facilities (one patient with aggressive behavior after TBI and the other with aggressive behavior after postanoxic encephalopathy) responded to an open trial of lithium (Bellus et al. 1996). Glenn et al. (1989) reported on their experience using lithium in the treatment of 10 "brain-injured patients with severe, unremitting, aggressive, combative, or self-destructive behavior or severe affective instability." Five patients had a "dramatic response," but only three of these individuals had a TBI.

Individuals with brain injury have increased sensitivity to the neurotoxic effects of lithium (Hornstein and Seliger 1989; Moskowitz and Altshuler 1991). Because of lithium's potential for neurotoxicity, we limit the use of lithium in patients whose aggression is related to manic effects and in patients whose recurrent irritability is related to cyclic mood disorders.

Antidepressants

The antidepressants that have been reported to control aggressive behavior are those that act preferentially (i.e., amitriptyline) or specifically (i.e., trazodone and fluoxetine) on serotonin. In open studies, Mysiw et al. (1988) and Jackson et al. (1985) reported that amitriptyline (maximum dose, 150 mg/day) was effective in the treatment of 20 patients with recent severe brain injury whose agitation had not responded to behavioral techniques. Improvement was documented in 12 of 17 patients with PTA within the first week of treatment. Szlabowicz and Stewart (1990) successfully treated a 43-year-old man with aggressive behavior subsequent to anoxic encephalopathy with amitriptyline, 75 mg at bedtime. Trazodone has also been reported to be effective in the treatment of aggression that occurs with organic mental disorders (Yudofsky et al. 1998). Kant et al. (1998) conducted a non-blind 8-week open trial of sertraline in 13 patients with irritability and aggression after TBI. Behaviors were monitored using the Overt Aggression Scale—Modified for outpatients), and sertraline was administered at up to 200 mg/day. Although there was a significant reduction in irritability and aggression, there were no changes in depressive symptoms.

Fluoxetine, a potent serotonergic antidepressant, has been reported to be effective in the treatment of aggressive behavior in a patient who experienced brain injury as well as in patients with personality disorders and depression and in adolescents with mental retardation and self-injurious behavior (Yudofsky et al. 1998). We have used selective serotonin reuptake inhibitors with considerable success in aggressive patients with brain lesions. The dosages used are similar to those for the treatment of mood lability and depression.

We have evaluated and treated many patients with emotional lability who enact the full symptomatic picture of neuroaggressive syndrome (characterized by frequent episodes of tearfulness and irritability). These patients, whose diagnoses according to DSM-IV-TR would be "Personality Change, Labile Type, Due to Traumatic Brain Injury," have responded well to SSRI antidepressants.

Stimulants

There have been several studies that have examined the role of dopaminergic medications and stimulants in the treatment of agitation and aggression. There have been case reports on the effects of amantadine by Nickels et al. (1994) (two of three subjects with postcoma agitation improved), Chandler et al. (1988) (two cases of agitation and aggression in the postacute stage improved), and Nichels et al. (1994) (two of three subjects with severe agitation improved). Mooney and Haas (1993) conducted a randomized, pretest and posttest, placebo-controlled, single-blind study of the effect of methylphenidate, 30 mg/day for 6 weeks, on brain-injury-related anger in 38 individuals with "serious" TBI 6 months or more after their injuries. Although those on methylphenidate had a lower level of anger after treatment, they also had greater levels of pretreatment anger.

Antihypertensive Medications: Beta-Blockers

Since the first report of the use of β-adrenergic receptor blockers in the treatment of acute aggression in 1977, over 25 articles have appeared in the neurologic and psychiatric literature reporting experience in using β-blockers with over 200 patients with aggression (Yudofsky et al. 1998). Most of these patients had been unsuccessfully treated with antipsychotics, minor tranquilizers, lithium, and/or anticonvulsants before treatment with β-blockers. The β-blockers that have been investigated in controlled prospective studies include propranolol (a lipid-soluble, nonselective receptor antagonist), nadolol (a water-soluble, nonselective receptor antagonist), and pindolol (a lipid-soluble, nonselective β receptor antagonist with partial sympathomimetic activity). The effectiveness of propranolol in reducing agitation has been demonstrated during the initial hospitalization after TBI in a double-blind, placebo-controlled study of 21 subjects with severe TBI (Brooke et al. 1992). Behavior was monitored using the OAS. The maximum intensity of episodes and the numbers of episodes were less after propranolol was given than they were after placebo was given. The authors of the study do not list the number of patients who dropped out at each time point during the study, thus diminishing the reliability of the conclusions. Greendyke et al. (1986) performed a double-blind, randomized, placebo-controlled crossover study of propranolol in 10 patients with aggression (mean dose, 520 mg). However, in the subgroup of five patients with TBI, the specific response to propranolol was not reported. This group (Greendyke and Kanter 1986) later performed a double-blind randomized placebo-controlled crossover study of pindolol (doses up to 60 mg/day) in 11 patients with behavioral problems, including aggression. It appears that most of these patients were in the earlier pro-

TABLE 14–8. Clinical use of propranolol

1. Conduct a thorough medical evaluation.

2. Exclude patients with the following disorders: bronchial asthma, chronic obstructive pulmonary disease, insulin-dependent diabetes mellitus, congestive heart failure, persistent angina, significant peripheral vascular disease, and hyperthyroidism.

3. Avoid sudden discontinuation of propranolol (particularly in patients with hypertension).

4. Begin with a single test dose of 20 mg/day in patients for whom there are clinical concerns with hypotension or bradycardia. Increase dose of propranolol by 20 mg/day every 3 days.

5. Initiate propranolol on a 20-mg-tid schedule for patients without cardiovascular or cardiopulmonary disorder.

6. Increase the dosage of propranolol by 60 mg/day every 3 days.

7. Increase medication unless the pulse rate is reduced below 50 beats/minute or systolic blood pressure is less than 90 mmHg.

8. Do not administer medication if severe dizziness, ataxia, or wheezing occurs. Reduce or discontinue propranolol if such symptoms persist.

9. Increase dose to 12 mg/kg body weight or until aggressive behavior is under control.

10. Doses of greater than 800 mg are not usually required to control aggressive behavior.

11. Maintain the patient on the highest dose of propranolol for at least 8 weeks before concluding that the patient is not responding to the medication. Some patients, however, may respond rapidly to propranolol.

12. Use concurrent medications with caution. Monitor plasma levels of all antipsychotic and anticonvulsive medications.

Source. Reprinted from Yudofsky SC, Silver JM, Schneider SE: "Pharmacologic Treatment of Aggression." *Psychiatric Annals* 17:397–407, 1987. Used with permission.

pranolol study. Only five of these patients had TBI. Although the group of patients demonstrated improvement in assaultiveness, hostility, and uncooperativeness, the authors of this chapter are unable to assess whether the TBI patients responded differentially. The study by Alpert et al. (1990) using nadolol was conducted with chronically hospitalized patients who did not have TBI. This literature suggests that β-adrenergic receptor blockers are effective agents for the treatment of aggressive and violent behaviors, particularly those related to organic brain syndrome.

TABLE 14–9. Pharmacotherapy of agitation/aggression

Presentation/drug	Primary indication
Acute agitation/severe aggression	
High-potency antipsychotic drugs (haloperidol, risperidone)	
Benzodiazepines (lorazepam)	
Chronic agitation	
Atypical antipsychotics (risperidone, olanzapine, quetiapine, clozapine)	Psychosis
Valproic acid, carbamazepine, ?gabapentin	Seizure disorder, severe aggression
Serotonergic antidepressants (selective serotonin reuptake inhibitors, trazodone)	Depression, mood lability
Buspirone	Anxiety
β-Blockers	Aggression without concomitant neuropsychiatry sequelae

Guidelines for the use of propranolol are listed in Table 14–8. When a patient requires the use of a once-a-day medication because of compliance difficulties, long-acting propranolol (i.e., Inderal LA) or nadolol (Corgard) can be used. When patients develop bradycardia that prevents prescribing therapeutic dosages of propranolol, pindolol (Visken) can be substituted, using one-tenth the dosage of propranolol. Pindolol's intrinsic sympathomimetic activity stimulates the β receptor and restricts the development of bradycardia.

The major side effects of β-blockers when they are used to treat aggression are a lowering of blood pressure and pulse rate. Because peripheral β receptors are fully blocked in doses of 300–400 mg/day, further decreases in these vital signs usually do not occur, even when doses are increased to much higher levels. Despite reports of depression with the use of β-blockers, controlled trials and our experience indicate that it is a rare occurrence (Ko et al. 2002; Yudofsky 1992). Because the use of propranolol is associated with significant increases in plasma levels of thioridazine, which has an absolute dosage ceiling of 800 mg/day, the combination of these two medications should be avoided whenever possible.

Table 14–9 summarizes our recommendations for the use of various classes of medications in the treatment of chronic aggressive disorders associated with TBI. Acute aggression may be treated by using the sedative properties of neuroleptics or benzodiazepines. In treating aggression, the clinician, when possible, should diagnose and treat underlying disorders and use, when possible, antiaggressive agents specific for those disorders. When there is partial response after a therapeutic trial with a specific medication, adjunctive treatment with a medication with a different mechanism of action should be instituted. For example, a patient with partial response to β-blockers can have additional improvement with the addition of an anticonvulsant.

Behavioral Treatment

It is clear that aggression can be caused and influenced by a combination of environmental and biological factors. Because of the dangerous and unpredictable nature of aggression, caregivers—both in institutions and at home—have intense and sometimes injudicious reactions to aggression when it occurs. Behavioral treatments have been shown to be highly effective in treating patients with organic aggression and may be useful when combined with pharmacotherapy. (A discussion of behavioral treatment is found in Chapter 37, Behavioral Treatment; for a review article, see Corrigan et al. 1993.)

Conclusion

Aggressive behavior after brain injury is common and can be highly disabling. Aggression often significantly impedes appropriate rehabilitation and reintegration into the community. There are many neurobiological factors that can lead to aggressive behavior after injury. After appropriate evaluation and assessment of possible etiologies, treatment begins with the documentation of the aggressive episodes. Psychopharmacologic strategies differ according to whether the medication is for the treatment of acute aggression or for the prevention of episodes in the patient with chronic aggression. Although the treatment of acute aggression involves the judicious use of sedation, the treatment of chronic aggression is guided by underlying diagnoses and symptomatologies. Behavioral strategies remain an important component in the comprehensive treatment of aggression. In applying this comprehensive approach, aggression can be controlled with minimal adverse cognitive sequelae.

References

Alexander RW, Davis JN, Lefkowitz RJ: Direct identification and characterization of β-adrenergic receptors in rat brain. Nature 258:437–440, 1979

Alexopoulos GS, Silver JM, Kahn DA, et al: The Expert Consensus Guideline Series: treatment of agitation in older persons with dementia. Postgrad Med, A Special Report. April 1998

Alpert M, Allan ER, Citrome L, et al: A double-blind, placebo-controlled study of adjunctive nadolol in the management of violent psychiatric patients. Psychopharmacol Bull 28:367–371, 1990

American Psychiatric Association: Diagnostic and Statistical Manual of Mental Disorders, 4th Edition, Text Revision. Washington, DC, American Psychiatric Association, 2000

Arango V, Ernsberger P, Marzuk P, et al: Autoradiographic demonstration of increased serotonin 5HT$_2$- and β-adrenergic binding sites in the brains of suicide victims. Arch Gen Psychiatry 47:1038–1047, 1990

Azouvi P, Jokic C, Attal N, et al: Carbamazepine in agitation and aggressive behaviour following severe closed-head injury: results of an open trial. Brain Inj 13:797–804, 1999

Bard P: A diencephalic mechanism for the expression of rage with special reference to the sympathetic nervous system. Am J Physiol 84:490–515, 1928

Bareggi SR, Porta M, Selenati A, et al: Homovanillic acid and 5-hydroxyindole-acetic acid in the CSF of patients after a severe head injury, I: lumbar CSF concentration in chronic brain post-traumatic syndromes. Eur Neurol 13:528–544, 1975

Bellus SB, Stewart D, Vergo JG, et al: The use of lithium in the treatment of aggressive behaviours with two brain-injured individuals in a state psychiatric hospital. Brain Inj 10:849–860, 1996

Beresin E: Delirium in the elderly. J Geriatr Psychiatry Neurol 1:127–143, 1988

Bogner JA, Corrigan JD, Strange M, et al: Reliability of the Agitated Behavior Scale. J Head Trauma Rehabil 14:91–96, 1999

Bogner JA, Corrigan JD, Fugate L, et al: Role of agitation in prediction of outcomes after traumatic brain injury. Am J Phys Med Rehabil 80:636–644, 2001

Brooke MM, Questad KA, Patterson DR, et al: Agitation and restlessness after closed head injury: a prospective study of 100 consecutive admissions. Arch Phys Med Rehabil 73:320–323, 1992

Brooks N, Campsie L, Symington C, et al: The five-year outcome of severe blunt head injury: a relative's view. J Neurol Neurosurg Psychiatry 49:764–770, 1986

Brower MC, Price BH: Neuropsychiatry of frontal lobe dysfunction in violent and criminal behaviour: a critical review. J Neurol Neurosurg Psychiatry 71:720–726, 2001

Brown G, Chadwick O, Shaffer D, et al: A prospective study of children with head injuries, III: psychiatric sequelae. Psychol Med 11:63–78, 1981

Brown GL, Goodwin FK, Ballenger JC, et al: Aggression in humans correlates with cerebrospinal fluid amine metabolites. Psychiatry Res 1:131–139, 1979

Carlsson GS, Svardsudd K, Welin L: Long-term effects of head injuries sustained during life in three male populations. J Neurosurg 67:197–205, 1987

Chandler MC, Barnhill JL, Gualtieri CT: Amantadine for the agitated head-injury patient. Brain Inj 2:309–311, 1988

Chatham-Showalter PE: Carbamazepine for combativeness in acute traumatic brain injury. J Neuropsychiatry Clin Neurosci 8:96–99, 1996

Cheetham S, Crompton M, Katona C, et al: Brain 5-HT$_2$ receptors binding sites in depressed suicide victims. Brain Res 443:271–280, 1988

Childers MK, Holland D: Psychomotor agitation following gabapentin use in brain injury. Brain Inj 11:537–540, 1997

Clifton GL, Ziegler MG, Grossman RG: Circulating catecholamines and sympathetic activity after head injury. Neurosurgery 8:10–14, 1981

Cooper JR, Bloom FE, Roth RH: The Biochemical Basis of Neuropharmacology, 6th Edition. New York, Oxford University Press, 1991

Corrigan PW, Yudofsky SC, Silver JM: Pharmacological and behavioral treatments for aggressive psychiatric inpatients. Hosp Community Psychiatry 44:125–133, 1993

De Deyne PP, Rabheru K, Rasmussen A, et al: A randomized trial of risperidone, placebo, and haloperidol for behavioral symptoms of dementia. Neurology 53:946–955, 1999

Dietch JT, Jennings RK: Aggressive dyscontrol in patients treated with benzodiazepines. J Clin Psychiatry 49:184–189, 1988

Dikmen S, McLean A, Termkin N: Neuropsychological and psychosocial consequences of minor head injury. J Neurol Neurosurg Psychiatry 49:1227–1232, 1986

Eichelman B: Neurochemical and psychopharmacologic aspects of aggressive behavior, in Psychopharmacology: The Third Generation of Progress. Edited by Meltzer HY. New York, Raven, 1987, pp 697–704

Elliott FA: Violence: The neurologic contribution: an overview. Arch Neurol 49:595–603, 1992

Engel J Jr, Bandler R, Griffith NC, et al: Neurobiological evidence for epilepsy-induced interictal disturbances, in Advances in Neurology, Vol 55: Neurobehavioral Problems in Epilepsy. Edited by Smith D, Trimble M. New York, Raven, 1991, pp 97–111

Feeney DM, Gonzalez A, Law WA: Amphetamine, haloperidol, and experience interact to affect rate of recovery after motor cortex injury. Science 217:855–857, 1982

Fernandez HH, Trieschmann ME, Burke MA, et al: Quetiapine for psychosis in Parkinson's disease versus dementia with Lewy bodies. J Clin Psychiatry 63:513–515, 2002

Freedman D, Hemenway D: Precursors of lethal violence: a death row sample. Soc Sci Med Vol 50:1757–1770, 2000

Freinhar JP, Alvarez WA: Clonazepam treatment of organic brain syndromes in three elderly patients. J Clin Psychiatry 47:525–526, 1986

Garyfallos G, Manos N, Adamopoulou A: Psychopathology and personality characteristics of epileptic patients: epilepsy, psychopathology and personality. Acta Psychiatr Scand 78:87–95, 1988

Geracioti TD Jr: Valproic acid treatment of episodic explosiveness related to brain injury. J Clin Psychiatry 55:416–417, 1994

Giakas WJ, Seibyl JP, Mazure CM: Valproate in the treatment of temper outbursts (letter). J Clin Psychiatry 51:525, 1990

Glenn MB, Wroblewski B, Parziale J, et al: Lithium carbonate for aggressive behavior or affective instability in ten brain-injured patients. Am J Phys Med Rehabil 68:221–226, 1989

Greendyke RM, Kanter DR: Therapeutic effects of pindolol on behavioral disturbances associated with organic brain disease: a double-blind study. J Clin Psychiatry 47:423–426, 1986

Greendyke RM, Kanter DR, Schuster DB, et al: Propranolol treatment of assaultive patients with organic brain disease: a double-blind crossover, placebo-controlled study. J Nerv Ment Dis 174:290–294, 1986

Greve KW, Sherwin E, Stanford MS, et al: Personality and neurocognitive correlates of impulsive aggression in long-term survivors of severe traumatic brain injury. Brain Inj 15:255–262, 2001

Grossman R, Beyer C, Kelly P, et al: Acetylcholine and related enzymes in human ventricular and subarachnoid fluids following brain injury (abstract). Proceedings of the 5th Annual Meeting for Neuroscience 76:3:506, 1975

Gualtieri CT: Buspirone for the behavior problems of patients with organic brain disorders. J Clin Psychopharmacol 11:280–281, 1991a

Gualtieri CT: Buspirone: neuropsychiatric effects. J Head Trauma Rehabil 6:90–92, 1991b

Hagen C, Malkmus D, Durham P: Rancho Los Amigos levels of cognitive functioning scale. Downey, CA, Professional Staff Association, 1972

Halgren E: Emotional neurophysiology of the amygdala within the context of human cognition, in The Amygdala: Neurobiological Aspects of Emotion, Memory, and Mental Dysfunction. Edited by Aggleton JP. New York, Wiley-Liss, 1992, pp 191–228

Hamill RW, Woolf PD, McDonald JV, et al: Catecholamines predict outcome in traumatic brain injury. Ann Neurol 21:438–443, 1987

Heinrichs RW: Frontal cerebral lesions and violent incidents in chronic neuropsychiatric patients. Biol Psychiatry 25:174–178, 1989

Hen R, Boschert U, Lemeur M, et al: 5-HT-1B receptor "knock out": pharmacological and behavioral consequences. Society for Neuroscience 23rd Annual Meeting Abstracts, Washington, DC, 19:632, 1993

Herrmann N, Lanctot K, Myszak M: Effectiveness of gabapentin for the treatment of behavioral disorders in dementia. J Clin Psychopharmacol 20:90–93, 2000

Herzberg JL, Fenwick PBC: The aetiology of aggression in temporal-lobe epilepsy. Br J Psychiatry 153:50–55, 1988

Hibbard MR, Uysal S, Kepler K, et al: Axis I psychopathology in individuals with traumatic brain injury. J Head Trauma Rehabil 13:24–39, 1998

Higley JD, Mehlman PT, Taum DM, et al: Cerebrospinal fluid monoamine and adrenal correlates of aggression in free-ranging Rhesus monkeys. Arch Gen Psychiatry 49:436–441, 1992

Horne M, Lindley SE: Divalproex sodium in the treatment of aggressive behavior and dysphoria in patients with organic brain syndromes. J Clin Psychiatry 56:430–431, 1995

Hornstein A, Seliger G: Cognitive side effects of lithium in closed head injury (letter). J Neuropsychiatry Clin Neurosci 1:446–447, 1989

Jackson RD, Corrigan JD, Arnett JA: Amitriptyline for agitation in head injury. Arch Phys Med Rehabil 66:180–181, 1985

Jorge RE, Robinson RG, Moser D, et al: Major depression following traumatic brain injury. Arch Gen Psychiatry 61:42–50, 2004

Kant R, Smith-Seemiller L, Zeiler D: Treatment of aggression and irritability after head injury. Brain Inj 12:661–666, 1998

Katz IR, Jeste DV, Mintzer JE, et al: Comparison of risperdone and placebo for psychosis and behavioral disturbances associated with dementia: a randomized, double-blind trial. Risperidone Study Group. J Clin Psychiatry 60:107–115, 1999

Kaufer D, Cummings JL, Christine D: Differential neuropsychiatric symptom responses to tacrine in Alzheimer's disease: relationship to dementia severity. J Neuropsychiatry Clin Neurosci 10:55–63, 1998

Keats MM, Mukherjee S: Antiaggressive effect of adjunctive clonazepam in schizophrenia associated with seizure disorder. J Clin Psychiatry 49:117–118, 1988

Knott P, Haroutunian V, Bierer L, et al: Correlations post-mortem between ventricular CSF and cortical tissue concentrations of MHPG, 5-HIAA, and HVA in Alzheimer's disease (abstract). Biol Psychiatry 25:112A, 1989

Ko DT, Hebert PR, Coffey CS, et al: Beta-blocker therapy and symptoms of depression, fatigue, and sexual dysfunction. JAMA 288:351–357, 2002

Kruesi MJ, Hibbs ED, Zahn TP, et al: A 2-year prospective follow-up study of children and adolescents with disruptive behavior disorders: prediction by cerebrospinal fluid 5-hydroxyindoleacetic acid, homovanillic acid, and autonomic measures? Arch Gen Psychiatry 49:429–435, 1992

Lammers AJ, van Rossum JM: Bizarre social behavior in rats induced by a combination of a peripheral decarboxylase inhibitor and dopa. Eur J Pharmacol 5:103–106, 1968

Levin HS, Grossman RG: Behavioral sequelae of closed head injury: a quantitative study. Arch Neurol 35:720–727, 1978

Levin HS, Grossman RG, Rose JE, et al: Long-term neuropsychological outcome of closed head injury. J Neurosurg 50:412–422, 1979

Levine AM: Buspirone and agitation in head injury. Brain Inj 2:165–167, 1988

Linnoila VMI, Virkkunen M: Aggression, suicidality, and serotonin. J Clin Psychiatry 53 (suppl 10):46–51, 1992

Malamud N: Psychiatric disorder with intracranial tumors of the limbic system. Arch Neurol 17:113–123, 1967

Mann JJ: Violence and aggression, in Psychopharmacology: The Fourth Generation of Progress. Edited by Bloom FE, Kupfer DJ. New York: Raven, 1995, pp 1919–1928

Mattes JA: Valproic acid for nonaffective aggression in the mentally retarded. J Nerv Ment Dis 180:601–602, 1992

McCracken JT, McGough J, Shah B, et al: Risperidone in children with autism and serious behavioral problems. N Engl J Med 347:314–321, 2002

McKinlay WW, Brooks DN, Bond MR, et al: The short-term outcome of severe blunt head injury as reported by the relatives of the injured person. J Neurol Neurosurg Psychiatry 44:527–533, 1981

McMillan TM, Glucksman EE: The neuropsychology of moderate head injury. J Neurol Neurosurg Psychiatry 50:393–397, 1987

Mendez MF, Cummings JL, Benson DF: Depression in epilepsy: significance and phenomenology. Arch Neurol 43:766–770, 1986

Michals ML, Crismon ML, Roberts S, et al: Clozapine response and adverse effects in nine brain-injured patients. J Clin Psychopharmacol 13:198–203, 1993

Mooney GF, Haas LJ: Effect of methylphenidate on brain injury-related anger. Arch Phys Med Rehabil 74:153–160, 1993

Moskowitz AS, Altshuler L: Increased sensitivity to lithium-induced neurotoxicity after stroke: a case report. J Clin Psychopharmacol 11:272–273, 1991

Muehlencamp F, Lucion A, Vogel WH: Effects of selective serotonin agonists on aggressive behavior in rats. Pharmacol Biochem Behav 50:671–674, 1995

Mysiw WJ, Jackson RD, Corrigan JD: Amitriptyline for posttraumatic agitation. Am J Phys Med Rehabil 67:29–33, 1988

New AS, Hazlett EA, Buchsbaum MS, et al: Blunted prefrontal cortical [18]fluorodeoxyglucose positron emission tomography response to *meta*-chlorophenylpiperazine in impulsive aggression. Arch Gen Psychiatry 59:621–629, 2002

Nielsen DA, Goldman D, Virkkunen M, et al: Suicidality and 5-hydroxyindoleacetic acid concentration associated with a tryptophan hydroxylase polymorphism. Arch Gen Psychiatry 51:34–38, 1994

Nichels JL, Schneider WN, Dombovy ML, et al: Clinical use of amantadine in brain injury rehabilitation. Brain Injury 8:709–718, 1994

Oddy M, Coughlan T, Tyerman A, et al: Social adjustment after closed head injury: a further follow-up seven years after injury. J Neurol Neurosurg Psychiatry 48:564–568, 1985

Olivier B, Mos J, Rasmussen DL: Behavioural pharmacology of the serenic, eltoprazine. Drug Metab Drug Interact 8:31–38, 1990

Patterson JF: Carbamazepine for assaultive patients with organic brain disease. Psychosomatics 28:579–581, 1987

Pietrini P, Guazzelli M, Basso G, et al: Neural correlates of imaginal aggressive behavior assessed by positron emission tomography in healthy subjects. Am J Psychiatry 157:1772–1781, 2000

Porta M, Bareggi SR, Collice M, et al. Homovanillic acid and 5-hydroxyindole-acetic acid in the CSF of patients after a severe head injury, II: ventricular CSF concentrations in acute brain post-traumatic syndromes. Eur Neurol 13:545–554, 1975

Post RM, Uhde TW, Putnam FW, et al: Kindling and carbamazepine in affective illness. J Nerv Ment Dis 170:717–731, 1982

Rao N, Jellinek HM, Woolston DC: Agitation in closed head injury: haloperidol effects on rehabilitation outcome. Arch Phys Med Rehabil 66:30–34, 1985

Ratey JJ, Leveroni C, Kilmer D, et al: The effects of clozapine on severely aggressive psychiatric inpatients in a state hospital. J Clin Psychiatry 54:219–223, 1993

Reis DJ: The relationship between brain norepinephrine and aggressive behavior. Res Publ Assoc Res Nerv Ment Dis 50:266–297, 1972

Rimel RW, Giordani B, Barth JT, et al: Disability caused by minor head injury. Neurosurgery 9:221–228, 1981

Roane DM, Feinberg TE, Meckler L, et al: Treatment of dementia-associated agitation with gabapentin. J Neuropsychiatry Clin Neurosci 12:40–43, 2000

Roberts WW: Escape learning without avoidance learning motivated by hypothalamic stimulation in cats. J Comp Physiol Psychol 51:391–399, 1958

Robertson MM, Trimble MR, Townsend HRA: Phenomenology of depression in epilepsy. Epilepsia 28:364–372, 1987

Roy A, Argen H, Pickar D, et al: Reduced CSF concentrations of homovanillic acid and homovanillic acid to 5-hydroxyindoleacetic acid ratios in depressed patients: relationship to suicidal behavior and dexamethasone suppression. Am J Psychiatry 143:1539–1545, 1986

Rutherford WH, Merrett JD, McDonald JR: Sequelae of concussion caused by minor head injuries. Lancet 1:1–4, 1977

Saint-Cyr JA, Taylor AE, Lang AE: Neuropsychological and psychiatric side effects in the treatment of Parkinson's disease. Neurology 43(suppl 6):S47–S52, 1993

Salzman C, Kochansky GE, Shader RI, et al: Chloridazepoxide-induced hostility in a small group setting. Arch Gen Psychiatry 31:401–405, 1974

Sandel ME, Olive DA, Rader MA: Chlorpromazine-induced psychosis after brain injury. Brain Inj 7:77–83, 1993

Schoenhuber R, Gentili M: Anxiety and depression after mild head injury: a case control study. J Neurol Neurosurg Psychiatry 51:722–724, 1988

Silver JM, Yudofsky SC: Documentation of aggression in the assessment of the violent patient. Psychiatric Ann 17:375–384, 1987

Silver JM, Yudofsky SC: The Overt Aggression Scale: overview and clinical guidelines. J Neuropsychiatry Clin Neurosci 3 (suppl):S22–S29, 1991

Sparadeo FR, Gill D: Effects of prior alcohol use on head injury recovery. Journal of Head Trauma Rehabilitation 4:75–82, 1989

Stanislav SW: Cognitive effects of antipsychotic agents in persons with traumatic brain injury. Brain Inj 11:335–341, 1997

Stanley M, Traskman-Bendz L, Dorovini-Zis K: Correlations between aminergic metabolites simultaneously obtained from human CSF and brain. Life Sci 37:1279–1286, 1985

Stevens JR, Hermann BP: Temporal lobe epilepsy, psychopathology, and violence: the state of the evidence. Neurology 31:1127–1132, 1981

Szlabowicz JW, Stewart JT: Amitriptyline treatment of agitation associated with anoxic encephalopathy. Arch Phys Med Rehabil 71:612–613, 1990

Tateno A, Jorge RE, Robinson RG: Clinical correlates of aggressive behavior after traumatic brain injury. J Neuropsychiatry Clin Neurosci 15:155–160, 2003

Thomsen IV: Late outcome of very severe blunt head trauma: a 10–15 year second follow-up. J Neurol Neurosurg Psychiatry 47:260–268, 1984

Tonkonogy TM: Violence and temporal lobe lesion: head CT and MRI data. J Neuropsychiatry Clin Neurosci 3:189–196, 1991

Traskman L, Asberg M, Bertilsson L, et al: Monoamine metabolites in CSF and suicidal behavior. Arch Gen Psychiatry 38:631–636, 1981

Tune L, Carr S, Hoag E, et al: Anticholinergic effects of drugs commonly prescribed for the elderly: potential means for assessing risk of delirium. Am J Psychiatry 149:1393–1394, 1992

Valzelli L: Psychobiology of Aggression and Violence. New York, Raven, 1981

van der Naalt, van Zomeren AH, Sluiter WJ, et al: Acute behavioural disturbances related to imaging studies and outcome in mild-to-moderate head injury. Brain Inj 14:781–788, 2000

Van Woerkom TCAM, Teelken AW, Minderhoud JM: Difference in neurotransmitter metabolism in frontotemporal-lobe contusion and diffuse cerebral contusion. Lancet 1:812–813, 1977

Van Zomeren A, Van Den Burg W: Residual complaints of patients two years after severe head injury. J Neurol Neurosurg Psychiatry 48:21–28, 1985

Vanier M, Mazaux J-M, Lambert J, et al: Assessment of neuropsychologic impairment after head injury: interrater reliability and factorial and criterion validity of the neurobehavioral rating scale-revised. Arch Phys Med Rehabil 81:796–806, 2000

Vecht CJ, Van Woerkom TCAM, Teelken AW, et al: Homovanillic acid and 5-hydroxyindoleacetic acid cerebrospinal fluid levels. Arch Neurol 32:792–797, 1975

Weiger WA, Bear DM. An approach to the neurology of aggression. J Psychiatr Res 22:85–98, 1988

Wolf AP, Gleckman AD, Cifu DX, et al: The prevalence of agitation and brain injury in skilled nursing facilities: a survey. Brain Inj 10:241–245, 1996

Wroblewski BA, Joseph AB, Kupfer J, et al: Effectiveness of valproic acid on destructive and aggressive behaviours in patients with acquired brain injury. Brain Inj 11:37–47, 1997

Yudofsky SC: β-blockers and depression: the clinician's dilemma. JAMA 267:1826–1827, 1992

Yudofsky SC, Kopecky HJ, Kunik ME, et al: The Overt Agitation Severity Scale for the objective rating of agitation. J Neuropsychiatry Clin Neuroscience 9:541–548, 1997

Yudofsky SC, Silver JM, Jackson W, et al: The Overt Aggression Scale for the objective rating of verbal and physical aggression. Am J Psychiatry 143:35–39, 1986

Yudofsky SC, Silver JM, Hales RE: Treatment of agitation and aggression, in American Psychiatric Press Textbook of Psychopharmacology, 2nd Edition. Edited by Schatzberg AF, Nemeroff CB. Washington, DC, American Psychiatric Press, 1998, pp 881–900

15 Mild Brain Injury and the Postconcussion Syndrome

Thomas W. McAllister, M.D.

Definitions

Severity of brain injury exists along a broad continuum clinically and pathophysiologically. Different schemes have been proposed for categorizing injury severity, but there is no universally accepted definition of *mild traumatic brain injury* (MTBI) (Tables 15–1 and 15–2). Injuries in which duration of unconsciousness is less than 30 minutes and Glasgow Coma Scale (GCS) (Teasdale and Jennett 1974) scores are 13 or greater are usually considered consistent with mild brain injury. When initially seen, these patients may be confused or disoriented and appear lethargic (Table 15–1). There have been several efforts to standardize the definition of MTBI. One of the more commonly used definitions is that proposed by the special task force of the American Congress of Rehabilitation Medicine. They defined an MTBI as a traumatically induced disruption of brain function that results in loss of consciousness (LOC) of less than 30 minutes' duration or in an alteration of consciousness manifested by incomplete memory of the event or being dazed and confused. The period of posttraumatic amnesia (PTA) should not last longer than 24 hours, and the individual may or may not have focal neurological findings (Kay et al. 1993).

The International Classification of Diseases, 9th Revision, Clinical Modification (World Health Organization 1989) includes a diagnostic category of concussion

defined as "transient impairment of function as a result of a blow to the brain" and distinguishes between concussion without LOC (with mental confusion), brief LOC (<1 hour), and more prolonged LOC.

The Centers for Disease Control and Prevention adopted the following definition for traumatic brain injury in 1995 (Thurman et al. 1995): "an occurrence of injury to the head that is documented in a medical record, with one or more of the following conditions attributed to head injury:

- observed or self-reported decreased level of consciousness,
- amnesia,
- skull fracture,
- objective neurological or neuropsychological abnormality, or
- diagnosed intracranial lesion."

Efforts to categorize severity of brain injury have also been a recent focus in sports medicine, and a variety of schemes have been proposed for the grading of concussions (see Echemendia and Julian 2001 and Chapter 26, Sports Injuries, for reviews). The American Academy of Neurology grading system (Practice parameter 1997) defines a grade 1 concussion as an injury resulting in confusion without LOC, with symptoms clearing within 15 minutes. A grade 2 concussion results in confusion without LOC, with symptoms that last longer than 15 min-

Supported in part by National Institute on Disability and Rehabilitation Research grants H133G70031 and H133000136, National Institutes of Health grant R01 NS40472–01, the Ira DeCamp Foundation, and New Hampshire Hospital.

TABLE 15–1.   Indicators of mild brain injury

Duration of loss of consciousness	None to 30 minutes
Duration of posttraumatic amnesia	Minutes to 24 hours (can be longer)
Glasgow Coma Scale[a] score	13–15
Clinical condition	May appear stunned or dazed
	May appear drowsy or indifferent
	May be disoriented or have trouble with complex commands
	May complain of headache or nausea or vomit

[a]See Teasdale and Jennett 1974.

utes. A grade 3 concussion is one in which there is LOC (see Table 15–2). DSM-IV-TR (American Psychiatric Association 2000) does not define *concussion* but does include "Postconcussional Disorder" in an appendix of proposals for new categories that need further research and clarification before they are included as official diagnoses. To meet criteria for postconcussional disorder, one must have a "significant cerebral concussion" manifested by LOC, evidence of deficits in attention and memory, and at least three other symptoms that have lasted at least 3 months.

There have been few studies that explore the clinical differences and diagnostic validity of these different diagnostic schemes. Ruff and Jurica (1999) evaluated 76 individuals with MTBI diagnosed using the American Congress of Rehabilitation Medicine criteria. Only 34% of these patients met the criteria for a significant cerebral concussion suggested by DSM-IV-TR. There were no significant between-group differences with respect to number of subjective complaints, neurocognitive performance, or preexisting emotional risk factors, suggesting the need for further research to define the population more clearly.

One of the reasons to clarify injury severity is to inform patients and family about likely outcome. However, using most common definitions of MTBI, the prognosis

TABLE 15–2.   Different definitions of mild traumatic brain injury in the literature

Study	Definition of mild traumatic brain injury
Gronwall and Wrightson 1974	Posttraumatic amnesia <24 hours.
Minderhoud et al. 1980	LOC <30 minutes and some posttraumatic amnesia.
Rimel et al. 1981	LOC <20 minutes, GCS score 13–15, hospitalization <24 hours.
Barth et al. 1983	LOC <20 minutes, GCS score 13–15, hospitalization <24 hours.
Levin et al. 1987b	LOC <30 minutes, GCS score 13–15 when hospitalized, without deterioration, normal computed tomography scan and neurological examination.
ICD-9-CM (World Health Organization 1989)	Concussion defined as "transient impairment of function as a result of a blow to the brain" and distinguishes between concussion without LOC (with mental confusion), brief LOC (<1 hour), and more prolonged LOC.
Leininger et al. 1990	Alteration in consciousness or LOC <20 minutes, GCS 13–15, no deterioration or surgical intervention.
Bohnen et al. 1993	LOC <15 minutes, posttraumatic amnesia <60 minutes, GCS=15, no focal neurological findings.
American Congress of Rehabilitation Medicine (Kay et al. 1993)	Alteration in consciousness (incomplete memory or confusion) or LOC <30 minutes, posttraumatic amnesia <24 hours, may have focal neurological deficits that may or may not be transient.
Practice parameter 1997	Grades of concussion—grade 1: confusion, no LOC, symptoms <15 minutes; grade 2: confusion, no LOC, symptoms >15 minutes; grade 3: LOC of any duration.
DSM-IV-TR (American Psychiatric Association 2000)	To make diagnosis of postconcussional disorder, must have "significant cerebral concussion" manifested by LOC, posttraumatic amnesia, or seizures. Evidence of deficits in memory and attention. At least three other symptoms of at least 3 months' duration (fatigues easily, disordered sleep, headache, dizziness, irritability, anxiety/depression/lability, apathy).

Note.   LOC = loss of consciousness; GCS = Glasgow Coma Scale.
Source.   Adapted from Brown SJ, Fann JR, Grant I: "Postconcussional Disorder: Time to Acknowledge a Common Source of Neurobehavioral Morbidity." *The Journal of Neuropsychiatry and Clinical Neurosciences* 6:15–22, 1994.

is clearly better than that for moderate and severe injury (Frencham et al., in press; Levin et al. 1990; Rees 2003; Rimel et al. 1982; Schretlen and Shapiro 2003; Williams et al. 1990). However, there is controversy about the nature, severity, and etiology of short- and long-term sequelae in these patients (Frencham et al., in press; Levin et al. 1990; Rees 2003; Schretlen and Shapiro 2003; Williams et al. 1990). This may reflect the inadequacy of the measures used to assess both severity and outcome. For example, Williams et al. (1990), in a careful study, suggested that GCS scores alone might be insufficient predictors of outcome in certain patients with mild brain injury. Patients with GCS scores in the mild range (13–15) with or without focal brain lesions, depressed skull fractures, or both, were compared with patients with moderate brain injury. The group with mild injury and associated focal lesions or depressed skull fractures was similar to the moderate injury group in terms of neuropsychological and outcome measures. Thus, the combination of clinical signs and symptoms shortly after injury and initial radiological findings may be a better scheme for predicting outcome.

In terms of the literature to be reviewed, *MTBI* is used in this chapter to signify injury with brief (<30 minutes) or no LOC and with GCS scores, when available, of 13–15. Typically, the duration of PTA is in the range of less than 1–24 hours, and many groups exclude patients hospitalized for more than 48 hours.

Epidemiology

There are relatively few good epidemiological studies on the incidence of mild brain injury, especially given the magnitude of the problem, the age groups affected, and the potential for significant sequelae. In 1981, Kraus and Nourjah (1988) studied all individuals admitted with brain injuries in San Diego County, California, and found that mild brain injury accounted for 82% of all patients hospitalized with TBI; 75% of this group had GCS scores of 15. These figures are similar to those reported by Whitman et al. (1984) in two Chicago area communities and somewhat higher than those reported by Annegers et al. (1980) and Rimel (1981), who found that mild brain injury accounted for 60% and 49% of all brain injuries, respectively. As Kraus and Nourjah (1989) noted, differences in definition of *mild brain injury*, time periods over which the data were collected, and patient referral sources may account for the discrepancies. On the basis of their data from the San Diego County study, hospitalization for mild brain injury occurs at a rate of 131 per 100,000 population or between 300,000 and 400,000 people per year

TABLE 15–3. Epidemiology of mild brain injury in the United States

Incidence	130–150 per 100,000 hospitalized patients (perhaps 4–5 times this number treated as outpatients)
Age distribution (years)	15–24 (peak range)
Sex distribution (male:female)	2:1 (peak for females: age >75 years)
Etiology (%)	Motor vehicle accidents: 40–45
	Falls: 20–25
	Assaults: 10–15
	Sports and recreation: 10–15
Treatment costs	More than $1 billion/year

in the United States. Probably four to five mild brain injuries occur for each one that results in hospitalization (U.S. Department of Health and Human Services 1989; Table 15–3). This is particularly true now because criteria for hospitalization of patients have become more strict.

More recently, Sosin et al. (1996) reported on a household survey of a national sample conducted in conjunction with the U.S. Census Bureau. Individuals were asked to report trauma to the head that resulted in LOC but not death or institutionalization; thus, the data probably include both mild and moderate TBI. Per 100,000 population, 460 reported LOC without hospitalization, and an additional 59 reported overnight hospitalization. Using 250 million as the approximate United States population, this translates into approximately 1.3 million mild brain injuries per year that result in a LOC. This does not take into account those injuries resulting in an altered level of consciousness (Centers for Disease Control and Prevention 1999; Malec 1999).

Mirroring the demographic profile of TBI in general, mild injury occurs twice as frequently in males, with a peak age distribution of 15–24 years (Kraus and Nourjah 1988). Causes of mild brain injury are also similar to those of brain injury in general, with motor vehicle accidents, falls, assaults, and sports or recreation accidents accounting for 40%–50%, 20%–25%, 15%–20%, and 10%–15% of injuries, respectively (Dacey and Dikmen 1987; Kraus and Nourjah 1988; Kraus and Nourjah 1989; Kraus et al. 1994). Assaults account for a higher percentage of mild brain injuries in some areas, especially in large urban centers (Sorenson and Kraus 1991). It is also probably true that the vast majority of sports-related mild brain injuries go unreported. Falls account for a larger percentage in children younger than 10 years and adults older than 65 years (Goleburn and Golden 2001; Luerssen et al. 1988).

Kraus and Nourjah (1988) estimated the cost to treat hospitalized patients with mild brain injury alone at well over $1 billion per year (1988 dollars). This does not include the nonhospitalized patients, nor does it include costs of ongoing care for patients. It is of some interest, given the known neuropsychiatric sequelae of mild brain injury, that only 15 of 2,435 patients with mild brain injury in the San Diego County study were discharged with planned medical follow-up.

Thus, in many respects, the term *mild* brain injury is a misnomer. Sequelae include problems in cognition, behavior, the constellation of signs and symptoms that make up the postconcussive syndrome, other psychopathology, and a surprisingly high rate of disability. Though the initial clinical picture may be mild relative to the spectrum of possible neuropathological and functional outcomes such as death or persistent minimally responsive state, the extent of the problem and the frequency and intensity of certain predictable sequelae make mild brain injury anything but a minor problem.

Pathophysiology

The structural concomitants of mild brain injury have been the subject of some discussion. The alteration in level of consciousness, even if brief, suggests widespread neuronal dysfunction (Gennarelli 1987; Peerless and Newcastle 1967). There is evidence that structural neuronal damage can accompany even very mild brain injury. Animal models of brain injury using the fluid percussion model in cats (Povlishock and Coburn 1989) and controlled angular acceleration devices in nonhuman primates (Jane et al. 1985) strongly suggest that mild brain injury is often associated with evidence of axonal injury. Although axotomy may occur at the time of injury, delayed axotomy also contributes significantly to the neuropathological outcome. Delayed axotomy is believed to occur subsequent to initial changes in the permeability of the axolemma (axonal membrane) and disruption of certain elements of the cytoskeleton, particularly axonal neurofilaments. This in turn can lead to axonal distortion, disruption of axoplasmic transport (see Povlishock and Christman 1995 for review), and eventual separation of the proximal and distal portion of the axon even in the absence of an overt tear at the time of injury. Wallerian degeneration (with beadlike swelling and eventual degeneration of the distal axon and its terminals) can occur. Secondary deafferentation (structural changes and sometimes neuronal death due to loss of synaptic input) in target areas of the afflicted axon can follow (Povlishock and Christman 1995; Povlishock and Coburn 1989).

These changes in axon structure evolve over a 12- to 24-hour period in the cat model and can be seen in the absence of structural damage to neighboring supportive or vascular tissue. The wallerian changes take place over the subsequent 2–60 days (Povlishock and Coburn 1989). Identification of the molecular mechanisms involved may eventually suggest interventions to block or reduce neuronal damage (see Chapter 2, Neuropathology, and Chapter 39, Pharmacotherapy of Prevention). Regenerative activity (including sprouting and enlarged axonal areas at the tip of growing axons) over a period of weeks to several months subsequent to the trauma can be seen, perhaps mirroring the recovery process observed in humans (Povlishock and Christman 1995; Povlishock and Coburn 1989). Povlishock and Christman (1995) suggested that the success or functional outcome of such regenerative activity may depend on the severity of injury.

There is evidence that MTBI results in neuropathological changes in humans similar to those described in animal models. For example, Oppenheimer (1968) reported destruction of myelin, axonal retraction bulbs (beadlike structures at the proximal end of a ruptured axon), and aggregates of small reactive glial cells (indicating recent tissue injury) in a variety of brain regions in five patients with minor or trivial injuries. One such patient had been knocked down by a motor scooter and had no LOC but was described as "stunned." PTA lasted approximately 20 minutes. Using immunostaining for amyloid precursor protein as a marker for axonal injury, Blumbergs et al. (1994) reported multifocal axonal injury in five individuals who had sustained very mild injuries with periods of unconsciousness as brief as 1 minute.

In addition to the microscopic structural changes described above, both animal models and human studies suggest that MTBI can result in at least temporary alteration of the normal balance between cellular energy demand and energy supply. Under normal circumstances, energy consumption roughly matches energy supply at the neuronal level, and alterations in energy demand (i.e., increased neuronal metabolic activity) can be accommodated by utilization of intracellular stores, and subsequently by increased blood flow to facilitate the supply of oxygen and glucose. However, even MTBI can result in significant changes in intracellular and extracellular concentrations of ions such as potassium, sodium, calcium, and magnesium. Restoration of the normal intracellular and extracellular milieu requires a significant increase in energy expenditure that is initially met by hyperglycolysis. However, ongoing energy demands require an increase in blood flow, and this normal coupling of increased energy demand to increased energy supply can be disrupted after MTBI (Bergsneider et al. 2000; Giza and

Hovda 2001; Lee et al. 1999). Both animal and human studies have shown an increase in glucose utilization shortly after MTBI associated with a reduction in cerebral blood flow (Arvigo et al. 1985; Junger et al. 1997; Strebel et al. 1997).

Injury does not always occur at the axonal level alone. Although cerebral concussion was the diagnosis in 80% of patients with mild brain injury in the San Diego County study (Kraus and Nourjah 1988), almost 5% had cerebral contusions, approximately 1% had intracerebral hemorrhages, and 14% had some other form of intracranial lesion. In Williams et al.'s (1990) study, of 155 consecutive patients with mild brain injury 32 had parenchymal contusions or hemorrhages (20%) and 27 (17%) had subdural or epidural hematomas. Three recent large cohort studies (Borczuk 1995; Haydel et al. 2000; Miller et al. 1997) assessed predictors of surgical lesions and abnormal computed tomography (CT) scans in MTBI patients with GCS scores of 15 representing more than 4,000 patients. The findings suggest that in individuals with very mild TBI as defined by GCS score alone, 5%–10% have abnormal CT scans. Clinical features such as headache, vomiting, increased age, alcohol or drug intoxication, short-term memory impairment (anterograde amnesia), head and neck trauma, or seizures appear to predict those patients more likely to have abnormal scans, although not necessarily in children (Quayle 1999).

Individuals who have GCS scores of 13 or 14 have a higher frequency of abnormal findings on CT scans, ranging from 20% to 35% (Harad and Kerstein 1992; Schynoll et al. 1993; Shackford et al. 1992; Stein and Ross 1992). Furthermore, the presence of structural lesions in MTBI, whether on CT or magnetic resonance imaging (MRI), is associated with outcomes more consistent with those seen in moderate TBI (van der Naalt et al. 1999; Williams et al. 1990), at least from a cognitive standpoint. Other neuropsychiatric outcome indices may be more closely associated with the duration of PTA and less closely associated with GCS scores (McCullagh et al. 2001).

Special concerns have been raised about a rare complication of MTBI known as *diffuse cerebral swelling*. In this condition, catastrophic decline in neurological function resulting in death or persistent vegetative state occurs hours to days after a seemingly mild brain injury (McCrory and Berkovic 1998). The majority of these events has occurred in children and adolescents, often in sports-related activities. In some instances, these precipitous declines have occurred after an earlier mild injury, giving rise to the term *second impact syndrome*, although the relationship to repetitive injuries is not clear cut (McCrory and Berkovic 1998).

The above suggests that brain injury considered trivial on the basis of the degree and duration of altered consciousness has demonstrable neuropathological effects, starting at the moment of impact and evolving over several hours to days and longer. The types of injuries seen, both macroscopically and microscopically, are similar in quality and location to those seen with moderate and severe degrees of brain injury.

Cognitive Sequelae

In considering the literature addressing cognitive deficits after MTBI it is important to take into account the criteria used for mild brain injury, the interval from injury to evaluation, and the measures used to assess cognitive function. With more uniformity in the definition of the mild brain injury, a better appreciation of the types of deficits seen, and more consistent use of measures that probe attention, speed of information processing, and memory, several factors have become clear.

Short-Term Effects

Most investigators agree that individuals with mild brain injury can be distinguished from healthy control subjects on measures of speed of information processing, selected tests of attention and memory, and performance consistency in the first week or so subsequent to the injury (Gentilini et al. 1989; Gronwall 1989; Levin et al. 1987b; McMillan and Glucksman 1987; Ruff et al. 1989b; Stuss et al. 1989). Even individuals who are asymptomatic several days after mild concussion with no LOC can have impaired processing speed (Warden et al. 2001). The usual course of recovery is fairly rapid. Studies of cognitive testing 1 month and 3 months after injury tend to show progressive diminution of cognitive deficits, although when differences persist they are also usually in the domains of memory, attention, and processing speed (Bohnen et al. 1993; Dikmen et al. 1986a, 1986b; Gentilini et al. 1989; Gronwall 1989; Ruff et al. 1989b). The study by Williams et al. (1990) suggests that those individuals with complications such as depressed skull fractures, contusions, and subdural or epidural hematomas may be those who are more likely to have persistent deficits in speed of information processing, verbal and recognition memory, and verbal fluency.

Long-Term Effects

The long-term cognitive sequelae of mild brain injury are a controversial area. In a careful study of 20 individuals with mild injury (GCS ≥12, LOC ≤1 hour) who were compared on a variety of neuropsychological measures taken largely from the Halstead-Reitan battery with 20 noninjured friends, Dikmen et al. (1986b) were unable to find significant differences between the two groups 12 months after the injury. It is also important to be aware that not all persistent deficits after MTBI are related to neuronal injury occurring at the time of the trauma. Several authors have demonstrated that cognitive deficits and postconcussive-like symptoms can be associated with accidents and injuries that do not involve the brain. There is an emerging literature on the use of "other-injury" control subjects (e.g., those with orthopedic injuries but without TBI) to control for nonspecific effects of injury on cognition. For example, Dikmen et al. (1995a), in a carefully designed study of the cognitive effects of TBI, compared 436 TBI participants with 121 general-trauma participants on a cognitive battery 1 year after injury. Their results showed very little effect of MTBI on cognition but a significant effect of moderate TBI. The researchers pointed out that these results did not rule out the existence of a well-described minority of MTBI patients with significant and persistent cognitive deficits. On the other hand, two recent meta-analyses of the effects of MTBI (Frencham et al., in press) and/or more severe TBI (Schretlen et al. 2003) confirm that most spontaneous recovery after MTBI is complete by 3 months postinjury; however, these researchers found very little difference in TBI-related effect sizes on cognition, whether compared with healthy control subjects or other-injury control subjects. For studies using other-injury control subjects in the follow-up interval of 1 year after injury, the effect size attributable to TBI was in the range of 0.1 (Schretlen et al. 2003) to 0.35 (Frencham et al., in press) for MTBI and 0.6–0.9 for moderate to severe TBI (Schretlen et al. 2003). These values represent effect sizes of 0.08 for MTBI and 0.91 for moderate to severe TBI in studies using healthy noninjured control subjects (Schretlen et al. 2003).

Studies of individuals with persistent symptoms are less encouraging. Leininger et al. (1990) found significant impairment on four of eight neuropsychological tests (Category Test, Paced Auditory Serial Addition Task—Revised, Auditory Verbal Learning Test, Complex Figure—Copy) in a group of persistently symptomatic individuals with mild brain injury (GCS 13 or greater, LOC less than 20 minutes) tested an average of 6–8 months after the injury. In this study, 53 individuals with MTBI who noted persistent complaints were compared with matched friends and relatives of TBI patients. Patients with a prior history of TBI were excluded. Of note is that a significant minority of the patients (40%) had no history of LOC, having sustained "dazing" injuries or mild concussions. Tests assess-

ing information processing, reasoning, and verbal learning were significantly different from the control group. There were no significant differences between those who did or did not lose consciousness, those tested before or after 3 months after the injury, or those who were or were not pursuing compensation claims. Guilmette and Rasile (1995) also found significant deficits in tests of verbal memory and learning in a sample of individuals with MTBI (LOC less than 30 minutes, PTA less than 24 hours) but with persistent complaints. These studies suggest that the persistently symptomatic group may have different characteristics from an otherwise unselected group who sustained an MTBI. However, this is not universally accepted, and a variety of explanations have been proposed to account for some of these group differences.

Binder and colleagues (Binder 1997; Binder et al. 1997) in a meta-analysis of data from eight studies of long-term (3 months to many years after injury) effects of MTBI found a small effect size on measures of attention and, in a review of additional studies, reported that approximately 8% of individuals remained symptomatic chronically and 14% had work-related disability. The small effect size across these several studies makes the large effects seen in the studies of symptomatic individuals by Leininger et al. (1990) and Guilmette and Rasile (1995) all the more remarkable and, as Larrabee (1999) suggests, raises the possibility that other factors might contribute to such discrepant findings. It is clear that MTBI is associated with increased rates of other psychiatric disorders such as depression, anxiety, and posttraumatic stress disorder (PTSD). The presence of these disorders can serve to accentuate or increase the degree of distress associated with lingering symptoms, and successful treatment of comorbid conditions can result in significant reduction of postconcussive symptoms (Fann et al. 2000, 2001).

Overall, the impression from these studies is that mild brain injury results in measurable deficits in speed of information processing, attention, and memory in the immediate postinjury period. Recovery from these deficits is the rule, occurring over a variable period ranging from 4 to 12 weeks. For a minority of patients, recovery may occur much more slowly or remain incomplete. Certain factors appear to predict a poorer prognosis. Barth et al. (1983) and Rimel et al. (1981) found significantly poorer outcomes in their studies that included a large percentage of individuals with a prior history of brain injury compared with studies (such as Dikmen et al. 1986b) that excluded those with a prior history of TBI. In the study by Leininger et al. (1990) of symptomatic mild brain injury, the study population was older than the typical brain injury population, perhaps consistent with the observation that age negatively influences a variety of outcome measures. Furthermore, it seems that novel or more difficult cognitive tasks, or tasks performed under mild degrees of physiological stress, can negatively influence the performance of patients with mild injury (Ewing et al. 1980; Gentilini et al. 1989; Gronwall 1989; Hugenholtz et al. 1988). Injury often occurs in the context of environmental and psychosocial upheaval, and such further injury may be a risk factor for persistent sequelae after MTBI (Fenton et al. 1993).

Methodological issues are critical in evaluating this literature. For example, excluding patients with a prior mild brain injury, history of alcohol abuse, or psychiatric illness is a double-edged sword; it makes it possible to better evaluate the pure contribution of the brain injury, and yet the results may not be easy to generalize to the mild brain injury population, most of whom have a history of one or more of these factors (Dicker 1989). It is also clear that studies that select for subjects with persistent subjective complaints are more likely to find indicators of cognitive impairment relative to control subjects or asymptomatic individuals after MTBI (Arcia and Gualtieri 1993; Bernstein 1999; Guilmette and Rasile 1995; Leininger et al. 1990). Many have raised questions about the roles of litigation and compensation, motivation, and malingering in explaining some of the discrepant results (discussed in the section Postconcussive Symptoms).

Behavioral Sequelae

In addition to the cognitive sequelae, a variety of significant emotional and behavioral sequelae are associated with mild brain injury. These sequelae take two broad forms, neuropsychiatric distress immediately or shortly after the injury that can be considered part of the natural course of injury and an increased vulnerability to psychiatric disorders during and subsequent to the acute recovery period (van Reekum et al. 2000).

Postconcussive Symptoms

The term *postconcussive syndrome* is generally used to refer to a constellation of symptoms experienced subsequent to brain injury. The most common symptoms encountered after a TBI can be grouped into three categories: cognitive complaints (decreased memory, attention, and concentration), somatic complaints (headache, fatigue, insomnia, dizziness, tinnitus, and sensitivity to noise or light), and affective complaints (depression, irritability, and anxiety). The symptoms are commonly reported subsequent to brain injury of varying severity and should not be considered synonymous with mild brain injury (Deb et al. 1998; Hinkeldey and Corrigan 1990; McKinlay et al. 1981; van Zomeron and van den Burg 1985). Furthermore, it may be helpful to distinguish different symptom patterns; someone who experiences intermittent headache and dizziness for several months after an MTBI may have a different disorder from the individual who presents 1–2 years after an astonishingly mild injury completely disabled by complaints of poor memory, fatigue, chronic pain, and balance problems. In fact, it is not at all clear if there is a postconcussive "syndrome" per se, or rather common symptoms that occur to greater or lesser degrees in a given individual as a function of his or her particular injury and relevant premorbid factors. Although it is common to see individuals who have subjective complaints in several different domains, it is not clear that it is helpful to conceptualize the sequelae of TBI or MTBI as a syndrome, as it may send one down the wrong treatment path. If one considers the multiple symptoms to be a syndrome with a common underlying mechanism (be it neural damage, depression, or malingering), one tends to attribute multiple symptoms to a single etiology (i.e., "postconcussive syndrome") and look for treatments that will ameliorate the syndrome. If one views the symptoms as having many different mechanisms (albeit the same initiating event), then one tends to take a more careful look at the typology of each symptom and is therefore better positioned to properly diagnose and treat the different sources of distress (e.g., dizziness related to labyrinthine trauma or headache due to cervical muscle strain). The more that is learned about the etiology of different symptoms commonly seen after TBI, the more it is clear that specific symptoms have specific underlying mechanisms and, by implication, treatments or potential treatments; thus, the less helpful the syndromic concept becomes. Common clinical experience suggests that individuals who experience multiple symptoms shortly after an injury can show improvement in all, some, or none of the symptoms over time, suggesting at the very least that the symptoms are not always tightly linked and can be uncoupled.

In the immediate postinjury period, 80%–100% of mild brain injury patients describe one or more symptoms (Levin et al. 1987b). The majority recover completely, although not immediately. Levin et al. (1987b) published a multicenter study of 57 individuals after a mild injury defined as a GCS of 13 or greater, LOC not exceeding 20 minutes, no focal neurological deficits, and without skull fracture or focal lesions on CT. Eighty-two percent of the patients said they had postconcussive complaints immediately after and 1 month subsequent to the injury. The most common complaints were headache, decreased energy, and dizziness. Dikmen et al. (1986b), in a study of 20 patients (GCS ≥12, LOC <1 hour) using age, sex, and educationally matched friends of patients as control subjects and eliminating patients with a prior history of brain injury, drug or alcohol abuse, or prior psychiatric illness, at 1 month found 55% of the patients complained of headache, 65% complained of fatigue, 40% complained of dizziness, and 65% complained of irritability. These percentages did not differ significantly from those in the control group, although the percentages were greater in each case for the mild brain injury patients. Furthermore, the study did not report the degree of symptom-related distress but rather considered whether the patients and control subjects simply endorsed any degree of the symptoms. Three complaints—sensitivity to noise, insomnia, and decreased memory—were endorsed by a significantly greater number of patients than control subjects. McLean et al. (1983) found that 65% of their 20 patients complained of persistent fatigue, 40% of decreased memory, and 45% of decreased concentration at 1 month subsequent to their mild brain injury. Forty-five percent of these individuals had not returned to their previous major daily activities and rated their overall level of function as significantly more impaired than control subjects.

Even at 3 months after injury, many studies suggest surprisingly high rates of symptoms. Rimel et al. (1981), in a widely quoted study of 424 individuals with mild brain injury (GCS ≥13, LOC<20 minutes), found that 78% complained of headache, 60% complained of decreased memory, and 50% and 25% either complained of decrease in financial status or were unemployed, respectively, at 3 months after their injury. Thirty-one percent of this population had a history of prior brain injuries. In the Levin et al. (1987b) multicenter study, 47%, 22%, and 22% of the individuals continued to complain of headache, decreased energy, and dizziness, respectively. Bohnen et al. (1993) studied 41 individuals who did not require hospitalization after an uncomplicated MTBI defined as GCS of 15, LOC of less than 15 minutes, and PTA of less than 60 minutes and who did not have focal neurological deficits, abnormal radiological findings, or prior injury. Three months after injury, 54% of the individuals remained symptomatic to some degree, and 25% of the sample had three or more symptoms. Headache, fatigue, dizziness, and concentration problems were the most common symptoms. Even 6 months after injury, almost 25% of the sample had three or more symptoms. At both 3 and 6 months, the group with three or more symptoms showed reduced performance on a measure of complex attention and reduced tolerance to light and sound relative to healthy control subjects. Postconcussive symptom base rates were not obtained or at least were not reported for the healthy control subjects. Ingebrigsten et al. (1998) evaluated 100 individuals hospitalized after MTBI defined as GCS of 13–15, some LOC (duration not defined), and without focal neurological deficits or CT findings. Sixty-two percent of the individuals had

one or more symptoms at 3 months after injury, and 40% had three or more symptoms. Once again, there was no ascertainment of base rates. Regardless of the exact percentage of individuals who are symptomatic 3 months after injury, it is readily apparent that there is a discrepancy between the message typically given to the individual with an MTBI in the emergency department ("You had a very mild injury or concussion. You will be fine...."), and the reality that many experience.

A recent study by McCullagh et al. (2001) found significant rates of persistent symptoms 5–6 months after MTBI, with virtually 50% of the 57 subjects reporting dizziness and headache and approximately 75% reporting fatigue. Furthermore, 50%–60% of those with GCS scores of 13–15 met General Health Questionnaire (Goldberg and Hebber 1979) criteria for psychiatric "caseness" indicative of significant psychological distress.

Even after 1 year, several studies have suggested a surprising rate of symptoms after MTBI. Deb et al. (1998, 1999) evaluated 140 individuals (134 face-to-face interviews) who had sustained MTBI 1 year earlier. The sample were those admitted to a hospital over a 1-year period with GCS scores of 13–15 and either some LOC (upper limit not specified), abnormal skull films or CT scan, or focal neurological signs on examination. Disability and outcome measures used included the Glasgow Outcome Scale (GOS) (Jennett 1976), the Edinburgh Rehabilitation Status Scale (Affleck et al. 1988), and the Barthel Index (Mahoney and Barthel 1965) as well as a postconcussion checklist. Almost 30% of the individuals had either moderate or severe disability measured by the GOS, and 33% showed some disability on the Edinburgh Rehabilitation Status Scale. Fifty-five percent had at least one ongoing postconcussional complaint—most commonly, irritability, sleep disturbance, or impatience. There was no control group that would allow for comparison of base rates in the general population.

A somewhat more encouraging picture is found if one limits the inquiry to those with uncomplicated MTBI. Alves et al. (1993) followed 587 consecutive admissions for MTBI defined as GCS scores of 13–15, no abnormal radiological findings (skull films and CT scans), and hospitalization less than 48 hours. Five hundred thirty-eight of the subjects had GCS scores of 15. Although two-thirds of the subjects were symptomatic (defined as two or more postconcussive symptoms) when discharged from the hospital, this percentage dropped to 40%–60% at 3 months, 25%–45% at 6 months, and 10%–40% at 1 year after injury. Again, headache was the most common complaint at all time points. Relatively few of the individuals experienced multiple complaints suggestive of a postconcussive syndrome (2%–5%). Interpretations must be tempered by the absence of a noninjured control group and the fact that in-

TABLE 15–4. Role of compensation and litigation in postconcussive symptoms—selected studies

Studies	Findings	Comments
Miller (1961)	Subsample of 47 individuals from medical-legal practice whose symptoms were "gross and unequivocally psychoneurotic."	Not representative of all patients with MTBI.
Cook (1972)	Survey of "mild head injury" admissions. Those with claims had increased absence from work.	"Mild" not defined. Poor compliance rate. Not controlled for other complications.
Keshavan et al. (1981)	Sixty TBI admissions, mixed severity followed at 1.5 and 3 months. Compensation unrelated to outcome measures.	Does not address mild brain injury specifically.
Rimel et al. (1981)	Four hundred twenty-four consecutive minor TBI patients. Litigation and compensation claims unrelated to symptoms or return to work.	Argues strongly against role of compensation in genesis or maintenance of symptoms.
Binder and Rohling (1996)	Meta-analysis of the effect of litigation on outcome in TBI. Found a mean weighted effect size of 0.47 across 18 studies.	Argues that litigation does have an impact on severity of symptoms and cognitive deficits in some individuals.
Feinstein et al. (2001)	Prospective study of 97 individuals with MTBI studied 6 weeks after injury. Litigants had poorer outcomes and increased anxiety and social dysfunction.	Argues that litigation can modulate outcome and symptoms presentation.
Others[a]	Various patient populations and sample sizes.	Numerous studies document similar symptoms in brain injuries of all severities, arguing against inverse relationship between severity of injury and severity of symptoms as suggested by Miller (1961).

Note. MTBI = mild traumatic brain injury.
[a]See Hinkeldey and Corrigan 1990; McKinlay et al. 1983; and Van Zomeren and Van Den Burg 1985.

dividuals were randomized to receive either routine discharge instructions, enhanced information about MTBI, or information and reassurance (weekly contact with a nurse clinician), although there were no dramatic differences in symptom frequency as a function of intervention. Attributing the cause of symptoms or cognitive impairment to an MTBI must be done with caution. As Satz et al. (1999) and others (Dacey et al. 1991; Dikmen et al. 1995a, 1995b) have pointed out, it is critical to take into account the effects of other system injuries, as well as the base rate of typical postconcussive symptoms in the general population. Ideally, studies looking at the longitudinal course of MTBI-related symptoms would include two control groups: one with another mild injury (not to the brain) and a noninjured group (Satz et al. 1999).

In some individuals, there can be a general sense that the severity of subjective distress is out of proportion to the usual injury severity indicators, prompting a variety of explanations. Several studies have attempted to address the role of compensation in the genesis of postconcussive symptoms (Table 15–4). Miller (1961) published a paper on this topic that is often quoted and almost as frequently misinterpreted. His experience was based on a medical-legal

practice, and thus cannot be generalized to all individuals with MTBI, although many try to make that leap. Furthermore, he was careful to point out that he was describing a small subsample of 47 patients with "indubitably psychoneurotic complaints" (p. 5230), and he distinguished these from his larger practice. Thus, he was focusing particularly on the small but puzzling group of individuals for whom sometimes astonishingly mild trauma is associated with persistent, often disabling sequelae. In this sample, he argued that many of the postconcussive symptoms, especially those of the more chronic, flamboyant variety, were linked to pending litigation and compensation cases. He observed an inverse relationship between severity of injury (primarily length of unconsciousness) and the severity of "psychoneurotic" symptoms. Forty-two percent of his patients without history of unconsciousness were thought to have "psychoneurotic" symptoms. He also reported that the vast majority of this subgroup of patients showed "symptomatic recovery" after settlement, and he attributed many postconcussive symptoms to malingering. Although some of the case studies suggest that conversion symptoms or malingering may have been present in those examples, there are few data in terms of diagnostic criteria, outcome criteria, and symptom picture supplied. However, this view has become enshrined in the literature and clinical lore, and generalized to all individuals with MTBI, such that some clinicians may even refuse to treat MTBI patients until their claims are settled.

In a survey of 63 poorly defined "mild head injury" patients, Cook (1972) found that patients pursuing compensation claims showed a threefold increase in absence from work compared with those not pursuing claims. He argued that these findings confirmed Miller's view. However, less than one-half of the patients returned the survey, there was no specific definition of mild head injury given, the results were not based on clinical interview, and no attempt was made to look at other complications (such as orthopedic injury) that often accompany head injury and have been shown to play a role in associated disability (Dikmen et al. 1986b).

Other studies have failed to confirm any significant linkage between compensation or litigation and frequency or severity of postconcussive symptoms. Merskey and Woodforde (1972) studied 27 patients with mild brain injury; 10 were not seeking compensation and 17 had already settled (favorably) their compensation claims. Thirty percent were either in a lower occupational status compared with their preinjury occupations or unemployed. Even in the compensated group, symptoms persisted for more than a year, and many of the patients were not fully recovered. Strauss and Savitsky (1934) cited several examples of significant disability independent of compensation claims. In a study of predictors of physical, social, and behavioral outcome in 60 TBI patients of varying severity, Keshavan et al. (1981) were unable to find a link between compensation issues and any outcome measure. Rimel et al. (1981), in their study of disability related to MTBI with a population of 424 patients, found no link between pursuit of compensation and disability; in fact, only 6 of their patients were involved in litigation at the time of follow-up. Furthermore, the observation that postconcussive symptoms occur in patients with varying degrees of severity (Hinkeldey and Corrigan 1990; McKinlay et al. 1983) suggests that compensation factors alone are not responsible for the genesis or maintenance of postconcussive symptoms.

Rutherford (1989) reported on a series of patients with mild brain injury involved in litigation that casts further doubt on many preconceptions about the relationship between compensation and symptoms. More than 40% of his group involved in litigation had no symptoms at the time of their medical-legal evaluation approximately 1 year after the injury. Approximately one-third of those who had symptoms at that time did not have symptoms at the time of settlement approximately 1 year later. Virtually all of the patients who were symptomatic at the time of settlement remained symptomatic 1 year later.

Thus, for many patients, improvement can occur before medical-legal evaluation, during the interval between evaluation and settlement, and may remain long after compensation issues have been settled.

This is not to say that compensation claims do not influence the clinical presentation of some individuals with persistent symptoms after an MTBI. Litigation and compensation proceedings are frequently highly adversarial, prolonged ordeals, and it would be naive to expect that this kind of psychosocial stress would not affect symptom presentation. Rees (2003) has in fact suggested that these issues may well cause sufficient stress to the hypothalamic pituitary adrenal axis to prolong or maintain symptoms. Binder et al. (1996) published a meta-analysis of some 18 studies that included 2,353 individuals with TBI of varying severity and found a weighted mean effect size of 0.47 and suggested that on the basis of these data, financial incentives could account for 20%–25% of the abnormal signs and symptoms associated with TBI. Feinstein et al. (2001) prospectively studied the role of litigation on symptoms in 97 consecutive individuals with MTBI seen approximately 6 weeks after injury. Even this early in the process, those involved in litigation were experiencing significantly more anxiety and social dysfunction and had poorer outcomes on the GOS and the Rivermead Head Injury Follow-up Questionnaire (Crawford et al. 1996) than did nonlitigants. The two groups did not differ demographically or with respect to other putative poor prognostic factors such as prior TBI, substance abuse, or premorbid psychiatric illness.

Other motivational factors may also play a role in functional level and cognitive performance. Keller et al. (2000) compared performance on a test of divided attention in 12 individuals with MTBI, 10 with more severe injuries, and 11 healthy control subjects before and after being told that test performance might affect ability to drive safely. The MTBI group did significantly better, and in fact test performance was within the published normal range with driving as a motivator. However, the healthy control subjects also improved and still outperformed the MTBI group. Thus, subjective complaint and objective performance should not be viewed as a simple linear relationship. Like the noninjured population, individuals with MTBI are subject to the influences of stress and complex motivations. Performance variation under various different conditions or worsening of symptoms in the context of heightened stress such as adversarial litigation is "normal" and should not be construed as evidence of malingering or of "real injury" not being present.

Anyone who evaluates and treats large numbers of individuals with MTBI will be faced with some individuals who present a clinical picture characterized by subjective complaints and apparent functional decline that appears way out of proportion to the severity of injury (judged by conventional criteria), and which evolves over a time course seemingly inconsistent with that of an uncomplicated MTBI (i.e., symptoms start several weeks after injury and become progressively worse). In the context of litigation, this frequently raises the question of malingering. A variety of tests have been developed to help with the assessment of these individuals (see Iverson and Binder 2000 for discussion). Many of these tests are based on a forced choice format in which performance is significantly worse than chance, or, in some cases, scores lower than norms obtained from populations with known severe neurological disorders suggest a negative response bias (Iverson and Binder 2000; Meyers et al. 1999). Rather than simply relying on one or more of these tests, it is important to assess consistency of performance over several tests that assess several cognitive domains such as memory, attention, and learning. Several points are worth noting. There are numerous reasons for apparent poor effort or negative response bias on tests of cognitive function, and malingering should not be immediately assumed. Inconsistent performance must be interpreted within the context of such factors as fatigue, medication effects, and medical or comorbid psychiatric conditions. With respect to the latter, somatoform disorders, depression, and factitious disorders need to be sorted out.

Other contributors to the distress after an MTBI may include the lack of education and information available to the public about mild injury, and the lack of consensus about the etiology and maintenance of symptoms among professionals who care for these individuals. Confusion exists among professionals as well (Evans et al. 1994). Two surveys (Harrington et al. 1993) done some 20 years apart suggest that the training and clinical practice of different specialists strongly influence views of the etiology of postconcussive symptoms, and, thus, the message that a physician is likely to communicate to his or her patients, increasing the chances of mixed messages. A recent Harris poll (2000) and several studies have shown that the lay public is ignorant about the nature and effects of MTBI (Aubrey et al. 1989) and that simple psychoeducational approaches aimed at adjusting expectations about common symptoms and the course of recovery, along with regular monitoring of clinical status, can reduce symptoms after injury (Kelly 1975; Minderhoud et al. 1980, 1997; Mittenberg et al. 1996; Paniak et al. 1998b; Wade et al. 1997, 1998; Wrightson 1989).

Another theory proposed to account for some of the disconnect between apparent injury severity and symptomatic distress is that the typical postconcussive symptoms both are relatively prevalent in the general population and are those that the lay public expect to experience after an MTBI. Mittenberg et al. (1992) asked a group of healthy control subjects who neither had a personal history of MTBI nor knew a brain-injured individual whether they were experiencing a variety of common, nonspecific symptoms such as headache and fatigue. They were then asked to imagine the symptoms they would experience 6 months after an MTBI. A group of MTBI patients were then asked to estimate the frequency of these common symptoms in the general population. The healthy control subjects expected a cluster of symptoms quite similar to those commonly reported by individuals with MTBI, and the MTBI group underestimated the frequency of these common symptoms in the general population. The authors suggested that the expectation of symptoms might play an etiological role in the symptoms some individuals experience after an MTBI (Mittenberg et al. 1992). However, if one expects something to happen and then it does, this in no way should suggest that the symptoms are not physiologically based. By this argument, because one might expect pain when slamming a finger in a car door, the pain experienced when this happens is caused by that expectation rather than the stimulation of pain fibers brought about by crushed tissue and related hemorrhaging and edema. A number of studies have documented high base rates of common postconcussive symptoms such as memory and concentration difficulties and headache in the general population. These complaints are also found frequently in personal injury litigants and in individuals with chronic pain. This suggests a lack of symptom specificity and that self-report of symptoms after MTBI should be judged carefully (Fox et al. 1995; Gouvier et al. 1988; Iverson and Mc-Cracken 1997; Lees-Haley and Brown 1993; Wong et al. 1994). However, the argument that because symptoms are common to a number of conditions one or more of those conditions does not exist or is a factitious or augmented caricature of that condition similarly makes little sense. The brain responds to a variety of disorders with similar signs and symptoms. In other words, certain symptoms are a final common pathway for a variety of disorders, much as fever is a sign of many disorders of different, discrete etiologies. Yet one rarely argues that because fever occurs commonly in many conditions the febrile individual is exaggerating, augmenting, or faking the condition. Psychotic syndromes are associated with schizophrenia, depression, mania, acute stress, and various medical and neurological conditions, yet one rarely argues that the psychotic signs and symptoms are not physiologically based. Furthermore, Gordon et al. (2000) have recently demonstrated that there appears to be a cluster of symptoms that are both sensitive and specific to a history of MTBI. The studies suggest that virtually all patients endorse symptoms generally thought to comprise the "postconcussive syndrome" within the immediate postinjury period. Significant resolution of these symptoms occurs in approximately one-half of the patients by 1 month and in roughly two-thirds at 3 months. It is important to take into account the preinjury vulnerabilities that may affect outcome, such as personality style, prior injuries, age at injury, and psychosocial support system, among others (see Kay 1992 for discussion). Several authors have suggested that "organic factors" are instrumental in the initial pathogenesis of the postconcussive symptoms and that, in patients in whom these symptoms do not resolve within a 2- to 3-month period, psychological "issues" are thought to be involved in the maintenance and elaboration of the symptoms (Alexander 1995; Goethe and Levin 1984; Leigh 1979; Lishman 1973, 1988). However, emotional factors may play a role early in the course of recovery. King (1996) and King et al. (1999) studied individuals hospitalized with MTBI and moderate TBI and explored the relationship between symptoms within 10 days of injury and persistent symptoms 3 and 6 months after injury. In their sample, measures of anxiety and depression and the impact of event scale score correlated highly with initial symptoms. Furthermore, the combination of these measures accounted for 53% and 23% of the variance in postconcussive symptoms at 3 and 6 months after injury, respectively. They suggest that psychological factors such as the degree of anxiety and depression and the meaning and impact of the injury play a role in symptom formation even before the development of "persistent" symptoms.

Thus, it is useful to separate the sequelae of MTBI into short- and long-term categories and subjective and objective categories. With respect to short-term sequelae, the evidence is good that both subjective and objective problems are the norm in the first month after injury. Most individuals note problems with the typical array of cognitive, somatic, and affective problems well described as "postconcussive" in nature. Studies addressing cognitive function after such injuries show group differences in attention, memory, and speed of information processing. These subjective and objective difficulties are often associated with abnormalities visible on newer MRI-based neuroimaging techniques and functional imaging such as positron emission tomography (PET), single-photon emission computed tomography (SPECT), and functional MRI (fMRI) (see the section Neuroimaging). Many of these complaints and deficits improve over the subsequent several months.

With respect to long-term sequelae, the evidence is good that the majority of unselected individuals with MTBI will be asymptomatic 1 year after injury and will have little if any cognitive deficit as a group. A small percentage (10%–20%) will have subjective postconcussive complaints. For some individuals, this will be a single complaint; in others, multiple complaints will be noted. Studies of groups selected with persistent long-term complaints have more frequently shown cognitive deficits and higher rates of abnormal findings on newer MRI-based imaging techniques, functional imaging, and electrophysiological techniques than those

studies of unselected individuals. The severity of subjective distress and disability in the persistently symptomatic group is subject to a variety of influences, including premorbid function, psychosocial stress, compensation/litigation, and psychiatric complications (see the section Disability). TBI in general and MTBI also appear to increase the risk for developing a variety of psychiatric disorders that can contribute to significant disability after the injury (Deb et al. 1998, 1999; Hibbard et al. 1998, 2000; Silver et al. 2001).

Psychotic Syndromes

Psychotic syndromes similar in presentation to those seen in schizophrenia and the affective disorders do occur subsequent to brain injury (see Chapter 11, Psychotic Disorders), although they are thought to be rare after mild brain injury (Merskey and Woodforde 1972). Both time-limited and chronic psychoses are described after TBI (Davison and Bagley 1969; Kwentus et al. 1985; Lishman 1973; Nasrallah et al. 1981) (Table 15–5). Even with more severe injuries, psychotic syndromes are thought to be a relatively rare though often devastating complication of brain injury, occurring in 0.07%–9.8% of brain-injured patients (Davison and Bagley 1969; Kwentus et al. 1985). In Lishman's (1968) study of penetrating brain injuries, only 5 of 144 patients with severe psychiatric disability were diagnosed with a psychotic disorder. It has been noted that up to 15% of individuals with schizophrenia have a history of brain injury (Nasrallah et al. 1981), which has led to questions about the interaction of brain injury with genetic vulnerability for psychosis. Few of the earlier studies addressed this in a rigorous way, and those that have suggest there is no clear linkage between a family history of or genetic predisposition to schizophrenia and the development of a psychotic syndrome after a brain injury (Nasrallah et al. 1981). However, Malaspina et al. (2001) recently reported that even MTBI can interact with genetic vulnerability to increase the risk of developing mental illness in general and schizophrenia in particular (see Chapter 11, Psychotic Disorders).

Depression

Depressive symptoms are a common complication of mild brain injury (see Busch and Alpern 1998 for review). Merskey and Woodforde (1972), in their study of 27 patients with mild brain injury, found that 7 patients had "endogenous" depressions, 9 others had a mixture of anxiety and depression, and another 4 had "reactive" depression in combination with a variety of other behavioral problems. Thus, depressive symptoms of some form were a part of the clinical picture in 20 of 27 patients. Schoenhuber and Gentilini (1988) studied 48 patients with mild

TABLE 15–5. Mild traumatic brain injury (TBI) and subsequent psychopathology

Syndrome	Comment
"Emotional distress"	General symptom inventories generally elevated in minor TBI. Mixed symptom picture.
Affective disorders	
Depression	Depression scales generally elevated (Schoenhuber and Gentilini 1988).
	Mobayed and Dinan (1990) found 20% of sample met DSM-III criteria.
	Federoff et al. (1992) and Jorge et al. (1993, 1994, 2002) found 25%–30% of their 66 patients depressed at 1 month and 1 year. Overall, almost 50% depression of some form in first year. Similar to Fann et al. (1995).
	Depression associated with poorer social and functional outcome.
	Many with persistent postconcussive symptoms are also depressed (McAllister and Flashman 1999).
	Increased rate of depression (van Reekum et al. 2000).
	Increased risk of depression and suicide associated with TBI (Hibbard et al. 1998; Silver et al. 2001).
Mania	May occur after very mild TBI, even without loss of consciousness (Bracken 1987; Nizamie et al. 1988; Pope et al. 1988; Reiss et al. 1987; Zwil et al. 1992, 1993).
	Increased relative risk of bipolar disorder (van Reekum et al. 2000).
	May have increased frequency of "irritable mania."
Psychotic disorders	Relatively rare complication. Can be associated with TBI-induced affective disorders.
	In genetically vulnerable individuals, even mild TBI associated with increased risk of psychotic disorders (Malaspina et al. 2001).
Anxiety disorders	Symptoms consistent with anxiety often endorsed, but may not be more frequent than in general population (Schoenhuber and Gentilini 1988). Generalized anxiety disorder found in ~25% (Fann et al. 1995). Increased rate of generalized anxiety disorder (van Reekum et al. 2000).
	Posttraumatic stress disorder seen in up to 20%–30% (Bryant and Harvey 1999a, 1999b; Mayou et al. 2000).

brain injury and matched control subjects drawn from friends and relatives (approximately 9 months after injury) with self-report anxiety and depression scales. The mild brain injury group had significantly elevated depression scores compared with control subjects. Studies of emotional distress after brain injury of varying severity and using a variety of instruments suggest that scale scores or clusters that access depressive symptoms are elevated (Burke et al. 1990; Fordyce et al. 1983; Hinkeldey and Corrigan 1990). Furthermore, many postconcussive symptoms such as subjective slowing, irritability, fatigue, and sleep disturbance can be consistent with a depressive syndrome, even when patients may not endorse explicit items such as "depressed mood." Gfeller et al. (1994) found a relationship between depression, increased rates of postconcussive symptoms, and impaired performance on some cognitive measures in their sample of 42 individuals with MTBI and headache. McAllister and Flashman (1999) reported a similar overlap in a sample of individuals with MTBI referred for cognitive evaluation.

Mobayed and Dinan (1990) reported that 30% of their 55 patients with mild brain injury had evidence of an affective disorder on the Leeds scale (Hamilton et al. 1976). Full psychiatric assessment of these 16 patients showed that 11 (20%) met DSM-III criteria for major depression and had mean Hamilton Rating Scale for Depression scores (Hamilton 1960) of 27. Saran (1985) studied 10 patients with depression after mild brain injury. Although the patients met DSM-III criteria for depression with melancholia, they differed from noninjured depressed patients, manifesting less diurnal variation, less anorexia or weight loss, and less psychomotor retardation or agitation. They did not differ with respect to the melancholic quality of depressed mood, presence of early morning awakening, and presence of excessive guilt.

Fann et al. (1995) reported on the neuropsychiatric sequelae of 50 individuals after TBI. Twenty-nine of this group had an MTBI, and 26% of the sample met criteria for major depression. This is similar to the results reported by Federoff et al. (1992) and Jorge et al. (1993) in their studies of 66 individuals with TBI, some 20% of whom had MTBI. In these studies, approximately 25%–30% of the group was depressed 1 month after the TBI, with a similar percentage depressed 1 year after the injury. They found a correlation between depression and left anterior and subcortical injury at the 1-month time point but less of a correlation with lesion location at 1 year. Outcome was adversely affected by depression (Jorge et al. 1994).

Thus, depressive symptoms are a common complication of an MTBI, with major depression occurring in between 20% and 30% of those with complicated mild injuries. Depressive symptoms can be a significant contributor to psychiatric disability subsequent to mild brain injury either as a component of many postconcussive symptoms or as a discrete major depressive episode. Patients with a prior history or family history of depression may be at greater risk to develop depressive symptoms subsequent to injury, although the majority of depressive episodes arises in patients with no such vulnerabilities.

Mania

Mania occurs subsequent to a wide array of neurological and medical disorders (Krauthammer and Klerman 1978). Secondary mania has been reported to occur in association with TBI of varying severity (Shukla et al. 1987). Phenomenologically, these manic syndromes are similar to "idiopathic" mania, demonstrating changes in mood, sleep, and activation level, and often associated with psychotic symptoms (Shukla et al. 1987). The course of illness can be bipolar, with both manic and depressed phases (Cohn et al. 1977; Hale 1982; Pope et al. 1988; Shukla et al. 1987; Stewart and Hemsath 1988); can be a rapid-cycling variant (Pope et al. 1988); and may be triggered by antidepressants (Stewart and Hemsath 1988).

TBI-related mania can occur after MTBI (Bracken 1987; Nizamie et al. 1988; Pope et al. 1988; Riess et al. 1987; Zwil et al. 1993), including in some patients in whom there is no documented LOC. The phenomenology of mania after TBI may differ somewhat from primary or idiopathic mania in having a higher rate of relapse (Hoff et al. 1988) and a higher percentage of irritable and violent behavior (Shukla et al. 1987). Quite commonly, patients have both personality changes secondary to their injury and a manic syndrome (Zwil et al. 1992). The latter can present as a periodic worsening of the irritability and impulsivity characteristic of the former. This periodicity may be mistaken for an integral part of the personality changes and may account for the lower frequency of mania diagnosed in these patients (Hale 1982; Stewart and Hemsath 1988).

It is not known what role genetic vulnerability plays in the development of bipolar illness after TBI. Most of the reports are small case series without adequate controls. One study (Shukla et al. 1987) failed to find bipolar illness in 85 first-degree relatives of 20 patients with TBI-related mania—although 30% of the patients had at least one relative with a history of depression. Studies of secondary mania with other underlying neurological causes suggest that genetic predisposition may be an important factor in the expression of manic syndromes (Robinson et al. 1988).

Anxiety and Posttraumatic Stress Disorder

Few studies have examined anxiety syndromes that occur after mild brain injury. There is a significant overlap between many postconcussive symptoms and core symptoms in generalized anxiety disorder (GAD). Thus, many patients endorse complaints of headache, dizziness, blurred vision, irritability, and sensitivity to noise or light after mild brain injury (Binder 1986; Dikmen et al. 1986b; Levin et al. 1987b). It is less clear how many patients actually experience anxiety and how many have diagnosable anxiety disorders. Although 55% of Dikmen's group (Dikmen et al. 1986b) of 20 patients with mild brain injury complained of subjective anxiety, 45% of the matched control subjects had similar complaints (a statistically nonsignificant difference). Schoenhuber and Gentilini (1988) were unable to find a significant difference in mean anxiety scores in their study of 35 patients with mild brain injury and matched control subjects. In the study by Fann et al. (1995), 24% of their sample (the majority of whom had MTBI) evaluated 2–3 years after injury met criteria for GAD. Hibbard et al. (1998) also found high rates of several different anxiety disorders (PTSD, 19%; obsessive-compulsive disorder, 15%; panic disorder, 14%; GAD, 9%) in their sample of individuals with mixed injury severity.

There is an increasing awareness of the relationship between PTSD and mild (or severe) brain injury. Certainly it is not uncommon in clinical practice to see patients with a history of mild brain injury who manifest signs and symptoms suggestive of PTSD. These may include sleep disturbance, recurrent nightmares, exaggerated startle responses, daytime flashbacks, and avoidant behaviors such as refusing to drive or leave home. Lishman (1973), in his review of the psychiatric sequelae of brain injury, refers to PTSD-like symptoms, including that "the circumstances of the accident may recur vividly in dreams, maintain states of anxiety, or become the focus for obsessional rumination or conversion hysteria" (p. 306). He goes on to suggest that these and other "neurotic disabilities" may be more likely to occur in milder degrees of injury, especially in the absence of PTA. However, McMillan (1991) described PTSD symptoms in a woman with a severe brain injury despite amnesia for the event itself and a PTA of approximately 6 weeks.

Bryant and Harvey have reported a series of studies of individuals hospitalized after motor vehicle accidents, some with and some without MTBI. They have shown that rates of acute stress disorder 1 month after an accident are comparable in the two groups, and that acute stress disorder is a good predictor of those who go on to develop PTSD 6 months after injury (Bryant and Harvey 1998; Harvey and Bryant 1998a, 1998b). For example, they studied 46 individuals admitted to a hospital after an MTBI (LOC with PTA <24 hours) and 59 survivors of motor vehicle accidents without evidence of TBI 6 months after their accidents (Bryant and Harvey 1999a, 1999b). Twenty percent of the TBI group and 25% of the non-TBI group had PTSD. The TBI group had more postconcussive symptoms than did the non-TBI group. Furthermore, the TBI group with PTSD was significantly more symptomatic than the TBI without PTSD group. This suggests that, like other psychiatric disorders such as depression, PTSD can amplify postconcussive symptoms after an MTBI and complicate recovery. In their MTBI sample (LOC <15 minutes), Mayou et al. (2000) found that an astonishing 48% of those with definite loss of consciousness had PTSD 3 months after injury, and one-third of their subjects with MTBI had PTSD 1 year after injury. Although it might at first seem strange that those with LOC could develop PTSD with intrusive memories, it has been suggested that the intrusive memories are of events immediately before or after the accident, or there may be patchy amnesia with some islands of preserved memory.

Disability

The overall disability caused by mild brain injury is not known. In the widely quoted study by Rimel et al. (1981), 34% of 310 patients gainfully employed before their mild brain injury were unemployed 3 months after the injury. Seventy-nine percent of these patients complained of persistent headaches, 59% complained of persistent memory deficits, and 15% noted difficulty with common household chores. This study included a high percentage of patients with a prior brain injury. Englander et al. (1992) found a much more encouraging picture, with 88% of their group of insured individuals with MTBI returning to work at 3 months. In their study of 20 individuals with mild brain injury and control subjects drawn from a pool of acquaintances of the injured subjects, Dikmen et al. (1986b) found significant impairment in many common daily activities such as work, sleep or rest, home management, and ambulation at 1 month after the injury. Only 4 of 19 subjects had returned to their major role (work, home management, studies) and leisure activities without limitations. However, much of this disability was not necessarily related to the brain injury per se, but was associated with injury to other body areas. Significant improvement in all of the above areas had occurred 12 months after the injury such that 15 of the 19 subjects had resumed their major activities without limitations. As noted,

the presence of other system injury (such as orthopedic injuries) appeared to account for some of the above disability. Ruffolo et al. (1999) studied return to work in 50 consecutive individuals hospitalized with MTBI sustained in motor vehicle accidents who were employed premorbidly, had no significant other injuries, and had no prior TBI, neurologic disease, or psychiatric illness requiring hospitalization. When assessed at a mean of 7 months after injury, 42% had returned to work of some sort; however, only 12% had returned to their premorbid level of employment. Twenty percent of those returning to modified employment reported cognitive limitations; 80% reported physical limitations. Binder et al. (1997), in a review of several studies of MTBI, reported a 14% rate of work-related disability.

Thus, it would seem that rates of overall disability mirror those of cognitive and behavioral dysfunction after mild brain injury, being quite high within the first 1–3 months and showing a significant drop over the subsequent 3–12 months. Again, it must be noted that a small percentage of patients continue to experience significant degrees of disability in various areas (cognitive, behavioral, psychosocial) at the 1-year mark and beyond.

Neurodiagnostic Findings

In an effort to clarify the clinical and theoretical underpinnings of the subjective and objective distress subsequent to MTBI, much attention has been directed to exploring what role a variety of neurodiagnostic techniques, particularly newer neuroimaging and electrophysiological techniques, should play in the evaluation and management of individuals with MTBI.

Neuroimaging

A wide array of neuropathological processes can be involved in TBI, including changes in bone (e.g., a skull fracture), tissue density and water content (edema), blood flow, white matter integrity and pathway connectivity (diffuse axonal injury), and subtle changes in the neuronal and extracellular biochemical milieu (Table 15–6). No single imaging technique is thus capable of addressing all of these processes. It is important to be aware of the advantages and limitations of various available imaging modalities and be clear on what question is being asked before choosing an imaging technique. In general, structural imaging techniques play a role in acute diagnosis and management, whereas functional imaging techniques show promise for clarification of pathophysiology, symptom genesis, and mechanisms of recovery (see McAllister et al. 2001b for review).

TABLE 15–6. Evidence of abnormal findings in mild traumatic brain injury (MTBI) with different imaging modalities

Modality	Possible role in MTBI	Strength of evidence
CT	Screening for structural and surgically correctable lesions, blood	Three recent prospective, blind, studies confirm numerous previous retrospective and cohort studies that CT scans abnormal in ~5%–10% of those with GCS of 15.
MRI	Overall increased sensitivity relative to CT for detecting variety of lesions	Numerous well-designed studies comparing CT and MRI.
	T1 and T2—acute hemorrhagic lesions	
	T2—non-hemorrhagic diffuse axonal injury lesions	
	Fluid-attenuated inversion recovery—shearing injuries, subarachnoid hemorrhage	
	Gradient echo and T2*—old hemorrhagic shear injuries	
Volumetry	Quantification of atrophy of various structures (e.g., corpus callosum, hippocampus)	No studies of MTBI alone.
		Several studies of mixed severity groups show atrophy of corpus callosum, hippocampus, and increased ventricular–brain ratio.
Magnetic resonance spectroscopy	Assessment of neuronal integrity Detection of dysfunctional tissue that otherwise appears normal	Three TBI studies with mixed injury severity showed N-acetylaspartate/creatinine differences.
Diffusion weighted imaging/Doppler tissue imaging	Assessment of white matter pathway integrity	Human TBI data limited to single case report and small case series (nine subjects) of mixed severity.
Magnetization transfer imaging	Characterization of dysfunctional neuronal tissue in both normal- and abnormal-appearing regions on conventional MRI	Three studies in TBI, two with mixed injury severity, one with mild TBI (13 patients).
SPECT	Assessment of localized perfusion, deficits especially in persistently symptomatic subjects	At least seven studies of mixed injury severity suggest SPECT shows perfusion deficits, some correlations with cognitive deficits, with normal structural scans.
Positron emission tomography	Assessment of regional glucose utilization in persistently symptomatic MTBI patients	Four small series suggesting areas of abnormal metabolic activity in symptomatic subjects with normal conventional scans (CT, MRI).
Functional MRI	Assessment of neurophysiological basis of cognitive complaints and deficits after MTBI	Prospective studies from overlapping samples show abnormalities of regional brain activation in MTBI on various memory tasks.
Magnetic source imaging	Assessment of abnormal regional dendritic electrical activity in persistently symptomatic patients	One cohort study of 30 subjects.

Note. CT = computed tomography; MRI = magnetic resonance imaging; SPECT = single-photon emission computed tomography.

Because of the ease of image acquisition, relatively low cost, and widespread availability, CT scanning remains the imaging modality of choice in the clinical arena to screen for life-threatening mass lesions that can complicate MTBI. As noted above, CT abnormalities are seen in approximately 10% of those with GCS scores of 15.

A variety of studies have demonstrated that conventional MRI detects more lesions than CT, particularly in MTBI and especially if performed shortly after injury

(Eisenberg and Levin 1989; Jenkins et al. 1986; Levin et al. 1987a). These typically take the form of cortical contusions or small areas of abnormal signal intensity in subcortical white matter. Levin and colleagues (Eisenberg and Levin 1989; Levin et al. 1987a) have shown a correspondence between lesion location, size, and neuropsychological performance and were able to demonstrate that resolution of structural lesions was associated with improvement of cognitive functioning (Levin et al. 1992). Godersky et al. (1990) found a similar relationship between cognitive function and MRI lesions. In general, the location of abnormalities seen with MRI is consistent with the distribution of neuropathological findings. Thus, cortical abnormalities are found primarily with milder injury, and injury to progressively deeper structures is associated with more severe injury, particularly with longer periods of unconsciousness (Eisenberg and Levin 1989; Levin et al. 1987a; Wilson et al. 1988). A variety of MRI-based techniques have been introduced over the last several years that enhance the ability to detect traumatic injuries (see Chapter 5, Structural Imaging). Most of these techniques manipulate or "weight" the image acquisition parameters (echo time and repetition time) or use various prepulses to suppress or enhance specific types of signals (see Table 15–6). The type of lesion and the interval from injury to imaging affect the sensitivity of a given sequence. The newer MRI-based techniques have yet to be systematically studied in MTBI, and the link between demonstrable abnormalities, neurobehavioral deficits, and outcome in MTBI remains to be determined. A recent report suggests that diffusion tensor imaging may be of particular interest in demonstrating abnormalities in white matter pathways and connectivity (Arfanakis et al. 2002). This technique capitalizes on the fact that the diffusion of water is nonrandom (shows anisotropy) because it is more rapid along the long axis of an axon. This allows the mapping of major white matter pathways and can show areas of axonal damage (regions of reduced anisotropy). Arfanakis et al. (2002) found regions of white matter abnormality in all five subjects with MTBI studied 24 hours after their injuries.

Functional imaging techniques such as PET, SPECT, and fMRI show promise in clarifying the underlying pathophysiology of the sequelae of MTBI. To date, most studies have focused on subjects with persistent neurobehavioral complaints, often a long time after injury, making it difficult to generalize the findings to the majority of patients with MTBI. More work is needed in consecutive, unselected MTBI populations followed over time, contrasted to appropriate control groups to further clarify the role that these techniques may play.

Several studies have explored the utility of SPECT in TBI (Abdel-Dayem et al. 1987; Nagamachi et al. 1995;

Newton et al. 1992; Reid et al. 1990; Roper et al. 1991). Many of these series consist of subjects with moderate, severe, or mixed injury severity, although some have included many subjects with MTBI (Jacobs et al. 1994; Roper et al. 1991). Most studies conclude that abnormalities in cortical perfusion can be shown even in the absence of structural abnormalities, and flow deficits observed with SPECT may more accurately reflect the size or extent of damaged tissue than CT (Choksey et al. 1991; Mitchener et al. 1997; Silverman et al. 1993). These results support the notion that SPECT demonstrates more abnormalities than do CT or conventional MRI and that a negative structural scan does not guarantee a normal functional brain. However, the clinical significance of perfusion deficits demonstrated on SPECT has not been clearly demonstrated. Wiedmann et al. (1989) suggested a good correspondence between SPECT abnormalities and neuropsychological performance in their TBI patients, most of whom had moderate to severe injuries. However, Goldenberg et al. (1992) were unable to confirm such a link in their study.

There is an emerging literature on the use of PET in TBI, although many of these studies have been conducted in patients with moderate and severe TBI (Alavi 1989; Alavi and Newberg 1996; Langfitt et al. 1986; Ruff et al. 1989a). Humayun et al. (1989) were among the first to use PET to explore the etiology of persistent cognitive and behavioral complaints after mild and moderate TBI. All three of their patients had normal MRI and CT scans but decreased glucose utilization in medial and posterior temporal cortex, posterior frontal cortex, and the left caudate nucleus during a visual vigilance task. Ruff et al. (1989b) studied six TBI subjects 2–4 years after their injuries; two had transient or momentary LOC, and one was described as unconscious for less than 1 hour. Despite normal CT scans, 18-fluorodeoxyglucose PET done while subjects performed a continuous performance test showed areas of focal frontal and fronto-temporal hypometabolism. This research group (Ruff et al. 1994), also reported the results of PET on nine symptomatic patients (two of whom were in the prior report) a mean of 29 months after an MTBI. All subjects had essentially normal ("generally negative") MRI or CT scans, or both. Compared with a group of 24 healthy control subjects, the TBI patients demonstrated temporal and frontal hypometabolism. Four of the nine patients had no LOC but had similar neuropsychological deficits and PET findings as those with a history of LOC. The authors correctly emphasize that these subjects were selected on the basis of persistent complaints and measurable cognitive deficits, and thus are not representative of the majority of individuals with MTBI.

Gross et al. (1996) reported a retrospective series of 20 patients in treatment for postconcussive symptoms after an MTBI who underwent PET a mean of 43 months postinjury. Injury severity in the majority of the group was quite mild by the usual criteria: 3 had no LOC ("stunned"), and 13 had very brief or momentary LOC. CT scans were normal in all but two subjects, showing a skull fracture in one and a possible small subarachnoid hemorrhage in another. All 20 patients had regions of abnormal activity, most commonly in the temporal area. Associations were found between the number of areas of abnormal activity and the number of postconcussive complaints and abnormal cognitive functions.

Although the above literature suggests that PET and SPECT may be more sensitive than MRI and CT scans in demonstrating brain dysfunction after MTBI, it is important to point out that many of these studies are single case reports or small case series, do not always report correlations between the functional imaging findings and more objective data such as standardized neuropsychological testing, and are limited by the absence of quantitative analytical techniques. Furthermore, many studies included patients with persistent postconcussive complaints—a group with significant relative risk for psychiatric comorbidity, which can also be associated with SPECT and PET abnormalities.

Another imaging modality that shows some promise in clarifying some of the underlying symptoms of TBI is fMRI. This technique capitalizes on the fact that oxygenated and deoxygenated hemoglobin differ in their magnetic properties. Thus, local changes in the ratio of oxygenated to deoxygenated hemoglobin can be used as an endogenous contrast agent. This is known as *blood oxygen level dependent* (BOLD) *fMRI*. Increases in local neuronal activity result in an initial drop in the level of oxygenated blood followed by an increase in oxygenated blood after several seconds. This relatively rapid response offers temporal resolution on the order of several seconds and when combined with the spatial resolution of MRI allows for the imaging of transient cognitive, motor, or sensory events. Two reports (McAllister et al. 1999, 2001a) of individuals with MTBI studied within 1 month of their injury showed different patterns of activation of working memory (WM) circuitry. Although cognitive performance was not different from that of healthy control subjects, the group with MTBI reported significantly more cognitive and memory complaints. This suggests the possibility that the MTBI group may have problems with the allocation of memory processing resources and may label this as memory trouble.

Two points should be highlighted from the above. The first point is that clear evidence of brain injury can be seen in many patients with a history of mild brain injury. This is more likely to be visualized by MRI, particularly with some of the newer pulse sequences, and may be less evident with time. The preliminary data suggest that the findings on

MRI correlate to some degree with functional deficits on neuropsychological measures. The second point is that many patients with a history of MTBI will not have abnormalities on structural imaging techniques, even the newer MRI-based modalities, but manifest evidence of functional impairment on neuropsychological measures and functional imaging modalities such as PET, SPECT, and fMRI. The presence of a normal CT or MRI scan cannot be equated with unequivocal absence of brain injury.

Electrophysiological Measures

A variety of electrophysiological techniques have been used to study brain function after MTBI (see Gaetz and Bernstein 2001 for review). These techniques can be usefully grouped into four broad categories: 1) standard electroencephalography (EEG), 2) computerized or quantitative EEG (QEEG), 3) evoked potentials (EPs) (usually using an auditory or visual stimulus), and 4) event-related potentials (ERPs). EEG and QEEG measure spontaneous electrical activity emanating from the brain. EP and ERP studies measure brain activity in response to specific stimuli (e.g., an auditory "click") and allow for repetitive measures and averaging of the stimulus-induced response. Specific components of the stimulus-induced electrical waveform reflect processing of that stimulus in different brain regions (e.g., brainstem vs. cortex) and other characteristics of the waveforms induced by the stimulus (e.g., latency between peaks or wave amplitude) can be used to infer characteristics of information processing in a given individual or population.

Schoenhuber and Gentilini (1989) suggested that approximately 10% of patients with mild brain injury have persistent abnormalities when studied with standard EEGs, although this opinion is not universally shared (Gaetz and Bernstein 2001; Voller et al. 1999). When present, conventional electroencephalographic abnormalities are typically nonspecific ones, such as mild disorganization of the background rhythms or a mild excess of slow wave frequencies.

Topographic brain electrical activity mapping and QEEG can demonstrate abnormalities not shown on routine EEG or EP studies, although this is not always the case (Garber et al. 1989). Thatcher et al. (1989) studied measures of electroencephalographic power spectral analyses in 608 patients with mild brain injury defined by GCS scores of 13–15 and LOC less than 20 minutes. They were able to develop a discriminant function that separated mild brain injury patients from age-matched control subjects with surprising accuracy. The location of the electroencephalographic abnormalities (frontal and frontotemporal, as well as changes in anterior–posterior patterns) was consistent with predictable areas of brain injury. Of note is that the patients were referred largely because of persistent complaints and thus may not be representative of all patients with a mild brain injury. This group has subsequently demonstrated correlations between certain electroencephalographic characteristics such as electroencephalographic coherence (a measure of homogeneity of electrical activity across different distances) and electroencephalographic amplitude within different wave frequencies (i.e., alpha, beta, delta, and theta) and the brain water proton relaxation times (T2) obtained with conventional MRI (Thatcher et al. 1998a, 1998b). The average T2 relaxation time is in part a function of the distribution of the H1 imaging agent in intracellular water, extracellular water, and protein/lipid membrane, and this distribution can, and often does, change after a tissue injury. Thus, changes in the T2 relaxation time can reflect past injury. Thatcher et al. (2001) compared a variety of electroencephalographic measures between groups with mild, moderate, and severe TBI and proposed an "EEG Severity Index" that showed promise in distinguishing MTBI from more severe forms. These reports suggest that quantitative electroencephalographic techniques may prove to be more valuable in the assessment of mild brain injury than standard EEGs, although they remain experimental and as yet are not recommended as routine diagnostic procedures in the guidelines put forth by the American Academy of Neurology and the American Clinical Neurophysiology Society (Gaetz and Bernstein 2001).

A similar picture emerges with respect to the EP and ERP literature. In their study of brainstem auditory evoked responses in 165 patients with mild brain injury (GCS, 13–15; LOC less than 20 minutes), Schoenhuber and Gentilini (1986) showed that approximately 10% of patients had at least one prolonged interpeak latency. However, these abnormalities did not correlate with the presence or absence of relevant postconcussion symptoms. Abd Al-Hady et al. (1990) also found prolongation of certain interpeak latencies in brainstem auditory responses in their group of 30 patients with mild brain injury. It was not clear whether these findings correlated with any subjective complaints. Pratrap-Chand et al. (1988) found increased P300 latencies in a group of 20 patients with mild brain injury compared with healthy control subjects when tested within 4 days after injury. The latencies were normal on retesting 30–250 days subsequent to initial testing. Only two of these patients were complaining of any postconcussive symptoms. Several studies have explored different EP paradigms, including aspects of the evoked response that represent subcortical and thalamocortical processing (Drake et al. 1996;

Soustiel et al. 1995) and visual evoked responses (Freed and Hellerstein 1997; Gaetz and Weinberg 2000; Gaetz et al. 2000; Papathanasopoulos et al. 1994). In general, a subsample of individuals with MTBI can be found with abnormal findings, the percentage of which varies with the range of "normal" that is used. This highlights the fact that there as yet are no established norms for many of these measures, or at least the ranges of norms are not universally agreed on. Thus, it is difficult to state with certainty what percentage of individuals with MTBI has abnormal findings.

Arciniegas et al. (2000a) have studied attentional gating mechanisms in individuals with persistent attentional complaints after TBI using a P50 auditory evoked response paradigm. In most healthy individuals, the evoked response to the second of a paired auditory stimulus is suppressed, implying the ability to screen out, or gate, auditory stimuli. A significantly higher percentage of persistently symptomatic individuals with TBI did not suppress the response to the second stimulus. These individuals were also found to have smaller hippocampal volumes (Arciniegas et al. 2001) and, in an open-label study, showed symptomatic improvement while taking donepezil, suggesting that cholinergic deficits may underlie some of the attentional complaints in this group (Arciniegas et al. 1999).

Thus, from a neurodiagnostic standpoint, both functional imaging techniques and some of the newer EPs and ERPs show promise for helping to clarify aspects of brain function after MTBI, particularly in those with persistent symptoms. However, none of these techniques can be considered part of a routine clinical evaluation at this time.

Treatment Issues

Evaluation

At the risk of stating the obvious, the foundation of the approach to patients with mild brain injury is a proper evaluation. Significant effort must be expended to clarify premorbid history. In particular, one must look for a prior history of brain injury, which can be seen in as many as 30% of patients (Rimel et al. 1981). The association of substance abuse with brain injury is well described (Sparadeo et al. 1990) and may contribute to postinjury sequelae. Interviews with significant others can be invaluable in gaining a clearer picture of these issues.

Signs and symptoms must be clearly defined, as well as any changes in symptom picture as a function of time from the injury. The profile of the injury itself must be outlined, including the type of injury, the presence or absence of LOC and its duration, and the presence, absence, and duration of any retrograde and anterograde amnesia. Corroborative information, including accounts from observers, emergency medical technicians, ambulance and emergency department personnel, and inpatient hospital records, can be invaluable. When evaluating these records, phrases such as "normal mental status" without sufficient documentation do not eliminate the possibility that there were cognitive changes. This is particularly true when the emergency team is distracted by other trauma such as injury to the spinal cord (Davidoff et al. 1985). The absence or presence and location of complications such as depressed skull fractures, cerebral contusions, and extradural hematomas should be noted because of the potential prognostic implications (Williams et al. 1990). The neurodiagnostic tests done and the timing in relation to the injury should be clarified and the reports or actual studies obtained.

All of the above information can then be integrated with findings from the clinical interview to determine the consistency of the history and examination with the known sequelae of mild brain injury. This process should determine the presence or absence of one or more of the specific syndromes outlined above, including postconcussive symptoms, depression, mania, anxiety syndromes (including PTSD), and psychotic syndromes. Treatment should then follow rationally from this diagnostic scheme.

Medication Approaches

Several general principles should be borne in mind when prescribing psychotropic agents in the population with MTBI. These patients seem to be more sensitive to common psychotropic side effects such as sedation, psychomotor slowing, and cognitive impairment (such as impairments of recent memory and attention). Although there are few actual data, most clinicians working with patients with TBI note this tendency toward increased side effects and a resultant narrowing of the benefit to toxicity ratio. In general, it is prudent to use lower starting and (often) final doses and prolong the titration intervals (Arciniegas et al. 2000b; Cope 1987; Gualtieri and Evans 1988; McAllister 1992c; McAllister and Price 1990; Silver et al. 1992).

Medication approaches to the sequelae of MTBI have generally taken three broad approaches: 1) amelioration of psychiatric complications, 2) amelioration of specific symptoms (e.g., headache, dizziness, and sleep disturbances; see Chapters 20, Fatigue and Sleep Problems; 21, Headaches; and 22, Balance Problems and Dizziness), and 3) approaches to cognitive complaints. With respect to amelioration of psychiatric complications, the same general approaches taken in the noninjured population

are typically used, although therapeutic efficacy studies are lacking in this group. An older study by Saran (1985) of 10 patients with mild brain injury and depression suggests that some of these patients may be less responsive to antidepressants than patients without a brain injury. On the other hand, Wroblewski et al. (1996) found a good response to desipramine in the treatment of their population of depressed individuals after TBI, and Fann et al. (2000) found a good antidepressant response to sertraline in 15 individuals with depression after an MTBI. In the Neuropsychiatry Clinic at Dartmouth Medical School, it is our experience is that there are no dramatic antidepressant efficacy differences in individuals with TBI relative to the noninjured population. Hoff et al. (1988) reported a higher relapse rate in patients with central nervous system secondary mania, although these were not patients with mild brain injury. The phenomenology of depressive and manic syndromes can also be altered by a brain injury (McAllister 1992b; McAllister and Price 1990; Saran 1985; Shukla et al. 1987; Silver et al. 1991), resulting in a mixed and atypical clinical presentation. Thus, psychotropic use is complicated by enhanced sensitivity to side effects, a mixed and atypical clinical picture (which can complicate assessment of target symptoms and drug response), and, perhaps, a reduced efficacy of certain standard agents, although the evidence for this is tentative.

The treatment of postconcussive cognitive symptoms is even less clear-cut. Work since the 1980s has focused more on the role of catecholaminergic and cholinergic mechanisms as mediators of the attentional and memory domains vulnerable to injury in TBI (McAllister and Arciniegas 2002). Catecholaminergic mechanisms, particularly through dopaminergic (DA) and α_2-adrenergic (A2A) systems, appear to play important roles in memory function, particularly WM function (see Arnsten 1998) both in healthy individuals and individuals with TBI. Luciana et al. (1992) and Luciana and Collins (1997) have found improvements in spatial WM tasks in healthy individuals treated with bromocriptine (a D2 agonist). Elliot et al. (1997) found improved performance on a spatial WM task after administration of methylphenidate. It is difficult to know whether the observed effect is strictly related to DA augmentation, because methylphenidate also results in release of norepinephrine (NE) and A2A stimulation is also known to improve WM performance in animals and healthy humans (Arnsten et al. 1998; Jakala et al. 1999a, 1999b).

There is some evidence that baseline WM capacity plays a role in DA enhancement. Kimberg et al. (1997) gave 2.5 mg of bromocriptine to 31 healthy human subjects and then administered several neurocognitive tasks, including a spatial WM task similar to that used by Luciana and Collins (1997). The subjects were divided into two groups (high- and low-WM capacity) on the basis of their performance on a reading span task. Administration of bromocriptine resulted in improvement in WM performance only in the low-capacity group. There are a few studies assessing the efficacy of DA agents on WM in individuals after TBI. McDowell et al. (1998) found significant improvement in tasks requiring "executive function" (e.g., dual-task paradigm) but not WM storage capacity or prefrontal tasks that did not require executive functions after a single dose of 2.5 mg bromocriptine to 24 subjects with TBI.

Several DA agonists, including bromocriptine and stimulants, particularly those with DA agonist properties such as methylphenidate, amphetamine, and levodopa, have been used to treat various cognitive and behavioral sequelae of TBI and other acquired brain injuries. Clinical observations suggested improvement in many subjects in areas as diverse as impulse control, attention, insight, cooperation, and memory (Arciniegas et al. 2000b; Crismon et al. 1988; Dobkin and Hanlon 1993; Glenn 1998; Gualtieri et al. 1989; Lal et al. 1988; McAllister 1992a, 1992c; Powell et al. 1996). Whyte et al. (1997) reported the results of a double-blind, placebo-controlled, crossover study of the effects of 0.25 mg/kg methylphenidate on measures of attention in 19 TBI subjects of mixed injury severity. Components of attention assessed included sustained arousal, phasic arousal, distraction, choice reaction time, and behavioral inattention. Methylphenidate was found to have a differential effect on different attentional performance variables.

There is limited but equally compelling evidence suggesting that A2A mechanisms play a prominent role in the activation and modulation of WM. Localized and global depletion of catecholamines (DA and NE) as well as aging impair performance on spatial WM tasks similarly to that seen with ablation of neural tissue in the prefrontal region (Arnsten 1998; Bartus et al. 1978; Brozoski et al. 1979; Cai et al. 1993; Luine et al. 1990). Infusion of A2A antagonists produces spatial WM impairment in both monkeys and rats (Steere and Arnsten 1997; Tanila et al. 1996). These performance deficits can be reversed by administration of A2A agonists (see Arnsten 1998). Of note is that adrenergic enhancement of WM appears to be relatively specific to manipulation of the α_2 receptors in that α_1- and β-adrenergic antagonists had no effect on WM performance (Li and Mei 1994). However, A1A agonists can impair WM function, suggesting 1) that different adrenergic receptors have opposing effects on cognitive function (Arnsten 1998) and 2) that it is important to clarify the different roles of these receptor families rather than simply administering broad-spectrum adrenergic agents such as stimulants. Thus,

broad-spectrum adrenergic agents, or agents that increase the endogenous release of NE such as methylphenidate, may have opposing effects on WM function. Jakala et al. (1999a, 1999b) gave healthy control subjects several different doses of clonidine or guanfacine (both A2A agonists). Guanfacine at the higher dose (29 μg/kg) was associated with significant improvement in several tasks, including a spatial WM task, paired associate learning, and Tower of London. They interpreted these results as consistent with guanfacine-enhanced frontal functioning in both spatial WM and planning.

Another hypothesis relates cognitive impairment after TBI to acute and long-term alterations in cortical cholinergic function (Arciniegas 2003). Animal studies (DeAngelis et al. 1994; Dixon et al. 1994; Saija et al. 1988) demonstrate chronic alterations in hippocampal cholinergic function after experimentally induced TBI and the relationship of such alterations to persistent cognitive impairments. Human postmortem studies (Dewar and Graham 1996; Murdoch et al. 1998) also demonstrate that TBI produces cortical cholinergic dysfunction via loss of cortical cholinergic afferents; these studies also demonstrate that postsynaptic muscarinic and nicotinic receptors are not reduced by TBI.

Multiple studies have demonstrated that cholinergic augmentation, generally using one of several cholinesterase inhibitors (e.g., physostigmine or donepezil) can improve TBI-induced memory deficits even in the late postinjury period (longer than 1 year) in some TBI survivors (Aigner 1995; Bogdanovitch et al. 1975; Cardenas et al. 1994; Eames and Sutton 1995; Goldberg et al. 1982; Levin et al. 1986; Tayerni et al. 1998; Whelan et al. 2000). Arciniegas and colleagues have advanced the theory that cholinergic mechanisms play a critical role, particularly in certain attentional deficits after TBI (Arciniegas et al. 1999) and have reported successful use of donepezil in some individuals with TBI (Arciniegas et al. 2001).

Thus, there appears to be increasing evidence, both theoretical and clinical, that suggests that the cautious, empiric use of cholinergic and catecholaminergic agents is warranted for the treatment of chronic memory and attentional deficits.

It is possible that specific genetic profiles contribute to response to neurotrauma and cognitive outcomes. As described above, the neuropathology of TBI and the neurochemistry of memory and attention suggest that genes that modulate cholinergic and catecholaminergic function and systems important to neural repair and plasticity are attractive candidate genes (McAllister and Summerall 2003). My group has hypothesized that individuals with alleles that reduce central catecholaminergic/cholinergic tone and neuronal repair/plasticity may well show greater cognitive deficits shortly after injury and less improvement in cognitive function over time than those with alternative alleles. Preliminary data for this hypothesis are encouraging (McAllister et al. 2004). Furthermore, the effect of these alleles may be additive, such that individuals with more of the "adverse" alleles may have poorer cognitive outcomes.

Psychoeducation

Often, the most effective intervention in patients with active neurobehavioral sequelae is a careful explanation of the pathophysiology, typical sequelae, and time course of recovery associated with minor brain injury (Kelly 1975; Minderhoud et al. 1980, 1997; Mittenberg et al. 1996; Paniak et al. 1998a; Wade et al. 1997, 1998; Wrightson 1989). Problems with slowing, attention, and memory, especially in the first 3–6 months, should be described. The potential for longer-term difficulties should be mentioned. This should be done soon after the injury and is best done in the presence of family, friends, or significant others (see Wrightson 1989). The realistic setting of goals for return to major activities is a difficult process that must be individualized for each patient. Psychiatrists often are involved in the later stages of the process, by which time there is frequently an unpleasant dynamic operating in which various individuals (including family, friends, employers, insurance carriers, and health care workers) are questioning the validity of complaints on the basis of the seemingly "minor" nature of the injury and the patient's healthy appearance. Validating the complaints of the patient without undue fostering of illness behavior can be a difficult and lengthy process.

Medical-Legal Issues

Psychiatrists increasingly are involved in the assessment of patients with mild brain injury, often at the request of attorneys or insurance carriers (see Chapter 33, Ethical and Clincal Legal Issues). Typically, an opinion is requested about whether the nature of the patient's complaints, as well as their severity and duration, is consistent with what is known about the injury.

The evaluation of such cases is time consuming and requires procurement and perusal of all pertinent records, including school and/or employment records, testing and evaluation, accident and emergency transport reports, and subsequent treatment records. When possible the clinician should interview the patient and others who knew the patient before the event.

Results of neurodiagnostic tests must be evaluated. If they have not been performed, an MRI, careful neuropsychological evaluation, EEG, and EPs can be helpful in establishing the presence of brain injury. All of these studies, as previously noted, are not always abnormal in the presence of obvious brain injury. Furthermore, even when abnormal, these studies may not reveal abnormalities that are pathognomonic for mild brain injury. Because few patients have these tests performed both before and after their injury, it is difficult to be certain that such abnormalities were caused by the traumatic event in question. Thus, the foundation of such evaluation remains the careful assessment of premorbid function; delineation of the type, location, and severity of the trauma; documentation of the profile and time course of subsequent changes in cognitive, behavioral, and somatic areas; and integration of this information with the appropriate neurodiagnostic studies. Many of the latter may not have been done until weeks to months after the injury, making the yield from such studies lower than if performed within a week or so of the trauma. Thus, even in the absence of positive neurodiagnostic findings, the history of a documented injury, with subsequent onset of the symptoms described above, should enable a reasonable opinion to be given about the relationship between the injury and the current clinical picture.

Summary

Mild brain injury is a significant public health problem. It can result in an array of common neurobehavioral sequelae. Several points in this chapter are worth highlighting:

- Well over a million people experience a mild TBI in the United States each year.
- Limited human data and more extensive animal data suggest that minor brain injury produces neuropathological changes to a lesser extent but of similar quality and location to those seen in more severe brain injury.
- Mild brain injury is associated with impairments in speed of information processing, attention, and memory. These deficits are most pronounced in the initial days to weeks after the injury. Most patients show a rapid, progressive improvement over the subsequent 1–3 months. A small percentage of patients have demonstrable long-term sequelae.
- A variety of predictable cognitive, somatic, and behavioral complaints, known as *postconcussive symptoms*, are seen subsequent to brain injury of all levels of severity. After mild brain injury, most patients show progressive resolution of these symptoms over the subsequent 1–6 months. A small but significant percentage has persistent symptoms 12 months or longer. A history of prior

brain injury, increased age at time of injury, certain complications (such as depressed skull fracture or computed tomography evidence of cerebral contusions or hemorrhages), injury to other body systems, and certain psychosocial factors may predict poorer outcomes. Compensation issues, although no doubt important factors in individual cases, are not consistently linked to the genesis or maintenance of symptoms.

• Mild brain injury has been associated with the new onset of discrete psychiatric disorders, including depression and mania, and psychotic and anxiety disorders. The brain injury may result in atypical clinical presentations, heightened sensitivity to standard psychotropic agents, and a somewhat more refractory course, although these observations must be considered tentative.

• Treatment of the neuropsychiatric sequelae involves careful assessment of premorbid function, psychosocial context, and injury profile. Psychoeducational strategies, supportive psychotherapy, and judicious use of appropriate psychotropic agents can be beneficial.

References

Abd Al-Hady MR, Shehata O, El-Mously M, et al: Audiological findings following head trauma. J Laryngol Otol 104:927–936, 1990

Abdel-Dayem HM, Sadek SA, Kouris K, et al: Changes in cerebral perfusion after acute head injury: comparison of CT with Tc-99m HM-PAO SPECT. Radiology 165:221–226, 1987

Affleck JW, Aitken RC, Hunter JA, et al: Rehabilitation status: a measure of medicosocial dysfunction. Lancet 1:230–233, 1988

Aigner TG: Pharmacology of memory: cholinergic-glutamatergic interactions. Curr Opin Neurobiol 5:155–160, 1995

Alavi A: Functional and anatomical studies of head injury. J Neuropsychiatry 1:S45–S50, 1989

Alavi A, Newberg AB: Metabolic consequences of acute brain trauma: is there a role for PET? (editorial; comment). J Nucl Med 37:1170–1172, 1996

Alexander MP: Mild traumatic brain injury: pathophysiology, natural history, and clinical management (see comments). Neurology 45:1253–1260, 1995

Alves W, Macciocchi SN, Barth JT: Postconcussive symptoms after uncomplicated mild head injury. J Head Trauma Rehabil 8:48–59, 1993

American Psychiatric Association: Diagnostic and Statistical Manual of Mental Disorders, 4th Edition, Text Revision. Washington, DC, American Psychiatric Association, 2000

Annegers JF, Grabow JD, Kurland LT, et al: The incidence, causes, and secular trends of head trauma in Olmstead County, Minnesota, 1935–1974. Neurology 30:912–919, 1980

Arcia E, Gualtieri CT: Association between patient report of symptoms after mild head injury and neurobehavioral performance. Brain Inj 7:481–489, 1993

Arciniegas DB, Adler LE, Topkoff J, et al: Attention and memory dysfunction after traumatic brain injury: cholinergic mechanisms, sensory gating, and a hypothesis for further investigation. Brain Inj 12:1–13, 1999

Arciniegas DB, Olincy A, Topkoff J, et al: Impaired auditory gating and P50 nonsuppression following traumatic brain injury. J Neuropsychiatry Clin Neurosci 12:77–85, 2000a

Arciniegas DB, Topkoff J, Silver JM: Neuropsychiatric aspects of traumatic brain injury. Curr Treat Options Neurol 2:169–186, 2000b

Arciniegas DB: The cholinergic hypothesis of cognitive impairment caused by traumatic brain injury. Curr Psychiatry Rep 5:391–399, 2003

Arciniegas DB, Topkoff J, Andersen HS, et al: Normalization of P50 physiology by donepezil hydrochloride in traumatic brain injury patients. J Neuropsychiatry Clin Neurosci 13:140, 2001

Arfakanis K, Haughton VM, Carew JD, et al: Diffusion tensor MR imaging in diffuse axonal injury. Am J Neuroradiol 23:794–802, 2002

Arnsten AFT: Catecholamine modulation of prefrontal cortical cognitive function. Trends Cogn Sci 2:436–447, 1998

Arnsten AF, Steere JC, Jentsch DJ, et al: Noradrenergic influences on prefrontal cortical cognitive function: opposing actions at postjunctional $\alpha 1$ versus $\alpha 2$-adrenergic receptors. Adv Pharmacol 42:764–767, 1998

Arvigo F, Cossu M, Fazio B, et al: Cerebral blood flow in minor cerebral contusion. Surg Neurol 24:211–217, 1985

Aubrey JB, Dobbs AR, Rule BG: Laypersons' knowledge about the sequelae of head injury and whiplash. J Neurol Neurosurg Psychiatry 52:842–846, 1989

Barth JT, Macciocri SN, Giordani B, et al: Neuropsychological sequelae of minor head injury. Neurosurgery 13:529–533, 1983

Bartus RT, Fleming D, Johnson HR: Aging in the rhesus monkey: debilitation effects on short-term memory. J Gerontol 33:858–871, 1978

Bergsneider M, Hovda DA, Lee SM, et al: Dissociation of cerebral glucose metabolism and level of consciousness during the period of metabolic depression following human traumatic brain injury. J Neurotrauma 17:389–401, 2000

Bernstein DM: Recovery from mild head injury. Brain Inj 13:151–172, 1999

Binder LM: Persisting symptoms after mild head injury: a review of the post-concussive syndrome. J Clin Exp Neuropsychol 8:323–346, 1986

Binder LM: A review of mild head trauma, II: clinical implications. J Clin Exp Neuropsychol. 19:432–457, 1997

Binder LM, Rohling ML: Money matters: a meta-analytic review of the effects of financial incentives on recovery after closed-head injury (see comments). Am J Psychiatry 153:7–10, 1996

Binder LM, Rohling ML, Larrabee J: A review of mild head trauma, I: meta-analytic review of neuropsychological studies. J Clin Exp Neuropsychol 19:421–431, 1997

Blumbergs PC, Scott G, Manavis J, et al: Staining of amyloid precursor protein to study axonal damage in mild head injury. Lancet 344:1055–1056, 1994

Bogdanovitch UJ, Bazarevitch GJ, Kirillov AL: The use of cholinesterase in severe head injury. Resuscitation 4:139–141, 1975

Bohnen N, Twijnstra A, Jolles J: Persistence of postconcussional symptoms in uncomplicated, mildly head-injured patients: a prospective cohort study. Neuropsychiatry Neuropsychol Behav Neurol 6:193–200, 1993

Borczuk P: Predictors of intracranial injury in patients with mild head trauma. Ann Emerg Med 25:731–736, 1995

Bracken P: Mania following head injury. Br J Psychiatry 150:690–692, 1987

Brown SJ, Fann JR, Grant I: Postconcussional disorder: time to acknowledge a common source of neurobehavioral morbidity. J Neuropsychiatry Clin Neurosci 6:15–22, 1994

Brozoski T, Brown RM, Rosvold HE, et al: Cognitive deficit caused by regional depletion of dopamine in prefrontal cortex of rhesus monkey. Science 205:929–931, 1979

Bryant RA, Harvey AG: Relationship between acute stress disorder and posttraumatic stress disorder following mild traumatic brain injury. Am J Psychiatry 155:625–629, 1998

Bryant RA, Harvey AG: The influence of traumatic brain injury on acute stress disorder and post-traumatic stress disorder following motor vehicle accidents. Brain Inj 13:15–22, 1999a

Bryant RA, Harvey AG: Postconcussive symptoms and posttraumatic stress disorder after mild traumatic brain injury. J Nerv Ment Dis 187:302–305, 1999b

Burke JM, Imhoff CL, Kerrigan JM: MMPI correlates among post-acute TBI patients. Brain Inj 4:223–231, 1990

Busch CR, Alpern HP: Depression after mild traumatic brain injury: a review of current research. Neuropsychol Rev 8:95–108, 1998

Cai JX, Xu L, Hu X: Reserpine impairs spatial working-memory performance in monkeys: reversal by the α_2-adrenergic agonist clonidine. Brain Res 614:191–196, 1993

Cardenas DD, McLean A, Farrell-Roberts L, et al: Oral physostigmine and impaired memory in adults with brain injury. Brain Inj 12:77–80, 1994

Centers for Disease Control and Prevention, National Center for Injury Prevention and Control: Traumatic brain injury in the United States: a report to Congress. Atlanta, GA, U.S. Department of Health and Human Services, 1999

Choksey MS, Costa DC, Iannotti F, et al: 99Tcm-HMPAO SPECT studies in traumatic intracerebral haematoma. J Neurol Neurosurg Psychiatry 54:6–11, 1991

Cohn CK, Wright JR, Vaul RAD: Post head trauma syndrome in an adolescent treated with lithium carbonate—case report. Dis Nerv Syst 38:630–631, 1977

Cook JB: The post-concussional syndrome and factors influencing recovery after minor head injury admitted to hospital. Scand J Rehabil Med 4:27–30, 1972

Cope DN: Psychopharmacologic consideration in the treatment of traumatic brain injury. J Head Trauma Rehabil 2:5, 1987

Crawford S, Wenden FJ, Wade DT: The Rivermead Head Injury Follow Up Questionnaire: a study of a new rating scale and other measures to evaluate outcome after head injury. J Neurol Neurosurg Psychiatry 60:510–514, 1996

Crismon ML, Childs A, Wilcox RE, et al: The effect of bromocriptine on speech dysfunction in patients with diffuse brain injury (akinetic mutism). Clin Neuropharmacol 11:462–466, 1988

Dacey RG, Dikmen SS: Mild head injury, in Head Injury. Edited by Cooper PR. Baltimore, MD, Williams & Wilkins, 1987, pp 125–140

Dacey R, Dickmen S, Temkin N, et al: Relative effects of brain and non-brain injuries on neuropsychological and psychosocial outcome. J Trauma 31:217–222, 1991

Davidoff G, Morris J, Roth E, et al: Closed head injury in spinal cord injured patients: retrospective study of loss of consciousness and post-traumatic amnesia. Arch Phys Med Rehabil 66:41–43, 1985

Davison K, Bagley CR: Schizophrenia-like psychosis associated with organic disorders of the central nervous system. Br J Psychiatry 114:113–184, 1969

DeAngelis MM, Hayes RL, Lyeth BG: Traumatic brain injury causes a decrease in M2 muscarinic cholinergic receptor binding in the rat brain. Brain Res 653:39–44, 1994

Deb S, Lyons I, Koutzoukis C: Neuropsychiatric sequelae one year after a minor head injury. J Neurol Neurosurg Psychiatry 65:899–902, 1998

Deb S, Lyons I, Koutzoukis C: Neurobehavioural symptoms one year after a head injury. Br J Psychiatry 174:360–365, 1999

Dewar D, Graham DI: Depletion of choline acetyltransferase activity but preservation of M1 and M2 muscarinic receptor binding sites in temporal cortex following head injury: a preliminary human postmortem study. J Neurotrauma 13:181–187, 1996

Dicker BG: Preinjury behavior and recovery after a minor head injury: a review of the literature. J Head Trauma Rehabil 4:73–81, 1989

Dikmen S, McLean A Jr, Temkin NR, et al: Neuropsychologic outcome at one-month postinjury. Arch Phys Med Rehabil 67:507–513, 1986a

Dikmen S, McLean A, Temkin N: Neuropsychological and psychosocial consequences of minor head injury. J Neurol Neurosurg Psychiatry 49:1227–1232, 1986b

Dikmen SS, Machamer JE, Winn HR, et al: Neuropsychological outcome at 1-year post head injury. Neuropsychology 9:80–90, 1995a

Dikmen SS, Ross BL, Machamer JE, et al: One year psychosocial outcome in head injury. J Int Neuropsychol Soc 1:67–77, 1995b

Dixon CE, Bao J, Bergman JS, et al: Traumatic brain injury reduces hippocampal high affinity [3H] choline uptake but not extracellular choline levels in rats. Neurosci Lett 180:127–130, 1994

Dobkin BH, Hanlon R: Dopamine agonist treatment of anterograde amnesia from a mediobasal forebrain injury. Ann Neurol 33:313–316, 1993

Drake ME Jr, Weate SJ, Newell SA: Auditory evoked potentials in postconcussive syndrome. Electromyogr Clin Neurophysiol 36:457–462, 1996

Eames P, Sutton A: Protracted post-traumatic confusional state treated with physostigmine. Brain Inj 9:729–734, 1995

Echemendia RJ, Julian LJ: Mild traumatic brain injury in sports: neuropsychology's contribution to a developing field. Neuropsychol Rev 11:69–88, 2001

Eisenberg HM, Levin HS: Computed tomography and magnetic resonance imaging in mild to moderate head injury, in Mild Head Injury. Edited by Levin HS, Eisenberg HM, Benton A. New York, Oxford University Press, 1989, pp 133–141

Elliot R, Sahakian BJ, Matthews K, et al: Effects of methylphenidate on spatial working memory and planning in healthy young adults. Psychopharmacology 131:196–206, 1997

Englander J, Hall K, Stimpson T, et al: Mild traumatic brain injury in an insured population: subjective complaints and return to employment. Brain Inj 6:161–166, 1992

Evans RW, Evans RI, Sharp MJ: The physician survey on the post-concussion and whiplash syndromes. Headache 34:268–274, 1994

Ewing R, McCarthy D, Gronwall D, et al: Persisting effects of mild head injury observable during hypoxic stress. J Clin Neuropsychol 2:147–155, 1980

Fann JR, Katon WJ, Uomoto JM, et al: Psychiatric disorders and functional disability in outpatients with traumatic brain injuries. Am J Psychiatry 152:1493–1499, 1995

Fann JR, Uomoto JM, Katon WJ: Sertraline in the treatment of major depression following mild traumatic brain injury. J Neuropsychiatry Clin Neurosci 12:226–232, 2000

Fann JR, Uomoto JM, Katon WJ: Cognitive improvement with treatment of depression following mild traumatic brain injury. Psychosomatics 42:48–54, 2001

Federoff JP, Starkstein SE, Forrester AW, et al: Depression in patients with acute traumatic brain injury. Am J Psychiatry 149:918–923, 1992

Feinstein A, Ouchterlony D, Somerville J, et al: The effects of litigation on symptom expression: a prospective study following mild traumatic brain injury. Med Sci Law 41:116–121, 2001

Fenton G, McClelland R, Montgomery A, et al: The postconcussional syndrome: social antecedents and psychological sequelae. Br J Psychiatry 162:493–497, 1993

Fordyce DJ, Roueche JR, Prigatano GP: Enhanced emotional reactions in chronic head trauma patients. J Neurol Neurosurg Psychiatry 46:620–624, 1983

Fox DD, Lees-Haley PR, Earnest K, et al: Post-concussive symptoms: base rates and etiology in psychiatric patients. Clin Neuropsychol 9:89–92, 1995

Freed S, Hellerstein LF: Visual electrodiagnostic findings in mild traumatic brain injury. Brain Inj 11:25–36, 1997

Frencham KAR, Fox AM, Maybery MT: Neuropsychological studies of mild traumatic brain injury: a meta-analytic review of research since 1995. J Clin Exp Neuropsychol, in press

Gaetz M, Bernstein DM: The current status of electrophysiologic procedures for the assessment of mild traumatic brain injury. J Head Trauma Rehabil 16:386–405, 2001

Gaetz M, Weinberg H: Electrophysiological indices of persistent post-concussion symptoms. Brain Inj 14:815–832, 2000

Gaetz M, Goodman D, Weinberg H: Electrophysiological evidence for the cumulative effects of concussion. Brain Inj 14:1077–1088, 2000

Garber HJ, Weilburg JB, Duffy FH, et al: Clinical use of topographic brain electrical activity mapping in psychiatry. J Clin Psychiatry 50:205–211, 1989

Gennarelli TA: Cerebral concussions and diffuse brain injuries, in Head Injury. Edited by Cooper PR. Baltimore, MD, Williams & Wilkins, 1987, pp 108–124

Gentilini M, Nichelli P, Schoenhuber R: Assessment of attention in mild head injury, in Mild Head Injury. Edited by Levin H, Eisenberg H, Benton A. New York, Oxford University Press, 1989, pp 163–175

Gfeller JD, Chibnall JT, Duckro PN: Postconcussion symptoms and cognitive functioning in posttraumatic headache patients. Headache 34:503–507, 1994

Giza CC, Hovda DA: The neurometabolic cascade of concussion. J Athl Train 36:228–235, 2001

Glenn MB: Methylphenidate for cognitive and behavioral dysfunction after traumatic brain injury. J Head Trauma Rehabil 13:87–90, 1998

Godersky JC, Gentry LR, Tranel D, et al: Magnetic resonance imaging and neurobehavioural outcome in traumatic brain injury. Acta Neurochir Suppl 51:311–314, 1990

Goethe KE, Levin HS: Behavioral manifestation during the early and long-term stages of recovery after closed head injury. Psychiatr Ann 14:540–546, 1984

Goldberg DP, Hebber VF: A scaled version of the general health questionnaire. Psychol Med 9:139–145, 1979

Goldberg E, Gerstman LJ, Hughes JE, et al: Selective effects of cholinergic treatment of verbal memory in posttraumatic amnesia. J Clin Neuropsychol 4:219–234, 1982

Goldenberg G, Oder W, Spatt J, et al: Cerebral correlates of disturbed executive function and memory in survivors of severe closed head injury: a SPECT study. J Neurol Neurosurg Psychiatry 55:362–368, 1992

Goleburn CR, Golden CJ: Traumatic brain injury outcome in older adults: a critical review of the literature. J Clin Gerontol 7:161–187, 2001

Gordon WA, Haddad L, Brown M, et al: The sensitivity and specificity of self-reported symptoms in individuals with traumatic brain injury. Brain Inj 14:21–33, 2000

Gouvier WD, Uddo-Crane M, Brown LM: Base rates of postconcussional symptoms. Arch Clin Neuropsychol 3:273–278, 1988

Gronwall D: Cumulative and persisting effects of concussion on attention and cognition, in Mild Head Injury. Edited by Levin H, Eisenberg H, Benton A. New York, Oxford University Press, 1989, pp 153–162

Gronwall D, Wrightson P: Delayed recovery of intellectual function after minor head injury. Lancet 2:605–609, 1974

Gross H, Kling A, Henry G, et al: Local cerebral glucose metabolism in patients with long-term behavioral and cognitive deficits following mild traumatic brain injury. J Neuropsychiatry Clin Neurosci 8:324–334, 1996

Gualtieri CT, Evans RW: Stimulant treatment for the neurobehavioral sequelae of traumatic brain injury. Brain Inj 2:273–290, 1988

Gualtieri CT, Chandler M, Coons TB, et al: Amantadine: a new clinical profile for traumatic brain injury. Clin Neuropharmacol 12:258–270, 1989

Guilmette TJ, Rasile D: Sensitivity, specificity and diagnostic accuracy of three verbal memory measures in the assessment of mild brain injury. Neuropsychology 9:338–344, 1995

Hale MS: Lithium carbonate in the treatment of organic brain syndrome. J Nerv Ment Dis 170:362–365, 1982

Hamilton MA: A rating scale for depressions. J Neurol Neurosurg Psychiatry 23:56–62, 1960

Hamilton MA, Smith RP, Bridge GW: The Leeds scale for the self-assessment of anxiety and depression. Br J Psychiatry 128:156–165, 1976

Harad FT, Kerstein MD: Inadequacy of bedside clinical indicators in identifying significant intracranial injury in trauma patients. J Trauma 32:359–61; discussion 361–363, 1992

Harrington DE, Malec J, Cicerone K, et al: Current perceptions of rehabilitation professionals towards mild traumatic brain injury. Arch Phys Med Rehabil 74:579–586, 1993

Harris poll: Public Perceptions of Brain and Head Injuries. New York, Harris Interactive, Study No. 11681, 2000

Harvey AG, Bryant RA: Acute stress disorder after mild traumatic brain injury. J Nerv Ment Dis 186:333–337, 1998a

Harvey AG, Bryant RA: Predictors of acute stress following mild traumatic brain injury. Brain Inj 12:147–154, 1998b

Haydel MJ, Preston CA, Mills TJ, et al: Indications for computed tomography in patients with minor head injury (see comments). N Engl J Med 343:100–105, 2000

Hibbard MR, Uysal S, Kepler K, et al: Axis I psychopathology in individuals with traumatic brain injury. J Head Trauma Rehabil 13:24–39, 1998

Hibbard MR, Bogdany J, Uysal S, et al: Axis II psychopathology in individuals with traumatic brain injury. Brain Inj 14:45–61, 2000

Hinkeldey NS, Corrigan JD: The structure of head injured patients' neurobehavioral complaints: a preliminary study. Brain Inj 4:115–133, 1990

Hoff AL, Shukla S, Cook BL, et al: Cognitive function in manics with associated neurologic factors. J Affect Disord 14:251–255, 1988

Hugenholtz H, Stuss DT, Stethem LL, et al: How long does it take to recover from a mild concussion? Neurosurgery 22:853–858, 1988

Humayun MS, Presty SK, Lafrance ND, et al: Local cerebral glucose abnormalities in mild closed head injured patients with cognitive impairment. Nucl Med Commun 10:335–344, 1989

Ingebrigtsen T, Waterloo K, Marup-Jensen S, et al: Quantification of post-concussion symptoms 3 months after minor head injury in 100 consecutive patients. J Neurol 245:609–612, 1998

Iverson GL, Binder LM: Detecting exaggeration and malingering in neuropsychological assessment. J Head Trauma Rehabil 15:829–858, 2000

Iverson GL, McCracken LM: "Postconcussive" symptoms in persons with chronic pain. Brain Inj 11:783–790, 1997

Jacobs A, Put E, Ingels M, et al: Prospective evaluation of technetium-99m-HMPAO SPECT in mild and moderate traumatic brain injury. J Nucl Med 35:942–947, 1994

Jakala P, Riekkinen M, Sirvio J, et al: Guanfacine, but not clonidine, improves planning and working memory performance in humans. Neuropsychopharmacology 20:460–470, 1999a

Jakala P, Sirvio J, Riekkinen M, et al: Guanfacine and clonidine, α2-agonists, improve paired associates learning, but not delayed matching to sample, in humans. Neuropsychopharmacology 20:119–130, 1999b

Jane JA, Steward O, Gennarelli T: Axonal degeneration induced by experimental noninvasive minor head injury. J Neurosurg 62:96–100, 1985

Jenkins A, Hadley MDM, Teasdale G, et al: Brain lesions detected by magnetic resonance imaging in mild and severe head injuries. Lancet 2:445–446, 1986

Jennett B: Assessment of the severity of head injury. J Neurol Neurosurg Psychiatry 39:647–655, 1976

Jorge RE, Robinson RG, Arndt S, et al: Depression following traumatic brain injury: a 1 year longitudinal study. J Affect Disord 27:233–243, 1993

Jorge RE, Robinson RG, Starkstein SE, et al: Influence of major depression on 1-year outcome in patients with traumatic brain injury. J Neurosurg 81:726–733, 1994

Jorge R, Robinson RG: Mood disorders following traumatic brain injury. Neurorehabilitation 17:311–324, 2002

Junger EC, Newell DW, Grant GA, et al: Cerebral autoregulation following minor head injury. J Neurosurg 86:425–432, 1997

Kay T: Neuropsychological diagnosis: disentangling the multiple determinants of functional disability after mild traumatic brain injury, in Physical Medicine and Rehabilitation: State of the Art Reviews. Philadelphia, PA, Hanley & Belfus, 1992, pp 109–127

Kay T, Harrington DE, Adams R, et al: Definition of mild traumatic brain injury. J Head Trauma Rehabil 8:86–87, 1993

Keller M, Hiltbrunner B, Dill C, et al: Reversible neuropsychological deficits after mild traumatic brain injury. J Neurol Neurosurg Psychiatry 68:761–764, 2000

Kelly R: The post-traumatic syndrome: an iatrogenic disease. Forensic Sci 6:17–24, 1975

Keshavan MS, Channabasavanna SM, Reddy GNN: Post-traumatic psychiatric disturbances: patterns and predictors of outcome. Br J Psychiatry 138:157–160, 1981

Kimberg DY, D'Esposito M, Farah MJ: Effects of bromocriptine on human subjects depend on working memory capacity. NeuroReport 8:3581–3585, 1997

King NS: Emotional, neuropsychological, and organic factors: their use in the prediction of persisting postconcussion symptoms after moderate and mild head injuries. J Neurol Neurosurg Psychiatry 61:75–81, 1996

King NS, Crawford S, Wenden FJ, et al: Early prediction of persisting post-concussion symptoms following mild and moderate head injuries. Br J Clin Psychol 38:15–25, 1999

Kraus JF, Nourjah P: The epidemiology of mild, uncomplicated brain injury. J Trauma 28:1637–1643, 1988

Kraus JF, Nourjah P: The epidemiology of mild head injury, in Mild Head Injury. Edited by Levin HS, Eisenberg HM, Benton AL. New York, Oxford University Press, 1989, pp 8–22

Kraus JF, McArthur DL, Silberman TA: Epidemiology of mild brain injury. Semin Neurol 14:1–7, 1994

Krauthammer C, Klerman GL: Secondary mania. Arch Gen Psychiatry 35:1333–1339, 1978

Kwentus JA, Hart RP, Beck E, et al: Psychiatric complications of closed head injury. Psychosomatics 26:8–17, 1985

Lal S, Merbtiz CP, Grip JC: Modification of function in head-injured patients with Sinemet. Brain Inj 2:225–233, 1988

Langfitt TW, Obrist WD, Alavi A, et al: Computerized tomography, magnetic resonance imaging, and positron emission tomography in the study of brain trauma: preliminary observations. J Neurosurg 64:760–767, 1986

Larrabee GJ: Current controversies in mild head injury: scientific and methodologic considerations, in The Evaluation and Treatment of Mild Traumatic Brain Injury. Edited by Varney NR, Roberts RJ. Mahwah, NJ, Erlbaum, 1999, pp 327–345

Lee SM, Wong MD, Samii A, et al: Evidence for energy failure following irreversible traumatic brain injury. Ann N Y Acad Sci 893:337–340, 1999

Lees-Haley PR, Brown RS: Neuropsychological complaint base rates of 170 personal injury claimants. Arch Clin Neuropsychol 8:203–209, 1993

Leigh D: Psychiatric aspects of head injury. Journal of Clinical and Experimental Psychiatry 40:21–33, 1979

Leininger BE, Gramling SE, Farrell AD, et al: Neuropsychological deficits in symptomatic minor head injury patients after concussion and mild concussion (see comments). J Neurol Neurosurg Psychiatry 53:293–296, 1990

Levin HS, Peters BH, Kalisky Z, et al: Effects of oral physostigmine and lecithin on memory and attention in closed head-injured patients. Cent Nerv Syst Trauma 3:333–342, 1986

Levin HS, Amparo E, Eisenberg HM, et al: Magnetic resonance imaging and computerized tomography in relation to the neurobehavioral sequelae of mild and moderate head injuries. J Neurosurg 66:706–713, 1987a

Levin HS, Mattis S, Ruff RM, et al: Neurobehavioral outcome following minor head injury: a three-center study. J Neurosurg 66:234–243, 1987b

Levin HS, Gary HE, Eisenberg HM, et al: Neurobehavioral outcome 1 year after severe head injury: experience of the traumatic coma data bank. J Neurosurg 73:699–709, 1990

Levin HS, Williams DH, Eisenberg HM, et al: Serial MRI and neurobehavioural findings after mild to moderate closed head injury. J Neurol Neurosurg Psychiatry 55:255–262, 1992

Li BM, Mei ZT: Delayed-response deficit induced by local injection of the α_2-adrenergic antagonist yohimbine into the dorsolateral prefrontal cortex in young adult monkeys. Behav Neural Biol 62:134–139, 1994

Lishman WA: Brain damage in relation to psychiatric disability after head injury. Br J Psychiatry 114:373–410, 1968

Lishman WA: The psychiatric sequelae of head injury: a review. Psychol Med 3:304–318, 1973

Lishman WA: Physiogenesis and psychogenesis in the "post-concussional syndrome." Br J Psychiatry 460–469, 1988

Luciana M, Collins PF: Dopaminergic modulation of working memory for spatial but not object cues in normal humans. J Cogn Neurosci 9:330–347, 1997

Luciana M, Depue RA, Arbisi P, et al: Facilitation of working memory in humans by a D_2 dopamine receptor agonist. J Cogn Neurosci 4:58–68, 1992

Luerssen TG, Klauber MR, Marshall L: Outcome from head injury related to patient's age: a longitudinal prospective study of adult and pediatric head injury. J Neurosurg 68:409–416, 1988

Luine V, Bowling D, Hearns M: Spatial memory deficits in aged rats: contributions of monoaminergic systems. Brain Res 537:271–278, 1990

Mahoney FI, Barthel DW: Functional evaluation: the Barthel index. Md State Med J 2:61–65, 1965

Malaspina D, Goetz RR, Friedman JH, et al: Traumatic brain injury and schizophrenia in members of schizophrenia and bipolar disorder pedigrees. Am J Psychiatry 158:440–446, 2001

Malec J: Mild traumatic brain injury: scope of the problem, in The Evaluation and Treatment of Mild Traumatic Brain Injury. Edited by Varney NR, Roberts RJ. Mahwah, NJ, Erlbaum, 1999, pp 15–37

Mayou RA, Black J, Bryant B: Unconsciousness, amnesia and psychiatric symptoms following road traffic accident injury. Br J Psychiatry 177:540–545, 2000

McAllister TW: Mixed neurologic and psychiatric disorders: pharmacological issues. Compr Psychiatry 33:296–304, 1992a

McAllister TW: Neuropsychiatric aspects of delusions. Psychiatr Ann 22:269–277, 1992b

McAllister TW: Neuropsychiatric sequelae of head injuries. Psychiatr Clin North Am 15:395–413, 1992c

McAllister TW, Arciniegas DB: Evaluation and treatment of postconcussive symptoms. NeuroRehabilitation 17:265–283, 2002

McAllister TW, Flashman LA: Mild brain injury and mood disorders: causal connection, assessment, and treatment, in The Evaluation and Treatment of Mild Traumatic Brain Injury. Edited by Varney NR, Roberts RJ. Mahwah, NJ, Erlbaum, 1999, pp 347–373

McAllister TW, Price TRP: Depression in the brain injured: phenomenology and treatment, in Depression: New Directions in Theory, Research, and Practice. Edited by Endler NS, McCann CD. Toronto, Canada, Wall & Emerson, 1990, pp 361–387

McAllister TW, Summerall L: Genetic polymorphisms in the expression and treatment of neuropsychiatric disorders. Curr Psychiatry Rep 5:400–409, 2003

McAllister TW, Saykin AJ, Flashman LA, et al: Differences in working memory-associated brain activation one month after mild traumatic brain injury: an fMRI study. Neurology 53:1300–1309, 1999

McAllister TW, Sparling MB, Flashman L, et al: Differential working memory load effects after mild traumatic brain injury. Neuroimage 14:1004–1012, 2001a

McAllister TW, Sparling MB, Flashman L, et al: Neuroimaging findings in mild traumatic brain injury. J Clin Exp Neuropsychol 23:775–791, 2001b

McAllister TW, McDonald BC, Flashman LA, et al: Differential effect of COMT allele status on frontal activation associated with a dopaminergic agonist. J Neuropsychiatry Clin Neurosci 16:238–239, 2004

McCrory PR, Berkovic SF: Second impact syndrome. Neurology 50:677–683, 1998

McCullagh S, Oucherlony D, Protzner A, et al: Prediction of neuropsychiatric outcome following mild trauma brain injury: an examination of the Glasgow Coma Scale. Brain Inj 15:489–497, 2001

McDowell S, Whyte J, D'Esposito M: Differential effect of a dopaminergic agonist on prefrontal function in traumatic brain injury patients. Brain 121:1155–1164, 1998

McKinlay WW, Brooks DN, Bond MR, et al: The short term outcomes of severe blunt head injury as reported by relatives of the injured persons. J Neurol Neurosurg Psychiatry 44:527–533, 1981

McKinlay WW, Brooks DN, Bond MR: Post-concussional symptoms, financial compensation and outcome of severe blunt head injury. J Neurol Neurosurg Psychiatry 46:1084–1091, 1983

McLean A, Temkin N, Dikmen S, et al: The behavioral sequelae of head injury. J Clin Neuropsychol 5:361–376, 1983

McMillan TM: Post-traumatic stress disorder and severe head injury. Br J Psychiatry 159:431–433, 1991

McMillan TM, Glucksman EE: The neuropsychology of moderate head injury. J Neurol Neurosurg Psychiatry 50:393–397, 1987

Merskey H, Woodforde JM: Psychiatric sequelae of minor head injury. Brain 95:521–528, 1972

Meyers JE, Galinsky AM, Volbrecht M: Malingering and mild brain injury: how low is too low. Appl Neuropsychol 6:208–216, 1999

Miller EC, Holmes JF, Derlet RW: Utilizing clinical factors to reduce head CT scan ordering for minor head trauma patients. J Emerg Med 15:453–457, 1997

Miller H: Accident neurosis. BMJ 1:919–925, 992–998, 1961

Minderhoud JM, Boelens ME, Huizenga J, et al: Treatment of minor head injuries. Clin Neurol Neurosurg 82:127–140, 1980

Minderhoud JM, Boelens ME, Huizenga J, et al: Treatment of minor head injuries. Clin Neurol Neurosurg 82:127–140, 1997

Mitchener A, Wyper D, Patterson J, et al: SPECT, CT, and MRI in head injury: acute abnormalities followed up at six months. J Neurol Neurosurg Psychiatry 62:633–636, 1997

Mittenberg W, DiGiulio DV, Perrin S, et al: Symptoms following mild head injury: expectation as aetiology. J Neurol Neurosurg Psychiatry 55:200–204, 1992

Mittenberg W, Tremont G, Zielinski RE, et al: Cognitive-behavioral prevention of postconcussion syndrome. Arch Clin Neuropsychol 11:139–145, 1996

Mobayed M, Dinan TG: Buspirone/prolactin response in post head injury depression. J Affect Disord 19:237–241, 1990

Murdoch I, Perry EK, Court JA, et al: Cortical cholinergic dysfunction after human head injury. J Neurotrauma 15:295–305, 1998

Nagamachi S, Nishikawa T, Ono S, et al: A comparative study of ^{123}I-IMP SPECT and CT in the investigation of chronic-stage head trauma patients. Nucl Med Commun 16:17–25, 1995

Nasrallah HA, Fowler RC, Judd LL: Schizophrenia-like illness following head injury. Psychosomatics 22:359–361, 1981

Newton MR, Greenwood RJ, Britton KE, et al: A study comparing SPECT with CT and MRI after closed head injury. J Neurol Neurosurg Psychiatry 55:92–94, 1992

Nizamie SH, Nizamie A, Borde M, et al: Mania following head injury: case reports and neuropsychological findings. Acta Psychiatr Scand 77:637–639, 1988

Oppenheimer DR: Microscopic lesions in the brain following head injury. J Neurol Neurosurg Psychiatry 31:299–306, 1968

Paniak C, MacDonald J, Toller-Lobe G, et al: A preliminary normative profile of mild traumatic brain injury diagnostic criteria. J Clin Exp Neuropsychol 20:852–855, 1998a

Paniak C, Toller-Lobe G, Durand A, et al: A randomized trial of two treatments for mild traumatic brain injury. Brain Inj 12:1011–1023, 1998b

Papathanasopoulos P, Konstantinou D, Flaburiari K, et al: Pattern reversal visual evoked potentials in minor head injury. Eur Neurol 34:268–271, 1994

Peerless SJ, Newcastle NW: Sheer injuries of the brain. Can Med Assoc J 96:577–582, 1967

Pope HG, McElroy SL, Satlin A, et al: Head injury, bipolar disorder, and response to valproate. Compr Psychiatry 29:34–38, 1988

Povlishock JT, Christman CW: The pathobiology of traumatically induced axonal injury in animals and humans: a review of current thoughts. J Neurotrauma 12:555–564, 1995

Povlishock JT, Coburn TH: Morphopathological change associated with mild head injury, in Mild Head Injury. Edited by Levin H, Eisenberg H, Benton A. New York, Oxford University Press, 1989, pp 37–53

Powell TJ, Collin C, Sutton K: A follow-up study of patients hospitalized after minor head injury. Disabil Rehabil 18:231–237, 1996

Practice parameter: the management of concussion in sports (summary statement). Report of the Quality Standards Subcommittee. Neurology 48:581–585, 1997

Pratrap-Chand R, Sinniah M, Salem FA: Cognitive evoked potential (P300): a metric for cerebral concussion. Acta Neurol Scand 78:185–189, 1988

Quayle KS: Minor head injury in the pediatric patient. Pediatr Clin North Am 46:1189–1199, 1999

Rees PM: Contemporary issues in mild traumatic brain injury. Arch Phys Med Rehabil 84:1885–1894, 2003

Reid RH, Gulenchyn KY, Ballinger JR, et al: Cerebral perfusion imaging with technetium-99m HMPAO following cerebral trauma: initial experience. Clin Nucl Med 15:383–388, 1990

Riess H, Schwartz CE, Klerman GL: Manic syndrome following head injury: another form of secondary mania. J Clin Psychiatry 48:29–30, 1987

Rimel RW: A prospective study of patients with central nervous system trauma. J Neurosurg Nurs 13:132–141, 1981

Rimel RW, Giordani B, Barth JT, et al: Disability caused by minor head injury. Neurosurgery 9:221–228, 1981

Rimel RW, Giordani B, Barth JT, et al: Moderate head injury: completing the clinical spectrum of brain trauma. Neurosurgery 11:344–351, 1982

Robinson RG, Boston JD, Starkstein SE, et al: Comparison of mania and depression after brain injury: causal factors. Am J Psychiatry 145:172–178, 1988

Roper SN, Mena I, King WA, et al: An analysis of cerebral blood flow in acute closed-head injury using technetium-99m HMPAO SPECT and computed tomography. J Nucl Med 32:1684–1687, 1991

Ruff RM, Jurica P: In search of a unified definition for mild traumatic brain injury. Brain Inj 13:943–952, 1999

Ruff RM, Buchsbaum MS, Troster AI, et al: Computerized tomography, neuropsychology, and positron emission tomography in the evaluation of head injury. Neuropsychiatry Neuropsychol Behav Neurol 2:103–123, 1989a

Ruff RM, Levin HS, Mather S, et al: Recovery of memory after mild head injury: a three center study, in Mild Head injury. Edited by Levin HS, Eisenberg HM, Benton AL. New York, Oxford University Press, 1989b, pp 176–188

Ruff RM, Crouch JA, Troster AI, et al: Selected cases of poor outcome following a minor brain trauma: comparing neuropsychological and positron emission tomography assessment. Brain Inj 8:297–308, 1994

Ruffolo CF, Friedland JF, Dawson DR, et al: Mild traumatic brain injury from motor vehicle accidents: factors associated with return to work. Arch Phys Med Rehabil 80:392–398, 1999

Rutherford WH: Postconcussive symptoms: relationship to acute neurological indices, individual differences, and circumstances of injury, in Mild Head Injury. Edited by Levin HS, Eisenberg HM, Benton AL. New York, Oxford University Press, 1989, pp 217–228

Saija A, Robinson SE, Lyeth BG, et al: The effects of scopolamine and traumatic brain injury on central cholinergic neurons. J Neurotrauma 5:161–170, 1988

Saran AS: Depression after mild closed head injury: role of dexamethasone suppression test and antidepressants. J Clin Psychiatry 1985:335–338, 1985

Satz PS, Alfano MS, Light RF, et al: Persistent post-concussive syndrome: a proposed methodology and literature review to determine the effects, if any, of mild head and other bodily injury. J Clin Exp Neuropsychol 21:620–628, 1999

Schoenhuber R, Gentilini M: Auditory brain stem responses in the prognosis of late postconcussional symptoms and neuropsychological dysfunction after minor head injury. Neurosurgery 19:532–534, 1986

Schoenhuber R, Gentilini M: Anxiety and depression after mild head injury: a case control study. J Neurol Neurosurg Psychiatry 51:722–724, 1988

Schoenhuber R, Gentilini M: Neurophysiological assessment of mild head injury, in Mild Head Injury. Edited by Levin HS, Eisenberg HM, Benton AL. New York, Oxford University Press, 1989, pp 142–150

Schretlen DJ, Shapiro AM: A quantitative review of the effects of traumatic brain injury on cognitive functioning. Int Rev Psychiatry 15:341–349, 2003

Schynoll WK, Overton D, Krome R, et al: A prospective study to identify high-yield criteria associated with acute intracranial computed tomography findings in head-injured patients. Am J Emerg Med 11:321–326, 1993

Shackford SR, Wald SL, Ross SE, et al: The clinical utility of computed tomographic scanning and neurologic examination in the management of patients with minor head injuries (see comments). J Trauma 33:385–394, 1992

Shukla S, Cook BL, Mukherjee S, et al: Mania following head trauma. Am J Psychiatry 144:93–96, 1987

Silver JM, Yudofsky SC, Hales RE: Depression in traumatic brain injury. Neuropsychiatry Neuropsychol Behav Neurol 4:12–23, 1991

Silver JM, Hales RE, Yudofsky SC: Neuropsychiatric aspects of traumatic brain injury, in The American Psychiatric Press Textbook of Neuropsychiatry. Edited by Yudofsky SC, Hales RE. Washington, DC, American Psychiatric Press, 1992, pp 179–190

Silver JM, Kramer R, Greenwald S, et al: The association between head injuries and psychiatric disorders: findings from the New Haven NIMH Epidemiologic Catchment Area Study. Brain Inj 15:935–945, 2001

Silverman I, Galetta SL, Gray LG, et al: SPECT in patients with cortical visual loss. J Nucl Med 34:1447–1451, 1993

Sorenson SB, Kraus JF: Occurrence, severity, and outcome of brain injury. J Head Trauma Rehabil 5:1–10, 1991

Sosin DM, Sniezek J, Thurman D: Incidence of mild and moderate brain injury in the United States, 1991. Brain Inj 10:47–54, 1996

Soustiel JF, Hafner H, Chistyakov AV, et al: Trigeminal and auditory evoked responses in minor head injuries and postconcussion syndrome. Brain Inj 9:805–813, 1995

Sparadeo FR, Strauss D, Bartels JT: The incidence, impact, and treatment of substance abuse in head trauma rehabilitation. J Head Trauma Rehabil 5:1–8, 1990

Steere JC, Arnsten AF: The alpha-2A noradrenergic receptor agonist guanfacine improves visual object discrimination reversal performance in aged rhesus monkeys. Behav Neurosci 111:883–891, 1997

Stein SC, Ross SE: Mild head injury: a plea for routine early CT scanning (see comments). J Trauma 33:11–13, 1992

Stewart JT, Hemsath RN: Bipolar illness following traumatic brain injury: treatment with lithium and carbamazepine. J Clin Psychiatry 49:74–75, 1988

Strauss J, Savitsky N: Head injury: neurologic and psychiatric aspects. Arch Neurol Psychiatry 31:893–955, 1934

Strebel S, Lam AM, Matta BF, et al: Impaired cerebral autoregulation after mild brain injury. Surg Neurol 47:128–131, 1997

Stuss DT, Stethem LL, Hugenholtz H, et al: Reaction time after head injury: fatigue, divided and focused attention, and consistency of performance. J Neurol Neurosurg Psychiatry 52:742–748, 1989

Tanila H, Rama P, Carlson S: The effects of prefrontal intracortical microinjections of an alpha-2 agonist, alpha-2 antagonist and lidocaine on the delayed alternation performance of aged rats. Brain Res Bull 40:117–119, 1996

Tayerni JP, Seliger G, Lichtman SW: Donepezil mediated memory improvement in traumatic brain injury during post acute rehabilitation. Brain Inj 12:77–80, 1998

Teasdale G, Jennett B: Assessment of coma and impaired consciousness: a practical scale. Lancet 2:81–84, 1974

Thatcher RW, Walker RA, Gerson I, et al: EEG discriminant analyses of mild head trauma. Electroencephalogr Clin Neurophysiol 73:94–106, 1989

Thatcher RW, Biver C, McAlaster R, et al: Biophysical linkage between MRI and EEG amplitude in closed head injury. Neuroimage 7:352–367, 1998a

Thatcher RW, Biver C, McAlaster R, et al: Biophysical linkage between MRI and EEG coherence in closed head injury. Neuroimage 8:307–326, 1998b

Thatcher RW, North DM, Curtin RT, et al: An EEG severity index of traumatic brain injury. J Neuropsychiatry Clin Neurosci 13:77–87, 2001

Thurman DJ, Sniezek JE, Johnson D, et al: Guidelines for Surveillance of Central Nervous System Injury. Atlanta, GA, Centers for Disease Control and Prevention, 1995

U.S. Department of Health and Human Services: Interagency Head Injury Task Force Report, Washington DC, U.S. Department of Health and Human Services 1989

van der Naalt J, Hew JM, van Zomeren AH, et al: Computed tomography and magnetic resonance imaging in mild to moderate head injury: early and late imaging related to outcome. Ann Neurol 46:70–78, 1999

van Reekum R, Cohen T, Wong J: Can traumatic brain injury cause psychiatric disorders? J Neuropsychiatry Clin Neurosci 12:316–327, 2000

van Zomeron AH, van Den Burg W: Residual complaints of patients two years after severe head injury. J Neurol Neurosurg Psychiatry 48:21–28, 1985

Voller B, Benke T, Benedetto K, et al: Neuropsychological, MRI and EEG findings after very mild traumatic brain injury. Brain Inj 13:821–827, 1999

Wade DT, Crawford S, Wenden FJ, et al: Does routine follow up after head injury help? A randomised controlled trial. J Neurol Neurosurg Psychiatry 62:478–484, 1997

Wade DT, King NS, Wenden FJ, et al: Routine follow up after head injury: a second randomised controlled trial. J Neurol Neurosurg Psychiatry 65:177–183, 1998

Warden DL, Bleiberg J, Cameron KL, et al: Persistent prolongation of simple reaction time in sports concussion. Neurology 57:524–526, 2001

Weidmann KD, Wilson JTL, Wyper D, et al: SPECT cerebral blood flow, MR imaging, and neuropsychological findings in traumatic head injury. Neuropsychology 3:267–281, 1989

Whelan FJ, Walker MS, Schultz SK: Donepezil in the treatment of cognitive dysfunction associated with traumatic brain injury. Ann Clin Psychiatry 12:131–135, 2000

Whitman S, Coonley-Hoganson R, Desai BT: Comparative head trauma experiences in two socioeconomically different Chicago area communities—a population study. Am J Epidemiol 119:570–580, 1984

Whyte J, Hart T, Schuster K, et al: Effects of methylphenidate on attentional function after traumatic brain injury: a randomized, placebo-controlled trial. Am J Phys Rehabil 76:440–450, 1997

Williams DH, Levin HS, Eisenberg HM: Mild head injury classification. Neurosurgery 27:422–428, 1990

Wilson JTL, Wiedman KD, Hadley DM, et al: Early and late magnetic resonance imaging and neuropsychological outcome after head injury. J Neurol Neurosurg Psychiatry 51:391–396, 1988

Wong JL, Regennitter RP, Barrios P: Base rate and simulated symptoms of mild head injury among normals. Arch Clin Neuropsychol 9:411–425, 1994

World Health Organization: International Classification of Diseases, 9th Revision, Clinical Modification, 3rd Edition. Washington, DC, U.S. Department of Health and Human Services, 1989

Wrightson P: Management of disability and rehabilitation services after mild head injury, in Mild Head Injury. Edited by Levin HS, Eisenberg HM, Benton AL. New York, Oxford University Press, 1989, pp 245–256

Wroblewski BA, Joseph AB, Cornblatt RR: Antidepressant pharmacotherapy and the treatment of depression in patients with severe traumatic brain injury: a controlled, prospective study. J Clin Psychiatry 57:582–587, 1996

Zwil AS, McAllister TW, Raimo E: The expression of bipolar affective disorders in brain injured patients. Int J Psychiatry Med 22:377–395, 1992

Zwil AS, McAllister TW, Cohen I, et al: Ultra-rapid cycling bipolar affective disorder following a closed head injury. Brain Inj 7:147–152, 1993

16 Seizures

Gary J. Tucker, M.D.

THE PRESENCE OF posttraumatic seizures is a major complication in the recovery of the brain injury patient. It not only adds further cognitive and behavioral changes (in addition to the brain injury itself), it also connotes a worse prognosis.

The many cognitive problems faced by the patient with traumatic brain injury (TBI), such as the inability to sustain attention (Parasuraman et al. 1991) and impairments in social interaction (Marsh and Knight 1991; Sarna 1980), are further exacerbated by the presence of seizures. Seizures in themselves can cause marked effects on cognitive functions and social performance (Matthews 1992). In addition, anticonvulsant medications can also cause cognitive changes (Farwell et al. 1990; Gillham et al. 1988; Meador et al. 1990). Aside from the cognitive effects, seizures have an enormous psychological impact on the patient's self-confidence in social interactions because of the stigma that has been associated with seizure disorders (Temkin 1971). Seizures, the medications used to treat them, and the psychological impact of seizures significantly complicate the rehabilitation of the brain-injured patient.

Epidemiology

Several studies have examined the occurrence of seizures after TBI. TBI associated with closed head injuries (i.e., when the dura has not been penetrated) has a 5% incidence of posttraumatic seizures that can occur any time after brain injury; however, with open head injury (when the dura has been penetrated), 30%–50% of the patients develop posttraumatic seizures (Jennett 1975; Lishman 1987). Jennett (1975) estimated that only 1% of patients will develop seizures if no seizure occurs during the first week after injury; however, if a seizure occurs during the first week, the lifetime incidence increases to 25%. Tech-

nically, if seizures occur after the first week postinjury and are recurrent, the term *posttraumatic epilepsy* should be used, but the literature uses the terms *posttraumatic seizures* and *posttraumatic epilepsy* interchangeably, and most seem to favor the use of *posttraumatic seizures*. Whatever term is used, there is almost no information in the literature on how many seizures a particular patient will have post-TBI. In those patients who develop seizures post-TBI, the long-term prognosis is good. Fifty percent of patients with posttraumatic seizures will no longer have seizures 5–10 years postinjury, 25% will have good seizure control while taking medication, and only 25% will continue to have seizures. The occurrence of seizures depends on the severity and type of the brain injury. Annegers et al. (1980) provided the best available epidemiological data on posttraumatic seizures from a large community-based survey using the community database developed by the Mayo Clinic. They surveyed all medical records of patients with reported brain injury in Olmsted County, Minnesota, from 1935 to 1974. This included all patients with head trauma who were admitted to a hospital or emergency department, who were seen as outpatients, or for whom a home visit was made. In this manner, they collected a total sample of 3,587 patients with TBI, 840 of whom were excluded either because of death within the first month or a prior history of epilepsy or TBI, or because the seizure was the result of other conditions. The remaining 2,747 patients with brain injuries were followed longitudinally for the development of posttraumatic seizures. Thus, the authors avoided one of the major pitfalls in many of the studies of patients with brain injury—that is, the lack of data on those patients lost to follow-up. However, this study was not without methodological problems. First, the authors noted the extreme complexity in estimating the risk of seizures due to the absence, at that time, of standardized definitions of brain trauma or severity of injury. (This lack of definition is present in most of the literature before the development of the standardized rating scales for TBI.) Second, there is the possibility that this was an atypical sample because it was obtained from a major neurosurgical center. Third, the authors noted the poor follow-up for most patients with brain trauma. Last, it was often unclear whether the patient had a history of seizures before the injury.

In spite of these methodological concerns, this community-based study is still valuable in presenting a most complete picture of the longitudinal course of patients with brain trauma. The patients were grouped into the following three categories:

- *Mild brain trauma* (1,640 patients)—defined as those without skull fractures and without loss of consciousness, or with a period of posttraumatic amnesia of less than 30 minutes.
- *Moderate brain trauma* (912 patients)—those patients who had more than a 30-minute period of unconsciousness or posttraumatic amnesia or had a skull fracture, or both.
- *Severe brain trauma* (195 patients)—evidence of brain contusion, hematoma, or more than 24 hours of unconsciousness.

With this classification, Annegers et al. (1980) followed the patients over the 40-year period from 1935 to 1974. Seizures developed in 51 patients during the first 4 years after injury. The risk for patients with severe injury (7.1% in the first year and 11.5% within the next 5 years) was much greater than for those with moderate (0.7% in the first year and 1.6% within 5 years) or mild injury (0.1% in the first year and 1.6% within 5 years). In children (younger than 14 years) with severe injury, the incidence of posttraumatic seizures was 30% compared with only 10% in adults with severe brain injury. Thus, the age of the patient and the severity of the injury are crucial determinants of the subsequent development of posttraumatic seizures.

In 1998, Annegers et al. reported the results of an extension of this study involving those who experienced TBI up to 1984, with a follow-up of these additional cases through 1994; in this manner, the sample was increased to 4,541 patients. In the total sample, 97 patients had unprovoked seizures post-TBI; 22 of these had single seizures, and 75 had multiple seizures. The 30-year cumulative incidence for seizures post mild TBI was 2.1% (3.1% for the first year and 2.1% for the next 4 years), 4.2% for moderate TBI, and 16.7% for severe TBI. Brain contusion, subdural hematoma, and age older than 65 years were the major risk factors for seizures, whereas skull fracture and prolonged unconsciousness were slightly less so.

Apparently, the early treatment of TBI can affect the occurrence of seizures as well. Temkin et al. (1990) treated patients with severe brain trauma with either phenytoin or a placebo immediately after the injury. Between drug loading and the seventh day after the trauma, 3.6% of the phenytoin group and 14.2% of the control group developed seizures. In the group in whom phenytoin was continued after day 8 through the end of the first year, 21.5% of the phenytoin group but only 15.7% of the placebo group had seizures. At the end of the second year, the seizure rates were 27.5% for the phenytoin group and 21.1% for the control group (these differences were statistically significant). The authors hypothesized that phenytoin exerts a prophylactic effect on reducing seizures during the first week post severe brain injury but may increase seizure frequency with prolonged treatment. In addition, patients who continued taking phenytoin longer than 1 week posttrauma had more cognitive deficits than those whose phenytoin was discontinued after the first week. The authors concluded that the drug has an early suppressive effect but not a true prophylactic one. In 1999, Temkin et al. repeated this study. Within 24 hours postinjury, 132 patients received 1-week treatment with phenytoin, 120 patients received 1-month treatment with valproate, and 127 received a 6-month course of treatment with valproate. The rate of early seizures was low and similar to that in the study by Annegers et al. (1998). The rates of late seizures (after 1 week) did not differ in the treatment groups (15% of the group taking phenytoin, 16% of the group taking valproate for 1 month, and 24% of the group taking valproate for 6 months). Although there was no difference in the treatment groups in the occurrence of side effects (e.g., coagulation problems or liver impairments), there was a trend toward a higher mortality rate in the valproate groups (7.2% vs. 13.4%). A study by Dikmen et al. (2000) also showed few cognitive effects of valproate but found a trend toward increased mortality with the use of valproate. A subsequent meta-analysis of controlled trials of post-TBI seizure prevention in late-occurring seizures (Temkin 2001) showed effectiveness for phenytoin and carbamazepine but not for valproate. There have been no studies to date evaluating the use of the more recently developed anticonvulsants such as gabapentin, lamotrigine, or topiramate for the treatment of posttraumatic seizures (Bazil 2001; Martin et al. 1999). In light of the findings with valproate, the newer drugs probably should be used with caution until detailed studies in patients with TBI are available.

In view of the cognitive changes associated with phenytoin and other anticonvulsants, their continued use after the first week following brain injury may be contraindicated. The American Academy of Physical Medicine and Rehabilitation (Brain Injury Special Interest Group of the American

Academy of Physical Medicine and Rehabilitation 1998) and the American Association of Neurological Surgeons (Brain Trauma Foundation 2000) recommend that only phenytoin, phenobarbital, or carbamazepine be used to prevent early (1 week post-TBI) seizures in patients without penetrating injuries of the dura and that no antiepileptic drug be used prophylactically in anticipation of late seizures.

Diagnosis

A major diagnostic indicator of a seizure disorder is an abnormal electroencephalogram (EEG), generally involving paroxysms or spikes, either focal or generalized (Tucker 2002). The presence of an epileptiform EEG pattern occurs more frequently with penetrating brain injury. It is important to emphasize, however, that even several EEGs will reveal seizure activity in only 41% of patients with symptomatic seizures (Desai et al. 1988). Consequently, this relatively low sensitivity of the EEG suggests that the presence or absence of an epileptiform spike should not be the sole factor in determining disability benefits for individuals with epilepsy, and one should not use such abnormalities as an entry criterion for research (Desai et al. 1988). Jabbari et al. (1986) performed EEG evaluations on 515 Vietnam War veterans 12–16 years after penetrating brain injury. They found that 42% of the subjects had abnormal EEGs, but only 9% demonstrated epileptiform findings. There was a significant correlation between EEG findings and the extent of brain volume loss visualized by computed tomography. All patients with anterior temporal or central spike foci experienced posttraumatic seizures. Focal slowing, as would be expected, correlated significantly with localized neurological deficits such as hemiplegia (Jabbari et al. 1986). Salazar et al. (1985) studied 421 Vietnam veterans with penetrating brain injuries. Posttraumatic seizures developed in 53% of these patients. However, only 12% of patients with seizures had EEG results diagnostic of a seizure disorder. The authors concluded that the EEG might not always be diagnostically helpful.

The severity of the injury increases the probability of EEG abnormality. Koufen and Hagel (1987) evaluated 100 patients with posttraumatic late seizures who also had at least 1 week of amnesia after brain injury and found that 95% had focal EEG abnormalities, 70% of which were bilateral. Many of these patients had focal neurological symptoms and skull fractures as well. The EEG normalized in 48% of patients after 2 years, but foci persisted in 22% of the patients, and 30% remained diffusely abnormal. The most common abnormalities were delta rhythms (85%) and focal dysrhythmias with temporal localization (58%–82%, depending on criteria).

Although many clinicians have the impression that most posttraumatic seizures are generalized, all types of partial seizures can also occur (Salazar et al. 1985) and, in fact, are equal in presentation to the generalized seizures. The diagnosis of seizure disorders is a clinical diagnosis because the best diagnostic test is to observe someone having a seizure. All evaluations of suspected seizure disorders should include regular EEGs, especially a sleep EEG, which is four times more likely to show an abnormality than a waking EEG (Bazil et al. 2000; Crespel et al. 2000; Foldvary et al. 2000; Gibbs and Gibbs 1952; Malow et al. 2000).

Although some researchers advocate the use of nasopharyngeal leads, these actually increase the rate of abnormal findings by only 10% (Bickford 1979). Although a recent study by Pacia et al. (1998) reports an increased diagnostic yield for the diagnosis of temporal lobe seizures with sphenoidal leads, a previous study (Sadler and Goodwin 1989) shows that submandibular notch placement on the buccal skin surface is as effective as either nasopharyngeal or sphenoidal leads.

Prolactin levels have been shown to rise in patients with seizures and may be of some use in diagnosis (Dana-Haer and Trimble 1984). Recent studies using single-photon emission tomography show approximately a 30%–40% chance of demonstrating a seizure focus interictally and a 70%–80% chance if the study is done ictally (Lassen and Holm 1992; Lee et al. 1988). This may prove to be a useful technique for the confirmation of seizure foci in patients with TBI.

Pathogenesis

Although the etiology of posttraumatic seizures is not certain, the most frequently associated factor is the actual disruption of brain tissue. Almost any injury that penetrates the dura and the cortex results in a higher incidence of posttraumatic seizures. The incidence of posttraumatic seizures in penetrating injuries reported in the literature varies from 28% to 50% (Salazar et al. 1985). Some seizure disorders can be treated successfully by the surgical removal of cortical scar tissue (Spencer and Katz 1990). We can infer that cortical disruption, scarring, or irritability and the release of various endogenous neurotoxins (e.g., glutamate) can lead to the onset of posttraumatic seizures. Vespa et al. (1998), using implanted extracellular microdialysis probes, studied 17 patients with severe TBI. They found that extracellular glutamate was increased in these patients, particularly in relation to seizure activity.

Heikkmen et al. (1990) noted that although the severity of injury was most predictive of the development of early seizures (within the first 7 days postinjury), other specific factors were also associated with the onset of seizures, including periods of unconsciousness over 24 hours, skull fracture with dural tears, contusions, hematomas, and/or hemorrhage. The presence of subcortical atrophy or impaired local cerebral blood flow was most predictive of late-onset seizures occurring in the 3- to 12-month period after injury (Table 16–1). There is some recent evidence that mesial temporal sclerosis may be important in the development of post-TBI seizures (Marks et al. 1998). Diaz-Arrastia et al. (2000) studied 23 patients with intractable epilepsy after TBI and found that 35% had hippocampal sclerosis, and 2 of the patients had temporal lobectomies with relief of seizures.

In a prospective, observational study of 647 individuals admitted to trauma centers after TBI who had abnormal CT findings or a Glasgow Coma Scale score of 10 or lower during the first 24 hours, 66 patients developed a late seizure during a 24-month follow-up period. Patients with biparietal contusions (66%), dural penetration with bone and metal fragments (62.5%), multiple intracranial operations (36.5%), multiple subcortical contusions (33.4%), subdural hematoma with evacuation (27.8%), midline shift greater than 5 mm (25.8%), or multiple or bilateral cortical contusions (25%) (Englander et al. 2003) had the highest cumulative probability for the development of seizures.

Mazzini et al. (2003) found that the degrees of hydrocephalus and temporal lobe hypoperfusion (found on single-photon emission tomography) were risk factors for the development of late posttraumatic seizures.

After severe brain injury, hyperexcitable neurons may produce an epileptic focus between the time of the trauma and the seizure occurrence (Kuhl et al. 1990). There is biochemical evidence from animal studies (Mori et al. 1990) that the occurrence of posttraumatic seizures may be related to a breakdown of red blood cells and hemoglobin in the cerebral cortex, leading to release of free hydroxyl radicals into the central nervous system, subsequently affecting the neuronal membranes and leading to seizures. Although a recent review (Maas 2001) found that no study had demonstrated any positive effect with any neuroprotective antioxidants, it was also noted that the heterogeneity of the brain trauma group may prevent the demonstration of effectiveness. Weiss et al. (1982) noted a higher incidence of cerebral vascular accidents in patients with posttraumatic epilepsy. Proctor et al. (1988) used an experimental model for seizure development in closed head injury. Their research involved cats subjected to significant atmospheric fluid percussion impact (3.5 atmospheres administered to the cerebral cortex). They found that there were significant differences in seizure development related to measures of oxygenation and cytochrome A and adenosine triphosphate.

It remains unclear why one person develops seizures and another, with the same degree of brain trauma, does not. Weiss et al. (1982) and Salazar et al. (1985) reported no genetic predisposition or a family history of seizures in those who developed seizures. Inheritance of the APOE ε4 allele was found to be associated with increased risk of late posttraumatic seizures (Diaz-Arrastia et al. 2003). Two recent animal studies (Koh et al. 1999; Schmid et al. 1999) demonstrated that neonatal seizures, even though they did not cause cellular injury, predisposed the animals to brain-damaging effects of seizures in later life. Certainly age, as noted in the section Epidemiology, seems to be a factor, with both younger patients (younger than 14 years) and older patients (older than 65 years) being more prone to posttraumatic seizures (Annegers et al. 1998). It is also unclear why the prolonged prophylactic use of anticonvulsants leads to a greater incidence of seizures (Temkin et al. 1999).

Prognosis

What are the implications of seizures for the person with TBI? In most cases, seizures indicate that the person has had a more severe brain injury. This factor constantly leaves one with the question of whether the seizures further complicate the clinical course of a patient with severe brain injury or simply reflect the more extensive injury. In favor of the latter, Dikmen and Reitan (1978) reported

TABLE 16–1. Factors associated with early and late seizures after traumatic brain injury

Early seizures (within the first week)	Late seizures (after the first week)
Younger age (especially <5 years)	Age >65 years
Posttraumatic amnesia >24 hours	Posttraumatic amnesia >24 hours
Skull fracture (especially depressed)	Depressed skull fracture
Intracranial hemorrhage	Hematoma
Seizures during first week posttrauma	Early seizures
Penetrating injury	Penetrating injury
	High Glasgow Coma Scale score

Source. Data from Heikkmen ER, Routy HS, Tolonen H, et al: "Development of Posttraumatic Epilepsy." *Stereotactic and Functional Neurosurgery* 54/55:25–33, 1990.

that a group of posttraumatic epilepsy patients with cortical defects on neuropsychological testing had a worse prognosis than those with posttraumatic epilepsy who showed no cortical deficits. The patients with cortical deficits and seizures would be expected to do poorly because they are usually the most severely injured. Corkin et al. (1984) showed that patients with posttraumatic epilepsy had shorter life expectancies than brain-injured patients without seizures. Walker and Blumer (1989) followed, over a 40-year period, 244 World War II veterans who had penetrating brain injuries and seizure disorders and found that 101 had died (a figure much higher than expected in a general population). Thus, patients with posttraumatic epilepsy have an increased mortality. Weiss et al. (1982) confirmed this increased mortality in patients with post-TBI seizures and also demonstrated that 25% of all brain injury survivors showed deterioration in cognitive functions and earlier signs of aging.

The prognosis for posttraumatic seizures is good. Walker and Blumer (1989) studied a group of World War II veterans with TBI and noted that in those with seizures, 75% had no seizures after 10 years. They also pointed out that the type of injury that occurs in the military differs from civilian brain injuries. Civilian brain injuries are usually in the frontal-temporal region, whereas those associated with military injuries are usually penetrating and in rolandic (motor) and parietal regions and involve several lobes. Thus, the mortality and neurological deficit studies may not be generalizable to civilian populations. Weiss et al. (1986), in a 15-year follow-up study of 520 veterans, noted that 95% of the patients were seizure free 3 years after the trauma. The presence of substance or alcohol abuse was not a factor in the cessation of seizure activity. However, Salazar et al. (1985) noted that seizures could occur up to 15 years posttrauma in a group of Vietnam veterans. Although the majority of veterans (57%) developed seizures within the first year of injury, 15% did not develop seizures until 2 years after brain injury, and 18% developed seizures within 5 years (Weiss et al. 1986).

Armstrong et al. (1990) surveyed 300 consecutive brain trauma admissions to a rehabilitation hospital and, after excluding those with penetrating brain injuries or prior histories of epilepsy, found 87 patients with posttraumatic epilepsy (37%) and 151 patients (63%) with brain trauma and no posttraumatic epilepsy. In comparing these patients, they noted that the posttraumatic epilepsy group had a greater incidence of males than females. There were no differences between the two groups in frequency of skull fractures, hematomas, or hemorrhages, or in Halstead-Reitan Neuropsychological Test Battery results; however, there were marked differences in outcome in the patients

TABLE 16–2. Factors associated with the presence of seizures in brain-injured patients

Increased levels of	Decreased levels of
Rehabilitation hospital stays	Communicative ability
Mood and affective disorders	Motor function
Cerebrovascular accidents	Activities of daily living
	Orientation
	Life expectancy

who had posttraumatic epilepsy. Patients with posttraumatic epilepsy had a longer stay in the hospital, more difficulty with receptive language and intelligibility, decreased ability to perform activities of daily living, decreased motor function, and more mood and affective changes, as well as more problems with orientation. Although all of the patients made gains from admission to discharge, the posttraumatic epilepsy group started lower and ended lower, a further indication that posttraumatic seizures may simply be a marker of TBI severity.

Table 16–2 summarizes factors associated with the presence of seizures in patients with brain injury. The onset of seizures after TBI is a poor prognostic sign for general recovery, although, as noted, the seizures themselves often remit during the recovery years. The presence of focal neurological and cognitive deficits markedly worsens the prognosis. However, it is difficult to determine the exact contribution of the seizures to this poor prognosis because, as noted, these patients usually have had more severe initial brain injuries.

Psychopathology

Seizure disorders are associated with increases in psychopathology (McKenna et al. 1985; Trimble 1991; Tucker 2002) as is TBI (van Reekum et al. 2000). It is not clear if the presence of seizures in patients with TBI increases the risk for the development of psychopathology. The psychopathology associated with seizure disorders can range from personality changes to frank episodic or chronic psychosis. Patients with seizure disorders, when assessed in large studies, often show statistically significant increased incidence of such personality traits as impulsiveness and irritability, emotional lability, hyposexuality, hypergraphia, viscosity, paranoia, nightmares, fluidity of thinking, chronic pain, aggression, and philosophical or religious preoccupation. Those individuals who developed posttraumatic seizures had a significantly higher incidence of personality disorders, including uninhibited

---

TABLE 16–3. Psychopathological disorders that have been reported in traumatic brain injury patients with seizure disorders

---

Mood disorders (dysphoric, euphoric, rapid cycling, and mixed)

Irritable-impulsive disorders

Schizophreniform disorders (paranoid, delusional, and hallucinatory)

Anxiety disorders (panic, phobic, and generalized)

Amnestic-confusional disorders

Somatoform disorders (pseudoseizures and pain)

Personality disorders (viscous, hyperemotional, and changes in sexual behavior)

---

behavior, irritability, agitated behavior, and aggressive behavior than did patients with TBI who did not have seizures (Mazzini et al. 2003). Almost every psychopathological symptom (Table 16–3) has been well noted in patients with seizure disorders (Blumer et al. 1990; Tucker 2002). These characteristics also occur in patients with abnormal EEGs and probably relate to a general dysfunction of the central nervous system, rather than specifically to seizures.

Affective disturbances, primarily depression, with suicidal thoughts and even suicidal attempts are common in both patients with seizure disorders and patients with TBI (see Chapter 10, Mood Disorders). Shukla et al. (1987) analyzed 20 cases of patients who developed mania after brain injury and found an association with posttraumatic seizures. They emphasized that this type of mania involved irritable mood and aggressive behavior, rather than euphoria. They postulated that the predisposition to mania may result from the posttraumatic seizures, particularly because the study group had no family history of affective disorder, only 30% had any prior depressive episodes, and only 15% had prior mania.

Treatment of Behavioral Conditions

The basic initial treatment of the behavioral complications of seizure disorders in patients with brain trauma is the treatment of the seizures themselves. The seizures and often the psychopathology respond to traditional anticonvulsant medications (phenytoin, carbamazepine, sodium valproate, ethosuximide, primidone, clonazepam, and phenobarbital); however, the barbiturate derivatives seem to have more cognitive and depressive effects than the others (Brent et al. 1990; Farwell et al. 1990) (Table 16–4). Because physicians often use anticonvulsants in a

prophylactic manner in brain-injured patients, one must first assess whether the behavioral and cognitive problems are not due to the anticonvulsant. Consequently, in the patient without seizures, one should consider stopping the anticonvulsants if no seizures are present. This is particularly important because studies have repeatedly shown little benefit of prophylactic anticonvulsant treatment in preventing the occurrence of seizures in patients with brain injury (McQueen et al. 1983; Perry et al. 1979; Temkin et al. 1990; Young et al. 1983). In the depressed, psychotic, or agitated patient with TBI with no posttraumatic seizures, one should first use the appropriate psychopharmacological agents for these conditions. However, even if a seizure disorder cannot be documented and there is no response to appropriate pharmacotherapy treatments, it would be appropriate to try anticonvulsants, hypothesizing that some occult seizure disorder or cerebral dysrhythmia may be present.

When seizures are present with behavioral symptoms, particularly episodic symptoms of psychosis, depressive feelings, or impulsive behavior, the first approach is to re-evaluate the existing anticonvulsants or begin anticonvulsant treatment. The behavioral symptoms seem to respond best to anticonvulsant blood levels in the mid to upper therapeutic ranges. It is important to keep the blood levels of anticonvulsants within the therapeutic window because there can be an increased occurrence of behavioral and cognitive impairments with levels beyond the therapeutic window and even an increased risk of seizures with toxic phenytoin levels. However, if there is no symptomatic response to anticonvulsants in the therapeutic blood level range, then medicating beyond the usual therapeutic range may be attempted to determine whether the targeted behavioral symptoms decrease in frequency or occurrence. Although earlier studies have noted that carbamazepine is associated with less cognitive impairment (Dodrill and Troupin 1977; Trimble 1987), recent studies have shown that there is cognitive impairment with all anticonvulsants when used in therapeutic ranges (Dodrill and Troupin 1991; Gillham et al. 1988; Massagli 1991; Meador et al. 1990); however, there is some evidence that such side effects are less with gabapentin and lamotrigine (Martin et al. 1999; Meador et al. 1999). The cognitive impairments noted with these anticonvulsants are in the area of attention and concentration, memory, information processing, and motor speed, all of which are frequently encountered in brain trauma. Consequently, it is clear how these medications in themselves may exacerbate certain deficits. Therefore, if the anticonvulsant-treated patient worsens, consider a decrease in these medications, which may improve some of the behavioral symptoms. Although most of the cognitive

TABLE 16–4. Daily doses, effective blood levels, and serum half-lives of anticonvulsants

Anticonvulsant	Usual daily dose (mg)	Effective blood level (µg/mL)	Serum half-life (hours)
Carbamazepine	200–2,000	6–12	12
Clonazepam	1–10	0.01–0.07	18–50
Ethosuximide	1,500–2,000	40–100	40
Gabapentin	1,800–3,600	4–16	5–7
Lamotrigine	100–500	2–16	12–60
Phenobarbital	60–200	10–40	96
Phenytoin	100–600	10–20	24
Primidone	250–1,500	5–15	12
Topiramate	200–400	4–10	19–25
Valproic acid	500–3,000	50–100	8

effects are dose dependent, they may occur in therapeutic blood level ranges. Some patients' seizures respond better to one anticonvulsant than another, and, if there is no response, serial medication trials should be undertaken. If the cognitive or other side effects are considerable with one anticonvulsant, it is worth attempting a change. The main anticonvulsants that have been used in the treatment of seizure disorders in posttraumatic epilepsy are listed in Table 16–4; there have been no controlled studies of the more recently marketed antiepileptic drugs (Temkin 2001). The drug interactions of these medications, not only with each other but also with psychotropic medications, are complex and varied (Duncan et al. 1991). As a result, frequent blood level checks are useful when anticonvulsants are combined either with each other or with other medications.

If the behavioral symptoms, particularly those of an affective or psychotic nature, do not respond to manipulation of the anticonvulsants, it is appropriate to use low doses of either neuroleptics or antidepressant medication. These patients are extremely sensitive to medication changes, so any adjustments should be done slowly and gradually. Although neuroleptics and many of the antidepressant medications may lower seizure threshold, in small doses they can be extremely helpful for the behavioral symptoms of these patients.

A number of patients will respond to surgical intervention, such as scar excision or lobectomy. With surgical treatment, it has been noted that after 40 years 51% of patients had no significant seizures and 11% had focal seizures. Of those medically treated, 63% of patients had no seizures after 40 years and only 8% had minor seizures; the rest continued to have seizures (Walker and Blumer 1989).

As noted in the section Psychopathology, the emotional burden of having seizures often complicates the clinical course for patients already coping with serious brain injury. The emotional impact on the patient and the family is considerable and adds significantly to the rehabilitation task. Certainly, patients with TBI and seizures can have the same emotional problems that any person with a seizure disorder has. However, the brain-injured patient has additional problems that Lezak (1978) clearly defined in what has now become a classic article. She noted the following five broad areas where behavior may become impaired:

1. Social and interpersonal perceptiveness
2. Capacity for self-regulation and control
3. Stimulus-bound behavior
4. Emotional control (e.g., apathy, irritability, lability)
5. Ability to profit from experience

These problems are compounded by the seizure disorder because seizures still carry a tremendous stigma as well as the potential to cause actual, often dangerous, lapses in behavior and attention. These two factors combine to mandate a psychotherapeutic approach that is first psychoeducational (Helgeson et al. 1990; Whitman and Hermann 1986). The patient, and particularly the family or the caregivers, must be educated about the behavioral and cognitive effects of TBI, seizures, and anticonvulsants. The family must learn what behaviors are associated with TBI and seizures and that any anger or apathy demonstrated by the patient is not related to the patient's feelings about them but to his or her illness. They must also learn behavioral strategies to deal with these behaviors and be counseled about how to take care of themselves and how to take time off from their care-taking responsibilities.

Conclusion

TBI is an etiologic cause of convulsive seizures. The primary treatment of these seizures is the use of anti-convulsants. Because there are many different anticon-vulsants, the clinician may try different anticonvulsants in a sequential fashion until seizure control is achieved. All of the anticonvulsants have blood levels for which therapeutic ranges have been established, so the clini-cian can titrate the clinical response to the dose by fol-lowing the anticonvulsant blood levels (see Table 16–4). At times, if there is no response from monotherapy, two anticonvulsants can be combined, again maintaining the appropriate blood levels of both drugs. In the patient with seizures, behavioral symptoms should be treated initially with anticonvulsants, again trying to keep the blood levels in the higher therapeutic range. Of course, even without overt seizures, if the patient has the onset of clear episodic behavioral symptoms, such as hallucinations, affective symptoms, and panic attacks, it may be appropriate to try anticonvulsants first. However, in the patient with post-TBI seizures, once adequate seizure control has been achieved the behavioral symptoms should be treated with appropri-ate pharmacotherapy. However, each TBI patient with seizures presents a unique therapeutic problem. Because there are so few of these patients, there are almost no large-scale studies of the systematic use of psychopharmacological agents in their treatment. As a result, each patient becomes a unique therapeutic chal-lenge or experiment and one must often try many dif-ferent agents or combinations of agents to achieve behavioral improvement.

It is clear that the presence of seizures is an added bur-den psychologically, socially, and cognitively for the pa-tient with TBI. Whether seizures are simply related to more severe brain injury or whether some patients just have a predisposition to seizures, they certainly compli-cate the rehabilitation task.

References

Annegers JF, Grabow J, Groover RV, et al: Seizures after head trauma: a population study. Neurology 30:683–689, 1980

Annegers J, Hauser W, Coan S, et al: A population-based study of seizures after traumatic brain injury. N Engl J Med 338:20–24, 1998

Armstrong KK, Sahgal V, Block R, et al: Rehabilitation out-comes in patients with post-traumatic epilepsy. Arch Phys Med Rehabil 71:156–160, 1990

Bazil C: Antiepileptic drugs in the 21st century. CNS Spectr 6:756–765, 2001

Bazil C, Castro L, Walczak T: Reduction of rapid eye movement sleep by diurnal and nocturnal seizures in temporal lobe ep-ilepsy. Arch Neurol 57:363–368, 2000

Bickford RG: Activation procedures and special electrodes, in Current Practice of Clinical Electroencephalography. Ed-ited by Kass D, Daly DD. New York, Raven, 1979

Blumer D, Neppe V, Benson DF: Diagnostic criteria for epilepsy-related mental changes. Am J Psychiatry 147:676–677, 1990

Brain Injury Special Interest Group of the American Academy of Physical Medicine and Rehabilitation: Practice parame-ter: antiepileptic drug treatment of posttraumatic seizures. Arch Phys Med Rehabil 79:594–597, 1998

Brain Trauma Foundation: The American Association of Neu-rological Surgeons: role of antiseizure prophylaxis follow-ing head injury. J Neurotrauma 17:549–553, 2000

Brent DA, Crumrine PK, Varma R, et al: Phenobarbital treat-ment and major depressive disorder in children with epi-lepsy. Pediatrics 85:1086–1091, 1990

Corkin S, Sullivan EV, Carr A: Prognostic factors for life expec-tancy after penetrating head injury. Arch Neurol 41:975–977, 1984

Crespel A, Coubes P, Bald-Moulinier: Sleep influence on seizures and epilepsy effects on sleep in partial frontal and temporal lobe seizures. Clin Neurophysiol 111 (suppl 2): S54–59, 2000

Diaz-Arrastia R, Gong Y, Fair S, et al: Increased risk of late post-traumatic seizures associated with inheritance of APOE e4 allele. Arch Neurol 60:818–822, 2003

Dana-Haer J, Trimble MR: Prolactin and gonadotropin changes following partial seizures in epileptic patients with and without psychopathology. Biol Psychiatry 19:329–336, 1984

Desai B, Whitman S, Bouffard DA: The role of the EEG in ep-ilepsy of long duration. Epilepsia 29:601–606, 1988

Diaz-Arrastia R, Agostini M, Frol A, et al: Neurophysiologic and neuroradiologic features of intractable epilepsy after traumatic brain injury in adults. Arch Neurol 57:1611–1616, 2000

Dikmen S, Reitan R: Neuropsychological performance in post-traumatic epilepsy. Epilepsia 19:177–183, 1978

Dikmen S, Machamer M, Winn H, et al: Neuropsychological effects of valproate in traumatic brain injury. Neurology 54:895–902, 2000

Dodrill CB, Troupin AS: Psychometric effects of carbamazepine in epilepsy. Neurology 27:1023–1028, 1977

Dodrill CB, Troupin AS: Neuropsychological effects of carba-mazepine and phenytoin: a reanalysis. Neurology 41:141–143, 1991

Duncan J, Potsalas P, Ghorvan S: Effects of discontinuation of phenytoin, carbamazepine, and valproate on concom-itant antiepileptic medication. Epilepsia 32:101–115, 1991

Englander J, Bushnik T, Duong TT, et al: Analyzing risk factors for late posttraumatic seizures: a prospective, multicenter investigation. Arch Phys Med Rehabil 84:365–373, 2003

Farwell J, Lee YJ, Hirtz DG, et al: Phenobarbital for febrile seizures: effects on intelligence and seizure recurrence. N Engl J Med 332:364–370, 1990

Foldvary H, Caruso A, Mascha E, et al: Identifying montages that best detect electrographic seizure activity during polysomnography. Sleep 15:221–229, 2000

Gibbs FA, Gibbs EL: Atlas of Electroencephalography. Cambridge, MA, Addison-Wesley, 1952

Gillham RA, Williams N, Wiedmann, et al: Concentration-effect relationships with carbamazepine and its epoxide on psychomotor and cognitive function in epileptic patients. J Neurol Neurosurg Psychiatry 51:929–933, 1988

Heikkmen ER, Routy HS, Tolonen U, et al: Development of posttraumatic epilepsy. Stereotact Funct Neurosurg 54/55:25–33, 1990

Helgeson DC, Mittan R, Tan SY, et al: Sepulveda Epilepsy Education: the efficacy of a psychoeducational treatment program in treating medical and psychosocial aspects of epilepsy. Epilepsia 31:75–82, 1990

Jabbari B, Vengrow MI, Salazar AM, et al: Clinical and radiological correlates of EEG in the late phase of head injury: a study of 515 Vietnam veterans. Electroencephalogr Clin Neurophysiol 64:285–293, 1986

Jennett WB: Epilepsy after Non-Missile Injuries, 2nd Edition. Chicago, IL, Year Book Medical, 1975

Koh S, Storey T, Santos B, et al: Early seizures in rats increase susceptibility to seizure-induced brain injury in adulthood. Neurology 53:915, 1999

Koufen H, Hagel KH: Systematic EEG follow-up study of traumatic psychosis. Eur Arch Psychiatry Neurol Sci 237:2–7, 1987

Kuhl DA, Boucher BA, Buhlbauer MS: Prophylaxis of post-traumatic seizures. DICP 24:277–285, 1990

Lassen NA, Holm S: Single photon emission computerized tomography (SPECT), in Clinical Brain Imaging. Edited by Mazziotta JC, Gilman S. Philadelphia, PA, FA Davis, 108–134, 1992

Lee BI, Markland ON, Wellman HN, et al: HIDPM-SPECT in patients with medically intractable complex partial seizures. Arch Neurol 45:397–402, 1988

Lezak M: Living with the characterologically altered brain injured patient. J Clin Psychiatry 39:592–598, 1978

Lishman WA: Organic Psychiatry, 2nd Edition. Oxford, UK, Blackwell, 1987

Maas A: Neuroprotective agents in traumatic brain injury. Expert Opin Investig Drugs 10:753–767, 2001

Malow A, Bowes R, Ross D: Relationship of temporal lobe seizures to sleep and arousal: a combined scalp-intracranial electrode study. Sleep 15:231–234, 2000

Marks D, Kim J, Spencer D, et al: Seizure localization and pathology following head injury in patients with uncontrolled epilepsy. Neurology 45:2051–2057, 1995

Marsh NV, Knight R: Behavioral assessment of social competence following severe head injury. J Clin Exp Neuropsychol 13:729–740, 1991

Martin R, Kusniecky S, Hetherington J, et al. Cognitive effects of topiramate, gabapentin, lamotrigine in healthy young adults. Neurology 52:321–327, 1999

Massagli T: Neurobehavioral effects of phenytoin, carbamazepine, and valproic acid: implications for use in traumatic brain injury. Arch Phys Med Rehabil 72:219–226, 1991

Matthews CG: The neuropsychology of epilepsy. J Clin Exp Neuropsychol 14:133–143, 1992

Mazzini L, Cossa FM, Angelino E, et al: Posttraumatic epilepsy: neuroradiologic and neuropsychological assessment of long-term outcome. Epilepsia 44:569–574, 2003

McKenna PJ, Kane JM, Parrish K: Psychotic syndromes in epilepsy. Am J Psychiatry 142:895–904, 1985

McQueen JK, Blackwood DNR, Harris P, et al: Low risk of late post-traumatic seizures following severe head injury. J Neurol Neurosurg Psychiatry 46:899–904, 1983

Meador KJ, Loring D, Huh BB, et al: Comparative cognitive effects of anticonvulsants. Neurology 40:391–394, 1990

Meador K, Loring D, Ray P, et al: Differential cognitive effects of carbamazepine and gabapentin. Epilepsia 40:1279–1285, 1999

Mori A, Hiromatsu M, Yoko I, et al: Biochemical pathogenesis of post-traumatic epilepsy. Pavlov J Biol Sci 25:54–62, 1990

Pacia S, Jung W, Devinsky O: Localization of mesial temporal lobe seizures with sphenoidal electrodes. J Clin Neurophysiol 15:256–261, 1998

Parasuraman R, Mutter S, Malloy R: Sustained attention following mild closed-head injury. J Clin Exp Neuropsychol 13:789–811, 1991

Perry JK, While BG, Brackett CE: A controlled prospective study of the pharmacologic prophylaxis of post-traumatic epilepsy. Neurology 29:600–601, 1979

Proctor HJ, Palladino GW, Fillipo D: Failure of autoregulation after closed head injury: an experimental model. J Trauma 28:347–352, 1988

Sadler M, Goodwin J: Multiple electrodes for detecting spikes in partial complex seizures. Can J Neurol Sci 16:326–329, 1989

Salazar AM, Jabbari B, Vance SC, et al: Epilepsy after penetrating head injury. Neurology 35:1406–1414, 1985

Sarna MT: The nature of verbal impairment after closed head injury. J Nerv Ment Dis 168:685–692, 1980

Schmid R, Tandon P, Stafstrom C, et al: Effects of neonatal injury on subsequent seizure-induced brain injury. Neurology 53:1754, 1999

Shukla S, Cook BL, Mukherjee S, et al: Mania following head trauma. Am J Psychiatry 144:93–96, 1987

Spencer S, Katz A: Arriving at the surgical options for intractable seizures. Senior Neurology 4:422–430, 1990

Temkin N: Antiepileptogenesis and seizure prevention trials with antiepileptic drugs: meta-analysis of controlled trials. Epilepsia 42:515–524, 2001

Temkin N, Dikmen S, Wilensky S, et al: A randomized double-blind study of phenytoin for the prevention of post-traumatic seizures. N Engl J Med 323:497–502, 1990

Temkin N, Dikmen S, Anderson O, et al: Valproate therapy for prevention of posttraumatic seizures: a randomized trial. J Neurosurg 91:593–600, 1999

Temkin O: The Falling Sickness, 2nd Edition. Baltimore, MD, Johns Hopkins University Press, 1971

Trimble MR: Anticonvulsant drugs and cognitive function: a review of the literature. Epilepsia 28 (suppl):S37–S45, 1987

Trimble MR: The Psychosis of Epilepsy. New York, Rover, 1991

Tucker G: Neuropsychiatric aspects of seizure disorders, in The American Psychiatric Textbook of Neuropsychiatry, 4th Edition. Edited by Yudofsky S, Hales R. Washington, DC, American Psychiatric Press, 2002

van Reekum R, Cohen T, Wong J: Can traumatic brain injury cause psychotic disorders? J Neuropsychiatry Clin Neurosci 12:316–327, 2000

Vespa P, Prinz M, Ronne-Engstrom E, et al: Increase in extracellular glutamate caused by reduced cerebral perfusion pressure and seizures after human traumatic brain injury: a microdialysis study. J Neurosurg 89:971–982, 1998

Walker AE, Blumer D: The fate of World War II veterans with post-traumatic seizures. Arch Neurol 46:23–26, 1989

Weiss GH, Caveness WF, Eisiedei-Lechtape H, et al: Life expectancy and courses of deaths in a group of head injured veterans of World War I. Arch Neurol 39:741–743, 1982

Weiss GH, Salazar AM, Vance SC, et al: Predicting post-traumatic epilepsy in penetrating brain injury. Arch Neurol 43:771–773, 1986

Whitman S, Hermann BP: Psychopathology in Epilepsy. New York, Oxford University Press, 1986

Young B, Rapp RP, Norton J, et al: Failure of prophylactically administered phenytoin to prevent late post-traumatic seizures. Neurosurgery 58:236–241, 1983

PART III

Neuropsychiatric Symptomatologies

17 Cognitive Changes

Scott McCullagh, M.D.

Anthony Feinstein, M.D., Ph.D.

COGNITIVE CHANGES ARE often the most salient features after closed traumatic brain injury (TBI) of any severity. After more severe injuries, disturbed cognition is the most commonly cited problem by patients and caregivers years later (Oddy et al. 1985; van Zomeren and van den Burg 1985), and it typically contributes more to persisting disability than physical impairment (Brooks et al. 1987).

The extent of cognitive deficit after TBI reflects a number of factors, the most important being 1) the severity of diffuse axonal injury, as indicated by the length of posttraumatic amnesia (PTA), the extent of generalized atrophy; and 2) the location, depth, and volume of focal cerebral lesions (Katz and Alexander 1994; Wilson et al. 1995). Other critical factors include the patient's age, preexisting morbidities, and the occurrence of significant extracranial or systemic injury (e.g., hypoxia or hypotension). The apolipoprotein E genotype may also contribute, but the evidence to date is somewhat mixed (Millar et al. 2003; Sundstrom et al. 2004). Despite a wide range of potential deficits after TBI, there is a degree of consistency as to the nature and frequency of difficulties observed. This occurs because of the concentration of damage in the anterior regions of the brain (Gentry et al. 1988). With more severe diffuse injury, involvement of more central regions such as the rostral brainstem is increasingly seen. Although discrete focal lesions may produce classic neurobehavioral syndromes such as aphasia, these are commonly superimposed on the more global dysfunction resulting from diffuse injury (Katz 1992).

This chapter emphasizes four cognitive domains that are commonly impaired after closed TBI: attention, memory, executive function, and language/communication. Particular implications for psychosocial/functional recovery exist for impairment within each area. The sim-

ilarity between mild and more severe brain injury is discussed—the two represent different locations on a continuum of cerebral involvement (Reitan and Wolfson 2000). However, the former generally has a much better prognosis. This chapter concludes with a review of the evidence supporting pharmacological interventions to enhance cognitive function after TBI.

Impairments of Attention

Impaired attentional processes are prevalent, if not universal, after TBI at all levels of injury severity (Gronwall 1987; Table 17–1).

During PTA, patients may demonstrate impaired awareness and wandering attention, whereas inability to concentrate for more than a few minutes and distractibility characterize the early phases of recovery (Katz 1992). At later stages, impairments may only be revealed with rigorous testing. Because attention underpins all aspects of cognition, even mild impairments can restrict other processes such as the capacity for new learning. Common subjective complaints include mental slowing, trouble following conversation, loss of train of thought, and difficulty attending to two things at once (Gronwall 1987; van Zomeren and Brouwer 1994).

Attention is not a unitary phenomenon; it can be subdivided using a commonly applied taxonomy that includes selective, sustained, and divided components, as well as information-processing speed and supervisory or executive aspects (see Table 17–1; van Zomeren and Brouwer 1994). These elements reflect the interactions of several widely dispersed networks (Fernandez-Duque and Posner 2001). For example, a network for spatial selective attention has been described that includes the posterior

TABLE 17–1.   Aspects of attention potentially impaired after traumatic brain injury

Arousal/alertness: general receptivity to sensory information and readiness to make a response

Selective attention: ability to select target information from a broad field of stimuli and inhibit irrelevant stimuli

Sustained attention: ability to sustain attention toward a source of information or task over a prolonged period (i.e., vigilance)

Divided attention: ability to share or divide attention between two or more sources of information or task demands at the same time

Information processing speed: rate at which information is processed within the central nervous system to allow cognitive activities to occur

"Supervisory control" aspects: involve the "top-down" coordination of lower-level attentional processes to perform complex, nonroutine tasks consistent with drives and intentions; the allocation of limited attentional resources is an essential feature at this level

Note.   "Components" of attention, as with other cognitive domains, are hypothetical constructs devised to integrate clinical observations, neuropsychological test results, and theoretical models of cognition. As such, they refer to interrelated rather than discrete processes and also overlap with other domains such as memory.

parietal, dorsal frontal, and cingulate regions, in concert with components of the basal ganglia, thalamus, and superior colliculi. These cortical regions may respectively provide sensory, motor-exploratory, and limbic-motivational "maps" to guide the targeting of attention. The brainstem reticular formation supports the overall attentional "tone" or degree of responsiveness to stimuli (Mesulam 2000).

It is thus apparent that focal or diffuse injury during TBI may disrupt these circuits, potentially impairing different aspects of attention. Although there is some debate as to the precise nature of the deficits after TBI, the greatest unanimity exists with respect to reduced information-processing speed. This frequent complaint corresponds with robust psychometric findings after TBI. Compared with control subjects, TBI patients demonstrate a slowing of reaction time (RT) that is proportional to task complexity. Choice RT paradigms, which require decision making among a number of alternative responses, have proved very sensitive to brain injury (Gronwall 1987; van Zomeren and Deelman 1978). Choice RT tasks can discriminate between grades of TBI severity and demonstrate improvement over time, although persisting deficits in patients with severe TBI are observed at 2 years or more (van Zomeren and Deelman 1978). Although it taps

a number of cognitive processes, the Paced Auditory Serial Addition Task (Gronwall 1977) has been used extensively to study processing efficiency after TBI. In this task, subjects are presented with a series of single-digit numbers verbally and instructed to add each new digit to the one immediately preceding it. Task difficulty is varied by adjusting the time interval between the items presented. Performance on this measure has been shown to correlate with injury severity, to track recovery of attentional capacities, and to predict return to vocational activities (Lezak 1995). Reduction in cognitive efficiency is thought to result from diffuse white matter dysfunction incurred during TBI.

In addition to cognitive slowing, deficits have been examined with respect to selective, sustained, and divided attentional components. Results are at times contradictory and may differ regarding the precise mechanisms underlying a particular deficit (Rios et al. 2004). For example, some investigators have hypothesized that slowed processing after TBI may explain many of the other attentional difficulties that are observed (Ponsford and Kinsella 1992; Spikman et al. 1996).

Notwithstanding, abnormalities of selective attention (i.e., the ability to inhibit processing of irrelevant stimuli, or distractions) and sustained attention (i.e., the ability to maintain performance over extended periods, or vigilance) have been reported in moderate to severe TBI (Kewman et al. 1988; Loken et al. 1995; Schmitter-Edgecombe and Kibby 1998). In a simulated classroom setting, Whyte et al. (2000) found that TBI patients demonstrated a greater rate of "off-task" behavior compared with control subjects when completing a task in the face of distracting stimuli.

The findings are quite consistent in the case of divided attention (Brouwer et al. 2001; Park et al. 1999; Zoccolotti et al. 2000), which is a frequent complaint. Impairments in this area appear to characterize TBI patients at all levels of severity (Cicerone 1996; Zoccolotti et al. 2000). More recently, the assessment of divided attention under dual task conditions (i.e., performing simultaneous tasks) has proved to be a sensitive means to probe deficits that may go otherwise undetected. Using paradigms that have controlled for slowed processing, recent dual-task studies point toward limitations of executive or "supervisory control" aspects of attention (Dell'Acqua et al. 2001; Park et al. 1999; Spikman et al. 2001). This component of the attentional system is hypothesized to govern lower-level attentional processes and includes the allocation of attentional resources, target selection, interference control, switching between tasks, error monitoring, and so forth (Rios et al. 2004). It is conceived as a limited-capacity component that is involved in the "effortful" or "stra-

---

TABLE 17–2. Aspects of learning and memory potentially impaired after traumatic brain injury

---

Declarative memory

  Episodic memory for events: encoding, consolidation, and retrieval

  Semantic memory for general facts

Implicit memory[a]

  Procedural learning

  Priming

  Conditioning

Aspects of memory related to executive functions

  Working memory

  Strategic memory

  Prospective memory

  Metamemory

  Source (or context) memory

---

[a]This memory component appears much less vulnerable to the effects of traumatic brain injury.

tegic" processing of nonroutine tasks—as opposed to those in which information is processed automatically. Thus, TBI patients perform significantly worse than control subjects when two tasks require *working memory* (see section Impairments of Learning and Memory), which is considered an essential component of controlled attentional processing (Park et al. 1999).

On balance, the weight of evidence clearly supports abnormalities in a number of aspects of attention, irrespective of TBI severity. Thus, even in patients with mild TBI, deficits in information processing and attention are considered principal features of the early postconcussional phase (Gronwall 1991). Nonetheless, studies of uncomplicated mild TBI demonstrate that resolution of cognitive deficits within 1–3 months is the norm (Gronwall 1991). This is not the case after more severe injuries, in which residual deficits of attentional functions can be expected.

Impairments of Learning and Memory

Memory dysfunction is a cardinal feature after TBI (Table 17–2). It is most dramatically apparent during the early intervals of retrograde amnesia and PTA, the duration of which strongly predicts eventual outcome. Yet, in the post-acute stage and beyond, it remains perhaps the most common subjective complaint (King et al. 1995; van Zomeren and van den Burg 1985). Using objective measures, both

verbal and nonverbal memory dysfunction have been repeatedly shown across the range of severity (Richardson 2000). In moderately to severely injured patients, dysfunction may persist despite the normalization of IQ scores over the course of recovery (Levin et al. 1988). The importance of concurrently assessing other processes that influence learning and memory, such as attention and executive function, has been emphasized (Lezak 1995).

Memory can be divided into two components: declarative (including episodic memory for personal events and semantic memory for facts) and implicit (occurring outside of conscious awareness, including procedural learning, priming, and conditioning) (Markowitsch 2000; see Table 17–2). After TBI, impairment of episodic memory is a hallmark feature (Richardson 2000). Some investigators report dysfunction at all stages of episodic processing, including encoding, consolidation, and retrieval (Curtiss et al. 2001), whereas others posit deficits at specific stages (Vanderploeg et al. 2001). For example, failure to apply strategies when learning—such as grouping words by semantic category (e.g., "fruit")—has often been described (Curtiss et al. 2001; Levin and Goldstein 1986). The significant heterogeneity observed among patients suggests that distinct patterns of memory deficit may characterize subgroups of patients (Curtiss et al. 2001). In general, tasks that require effortful, controlled, and generally conscious processing—as opposed to automatic processes that occur unconsciously—show the greatest degree of disruption. Thus, implicit memory is relatively spared after TBI (Shum et al. 1996).

Other aspects of memory associated with executive processing are vulnerable to injury. TBI affects working memory, which is considered a temporary, limited-capacity storage system required during activities such as language comprehension and problem solving (Markowitsch 2000). The control aspects of working memory are mediated by frontal systems. Dysfunction of these aspects may only be revealed by using more complex procedures such as dual-task paradigms (Park et al. 1999). A related construct known as *prospective memory*, or the ability to remember one's future intentions, is a frequent difficulty after TBI (Kinsella et al. 1996). Thus, forgetting appointments, payment of bills, and so on may occur despite relatively normal scores on tests of new learning (Kinsella et al. 1996). Additionally, TBI patients often regard their memory function as better than that suggested by reports of caregivers. This discrepancy indicates a deficit of *metamemory*, or self-awareness of memory efficiency. In a recent study, moderate- to severe-TBI patients showed reduced ability to gauge their performance during formal memory testing compared with control subjects (Kennedy and Yorkston 2000). A more accurate picture of function may be obtained by using a measure of "everyday memory" (Wills et al. 2000), which includes analogues of daily tasks such as remembering to deliver a message, remembering the location of belongings, and remembering people's names.

Neuroimaging studies provide a basis for understanding memory impairments post-TBI. The consistent magnetic resonance imaging (MRI) finding of hippocampal atrophy (Tate and Bigler 2000), the sensitivity of this structure to multiple injury effects, and the crucial role it plays in declarative memory strongly implicate damage to the hippocampal network as a major contributor to memory deficits after TBI. However, Bigler and colleagues (Tate and Bigler 2000) note that only modest correlations between hippocampal size and reduced memory performance are observed, pointing to the significance of injury elsewhere. The prefrontal areas represent another susceptible region, given the mounting evidence for their involvement in the tasks of encoding and retrieval (Cabeza and Nyberg 2000). The contribution of diffuse injury is further emphasized by the fact that memory deficit has shown greater correlation with severity indicators such as PTA duration and Glasgow Coma Scale score than with the presence of specific focal lesions on neuroimaging (Levin et al. 1992; Richardson 2000).

In mild TBI, prospective studies demonstrate that, as with attention, early impairment on formal memory tests tends to resolve fully over 1–3 months (Ruff et al. 1989). However, a discrepancy between neuropsychological recovery and persisting subjective complaints has been described (Ruff et al. 1989). It is possible that residual memory inefficiency contributes to a sense of "forgetfulness" that is not tapped by standard tests of episodic memory. A study of working memory using functional MRI offers some support for this idea (McAllister et al. 1999). Despite test performance similar to that of control subjects, mild TBI patients examined at 1 month postinjury showed more extensive cerebral activation as working memory load increased. This finding suggests that mild TBI patients may have to work harder to maintain premorbid levels of cognitive performance (McAllister et al. 1999).

In contrast to the spontaneous recovery seen in mild TBI, a recent longitudinal study of moderate to severe TBI confirmed the presence of substantial memory impairments in 50% of subjects at 5 years postinjury (Millis et al. 2001).

Impairments of Frontal Executive Functions

The term *executive functions* refers to a set of higher-order capabilities that are considered the domain of the frontal

---

TABLE 17–3.   Aspects of executive functions potentially impaired after traumatic brain injury

Goal establishment, planning, and anticipation of consequences

Initiation, sequencing, and inhibition of behavioral responses

Generation of multiple response alternatives (in contrast to preserverative or stereotyped responses)

Conceptual/inferential reasoning, problem solving

Mental flexibility/ease of mental and behavioral switching

Transcending the immediately salient aspects of a situation (in contrast to "stimulus bound behavior" or "environmental dependency")

Executive attentional processes

Executive memory processes

Self-monitoring and self-regulation, including emotional responses

Social adaptive functioning[a]: sensitivity to others, using social feedback, engaging in contextually appropriate social behavior

[a]For further discussion, see Eslinger et al. (1996) and Chapter 13, Personality Disorders, in this volume.

---

lobes and their projections (Stuss and Levine 2002). They govern and use subordinate mental activities such as attention, memory, language, and perceptual functions in the mediation of real-world problems. Specific frontal executive "tasks" include establishing goals and planning; initiating, sequencing, and inhibiting responses; conceptual reasoning; decision making; as well as the activities of self-monitoring and self-regulation (Stuss and Levine 2002; Table 17–3).

Deficits in executive function are a critical determinant of functional outcome after TBI (Crepeau and Scherzer 1993). Historically, a parallel has been noted between the pattern of deficit seen after severe TBI and that resulting from focal frontal lobe damage (Stuss and Gow 1992). This association is strengthened by the fact that TBI has a strong predilection for the anterior portions of the brain, with polar and ventral frontal and temporal regions being particularly prone to contusional damage (Adams et al. 1985; Levin et al. 1992). Additionally, although diffuse axonal injury is observed throughout the neuraxis, it too may be more concentrated in the anterior regions (Gentry et al. 1988).

The understanding of frontal lobe functions has been advanced with the identification of several frontal-subcortical circuits and their neurobehavioral correlates (Alexander and Crutcher 1990; Cummings 1993). The dorsolateral prefrontal circuit, in particular, is considered important for executive function because impairments of planning, organization, and working memory follow focal injury to this cortical region. Notably, a similar picture may result from damage at other points along this network, which involves sequential projections to regions of striatum, pallidum, and thalamus that ultimately return to the prefrontal cortex (Cummings 1993).

Studies in patients with moderate to severe TBI have found deficits of verbal/design fluency (Levin et al. 1991; Millis et al. 2001), conceptual reasoning/flexibility on the Wisconsin Card Sorting Test (Gansler et al. 1996; Millis et al. 2001; Stuss et al. 1985), working memory (Stuss et al. 1985), application of strategic memory (Levin and Goldstein 1986), planning (Leon-Carrion et al. 1998), and executive attentional processes (Levin et al. 1991; Zoccolotti et al. 2000). When examining the neuroanatomical basis for these findings, however, several investigators have found stronger correlations with indicators of diffuse injury (e.g., coma depth and generalized atrophy) than with the presence or absence of a demonstrable frontal lesion (Anderson et al. 1995; Vilkki et al. 1996). Thus, marked executive impairment may occur in the absence of an identifiable "frontal" lesion (Goldberg et al. 1989), a circumstance that emphasizes the need to consider dysfunction of wider networks because of axonal injury.

Another important issue is that performance on traditional tests of executive function may fail to capture the substantial deficits in real-life decision-making and interpersonal function that often follow severe TBI (Levine et al. 2000; Pachalska et al. 2002; Sbordone 2001). These vital aspects of behavior are linked to the integrity of ventral frontal regions, which often bear the brunt of TBI-related damage and yet fall outside the domain of routine cognitive testing. Given the prominence of the orbitofrontal cortex in emotional processing and mediation of stimulus-reward associations (Rolls 2000), marked impairment of self-regulation may follow disruption of networks associated with this region. Novel measures have been devised that may tap these aspects of executive function (Bechara et al. 1994; Levine et al. 2000). In these paradigms, subjects must discern strategies in relatively unstructured situations in which the "correct" responses are not readily suggested by the task itself. Thus, Levine et al. (2000) found that deficits of self-regulation correlated with TBI severity as well as current social/occupational dysfunction. These relationships appeared to be independent of performance on other neuropsychological tests, including the Wisconsin Card Sorting Test.

There is evidence for dysfunction of executive processes in mild TBI, at least early in the course of recovery, with reduced verbal fluency a frequent finding (J. Brooks et al. 1999; Mathias and Coats 1999). As noted, deficits of higher-order functions may be apparent only under certain circumstances (e.g., during dual task conditions) (Stablum et al. 1996) or by using functional MRI activation

TABLE 17–4. Aspects of language/ communication potentially impaired after traumatic brain injury

Language impairment

Classic aphasia syndromes: anomic aphasia; Wernicke's aphasia; other forms rare

"Subclinical" aphasia or language processing deficits: object naming, verbal associative fluency, comprehension of complex commands, writing to dictation

Discourse and pragmatic use of language

Less productive, less efficient speech; greater fragmentation

Difficulty initiating/maintaining topic of conversation, meeting a listener's needs, interpreting indirect communication

Other speech disorders

Mutism, stuttering, echolalia, palilalia

Dysarthria

paradigms (McAllister et al. 1999). In these situations, effective performance appears to be sustained at a cost (e.g., sacrificing speed of performance for accuracy). This circumstance may contribute to ongoing subjective complaints, despite recovery that is shown on standard neuropsychological tests.

Impairments of Language and Communication

Although complaints of "word finding" difficulty are frequent after any TBI, objective disturbance of language and communication more typically attends moderate to severe TBI (Levin and Chapman 1998). For example, relatives of severely injured patients identified "difficulty speaking" in 50% of cases reviewed at 7 years post-TBI (Oddy et al. 1985). The ability to communicate, or transmit and exchange information, is a fundamental determinant of psychosocial well-being (Prigitano et al. 1986). It reflects the complex interplay between primary receptive/expressive language functions, other nonlinguistic cognitive processes, and higher-order executive functions (Hinchliffe et al. 1998). The neural substrate involves distributed networks linking dominant prefrontal, perisylvian, and parietal language areas as well as other cerebral regions that mediate broader aspects of communication, such as the nondominant hemisphere. The vulnerability of communicative functions to diffuse or focal injury incurred during TBI is thus apparent (Table 17–4).

Classic aphasia syndromes are intermittently seen among consecutive samples of TBI patients (Heilman et al. 1971; Levin et al. 1976). Anomic aphasia is the most frequent type, manifesting as a fluent aphasia with marked inability to identify objects and proper names, frequent paraphasias and circumlocution, and preserved comprehension and repetition. Wernicke's, or receptive, aphasia is also observed; other forms are rare (Richardson 2000). The prognosis in acute aphasia syndromes is reasonably good. In a series of 21 patients examined at 8 months postinjury, full recovery of linguistic ability occurred in 43%, and 29% had a deficit confined to a single language function, predominantly anomia (Levin et al. 1981). Additional speech disorders such as mutism, stuttering, and echolalia have been occasionally observed (Levin and Chapman 1998). In contrast, dysarthria is relatively common after severe TBI and may persist after resolution of other language deficits (Richardson 2000).

Although frank aphasia is uncommon, impairments of basic language functions has been repeatedly demonstrated using psychometric testing. These impairments include deficits of object naming, verbal associative fluency, and—to a lesser extent—comprehension of complex commands (Levin et al. 1976; Sarno et al. 1986). However, these measures are insufficiently sensitive to the broader difficulties experienced by many patients after TBI (Coelho 1995). Thus, patients may appear functionally intact on the basis of results from a traditional aphasia battery, despite the presence of a variety of communication difficulties.

Some studies have examined naturalistic language production or "discourse," such as retelling a story or describing how to perform a task. Patients with severe TBI demonstrate less productive and efficient speech, convey less content with longer utterances, and use fewer "cohesive ties," leading to fragmented discourse (Hartley and Jensen 1991). Further work examining interactive conversation has disclosed difficulties in the pragmatic use of language, including problems initiating and maintaining a topic of conversation, meeting the needs of a listener, and interpreting or using indirect communication, such as sarcasm (Snow and Douglas 2000). (See Chapter 13, Personality Disorders.)

It is thus evident that communicative functions cannot be viewed in isolation. Associated relationships between basic linguistic faculties and divided attention, working memory, and—in particular—frontal control functions are germane. Stuss and Levine (2002) summarized that left prefrontal injury is associated with simplified, repetitive, and impoverished discourse. In contrast, right prefrontal lesions may produce amplification of detail, insertion of irrelevant elements, and a tendency toward

TABLE 17–5. Medications reported to improve cognition after closed traumatic brain injury

Cholinergic agents

  Physostigmine (not recommended)

  Cytidine-5'-diphosphocholine

  Cholinesterase inhibitors (donepezil)

Catecholaminergic agents

  Psychostimulants

  Amantadine

  Bromocriptine

  Levodopa

  Selegiline

Other agents

  Tricyclic antidepressants

  ? Selective serotonin reuptake inhibitor antidepressants

  ? Lamotrigine

  ? Pergolide, pramipexole, ropinirole (other dopamine receptor agonists)

  ? Atomoxetine (selective norepinephrine reuptake inhibitor)

  ? Guanfacine (selective α_{2A}-adrenergic agonist)

Treatment of Cognitive Impairments

Attempts to ameliorate cognitive impairments after TBI have broadly focused on neurocognitive rehabilitation, including a combination of restorative and compensatory approaches for damaged or lost functions (see Chapter 36, Cognitive Rehabilitation). Increasingly, these efforts have included pharmacological strategies to augment rehabilitation and influence functional recovery (Table 17–5). In this section, the literature supporting such interventions is surveyed. When possible, studies that used at least some degree of experimental control are highlighted. Specific details regarding the prescription and monitoring of these agents is provided in Chapter 34, Psychopharmacology.

The rationale for treatment has derived from two principal sources. First, there is growing evidence for perturbation of multiple neurotransmitter pathways after brain injury, both focal and diffuse. This suggests that agents with known effects on these systems may have an important role in facilitating recovery (Donnemiller et al. 2000; McIntosh 1994; Murdoch et al. 1998; Van Woerkom et al. 1982; Yan et al. 2002). As a result, testable hypotheses regarding the impact of TBI on aspects of cholinergic (Arciniegas 2003) and catecholaminergic

(McAllister et al. 2004) neurotransmission are being currently explored.

Second, some of the neurobehavioral features after TBI show considerable resemblance to those in other neuropsychiatric conditions, for which there are well-established treatments. These include deficiencies of concentration in attention-deficit/hyperactivity disorder (ADHD), memory in Alzheimer's disease, alertness/arousal in narcolepsy, and mental speed in Parkinson's disease. Such similarities have led to the use of drugs in TBI patients that have shown benefit in the treatment of analogous neuropsychiatric syndromes, despite the lack of comprehensive research in the area.

Two other areas of pharmacotherapy should be mentioned, although beyond the scope of this chapter. Much research has been aimed at reducing the damage resulting from the initial injury; for example, by administering agents such as glutamate antagonists or free radical scavengers to limit the initial neurotoxic cascades. The interested reader is referred to Chapter 39, Pharmacotherapy of Prevention, as well as Royo et al. (2003), for reviews. Another potential application for drug therapy is in the promotion of recovery from coma and minimally responsive states. Despite being a frequent intervention, there has been only limited research in this area (Giacino and Trott 2004).

Cholinergic Medication

The importance of cortical acetylcholine in attention, memory, and other cognitive processes is well established (Pepeu and Giovannini 2004; Sarter and Bruno 1997). Procholinergic agents are currently the mainstay of treatment in patients with Alzheimer's disease (Gauthier 2002). Animal models (Dixon et al. 1997; Pike and Hamm 1997) and human data (Arciniegas 2003; Murdoch et al. 1998) support the rationale that cholinergic augmentation after TBI might be of benefit.

A small clinical literature, which comprises single-case reports, small open-label trials, and a number of controlled studies with varying methodology (reviewed by Griffin et al. 2003), provides support for cholinergic augmentation. Among the controlled trials, almost all report some degree of improved cognition, although translation into functional improvement is not always noted. For example, physostigmine, an acetylcholinesterase inhibitor, was shown by Cardenas et al. (1994) to have positive effects on memory and attention measures in a subset of 36 patients with severe TBI. Levin et al. (1986) also observed benefit in sustained attention in 16 patients using this agent. The drug's usefulness is limited, however, by the risk of systemic cholinergic toxicity.

Similarly, treatment with cytidine 5'-diphosphocholine (CDP-choline), a choline precursor, has also shown some benefit with memory tasks when used early in recovery (Levin et al. 1991). Leon-Carrion et al. (2000) examined 10 patients with "severe" memory deficits (more than 6 months postinjury) who were randomized to either placebo or CDP-choline as an adjunct to cognitive rehabilitation. The latter group showed significant gains on measures of memory and verbal fluency, unlike the placebo group, leading the authors to conclude that CDP-choline facilitates neurorehabilitation.

Since its approval for Alzheimer's disease treatment, the selective acetylcholinesterase inhibitor donepezil has been the subject of several reports. Case reports and open-label trials describe improvement on cognitive measures, including measures of memory (Bourgois et al. 2002; Masanic et al. 2001; Taverni et al. 1998; Whitlock 1999). Of note, Whitlock (1999) described an adverse behavioral reaction in two patients (agitation and aggression) requiring drug discontinuation. Another open-label study of 10 patients by Kaye et al. (2003) is of interest because 6 had experienced mild TBI (mean, 1.2 years postinjury). Although objective change on memory testing was not shown, patients were rated as globally improved by the investigators. The patients were also in agreement, and reported "improved focus, attention, and clarity of thought…[but] not necessarily in the domain of memory." In another open-label trial, Whelan et al. (2000) treated 53 patients with a history of TBI using donepezil (severity and time postinjury not given). The authors reported that benefit was most apparent on a global, clinician-rated assessment of functional ability, although improvement of the Wechsler Adult Intelligence Scale—Revised IQ scores was also noted.

Three controlled studies of donepezil in TBI patients have been published. Morey et al. (2003) used a within-subjects design to evaluate seven patients with severe TBI with persisting memory dysfunction in the late recovery phase. Treatment phases included donepezil (titrated rapidly to 10 mg) for 6 months, a subsequent 6-week washout period, and a second 6-month treatment trial at 5 mg. Significant benefit on a visual memory measure was observed in the 10-mg phase only. No other effects were found, including measures tapping other aspects of memory. Nor did the improvement in visual memory appear to correlate with the patients' self-report on a memory complaints questionnaire. Those choosing to continue taking donepezil at the end of the study cited nonspecific cognitive benefits that could not be fully characterized.

Walker et al. (2004) obtained negative results using a retrospective case-control design among 36 patients with severe TBI in an acute rehabilitation setting (mean, 34.5 days postinjury). Eighteen patients receiving donepezil were contrasted with control subjects, matched for age and severity of injury. No difference was found on the primary outcome tool, the Functional Independence Measure—Cognitive Scale. As the authors note, however, this measure may be insufficiently sensitive to drug-induced changes. Additionally, only 25% of the treatment sample achieved a dose of 10 mg over the relatively short study period (mean, 33.8 days).

Zhang et al. (2004) examined 18 patients with moderate to severe TBI (mean, 4–5 months postinjury) using two indices of immediate memory (verbal and nonverbal subtests from the Weschler Memory Scale—Revised) and the Paced Auditory Serial Addition Task (as described in the section Impairments of Attention). Patients were randomly assigned to receive donepezil (increased rapidly to 10 mg) or placebo. After a 4-week washout phase, patients were crossed over to the alternate condition. Significant differences in favor of donepezil on all measures were observed, indicating improvement of immediate memory and attention/processing speed. Whether these test improvements led to functional gains or clinical improvement was not examined in the study.

In summary, although promising, the data with respect to cholinergic agents after TBI remain somewhat equivocal. Nonetheless, there does appear to be evidence supporting cognitive improvement in some patients.

Catecholaminergic Agents

There is accumulating evidence that both norepinephrine and dopamine have a powerful influence on cognitive activities, particularly those tasks associated with the prefrontal cortex (Arnsten and Robbins 2002).

Psychostimulants

Psychostimulants include methylphenidate and dextroamphetamine, considered indirect sympathomimetic agonists, in that they do not act directly on receptors, but rather increase the synaptic release and reuptake of catecholamines.

Until recently, rationale for their use after TBI was based on their efficacy for conditions such as ADHD, narcolepsy, and depression/apathy attending medical/neurological conditions. There were only a handful of published cases in the TBI population (Evans et al. 1987; Gualtieri and Evans 1988). Since the 1980s, however, several controlled studies of methylphenidate have been reported (see Whyte et al. 2002, for detailed review). Although the results are somewhat equivocal and studies of varying experimental rigor, there is evidence that methylphenidate can have positive effects on attention after TBI, particularly with respect to mental processing speed (Whyte et al. 2002). This may also be true for some aspects of memory, but the results to date

are more mixed (Whyte et al. 2002). In general, benefits of stimulants appear quite modest when compared to the robust effects observed in primary ADHD.

In an effort to circumvent the shortcomings of earlier work, Whyte's group systematically explored the domain of attention in two studies of patients with residual cognitive complaints (almost all severe TBI and in the late phase of recovery) (Whyte et al. 1997, 2004). Both used a controlled, randomized, double-blind protocol. Results for the two studies were similar, showing significant positive effects on measures tapping information processing speed, but not for other facets of attention, such as susceptibility to distraction or sustained attention. The second study also found a reduction in off-task behavior in a simulated classroom setting, as well as on caregiver ratings of attention, suggesting that better test scores may translate into demonstrable functional improvements (Whyte et al. 2004). It is notable, however, that despite positive results, treatment effect sizes were modest, at best. The fact that methylphenidate appears to have differential effects on attentional processes, perhaps with greater efficacy in some individuals but not others, may not be surprising given similar findings in the ADHD literature (Konrad 2004).

Reports of dextroamphetamine treatment for cognitive sequelae after TBI have been limited to single case studies (Blieberg et al. 1993; Evans et al. 1987), which indicate positive results. This agent has been of particular interest due to evidence that it may enhance the rate and extent of recovery if given early after ischemic stroke—perhaps by modulating central noradrenergic transmission (Goldstein 2003). This suggests a "temporal window" for the administration of treatment to optimize long-term benefit. Similar studies with dextroamphetamine have yet to be done in TBI patients; however, Plenger et al. (1996) examined the effects of methylphenidate in the acute setting. Although some benefits were noted at 30 days after drug discontinuation (better performance on two measures of vigilance and procedural learning, respectively; but not on other measures of attention or memory), these effects were not sustained at 90 days. The authors concluded that early methylphenidate perhaps improved the rate but not the ultimate level of recovery. However, these conclusions are difficult to disentangle from the effects of stimulants on general arousal during this period as well as the significant impact of spontaneous recovery (Whyte et al. 2002).

Although encouraging, further data are needed to carefully delineate the role of psychostimulants in treating cognitive impairment. It is unknown if enhancement of processing speed translates into improvement in other cognitive domains (e.g., memory) or whether a "window" of treatment opportunity exists for dextroamphetamine, as in some studies of outcome after stroke.

Amantadine

Amantadine is frequently used in the TBI population, although more commonly in the setting of reduced arousal or marked behavioral disturbance after severe TBI (Gualtieri et al. 1989). It appears to have effects on both pre- and postsynaptic dopamine transmission and is also an N-methyl-D-aspartate antagonist. In a number of uncontrolled case reports and case series, improvements with respect to attentional processes and speed of processing (Andersson et al. 1992; Nickels et al. 1994), behavioral initiation (Nickels et al. 1994; van Reekum et al. 1995), verbal fluency, and mental flexibility (Kraus and Maki 1997b) have been noted.

However, two controlled studies have shown contrasting results. Schneider et al. (1999) studied 10 TBI patients of mixed severity in early recovery (time unspecified) using measures of attention, memory, and executive function. A randomized, placebo-controlled crossover design was used to evaluate a 2-week trial of amantadine. Although all patients "generally improved" over time, there was no difference in the rate of improvement between amantadine and the placebo condition.

In a second study, Meythaler et al. (2002) examined 35 severe TBI patients within 6 weeks of injury who were randomized to receive either amantadine or placebo for 6 weeks. Crossover to the alternate condition occurred for a second 6-week period. Patients showed more rapid improvement when taking amantadine verses placebo on both screening cognitive tests and measures of functional ability, although not all comparisons reached statistical significance. Of note, the exact timing of active treatment (i.e., whether patients received amantadine in the first 6 weeks verses the second) had no impact on the ultimate level of recovery. Thus, at 3 and 6 months there were no differences between the groups on any measure, lending no support to the notion of a treatment "window" within the first 3 months postinjury.

As with other agents, data regarding amantadine require confirmation as well as extension to different phases of recovery and levels of severity. The limited research in the early recovery phase cannot rule out general improvements in arousal, or "behavioral" improvements in initiation or agitation, as alternate explanations for the apparent cognitive improvement. Nor can the research fully separate out the effects of spontaneous recovery.

Other Dopaminergic Agents

Direct dopamine agonists, the dopamine precursor levodopa, and selegiline may also be of benefit. Several case

reports describe the use of the selective D_2 agonist bromocriptine after TBI, as summarized by Muller et al. (1994), who also described seven TBI cases of their own. They reported that bromocriptine led to clear benefit in some patients and proposed that reduced responsiveness and initiation in markedly apathetic states (i.e., akinetic mutism) may be the principal applications after acquired cerebral trauma. In their series, the authors did not, however, observe "consistent improvement" on standard measures of attention, memory, or problem solving with bromocriptine, and also noted that relatively high doses might be required (Muller et al. 1994).

Two subsequent reports provide additional support for this treatment. Powell et al. (1996) described a series of 11 postacute patients with abulia (8 with TBI, 3 with subarachnoid hemorrhage), all of whom improved while taking bromocriptine with respect to abulia, as well as on measures of digit span, verbal list learning, and fluency. In the only controlled trial to date, McDowell et al. (1998) examined the impact of low-dose bromocriptine on cognition in 24 patients who were generally in the postacute phase after severe TBI. In contrast to earlier reports, these patients were not selected on the basis of apathy. Drug treatment was found to enhance performance on tests of executive function and a dual task paradigm, although not on measures tapping basic processes, such as information processing speed, or on a working memory task with minimal executive demands. The authors hypothesized that bromocriptine might selectively target deficits in executive control rather than simple attention, arousal, or processing speed. Further study is needed, however, because these investigators used a relatively low dose of bromocriptine in their cohort.

Despite preclinical evidence for a unique contribution of the D_1 receptor to working memory (Arnsten and Robbins 2002), the potential role of pergolide, a mixed D_1/D_2 agonist, has not been explored in cognitively impaired TBI patients. The newer dopamine agonists pramipexole and ropinirole—which act preferentially at the D_3 and D_2 receptors, respectively—may also prove useful, but have not yet been tried. These latter two agents may offer additional neuroprotective benefit.

Other dopaminergic agents have shown positive results, according to case reports. Lal et al. (1988) gave levodopa to 12 TBI patients who had "plateaued" in their recovery after severe TBI. Improved arousal, attention, and initiation were noted. Kraus and Maki (1997a) reported enhanced cognition in a severe TBI patient when levodopa was added to amantadine treatment. Selegiline, a selective monoamine oxidase-B inhibitor, may also mitigate some of the cognitive impairment in TBI patients (Marin et al. 1995; Zhu et al. 2000).

Antidepressants and Other Drugs

Antidepressants of the tricyclic class have been reported to display "stimulant-like" effects on arousal and initiation in two case series (Reinhard et al. 1996; Wroblewski et al. 1993). The authors attributed the positive effects to the enhancement of catecholaminergic transmission. In contrast, the selective serotonin reuptake inhibitor class has shown mixed results. Sertraline failed to improve cognition in 11 patients treated at 2 weeks after severe TBI (Meythaler et al. 2001). Horsfield et al. (2002) reported improvement on a single working memory task, but not on other measures, in a series of five patients treated with fluoxetine in the late recovery phase. However, all had been referred concerning "mental health problems" and improved with respect to depressive symptoms over the study period. Moreover, the notion that working memory might specifically be enhanced by selective serotonin reuptake inhibitor treatment appears to conflict with research showing working memory decrements in volunteers given either tryptophan, a 5-hydroxytryptamine (5-HT) precursor, or fenfluramine, a 5-HT agonist (Luciana et al. 2001). The role of the 5-HT system in opposing certain dopamine-mediated cognitive functions, such as working memory, was cited to explain these findings (Luciana et al. 2001).

Two reports have indicated positive effects of lamotrigine on cognition after TBI. This agent alters neuronal excitability by modulating ion channels and inhibits the release of glutamate. It has also been noted to improve alertness in those with seizure disorders. Showalter and Kimmel (2000) noted greater than expected cognitive improvement in 9 of 13 patients with a persistently reduced level of arousal at 3 months postinjury (6 with severe TBI; 5 with subarachnoid hemorrhage). A single case study described "pronounced" improvement on the cognitive dimensions of two functional assessment measures at 6 months after severe closed TBI (Pachet et al. 2003). However, in each of these reports, lamotrigine was initially prescribed as an add-on treatment for posttraumatic seizures. This raises the question of whether the apparent cognitive benefit could have derived from better seizure control.

Summary

Patients with TBI may exhibit diverse neurobehavioral impairments as a consequence of injury to the frontotemporal regions of the brain and the associated neural networks that subserve complex, adaptive behavior. This chapter has addressed the cognitive changes that are fre-

TABLE 17–6. Methodological obstacles to drug treatment of cognitive impairment

Lack of randomized controlled studies: support for some agents remains limited to single case reports. Larger sample sizes are also required.

Adequate control is needed for confounding factors such as spontaneous neurological recovery, drug carryover effects (i.e., into placebo phase), practice effects, and the impact of concurrent treatments (ideally via parallel group designs).

The issue of patient heterogeneity has been minimally addressed to date. Little is known about the contribution of factors such as premorbid cognitive function, type of neuropathology (diffuse vs. focal), and severity of diffuse axonal injury to drug response.

Treatment groups should be well balanced with respect to factors known to independently predict outcome (e.g., severity of injury). This ensures that alternate factors do not create or mask apparent differences between groups.

Standardized outcome measures are necessary to assess treatment-related changes that have proven sensitivity for the types of cognitive difficulties observed after traumatic brain injury. This may be difficult because the nature of complex cognitive processes and their underpinnings has yet to be fully understood/agreed on (e.g., how best to measure the effects of treatment on attentional processes).

Outcome measures should assess the functional relevance of apparent cognitive change: what, if any, is the relationship between neurocognitive test scores and task performance?

Note. For further discussion, see Whyte (2002), Whyte et al. (2002), Griffin et al. (2003), and Forsyth and Jayamoni (2003).

quently observed, at least to some degree, across the range of TBI severity. Although at times these impairments may be readily appreciable during an office or bedside interview, formal neuropsychological assessment is often required to elicit and carefully map out the deficits. Some aspects of cognition, such as mental processing speed and episodic memory, appear to be particularly susceptible to disruption after TBI. Further work is needed to delineate the effects of TBI on complex cognitive constructs such as executive control processes and to determine the extent to which neurocognitive test results capture real-world performance (e.g., the ability to operate a vehicle or suitability for a rehabilitation program). Remediation of cognitive impairment remains an important challenge because it is frequently associated with long-term disruption in social and vocational function.

The literature provides support for a number of pharmacological interventions that can potentially facilitate rehabilitative efforts. Despite methodological shortcomings (Table 17–6), the accumulated data indicate fairly clear ben-

TABLE 17–7. Clinical questions yet to be addressed

What are the patient and injury characteristics that predict a treatment response?

Which cognitive functions may or may not be facilitated by treatment?

What is the optimal dose and timing of treatment?

What is the duration of effect? Can medications improve the ultimate level of outcome?

What is the comparative efficacy of different drugs? Are there particular indications for a specific agent?

What is the significance/extent of adverse effects (e.g., the negative impact on behavior that is not uncommon with some of the agents)?

Might there be deleterious effects from the use of these agents in the early recovery phase?

efit in some individuals with respect to alertness and mental processing speed using agents that alter catecholaminergic transmission. Cholinergic agents also appear useful, although evidence for definite improvement in the domain of memory with these (or any other agent) appears limited to date. Similarly, the extent to which executive cognitive functions can be shown to improve with drug therapy remains unclear. It may be difficult to demonstrate enhancement of these higher-order functions because they do not operate in isolation from "subordinate" processes such as attention, memory, and perception. Additionally, because most of the agents used to date influence neurobehavioral parameters such as basic arousal, motivational tone, psychomotor activation, as well as affective lability and mood, it is clear that a multifaceted assessment approach will be necessary to fully determine which aspects of cognition and behavior respond to a specific treatment intervention. In this manner, the relationship between improved mood or apathy and enhanced cognitive function can be explored.

Despite the evidence supporting drug treatment, many questions remain (Table 17–7). No firm conclusions can be drawn concerning the relationship of TBI severity, location of focal lesions, or other patient-specific variables to drug response as yet; and there are no data regarding the differential effects of various pharmacological agents. It is apparent that not all patients will respond to a given agent. Presumably, this reflects variations in the degree to which any one neurotransmitter is disrupted within an individual (Arciniegas 2003). Principles regarding the clinical use of agents reviewed are provided in Chapter 34 (see also Arciniegas et al. 2002). Where there is any uncertainty, a clinical "N of 1" experiment may be the best means to answer

individual-specific questions concerning treatment (Evans et al. 1987; Van Reekum et al. 1995; Whyte 2002).

In conclusion, further work is necessary to firmly establish the efficacy and specific indications for these agents. There remains an urgent need to explore the potential for these (and other) treatments to enhance late cognitive outcome or ultimate level of recovery after TBI. Although knowledge is incomplete, there is no evidence to suggest that the use of these medications should be discontinued. Medications clearly assist some individuals with TBI, and side effects do not appear prohibitively greater than in other populations.

References

Adams JH, Doyle D, Graham DI, et al: The contusion index: a reappraisal in human and experimental non-missile head injury. Neuropathol Appl Neurobiol 11:299–308, 1985

Alexander GE, Crutcher MD: Functional architecture of basal ganglia circuits: neural substrates of parallel processing. Trends Neurosci 13:266–271, 1990

Anderson CV, Bigler ED, Blatter DD: Frontal lobe lesions, diffuse damage, and neuropsychological functioning in traumatic brain-injured patients. J Clin Exp Neuropsychol 17:900–908, 1995

Andersson S, Berstad J, Finset A, et al: Amantadine in cognitive failure in patients with traumatic head injuries. Tidsskr Nor Laegeforen 112:2070–2072, 1992

Arciniegas DB: The cholinergic hypothesis of cognitive impairment caused by traumatic brain injury. Curr Psychiatry Rep 5:391–399, 2003

Arciniegas DB, Held K, Wagner P: Cognitive impairment following traumatic brain injury. Curr Treat Options Neurol 4:43–57, 2002

Arnsten AFT, Robbins TW: Neurochemical modulation of prefrontal cortical function in humans and animals, in Principals of Frontal Lobe Function. Edited by Stuss DT, Knight RT. New York, Oxford University Press, 2002, pp 51–84

Bechara A, Damasio AR, Damasio H, et al: Insensitivity to future consequences following damage to human prefrontal cortex. Cognition 50:7–15, 1994

Bleiberg J, Garmoe W, Cederquist J, et al: Effect of Dexedrine on performance consistency following brain injury: a double-blind placebo crossover case study. Neuropsychiatry Neuropsychol Behav Neurol 6:245–248, 1993

Bourgeois JA, Bahadur N, Minjares S: Donepezil for cognitive deficits following traumatic brain injury: a case report. J Neuropsychiatry Clin Neurosci 14:463–464, 2002

Brooks J, Fos LA, Greve KW, et al: Assessment of executive function in patients with mild traumatic brain injury. J Trauma 46:159–163, 1999

Brooks N: Mental deterioration late after head injury—does it happen? J Neurol Neurosurg Psychiatry 74:1014, 2003

Brooks N, McKinlay W, Symington C, et al: Return to work within the first seven years of severe head injury. Brain Inj 1:5–19, 1987

Brouwer W, Verzendaal M, van der Naalt J, et al: Divided attention years after severe closed head injury: the effect of dependencies between the subtasks. Brain Cogn 46:54–56, 2001

Cabeza R, Nyberg L: Imaging cognition II: an empirical review of 275 PET and fMRI studies. J Cogn Neurosci 12:1–47, 2000

Cardenas DD, McLean A Jr, Farrell-Roberts L, et al: Oral physostigmine and impaired memory in adults with brain injury. Brain Inj 8:579–587, 1994

Cicerone KD: Attention deficits and dual task demands after mild traumatic brain injury. Brain Inj 10:79–89, 1996

Coelho CA: Discourse production deficits following traumatic brain injury: a critical review of the recent literature. Aphasiology 9:409–429, 1995

Crepeau F, Scherzer P: Predictors and indicators of work status after traumatic brain injury: a meta-analysis. Neuropsychological Rehabilitation 3:5–35, 1993

Cummings JL: Frontal-subcortical circuits and human behavior. Arch Neurol 50:873–880, 1993

Cummings JL: Cholinesterase inhibitors: a new class of psychotropic compounds. Am J Psychiatry 157:4–15, 2000

Curtiss G, Vanderploeg RD, Spencer J, et al: Patterns of verbal learning and memory in traumatic brain injury. J Int Neuropsychol Soc 7:574–585, 2001

Dell'Acqua R, Stablum F, Galbiati S, et al: Selective effect of closed-head injury on central resource allocation: evidence from dual-task performance. Exp Brain Res 136:364–378, 2001

Dixon CE, Ma X, Marion DW: Effects of CDP-choline treatment on neurobehavioral deficits after TBI and on hippocampal and neocortical acetylcholine release. J Neurotrauma 14:161–169, 1997

Donnemiller E, Brenneis C, Wissel J, et al: Impaired dopaminergic neurotransmission in patients with traumatic brain injury: a SPECT study using 123i-beta-cit and 123i-ibzm. Eur J Nucl Med 27:1410–1414, 2000

Eslinger PJ, Grattan LM, Geder L: Neurologic and neuropsychologic aspects of frontal lobe impairments in postconcussive syndrome, in Head Injury and Postconcussive Syndrome. Edited by Rizzo M, Traniel D. New York, Churchill Livingstone, 1996, pp 415–440

Evans RW, Gualtieri CT, Patterson D: Treatment of chronic closed head injury with psychostimulant drugs: a controlled case study and an appropriate evaluation procedure. J Nerv Ment Dis 175:106–110, 1987

Fernandez-Duque D, Posner MI: Brain imaging of attentional networks in normal and pathological states. J Clin Exp Neuropsychol 23:74–93, 2001

Forsyth R, Jayamoni B: Noradrenergic agonists for acute traumatic brain injury. Cochrane Database Syst Rev CD003984, 2003

Gansler DA, Covall S, McGrath N, et al: Measures of prefrontal dysfunction after closed head injury. Brain Cogn 30:194–204, 1996

Gauthier S: Advances in the pharmacotherapy of Alzheimer's disease. Can Med Assoc J 166:616–623, 2002

Gentry LR, Godersky JC, Thompson B: MR imaging of head trauma: review of the distribution and radiopathologic features of traumatic lesions. AJR Am J Roentgenol 150:663–672, 1988

Giacino JT, Trott CT: Rehabilitative management of patients with disorders of consciousness: grand rounds. J Head Trauma Rehabil 19:254–265, 2004

Goldberg E, Bilder RM, Hughes JE, et al: A reticulo-frontal disconnection syndrome. Cortex 25:678–695, 1989

Goldstein LB: Neuropharmacology of TBI-induced plasticity. Brain Inj 17:685–694, 2003

Griffin SL, van Reekum R, Masanic C: A review of cholinergic agents in the treatment of neurobehavioral deficits following traumatic brain injury. J Neuropsychiatry Clin Neurosci 15:17–26, 2003

Gronwall D: Paced Auditory Serial Addition Task: a measure of recovery from concussion. Percept Mot Skills 44:367–373, 1977

Gronwall D: Advances in the assessment of attention and information processing after head injury, in Neurobehavioral Recovery from Head Injury. Edited by Levin HS, Grafman J, Eisenberg HM. New York, Oxford University Press, 1987, pp 355–371

Gronwall D: Minor head injury. Neuropsychology 5:253–265, 1991

Gualtieri CT, Evans RW: Stimulant treatment for the neurobehavioural sequelae of traumatic brain injury. Brain Inj 2:273–290, 1988

Gualtieri CT, Chandler M, Coons T, et al: Amantadine: a new clinical profile for traumatic brain injury. Clin Neuropharmacol 12:258–279, 1989

Hartley LL, Jensen PJ: Narrative and procedural discourse after closed head injury. Brain Inj 5:267–285, 1991

Heilman KM, Safran A, Geschwind N: Closed head trauma and aphasia. J Neurol Neurosurg Psychiatry 34:265–269, 1971

Hinchliffe FJ, Murdoch BE, Chenery HJ: Towards a conceptualization of language and cognitive impairment in closed-head injury: use of clinical measures. Brain Inj 12:109–132, 1998

Horsfield SA, Rosse RB, Tomasino V, et al: Fluoxetine's effects on cognitive performance in patients with traumatic brain injury. Int J Psychiatry Med 32:337–344, 2002

Katz DI: Neuropathology and neurobehavioral recovery from closed head injury. J Head Trauma Rehabil 7:1–15, 1992

Katz DI, Alexander MP: Traumatic brain injury: predicting course of recovery and outcome for patients admitted to rehabilitation. Arch Neurol 51:661–670, 1994

Kaye NS, Townsend JB, Ivins R: An open-label trial of donepezil (Aricept) in the treatment of persons with mild traumatic brain injury. J Neuropsychiatry Clin Neurosci 15:383–384; author reply 384–385, 2003

Kennedy MRT, Yorkston KM: Accuracy of metamemory after traumatic brain injury: predictions during verbal learning. J Speech Lang Hear Res 43:1072–1086, 2000

Kewman DG, Yanus B, Kirsch N: Assessment of distractibility in auditory comprehension after traumatic brain injury. Brain Inj 2:131–137, 1988

King NS, Crawford S, Wenden FJ, et al: The Rivermead Post Concussion Symptoms Questionnaire: a measure of symptoms commonly experienced after head injury and its reliability. J Neurol 242:587–592, 1995

Kinsella G, Murtagh D, Landry A, et al: Everyday memory following traumatic brain injury. Brain Inj 10:499–507, 1996

Konrad K, Gunther T, Hanisch C, et al: Differential effects of methylphenidate on attentional functions in children with attention-deficit/hyperactivity disorder. J Am Acad Child Adolesc Psychiatry 43:191–198, 2004

Kraus MF, Maki PM: The combined use of amantadine and L-dopa/carbidopa in the treatment of chronic brain injury. Brain Inj 11:455–460, 1997a

Kraus MF, Maki PM: Effect of amantadine hydrochloride on symptoms of frontal lobe dysfunction in brain injury: case studies and review. J Neuropsychiatry Clin Neurosci 9:222–230, 1997b

Lal S, Merbitz CP, Grip JC: Modification of function in head-injured patients with Sinemet. Brain Inj 2:225–233, 1988

Leon-Carrion J, Alarcon JC, Revuelta M, et al: Executive functioning as outcome in patients after traumatic brain injury. Int J Neurosci 94:75–83, 1998

Leon-Carrion J, Dominguez-Roldan JM, Murillo-Cabezas F, et al: The role of citicholine in neuropsychological training after traumatic brain injury. NeuroRehabilitation 14:33–40, 2000

Levin HS: Treatment of postconcussional symptoms with CDP-choline. J Neurol Sci 103 (suppl):S39–42, 1991

Levin HS, Chapman SB: Aphasia after traumatic brain injury, in Acquired Aphasia, 3rd Edition. Edited by Sarno MT. San Diego, CA, Academic Press, 1998, pp 481–529

Levin HS, Goldstein FC: Organization of verbal memory after severe closed-head injury. J Clin Exp Neuropsychol 8:643–656, 1986

Levin HS, Grossman RG, Kelly PJ: Aphasic disorder in patients with closed head injury. J Neurol Neurosurg Psychiatry 39:1062–1070, 1976

Levin HS, Grossman RG, Sarwar M, et al: Linguistic recovery after closed head injury. Brain Lang 12:360–374, 1981

Levin HS, Peters BH, Kalisky Z, et al: Effects of oral physostigmine and lecithin on memory and attention in closed head-injured patients. Cent Nerv Syst Trauma 3:333–342, 1986

Levin HS, Goldstein FC, High WM Jr, et al: Disproportionately severe memory deficit in relation to normal intellectual functioning after closed head injury. J Neurol Neurosurg Psychiatry 51:1294–1301, 1988

Levin HS, Goldstein FC, Williams DH, et al: The contribution of frontal lobe lesions to the neurobehavioral outcome of closed head injury, in Frontal Lobe Function and Dysfunction. Edited by Levin HS, Eisenberg HM, Benton AL. New York, Oxford University Press, 1991, pp 318–338

Levin HS, Williams DH, Eisenberg HM, et al: Serial MRI and neurobehavioural findings after mild to moderate closed head injury. J Neurol Neurosurg Psychiatry 55:255–262, 1992

Levine B, Dawson D, Boutet I, et al: Assessment of strategic self-regulation in traumatic brain injury: its relationship to injury severity and psychosocial outcome. Neuropsychology 14:491–500, 2000

Lezak M: Neuropsychological assessment. New York, Oxford University Press, 1995, pp 176–193; 429–465

Loken WJ, Thornton AE, Otto RL, et al: Sustained attention after severe closed head injury. Neuropsychology 9:592–598, 1995

Luciana M, Burgund ED, Berman M, et al: Effects of tryptophan loading on verbal, spatial and affective working memory functions in healthy adults. J Psychopharmacol 15:219–230, 2001

Marin RS, Fogel BS, Hawkins J, et al: Apathy: a treatable syndrome. J Neuropsychiatry Clin Neurosci 7:23–30, 1995

Markowitsch HJ: Memory and amnesia, in Principles of Behavioral and Cognitive Neurology, 2nd Edition. Edited by Mesulam MM. New York, Oxford University Press, 2000, pp 257–293

Masanic CA, Bayley MT, VanReekum R, et al: Open-label study of donepezil in traumatic brain injury. Arch Phys Med Rehabil 82:896–901, 2001

Mathias JL, Coats JL: Emotional and cognitive sequelae to mild traumatic brain injury. J Clin Exp Neuropsychol 21:200–215, 1999

McAllister TW, Flashman LA, Sparling MB, et al: Working memory deficits after traumatic brain injury: catecholaminergic mechanisms and prospects for treatment—a review. Brain Inj 18:331–350, 2004

McAllister TW, Saykin AJ, Flashman LA, et al: Brain activation during working memory 1 month after mild traumatic brain injury: a functional MRI study. Neurology 53:1300–1308, 1999

McDowell S, Whyte J, D'Esposito M: Differential effect of a dopaminergic agonist on prefrontal function in traumatic brain injury patients. Brain 121:1155–1164, 1998

McIntosh TK: Neurochemical sequelae of traumatic brain injury: therapeutic implications. Cerebrovasc Brain Metab Rev 6:109–162, 1994

Mesulam MM: Attentional networks, confusional states, and neglect syndromes, in Principles of Behavioral and Cognitive Neurology, 2nd Edition. Edited by Mesulam MM. New York, Oxford University Press, 2000, pp 174–256

Meythaler JM, Depalma L, Devivo MJ, et al: Sertraline to improve arousal and alertness in severe traumatic brain injury secondary to motor vehicle crashes. Brain Inj 15:321–331, 2001

Meythaler JM, Brunner RC, Johnson A, et al: Amantadine to improve neurorecovery in traumatic brain injury-associated diffuse axonal injury: a pilot double-blind randomized trial. J Head Trauma Rehabil 17:300–313, 2002

Millar K, Nicoll JA, Thornhill S, et al: Long term neuropsychological outcome after head injury: relation to APOE genotype. J Neurol Neurosurg Psychiatry 74:1047–1052, 2003

Millis RS, Rosenthal M, Novack TA, et al: Long-term neuropsychological outcome after traumatic brain injury. J Head Trauma Rehabil 16:343–355, 2001

Morey CE, Cilo M, Berry J, et al: The effect of Aricept in persons with persistent memory disorder following traumatic brain injury: a pilot study. Brain Inj 17:809–815, 2003

Muller U, von Cramon DY: The therapeutic potential of bromocriptine in neuropsychological rehabilitation of patients with acquired brain damage. Prog Neuropsychopharmacol Biol Psychiatry 18:1103–1120, 1994

Murdoch I, Perry EK, Court JA, et al: Cortical cholinergic dysfunction after human head injury. J Neurotrauma 15:295–305, 1998

Nickels JL, Schneider WN, Dombovy ML, et al: Clinical use of amantadine in brain injury rehabilitation. Brain Inj 8:709–718, 1994

Oddy M, Coughlan T, Tyerman A, et al: Social adjustment after closed head injury: a further follow-up seven years after injury. J Neurol Neurosurg Psychiatry 48:564–568, 1985

Pachalska M, Kurzbauer H, Talar J, et al: Active and passive executive function disorder subsequent to closed-head injury. Med Sci Monit 8:CS1–CS9, 2002

Pachet A, Friesen S, Winkelaar D, et al: Beneficial behavioural effects of lamotrigine in traumatic brain injury. Brain Inj 17:715–722, 2003

Park NW, Moscovitch M, Robertson IH: Divided attention impairments after traumatic brain injury. Neuropsychologia 37:1119–1133, 1999

Pepeu G, Giovannini MG: Changes in acetylcholine extracellular levels during cognitive processes. Learn Mem 11:21–27, 2004

Pike BR, Hamm RJ: Activating the posttraumatic cholinergic system for the treatment of cognitive impairment following traumatic brain injury. Pharmacol Biochem Behav 57:785–791, 1997

Plenger PM, Dixon CE, Castillo RM, et al: Subacute methylphenidate treatment for moderate to moderately severe traumatic brain injury: a preliminary double-blind placebo-controlled study. Arch Phys Med Rehabil 77:536–540, 1996

Ponsford J, Kinsella G: Attentional deficits following closed-head injury. J Clin Exp Neuropsychol 14:822–838, 1992

Powell JH, al-Adawi S, Morgan J, Greenwood RJ: Motivational deficits after brain injury: effects of bromocriptine in 11 patients. J Neurol Neurosurg Psychiatry 60:416–421, 1996

Prigatano GP, Roueche JR, Fordyce DJ: Nonaphasic language disturbances after brain injury, in Neuropsychological Rehabilitation after Brain Injury. Edited by Prigatano GP. Baltimore, MD, Johns Hopkins University Press, 1986, pp 18–28

Reinhard DL, Whyte J, Sandel ME: Improved arousal and initiation following tricyclic antidepressant use in severe brain injury. Arch Phys Med Rehabil 77:80–83, 1996

Reitan RM, Wolfson D: The neuropsychological similarities of mild and more severe head injury. Arch Clin Neuropsychol 15:433–442, 2000

Richardson JTE: Clinical and Neuropsychological Aspects of Closed Head Injury. East Sussex, UK, Psychology Press, 2000, pp 97–124; 146–156

Rios M, Perianez JA, Munoz-Cespedes JM: Attentional control and slowness of information processing after severe traumatic brain injury. Brain Inj 18:257–272, 2004

Rolls ET: The orbitofrontal cortex and reward. Cereb Cortex 10:284–294, 2000

Royo NC, Shimizu S, Schouten JW, et al: Pharmacology of traumatic brain injury. Curr Opin Pharmacol 3:27–32, 2003

Ruff RM, Levin HS, Mattis S, et al: Recovery of memory after mild head injury: a three-center study, in Mild Head Injury. Edited by Levin HS, Eisenberg HM, Benton AL. New York, Oxford University Press, 1989, pp 176–188

Sarno MT, Buonaguro A, Levita E: Characteristics of verbal impairment in closed head injured patients. Arch Phys Med Rehabil 67:400–405, 1986

Sarter M, Bruno JP: Cognitive functions of cortical acetylcholine: toward a unifying hypothesis. Brain Res Brain Res Rev 23:28–46, 1997

Sbordone RJ: Limitations of neuropsychological testing to predict the cognitive and behavioral functioning of persons with brain injury in real-world settings. NeuroRehabilitation 16:199–201, 2001

Schmitter-Edgecombe M, Kibby MK: Visual selective attention after severe closed head injury. J Int Neuropsychol Soc 4:144–159, 1998

Schneider W, Drew-Cates J, Wong T, et al: Cognitive and behavioral efficacy of amantadine in acute traumatic brain injury: an initial double-blind placebo controlled study. Brain Inj 13:863–872, 1999

Showalter PE, Kimmel DN: Stimulating consciousness and cognition following severe brain injury: a new potential clinical use for lamotrigine. Brain Inj 14:997–1001, 2000

Shum D, Sweeper S, Murray R: Performance on verbal implicit and explicit memory tasks following traumatic brain injury. J Head Trauma Rehabil 11:43–53, 1996

Snow PC, Douglas JM: Conceptual and methodological challenges in discourse assessment with TBI speakers: towards an understanding. Brain Inj 14:397–415, 2000

Spikman JM, van Zomeren AH, Deelman BG: Deficits of attention after closed-head injury: slowness only? J Clin Exp Neuropsychol 18:755–767, 1996

Spikman JM, Kiers HA, Deelman BG, et al: Construct validity of concepts of attention in healthy controls and patients with CHI. Brain Cogn 47:446–460, 2001

Stablum F, Mogentale C, Umilta C: Executive functioning following mild closed head injury. Cortex 32:261–278, 1996

Stuss DT, Gow CA: "Frontal dysfunction" after traumatic brain injury. Neuropsychiatry Neuropsychol Behav Neurol 5:272–282, 1992

Stuss DT, Levine B: Adult clinical neuropsychology: lessons from studies of the frontal lobes. Annu Rev Psychol 53:401–433, 2002

Stuss DT, Ely P, Hugenholtz H, et al: Subtle neuropsychological deficits in patients with good recovery after closed head injury. Neurosurgery 17:41–47, 1985

Sundstrom A, Marklund P, Nilsson LG, et al: APOE influences on neuropsychological function after mild head injury: within-person comparisons. Neurology 62:1963–1966, 2004

Tate DF, Bigler ED: Fornix and hippocampal atrophy in traumatic brain injury. Learn Mem 7:442–446, 2000

Taverni JP, Seliger G, Lichtman SW: Donepezil mediated memory improvement in traumatic brain injury during post acute rehabilitation. Brain Inj 12:77–80, 1998

Van Reekum R, Bayley M, Garner S, et al: N of 1 study: amantadine for the amotivational syndrome in a patient with traumatic brain injury. Brain Inj 9:49–53, 1995

van Woerkom TC, Minderhoud JM, Gottschal T, et al: Neurotransmitters in the treatment of patients with severe head injuries. Eur Neurol 21:227–234, 1982

Van Zomeren AH, Brouwer WH: Clinical Neuropsychology of Attention. New York, Oxford University Press, 1994, pp 63–94

Van Zomeren AH, Deelman BG: Long-term recovery of visual reaction time after closed head injury. J Neurol Neurosurg Psychiatry 41:452–457, 1978

Van Zomeren AH, Van den Burg W: Residual complaints of patients two years after severe head injury. J Neurol Neurosurg Psychiatry 48:21–28, 1985

Vanderploeg RD, Crowell TA, Curtiss G: Verbal learning and memory deficits in traumatic brain injury: encoding, consolidation, and retrieval. J Clin Exp Neuropsychol 23:185–195, 2001

Vilkki J, Virtanen S, Surma-Aho O, et al: Dual task performance after focal cerebral lesions and closed head injuries. Neuropsychologia 34:1051–1056, 1996

Walker W, Seel R, Gibellato M, et al: The effects of donepezil on traumatic brain injury acute rehabilitation outcomes. Brain Inj 18:739–750, 2004

Whelan FJ, Walker MS, Schultz SK: Donepezil in the treatment of cognitive dysfunction associated with traumatic brain injury. Ann Clin Psychiatry 12:131–135, 2000

Whitlock JA: Brain injury, cognitive impairment, and donepezil. J Head Trauma Rehabil 1:424–427, 1999

Whyte J: Methodological issues in the study of drug treatment for traumatic brain injury, in Neuropsychological Interventions: Clinical Research and Practice. Edited by Eslinger S. New York, Guilford, 2002, pp 59–79

Whyte J, Hart T, Schuster K, et al: Effects of methylphenidate on attentional function after traumatic brain injury: a randomized, placebo-controlled trial. Am J Phys Med Rehabil 76:440–450, 1997

Whyte J, Schuster K, Polansky M, et al: The frequency and duration of inattentive behavior after traumatic brain injury: effects of distraction, task, and practice. J Int Neuropsychol Soc 6:1–11, 2000

Whyte J, Vaccaro M, Grieb-Neff P, et al: Psychostimulant use in the rehabilitation of individuals with traumatic brain injury. J Head Trauma Rehabil 17:284–299, 2002

Whyte J, Hart T, Vaccaro M, et al: Effects of methylphenidate on attention deficits after traumatic brain injury: a multidimensional, randomized, controlled trial. Am J Phys Med Rehabil 83:401–420, 2004

Wills P, Clare L, Shiel A, et al: Assessing subtle memory impairments in the everyday memory performance of brain injured people: exploring the potential of the Extended Rivermead Behavioural Memory Test. Brain Inj 14:693–704, 2000

Wilson JT, Hadley DM, Wiedmann KD, et al: Neuropsychological consequences of two patterns of brain damage shown by MRI in survivors of severe head injury. J Neurol Neurosurg Psychiatry 59:328–331, 1995

Wroblewski B, Glenn MB, Cornblatt R, et al: Protriptyline as an alternative stimulant medication in patients with brain injury: a series of case reports. Brain Inj 7:353–362, 1993

Yan HQ, Kline AE, Ma X, et al: Traumatic brain injury reduces dopamine transporter protein expression in the rat frontal cortex. Neuroreport 13:1899–1901, 2002

Zhang L, Plotkin RC, Wang G, et al: Cholinergic augmentation with donepezil enhances recovery in short-term memory and sustained attention after traumatic brain injury. Arch Phys Med Rehabil 85:1050–1055, 2004

Zhu J, Hamm RJ, Reeves TM, et al: Postinjury administration of L-deprenyl improves cognitive function and enhances neuroplasticity after traumatic brain injury. Exp Neurol 66:136–52, 2000

Zoccolotti P, Matano A, Deloche G, et al: Patterns of attentional impairment following closed head injury: a collaborative European study. Cortex 36:93–107, 2000

18 Disorders of Diminished Motivation

Robert S. Marin, M.D.

Sudeep Chakravorty, M.D.

MOTIVATION IS ESSENTIAL to adaptive functioning and quality of life. This is as much true for individuals with traumatic brain injury (TBI) as those with stroke, dementia, or any other neuropsychiatric illness. Clinicians understand intuitively the importance of motivation. We know that without motivation individuals with TBI will fail to keep appointments, stay on their medications, devote themselves to friends and family, or return to their jobs. Motivational loss handicaps physical rehabilitation and coping skills (Finset and Andersson 2000) and is an important source of burden for families of individuals with TBI (Marsh et al. 1998).

Western psychology has long recognized the place of motivation in human behavior (Hillgard 1980). Motivation is an ever-present, essential determinant of behavior and adaptation. Motivation, like attention, emotion, and other state variables, is not a single function of the brain. Psychologically and biologically, motivation is a complex of capacities, and the neural systems subserving it are themselves both delimited and distributed, integrated and interdependent.

In this chapter, we present an approach to motivational impairments in TBI. We provide definitions of motivation and disorders of diminished motivation (DDMs) and descriptions of their assessment and management that are based on a biopsychosocial approach to the causes of motivational loss (Marin 1996a). We then discuss the neural mechanisms of motivation and the ways in which the DDMs reflect selective dysfunction of these systems. Readers should expect the clinical material to be familiar in some ways—because neuropsychiatric assessment of motivation builds on everyday clinical skills and experiences—and unfamiliar in others—because most clinicians are not in the habit of making explicit our intuitive understanding of motivation in clinical practice. As we proceed, we reference the modest literature that addresses diminished motivation and its mechanisms in TBI.

Investigators from the fields of psychiatry (Kant et al. 1998), neuropsychology (al-Adawi et al. 1998), rehabilitative medicine (Mazaux et al. 1997), and occupational therapy (Giles and Clark-Wilson 1988) agree that DDMs are an important source of disability for patients with TBI. Diminished motivation in TBI contributes to loss of social autonomy (Mazaux et al. 1997), financial and vocational loss, and family burden (Marsh et al. 1998). Given the frequency of diminished motivation in TBI—estimates vary from 5% to 67% (Andersson et al. 1999a; Dunlop et al. 1991; Kant et al. 1998)—effective treatment for DDMs has enormous potential to alleviate the personal and social burden of TBI.

Motivation

Because motivation is largely ignored in formal psychiatric education, we begin by saying a few words about the meaning of *motivation*. *Motivation* refers to the characteristics and determinants of goal-directed behavior. Theories of motivation are intended to account for the "direction, vigor, and persistence of an individual's actions" (Atkinson and Birch 1978, p. 4)—that is, for how behavior "gets started, is energized, is sustained, is directed, is stopped and what kind of subjective reaction is present in the organism when all this is going on" (Jones 1955).

Disorders of Motivation

Disorders of motivation are a "third domain of psychopathology" (Marin 1996a); disorders of cognition and emotion are the other two. Disorders of motivation may be classified by increase, decrease, or dysregulation of motivation. Increased motivation is exemplified by the hyperconnection symptoms of interictal personality in temporal lobe epilepsy and by appetitive disorders such as aggression and hyperphagia. Dysregulation of motivation is exemplified by impulse control disorders or obsessive-compulsive disorder. Disorders of diminished motivation include akinetic mutism, abulia, and apathy, which are the focus of this chapter.

The essential feature of apathy, abulia, and akinetic mutism is diminished motivation. Recent literature (American Congress of Rehabilitation Medicine 1995; Fisher 1983; Marin 1997b; Mega and Cohenour 1997) places them on a continuum of motivational loss, with apathy at the minor pole and akinetic mutism at the major pole of severity. The three result from dysfunction of the neural machinery that mediates motivation. Apathy, however, is a more complex clinical problem because it may also result from a variety of psychiatric disorders and psychosocial problems.

Akinetic mutism was first described (Cairns et al. 1941) in a 14-year-old girl with a craniopharyngioma cyst of the third ventricle. Her presentation was characteristic (Mega and Cohenour 1997). She was essentially mute and motionless despite full wakefulness. Her visual tracking was intact. The mutism and inactivity were not attributable to elementary neurological deficits (e.g., quadriparesis). Intact visual tracking is essential for the diagnosis; its presence excludes more extensive damage involving the brainstem. Meaningful responses occur in akinetic mutism, but they are erratic and infrequent. Therefore, impaired initiation of behavior and cognition as well as preservation of visual tracking are the essential features of akinetic mutism (American Congress of Rehabilitation Medicine 1995). TBI may cause akinetic mutism, although there are few reported cases of akinetic mutism in the TBI literature (Campbell and Duffy 1997).

The term *abulia* was coined in the 19th century to reference diverse disorders of diminished will (*bul* in Latin) (Berrios and Gili 1995). The term is used in recent literature (Fisher 1983; Mega and Cohenour 1997) for symptoms less severe than but qualitatively identical to akinetic mutism: poverty of behavior and speech output, lack of initiative, loss of emotional responses, psychomotor slowing, and prolonged speech latency. Abulia shades into akinetic mutism when it worsens and into apathy when it improves.

Apathy indicates diminished motivation that occurs in the presence of normal consciousness, attention, cognitive capacity, and mood. Patients with apathy are generally able to initiate and sustain behavior; describe their plans, goals, and interests; and react emotionally to significant events and experiences. However, these features are less common, less extensive, less intense, and shorter in duration than they are in individuals who are not apathetic. In other words, apathy differs from normality quantitatively instead of qualitatively.

The boundary between apathy and abulia is also relative. In abulia, the presentation is dominated by the near absence of goal-directed activity (e.g., walking, talking, gesturing). In apathy, activity and initiative are also diminished, but the poverty of motivation requires attending as well to the changes in thought content and emotional responding, as we describe next.

Recognition

How do we recognize a DDM? Because motivation is the psychological domain concerned with *goal-directed* behavior, the detection of diminished motivation requires examining *goal-related* aspects of overt behavior, cognition, and emotion. Thus, DDMs present with diminution in each of these three aspects of behavior:

1. *Diminished overt behavior* may range from subtle attenuation in social or occupational functioning (in apathy) to profound deficits in the capacity to initiate any movement whatsoever (in abulia and akinetic mutism).
2. *Diminished goal-related cognition*, if mild, is indicated by thought content revealing attenuation of interests, plans, or goals for the future. If severe, there is virtual absence of goal-related thought content: no interests, no intentions, no plans. The latter characterizes abulia and, of course, akinetic mutism.
3. *Diminished emotional responses to goal-related events* simply means that when something of importance happens, emotional responses are decreased: they are brief, shallow, or restricted in range. Note that this decrease does not mean absence of depressed mood or anxiety but only that the affect is attenuated. Clinically, this usually means flattened, labile, or shallow affect; lack of emotions; emotional indifference; and so on.

To summarize, we can say that diminished motivation is present if a patient with intact level of consciousness, attention, language, and sensorimotor capacity presents with simultaneous decrease in the overt behavioral, cognitive, and emotional concomitants of goal-directed behavior. This is an operational definition of diminished motivation and thus is a guideline for identifying the features that define DDMs and differentiate them from other disorders.

Differential Diagnosis

Differential diagnosis of DDMs depends on the acuity and severity of the TBI. For acute and severe cases, differential diagnosis focuses on TBI complications that produce profound impairment in level of consciousness, attention, speech, or motor capacity (e.g., vegetative states, delirium and stupor, locked-in syndrome, or quadriparesis) (American Congress of Rehabilitation Medicine 1995; Celesia 1997). Chronic or less severely impaired patients should be evaluated for depression and dementia as well as frontal-subcortical syndromes that affect personality and executive cognitive dysfunction.

Clinicians should proceed with differential diagnosis with the awareness that if DDMs are overdiagnosed, reversible or more readily treated causes of inactivity such as stupor or delirium are overlooked. Underdiagnosis leads to premature attempts at physical rehabilitation or other interventions whose success depends on strong motivation. Antidepressant treatment may also fail, not because a reversible mood disorder is absent but rather because it is overshadowed by a DDM that requires treatment first.

Patients with diminished motivation all show diminished activity. Inactivity—whether motor, cognitive, or emotional—may result from changes in virtually any domain of mental status. *Attentional changes* associated with coma, stupor, or mild delirium suggest diminished motivation because they are often associated with diminished activity. *Memory loss* may suggest diminished motivation when there is increased latency of response or when patients have poverty of speech because they have poverty of recall. *Perceptual changes*—illusions, hallucinations, and reduplicative phenomena—may lead to bewilderment and preoccupation, which also may bring apathy and abulia to mind. *Mood changes* operate similarly. In addition, complications of depression—for example, psychomotor retardation or catatonia—also resemble diminished motivation because motor activity, speech, and emotional expressivity are often reduced. *Disorder of thought content and form* may be particularly misleading. Psychotic thought content may lead to autistic or self-absorbed presentation of self. Thought blocking, circumstantiality, and impaired coherence of thought may appear as reduced goal-directedness or drive.

In light of these factors, the two groups of disorders to distinguish in differential diagnosis are those in which the following occur:

1. *Diminished activity suggests diminished motivation but is actually due to other impairment.* In *stupor* and *coma*, the essential impairment is diminished level of consciousness. *Delirium* may involve a diminished level of consciousness but is primarily a disorder of attention (impaired ability to establish, shift, or maintain attention) accompanied by some other cognitive, perceptual impairment. *Aprosodia* is a disorder of emotion information; there is impairment in the ability to understand, process, or express emotion (Ross 2000). Aprosodia may be mistaken for apathy because both may be associated with truncated emotional responses. Diminished motivation is not a feature of aprosodia, however (Marin 1996a). *Catatonia and psychomotor retardation* resemble DDMs because of the presence of reduced motor and speech activity. Executive cognitive impairments may be seen in catatonia. Waxy flexibility, if present, points to catatonia (Fink and Taylor 2001). Slowing of thought and activity, the essential features of psychomotor retardation, may occur in many disorders, including DDMs. Therefore, psychomotor retardation should not be viewed as a pathognomonic feature of depression or any other diagnosis (Benson 1990; Widlocher 1983). *Akinesia* is a disorder of movement rather than motivation. Akinesia involves diminished initiation of activity due to extrapyramidal motor dysfunction. Akinesia may be associated with apathy, however (Rifkin et al. 1975).

2. *Diminished activity is associated with diminished motivation, but both are due to some other disorder. Depression* is a disorder of mood. By definition, it is a dysphoric state. Negative thoughts about the self, the present, and the future (Beck's triad of depression) are characteristic. Consequently, one *suffers* from depression. By contrast, one does not *suffer* from apathy or other DDMs. In other words, DDMs are not dysphoric states. However, motivational symptoms are commonplace in depression; it is dysphoria and negative thought content that distinguish depression. *Demoralization*, like depression, is a dysphoric state. Demoralization is distinguished by a sense of futility, resignation, or a sense of powerlessness to realize some goal that is still desired. *Dementia* is, by definition, a disorder of intellect. Memory, executive capacity, or other cognitive impairments are essential to diagnosis.

Mechanism

A model for the mechanism of motivation aids in the assessment and treatment of DDMs. It also provides a framework for defining research questions and integrating new knowledge. The essential feature of the model presented here is the *core circuit* (Marin 1996b), a postulated subsystem of the forebrain, composed of the anterior cingulum, nucleus accumbens (NA), ventral pallidum (VP), and ventral tegmental area (VTA) (Figure 18–1). One hypothesis, based on a growing body of research

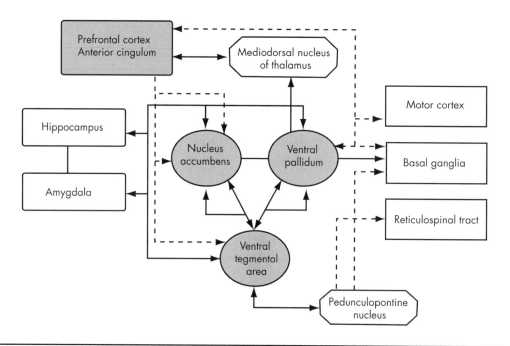

FIGURE 18–1.   Motivational circuitry.

The core circuit (shaded) consists of anterior cingulum, nucleus accumbens (NA), ventral pallidum (VP), and the ventral tegmental area (VTA) (NA, VP, and VTA correspond to the "motive circuit" of Kalivas et al. 1993). NA and VP are divided into 1) more medial portions that are associated with limbic input from amygdala and hippocampus, and 2) more lateral portions associated with output circuits. Output is via motor cortex, basal ganglia, reticulospinal tract, and pedunculopontine nucleus. The amygdala and hippocampus, as well as the prefrontal cortex, modulate information in the core circuit based on the current environment and the drive state of the organism. VP output reaches the prefrontal cortex via the mediodorsal nucleus of the thalamus. Current motivational state is represented by the pattern of activity distributed within the core circuit. The flow of information within and through the core circuit permits the translation of motivation into action. The structures illustrated are interconnected in two distinct ways, as exemplified by solid versus dotted lines.

Source.   From Kalivas et al. 1993, Figures 1 and 2, pp. 239 and 242, respectively. Modified with permission from CRC Press, LLC.

(Kalivas and Barnes 1993; Kalivas et al. 1993; Marin 1996b; Mega and Cummings 1994), is that an organism's current motivational state is represented by the pattern of information in the core circuit. The function of other limbic structures (e.g., amygdala, hippocampus, prefrontal cortex [PFC]) is continuous modulation of the core circuit on the basis of the motivational significance of the internal and external environment.

One should keep in mind that before engaging the motivational systems, information about the environment is first decoded, recognized, and integrated cross-modally via posterior hemispheric systems that appraise *what* is there and *where* it is (Ungerleider and Mishkin 1982). This *what* and *where* information is represented in a highly processed form in the anterior temporal lobe and insular cortex (Rolls 1999; Scheel-Kruger and Willner 1989). As a first approximation, motivational processes begin with projection of this information to the amygdala, hippocampus, and PFC (Rolls 1992).

It is also important to note that there are several ways in which the motivational significance of the environment

is influenced by nonmotivational processes. First, determining *what* and *where* requires integrity of the sensory apparatus and the peripheral nervous system. If one is unable to perceive what is there, one's appraisal of its motivational significance suffers or, at least, is altered. Therefore, the reward potential of the environment depends not only on the objective status of the environment but also on the organism's sensorimotor capacities. Sensorimotor capacity also modifies behavior because motivation depends on the individual's subjective assessment of the likelihood that behavior will lead to goal attainment. This appraisal may be characterized as perceived inability to control the environment or diminished subjective probability of success (Atkinson and Birch 1978). It applies equally to patients adapting to hip fracture, hemiparesis, or executive cognitive impairment: motivation suffers if the individual judges that effort will be fruitless.

In evaluating motivational loss and its neural basis, it is helpful to divide the motivational process into these five steps (Marin 1996b): 1) represent the current motivational state of the organism, 2) determine the reward potential of the environment, 3) modify current motivational state on the basis of changes in the environment and the drive state of the organism (e.g., hunger, thirst, sex, sleep), 4) select a new behavioral response, 5) implement the new behavioral response—that is, "translate motivation into action" (Mogenson et al. 1980).

1. *Represent current motivational state*: As introduced earlier in this section, the current motivational state of the organism is represented by the pattern of information in the core circuit composed of the anterior cingulum, NA, VP, and VTA. Viewing these structures as a functional unit is based in part on experimental studies (Kalivas et al. 1993) showing that NA, VP, and VTA (the "motive circuit" according to Kalivas et al.) must be intact for normal activity to occur. Electrical or chemical inactivation of any of its components eliminates the ability to elicit activity normally.

2. *Determine the reward potential of the current environment*: The central mechanisms for determining the reward potential of the environment involve circuits within the basal ganglia, limbic system, and right cerebral hemisphere. Single-cell recording has identified reward-related inputs within the ventral striatum (Schultz et al. 1992), VTA, and substantia nigra of the basal ganglia (Alexander 1994; Schultz 1997). However, classic limbic structures, especially the amygdala and orbitofrontal cortex (Rolls 1992, 1999), seem particularly important for determining reward potential. Single-cell recording within the amygdala and orbitofrontal cortex demonstrates selective firing in response to conditioned stimuli. The amygdala seems preferentially involved in establishing stimulus-reward associations (i.e., in learning motivational associations). The orbitofrontal cortex seems more engaged in determining the moment-to-moment significance of the current environment (Rolls 1992, 1999; Wilson and Rolls 1990). A related motivational task may be to establish a "motivational map" of the environment—a representation of the motivational significance of "what's out there" (i.e., of extracorporeal space). This motivational map is hypothesized to reflect integrated activity of the anterior cingulum, inferior parietal lobule of the right hemisphere, and reticular activating system (Mesulam 2000a).

3. *Modify the current motivational state*: When the environment or the drive state of the organism changes, activity in the core circuit is modified. There are limbic and PFC sources of input to the core circuit. Limbic input is from the amygdala, hippocampus, and other limbic structures (Mesulam 2000b). PFC activity is integrated with the core circuit by two subcircuits: the medial, motivation subcircuit involving the anterior cingulum, NA, VP, and mediodorsal nucleus of the thalamus (Mega and Cummings 1994); and a subcircuit involving the PFC and VTA (Kalivas et al. 1993, 1999).

4. *Select a new behavioral response*: The mechanisms underlying response selection are least understood. Undoubtedly, selection of a new behavior reflects processes occurring at multiple sites in the forebrain and brainstem. The amygdala, hippocampus, and orbitofrontal cortex contribute implicitly to response selection because they participate in circuits that indicate the association of current environmental stimuli with sources of reward (Kalivas et al. 1993). The amygdala provides a major input to the anterior cingulum, which participates in developing the motivational map of the current environment. Clinical and positron emission tomography studies (Bush et al. 1999; Raichle et al. 1994) suggest extensive involvement of the anterior cingulum in response selection and organization of emotional, autonomic, and behavioral motor responses. The NA is clearly a crucial area for selecting and focusing limbic activity. Extensive work in animals (Schultz 1997), supported by functional magnetic resonance imaging in humans (Pagnoni et al. 2002), indicates that activity in the NA is strongly affected by events signaling unexpected outcomes and, thus, events of potential importance for changing current motivational state. These changes in NA activity are modulated by the mesolimbic dopaminergic systems projecting from the VTA. Therefore, the VTA and its inputs are postulated to serve a crucial, integrative role in response selection. These inputs include the PFC, NA, VP, septum, and central nucleus of the amygdala (Scheel-Kruger and Willner 1989).

5. *Translate motivation into action*: Finally, motivation must be translated into action, a function reflected in the connectivity of the core circuit and in its outputs to several regions of the basal ganglia and upper brainstem (Mogenson et al. 1993) (Figure 18–1, shaded regions). The internal organization and connectivity of the core circuit transfers information about current motivational state into the cognitive, motor, emotional, and autonomic output systems that organize and integrate goal-directed behavior (Kalivas et al. 1993). This "translation of motivation into action" (Mogenson et al. 1993) depends on the mediolateral differentiation of the core circuit nuclei (NA, VP, and VTA) (Kalivas and Barnes 1993) (Figure 18–1). The NA is subdivided into a more medially located *shell region*, primarily affiliated with the limbic inputs to the core circuit, and a more lateral *core region*, affiliated in its connectivity with output regions in the basal ganglia and brainstem. The VP and VTA show similar functional differentiation into limbic-motive and motor-

output regions. Internal and external connections among core circuit nuclei and with other regions (e.g., PFC) provide multiple routes for this transfer. Connections within and between the core circuit nuclei permit direct transfer from limbic to motor parts of the motive circuit. Direct translation involves intranuclear and internuclear connections within and between nuclei of the core circuit. Indirect translation occurs when information leaves the medial circuit, projects to other regions (e.g., PFC), and is then projected back to the lateral division of the core circuit (Kalivas et al. 1993).

Clinical Pathogenesis

Neurobehavioral Mechanisms

Understanding the pathogenesis of DDMs requires considering the location, behavioral function, and neurochemistry of the neural systems that mediate them (Marin 1996b). The anatomical and physiological changes that affect these systems are a result of the complex mechanical and physiological effects of TBI. Gross pathology, such as contusion and hemorrhage, or more subtle changes, such as diffuse axonal injury, hypoxia, and microvascular changes (see Chapter 2, Neuropathology) (Levin and Kraus 1994), may damage cortical, subcortical, or deep parenchymal structures. Pathogenesis of TBI symptoms also may be understood in terms of the neurochemistry of the motivational circuitry (e.g., dopaminergic or glutamatergic pathways) (Levin and Kraus 1994).

Disruption of the core circuit undermines all of the major motivational functions described above in steps 1–5. Severe dysfunction leaves patients unable to establish or modify motivational state, select among alternative response options, or initiate behavior. If severe, this dysfunction presents as akinetic mutism or abulia. If less severe—either because the initial insult is less severe or because a patient with severe injury is improving—the patient shows apathy. These cases of apathy may be described as *pure* or affective apathy, because motivation is lost without impairment of extrapyramidal motor or executive cognition. This interpretation of pathogenesis is supported by clinical reports of DDMs in association with coarse brain disease affecting the anterior cingulum, ventral striatum, VP, and midbrain (Campbell and Duffy 1997; Mega and Cohenour 1997; Stuss et al. 2000). Cases of pure or affective apathy also result from dysfunction of other limbic structures that modify current motivational state (e.g., the amygdala, orbitofrontal cortex, and hippocampus). Therefore, patients with affective apathy should be evaluated for the features associated with dysfunction of these structures (e.g., Klüver-Bucy syndrome, "frontal personality," or amnestic syndrome) (Marin 1996a).

If dysfunction simultaneously affects the core circuit and the striatonigral system, motivational loss and extrapyramidal symptoms occur together. This presents as akinesia or *motor apathy*, depending on whether the extrapyramidal or motivational symptoms predominate, respectively. *Cognitive apathy*, the association of motivational loss with executive cognitive dysfunction, may have a neurological or behavioral mechanism, as described in the following sections.

A functional analysis of patients with diminished motivation suggests several ways in which loss of behavioral capacity may contribute to motivational loss. Although motivation is said to be the function of the medial circuit, clinical observations have long suggested that DDMs may result from dysfunction of the dorsolateral and orbitofrontal circuits as well (Marin 1996a, 1997b; Stuss et al. 2000). Cognitive apathy may be due to simultaneous damage to the dorsolateral cortex and the contiguous structures of the medial "motivation" circuit. However, the association of dorsolateral circuit dysfunction with apathy may have another explanation: it may be a psychological response to the perceived inability to organize behavior. In other words, lacking executive cognitive capacity, patients are less motivated to make an effort because they recognize that their efforts are not likely to succeed. Orbitofrontal dysfunction is also associated with a "background of apathy and abulia" (Hecaen and Albert 1975). Such motivational loss may result from loss of the capacity to establish the reward potential of current environmental stimuli.

These are not the only neurobehavioral mechanisms for motivational loss in DDMs. Loss of awareness of impairment, another symptom of prefrontal cortical damage, is predictive of return to work and rehabilitation potential of individuals with TBI (Sherer et al. 1998b). Although not yet demonstrated empirically, impaired awareness is thought to mediate these functional problems at least in part because of its impact on motivation (Andersson et al. 1999a; Sherer et al. 1998a). Incentive motivation can be operationalized by neuropsychological procedures that measure the effect of financial incentive on the speed of performing a simple psychomotor task (al-Adawi et al. 1998). Novelty seeking in Alzheimer's disease has been shown to discriminate between patients with and without apathy (Daffner et al. 1999). The validity of novelty seeking as a neurobehavioral mechanism for apathy is strengthened by physiological observations: Apathy in patients with frontal lobe damage was associated with diminished amplitude of P3 event-related potentials, which are correlates of stimulus novelty (Daffner et al. 2000). Other mechanisms of apathy are also possible. For example, in a sample of TBI and other neurological disorders, apathy was associated with diminished heart rate reactivity to emotional arousal (Andersson et al. 1999b).

Neurochemical Mechanisms

Neurochemical sequelae of TBI provide another way to understand DDMs. There is some evidence (van Woerkom et al. 1977; Vecht et al. 1975) that dopaminergic activity is affected in TBI. This is of particular importance given the essential role of dopamine systems in mediating responses to reward, novelty, and other elements of motivated behavior (McAllister 2000). Several other biochemical changes have been described in TBI, including changes in levels of glutamate, acetylcholine, neuropeptides, and oxygen-free radicals (see Chapter 2, Neuropathology). Their direct or indirect participation in the motivational circuitry provides a theoretical basis for them to alter motivation in TBI. This, in turn, provides a rationale for other pharmacological therapies in the treatment of DDMs (e.g., glutamatergic and cholinergic agents).

Assessment of Diminished Motivation

The assessment of patients with diminished motivation depends on knowledge of the etiology of diminished motivation and the confluence of biological, psychosocial, and socioenvironmental factors that control motivated behavior. Table 18–1 lists conditions associated with apathy, abulia, and akinetic mutism (Marin 1996a; Stuss et al. 2000). When less severe, the diseases that cause akinetic mutism cause abulia and apathy. In addition, there are many psychiatric disorders and psychosocial conditions that produce apathy. The information in the table implies that the assessment of patients with diminished motivation requires comprehensive and systematic neuropsychiatric assessment. This includes careful evaluation of the patient's social and physical environment. Differential diagnosis of diminished motivation, as discussed in the section Differential Diagnosis, guides the clinician to distinguish among these possibilities.

The psychosocial history indicates the baseline level of motivation (Marin 1996a) and coping skills (Finset and Andersson 2000) that characterize adult personality. This is particularly important in evaluating patients with subtle motivational loss. The clinician estimating an individual's premorbid or "normal" motivation must also consider cultural factors and diverse personal qualities and psychological features. It is important to keep in mind the enormous variability in individuals' accomplishments, interests, and goals and the way these are influenced by personal experience, education, social class, culture, and age cohort.

Personal loss, psychological trauma, and phase-of-life events may alter motivation. Occasionally, apathy is the primary symptom of an adjustment disorder (e.g., an

TABLE 18–1. Conditions associated with apathy, abulia, and akinetic mutism

Neurological disorders
  Frontal lobe
    Frontotemporal dementia
    Anterior cerebral artery infarction
    Tumor
    Hydrocephalus
    Trauma
  Right hemisphere
    Right middle cerebral artery infarction
  Cerebral white matter
    Ischemic white matter disease
    Multiple sclerosis
    Binswanger's encephalopathy
    Human immunodeficiency virus
  Basal ganglia
    Parkinson's disease
    Huntington's disease
    Progressive supranuclear palsy
    Carbon monoxide poisoning
  Diencephalon
    Degeneration or infarction of thalamus
    Wernicke-Korsakoff disease
  Amygdala
    Klüver-Bucy syndrome
  Multifocal disease
    Alzheimer's disease (apathy may be mediated by damage to prefrontal cortex, parietal cortex, amygdala)

Medical disorders
  Apathetic hyperthyroidism
  Hypothyroidism
  Pseudohypoparathyroidism
  Lyme disease
  Chronic fatigue syndrome
  Testosterone deficiency
  Debilitating medical conditions (e.g., malignancy, renal or heart failure)

Drug induced
  Neuroleptics, especially typical neuroleptics
  Selective serotonin reuptake inhibitors
  Marijuana dependence
  Amphetamine or cocaine withdrawal

Socioenvironmental (lack of reward, loss of incentive, lack of perceived control)
  Role change
  Institutionalism

Note. Akinetic mutism results from stroke, trauma, tumor, degenerative disease, or toxins (e.g., carbon monoxide poisoning) affecting the anterior cingulate gyrus (bilaterally) or paramedian structures of the diencephalon and midbrain (ascending reticular formation, medial forebrain bundle, or ventral pallidum). When improving or less severe, such cases present as abulia or apathy.

"empty nest syndrome" or retirement reaction) or the primary means for dealing with anxiety (i.e., a defense mechanism). The clinician should evaluate symptoms of personality disorder as well, keeping in mind the dynamics of motivation. The social withdrawal or emotional distance seen in Cluster A personality disorders may be mistaken for neurogenic motivational loss. Conversely, it is easy to err by attributing subtle motivational loss to Cluster A personality disorder when, in fact, one has encountered the first symptoms of neurogenic apathy (Marin 1996a).

Interactions of medical, psychological, and neurological variables are particularly relevant in elderly patients because they often have so many clinical problems. There is an extensive list of drugs whose use may alter motivation. Dopaminergic agents—agonists or antagonists—are most familiar as mediators of motivational change. But equally important are serotonergic, cholinergic, and adrenergic agents because of their interaction with dopamine systems. Pharmacokinetic variables, especially facilitation and inhibition of P450 enzymes, are an independent influence on motivation. For example, there are case reports suggesting that fluoxetine and other selective serotonin reuptake inhibitors (SSRIs) may dispose to apathy (Hoehn-Saric et al. 1990). Furthermore, SSRIs, particularly fluoxetine and paroxetine, are both potent 2D6 inhibitors. Therefore, if an irritable patient with TBI is treated with haloperidol and then, because apathy is misdiagnosed as depression, treated with one of these two SSRIs, motivation may worsen for two reasons: the SSRI may induce apathy directly, and haloperidol-induced motor apathy may worsen because the SSRI increases levels of haloperidol.

The neurological disorders affecting motivation and its neural machinery should direct the clinician's attention to several aspects of the neurological examination. Because frontal and diencephalic diseases figure prominently in the differential diagnosis of DDMs, it is important to know whether olfactory function, visual acuity, and visual fields are intact. Frontal release signs and paratonic rigidity (gegenhalten) are relevant for the same reason. Extrapyramidal motor signs clarify the evaluation of motor subtypes of DDMs. For example, chorea, micrographia, loss of associated movements, or loss of vertical eye movements suggest that diminished motivation may be due to Huntington's disease, Parkinson's disease, or progressive supranuclear palsy. Neuropsychological assessment clarifies the cognitive subtypes of motivational loss, often in intricate and unexpected ways. For example, the results of executive cognitive assessment may suggest that lack of activity in one patient reflects impairment in sequencing, whereas in another patient it reflects loss of verbal fluency and initiation. Each benefits from a different type of "psychological prosthesis," as discussed in the section Treatment.

A word is in order about formal rating of motivational loss. Clinicians, especially those unfamiliar with DDMs, may find it helpful to rate the severity of motivational loss. The rating process familiarizes one systematically with the clinical signs of motivation and its loss. Furthermore, ratings may aid differential diagnosis. For example, if a clinician is unsure of whether a psychomotor-retarded patient is apathetic or depressed, it may be helpful for the clinician to discover that ratings show high levels of apathy and low levels of depression. This would suggest the psychomotor retardation is better characterized as bradykinesia and akinesia. If so, the next clinical step may be to perform a neurological examination and obtain a magnetic resonance image of the head rather than to have the patient start taking an antidepressant.

Several rating methods are available for quantifying loss of motivation. Construct validity is strongest for the Apathy Evaluation Scale (AES; Figure 18–2) (Marin et al. 1991), an 18-item scale that can be administered as a self-rated scale, a caregiver pencil-and-paper test, or a clinician-rated semistructured inventory. Several papers document the feasibility of rating apathy with the Apathy Scale (Starkstein et al. 1992, 1993) that is derived from a preliminary version of the AES. Its content is close enough to that of the AES that there is little reason to doubt its validity. The Children's Motivation Scale (Gerring et al. 1996), also derived from the AES, uses developmentally appropriate behavioral anchors to permit rating of apathy in children and adolescents. The Neuropsychiatric Inventory (Cummings et al. 1994) is a multidimensional instrument administered to caregivers. It was developed specifically to assess noncognitive symptoms of dementia and devotes 1 of 10 item domains to apathy. Instruments (Reichman and Negron 2001) derived from the Schedule for the Assessment of Negative Symptoms (SANS) have also been presented to estimate negative symptoms in dementia by using information from caregiver interviews. Observations of patient participation by clinical staff also have been used to index motivation (al-Adawi et al. 1998). A test based on the effect of monetary incentive on psychomotor speed has also been described (al-Adawi et al. 1998), although it is intended more for experimental than clinical purposes.

Apathy may be the dominant feature of the mental status, or it may occur in association with symptoms of other syndromes. In the former instance, one diagnoses a *syndrome* of apathy or one of the other DDMs (Marin 1996a, 1997a). Criteria for the syndrome of apathy have been proposed (Marin 1991), and in Alzheimer's disease, evidence for their validity has been presented (Starkstein et al. 2001). When associated with depression, dementia, or, for that matter, any other syndrome, the presence of diminished motivation should be carefully discriminated

___ 1. She/he is interested in things.

___ 2. She/he gets things done during the day.

___ 3. Getting things started on his/her own is important to him/her.

___ 4. She/he is interested in having new experiences.

___ 5. She/he is interested in learning new things.

___ 6. She/he puts little effort into anything.

___ 7. She/he approaches life with intensity.

___ 8. Seeing a job through to the end is important to her/him.

___ 9. She/he spends time doing things that interest her/him.

___ 10. Someone has to tell her/him what to do each day.

___ 11. She/he is less concerned about her/his problems than she/he should be.

___ 12. She/he has friends.

___ 13. Getting together with friends is important to him/her.

___ 14. When something good happens, she/he gets excited.

___ 15. She/he has an accurate understanding of her/his problems.

___ 16. Getting things done during the day is important to her/him.

___ 17. She/he has initiative.

___ 18. She/he has motivation.

FIGURE 18–2.   The Apathy Evaluation Scale (AES).

Scoring the AES: All items are rated 1–4 as follows: 1=not at all characteristic, 2=slightly characteristic, 3=somewhat characteristic, 4=a lot characteristic. The AES rating is the total score for the AES *after* recoding items. Items are recoded so that a higher score on the AES indicates higher levels of apathy. Therefore, all positively worded items must be recoded as follows: 1=4, 2=3, 3=2, 4=1. *Thus, all items must be recoded except items 6, 10, and 11.* **Interpretation:** The minimum score for the AES is 18. A score of 36 suggests mild apathy. However, the AES is not well standardized. Age, social environment, diagnosis, and other factors should be considered in evaluating results. *Source.*   Reprinted from Marin RS, Biedrzycki RC, Firinciogullari S: "Reliability and Validity of the Apathy Evaluation Scale." *Psychiatry Research* 38:143–162, 1991. Used with permission.

and the question asked, Is apathy simply a feature of this other syndrome (e.g., depression), or does the patient have a second condition whose presence is signaled by motivational loss? This approach implies that it is appropriate to diagnose a DDM and some other syndrome simultaneously. Just as a patient with schizophrenia may have psychosis and negative symptoms, a patient with TBI may have depression and apathy simultaneously.

Treatment

Diminished motivation can cause a range of impairment, from subtle to serious, in biopsychosocial functioning. Physical rehabilitation, functional capacity, socialization, and family involvement all suffer when motivation falters. Therefore, treating DDMs requires psychosocial and bio-

logical interventions that are based on comprehensive assessment. This is as true for DDMs as it is for any other neuropsychiatric complication of TBI. The growing interest in apathy and related DDMs is leading to novel approaches to understanding coping impairments (Finset and Andersson 2000) and pathogenetic neuropsychological losses (al-Adawi et al. 1998) of patients with apathy. These and other new approaches are likely to lead to new therapies for DDMs.

Treatment of akinetic mutism and abulia is primarily pharmacological. Patients with apathy may require pharmacological interventions; however, their preservation of cognitive and communicative capacity calls increasingly for psychological and social interventions. Such interventions are based on careful and ongoing characterization of the patient's motivational and neuropsychological status. The general principle is to define the patient's losses and residual capacities and then design a "psychological prosthesis" that compensates for the deficits and makes the best possible use of residual abilities. Regardless of severity, treatment must consider the physical and psychosocial environment. Therefore, modifying the overall environment and attending to family and professional caregivers is an elementary but crucial dimension of treatment for DDMs.

As a preliminary step, treating a DDM requires optimizing the patient's general medical condition. This may mean controlling seizures or headaches, arranging physical or cognitive rehabilitation for cognitive and sensorimotor loss, or ensuring optimal hearing, vision, and speech. These are elementary steps for any treatment plan. However, they also increase motivation because improved physical status may enhance functional capacity, drive, and energy and thereby increase the patient's expectation that initiative and effort will be successful. In the terms offered in the section Mechanism, these steps increase the patient's sense of control or subjective probability of success.

Environmental Interventions

The purpose of environmental interventions is to increase the reward potential of the environment. Adaptive devices, such as motorized wheelchairs or voice-activated computers, compensate directly for the sensorimotor and neurological impairments that deny the patient the full benefit of the environment. In impoverished environments, either at home or in institutions, interventions may entail directly introducing new sources of pleasure, interest, and stimulation. Apathetic TBI patients in the intensive care unit or on general medical floors are particularly vulnerable to sensory deprivation, social isolation, and perceived loss of control. Sensory deprivation may be addressed by improving lighting, normalizing the diurnal pattern of lighting, and minimizing the impact of white noise and electrical devices. Social isolation and socialization may be improved by extending visiting hours and improving access to areas where patients gather for dining, groups, and informal socialization. For many, returning to the familiar personal and physical circumstances of their homes may be the fastest way to a healthier physical or social environment.

Psychological Interventions

General psychological status contributes to motivation in the same way that general medical condition does. Goal-directed behavior depends not only on motivation but also on other state variables: arousal, attention, mood, and cognition. Therefore, the psychological treatment for DDMs goes hand in hand with the treatment of con-

ditions—for example, stupor, delirium, depression, dementia—that lead to these disorders. Such treatments may include a variety of behavioral techniques (Campbell and Duffy 1997; Giles and Clark-Wilson 1988, 1993) or specialized cognitive rehabilitative approaches to accomplish, for example, enhancement of attention or performance speed (Palmese and Raskin 2000). Psychoeducation, vocational counseling, and psychotherapy should not be overlooked. Psychotherapy may focus on injury-related loss, interpersonal problems, or family stressors.

Behavioral Interventions

The clinician should introduce behavioral interventions methodically, making clear the tasks and skills required of the patient. Goals should be developed collaboratively to strengthen engagement and enhance the patient's sense of control and expectation of success. Once goals are developed, staff should be careful to follow through on the treatment plan. The countertransference response of care providers to patients with DDMs is becoming apathetic, expending less effort, and feeling resigned or depressed. Health care providers are all vulnerable to misinterpreting patients' lack of motivation as their own, because apathy and other DDMs can evoke futility, resignation, and depression in caregivers. Such countertransference inadvertently truncates efforts by the treatment team.

General supportive measures are obviously valuable for patients with DDMs. However, these general supportive measures have specific aims in patients with diminished motivation. These aims include improving diminished initiative, impersistence, lack of ambition, lack of awareness, diminished response to reward, perceived lack of control of environment, and absence of goals. Supportive therapy can be provided in many forms. Examples include encouraging, reassuring, helping the patient identify and maintain short-term objectives, providing reward for positive outcomes, and reframing the patient's goals as achieving an objective "for yourself" or "for your family's sake."

Finally, there is the integration of neuropsychological assessment with the treatment of motivational loss. Accurate assessment provides the template for developing an individualized plan for psychological treatment. The treatment can be thought of as a psychological or motivational prosthesis because it is precisely molded to the pattern of abilities lost as a result of injury. A few examples may be useful. Patients with affective apathy show deficits in initiation and perseveration. Therefore, their psychological prosthesis requires the caregiver to prompt the patient regarding when to begin or end a particular task. In other words, the psychological prosthesis is a specific substitute for the impairments in beginning and ending an activity. On the other hand, patients with cognitive apathy may be able to initiate behavior but fail to act because they are unable to sequence, plan, and monitor behavior. Their motivational prosthesis requires the caregiver to tell the patient, "Go into the kitchen…. Now open the refrigerator door…. Now take out the sour cream on the top shelf…. Bring the sour cream into the dining room…. Thank you very much." In this case, the motivational prosthesis is a specific substitute for the impairments in planning and sequencing.

Similar psychological prostheses aid DDM patients with other neurobehavioral impairments. Of particular importance is the association of diminished motivation with *environmental dependency* or *stimulus-bound behavior*. This is the tendency of the patient to respond automatically or concretely to environmental stimuli; it contrasts with actions that follow a verbal instruction or an internally generated plan. Because of environmental dependency, a patient who likes music may turn on a radio in his own home but will not do so in the hospital. A bland or unfamiliar environment aggravates this condition because there is nothing to trigger the old behaviors. Families complain, "All he does is sit around here and do nothing." Professional caregivers may have the same complaints. A variety of neuropsychological impairments contribute to environmental dependency. One is that the patient is unable to generate an idea or goal for behavior. The psychological prosthesis in this instance uses the pathology itself to treat the problem. Instead of trying to create new habits, the caregiver returns the person to an environment that habitually elicits the desired behavior. In most cases, this means returning the patient home or at least creating an environment that looks like home (e.g., by bringing in family photographs and favorite books). If tested in the psychiatrist's office (an unfamiliar environment), the patient may seem as apathetic as before. But to caregivers, behavior is improved. The old environment triggers old behaviors that make the patient "look better than he is."

The principle of a psychological prosthesis is, of course, not specific to DDMs. It can be applied to other problems that contribute to motivational loss. Memory aids help the amnestic patient and may enhance motivation in the process. These may be used by the patient directly, provided that memory problems are not simply due to forgetfulness. In either case, caregivers can devise methods to remind the patient of goals and plans, keeping the patient on track with short-term objectives and long-term goals. Organizational skills help the patient with attentional- and working-memory impairment. Here, too, increasing the subjective sense of competency may improve motivation.

Pharmacological Treatment

There are four steps to pharmacological treatment:

1. Optimize medical status.
2. Diagnose and treat other conditions more specifically associated with diminished motivation (e.g., apathetic hyperthyroidism, Parkinson's disease).
3. Eliminate or reduce doses of psychotropics and other agents that aggravate motivational loss (e.g., SSRIs, dopamine antagonists).
4. Treat depression in the most efficacious way possible. Because knowledge of depression treatment exceeds that of treatment of DDMs, treating depression usually takes preference when symptoms of both disorders are present. When apathy is associated with depression, consider using more activating antidepressants (e.g., sertraline, bupropion). Venlafaxine also may be useful, particularly at higher doses that are associated with noradrenergic as well as serotonergic reuptake inhibition. In some patients, a monoamine oxidase inhibitor may be indicated for treatment of depression. If so, tranylcypromine sulfate may be preferable to other monoamine oxidase inhibitors because of its stimulant or amphetamine-like property. If apathy persists after resolution of dysphoria and vegetative symptoms, it can be specifically targeted for further treatment, as described next. However, one should first reconsider the diagnosis. Apathy in this setting may be a symptom of a second, perhaps unrecognized, disorder whose diagnosis and treatment may be of consequence. For example, an individual with TBI may develop posttraumatic normal pressure hydrocephalus or parkinsonism.

When apathy or another DDM is the primary clinical problem, stimulants, dopamine agonists, and other agents are introduced (Table 18–2). These agents have been used for a variety of behavioral and cognitive impairments in TBI (Gualtieri 1988; Levin and Kraus 1994; Powell et al. 1996) (see Chapter 34, Psychopharmacology). For DDMs, stimulants and dopamine agonists may be clinically effective, sometimes dramatically so (Campbell and Duffy 1997; Crismon et al. 1988; Muller and von Cramon 1994). Well-designed studies evaluating these agents in large samples are not available for treatment of DDMs in TBI or other neuropsychiatric disorders. However, some systematic work has been reported (al-Adawi et al. 1998; Powell et al. 1996; van Reekum et al. 1995). There is a developing literature (Cummings 2000) suggesting that cholinesterase inhibitors (i.e., donepezil, galantamine, rivastigmine) may benefit patients with apathy, as well as other symptoms, who also have dementia of various causes. Given their relatively low risk for serious toxicity, cholinesterase inhibitors may have a place in the treat-

TABLE 18–2.   Drugs used in the treatment of apathy, abulia, and akinetic mutism

Agent	Usual total daily dosage in mg (range)
Stimulants	
Dextroamphetamine	20 (5–60)
Methylphenidate	20 (10–60)
Activating antidepressants	
Bupropion	200 (100–400)
Tranylcypromine sulfate	45 (30–90)
Protriptyline	40 (20–60)
Venlafaxine	150 (100–450)
Dopamine agonists (selective and mixed)	
Amantadine	200 (100–300)
Bromocriptine	10 (5–90)
Selegiline	10 (5–40)[a]
Levodopa/carbidopa	25/100 tid–25/250 qid
Pergolide	2 (1–5)
Other psychotropics	
Modafinil	200 (50–400)
Donepezil	5 (5–10)
Galantamine	8 bid (4–8 bid)
Rivastigmine	3 bid (1.5–6 bid)

[a]Requires diet low in tyramine, especially at doses above 10 mg; lower doses may produce serotonin syndrome if administered with agents that slow selegiline metabolism.

ment of TBI patients with apathy and, conceivably, more severe DDMs.

With stimulants and dopamine agonists, treatment is initiated at minimal doses. Once benefit begins, improvement is usually dose dependent. Therefore, slowly increasing the dose is indicated until the patient is clearly functioning better or until concerns about drug toxicity limit dose increases. Some patients respond to small doses. But when impairment is clear-cut and risk factors for treatment are few, higher doses should be considered.

There is little knowledge of how to manage stimulants and dopamine agonists once optimal benefit is achieved. The response to missed doses or discontinuation is variable. Some patients worsen promptly, even after missing single doses. The duration of dopaminergic and other pharmacotherapies for DDMs must be evaluated individually. In some patients, treatment must be continued indefinitely because discontinuation precipitates recurrence of

symptoms. In other patients, a gradual taper and discontinuation may be feasible, presumably reflecting neural plasticity or other processes that are part of recovery. Even when successful, the discontinuation may not be possible until after a year or more of treatment. Fortunately, tachyphylaxis seems unusual. In addition to ongoing risks of side effects, financial cost may obligate the physician to consider dose reduction (Campbell and Duffy 1997; Levin and Kraus 1994; Muller and von Cramon 1994).

Patients with cognitive apathy (apathy associated with executive cognitive dysfunction) may be treated with methylphenidate or amphetamine. There is a modest literature (Campbell and Duffy 1997; Muller and von Cramon 1994) describing significant and sometimes dramatic benefit of bromocriptine in the treatment of abulia and akinetic mutism. Presumably other and less-toxic dopamine agonists have comparable potential. Pramipexole may have some advantage for DDMs because it has selectivity for D_3 dopamine receptors, which are preferentially distributed in the limbic forebrain, but this remains to be proved. All of the dopaminergic drugs dispose to behavioral toxicity, including psychosis, motor activation and restlessness, sleep disturbance, and delirium. With the stimulants, care should be taken to monitor pulse and blood pressure, although serious problems are unusual. Amantadine may benefit patients with apathy (Kraus and Maki 1997; Schneider et al. 1999; van Reekum et al. 1995). However, amantadine's nonspecificity—it alters dopaminergic and glutamatergic receptors—may actually be a clinical advantage (Kraus and Maki 1997), because DDMs are not due to lack of dopaminergic activity only. In older patients, amantadine dosing must be adjusted for decreased creatinine clearance.

DDM associated with extrapyramidal motor symptoms (i.e., motor apathy) is treated with the same agents, including amantadine. What is distinctive in treating motor apathy is the goal of treatment: The aim is to manipulate dopaminergic function for the sake of motivation, not just to improve walking or speech. Overlooking this point may compromise outcome in the end, because the benefit of improved mobility is undercut by lack of motivation.

Newer psychotropic medications may be helpful for DDMs. Modafinil, introduced recently for the treatment of narcolepsy, has stimulating or arousing effects that may prove useful in some patients. Modafinil may cause headache and gastrointestinal symptoms but otherwise seems relatively free of major toxicity. Growing knowledge of glutamate systems raises the possibility that glutamatergic agents may prove useful as well (Goff and Coyle 2001).

The following case example illustrates the integration of psychological, socioenvironmental, and pharmacological treatments in DDM:

Mr. Q, a senior partner in a reputable law firm, sustained a closed head injury in a motor vehicle accident 2 years ago. Previously a typical type A personality, since the accident he had become socially disengaged and uninterested in his work or leisure activities. His family found him emotionally distant and uncommunicative. He seemed withdrawn but denied feeling depressed. He acknowledged others' complaints about him but was unable to state why he was this way. After participating in multiple antidepressant trials with no improvement, he was referred to the neuropsychiatry clinic, where he was recognized as having moderately severe apathy, mild dysphoria, and impairments in memory and executive cognitive capacity. While taking methylphenidate, 10 mg bid, he showed improved affective connection and communication with his wife and children. His work performance remained poor, however. In part, he was demoralized because his law firm, recognizing his impairments, removed him from challenging, high-pressure cases. In part, he lacked any meaningful way to make use of his experience and residual abilities. At an early point, it was recognized that the support of his wife and children was compromised by their belief that he had become "lazy and depressed."

Psychoeducational meetings made it possible for the family to understand that his personality changes were due to brain damage. Thereby, they became more understanding of his impairments and more tolerant of the unavoidable frustrations and fears they were all facing. When the patient considered resigning from his job, he was referred for individual therapy. Supportive measures focused his attention on the fact that he was still dedicated to being the financial provider and personal support to his wife and family. He was persuaded not to resign his position, even though the workplace offered him little incentive or satisfaction. Additional motivational benefit was gained through increase of methylphenidate to 60 mg/day. Cognitive rehabilitation addressed the impact of his cognitive deficits on his motivation to persevere at work. "Psychological prostheses" were created to compensate for cognitive and motivational deficits: Memory and planning aids were introduced to help him deal with personal and work responsibilities, and the reward potential of his work environment was improved by finding tasks that were better matched to his cognitive abilities. For the latter, the patient's business partners, prompted by his wife, shifted his work to taxation law (more use of rote memory) and away from his previous role as a trial lawyer so that there was less need to "think on his feet" (i.e., less demand for executive functions and working memory). Overall, the rewards of his work experience were enhanced by balancing the patient's residual strengths and capacities with the flexibility and resources of his work environment. As the patient spent more time "behind the scenes" than in the courtroom, his sense of stress and demoralization diminished, and his ability to see himself as a financial provider, spouse, and parent improved.

Conclusion

Motivation is fundamental for adaptive behavior. The major disorders of diminished motivation (DDMs) are apathy, abulia, and akinetic mutism. Depending on its etiology, a DDM may be the primary clinical disturbance, a symptom of some other disorder, or a coexisting second disorder requiring independent diagnosis and management. This makes assessment complicated and challenging. Differential diagnosis usually focuses on delirium, dementia, depression, demoralization, akinesia, catatonia, and aprosodia. Motivation is considered to be a distributed capacity. The neurology of motivation focuses on the representation of current motivational state in a core circuit (composed of the anterior cingulum, nucleus accumbens, ventral pallidum, and ventral tegmental area) and the modification of current motivational state by the prefrontal cortex, amygdala, and hippocampus. Current knowledge permits an approach to assessment and treatment of DDMs through an understanding of these systems. Treatment of DDMs includes the full range of biomedical, psychological, and socioenvironmental approaches available in neuropsychiatry. Treating DDMs is an essential part of TBI care, offering individuals with TBI a way to improve their functional abilities and quality of life. Because the neuropsychiatry of motivation is so new, there is limited knowledge for guidance. However, experience has shown that individuals with TBI and their families may benefit in many and sometimes dramatic ways from the treatment of DDMs.

References

al-Adawi S, Powell JH, Greenwood RJ: Motivational deficits after brain injury: a neuropsychological approach using new assessment techniques. Neuropsychology 12:115–124, 1988

Alexander GE: Basal ganglia-thalamocortical circuits: their role in control of movements. J Clin Neurophysiol 11:420–431, 1994

American Congress of Rehabilitation Medicine: Recommendations for use of uniform nomenclature pertinent to patients with severe alterations in consciousness. Arch Phys Med Rehabil 76:205–209, 1995

Andersson S, Gundersen PM, Finset A: Emotional activation during therapeutic interaction in traumatic brain injury: effect of apathy, self-awareness and implications for rehabilitation. Brain Inj 13:393–404, 1999a

Andersson S, Krogstad JM, Finset A: Apathy and depressed mood in acquired brain damage: relationship to lesion localization and psychophysiological reactivity. Psychol Med 29:447–456, 1999b

Atkinson JW, Birch D: An Introduction to Motivation. Princeton, NJ, Van Nostrand, 1978

Benson DF: Psychomotor retardation. Neuropsychiatry Neuropsychol Behav Neurol 3:36–47, 1990

Berrios GE, Gili M: Abulia and impulsiveness revisited: a conceptual history. Acta Psychiatr Scand 92:161–167, 1995

Bush G, Frazier JA, Rauch, SL, et al: Anterior cingulate cortex dysfunction in attention-deficit/hyperactivity disorder revealed by fMRI and the counting Stroop. Biol Psychiatry 45:1542–1552, 1999

Cairns H, Oldfield RC, Pennybacker JB, et al: Akinetic mutism with an epidermoid cyst of the third ventricle. Brain 64:273–290, 1941

Campbell JJ III, Duffy JD: Treatment strategies in amotivated patients. Psychiatr Ann 27:44–49, 1997

Celesia GG: Persistent vegetative state: clinical and ethical issues. Theor Med 18:221–236, 1997

Crismon ML, Childs A, Wilcox RE, et al: The effect of bromocriptine on speech dysfunction in patients with diffuse brain injury (akinetic mutism). Clin Neuropharmacol 11:462–466, 1988

Cummings JL: Cholinesterase inhibitors. Am J Psychiatry 157:4–15, 2000

Cummings JL, Mega M, Gray K, et al: The Neuropsychiatric Inventory: comprehensive assessment of psychopathology in dementia. Neurology 44:2308–2314, 1994

Daffner KR, Mesulam MM, Cohen LG, et al: Mechanisms underlying diminished novelty-seeking behavior in patients with probable Alzheimer's disease. Neuropsychiatry Neuropsychol Behav Neurol 12:58–66, 1999

Daffner KR, Mesulam MM, Scinto LFM, et al: The central role of the prefrontal cortex in directing attention to novel events. Brain 123:927–939, 2000

Dunlop TW, Udvarhelyi GB, Stedem AF, et al: Comparison of patients with and without emotional/behavioral deterioration during the first year after traumatic brain injury. J Neuropsychiatry Clin Neurosci 3:150–156, 1991

Fink M, Taylor MA: The many varieties of catatonia. Eur Arch Psychiatry Clin Neurosci 251 (suppl 1):I8–I13, 2001

Finset A, Andersson S: Coping strategies in patients with acquired brain injury: relationships between coping, apathy, depression and lesion location. Brain Inj 14:887–905, 2000

Fisher CM: Honored guest presentation: abulia minor vs. agitated behavior. Clin Neurosurg 31:9–31, 1983

Gerring JP, Freund L, Gerson AC, et al: Psychometric characteristics of the Children's Motivation Scale. Psychiatry Res 63:205–217, 1996

Giles GM, Clark-Wilson J: The use of behavioral techniques in functional skills training after severe brain injury. Am J Occup Ther 42:658–665, 1988

Giles GM, Clark-Wilson J: Brain Injury Rehabilitation: A Neurofunctional Approach. New York, Chapman and Hall, 1993

Goff DC, Coyle JT: The emerging role of glutamate in the pathophysiology and treatment of schizophrenia. Am J Psychiatry 158:1367–1377, 2001

Gualtieri CT: Pharmacotherapy and the neurobehavioral sequelae of traumatic brain injury. Brain Inj 2:101–129, 1988

Hecaen H, Albert M: Disorders of mental functioning related to frontal lobe pathology, in Psychiatric Aspects of Neurological Disease. Edited by Benson DF, Blumer D. New York, Grune & Stratton, 1975, pp 137–149

Hillgard ER: The trilogy of mind: cognition, affection and conation. J Hist Behav Sci 16:107–117, 1980

Hoehn-Saric R, Lipsey JR, McLeod DR: Apathy and indifference in patients on fluvoxamine and fluoxetine. J Clin Psychopharmacol 32:672–674, 1990

Jones MR: Introduction, in Nebraska Symposium on Motivation. Edited by Jones MR. Lincoln, NE, University of Nebraska Press, 1955, pp v–x

Kalivas PW, Barnes, CD: Limbic Motor Circuits and Neuropsychiatry. Boca Raton, FL, CRC Press, 1993

Kalivas PW, Churchill L, Klitenick MA: The circuitry mediating the translation of motivational stimuli into adaptive motor responses, in Limbic Motor Circuits and Neuropsychiatry. Edited by Kalivas PW, Barnes CD. Boca Raton, FL, CRC Press, 1993, pp 237–288

Kalivas PW, Churchill L, Romanides A: Involvement of the pallidal-thalamocortical circuit in adaptive behavior. Ann N Y Acad Sci 877:64–70, 1999

Kant R, Duffy JD, Pivovarnik A: Prevalence of apathy following head injury. Brain Inj 12:87–92, 1998

Kraus MF, Maki PM: Effect of amantadine hydrochloride on symptoms of frontal lobe dysfunction in brain injury: case studies and review. J Neuropsychiatry Clin Neurosci 9:222–230, 1997

Levin H, Kraus MF: The frontal lobes and traumatic brain injury. J Neuropsychiatry Clin Neurosci 6:443–454, 1994

Marin RS: Apathy: a neuropsychiatric syndrome. J Neuropsychiatry Clin Neurosci 3:243–254, 1991

Marin RS: Apathy and related disorders of diminished motivation, in American Psychiatric Press Review of Psychiatry, Vol. 15. Edited by Dickstein L, Riba MB, Oldham JM. Washington, DC, American Psychiatric Press, 1996a, pp 205–242

Marin RS: Apathy: concept, syndrome, neural mechanisms, and treatment. Semin Clin Neuropsychiatry 1:304–314, 1996b

Marin RS: Apathy—who cares? an introduction to apathy and related disorders of diminished motivation. Psychiatr Ann 27:18–23, 1997a

Marin RS: Differential diagnosis of apathy and related disorders of diminished motivation. Psychiatr Ann 27:30–33, 1997b

Marin RS, Biedrzycki RC, Firinciogullari S: Reliability and validity of the Apathy Evaluation Scale. Psychiatry Res 38:143–162, 1991

Marsh NV, Kersel DA, Havill JH, et al: Caregiver burden at 1 year following severe traumatic brain injury. Brain Inj 12:1045–1059, 1998

Mazaux JM, Masson F, Levin HS, et al: Long-term neuropsychological outcome and loss of social autonomy after traumatic brain injury. Arch Phys Med Rehabil 78:1316–1320, 1997

McAllister TW: Apathy. Semin Clin Neuropsychiatry 5:275–282, 2000

Mega MS, Cohenour RC: Akinetic mutism: disconnection of frontal-subcortical circuits. Neuropsychiatry Neuropsychol Behav Neurol 10:254–259, 1997

Mega MS, Cummings JL: Frontal-subcortical circuits and neuropsychiatric disorders. J Neuropsychiatry Clin Neurosci 6:358–370, 1994

Mesulam M-M: Attentional networks, confusional states, and neglect syndromes, in Principles of Behavioral and Cognitive Neurology. Edited by Mesulam M-M. New York, Oxford University Press, 2000a, pp 174–256

Mesulam M-M (ed): Principles of Behavioral and Cognitive Neurology, 2nd Edition. New York, Oxford University Press, 2000b

Mogenson GJ, Jones DL, Yim CY: From motivation to action: functional interface between the limbic system and the motor system. Prog Neurobiol 14:69, 1980

Mogenson GJ, Brudzynski SM, Wu M, et al: From motivation to action: a review of dopaminergic regulation of limbic—nucleus accumbens—ventral pallidum—pedunculopontine nucleus circuitries involved in limbic-motor integration, in Limbic Motor Circuits and Neuropsychiatry. Edited by Kalivas PW, Barnes CD. Boca Raton, FL, CRC Press, 1993, pp 193–207

Muller U, von Cramon DY: The therapeutic potential of bromocriptine in neuropsychological rehabilitation of patients with acquired brain damage. Prog Neuropsychopharmacol Biol Psychiatry 18:1103–1120, 1994

Pagnoni G, Zink CF, Montague PR, et al: Activity in human ventral striatum locked to errors of reward prediction. Nat Neurosci 5:97–98, 2002

Palmese CA, Raskin SA: The rehabilitation of attention in individuals with mild traumatic brain injury, using the APT-II programme. Brain Inj 14:535–548, 2000

Powell JH, al-Adawi S, Morgan J, et al: Motivational deficits after brain injury: effects of bromocriptine in 11 patients. J Neurol Neurosurg Psychiatry 60:416–421, 1996

Raichle ME, Fiez JA, Videen TO, et al: Practice-related changes in human brain functional anatomy during nonmotor learning. Cereb Cortex 4:8–26, 1994

Reichman WE, Negron A: Negative symptoms in the elderly patient with dementia. Int J Geriatr Psychiatry 16 (suppl 1):S7–S11, 2001

Rifkin A, Quitkin F, Klein D: Akinesia: a poorly recognized drug-induced extrapyramidal behavioral disorder. Arch Gen Psychiatry 32:672–674, 1975

Rolls ET: Neurophysiology and functions of the primate amygdala, in The Amygdala. Edited by Aggleton JD. New York, Wiley, 1992

Rolls ET: The Brain and Emotion. Oxford, Oxford University Press, 1999

Ross ED: Affective prosody and the aprosodias, in Principles of Behavioral and Cognitive Neurology, 2nd Edition. Edited by Mesulam M-M. New York, Oxford University Press, 2000, pp 316–331

Scheel-Kruger J, Willner P: The mesolimbic system: principles of operation, in The Mesolimbic Dopamine System: From Motivation to Action. Edited by Willner P, Scheel-Kruger J. Chichester, England, Wiley, 1989, p 559–597

Schneider WN, Drew-Cates J, Wong TM, et al: Cognitive and behavioural efficacy of amantadine in acute traumatic brain injury: an initial double-blind placebo-controlled study. Brain Inj 13:863–872, 1999

Schultz W: Dopamine neurons and their role in reward mechanisms. Curr Opin Neurobiol 7:191–197, 1997

Schultz W, Apicella P, Scamati E, et al: Neuronal activity in monkey ventral striatum related to the expectation of reward. J Neurosci 12:4595–4610, 1992

Sherer M, Bergloff P, Boake C, et al: The Awareness Questionnaire: factor structure and internal consistency. Brain Inj 12:63–68, 1998a

Sherer M, Bergloff P, Levin E, et al: Impaired awareness and employment outcome after traumatic brain injury. Brain Inj 13:52–61, 1998b

Starkstein SE, Mayberg HS, Preziosi TJ, et al: Reliability, validity, and clinical correlates of apathy in Parkinson's disease. J Neuropsychiatry Clin Neurosci 4:134–139, 1992

Starkstein S, Federoff JP, Price TR, et al: Apathy following cerebrovascular lesions. Stroke 24:1625–1630, 1993

Starkstein SE, Petracca G, Chemerisnki E, et al: Syndromic validity of apathy in Alzheimer's disease. Am J Psychiatry 158:872–877, 2001

Stuss DT, van Reekum R, Murphy KJ: Differentiation and states and causes of apathy, in The Neuropsychology of Emotion. Edited by Borod JC. New York, Oxford University Press, 2000, pp 340–366

Ungerleider LG, Mishkin M: Two cortical visual systems, in The Analysis of Visual Behavior. Edited by Ingle DJ, Mansfield RJW, Goodale MD. Cambridge, MA, MIT Press, 1982, pp 549–586

van Reekum R, Bayley M, Garner S, et al: N of 1 study: amantadine for the amotivational syndrome in a patient with traumatic brain injury. Brain Inj 9:49–53, 1995 van Woerkom TC, Teelken AW, Minderhoud JM, et al: Difference in neurotransmitter metabolism in frontotemporal lobe contusion and diffuse cerebral contusion. Lancet 1:812–813, 1977

Vecht CJ, van Woerkom CA, Teelken AW, et al: Homovanillic acid and 5-hydroxyindoleacetic acid cerebrospinal fluid levels. Arch Neurol 32:792–797, 1975

Widlocher DJ: Psychomotor retardation: clinical, theoretical, and psychometric aspects. Psychiatr Clin North Am 6:27–40, 1983

Wilson FA, Rolls ET: Neuronal responses related to reinforcement in the primate basal forebrain. Brain Res 502:213–231, 1990

19 Awareness of Deficits

Laura A. Flashman, Ph.D.

Xavier Amador, Ph.D.

Thomas W. McAllister, M.D.

INDIVIDUALS WHO EXPERIENCE a traumatic brain injury (TBI) may have multiple medical, physical, and cognitive limitations. They may also have reduced awareness of these deficits. In fact, up to 45% of individuals with moderate to severe TBI demonstrate awareness deficits (Freeland 1996). Deficits that are clearly evident to family or therapists are often not "seen" by the individual, are judged to be inconsequential, or are discounted. Such unawareness is often permanent and can be an enormous impediment to successful rehabilitation. Furthermore, deficits in awareness can be function specific. Some individuals with TBI can accurately assess their physical status (e.g., hemiplegia) but are less reliable in their assessment of their capacity for sound judgment, cognitive skills, interpersonal skills, and other aspects of social behavior. Lack of awareness of cognitive deficits, personality changes, and abnormal behavior is commonly observed in moderate to severe TBI (usually associated with loss of consciousness of more than 20–30 minutes), and the behavior that can result is frequently the most troublesome to families and caregivers and presents the most significant barrier to returning to a more normalized existence after an injury.

Definition of Lack of Awareness

Awareness of capabilities, or the absence of such awareness, is not a straightforward, unitary concept. Many terms are used in the scientific literature and in common parlance to convey different aspects of this concept. It is important to keep these different terms, characteristics, and distinctions in mind as one considers the literature addressing awareness, not only in patients with TBI, but in other forms of central nervous system (CNS) insults, because there has been some imprecision in the use of these terms. Terms such as *agnosia*, *anosognosia*, *unawareness*, and *denial* are often used interchangeably, and examination of the manner in which they are used often suggests various meanings, depending on the author or context. This is further complicated by the fact that awareness deficits may be attributable to neurological impairment, psychological denial of disability, or some combination of the two (Katz et al. 2002). For clarification, we briefly define a number of related terms in Table 19–1.

Dimensions of Awareness

To better understand the concept of lack of awareness, it is helpful to conceptualize several different dimensions to the problem. We have previously described a schema (Flashman and McAllister 2002; Flashman et al. 1998) proposing three distinct dimensions related to awareness. Briefly, the first dimension is whether an individual has knowledge of a specific deficit or difficulty. For example, it is common for individuals who have had a TBI to have

This work was supported in part by National Institute on Disability and Rehabilitation Research grants H133G70031 and H133000136, National Institutes of Health grant R01 NS40472–01, National Institute of Mental Health grant P20 MH50727, the Developing Schizophrenia Research Center, and a Young Investigator Award from the National Alliance for Research on Schizophrenia and Depression.

TABLE 19–1. Terms and definitions used when describing lack of awareness

Term	Definition
Agnosia	Denotes an impairment in recognition that cannot be explained on the basis of primary motor or sensory impairment; failure to recognize the significance of objects (e.g., visual agnosia).
Anosognosia	A lack of knowledge about a deficit. Usually used to describe an apparent loss of recognition or awareness of left hemiplegia after an abrupt brain insult (Babinski 1914). Currently used to describe the occurrence of frank denial of a neurological deficit. It is often used to refer to the inability to truly recognize one's strengths and deficits after a traumatic brain injury.
Denial of illness	Redescription of anosognosia (Weinstein and Kahn 1955); implies a psychological or psychodynamic level of explanation—that is, patients with anosognosia are thought to be motivated to block distressing symptoms from awareness by using a defense mechanism (denial).
Lack of insight	Has been used to describe a spectrum of concepts, ranging from a psychological defense mechanism to lack of cognitive skills that permit understanding of deficits; generally considered to be a multidimensional construct.
Anosodiaphoria	The absence of concern, or indifference to an acknowledged deficit or illness.

problems in several domains, including sensorimotor, cognitive, and behavioral difficulties. Although some individuals may accurately describe their postinjury changes, others with similar deficits may argue persuasively that they are no different from their preinjury state despite dramatic evidence to the contrary. The second dimension is the emotional response that an individual manifests to his or her difficulties or deficits. In patients who are aware of a given deficit, responses can range from complete indifference (anosodiaphoria) to bitter complaint. Similarly, patients unaware of their deficits can manifest responses ranging from indifference to angry denial when attempts are made to convince them of their impairment. The third dimension is the ability to comprehend the impact or consequence(s) of a deficit on day-to-day life. For example, some patients are aware that

they have significant deficits (e.g., memory impairment) and are concerned about them but believe that they can function at their premorbid level without difficulty.

The manner in which an individual accounts for admitted difficulties or deficits is a separate but related issue. Causal attribution of a particular deficit or difficulty requires two things: first, that a person acknowledge a deficit; and second, that he or she attribute it to the injury to a degree sufficient to have the trauma become part of his or her self-definition (Gordon et al. 1998). For example, many individuals acknowledge difficulties in certain areas but attribute those difficulties to factors other than their brain injury (e.g., "stress" or "tension"). Although these individuals have some awareness of a deficit, their inability to attribute the deficit to their injury can result in problems overcoming the deficit and engaging in specific therapeutic activities.

Awareness in Healthy Individuals

It is important to note that even healthy individuals engage in inaccurate self-representation at times, which is not always deliberate or conscious; this is a different phenomenon from "impression management," which has been defined as an intentional or deliberate form of socially desirable responding. The cognitive distortions displayed by healthy individuals are believed to represent a normal pattern of functioning and have been shown to be positively linked to well-being, positive effectivity, and self-esteem (Tournois et al. 2000). In addition, positive forms of self-deception (i.e., self-deceptive enhancement) may help serve to orient a person favorably toward the future (Trivers 2000). Research has suggested that self-deception is maximized when there is a lack of concrete information (i.e., making predictions about the future or recalling certain information from the past), and the motivation to self-deceive is high (i.e., a wish to make a good impression on someone or strong belief in one's own abilities and capabilities). Sackeim and Wegner (1986) examined aspects of self-evaluation in patients with depression and schizophrenia and in healthy control subjects. They found that the latter two groups used "self-serving biases" in their appraisals of their behaviors and outcomes, whereas the depressed patients did not. The self-serving biases were characterized as follows: "If an outcome is positive, I controlled it, I should be praised, and the outcome was very good. If an outcome is negative, I did not control it (as much), I should not be blamed, and it was not so bad anyway." Although individuals with TBI also use this defense mechanism in everyday life, the unawareness of symptoms manifested as part of their brain damage is a distinct, neurologically driven phenomenon, as described in the section Lack of Awareness After TBI.

Lack of Awareness in Other Neuropsychiatric Disorders

Bearing differences in meaning, terminology, and methodology in mind, it is helpful to review what is known about the different aspects of lack of awareness in other neurological disorders, as it can inform our understanding of the problem in individuals with TBI.

Anton's Syndrome

One of the more dramatic examples of awareness deficits in CNS injury occurs in Anton's syndrome. Individuals with this syndrome are cortically blind, usually from damage to the occipital cortex or optic radiations involving the primary visual or visual association cortex, or both (Anton 1898; Heilman 1991). They are unable to describe objects placed before them and stumble into walls or furniture when attempting to walk, but, remarkably, believe that they can see. A variety of mechanisms have been proposed to account for the lack of awareness seen in these patients (see Heilman 1991 for full discussion), including associated confusion and memory loss, an inability to monitor visual input, and a disconnection of visual processing from speech and language areas. Heilman (1991) has suggested another scheme in which visual imagery and visual processing compete for attention and "representation on a visual buffer" (p. 57). Destruction of visual processing results in unimpeded display of visual imagery, which is misinterpreted by the individual as the ability to see, and may relate to the confabulated responses frequently noted.

Anosognosia Related to Hemiplegia and Hemianopia

Another dramatic example of lack of awareness of deficits can be seen in individuals with sudden hemiplegia and hemianopia, most commonly of vascular origin, and typically in the nondominant hemisphere. Functionally, these individuals are unable to move the contralateral limb (usually the arm) or perceive stimuli in the contralateral hemifield, yet they proclaim that they are well and unimpaired in these functions. When the deficits are pointed out, emotional responses can range from denial ("anosognosia," often associated with confabulated explanations for the observed facts) to bland acceptance (anosodiaphoria). Most evidence suggests that involvement of the nondominant inferoparietal cortex is required (Critchley 1953; Gerstmann 1942); however, patients with lesions apparently restricted to the frontal lobes have

also been described (Zingerle 1913). Anosognosia related to left hemiplegia and left hemianopia with both cortico-subcortical lesions and lesions confined to deep structures has also been reported (Bisiach et al. 1986; Gerstmann 1942; Healton et al. 1982; Watson and Heilman 1979). Furthermore, although the most common examples of anosognosia occur after nondominant hemisphere lesions, the frequent occurrence of severe speech and language deficits associated with analogous lesions in the dominant hemisphere limits the conclusions that can be drawn. Notably, not all hemiplegic and hemianopic patients with large lesions involving the inferoparietal cortex develop anosognosia.

A related but separate phenomenon is that of neglect, which refers to the lack of attention directed to part of the body (usually one side, commonly the nondominant side) or space, or both. This can take the form of failure to orient to stimuli originating from the neglected region or the selective extinguishing of competing stimuli originating from different regions (e.g., left body and right body). This occurs in the context of intact visual fields and thus is a different phenomenon from hemianopia. Neglect is also more commonly seen after nondominant hemispheric injury, but not exclusively so. Neglect is often seen in patients with anosognosia, but there are individuals in whom these phenomena are dissociated (Bisiach and Geminiani 1991; Heilman 1991).

Anosognosia in Aphasia

Anosognosia has been reported to accompany jargon aphasias (e.g., Wernicke's aphasia, transcortical sensory aphasia, and global aphasia). Jargon aphasia is characterized by long, rambling sentences, meaningless utterances, phonemic or semantic paraphasias, and neologisms. Typically, patients with jargon aphasia do not appear to monitor their own utterances. They make few hesitations, pauses, or self-corrections. The patients' behaviors generally suggest that they are unaware both that listeners do not understand them and that they themselves do not comprehend what is said to them. Although some researchers have suggested that many patients appear to have at least some awareness of their speech and language deficits (e.g., Cohn and Neuman 1958), it should be noted that there is significant variability in the degree of awareness of aphasia in published cases of jargon aphasia.

The anatomical substrate of the lack of awareness associated with jargon aphasias is not clear. Weinstein et al. (1966) compared patients with jargon aphasia to those with aphasia without jargon. All of the patients with jargon aphasia had bilateral damage, whereas the remaining 24 patients with aphasia had mostly unilateral brain lesions. In addition to being seemingly unaware of their language deficits, the patients with jargon aphasia tended to deny other deficits such as hemiparesis or hemianopia. The authors concluded that jargon aphasia requires a left hemisphere lesion accompanied by further neurological damage, which is also required for anosognosia. Although Brown (1981) also reported bilateral lesions in patients with jargon aphasia, Gianotti (1972) found that 30% of his patients with Wernicke's aphasia with anosognosia had only left hemisphere damage, indicating that although bilateral involvement may be conducive to anosognosia in aphasia, it is not necessary.

Awareness of Deficits in Other Neuropsychiatric Disorders

Although the preceding syndromes provide the most dramatic examples of awareness deficits after CNS injury, other neurological disorders are frequently associated with more subtle awareness deficits. For example, many patients with Alzheimer's disease fail to recognize the cognitive impairments caused by their illness, as well as the impact that their deficits have on their lives and those who care for them. Although there is considerable variability in the degree of deficit awareness among patients (Neary et al. 1986), some findings (Feher et al. 1991; Reisberg et al. 1985; Santillan et al. 2003) suggest that the lack of insight in these patients increases with severity of dementia, correlates with executive dysfunction (Lopez et al. 1994), and may be associated with hypoperfusion of the right dorsolateral frontal lobe (Reed et al. 1993). Unawareness in dementia has also been identified as a multidimensional construct (Howorth and Saper 2003).

Individuals with schizophrenia also frequently demonstrate a lack of awareness of the deficits caused by their illness and its impact. Lack of awareness of illness in schizophrenia does not appear to be associated with epidemiological variables, neurological signs, or positive and negative symptoms (Amador et al. 1993; Cuesta and Peralta 1994; David et al. 1995; Peralta and Cuesta 1994). The relationship between severity of illness and lack of awareness of illness remains unclear, although there are a number of reports that suggest they are independent of each other (e.g., Amador et al. 1994; Bartko et al. 1988; David et al. 1995; McGlashan 1981).

The literature suggests that lack of awareness of illness is not simply a function of global cognitive deficits but perhaps is more related to frontal-executive dysfunction (Cuesta and Peralta 1994; Cuesta et al. 1995; David et al. 1995; Lysaker and Bell 1994, 1998; McEvoy et al. 1989; Mohamed et al. 1999; Rossell et al. 2003; Young et al. 1993). Our own work has suggested that lack of aware-

ness in schizophrenia is associated with selective structural brain changes, including smaller brain size and selective atrophy of certain subregions of the frontal lobes (Flashman et al. 2000, 2001).

It seems clear, then, that a variety of CNS disorders are commonly associated with deficits in awareness, and that the latter is more a final common pathway for certain profiles of brain damage than a problem unique to those with TBI. We now review what is known about awareness deficits in TBI and discuss how the profile of injury commonly seen in TBI fits with the disorders described in preceding sections to assist in understanding the neuroanatomical substrate of lack of awareness.

Lack of Awareness After TBI

As noted at the beginning of this chapter, lack of awareness is a common and disabling sequela of TBI (Freeland 1996). Furthermore, it has become clear that certain deficits are more commonly acknowledged than others after an injury. Several investigators (e.g., Ford 1976; Miller and Stern 1965; Ota 1969) have noted that, in contradistinction to those who care for them, individuals with TBI are much less likely to complain of changes in judgment, personality, and/or behavior. Fahy et al. (1967) evaluated ratings of 32 patients with severe TBI and their relatives (mean, 6 years postinjury). They found that, although patients exhibited some awareness of their intellectual, memory, and speech deficits, they rarely acknowledged changes in personality or behavior such as irritability, impulsivity, and affective instability that were reported by relatives. Others have also reported less patient awareness of changes in personality in the context of at least some awareness of cognitive deficits (McKinlay and Brooks 1984; Thomsen 1974). Furthermore, these individuals may not acknowledge, or may minimize, the severity of deficits for up to several years after the injury (Groswasser et al. 1977; Prigatano 1986). For example, Groswasser et al. (1977) reported that all patients who demonstrated unawareness of behavioral problems at 6 months postinjury continued to be unaware of these changes at a 30-month follow-up.

Tyerman and Humphrey (1984) assessed self-concept in 25 severely brain-injured patients at 7 months postinjury by evaluating their ratings of anxiety, depression, and attitude toward physical disability. They reported that although patients with TBI were aware of numerous changes in themselves compared with before their accidents (i.e., viewed themselves as quite different from their "past self"), the majority of subjects reported that they expected to recover completely within a year. In fact, ratings of their "present self" did not differ significantly in most domains from ratings of "a typical person," and were generally more positive than their ratings of "a typical head-injured person." This suggests that despite awareness of some degree of change resulting from their TBI, they were somewhat unrealistic about their prospects of recovery, because most severely brain-injured patients continue to have some degree of impairment.

Port et al. (2002) noted that most studies investigating self-awareness after TBI are conducted at least 2 years after the injury. They examined awareness deficits in 30 moderate to severe TBI patients who were less than 2 years postinjury, using ratings provided by the patients and their significant others on the Awareness of Deficit Questionnaire, which examines various domains of daily functioning. Although the researchers found substantial agreement between the patients and their significant others, the patients were less likely to acknowledge problems in executive functioning. This finding suggests that awareness is impaired even in the early recovery stages, which has significant implications for rehabilitation.

Measurement of Awareness

The methodology used to assess awareness is also important to consider. A number of strategies have been used to attempt to quantify awareness of deficits in patients with TBI. The most common strategy is comparison of patients' self-report of their function with another more objective measure. That is, comparisons can be made on the difference between patients' ratings and those made by their families, those made by rehabilitation staff, or by comparing patients' estimates of their abilities to actual performance measures. Additionally, self-report questionnaires have been used to gather quantitative data on other measures of function. The most frequently used of these questionnaires are described briefly in Table 19–2. Recent work has attempted to correlate some of these measures with each other and with cognitive measures (Bogod et al. 2003; Sherer et al. 2003b). An alternate means of quantitative assessment is use of structured interview questions, in which responses are scored by the interviewer according to a rating scale. In this case, the clinician is rating the patient's accuracy of self-perception (e.g., Ezrachi et al. 1991; Fleming et al. 1996; Levin et al. 1987).

There are some limitations to these methods. The use of questionnaires and structured interviews to quantify awareness of deficits relies predominantly on patients' ability to understand verbal questions and to verbalize their understanding of their deficits. A number of patients, due to speech and language disorders, are there-fore unable to be assessed using such methods. There is also literature that suggests that relatives also may deny disability (McKinlay and Brooks 1984; Romano 1974), another confounding variable to obtaining accurate information regarding changes after TBI. In addition, it has been noted that there are certain circumstances in which participants may rate themselves as having more difficulty than does their informant, who may simply not be familiar enough with the behavior to be aware of difficulties (Leathem et al. 1998). Finally, when ratings are made by rehabilitation or other clinical staff, information regarding how the person was before the TBI may not be available to the raters; this information could be important in accurately completing the objective assessment. Giacino and Cicerone (1998) use an open-ended interview with patients in which they assess the nature of their responses to confrontation or feedback regarding these deficits, or both, and suggest that this may provide additional information about the basis of the unawareness. They suggest that it may be possible to characterize individuals' reactions to objective performance feedback according to their cognitive response, their affective response, and the manner in which feedback is used.

In general, however, individuals with TBI have been shown to underestimate the severity of their cognitive and behavioral impairments when compared with ratings of family members, clinician ratings, and their performance on neuropsychological testing. These difficulties in accurately assessing strengths and weaknesses have a significant negative impact on overall outcome by decreasing motivation for treatment. Clinicians working to rehabilitate individuals with TBI report that unawareness is a major factor in determining long-term functional recovery (Gerstmann 1942; Trudel et al. 1996), including eventual return to employment, level of vocational achievement, and independent living status. Several studies have investigated the association between impaired awareness and functional outcome after TBI (Cavallo et al. 1992; Ezrachi et al. 1991; Fordyce and Roueche 1986; Rattok et al. 1992; Sherer et al. 1998a, 2003a; Trudel et al. 1996; Walker et al. 1987). These findings are summarized in Table 19–3 and provide strong, though not unqualified, evidence of a positive association between accurate self-awareness and favorable employment outcome after TBI.

Newman et al. (2000) studied self-awareness in 37 patients with TBI in an acute rehabilitation program using the Functional Self-Appraisal Scale, which compares patient and staff ratings of patient performance on tasks relevant for acute rehabilitation. There was a significant difference between ratings near admission, consistent with previous findings in acute settings that individuals with

TABLE 19–2. **Rating scales frequently used to assess unawareness of illness in traumatic brain injury**

Scale name	Authors	Purpose
Patient Competency Rating Scale	Prigatano and Fordyce 1986	Evaluates competency to perform various behavioral, cognitive, and emotional tasks, as well as providing insight into the level of awareness; 30 items scored on a 5-point Likert scale; informant and patient versions
The Awareness Questionnaire	Sherer et al. 1998b	Assesses awareness of motor/sensory, cognitive, and behavioral/affective deficits after traumatic brain injury; 18 items scored on a 5-point Likert scale; rated by patients and family/significant others or clinician
Head Injury Behaviour Scale	Godfrey et al. 1993	Rates 20 behavioral items on a 4-point Likert scale; generates two scores: number of problems and distress score; patient and relative versions
Functional Self-Assessment Scale	Newman et al. 2000	Rates abilities in functional areas related to physical, cognitive, and emotional capabilities; 12 items rated on a 4-point scale; can be self-administered or used in a structured interview format; patient and rehabilitation staff member version
Barrow Neurological Institute Screen for Higher Cerebral Functions	Prigatano et al. 1995	Samples a wide range of neuropsychological functions; scores range from 3 to 50 (all items passed successfully); provides quantitative and qualitative information
Self-Awareness of Deficits Interview	Fleming et al. 1996	Obtains both qualitative and quantitative data on self-awareness (of deficits, functional implications, and ability to set realistic goals); interview style with responses rated on a 4-point scale
Self/Other Rating Form	Sohlberg et al. 1998	Rates cognition, social/emotional issues, daily living skills, physical abilities, and leisure time management; 24 items rated on a 5-point scale; patient and caregiver versions, interview format used

TBI tend to overestimate their abilities relative to other raters (Allen and Ruff 1990; Prigatano et al. 1990; Sherer et al. 1995, 1998b). By time of discharge, there was no significant difference between patient and staff ratings. However, it was suggested that this convergence of ratings was due primarily to patient improvement on the rehabilitation tasks, rather than a reflection of increased awareness—that is, staff ratings changed from time 1 to time 2 assessments, whereas patient ratings did not. The authors noted that the difference between patients' and staffs' ratings did not correlate with neuropsychological performance on admission and suggested that this supports the notion that awareness early in the recovery process is a distinct construct.

Overview of the Neuroanatomical Substrate of Awareness

On the basis of the study of cognitive processes in patients with various unawareness syndromes, a variety of models have been proposed to explain how individuals are aware of deficits and how they respond to them. Most of the models suggest several key features are necessary to the proper functioning of these metacognitive processes.

TABLE 19–3. Studies investigating the relationship between impaired awareness and functional outcome after traumatic brain injury (TBI)

Study	Participants	Findings
Fordyce and Roueche 1986	Twenty-eight patients, severity unknown; three groups: one with ratings similar to clinicians, one rating themselves as less impaired; one group rating themselves as less impaired at admission but consistent with clinicians at discharge	No group differences in vocational outcome at follow-up. Reanalysis by Sherer et al. (1998a) found that final self-ratings indicating accurate awareness were more predictive of favorable vocational outcomes.
Walker et al. 1987	Twenty-five patients, severity unknown; compared patient self-ratings to ratings of family/significant others at admission to day treatment program	At follow-up, patients whose initial self-assessments agreed with assessments of family members were more productive than those who rated themselves as less impaired.
Ezrachi et al. 1991	Fifty-nine patients with moderate or severe TBI	Accuracy of self-appraisal was predictive of vocational status 6 months after discharge. Awareness and acceptance were most favorable predictors of successful return to work.
Cavallo et al. 1992	Thirty-four patients with mild to severe TBI; compared patient ratings to those of family/significant others	Accuracy of awareness ratings did not affect return-to-work rates.
Trudel et al. 1996	Compared patient and therapist ratings	Direct relationship between the size of discrepancy in ratings and poorer outcome. Awareness was primary predictor of vocational and independent living status.
Sherer et al. 1998a	Sixty-six individuals with mild to severe TBI; two ratings of awareness (direct clinician rating of patients' accuracy and comparison of patient ratings to those of family/significant other)	Positive relationship between accurate self-awareness of functioning after TBI and favorable long-term employment outcome, regardless of awareness rating used.

These include intact primary stimulus processing (e.g., visual or other sensory input), the ability to monitor properly the input (compare it to known templates), the ability to formulate a response or choose from a menu of responses to the input, the ability to monitor the response chosen, and the ability to compare the anticipated response with the actual response. For example, Heilman (1991) suggests that the reason many patients with Wernicke's aphasia do not self-correct is that they are unable to monitor their verbal output; they are thus unaware that what they say makes no sense and can become quite frustrated when others fail to understand what they are saying. In the instance of hemiplegia and associated anosognosia, Heilman (1991) suggests a different mechanism, namely that the usual right hemisphere lesion that produces the hemiplegia in some instances also disables the motor intention system. In the normal course of events, the motor intention circuits prepare the motor system for action and along with that the "expectation" that movement will take place. This expectation is subsequently compared with the actual results (i.e., movement does or does not take place in accordance with expectation), a function he terms "the comparator." In the presence of a disabled motor intention system, there is no intention fed into the "comparator," no expectation of movement set up, and thus no discrepancy noted by the comparator when no movement takes place. When confronted by the absence of movement and the observation by an observer that thus the arm must be paralyzed, the patient interprets the absence of such a discrepancy or mismatch as an intact motor system. In the case of the Wernicke's patient, the error is one of inadequate feedback; in the instance of the motor anosognosia, the error is improper "feedforward."

Stuss (1991; Stuss and Benson 1986) has suggested that the frontal lobes, or perhaps frontal systems, play a critical role in the maintenance of full awareness, whereas the knowledge of function, or conversely the knowledge of specific deficits, is associated with posterior brain functions. Lesions in specific posterior regions can lead to specific primary deficits (e.g., Anton's syndrome, neglect, and anosognosia). As noted in the section Lack of Awareness in Other Neuropsychiatric Disorders, patients with these disorders can have knowledge of some deficits and absence of knowledge about other deficits. This has been termed *modality-specific awareness*. Cases of modality-specific awareness argue against a central awareness mechanism. Rather, such cases suggest that the substrate underlying knowledge or awareness of specific deficits may be linked to modality-specific posterior (probably nondominant) brain regions. Thus, for example, awareness of visual deficits would seem to involve posterior regions, probably in the visual association cortex. On the basis of the anosognosia associated with hemiplegia findings, awareness of contralateral motor function has been linked to the region of the inferior parietal lobule.

The response to acknowledged deficits may well involve several different brain regions. The response to deficits most closely linked to lack of awareness is anosodiaphoria. An important component of this indifference to an obvious deficit may be selective inattention or neglect. Watson et al. (1981), for example, reported a patient with a right medial thalamic stroke who demonstrated contralateral neglect. He acknowledged his neurological deficits, including hemiparesis, but was quite unconcerned about the deficits. Watson et al. (1981) suggest that several interconnected regions, including the midbrain reticular formation, selected thalamic nuclei, and frontal cortex, facilitate attention and preparation of the brain for action (motor intention). Lesions in these areas may result in problems with neglect or the motor intention system, or both, and could result in an individual's appearing somewhat unconcerned by obvious deficits. The frontal lobes also may be important, because they play a role in the affective response to a given stimulus. Individuals with dorsolateral frontal injury often display muted, bland, apathetic responses to significant stimuli. This may well tie into the anosodiaphoria, or indifference to deficits, that brain-injured patients can manifest.

Stuss (1991; Stuss and Benson 1986) suggests that frontal systems generate self-awareness, self-reflectiveness, and self-monitoring. Because frontal systems also play a critical role in the modulation of key social skills and behaviors (e.g., initiation, motivation, problem solving, and affective modulation), frontal lobe damage can affect the ability to understand the impact that deficits have on day-to-day function and future function and how to apply that knowledge to a current situation. In individuals with TBI, this dimension is frequently the focus of concern. Irritability, disinhibited outbursts, childishness, and intrusiveness are extremely common behavioral traits, yet are often not recognized by individuals with TBI (Ford 1976; McAllister 1992; Miller and Stern 1965; Oddy et al. 1985; Ota 1969; Prigatano 1991). One frequently sees the malignant combination of severe social skills deficits and an inability to understand the ramifications of these deficits. Even when the individual admits to some difficulties, he or she is often unable to predict the implications of these deficits in current or future social situations.

The neuroanatomical substrate of properly attributing the cause of various acknowledged deficits or difficulties to the TBI is not known. Table 19–4 presents a brief summary of this information.

TABLE 19–4.   **Putative brain circuitry associated with components of unawareness**

Component	Putative brain mechanisms or neural circuitry	Sample references
Lack of knowledge of deficits	Posterior modality-specific primary sensorimotor cortex (e.g., impaired visual cortex in Anton's syndrome)	Anton 1898; Heilman 1991; Stuss 1991; Stuss and Benson 1986
Performance monitoring	Unknown; hypothesized "comparator" region that monitors fit between intention and action/output (e.g., people with Wernicke's aphasia unable to monitor own verbal output	Heilman 1991; Stuss 1991; Stuss and Benson 1986
Response to deficits	Loop involving midbrain reticular activating system, medial thalamus, and medial and dorsolateral prefrontal cortex	Stuss 1991; Stuss and Benson 1986; Watson et al. 1981
Generalizability/ application of knowledge to other contexts	Dorsolateral and mesial frontal-striatal-thalamic-frontal circuits	Cummings 1993; Stuss 1991; Stuss and Benson 1986
Attribution/cause of deficits	Unknown	

Relationship of the Typical Profiles of TBI Pathology to the Circuitry of Awareness

Given the preceding, it is not surprising that awareness deficits of various types are a common and challenging problem in individuals with TBI. As described by Gennarelli and Graham (1998; see Chapter 2, Neuropathology), the typical profile of brain injury in acceleration-deceleration injuries includes contusions in the orbitofrontal region, the anterior and inferior temporal regions, and beneath or contralateral to the site of impact (coup or contrecoup). Intracerebral hemorrhages are seen in a variety of regions, including the basal ganglia. In moderate and severe TBI, diffuse axonal injury occurs. Such diffuse injury is often particularly evident in the corpus callosum, the superior cerebellar peduncle, the basal ganglia, and the periventricular white matter.

As DeKosky et al. (1998) point out, not all injury occurs at the time of impact. "Secondary injury," or that injury that is set in motion by the primary impact but evolves over the subsequent minutes, hours, or even days, also plays a crucial role in the postinjury sequelae. The various cascades involved in secondary injury can result in significant and far-reaching sequelae removed in location and time from the primary injury (see Chapters 2, Neuropathology, and 39, Pharmacotherapy of Prevention).

Thus, there is significant overlap between the brain regions that play a role in awareness (broadly defined) and those regions most commonly injured in the typical TBI. There is a direct relationship between increased degree of diffuse axonal injury and injury severity; thus, it is not surprising that there is a correlation between injury severity and lack of awareness (Freeland 1996). The frontal lobes, both the dorsolateral and orbitofrontal areas, and related circuitry (subcortical white matter, basal ganglia, and thalamus) are also vulnerable to TBI. The known role these regions play in cognition and behavior, self-monitoring, self-awareness, and other metacognitive processes makes it readily apparent why challenging behaviors, along with failure to acknowledge the significance of those behaviors, inappropriate response to the behaviors, and difficulty comprehending the implications of these behaviors and other deficits, are such a common and vexing problem in individuals with TBI.

Impact of Lack of Awareness on Treatment and Rehabilitation

Individuals with TBI and impaired awareness can be challenging for both rehabilitation workers and families. Evidence suggests individuals with TBI are more likely to be aware of residual physical disabilities and often have a reduced appreciation of their limitations and impairments in the cognitive, functional, and psychosocial domains (Bond 1975; Brooks 1991). It has also been reported that in some circumstances significant others and family members are less aware of cognitive problems than are some individuals with TBI (Cavallo et al. 1992; Heilbronner et al. 1989; Hillier and Metzer 1997). Similarly, although family members may be less aware of more internal problems such as fatigue or pain, they are more likely than individuals with TBI to report personality and behavior problems (Hillier and Metzer 1997). This demonstrates that there can be a wide divergence of perceptions between the three groups of individuals—patients with TBI, family members, and clinical staff—involved in the recovery and outcomes after TBI, and this can cause significant conflict that can affect the course of rehabilitation. In fact, failure to recognize cognitive, emotional, and behavioral barriers may be one of the most disabling effects of TBI and represents the greatest impediment to rehabilitation.

Giacino and Cicerone (1998) suggest that the existence of different types of unawareness after TBI may have implications for prognosis and rehabilitation because unawareness of deficits is related to rehabilitation outcome. In their view, patients with unawareness of deficits secondary to impairment of cognitive subsystems such as attention, memory, or reasoning appear capable of increasing their awareness when they are provided with relevant feedback and information about their disability, in parallel with improvements in these cognitive domains. Patients with unawareness secondary to psychological denial are unlikely to modify their behavior and are likely to demonstrate reduced motivation and resistance to treatment with attempts to increase their awareness. Finally, patients with unawareness secondary to breakdown of a supraordinate monitoring system may also be incapable of modifying their behavior, despite intact intellectual knowledge of possible deficits.

There are various strategies for working with patients with unawareness of deficits secondary to TBI (Deaton 1978), although little empirical evidence exists to demonstrate their effectiveness (Fleming et al. 1996). From a theoretical standpoint, approaches generally can be categorized as those that address awareness as an overarching deficit that must be addressed before change can occur, and those that nest the treatment of awareness deficits in a broader, integrative program designed to maximize functional capacity. For example, some clinicians argue that neither a prerequisite level of awareness nor awareness training is an essential ingredient for behavior change (e.g., Sohlberg et al. 1998). That is, individuals with TBI can be trained to use compensatory strategies even when they do not understand why or believe that they do not need them. However, the fact that behavior can change without changed awareness does not imply that increased awareness cannot change behavior. As Kent (1999) points out, the deeper and more comprehensive an individual's awareness becomes, the more that person is able to apply his or her understanding to new and different situations. Although one can behaviorally train a person to use compensatory strategies, without some increase in awareness of the need for these strategies, it is difficult to get that person to continue to use the strategies or generalize to other situations.

Many different approaches have been attempted to increase the level of awareness in individuals with brain injury, including education regarding the consequences of brain injury (Fordyce and Roueche 1986), community activities designed to highlight limitations and barriers (Barin et al. 1985), videotaping individuals with brain injury and providing feedback regarding their behavior (Alexy et al. 1983), and development of an instructional game format (Zhou et al. 1996). For example, Chittum et al. (1996) used an individualized training package (educational discussion) in conjunction with the board game format to teach awareness of behavioral and cognitive difficulties to three adults with acquired brain injury. All three participants responded favorably to the training, which was assessed by percentage of questions answered correctly during the game sessions and in pre/postgeneralization probes in both domains.

As noted, others argue for what they conceptualize as a more comprehensive-integrative model. This model of treatment involves developing and working toward goals in several areas of everyday life. Patients work toward goals in a gradual, stepwise fashion. Each step involves increasingly greater levels of independence, with the overall goal being the highest level of functional independence for each individual. Significant changes have been reported in the vocational status and living situation of even severely injured TBI patients after several months of treatment (Ben-Yishay et al. 1987; Malec et al. 1993; Prigatano et al. 1984). Although it is not clear which aspects of the program are most crucial to successful outcome, level of awareness has been identified as an important component (Bergquist and Jacket 1993; Ezrachi et al. 1991; Prigatano et al. 1990).

We would argue that there are several components of any successful approach that should be attended to, including assessment, neuropsychological evaluation, development of a therapeutic alliance, supportive group and family therapy, and education of the patient and his or her support system. These components are outlined in Table 19–5 and discussed briefly in the following paragraphs.

First, it is helpful to delineate the extent and profile of the awareness deficit. One should clarify whether the problem is more a deficit in knowledge, an inappropriate response to an acknowledged deficit (e.g., anosodiaphoria), or an inability to understand the impact or consequences that the deficits will have on areas of day-to-day function. For those who acknowledge deficits, it is important to assess whether they accurately attribute those deficits to their TBI. This clarification process informs the treatment process.

A difficult issue is assessing to what extent lack of awareness in any of the preceding dimensions is related to cognitive deficits or to psychological denial, or both. Critical to this differentiation is information provided by the neuropsychological evaluation. Evidence of significant cognitive impairment makes it more likely that awareness deficits are related to actual brain injury as opposed to the psychological defense mechanism of denial. It should be remembered that individuals can have a combination of injury-induced awareness deficits and psychological responses to those deficits. They then present a mixed picture of "neurological" and "psychological" denial.

An important intervention is the establishment of a therapeutic relationship. This is particularly important for individuals in whom the very premise that they need assistance is disputed. The therapist must tread a difficult line between validation of the individuals' self and world view and not fostering unrealistic expectations and hopes. Even when there is a solid relationship between patient and therapist, it can be difficult to overcome some of the awareness deficits. Although some of the more dramatic knowledge deficits such as those seen in Anton's syndrome and the anosognosia associated with hemiplegia resolve over days to weeks, this is not a universal outcome. Many of the deficits associated with TBI, especially those in the areas of social skills and behavior, are permanent. However, these patients often comply with rehabilitation, especially if the rehabilitation is subtle and not called *rehabilitation*. Some individuals may be open to receiving help in certain areas (e.g., ambulation and speech) but may be resistant to the idea that they need help with interpersonal skills or anger management. When social skills and anger management rehabilitation can be integrated into rehabilitation in domains people are willing to consider, multiple goals can be met. Once an adequate therapeutic foundation is present, interventions should be geared toward gently confronting the individual with the discrepancy between the patient's own view of his or her strengths and abilities and the perceptions of others. Because of the usual associated memory and related cognitive deficits, this must usually be done repetitively and in small doses, taking cues from the individual with regard to his or her tolerance for this process (De-Luca et al. 1996).

TABLE 19–5.   Components of the treatment process

Component	Goal	Likely problems
Assessment	To delineate the extent and profile of the awareness deficit.	Deficits in knowledge. Inappropriate response to acknowledged deficit. Inability to understand impact/consequences of deficits on function.
Neuropsychological evaluation	To determine to what extent awareness deficits are related to cognitive deficits.	Frontal-subcortical system impairment. Right parietal lobe dysfunction.
Development of a therapeutic alliance	To develop a relationship in which therapists can validate individuals' self and world view without fostering unrealistic hopes/expectations. Individuals with TBI may comply with rehabilitation even when they do not agree they have deficits.	Individuals may become alienated from therapist and rehabilitation process if they feel assistance is being forced on them.
Education of individual with TBI	To provide individuals with some idea of the treatment goals.	Poor motivation in individuals who do not agree with identified problems. Difficulty with generalizing knowledge to real-life situations.
Group therapy	To provide individuals with TBI feedback from others who are or have been in similar circumstances.	Resistance to identifying with others as "similar."
Education of support system (family/significant others)	To provide family and significant others with better understanding of brain injury and issues related to awareness.	Family members and/or significant others may provoke catastrophic reactions in individuals with TBI by attempting to "force awareness" on them.
Supportive therapy for family/significant others	To facilitate coping skills and allow family/significant others to provide more support to individuals with TBI.	Family members and significant others may also be in denial regarding seriousness of deficits.

Note.   TBI=traumatic brain injury.

To maintain goals made during treatment, patients should be consulted and care taken to set goals that will motivate them. Although individuals are typically poorly motivated to pursue goals they see as irrelevant, rehabilitation becomes aimless without some appropriate set of goals (Bergquist and Jacket 1993). Creating a realistic set of goals that the patient is motivated to pursue represents a significant but crucial challenge. Making decisions regarding appropriate goals involves obtaining history and input from the patient and other informants and from direct observation. Group therapy may also be effective. Feedback from others who are or have been in similar circumstances can further assist people in recognizing that a problem behavior has occurred. Assistance may be required with generalization of skills as well, because even when an individual is aware of his or her deficits, or at least acknowledges them, he or she can have great difficulty applying that knowledge to real-life situations.

Education and supportive therapy for significant others also play a vital role in the process of improving the patient's awareness (Ergh et al. 2002). This therapy permits the family to gain a better understanding of brain injury and the issues related to awareness and leads to an appreciation of how that applies to their loved one. This facilitates improved coping skills and in turn allows the family to provide more support to the TBI survivor. Modeling the process of gentle teaching about deficits is often necessary to prevent significant others from provoking catastrophic reactions in the brain-injured individual.

Summary

Since the 1990s, the research literature on lack of awareness of deficits has burgeoned, primarily in the areas of dementia, other central nervous system diseases, and schizophrenia (Amador et al. 1991, 1994; McGlynn and Schacter 1989). Advances made in understanding lack of awareness in these disorders compared with similar deficits found in TBI can illuminate the nature, pathophysiology, and treatment approach needed in such patients. In this chapter, we describe dimensions and distinctions within the concept of lack of awareness and argue for the clinical, research, and theoretical value of making such discriminations. We review evidence suggesting that different aspects or dimensions of lack of awareness have differing neurological underpinnings and treatment implications. We argue that increased sensitivity to the multidimensional nature of TBI unawareness–related deficits will not only inform treatment interventions, but also shed light on the underlying pathology of lack of awareness in TBI patients.

We believe that the next steps in the understanding of unawareness may well come from the application of new functional imaging techniques to this critical clinical problem. Specifically, the development of tasks that will allow us to probe the different dimensions of unawareness discussed in the preceding sections will facilitate the better characterization of the circuitry underlying these distinct dimensions. It would not surprise us to learn that the different clinical dimensions (i.e., unawareness of deficits, reaction/response to deficits, generalizability/impact of deficits in daily functioning, attribution of deficits) have overlapping but distinct neural circuits that can be clarified with, for example, functional magnetic resonance imaging. We have identified several potential candidate functions that we hypothesize contribute to the neural and cognitive substrates underlying unawareness of illness, including working memory, episodic memory, source/reality monitoring, self-monitoring, and theory of mind. We and others are beginning to explore the utility of these constructs by developing tasks that assess the integrity of these functions and that can be used in functional magnetic resonance imaging paradigms.

References

Alexy WD, Foster M, Baker A: Audio-visual feedback: an exercise in self-awareness for the head injured patient. Cognitive Rehabilitation 1:8–10, 1983

Allen CC, Ruff RN: Self-rating versus neuropsychological performance of moderate versus severe head injured patients. Brain Inj 4:7–17, 1990

Amador XF, Strauss DH, Yale SA, et al: Awareness of illness in schizophrenia. Schizophr Bull 17:113–132, 1991

Amador XF, Strauss DH, Yale SA, et al: Assessment of insight in psychosis. Am J Psychiatry 150:873–879, 1993

Amador XF, Flaum M, Andreasen NC, et al: Awareness of illness in schizophrenia and schizoaffective and mood disorders. Arch Gen Psychiatry 51:826–836, 1994

Anton G: Ueber Herderkrankungen des Gehirnes, welche von Patienten selbst nicht wahrgenommen werden. Wien Klin Wochnschr 11:227–229, 1898

Babinski J: Contribution a l'etude des troubles mentaux dans l'hemiplegie organique cerebrale (anosognosie). Rev Neurol (Paris) 27:845–848, 1914

Barin JJ, Hanchett JM, Jacob WI, et al: Counseling the head injured patient, in Head Injury Rehabilitation: Children and Adolescents. Edited by Yivisaker M. San Diego, CA, College Hill Press, 1985, pp 362–379

Bartko G, Herczog I, Zador G: Clinical symptomatology and drug compliance in schizophrenic patients. Acta Psychiatr Scand 77:74–76, 1988

Ben-Yishay Y, Silver S, Piasetsky E: Relationship between employability and vocational outcome after intensive holistic cognitive rehabilitation. J Head Trauma Rehabil 2:35–48, 1987

Bergquist TF, Jacket MP: Programme methodology: awareness and goal setting with the traumatically brain injured. Brain Inj 7:275–282, 1993

Bisiach E, Geminiani G: Anosognosia related to hemiplegia and hemianopia, in Awareness of Deficit After Brain Injury. Edited by Prigatano GP, Schacter DL. New York, Oxford University Press, 1991, pp 17–39

Bisiach E, Vallar G, Perani D, et al: Unawareness of disease following lesions of the right hemisphere: anosognosia for hemiplegia and anosognosia for hemianopia. Neuropsychologia 24:471–482, 1986

Bond MR: Assessment of the psychosocial outcomes after severe head injury. CIBA Found Symp 34:141–155, 1975

Bogod NM, Mateer CA, MacDonald SW: Self-awareness after traumatic brain injury: a comparison of measures and their relationship to executive functions. J Int Neuropsychol Soc 9:450–458, 2003

Brooks N: The effectiveness of post-acute rehabilitation. Brain Inj 5:103–109, 1991

Brown J: Introduction, in Jargon Aphasia. Edited by Brown J. Orlando, FL, Academic Press, 1981, pp 1–8

Cavallo MM, Kay T, Ezrachi O: Problems and changes after traumatic brain injury: differing perceptions within and between families. Brain Inj 6:327–335, 1992

Chittum WR, Johnson K, Chittum JM, et al: Road to awareness: an individualized training package for increasing knowledge and comprehension of personal deficits in persons with acquired brain injury. Brain Inj 10:763–776, 1996

Cohn R, Neuman MA: Jargon aphasia. J Nerv Ment Dis 127:381–399, 1958

Critchley M: The Parietal Lobes. London, England, Hafner Press, 1953

Cuesta MJ, Peralta V: Lack of insight in schizophrenia. Schizophr Bull 20:359–366, 1994

Cuesta MJ, Peralta V, Caro F, et al: Is poor insight in psychotic disorders associated with performance on the Wisconsin Card Sorting Test? Am J Psychiatry 152:1380–1382, 1995

Cummings JL: Frontal-subcortical circuits and human behavior. Arch Neurol 50:873–880, 1993

David A, Van Os J, Jones P, et al: Insight and psychotic illness: cross-sectional and longitudinal associations. Br J Psychiatry 167:621–628, 1995

Deaton AV: Denial in the aftermath of traumatic brain injury: its manifestations, measurement and treatment. Rehabil Psychol 31:231–240, 1978

DeKosky ST, Kochanek PM, Clark RSB, et al: Secondary injury after head trauma: subacute and long-term mechanisms. Semin Clin Neuropsychiatry 3:176–185, 1998

DeLuca J, Tiersky L, Diamond BJ: Impaired awareness following brain injury: suggested remediation techniques. i.e. Magazine 4:14–20, 1996

Ergh TC, Rapport LJ, Coleman RD, et al: Predictors of caregiver and family functioning following traumatic brain injury: social support moderates caregiver distress. J Head Trauma Rehabil 17:155–174, 2002

Ezrachi O, Ben-Yishay Y, Kay T, et al: Predicting employment in traumatic brain injury following neuropsychological rehabilitation. J Head Trauma Rehabil 6:71–84, 1991

Fahy TJ, Irving MH, Millac P: Severe head injuries. Lancet 2:475–479, 1967

Feher EP, Mahurin RK, Inbody SB, et al: Anosognosia in Alzheimer's disease. Neuropsychiatry Neuropsychol Behav Neurol 4:136–146, 1991

Flashman LA, McAllister TW: Lack of awareness and its impact in traumatic brain injury. Neurorehabilitation 17:285–296, 2002

Flashman LA, Amador X, McAllister TW: Lack of awareness of deficits in traumatic brain injury. Semin Clin Neuropsychiatry 3:201–210, 1998

Flashman LA, McAllister TW, Andreasen NC, et al: Smaller brain size associated with unawareness in patients with schizophrenia. Am J Psychiatry 157:1167–1169, 2000

Flashman LA, McAllister TW, Saykin AJ, et al: Specific frontal lobe regions correlated with unawareness of illness in schizophrenia. J Neuropsychiatry Clin Neurosci 13:255–257, 2001

Fleming JM, Strong J, Ashton R: Self-awareness of deficits in adults with traumatic brain injury: How best to measure? Brain Inj 10:1–15, 1996

Ford B: Head injuries—what happens to survivors. Med J Aust 1:603–605, 1976

Fordyce DJ, Roueche JR: Changes in perspectives of disability among patients, staff, and relatives during rehabilitation of brain injury. Rehabil Psychol 31:217–229, 1986

Freeland J: Awareness of deficits: a complex interplay of neurological, personality, social and rehabilitation factors. i.e. Magazine 4:32–34, 1996

Genarelli TA, Graham DI: Neuropathology of the head injuries. Semin Clin Neuropsychiatry 3:160–175, 1998

Gerstmann J: Problems of imperception of disease and of impaired body territories with organic lesions. Arch Neurol Psychiatry 48:890–913, 1942

Giacino JT, Cicerone KD: Varieties of deficit unawareness after brain injury. J Head Trauma Rehabil 13:1–15, 1998

Gianotti G: Emotional behavior and hemispheric side of lesion. Cortex 8:41–55, 1972

Godfrey HP, Partridge FM, Knight RG, et al: Course of insight disorder and emotional dysfunction following closed head injury: a controlled cross-sectional follow-up study. J Clin Exp Neuropsychol 15:503–515, 1993

Gordon WA, Brown M, Sliwinski M, et al: The enigma of "hidden" traumatic brain injury. J Head Trauma Rehabil 13:39–56, 1998

Groswasser Z, Mendelson L, Stern MJ, et al: Re-evaluation of prognostic factors in rehabilitation after severe head injury. Scand J Rehabil Med 9:147–149, 1977

Healton EB, Navarro C, Bressman S, et al: Subcortical neglect. Neurology 32:776–778, 1982

Heilbronner RL, Roueche JR, Everson SA, et al: Comparing patient perspectives of disability and treatment effects with quality of participation in a post-acute brain injury rehabilitation programme. Brain Inj 3:387–395, 1989

Heilman KM: Anosognosia: possible neuropsychological mechanisms, in Awareness of Deficit After Brain Injury. Edited by Prigatano GP, Schacter DL. New York, Oxford University Press, 1991, pp 53–62

Hillier SL, Metzer J: Awareness and perceptions of outcomes after traumatic brain injury. Brain Inj 11:525–536, 1997

Howorth P, Saper J: The dimensions of insight in people with dementia. Aging Ment Health 7:113–122, 2003

Katz N, Fleming J, Keren N, et al: Unawareness and/or denial of disability: implications for occupational therapy intervention. Can J Occup Ther 69:281–292, 2002

Kent H: Letter to the editor (comment on Awareness Intervention: Who needs it? by Sohlberg et al. J Head Trauma Rehabil 13:62–78, 1998). J Head Trauma Rehabil 1999

Leathem JM, Murphy LJ, Flett RA: Self- and informant-ratings on the Patient Competency Rating Scale in patients with traumatic brain injury. J Clin Exp Neuropsychol 20:694–705, 1998

Levin HS, High WM, Goethe KE, et al: The neurobehavioral rating scale: assessment of the behavioral sequelae of head injury by the clinician. J Neurol Neurosurg Psychiatry 50:183–193, 1987

Lopez OL, Becker JT, Somsak D, et al: Awareness of cognitive deficits and anosognosia in probable Alzheimer's disease. Eur Neurol 34:277–282, 1994

Lysaker P, Bell M: Insight and cognitive impairment in schizophrenia: performance on repeated administrations of the Wisconsin Card Sorting Test. J Nerv Ment Dis 182:656–660, 1994

Lysaker P, Bell M: Impaired Insight in Schizophrenia: Advances from Psychosocial Treatment Research. Oxford, England, Oxford University Press, 1998

Malec J, Smigielski J, DePompolo R, et al: Outcome evaluation and prediction in a comprehensive-integrated post-acute outpatient brain injury rehabilitation programme. Brain Inj 7:15–29, 1993

McAllister TW: Neuropsychiatric sequelae of head injuries. Psychiatr Clin North Am 15:395–413, 1992

McEvoy JP, Freter S, Everett G, et al: Insight and the clinical outcome of schizophrenics. J Nerv Ment Dis 177:48–51, 1989

McGlashan T: Does attitude toward psychosis related to outcome? Am J Psychiatry 138:797–801, 1981

McGlynn SM, Schacter DL: Unawareness of deficits in neuropsychological syndromes. J Clin Exp Neuropsychol 11:143–205, 1989

McKinlay WW, Brooks DN: Methodological problems in assessing psychosocial recovery following severe head injury. J Clin Neuropsychol 6:97–99, 1984

Miller H, Stern G: The long-term prognosis of severe head injury. Lancet 1:225–229, 1965

Mohamed S, Fleming S, et al: Insight in schizophrenia: its relationship to measures of executive functions. J Nerv Ment Dis 187:525–531, 1999

Neary D, Snowden JS, Bowen DM, et al: Neuropsychological syndromes in presenile dementia due to cerebral atrophy. J Neurol Neurosurg Psychiatry 49:163–174, 1986

Newman AC, Garmoe W, Beatty P, et al: Self-awareness of traumatically brain injured patients in the acute inpatient rehabilitation setting. Brain Inj 14:333–344, 2000

Oddy M, Coughlan T, Tyerman A, et al: Social adjustment after closed head injury: a further follow-up seven years after injury. J Neurol Neurosurg Psychiatry 48:564–568, 1985

Ota Y: Psychiatric studies on civilian head injuries, in The Late Effects of Head Injury. Edited by Walker AE, Caveness WF, Critchley M. Springfield, IL, Charles L. Thomas, 1969, pp 110–119

Peralta V, Cuesta MJ: Lack of insight: its status within schizophrenic psychopathology. Biol Psychiatry 36:559–561, 1994

Port A, Willmott C, Charlton J: Self-awareness following traumatic brain injury and implications for rehabilitation. Brain Inj 16:277–289, 2002

Prigatano GP: Personality and psychosocial consequences of brain injury, in Neuropsychological Rehabilitation After Brain Injury. Edited by Prigatano GP. Baltimore, MD, Johns Hopkins University Press, 1986, pp 96–118

Prigatano GP: Disturbances of self-awareness of deficit after traumatic brain injury, in Awareness of Deficit After Brain Injury. Edited by Prigatano GL, Schacter DL. New York, Oxford University Press, 1991, pp 111–126

Prigatano GL, Fordyce DJ: Cognitive dysfunction and psychosocial adjustment after brain injury, in Neuropsychological Rehabilitation after Brain Injury. Edited by Prigatano GL, Fordyce DJ, Zeiner HK, et al. Baltimore, MD, Johns Hopkins University Press, 1986, pp 96–118

Prigatano GP, Fordyce D, Zeiner H, et al: Neuropsychological rehabilitation after closed head injury. J Neurol Neurosurg Psychiatry 47:505–513, 1984

Prigatano GL, Amin K, Rosenstein LD: Administration and scoring manual for the BNI screen for higher cerebral functions. Phoeniz, AZ, Barrow Neurological Institute, 1995

Prigatano GP, Altman IM, O'Brien KP: Behavioral limitations that brain injured patients tend to underestimate. Clin Neuropsychol 4:163–176, 1990

Rattok J, Ben-Yishay Y, Lakin P, et al: Outcome of different treatment mixes in a multidimensional neuropsychological rehabilitation program. Neuropsychology 6:395–415, 1992

Reed BR, Jagust WJ, Coulter L: Anosognosia in Alzheimer's disease: relationships to depression, cognitive function, and cerebral perfusion. J Clin Exp Neuropsychol 15:231–244, 1993

Reisberg B, Gordon B, McCarthy M, et al: Clinical symptoms accompanying progressive cognitive decline and Alzheimer's disease, in Alzheimer's Dementia. Edited by Melnick VL, Dubler NN. Clifton, NJ, Humana Press, 1985, pp 19–31

Romano MD: Family response to traumatic head injury. Scand J Rehabil Med 6:1–4, 1974

Rossell SL, Coakes J, Shapleske J, et al: Insight: its relationship with cognitive function, brain volume and symptoms in schizophrenia. Psychol Med 33:111–119, 2003

Sackeim HA, Wegner AZ: Attributional patterns in depression and euthymia. Arch Gen Psychiatry 43:553–560, 1986

Santillan CE, Fritsch T, Geldmacher DS: Development of a scale to predict decline in patients with mild Alzheimer's disease. J Am Geriatr Soc 51:91–95, 2003

Sherer M, Boake C, Silver BV: Assessing awareness of deficits following acquired brain injury: the Awareness Questionnaire. J Int Neuropsychol Soc 1:163, 1995

Sherer M, Bergloff P, Levin E, et al: Impaired awareness and employment outcome after traumatic brain injury. J Head Trauma Rehabil 13:52–61, 1998a

Sherer M, Boake C, Levin E, et al: Characteristics of impaired awareness after traumatic brain injury. J Int Neuropsychol Soc 4:380–387, 1998b

Sherer M, Hart T, Nick TG, et al: Early impaired self-awareness after traumatic brain injury. Arch Phys Med Rehabil 84:168–176, 2003a

Sherer M, Hart T, Nick TG: Measurement of impaired self-awareness after traumatic brain injury: a comparison of the patient competency rating scale and the awareness questionnaire. Brain Inj 17:25–37, 2003b

Sohlberg MM, Mateer C, Penkman L, et al: Awareness intervention: who needs it? J Head Trauma Rehabil 13:62–78, 1998

Stuss DT: Disturbance of self-awareness after frontal system damage, in Awareness of Deficit After Brain Injury. Edited by Prigatano GP, Schacter DL. New York, Oxford University Press, 1991, pp 63–83

Stuss DT, Benson DF: The Frontal Lobes. New York, Raven, 1986

Thomsen IV: The patient with severe head injury and his family. Scand J Rehabil Med 6:180–183, 1974

Tournois J, Mesnil F, Kop J-L: Self-deception and other-deception: a social desirability questionnaire. Eur Rev Appl Psychol 50:219–233, 2000

Trivers R: The elements of a scientific theory of self-deception, in Evolutionary Perspectives on Human Reproductive Behavior. Annals of the New York Academy of Science. Edited by LeCroy D, Moller P. New York, New York Academy of Science, 2000, pp 114–131

Trudel TM, Tryon WW, Purdum CM: Closed head injury, awareness of disability and long term outcome. New Hampshire Brain Injury Association Annual Meeting, Center of New Hampshire Convention Center, Manchester, NH, May 1996

Tyerman A, Humphrey M: Changes in self-concept following severe head injury. Int J Rehabil Res 7:11–23, 1984

Walker DE, Blankenship V, Ditty JA, et al: Prediction of recovery for closed-head-injured adults: an evaluation of the MMPI, the Adaptive Behavior Scale, and a "Quality of Life" rating scale. J Clin Psychol 43:699–707, 1987

Watson RT, Heilman KM: Thalamic neglect. Neurology 29:690–694, 1979

Watson RT, Valenstein E, Heilman KM: Thalamic neglect: possible role of the medial thalamus and nucleus reticularis in behavior. Arc Neurol 38:501–506, 1981

Weinstein EA, Kahn RL: Denial of Illness. Symbolic and Physiological Aspects. Springfield, IL, Charles C. Thomas, 1955

Weinstein EA, Lyerly OG, Cole M, et al: Meaning in jargon aphasia. Cortex 2:165–187, 1966

Young DA, Davila R, Scher H: Unawareness of illness and neuropsychological performance in chronic schizophrenia. Schizophr Res 10:117–124, 1993

Zhou J, Chittum WR, Johnson-Tompkins K, et al: The utilization of a game format to increase knowledge or residuals among people with acquired brain injury. J Head Trauma Rehabil 11:51–61, 1996

Zingerle H: Ueber Stoerungen der Wahrnehmung des eigenen Koerpers bei organischen Gehirnerkrankungen. Monatsschr Psychiatr Neurol 34:13–36, 1913

20 Fatigue and Sleep Problems

Vani Rao, M.D.

Pamela Rollings, M.D.

Jennifer Spiro, M.S.

FATIGUE AND SLEEP disturbances are two common disabling symptoms that affect the recovery course and disrupt rehabilitation in patients who survive traumatic brain injury (TBI). Despite the ubiquity of these problems, objective data are scarce on the prevalence, pathophysiology, and treatment of these conditions in the TBI literature. The exact etiology of these disturbances is also unclear. Sleep disturbance and fatigue after TBI can be best conceptualized as primary effects of the trauma itself, which can cause neurohormonal and neurotransmitter dysfunction in the central nervous system, or as secondary effects of neuropsychiatric disturbances associated with the TBI. Side effects of medications used to treat TBI and psychological distress associated with trauma may also cause sleep disturbance. Sleep disturbance and fatigue are common and have important rehabilitation implications for patients with TBI.

Fatigue is a nonspecific and highly subjective symptom often reported as a feeling of exhaustion, tiredness, or weakness. Bigland-Ritchie et al. (1978) defined *fatigue* physiologically as the inability of a muscle or groups of muscle to sustain the expected or required force of work. This inability could either be due to a central mechanism decrease or inability to sustain the central drive to the spinal motor neurons, or due to a peripheral mechanism failure of force-generating capacity within the muscle (Comi et al. 2001). Chandhuri and Beehan (2000) have also defined *central fatigue* as the failure to initiate and/or sustain attentional tasks and physical activities requiring self-motivation.

Sleep disturbances may be broadly divided into insomnia (difficulty in initiating or maintaining sleep), hypersomnia (excessive daytime sleepiness), and alterations of the sleep-wake schedule (displacement of sleep from its original circadian pattern).

Prevalence

The exact prevalence of fatigue in individuals with TBI is unknown. Kreutzer et al. (2001) studied 722 outpatients with an average of 2.5 years post–brain injury who were referred for comprehensive assessment at a regional level 1 trauma center. Of the 42% of patients who met DSM-IV (American Psychiatric Association 1994) criteria for major depression, 46% complained of fatigue, the most commonly cited symptom of depression. Clinchot et al. (1998), in a study of 145 brain-injured subjects admitted to a rehabilitation facility, noted that 50% of subjects had difficulty sleeping and 80% of subjects who reported sleep problems also reported fatigue. Fatigue is one of the symptoms included in the postconcussion syndrome (see Chapter 15, Mild Brain Injury and the Postconcussion Syndrome). Fatigue is the third most common symptom of postconcussion syndrome (Middelboe et al. 1992): 29%–47% of patients complain of fatigue within the first month after TBI (Keshavan et al. 1981; Minderhoud et al. 1980), and fatigue continues to be reported frequently (22%–37% of patients) after 3 months (Keshavan et al. 1981; Levin et al. 1987). After 1 year postinjury, approximately 20% of patients still report fatigue (Middelboe et al. 1992). Although there is a trend toward improvement over time, a significant number of TBI survivors still experience fatigue after the first year of injury. In an outcome study of 67 brain-injured subjects interviewed 5 years after TBI, 37% continued to report fatigue (Hillier et al. 1997). Thus, studies indicate that 20%–50% of individuals with TBI complain of fatigue sometime during the recovery period.

Sleep disturbances are equally common after TBI, occurring in 36%–70% of patients (Keshavan et al. 1981; McLean et al. 1984). In a prospective study of 50 consecutive postacute TBI patients, Mann et al. (1997) found that 30% reported insomnia. Cohen et al. (1992) have suggested that sleep complaints may vary temporally; difficulty in initiating and maintaining sleep occurs soon after injury, and excessive daytime somnolence occurs months to years after injury. In their study of 22 hospitalized patients 3–5 months after injury, 81% had difficulty in initiating and maintaining sleep (early and middle insomnia) and 14% had excessive daytime sleepiness. In a study of 77 outpatients who had sustained TBI 2–3 years previously, 73% complained of excessive daytime sleepiness and only 8% complained of difficulty in initiating and maintaining sleep (Cohen et al. 1992). There is little literature available on sleep-wake schedule disturbances, although symptoms such as "difficulty in going to sleep until later than usual, but able to have normal amount of sleep" are commonly reported.

Pathophysiology

Normal Sleep Cycle

Only a brief review of the normal sleep cycle is provided here. For an in-depth understanding, the reader is encouraged to read a standard textbook on sleep disorders (Kryger et al. 2000).

Sleep is an active, complex, and vital process, with multiple regulating factors. Homeostasis determines the amount of prior sleep and waking states. The circadian mechanism organizes sleep and waking over 24 hours. The ultradian mechanism controls the alteration between rapid eye movement (REM) and nonrapid eye movement (NREM) sleep. Several regions in the central nervous system, including the brainstem, basal forebrain, and hypothalamus, regulate the sleep-wake cycle. Serotonin and acetylcholine are two common neurotransmitters involved, although other hormones and endogenous products such as substances C and S, dopamine, and norepinephrine also play important roles.

Sleep consists of two distinct states, REM and NREM sleep, which affect physiological functions and behavior (Table 20–1). REM periods occur approximately every 90–100 minutes and last about 10–40 minutes. The first REM period occurs approximately 90 minutes after sleep onset (REM latency). REM sleep is

TABLE 20–1.   Sleep states

State	General characteristics
Rapid eye movement	High level of brain activity
	Physiological activity similar to wakefulness
	Episodic bursts of rapid eye movement
	Dreaming associated with vivid dream recall
	Poikilothermia
	Absence of body movement but partial or full penile erection
	Increase in pulse rate, blood pressure, and respiratory rate
	Decreased ventilatory response to increased levels of carbon dioxide
	Cortical electroencephalogram reveals low-voltage mixed-frequency waves
Nonrapid eye movement	Low level of brain activity
	Physiological activity markedly reduced
	No rapid eye movement activity
	Four stages present
	Hypothermia
	Slight decrease in pulse rate, blood pressure, and respiratory rate
	Decrease in blood flow through all tissues
	Intermittent involuntary body movement
	Cortical electroencephalogram reveals increased-voltage slowed-frequency waves
	Four stages present, with arousal threshold lowest in stage 1 and highest in stage 4

characterized by increased brain and physiological activity similar to that of wakefulness. NREM sleep is a more peaceful state. There are four stages of NREM sleep with typical electroencephalographic patterns (Table 20–2).

The sleep-wake cycle is regulated by the interaction of internal "biological clocks" and environmental influences. The two important internal synchronizers are the suprachiasmatic nucleus of the hypothalamus and the endogenous production of a substance—process S. The external synchronizers, also called "Zeitgebers," are light-darkness alteration, eating and social schedule, temperature, and relative humidity. Dysfunction or maladjustment of these internal and external time markers due to brain damage, cognitive deficits, and/or sensory deprivation may be responsible for disorders of sleep in TBI patients (Espinar-Sierra 1997).

TABLE 20–2. Stages of nonrapid eye movement sleep

Stage	General characteristics	Electroencephalographic findings
1	Light stage of sleep. Lasts for a brief period. Occupies approximately 5% of total sleep.	3–7 cycles/second, low-voltage mixed-frequency waves.
2	Occupies approximately 50% of total sleep.	Spindle-shaped tracings at 12–14 cycles per second. K complexes characterized by slow triphasic waves.
3	Slow wave sleep. Disorganization during arousal.	High-voltage delta waves at 0.5–2.0 cycles/second. Occupies 20%–50% of the tracing.
4	Slow wave sleep. Disorganization during arousal.	High-voltage delta waves. Occupies more than 50% of sleep.

Relationship Between TBI, Sleep Disturbances, and Fatigue

The cause-and-effect relationship between TBI and sleep disturbance and fatigue is not well delineated (Figure 20–1). The understanding of the pathophysiology of these disturbances is based on knowledge of the neuropathology of TBI and the physiology of the sleep-wake schedule. Both fatigue and sleep disturbances may be the primary effect of trauma to the brain or secondary to other neuropsychiatric sequelae of TBI such as depressive disorder, anxiety disorder, substance abuse, chronic pain, and/or medications. In addition, fatigue can cause sleep disturbance and vice versa.

Brain injury of any degree of severity is a complex process that affects multiple brain regions (see Chapter 2, Neuropathology). Therefore, it is not surprising that sleep disturbance is a common occurrence after TBI because maintenance of the sleep-wake cycle is dependent on the proper functioning of multiple levels of the central nervous system—the brainstem, basal forebrain, hypothalamus, and the frontal-subcortical system (Parmeggiani 2000).

Much less is known about fatigue in TBI. Chandhuri and Beehan (2000) have proposed that central fatigue is due to failure in the integration of the limbic input and

the motor functions affecting the striatal-thalamic-frontal cortical system. Studies in patients with multiple sclerosis (MS) suggest that fatigue is often due to "central abnormalities," even though peripheral mechanisms may have some role in the pathogenesis (Comi et al. 2001). A study by Attarian et al. (2004) demonstrated a significant correlation between fatigue in MS patients and sleep disturbances. This study suggested that circadian rhythm abnormalities and sleep disruptions play a role in the pathophysiology of fatigue. Other studies (Tartaglia et al. 2004) have found, using proton magnetic resonance spectroscopy imaging, that widespread cerebral axonal dysfunction is associated with fatigue in MS. Metabolic abnormalities have been found in the frontal cortex and basal ganglia by positron emission tomography in the brains of MS patients with fatigue compared with those patients without fatigue (Roecke et al. 1997). Certain cytokines such as tumor necrosis factor and interleukin-1 have also been implicated in the pathogenesis of fatigue in MS patients (Bertolone et al. 1993; Chao et al. 1992). Similar central and immune mechanisms may also be responsible for fatigue in TBI patients because trauma produces injury to multiple levels of the brain and causes secondary inflammatory reactions, with production of tumor necrosis factor and interleukins (Gennarelli and Graham 1998; see Chapters 2, Neuropathology, and 39, Pharmacotherapy of Prevention).

Evaluation of Fatigue and Sleep Disturbances

Clinical Presentation

Fatigue

Fatigue is one of the common and earliest signs of brain injury, yet there is a paucity of literature on the clinical presentation and evaluation of fatigue in TBI patients.

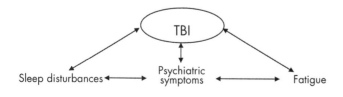

FIGURE 20–1. Algorithm showing possible cause-and-effect relationship between traumatic brain injury (TBI), sleep disturbances, psychiatric symptoms, and fatigue.

Lezak (1978) has suggested that soon after TBI patients tend to tire more easily and require more concentration and effort for their performance. Years after brain injury, however, fatigue gradually diminishes, and the person learns to cope and adjust to his or her new level of performance.

In our clinical experience, patients rarely complain of "fatigue." They are more likely to describe their experiences in negativistic terms such as, "I don't feel like working," "I can't concentrate," "I feel drained," or "I have no energy." This may either occur as an isolated symptom or in association with other symptoms such as pain; changes in mood, sleep, appetite, and ability to enjoy activities; or other physical and neurological symptoms.

Because fatigue is a subjective experience, self-report scales are more appropriate for assessing the severity of this symptom, although they have obvious limitations. Both unidimensional and multidimensional fatigue scales are available (Comi et al. 2001). LaChapelle and Finlayson (1998) examined three self-report scales and performed an objective test to assess fatigue in 30 brain-injured subjects and 30 healthy control subjects. The scales were the Fatigue Impact Scale (FIS), which has 64 questions and three sections that assess the incidence and onset of fatigue, factors modulating the fatigue experience, and the impact of fatigue on cognitive, physical, and social functioning; the Visual Analogue Scale for Fatigue (VAS-F); and the Fatigue Severity Scale (FSS), a nine-item scale to assess the impact of fatigue on patients' functioning over the past month. A continuous thumb-pressing task was used as an objective measure of fatigue. Overall, individuals with brain injury were found to experience significant levels of fatigue. Significant group differences were found on the FIS and the FSS but not the VAS-F, probably because of the latter's failure to differentiate between fatigue and sleepiness. The objective motor task found that patients with brain injury fatigued more easily than control subjects and correlated positively with the subjective rating scales.

The VAS-F, although easy to administer, has been criticized for not being able to distinguish between sleepiness and fatigue. The overall score of the FSS was able to differentiate between the group of brain-injured patients and a group of healthy control subjects, but not all of the nine questions were able to do so. Also, the FSS does not address the impact of fatigue on patients' social experiences. In the study by LaChapelle and Finlayson (1998), data from the section regarding the onset of fatigue were not used because brain injury has a sudden onset. There was no significant difference between the patient and control groups on the results from the section of the FIS that included "fatigue modulating factors." There was,

however, a significant difference on the section of the FIS that focused on "the impact of fatigue on social, cognitive, and physical functioning." This provides a broad indication of what aspects of the patient's life are most impaired by fatigue. The Revised Version of the FIS is shorter and is designed to evaluate the perceived impact of fatigue, factors that affect patients' perception of fatigue, and how fatigue affects the mental and general health of patients. The scale was first designed to study patients with MS (Fisk et al. 1994) but has also been found to be useful in stroke patients (Ingles et al. 1999). We propose using the FIS to assess fatigue in TBI because it is a multidimensional scale that determines the effects of fatigue on the physical, cognitive, and social domains of a patient's life (Figure 20–2).

Sleep Disturbances

Few studies are available reviewing sleep disturbances after TBI. Insomnia, hypersomnia, sleep-wake cycle abnormalities, and parasomnia are some of the common sleep disturbances and are described in the following sections. Similar to fatigue, sleep disturbance may occur as an isolated feature or as a symptom of other psychiatric, medical, or neurological syndromes. Sleep disorder may also be a preexisting condition; it is found in approximately 30% of the adult population (Rosekind 1992).

Some researchers have suggested that patients with injury of recent onset have problems initiating and maintaining sleep, whereas patients with chronic injuries experience excessive sleep (Cohen et al. 1992). The pathophysiological changes that occur in the brain during the recovery process and the severity of injury have been postulated to be some of the factors responsible for this temporally related change of sleep complaints (Cohen et al. 1992).

Insomnia. Insomnia, defined as difficulty in initiating or maintaining sleep associated with daytime fatigue or impaired functioning, is common in patients with acute TBI. The prevalence in this patient group ranges from 36% (McLean et al. 1984) to approximately 70% (Keshavan et al. 1981). Using DSM-IV criteria for insomnia, Mann et al. (1997) noted a prevalence of 30% in postacute TBI patients.

Even though clinical evidence reveals that insomnia is a common complaint in individuals after TBI who are also depressed, there are few studies that have documented the relationship between the two. Fichtenberg et al. (2000) evaluated 91 consecutive patients with brain injury admitted to an outpatient rehabilitation center an average of 3 months after injury. They found a significant positive correlation between insomnia, depression as measured by the Beck Depression Inventory, and mild

Name/Study Number: _____   Date: _____

Below is a list of statements that describe how fatigue may cause problems in people's lives. Please read each statement carefully. Circle the number that indicates best how much of a problem fatigue has been for you these **past four (4) weeks**, including today. Please check one box for each statement and do not skip any statements.

Circle one number on each line	No Problem	Small Problem	Moderate Problem	Big Problem	Extreme Problem
1. *Because of my fatigue...* **I feel less alert.**	0	1	2	3	4
2. *Because of my fatigue...* **I feel that I am more isolated from social contact.**	0	1	2	3	4
3. *Because of my fatigue...* **I have to reduce my workload or responsibilities.**	0	1	2	3	4
4. *Because of my fatigue...* **I am more moody.**	0	1	2	3	4
5. *Because of my fatigue...* **I have difficulty paying attention for a long period of time.**	0	1	2	3	4
6. *Because of my fatigue...* **I feel like I cannot think clearly.**	0	1	2	3	4
7. *Because of my fatigue...* **I work less effectively. (this applies to work inside or outside the home).**	0	1	2	3	4
8. *Because of my fatigue...* **I have to rely more on others to help me or do things for me.**	0	1	2	3	4
9. *Because of my fatigue...* **I have difficulty planning activities ahead of time because my fatigue may interfere with them.**	0	1	2	3	4
10. *Because of my fatigue...* **I am more clumsy and uncoordinated.**	0	1	2	3	4
11. *Because of my fatigue...* **I find that I am more forgetful.**	0	1	2	3	4
12. *Because of my fatigue...* **I am more irritable and more easily angered.**	0	1	2	3	4
13. *Because of my fatigue...* **I have to be careful about pacing my physical activities.**	0	1	2	3	4
14. *Because of my fatigue...* **I am less motivated to do anything that requires physical effort.**	0	1	2	3	4
15. *Because of my fatigue...* **I am less motivated to engage in social activities.**	0	1	2	3	4
16. *Because of my fatigue...* **my ability to travel outside my home is limited.**	0	1	2	3	4
17. *Because of my fatigue...* **I have trouble maintaining physical effort for long periods.**	0	1	2	3	4
18. *Because of my fatigue...* **I find it difficult to make decisions.**	0	1	2	3	4
19. *Because of my fatigue...* **I have few social contacts outside of my own home.**	0	1	2	3	4
20. *Because of my fatigue...* **Normal day-to-day events are stressful for me.**	0	1	2	3	4

FIGURE 20–2.   Fatigue Impact Scale (continues).

Source.   Adapted from the Fatigue Impact Scale with permission of John D. Fisk. Copyright 1991 J.D. Fisk, P.G. Ritvo, and C.J. Archibald.

brain injury, but no association between insomnia and age, gender, education, and time since the injury.

Frieboes et al. (1999) studied 13 men with severe brain injury (age range, 19–36 years) and 13 age-matched control subjects. They found abnormal sleep electroencephalographic parameters (reduction in stage 2 sleep in the first half of the night and an increase in REM during the second half of the night) and nocturnal hormone secretion (decrease in growth hormone secretion compared with control subjects) similar to that in patients with remitted depression. The significant relationship between depression and insomnia post-TBI is consistent with the increased frequency of insomnia

Circle one number on each line	No Problem	Small Problem	Moderate Problem	Big Problem	Extreme Problem
21. *Because of my fatigue...* **I am less motivated to do anything that requires thinking.**	0	1	2	3	4
22. *Because of my fatigue...* **I avoid situations that are stressful for me.**	0	1	2	3	4
23. *Because of my fatigue...* **My muscles feel much weaker than they should.**	0	1	2	3	4
24. *Because of my fatigue...* **My physical discomfort is increased.**	0	1	2	3	4
25. *Because of my fatigue...* **I have difficulty dealing with anything new.**	0	1	2	3	4
26. *Because of my fatigue...* **I am less able to finish tasks that require thinking.**	0	1	2	3	4
27. *Because of my fatigue...* **I feel unable to meet the demands that people place on me.**	0	1	2	3	4
28. *Because of my fatigue...* **I feel less able to provide financial support for myself and my family.**	0	1	2	3	4
29. *Because of my fatigue...* **I engage in less sexual activity.**	0	1	2	3	4
30. *Because of my fatigue...* **I find it difficult to organize my thoughts when I am doing things at home or at work.**	0	1	2	3	4
31. *Because of my fatigue...* **I am less able to complete tasks that require physical effort.**	0	1	2	3	4
32. *Because of my fatigue...* **I worry about how I look to other people.**	0	1	2	3	4
33. *Because of my fatigue...* **I am less able to deal with emotional issues.**	0	1	2	3	4
34. *Because of my fatigue...* **I feel slowed down in my thinking.**	0	1	2	3	4
35. *Because of my fatigue...* **I find it hard to concentrate.**	0	1	2	3	4
36. *Because of my fatigue...* **I have difficulty participating fully in family activities.**	0	1	2	3	4
37. *Because of my fatigue...* **I have to limit my physical activities.**	0	1	2	3	4
38. *Because of my fatigue...* **I require more frequent or longer periods of rest.**	0	1	2	3	4
39. *Because of my fatigue...* **I am not able to provide as much emotional support to my family as I should.**	0	1	2	3	4
40. *Because of my fatigue...* **Minor difficulties seem like major difficulties.**	0	1	2	3	4

Total Score: _____

FIGURE 20–2. **Fatigue Impact Scale (continued).**

Source. Adapted from the Fatigue Impact Scale with permission of John D. Fisk. Copyright 1991 J.D. Fisk, P.G. Ritvo, and C.J. Archibald.

in patients with primary depression (Breslau et al. 1996). Evaluation of patients with insomnia should therefore include careful screening for depression and/or other psychiatric disturbances (Fichtenberg et al. 2000).

There are conflicting results concerning the relationship between severity of brain injury and insomnia. Cohen et al. (1992) found increased prevalence of insomnia

in patients with severe brain injury, whereas Clinchot et al. (1998) and Fichtenberg et al. (2000) noted a decreased prevalence in this population. The reason for the decreased prevalence after severe TBI could either be underreporting of sleep problems (Clinchot et al. 1998) or increased awareness of symptoms in the subjects with mild brain injury (Fichtenberg et al. 2000).

There have been inconsistent results when the relationship between pain and insomnia has been examined. Beetar et al. (1996) found a positive correlation between the two, whereas other research workers have not found a significant relationship between insomnia and pain (Fichtenberg et al. 2000). More studies are necessary to establish this association, although clinical evidence reveals that pain is closely associated with insomnia in the general population (Peres et al. 2001; Sutton et al. 2001).

Early diagnosis and treatment of insomnia are important because they may improve cognitive difficulties, psychosocial distress, and overall quality of life. The Pittsburgh Sleep Quality Index has been found to be a valid and reliable instrument for assessing insomnia among postacute patients after TBI (Fichtenberg et al. 2001). The scale examines a wide range of sleep disturbances; provides information about basic sleep variables such as sleep efficiency, latency, and duration; and is brief and comprehensible, making it uniquely advantageous for brain-injured individuals.

Hypersomnia.   Hypersomnia, defined as subjective complaints of excessive daytime sleepiness and objective finding of a score less than 10 on the multiple sleep latency test (MSLT; described in the section Multiple Sleep Latency Test), has been reported in individuals after brain injury (Castriotta and Lai 2001; Masel et al. 2001). In a study of 184 patients referred to a sleep clinic approximately 15 months after brain trauma, 98% reported excessive daytime sleepiness (Guilleminault et al. 2000). Approximately 82% of the patients were found to have hypersomnia with a multiple sleep latency score of less than 10, and 32% were found to have sleep-disordered breathing problems. Prolonged coma of longer than 24 hours, neurosurgical intervention, pain, and skull fracture were commonly associated with hypersomnia. Eight of these patients were found to be "apathetic" (complained of sleepiness but were found to have normal MSLT) and were described as having "pseudohypersomnia" (Guilleminault et al. 2000).

In a study of 71 subjects with brain injury (traumatic and nontraumatic) referred to a rehabilitation facility, hypersomnia (defined as a mean sleep latency score of less than 10) was observed in 47% (Masel et al. 2001). Within this group, 17% had abnormal respiratory indices and periodic leg movements as detected by polysomnography. No differences were found between the hypersomnolent and the nonhypersomnolent group in Glasgow Coma Scale score, length of coma, time since brain injury, nature of injury, gender, or medications. No significant correlation was noticed between the results of the objective MSLT and self-reported sleep questionnaires such as the Epworth Sleepiness Scale (Figure 20–3) and the Pittsburgh Sleep Quality Index, suggesting the inability of subjects with significant hypersomnia to perceive their hypersomnolence (Masel et al. 2001).

Therefore, the individual who has had a TBI and complains of excessive daytime sleepiness should be evaluated for sleep apnea and narcolepsy. Sleep apnea is classified as obstructive (cessation of breathing with continued efforts to breathe caused by collapse of upper airway), central (cessation of breathing with no effort to breathe caused by abnormal respiratory drive), or mixed. Narcolepsy is a disorder of REM sleep with hypersomnia, sleep attacks, early-onset REM, and the intrusion of REM sleep into wakefulness. A type of human leukocyte antigen (HLA) called *HLA-DR2* is found in 90%–100% of patients with narcolepsy and only in 10%–35% of unaffected individuals. TBI can cause alterations of the respiratory control systems and cause or exacerbate obstructive sleep apnea (Chokroverty 1994). Similarly, other factors associated with TBI such as injury to the upper airways, cervical cord lesions, sedative drugs (often given to patients for control of aggression), and weight gain (which often occurs in relatively immobile patients) are risk factors for the development of sleep apnea (Mahowald and Mahowald 1996).

In a study of 10 adult subjects with a history of chronic mild to severe closed head injury and complaints of excessive sleepiness, all were found to have a sleep disorder. Eight individuals were found to have obstructive sleep apnea. Upper airway resistance syndrome (hypersomnia secondary to sleep disturbance due to increased effort of breathing through a narrow airway without measurable apnea or hypopnea) was found in one subject, and narcolepsy was diagnosed in two subjects (Castriotta and Lai 2001). Sleep apnea has also been described in the postacute phase. In a prospective study of 28 patients with mild to severe TBI and a mean age of 34 years within 3 months of injury, 47% were found to have sleep apnea during overnight sleep studies. No correlation was found between the occurrence of sleep apnea and TBI severity or other demographic variables. Sleep-related breathing episodes were also found to be primarily more central than obstructive, which is in contrast to those seen in the general population. This also suggests that trauma to the brain may be partly responsible for this phenomenon (Webster et al. 2001).

Narcolepsy has also been reported after TBI. Good et al. (1989) reported on a patient with posttraumatic narcolepsy who had both subjective complaints of sleepiness and HLA typing that indicated a genetic predisposition to narcolepsy. Lankford et al. (1994) studied a small group of patients with mild to moderate TBI with persistent sleep

Epworth Sleepiness Scale

Name: ______________________________ Today's date: __________

Your age (yrs): ____________ Your sex (Male = M, Female = F): ______

How likely are you to doze off or fall asleep in the following situations, in contrast to feeling just tired?

This refers to your usual way of life in recent times.

Even if you haven't done some of these things recently, try to work out how they would have affected you.

Use the following scale to choose the **most appropriate number** for each situation:

0 = would **never** doze
1 = **slight chance** of dozing
2 = **moderate chance** of dozing
3 = **high chance** of dozing

It is important that you answer each question as best you can.

Situation	**Chance of Dozing (0–3)**
Sitting and reading	___
Watching TV	___
Sitting, inactive in a public place (e.g., a theater or a meeting)	___
As a passenger in a car for an hour without a break	___
Lying down to rest in the afternoon when circumstances permit	___
Sitting and talking to someone	___
Sitting quietly after a lunch without alcohol	___
In a car, while stopped for a few minutes in the traffic	

THANK YOU FOR YOUR COOPERATION

FIGURE 20–3. Epworth Sleepiness Scale.
Source. From Johns MW: "A New Method for Measuring Daytime Sleepiness: The Epworth Sleepiness Scale." *Sleep* 14:540–545, 1991. Revised 1997. Used with permission of M.W. Johns. Copyright M.W. Johns 1991–1997.

complaints and diagnosed posttraumatic narcolepsy using formal sleep studies such as the polysomnogram (PSG) and MSLT.

We recommend that clinical diagnosis of narcolepsy should always be accompanied by formal sleep studies and HLA typing. However, even if a patient is confirmed to have the appropriate HLA haplotype, the question always exists whether TBI was the causative factor or a precipitating event.

Post-TBI hypersomnia is an understudied area. The prevalence, varieties, associated psychiatric disturbances, and effect on rehabilitation and physical, cognitive, and social level of functioning are yet to be identified. Such identification is important because effective management of treatable disorders can have far-reaching results for the rehabilitative process.

Sleep-wake cycle disturbances. Sleep-wake cycle disturbance, or circadian rhythm sleep disorder, is defined as inability to go to sleep or stay awake at a desired clock time. Both the duration and pattern of sleep are normal when patients with this disorder do fall asleep (Kryger et al. 2000). There are several varieties of sleep-wake cycle disturbances, including the delayed, advanced, and disorganized types. The pathogenesis remains unclear, although dysfunction of the suprachiasmatic nucleus has been postulated (Okawa et al. 1987). Other factors often associated with this disorder in the general population include shift work and travel through different time zones (Patten and Lauderdale 1992). There is little literature available on the prevalence of this disorder in the TBI population.

Schreiber et al. (1998) described circadian rhythm and sleep-wake cycle abnormalities in all 15 individuals evaluated after mild TBI using actigraphy (described in the section Evaluation of Fatigue and Sleep Disturbances in TBI) and PSG recordings. None had past history of neurological illness, psychiatric history, or sleep apnea syndrome. More than one-half of the patients were diagnosed with delayed-phase type and the rest disorganized-type sleep-wake cycle disturbance.

Quinto et al. (2000) described the case of a 48-year-old man who presented with sleep-onset insomnia after a severe closed head injury. His complaints included difficulty in initiating sleep, being able to finally fall asleep around 3:00–5:00 A.M., and waking up around noon. His attempts to wake up earlier resulted in poor functioning. Before the injury, he was reportedly high functioning and denied problems with sleep. A diagnosis of delayed sleep phase syndrome was confirmed by sleep logs and actigraphy. Patten and Lauderdale (1992) also reported delayed sleep phase disorder in a 13-year-old boy after mild closed head injury.

Complaints of sleep disturbance in TBI patients are common, and therefore awareness and diagnosis of this disorder are important; some patients may respond to simple therapies such as adjusting the time of sleep (described in the section Chronotherapy) or exposure to bright light (described in the section Phototherapy).

Parasomnias. Parasomnias are undesirable motor or behavioral events that occur during sleep that can result in physical injuries to the patient and mental agony to the caregivers (Mahowald and Mahowald 1996). Sleepwalking, sleep terrors, REM sleep behavior disorders, and nocturnal seizures are some of the varieties of parasomnias. Other than occasional case studies (Drake 1986), there is no literature available on the prevalence and clinical presentation of this condition after TBI.

Evaluation of Fatigue and Sleep Disturbances in TBI

Evaluation of a brain-injured individual with fatigue or sleep disturbances should be complete and comprehensive (Table 20–3). It is important to differentiate between fatigue and sleep disturbance if possible and determine if these symptoms are occurring in isolation or are secondary to other

TABLE 20–3. Evaluation of fatigue and sleep disturbances in traumatic brain injury

Detailed history from patient and collateral informants

Key questions:

Level of physical and mental functioning pre- and postinjury

Sleep pattern and duration pre- and postinjury

Type and severity of brain injury

Various treatments received since injury

Alcohol and substance abuse history

Medical history, including chronic pain, dizziness

Current medications and dosages

Past psychiatric history

Duration and description of current problems

Neuropsychiatric evaluation

Includes physical, neurological, and mental status examination

Neuropsychological tests in subjects with cognitive deficits

Laboratory tests

Blood count, comprehensive metabolic panel, vitamin B_{12} and folate levels, thyroid function test, and erythrocyte sedimentation rate

Brain scans

Computed tomography and/or magnetic resonance imaging

Specific sleep studies

Polysomnography

Multiple sleep latency test

neuropsychiatric disturbances such as mood disorder, anxiety disorder, substance abuse, chronic pain, or dizziness. Patients with cognitive deficits, especially pertaining to attention and concentration, often complain of fatigue. Medical illnesses such as idiopathic sleep disorders, chronic viral illness, malignancies, and medication side effects should always be ruled out. The key elements include obtaining a detailed history from the patient and collateral information from family members with the patient's consent, reviewing old medical records, and performing medical, neurological, and psychiatric examinations.

If the sleep disturbance is not considered to be secondary to another clinical syndrome, sleep studies should be performed. These studies not only help in identifying the type of sleep disturbance but also may be helpful in differentiating fatigue (normal sleep studies) from sleep disturbances. The most commonly used objective tests include the PSG and the MSLT (described in the section Multiple Sleep Latency Test). Actigraphy is a recently developed measure to obtain objective data regarding activity during sleep and wakeful state and helps supplement the subjective sleep log. An actigraph is a small device worn around the wrist or ankle that quantifies and records movements and thus detects activity during wakefulness and sleep.

Detailed information on these tests can be found in comprehensive texts on sleep disorders (Kryger et al. 2000).

Polysomnography

The PSG is the standard tool for measurement of sleep disturbances and includes assessment of breathing, respiratory muscle effort, muscle tone, REM sleep, and the four stages of NREM sleep (Castriotta and Lai 2001). Standard electrophysiologic recording systems are used in polysomnography. Polysomnography includes at least one channel of electroencephalography, electrocardiography, submental and anterior tibialis electromyography, and continuous monitoring of eye movements. If clinically indicated, multiple respiratory parameters are monitored to evaluate breathing problems during sleep, extensive electroencephalography is monitored for parasomnias, esophageal pH is monitored for gastroesophageal reflux, and penile tumescence is monitored for erectile functions. An all-night PSG will help to accurately quantify sleep and its different stages. In addition, other abnormalities such as disruption of sleep architecture, motor activity, or any other abnormality associated with sleep and cardiopulmonary irregularities can also be determined (Mahowald and Mahowald 1996). Polysomnography aids in the diagnosis of sleep disorders such as obstructive sleep apnea, central sleep apnea, upper airway resistance syndrome, nocturnal seizures, and periodic limb movements.

Multiple Sleep Latency Test

The MSLT is a well-validated measure of physiological sleep and provides objective measurement of daytime sleepiness. It is a useful tool to quantify daytime sleepiness and differentiate pathological sleep abnormalities from subjective complaints of sleepiness and fatigue (Mahowald and Mahowald 1996). It consists of four or five 20-minute naps at two hourly intervals and quantifies sleepiness by measuring how quickly one falls asleep during the day and also identifies abnormal occurrence of REM during the nap. A mean sleep latency of 5 minutes or less indicates abnormality. The diagnosis of narcolepsy is based on an MSLT score of less than 5 minutes, with REM sleep during at least two of the naps. Posttraumatic hypersomnia is diagnosed on the basis of a history of trauma, exclusion of other sleep disorders, excessive daytime sleepiness, MSLT of less than 10 minutes without sleep-onset REM periods, and a relatively normal PSG (Castriotta and Lai 2001).

TABLE 20–4. **Management of fatigue**

Pharmacological measures

    Psychostimulants

    Dopamine agonists

    Amantadine

    Modafanil

Nonpharmacological measures

    Balanced diet and lifestyle

    Sleep hygiene

    Regular exercise

    Psychotherapy

Always treat underlying medical and psychiatric disorders

Treatment

Treatment of fatigue and sleep disturbances includes pharmacological and nonpharmacological measures. Knowledge regarding pharmacotherapy in brain-injured patients is derived mainly from our experience in taking care of patients with primary psychiatric disorders and from case reports or small case series. Pharmacological interventions should target the observable symptom and any other coexisting psychiatric disorder, if present. If fatigue or sleep disturbance, or both, is secondary to any other psychiatric or medical disorder, the underlying disease should be treated. Because individuals with TBI may be sensitive to medications, it is important to start at the lowest dose and gradually increase, if necessary. Although there is overlap both pharmacologically and nonpharmacologically between fatigue and sleep disorders, we describe each of them separately (Tables 20–4 through 20–6).

TABLE 20–5. **Sleep hygiene**

Keep a regular sleep schedule of going to bed and awakening around the same time every day, including holidays and weekends.

Avoid lengthy naps during the day.

If unable to fall asleep within 10 minutes of lying in bed, get up and stay awake.

Avoid coffee, sodas, alcohol, and strenuous exercise late in the day, as they may be too stimulating and delay sleep.

Avoid bright lights and loud noise in the bedroom, especially before bedtime.

Maintain a sleep log, noting duration and quality of sleep.

TABLE 20–6. **Management of sleep disturbances**

Pharmacological measures

    Benzodiazepine sedative-hypnotics

    Nonbenzodiazepine sedative-hypnotics

    Modafinil

    Melatonin

Nonpharmacological measures

    Balanced diet and lifestyle

    Sleep hygiene

    Phototherapy

    Chronotherapy

    Psychotherapy

Always treat underlying medical and psychiatric disorders

Treatment of Fatigue

Pharmacological Measures

There are only a few studies available on the treatment of fatigue specifically after TBI. Psychostimulants, amantadine, and dopamine agonists have been used to treat impaired arousal, fatigue, inattention, and hypersomnia after brain injury (Gualtieri and Evans 1988; Neppe 1988). However, there are no studies available specifically for the treatment of fatigue in the TBI population.

Psychostimulants. Psychostimulants exert their effect by augmenting the release of catecholamines into the synapses. Methylphenidate (10–60 mg/day) and dextroamphetamine (5–40 mg/day) are the commonly used stimulants. Pemoline (18.75–75.0 mg/day), which is another stimulant, is less commonly used because of its potential for hepatotoxicity as well as its long half-life that prevents rapid clearance from the body in the event of an adverse reaction (Gualtieri and Evans 1988). Psychostimulants are usually taken twice a day, with the second dose taken approximately 6–8 hours before sleep to prevent initial insomnia. Treatment is usually begun at the lowest dose and gradually increased if necessary. Possible side effects include paranoia, dysphoria, agitation, dyskinesia, anorexia, and irritability. There is a potential for abuse, and, hence, patients taking these drugs should be closely monitored.

    The efficacy of psychostimulants in the treatment of cancer, human immunodeficiency virus infection, and MS has been studied. In a prospective, open-label pilot study, methylphenidate was used successfully to treat cancer fatigue in seven of the nine patients (Sarhill et al. 2001). In another randomized, double-blind, placebo-controlled trial of psychostimulants such as methylphenidate and pemoline for the treatment of fatigue associated with human immunodeficiency virus infection, both of the psychostimulants were found to be equally effective and superior to placebo in decreasing fatigue severity and improving quality of life (Breitbart et al. 2001). Studies of MS patients have not favored pemoline over placebo for the treatment of fatigue (Branas et al. 2000).

Dopaminergic agonists. Carbidopa/levodopa (10/100 mg to 25/100 mg qid) and bromocriptine (2.5–10.0 mg/day) are both dopamine agonists that have been studied in small uncontrolled case studies for the treatment of mood, cognition, and behavior problems in TBI patients (Dobkin and Hanlon 1993; Lal et al. 1988). Bruno et al. (1996), in a study of five postpolio patients with history of moderate to severe fatigue, noted significant improvement in fatigue and cognitive tests of attention and information processing in three patients when treated with bromocriptine up to a maximum of 12.5 mg/day.

Amantadine. Amantadine was first used in the treatment of influenza in the 1960s and was later found to have antiparkinsonian effects. It enhances release of dopamine, inhibits reuptake, and increases dopamine activity at the postsynaptic receptors (Nickels et al. 1994). Case reports have found amantadine to be useful in the treatment of mutism, apathy, inattention, and impulsivity. The usual doses are 100–400 mg/day. Confusion, hallucinations, pedal edema, and hypotension are common side effects. Krupp et al. (1995) conducted a double-blind, randomized parallel trial of amantadine, pemoline, and placebo in 93 patients with MS who complained of fatigue. Amantadine-treated patients improved significantly (both by verbal report and on the MS-specific Fatigue Severity Scale) compared with pemoline and placebo. The benefit was not due to changes in sleep, depression, or physical disability. Studies on the efficacy of amantadine for the treatment of fatigue in TBI patients are warranted.

Modafinil. Modafinil is a new agent with unclear mechanism of action but appears to activate the brain in a pattern different from that of the classic psychostimulants (Elovic 2000). Lin et al. (1996), in studies of cats given equivalent doses of modafinil, amphetamines, and methylphenidate, noted that although the latter two drugs brought about widespread increase in activation of the cerebral cortex and dopamine-rich areas such as the striatum and mediofrontal cortex, modafinil was associated with activity in the anterior hypothalamus, hippocampus, and amygdala. Modafinil's effect was supposed to be more selective on the pathways that regulate sleep. With regards to the neurotransmitter activity, modafinil has been shown to inhibit γ-aminobutyric acid levels and increase glutamate levels (Ferraro et al. 1999). It has been found to have little activity on the catecholamine system, cortisol, melatonin, and growth hormone (Brun et al. 1998; Elovic 2000). The addictive potential of modafinil is much less than the classic stimulants.

Currently, there are no specific data on the use of modafinil for the treatment of fatigue in TBI patients. Teitelman (2001) conducted an open-label study in 10 individuals with closed head injury who complained of excessive daytime sleepiness and in two individuals with somnolence secondary to sedating psychiatric drugs. Modafinil was well tolerated at a dose of 100–400 mg given once a day. All patients reported improvement in daytime sleepiness. No adverse effects were encountered.

Modafinil has been studied for the treatment of fatigue in MS. Rammohan (2002) conducted a single-blind Phase II study in MS patients and found that modafinil effectively treated fatigue. Similar results were found by Zifko et al. (2002) in an open-label study of modafinil and fatigue in MS patients. Side effects were minimal in both studies.

Nonpharmacological Measures

Education.   Patient and family members should be educated about the frequent occurrence of fatigue in TBI as an isolated problem or secondary to other psychiatric disturbances, or both. Often, it enhances the patient's self-esteem to be told that the "feeling of tiredness" is not a sign of laziness but a symptom of the brain injury.

Diet and lifestyle.   Good nutrition and a balance between regular exercise and adequate rest are important measures to combat fatigue. Patients should be encouraged to have three well-balanced meals a day. Regular exercise is important because it prevents deconditioning and promotes normalization of physical efficiency and performance, both physically and mentally. The exercise protocol should be individualized because too much or too little exercise can be detrimental. In addition, adequate rest is also important, and patients should be encouraged to practice good sleep hygiene measures (see Table 20–5). Lezak (1978) has suggested that individuals who have difficulty with fatigue should be encouraged to perform most important activities in the morning or at a time when they feel best.

Psychotherapy and behavioral therapy.   Cognitive-behavioral therapy has been found to be useful in patients with chronic fatigue syndrome (Prins et al. 2001). In a large multicenter randomized, controlled trial, cognitive-behav-

ioral therapy was found to be significantly more effective than control conditions both for fatigue improvement and functional performance. Studies of this approach are lacking for the treatment of fatigue after brain injury.

Treatment of Sleep Disturbances

The general guidelines for the management of sleep disturbances are similar to those for fatigue. Establishing a diagnosis is crucial. Recognition and treatment of other coexisting psychiatric and medical disorders are important because they could be contributing to or exacerbating the sleep disturbance. Management includes pharmacological interventions and an array of nonpharmacological measures such as sleep hygiene techniques, phototherapy, chronotherapy, and psychotherapy.

Pharmacological Measures

Even though sleep disturbances are commonly seen in TBI patients, there are only a few drug trial studies available in the TBI literature. Medications are mentioned here based on our knowledge of treatment of primary psychiatric disorders and sleep disturbances in the general population.

Benzodiazepine sedative-hypnotics.   The mechanism of action of benzodiazepines in the treatment of insomnia is unclear, although there is subjective and objective evidence of improvement in sleep (Chokroverty 2000). However, animal studies reveal impairment of neuronal recovery with the administration of benzodiazepines after laboratory-induced brain injury (Schallert et al. 1986; Simantov 1990). Similarly, studies in humans have shown poorer sensorimotor functioning in stroke patients who received benzodiazepines compared with those who did not (Goldstein and Davies 1990). Therefore, benzodiazepines should be used with caution in individuals with brain injury because they theoretically may impair neuronal recovery. Benzodiazepines commonly used as hypnotics include lorazepam (0.5–2.0 mg at bedtime), temazepam (7.5–30.0 mg at bedtime), and clonazepam (0.25–2.0 mg at bedtime). The main indication is for the treatment of transient insomnia or insomnia of short duration. Benzodiazepines should not be used for more than a few days to a couple of weeks because of the risk of dependence.

Nonbenzodiazepine sedative-hypnotics.   Zolpidem (5–10 mg at bedtime) and zaleplon (5–10 mg at bedtime) are two nonbenzodiazepines also used in the treatment of transient insomnia. They are structurally different from the benzodiazepines but act on the benzodiazepine receptor complex with more selectivity to the type 1 receptors that are involved in the mediation of sleep (Damgen and Luddens 1999; Wagner et al. 1998). Because of nonbenzodiazepines' selectivity, they are less likely to produce cognitive side effects. They also have short half-lives and are less likely to cause daytime drowsiness. Common side effects include anxiety, nausea, and dysphoric reactions, although rebound insomnia and anterograde amnesia have also been reported.

In a randomized, placebo-controlled, double-blind study comparing a 10-mg dose of zolpidem with a 10-mg dose of zaleplon given 5, 4, 3, and 2 hours before awakening in the morning to 36 healthy subjects, zaleplon was found to be free of hypnotic or sedative effects when administered as late as 2 hours before awakening (Danjou et al. 1999). Zaleplon was found to be indistinguishable from placebo in terms of subjective and objective assessment of memory and even adverse reactions. Zolpidem, in contrast, produced results different from that of placebo. Memory problems (immediate and delayed recall) were detected up to 5 hours after nocturnal administration. The differences between the two drugs are more likely to be due to their pharmacokinetic profiles than to their pharmacology (Danjou et al. 1999). Vermeeren et al. (2002), in their study of 30 healthy volunteers, demonstrated that zaleplon, 10–20 mg, could be taken at bedtime or even later (up to 5 hours before driving) with no serious risk of impairment. No studies are currently available on the use of zaleplon or zolpidem in TBI subjects.

Modafinil.   Modafinil has been found to be both safe and efficacious in the treatment of narcolepsy at a dosage of 200–400 mg/day. However, in patients with liver dysfunction, one-half of the recommended dose should be provided because there is a rare chance it can cause liver toxicity (Elovic 2000). Beusterien et al. (1999) performed a double-blind, placebo-controlled study and looked at quality-of-life issues in patients with narcolepsy. The treatment group reported improvement in energy level and in overall social functioning, increased productivity, and improved psychological well-being. Headache was the only common side effect in clinically therapeutic doses of 200–400 mg/day. Although modafinil appears to be useful in the treatment of hypersomnia, controlled studies need to be conducted to determine efficacy and side effects after brain injury in individuals with complicated and uncomplicated sleep disorders.

Melatonin.   Melatonin is a hormone secreted by the pineal gland. It is a metabolite of serotonin. Darkness augments the production of melatonin, and light suppresses its secretion. It plays an important role in maintaining the body's biological rhythm and synchronizing the sleep-wake cycle with the environment. The suprachiasmatic nucleus, which mediates the circadian rhythm, has several melatonin receptors, suggesting the importance of melatonin in maintaining the body's internal clock (Reppet et al. 1988). Studies in the general population have shown that exogenous melatonin may be useful in improving duration and quality of sleep and altering the biological rhythm (Lewy et al. 1992).

Information on this drug is limited. Although some people report improvement in sleep while taking a dose of 1.5 mg, the actual therapeutic dose is unknown. Its manufacture is not regulated by government agencies. Because of its vascular constriction property, melatonin should be avoided in patients with atherosclerosis, heart disease, and stroke. Drowsiness is a common side effect of melatonin.

Herbal supplements.   Herbs and natural remedies have been widely used to treat numerous ailments, including sleep disturbances (Tariq 2004). A number of these natural remedies have been purported to be effective in the treatment of insomnia. However, there is a paucity of studies in this area (Sateia et al. 2004).

Valerian is one of the traditional herbal sleep remedies that has been studied. Ziegler et al. (2002) conducted a randomized, double-blind, comparative clinical study in which insomnia patients (ages 18–65 years) took either 600 mg/day valerian extract LI 156 or 10 mg/day oxazepam for 6 weeks. The results found that valerian was as safe and efficacious as oxazepam. However, Glass et al. (2003) conducted a placebo-controlled, double-blind, crossover study comparing single doses of temazepam (15 mg and 30 mg), diphenhydramine (50 mg and 75 mg), and valerian (400 mg and 800 mg) in 14 healthy elderly volunteers (mean age, 71.6 years; range, 65–89 years). Valerian was comparable to placebo in measures of both sedation and psychomotor performance.

Nonpharmacological Measures

Diet and lifestyle.   Diet, rest, exercise, and sleep hygiene programs, as mentioned in the section Treatment of Fatigue, should be recommended to patients with sleep disturbance. Patients and their families should also be educated about their symptoms and the treatment options available.

Phototherapy.   Circadian rhythm disorders may respond to phototherapy. The actual mechanism of action is unknown, but exposure to bright light at strategic times of the sleep-wake cycle produces a shift of the underlying biological rhythm (Mahowald and Mahowald 1996). The timing of light exposure depends on the diagnosis because morning exposure results in phase advance, and there is phase delay with evening exposure. Bright light of 10,000 lux is commonly used. The duration of exposure varies from half an hour to 2–3 hours. Common side effects of phototherapy include headache and eye strain. Light therapy should be avoided in photosensitive patients or those who have eye diseases. There is a still lot to be learned about the indications, risks, and benefits of phototherapy.

Chronotherapy.   Chronotherapy involves obtaining a new sleep schedule by advancing or delaying sleep onset by a few hours every day until the desired sleep onset time is obtained. This requires much determination on the part of the patient, not only to obtain the "new" sleep schedule but also to maintain it thereafter. Similarly, the setting is also important, as hospitalized patients with strict ward rules may not be able to implement chronotherapy effectively (Mahowald and Mahowald 1996). Systematic studies on the indications and effectiveness of chronotherapy are lacking.

Psychotherapy.   There are few studies available on the effectiveness of behavioral therapies such as progressive deep muscle relaxation in the treatment of initial and middle insomnia in the general population (Morin et al. 1994; Vaughn 2001). No such studies are available in the TBI literature.

Summary and Future Directions

Fatigue and sleep disturbances are common in TBI patients. The etiopathology is unclear. They are probably due to a combination of factors: biological effects of the injury, psychosocial stressors, and environmental factors. In TBI subjects, fatigue and sleep disturbance may occur as isolated entities or as symptoms of another medical or psychiatric syndrome. Establishing the correct diagnosis is important because treatment differs. However, diagnosis may not always be possible. The relationship between fatigue and sleep disturbance is both complex and controversial. They may be related to each other or occur independently. Subjective sleep logs, fatigue scales, and objective laboratory sleep tests such as the polysomnogram and the multiple sleep latency test may help in differentiating the two conditions. Management of these disorders is multidimensional and includes both pharmacological and nonpharmacological interventions.

Despite the wide prevalence of fatigue and sleep disturbances, there is a marked paucity of objective data on the epidemiology, pathophysiology, clinical presentation,

diagnosis, and treatment of these conditions. The TBI literature requires more research. Identification and early, adequate treatment of these disorders will improve rehabilitation potential and enhance productivity personally, socially, and occupationally for TBI patients.

References

American Psychiatric Association: Diagnostic and Statistical Manual of Mental Disorders, 4th Edition. Washington, DC, American Psychiatric Association, 1994

Attarian HP, Brown KM, Duntley SP, et al: The relationship of sleep disturbances and fatigue in multiple sclerosis. Arch Neurol 61:525–528, 2004

Beetar JT, Guilmette TJ, Sparadeo FR: Sleep and pain complaints in symptomatic traumatic brain injury and neurologic populations. Arch Phys Med Rehabil 77:1298–1302, 1996

Bertolone K, Coyle PK, Krupp LB, et al: Cytokine correlates of fatigue in multiple sclerosis. Neurology 43:A356, 1993

Beusterien KM, Rogers AE, Walsleben JA, et al: Health-related quality of life effects of modafinil for treatment of narcolepsy. Sleep 22:757–765, 1999

Bigland-Ritchie B, Jones DA, Hosking GP, et al: Central and peripheral fatigue in sustained maximum voluntary contraction of human quadriceps muscle. Clin Sci Mol Med 54:609–614, 1978

Branas P, Jordan R, Fry-Smith A, et al: Treatment for fatigue in multiple sclerosis: a rapid and systematic review. Health Technol Assess 4:1–61, 2000

Breitbart W, Rosenfeld B, Kaim M et al: A randomized, double-blind placebo-controlled trial of psychostimulants for the treatment of fatigue in ambulatory patients with human immunodeficiency virus disease. Arch Intern Med 161:411–420, 2001

Breslau N, Roth T, Rosenthal L, et al: Sleep disturbance and psychiatric disorders: a longitudinal epidemiological study of young adults. Biol Psychiatry 39:411–418, 1996

Brun J, Chamba G, Khalfallah Y, et al: Effect of modafinil on plasma melatonin, cortisol and growth hormone rhythms, rectal temperature and performance in healthy subjects during a 36 h sleep deprivation. J Sleep Res 7:105–114, 1998

Bruno RL, Zimmerman JR, Creange SJ, et al: Bromocriptine in the treatment of post-polio fatigue: a pilot study with implications for the pathophysiology of fatigue. Am J Phys Med Rehabil 75:340–347, 1996

Castriotta RJ, Lai JM: Sleep disorders associated with traumatic brain injury. Arch Phys Med Rehabil 82:1403–1406, 2001

Chandhuri A, Behan PO: Fatigue and basal ganglia. J Neurol Sci 179:34–42, 2000

Chao CC, DeLa Hunt M, Hu S, et al: Immunologically mediated fatigue: a murine model. Clin Immunol Immunopathol 64:161–165, 1992

Chokroverty S: Sleep, breathing and neurological disorders, in Sleep Disorders Medicine. Edited by Chokroverty S. Boston, MA, Butterworth–Heinemann, 1994, pp 295–335

Chokroverty S: Diagnosis and treatment of sleep disorders caused by co-morbid disease. Neurology 54 (suppl 1):S8–S15, 2000

Clinchot D, Bogner J, Mysiw J, et al: Defining sleep disturbance after brain injury. Am J Phys Med Rehabil 77:291–295, 1998

Cohen M, Oksenberg A, Snir D, et al: Temporally related changes of sleep complaints in traumatic brain injured patients. J Neurol Neurosurg Psychiatry 55:313–315, 1992

Comi G, Leocani L, Rossi P, et al: Physiopathology and treatment of fatigue in multiple sclerosis. J Neurol 248:174–179, 2001

Damgen K, Luddens H: Zaleplon displays a selectivity to recombinant $GABA_A$ receptors different from zolpidem, zopiclone and benzodiazepines. Neurosci Res Commun 25:139–148, 1999

Danjou P, Paty I, Fruncillo R, et al: A comparison of the residual effects of zaleplon and zolpidem following administration 5–2 h before awakening. Br J Clin Pharmacol 48:367–374, 1999

Dobkin BH, Hanlon R: Dopamine agonist treatment of anterograde amnesia from a mediobasal forebrain injury. Ann Neurol 33:313–316, 1993

Drake ME Jr: Jactatio nocturna after head injury. Neurology 36:867–868, 1986

Elovic E: Use of Provigil for underarousal following TBI. J Head Trauma Rehabil 15:1068–1071, 2000

Espinar-Sierra J: Treatment and rehabilitation of sleep disorders in patients with brain damage, in Neuropsychological Rehabilitation. Fundamentals, Innovations and Directions. Edited by Leon-Carrion J. Delray Beach, FL, Lucie, 1997, pp 263–281

Ferraro L, Antonelli T, Tanganelli S, et al: The vigilance promoting drug modafinil increases extracellular glutamate levels in the medial preoptic area and posterior hypothalamus of the conscious rat: prevention by local GABA receptor blockade. Neuropsychopharmacology 4:346–356, 1999

Fichtenberg NL, Millis SR, Mann RN, et al: Factors associated with insomnia among post-acute traumatic brain injury survivors. Brain Inj 7:659–667, 2000

Fichtenberg NL, Putnam SH, Mann NR, et al: Insomnia screening in postacute traumatic brain injury: utility and validity of the Pittsburgh Sleep Quality Index. Am J Phys Med Rehabil 80:339–345, 2001

Fisk JD, Ritvo PG, Ross L, et al: Measuring the functional impact of fatigue: initial evaluation of the Fatigue Impact Scale. Clin Infect Dis 18 (suppl 1):S79–S83, 1994

Frieboes RM, Muller U, Murck H, et al: Nocturnal hormone secretion and the sleep EEG in patients several months after traumatic brain injury. J Neuropsychiatry Clin Neurosci 11:354–360, 1999

Gennarelli TA, Graham DI: Neuropathology of the head injuries. Semin Clin Neuropsychiatry 3:160–175, 1998

Glass JR, Sproule BA, Herrmann N, et al: Acute pharmacological effects of temazepam, diphenhydramine, and valerian in healthy elderly subjects. J Clin Psychopharmacol 23:260–268, 2003

Good JL, Barry E, Fishman PS: Posttraumatic narcolepsy: the complete syndrome with tissue typing. J Neurosurg 71:765–767, 1989

Goldstein LB, Davies JN: Clonidine impairs recovery of beam-walking after a sensorimotor cortex lesion in the rat. Brain Res 508:305–309, 1990

Gualtieri CT, Evans RW: Stimulant treatment for the neurobehavioral sequelae of traumatic brain injury. Brain Inj 2:273–290, 1988

Guilleminault C, Yuen KM, Gulevich BA, et al: Hypersomnia after head-neck trauma: a medico-legal trauma. Neurology 54:653–659, 2000

Hillier SL, Sharpe MH, Metzer J: Outcomes 5 years post–traumatic brain injury (with further reference to neurophysical impairment and disability). Brain Inj 11:661–675, 1997

Ingles JL, Eskes GA, Phillips SJ: Fatigue after stroke. Arch Phys Med Rehabil 80:173–178, 1999

Keshavan MS, Channabasavanna SM, Reddy GN: Post-traumatic psychiatric disturbances: patterns and predictions of outcome. Br J Psychiatry 138:157–160, 1981

Kreutzer JS, Seel RT, Gourley E: The prevalence and symptom rates of depression after traumatic brain injury: a comprehensive examination. Brain Inj 15:563–576, 2001

Krupp LB, Coyle PK, Doscher C, et al: Fatigue therapy in multiple sclerosis: results of a double-blind, randomized parallel trial of amantadine, pemoline and placebo. Neurology 45:1956–1961, 1995

Kryger MH, Roth T, Dement WC (eds): Sleep Medicine. Philadelphia, PA, WB Saunders, 2000

LaChapelle DL, Finlayson MA: An evaluation of subjective and objective measures of fatigue in patients with brain injury and healthy controls. Brain Inj 12:649–659, 1998

Lal S, Merbitz CP, Gripp JC: Modification of function in a head injury patient with Sinemet. Brain Inj 2:225–233, 1988

Lankford DA, Wellman JJ, O'Hara C: Posttraumatic narcolepsy in mild to moderate closed head injury. Sleep 17:S25–S28, 1994

Levin HS, Mattis S, Ruff RM, et al: Neurobehavioral outcome following minor head injury: a three center study. J Neurosurg 66:234–243, 1987

Lewy AJ, Ahmed S, Latham Jackson JM, et al: Melatonin shifts human circadian rhythms according to a phase response curve. Chronobiol Int 9:380–392, 1992

Lezak MD: Subtle sequelae of brain damage: perplexity, distractibility and fatigue. Am J Phys Med 57:9–15, 1978

Lin JS, Hou Y, Jouvet M: Potential brain neuronal targets for amphetamine, methylphenidate and modafinil induced wakefulness, evidenced by c-fos immunocytochemistry in the cat. Proc Natl Acad Sci U S A 93:14128–14133, 1996

Mahowald MW, Mahowald ML: Sleep disorders, in Head Injury and Postconcussive Syndrome. Edited by Rizzo M, Tranel D. New York, Churchill Livingstone, 1996, pp 285–304

Mann NR, Fichtenberg NL, Putnam SH, et al: Sleep disorders among TBI survivors: a comparison study. Arch Phys Med Rehabil 78:1055, 1997

Masel BE, Scheibel RS, Kimbark T, et al: Excessive daytime sleepiness in adults with brain injuries. Arch Phys Med Rehabil 82:1526–1532, 2001

McLean A, Dikmen S, Temkin NR, et al: Psychosocial functioning at one month after head injury. Neurosurgery 14:393–399, 1984

Middelboe T, Anderson HH, Birket-Smith M, et al: Minor head injury: impact on general health after 1 year: a prospective follow-up study. Acta Neurol Scand 85:5–9, 1992

Minderhoud JM, Boelens MEM, Huizenga J, et al: Treatment of minor head injuries. Clin Neurol Neurosurg 82:127–140, 1980

Morin CM, Culbert JP, Schwartz SM: Non-pharmacologic interventions for insomnia: a meta-analysis of treatment efficacy. Am J Psychiatry 151:1172–1180, 1994

Neppe VM: Management of catatonic stupor with L-dopa. Clin Neuropharmacol 11:90–91, 1988

Nickels JL, Schneider WN, Dombovy ML, et al: Clinical use of amantadine in brain injury rehabilitation. Brain Inj 8:709–718, 1994

Okawa M, Nanami T, Wada S, et al: Four congenitally blind children with circadian sleep-wake rhythm disorder. Sleep 10:101–110, 1987

Parmeggiani PL: Physiological regulation in sleep, in Principles and Practice of Sleep Medicine. Edited by Kryger MH, Roth T, Dement WC. Philadelphia, PA, WB Saunders, 2000, pp 169–178

Patten SB, Lauderdale WM: Delayed sleep phase disorder after traumatic brain injury. J Am Acad Child Adolesc Psychiatry 31:100–102, 1992

Peres MF, Young WB, Kaup AO, et al: Fibromyalgia is common in patients with transformed migraine. Neurology 57:1326–1328, 2001

Prins JB, Bleijenberg G, Bazelmans E, et al: Cognitive behavior therapy for chronic fatigue syndrome: a multicentre randomised controlled trial. Lancet 357:841–847, 2001

Quinto C, Gellido C, Chokroverty S, et al: Posttraumatic delayed sleep phase syndrome. Neurology 54:250–252, 2000

Rammohan KW, Rosenberg JH, Lynn DJ, et al: Efficacy and safety of modafinil (Provigil) for the treatment of fatigue in multiple sclerosis: a two centre phase 2 study. J Neurol Neurosurg Psychiatry 72:179–183, 2002

Reppet SM, Weaver DR, Rivkees SA, et al: Putative melatonin receptors in a human biological clock. Science 242:78–81, 1988

Roecke U, Kappos L, Lechner-Scott J, et al: Reduced glucose metabolism in the frontal cortex and basal ganglia of multiple sclerosis patients with fatigue. Neurology 48:1566–1571, 1997

Rosekind MR: The epidemiology and occurrence of insomnia. J Clin Psychiatry 53:S4–S6, 1992

Sarhill N, Walsh D, Nelson KA, et al: Methylphenidate for fatigue in advanced cancer: a prospective open-label pilot study. Am J Hosp Palliat Care 18:187–192, 2001

Sateia MJ, Pigeon WR: Identification and management of insomnia. Med Clin North Am 88:567–596, 2004

Schallert T, Hernandez TD, Barth TM: Recovery of function after brain damage: severe and chronic disruption by diazepam. Brain Res 379:104–111, 1986

Schreiber S, Klag E, Gross Y, et al: Beneficial effect of risperidone on sleep disturbance and psychosis following traumatic brain injury. Int Clin Psychopharmacol 13:273–275, 1998

Simantov R: Gamma-aminobutyric acid (GABA) enhances glutamate cytotoxicity in a cerebellar cell line. Brain Res Bull 24:711–715, 1990

Sutton DA, Moldofsky H, Badley EM: Insomnia and health problems in Canadians. Sleep 24:665–670, 2001

Tariq SH: Herbal therapies. Clin Geriatr Med 20:237–257, 2004

Tartaglia MC, Narayanan S, Francis SJ, et al: The relationship between diffuse axonal damage and fatigue in multiple sclerosis. Arch Neurol 61:201–207, 2004

Teitelman E: Off-label uses of modafinil. Am J Psychiatry 158:970–971, 2001

Vaughn MW. A psychiatric perspective on insomnia. J Clin Psychiatry 62 (suppl 10):27–32, 2001

Veermeerer A, Riedel WJ, van Boxtel MP, et al: Differential residual effects of zaleplon and zopiclone on actual driving: a comparison with low dose of alcohol. Sleep 25:224–231, 2002

Wagner J, Wagner ML, Hening WA: Beyond benzodiazepines: alternative pharmacologic agents for the treatment of insomnia. Ann Pharmacother 32:680–691, 1998

Webster JB, Bell KR, Hussey JD, et al: Sleep apnea in adults with traumatic brain injury: a preliminary investigation. Arch Phys Med Rehabil 82:316–321, 2001

Ziegler G, Ploch M, Miettinen-Baumann A, et al: Efficacy and tolerability of valerian extract LI 156 compared with oxazepam in the treatment of non-organic insomnia: a randomized, double-blind, comparative clinical study. Eur J Med Res 7:480–486, 2002

Zifko UA, Rupp M, Schwarz S, et al: Modafinil in treatment of fatigue in multiple sclerosis. Results of an open-label study. J Neurol 249:983–987, 2002

21 Headaches

Thomas N. Ward, M.D.

Morris Levin, M.D.

POSTTRAUMATIC HEADACHE (PTH) affects millions of people annually. It is the most common presenting complaint of postconcussion syndrome (see Chapter 15, Mild Brain Injury and the Postconcussion Syndrome). PTH is defined as a new headache beginning after brain injury. Headache associated with brain or neck injury usually is short-lived; when it persists for months to years after the event, it is termed *chronic*. Awareness of this phenomenon allows proper evaluation, diagnosis, treatment, and ascertainment of prognosis.

Prevalence

Estimates of PTH after injury to the brain or neck vary from 30% to 90% (Gfeller et al. 1994; Rimel et al. 1981). However, definitions are inconsistent, making comparisons of reports problematic. For example, the current International Headache Society (IHS) criteria for PTH do not recognize late-onset headaches (headaches beginning more than 7 days after the injury or after regaining consciousness therefrom) (International Headache Society 2004). However, such headaches are described. Brain injury may also occur as part of "whiplash" injuries. Just as headache is the most frequent symptom of postconcussion syndrome, occurring in up to 90% of patients, more than 90% of patients evaluated medically after whiplash events complain of headaches (Machado et al. 1988). Precise numbers are elusive because most whiplash events are not reported. Given the common co-occurrence of brain injury and whiplash, an estimate of 4 million cases of PTH annually in the United States is conservative.

PTH seems to occur more frequently in milder brain injuries. There appears to be no clear relationship between the severity or duration of PTH and gender, age,

intelligence, occupation, or conditions under which the injury occurred (Guttman 1943).

Definitions

The IHS criteria defines acute PTH as beginning within 7 days of the trauma (or of awakening therefrom) and resolving within 3 months. Chronic PTH is defined as persisting beyond 3 months (International Headache Society 2004). In that the majority of PTH resolves within 6 months, it has been proposed that persistence beyond 6 months is a more practical definition of chronic PTH (Packard and Ham 1993). The IHS criteria additionally specify two subtypes of acute PTH. First is acute PTH with significant head trauma (having at least one of the following: loss of consciousness; posttraumatic amnesia lasting longer than 10 minutes; and at least two abnormalities among the clinical neurological examination, including skull X ray, neuroimaging, evoked potentials, and cerebrospinal fluid [CSF], vestibular function, and neuropsychological tests). Acute PTH after minor head trauma and no confirmatory signs is the other subtype.

Whiplash injuries refer to flexion-extension and lateral motions of the neck related to acceleration-deceleration injuries. Because these movements also affect the head and brain, it is not surprising that both are injured concomitantly and that there is great overlap between postconcussion syndrome and whiplash syndrome.

Pathophysiological Changes

The mechanism(s) of PTH are not fully understood. Most cases of PTH clinically resemble tension-type

TABLE 21–1. International Headache Society criteria for episodic tension-type headache

A. At least 10 previous episodes occurring <15/month, fulfilling criteria B through D

B. Headache lasting from 30 minutes to 7 days

C. At least two of the following pain characteristics:

  1. Bilateral location

  2. Pressing/tightening (nonpulsating) quality

  3. Mild or moderate intensity

  4. Not aggravated by routine physical activity such as walking or climbing stairs

D. Both of the following:

  1. No nausea and vomiting (anorexia may occur)

  2. No more than one of photophobia or phonophobia

Source. Reprinted from Headache Classification Subcommittee of the International Headache Society: "The International Classification of Headache Disorders: Second Edition." *Cephalalgia* 24 (suppl 1):9–160, 2004. Used with permission.

headache (TTH) (Table 21–1), which also is poorly understood. The spinal trigeminal nucleus caudalis is thought to be a point of physiological and anatomical convergence relevant to the genesis of headache. It receives input from the distribution of the trigeminal nerve as well as upper cervical segments. This arrangement explains how neck pain might be referred to the head and vice versa.

It has been speculated that PTH may be due to "central sensitization." It is suggested that persistent peripheral input through the spinal trigeminal nucleus caudalis results in permanently altered function of second- and third-order neurons along the pain pathway in the spinal trigeminal nucleus and thalamus (Post and Silberstein 1994). If correct, this concept might explain how persistent musculoskeletal injuries could generate chronic PTH.

During head injury or whiplash, shear forces affect the brain. Asynchronous movements occur between the contents of the posterior fossa (i.e., brainstem and cerebellum) and the cerebral hemispheres. Direct impact is unnecessary (Gennarelli 1993). Acceleration-deceleration and/or rotational forces can result in stretching, compression, even anatomical disruption of axons (diffuse axonal injury). These pathological changes most often occur in the internal capsule, corpus callosum, fornices, dorsolateral midbrain, and pons (Blumbergs et al. 1989). Axons traversing the upper brainstem seem to be particularly at risk for axonal injury in this setting. The area encompassing the periaqueductal gray/dorsal raphe nucleus is in this

region and has been implicated in headache (migraine) activity. Also in the midbrain/upper pons is the ascending reticular activating system. Damage to the ascending reticular activating system might explain the sleep-wake disturbances and attentional and concentration problems frequently described in postconcussion syndrome.

Severe brain injury may result in ischemic brain damage, but even with lesser degrees of insult posttraumatic vasospasm or abnormal cerebrovascular autoregulation may occur (Junger et al. 1997; Zubkov et al. 1999). Abnormalities demonstrated on cerebral blood flow studies and single-photon emission computed tomography (SPECT) have been reported to persist up to 3 years after the trauma (Taylor and Bell 1996). Similarly, positron emission tomography (PET) studies may be abnormal. However, PTH patients generally have not had such studies before their injuries, and SPECT and PET studies are also abnormal during headache.

Packard and Ham (1997) have noted similarities in neurochemical changes between experimental brain injury and migraine. These include increased extracellular potassium; increased intracellular sodium, calcium, and chloride; increased release of excitatory amino acids (glutamate); decreased intracellular and total brain magnesium; and possible changes in nitric oxide.

There seems to be an inverse relation between the severity of the brain injury or whiplash and the severity of postconcussion syndrome. Perhaps dysfunction or damage to brain systems allows the genesis of headache, whereas more severe injury (destruction) does not (Packard and Ham 1997).

Assessment

The evaluation of acute posttraumatic headache usually transpires in the emergency department setting. A thorough history and general physical and neurological examinations need to be performed expeditiously to rule out potentially life-threatening conditions (Table 21–2) (Ward et al. 2001). Cervical spine injury should be considered and evaluated and treated as part of the initial examination. Patients requiring immediate treatment or in whom a period of observation is deemed prudent are hospitalized. Otherwise, patients may be sent home with supervision and instructions regarding under what circumstances to return for reevaluation. Arrangements for appropriate follow-up appointments should be made.

When patients are evaluated for chronic PTH, the strategy is somewhat different. The possible causes of chronic PTH are slightly different from the acute situation (Table 21–3). Trauma can trigger the development of

TABLE 21–2. Secondary ("threatening") causes of acute posttraumatic headache

Condition	Useful tests
Epidural hematoma	CT scan
Subdural hematoma	CT scan
Vascular dissection	Magnetic resonance angiography, angiography
Subarachnoid hemorrhage	CT scan, lumbar puncture, angiography
Intracerebral hematoma	CT scan
Cerebral venous sinus thrombosis	Magnetic resonance venography, angiography
Ischemic stroke	Magnetic resonance imaging, CT scan
Cervical spine fracture	X ray, CT scan

Note. CT=computed tomography.

headaches that mimic primary headaches, but obvious structural etiologies still should be considered. One needs to ensure that nothing was overlooked during the initial evaluation and that a new problem has not declared itself, and to remember that some patients have more than one type of headache.

The patient should be examined again, without preconceptions. It is not sufficient simply to rely on prior normal neuroimaging and other evaluations. An adequate assessment includes a neurological examination (with mental status examination) and attention to the head and

TABLE 21–3. Causes and triggers of chronic posttraumatic headache

Whiplash or cervical spine injury

Upper cervical root entrapment

Temporomandibular joint injury

Dysautonomic cephalgia

Vascular dissection (carotid, vertebral arteries)

Subdural hematoma (rarely, epidural hematoma)

Neuromas

Neuralgias (e.g., Eagle's syndrome)

CSF hypotension (CSF leak)

Intracranial hypertension or hydrocephalus

Venous sinus thrombosis, cerebral vein thrombosis

Posttraumatic seizures

Note. CSF=cerebrospinal fluid.

neck. Any abnormality should prompt consideration of further investigation.

The cranial examination should include inspection for local residua of trauma. Posttraumatic temporomandibular joint syndrome may be a source of discomfort as well as a headache trigger. Typically, there are clicking and popping of the joint, pain with use, and restriction of jaw opening. One may appreciate associated masseter muscle spasm. The head should be inspected and palpated for the possible presence of painful scars and neuromas. The finding of otorrhea or rhinorrhea suggests a CSF leak, which could cause orthostatic headache (CSF hypotension) or predispose the patient to acquiring meningitis. A Tinel's sign over the occipital nerve may suggest occipital neuralgia. However, if there is a persistent side-locked headache with decreased sensation in the ipsilateral C2 or C3 dermatome, the possibility of an upper cervical root entrapment should be considered (Pikus and Phillips 1996).

An abnormality on the examination, or even a worrisome history (worsening headache pattern), should prompt further testing. Otherwise, the patient's description of the head pain should allow a diagnosis to be assigned. Though PTH may mimic the primary headaches described by the IHS, posttraumatic neuralgia may also occur. For example, injury or fracture to the styloid process may cause Eagle's syndrome, which is essentially a symptomatic form of glossopharyngeal neuralgia (Young et al. 2001). Paroxysms of pain occur in the oropharynx or radiate toward the ear. The diagnosis requires a careful description of the head pain(s).

In our experience, the most likely causes of symptomatic, chronic PTH are chronic subdural hematoma, late-onset hydrocephalus, upper cervical root entrapment, unsuspected vascular dissection, and cerebral vein or venous sinus thrombosis. It is important to remember that increased intracranial pressure may occur (with or without hydrocephalus) and papilledema need not always be present (Mathew et al. 1996). Last, it has been reported that PTH may be perpetuated by overuse of symptomatic medications, so-called analgesic rebound headache (Warner and Fenichel 1996). In this situation, symptomatic pain medications used daily or nearly daily actually lead to a worsening of the headache pattern. Getting the patient out of this pattern may lead to dramatic improvement.

If the history or examination, or both, suggests the need for further testing, test selection for chronic PTH is somewhat different from that in the emergency department. Although brain computed tomography scanning is often preferred in the acute setting because it is usually more readily available and detects acute hemorrhage well, magnetic resonance imaging, angiography, or venography is usually desired to search for diffuse axonal injury, subdural hematoma, vascular dissection, hydrocephalus, or venous sinus thrombosis. After mass lesion has been ruled out, lumbar puncture may be performed if increased or decreased (by CSF leak) intracranial pressure is being considered. Further tests, such as bloodwork, are selected in accordance with diagnostic possibilities suggested by the history and examination. If upper cervical root entrapment is suspected on clinical grounds, a deep computed tomography–guided root block may be diagnostic.

Electroencephalography (EEG) is frequently abnormal in patients with PTH; however, the findings are not specific. If seizures are a diagnostic possibility, then EEG is appropriate. Many other tests are often abnormal in PTH. These include evoked potentials, quantitative EEG (brain mapping), SPECT, and PET. Again, the findings are generally not specific for brain injury and are not directly useful for patient management. For example, the American Academy of Neurology (1996) labels the use of SPECT in the evaluation of PTH "investigational." Although of interest in a research setting, these investigations should not be routinely performed.

Many patients with PTH have other symptoms of postconcussion syndrome (Table 21–4). If vertigo is a prominent symptom, ear, nose, and throat referral, including electronystagmography, may document dysfunction of the vestibular apparatus. If psychiatric or cognitive complaints, or both, are found, psychiatric consultation and/or neuropsychological testing may be invaluable. If sleep dysfunction is evident, evaluation by a sleep specialist, and possibly polysomnography, might be helpful.

Natural History

Approximately 80% of patients with PTH improve by the end of the first year. Studies show that 1 year after mild traumatic brain injury, 8%–35% of patients had persistent headache (Dencker and Lofving 1958; Rutherford et al. 1978). However, after the passage of another 3 years, 20%–24% still had headache. Therefore, Packard (1994) suggests that if reasonable therapeutic maneuvers have been attempted, PTH is likely to be permanent if it lasts longer than 12 months, or longer than 6 months with a lack of further improvement for 3 months.

Much has been made of the potential confounding effects of litigation and financial compensation on resolution of PTH. Financial settlement does not seem to predict persistence or resolution of symptoms in most cases. Although malingering occasionally occurs, probably fewer than 10% of patients are thought to be manipulating the situation for financial reasons (Gutkelch 1980).

TABLE 21–4. Symptoms of postconcussion syndrome

Headaches

Psychiatric symptoms

    Anxiety

    Depression

    Irritability

    Mania

    Difficulty concentrating

Sleep disturbances

Seizures

Dystonia

Tremor

Vertigo, tinnitus, hearing loss

Blurred vision, double vision

Anosmia

Neuralgia

Temporomandibular joint dysfunction

Complications

It is difficult to discuss complications of PTH without including those of postconcussion syndrome (see Table 21–4). In approximately one-fifth of patients, the headaches fail to resolve. Beyond the head pain itself, the cognitive and psychiatric problems occurring as part of postconcussion syndrome lead to significant disability. These symptoms may actually become more prominent clinically as the headaches improve (Packard 1994).

Many of the complications of PTH are related to drug therapy. Overuse of narcotics can lead to dependence, and overuse of other analgesics has led to untold numbers of cases of renal failure, hepatic damage, and gastrointestinal bleeding.

Treatment

The approach to the patient with PTH must be individualized. Although the type(s) of headache must be diagnosed, all of the patient's symptoms must be inventoried to select the appropriate treatments. Comorbid and coexistent conditions impose therapeutic limitations but may also suggest therapeutic opportunities (Table 21–5). Many associated symptoms may be quite disabling in their own right, such as vestibular symptoms, cognitive

TABLE 21–5. Therapeutic opportunities and constraints in posttraumatic headache

Comorbid or coexistent conditions	Possibly useful	Relatively contraindicated
Raynaud's phenomenon	Calcium channel agents	β-Blockers
Epilepsy	Sodium valproate, gabapentin, topiramate	Tricyclic antidepressants
Mitral valve prolapse	β-Blockers	—
Depression	Tricyclic antidepressants, MAOIs	β-Blockers
Bipolar disorder	Sodium valproate	Tricyclic antidepressants, MAOIs
Hypertension	β-Blockers, calcium channel drugs	—
Asthma	Leukotriene inhibitors (montelukast, zafirlukast)	β-Blockers

Note. MAOIs=monoamine oxidase inhibitors.

dysfunction, and mood changes, and failure to recognize them may impair compliance and delay recovery.

For headaches due to an obvious underlying etiology, treatment is directed against the underlying condition. This is particularly true for headache in the acute posttraumatic period. Many cases of chronic PTH mimic primary headache (e.g., migraine and TTH), and in these cases treatment is directed at that type of headache. Options include nonpharmacological measures such as physical therapy, cognitive-behavioral therapy, and biofeedback. Pharmacological measures include acute medications for specific episodes and preventive drugs to attempt to lessen the frequency, duration, and severity of the headaches (Ward 2000).

An essential first step in the treatment of PTH is to educate the patient about the diagnosis and integrate his or her participation into the headache plan. The patient's condition should be clearly explained and the natural history of likely substantial clinical improvement emphasized. Patient preferences regarding therapy should be considered to enhance compliance. Limits on acute medication intake should be set to avoid causing analgesic rebound and inadvertently prolonging the clinical course. The patient's progress should be monitored regularly and

any new problems or setbacks dealt with promptly. The use of headache calendars or diaries is very important. Patients must understand that optimal treatment is often a team effort, with various consultants involved for the management of specific problems as they are identified.

In general, nonpharmacological measures are nearly always indicated. These treatments may enhance compliance, help identify problems, and may reduce the need for medication. Lifestyle adjustments such as sleep regulation, avoidance of trigger activities, discontinuation of nicotine and alcohol, and regular appropriate exercise should be encouraged. Relaxation techniques, including thermal and myographic biofeedback, imagery, and hypnotherapy, have proven helpful for many patients. Cognitive-behavioral programs can also be highly effective but are clearly limited in patients with significant cognitive impairment. Individual (as well as family or group) psychotherapy can address associated posttraumatic mood and behavioral changes, but can also provide effective pain-coping strategies. Massage, mobilization techniques, and myofascial release can be effective in management of PTH, particularly in patients in whom cervicogenic headache seems significant. Transcutaneous electrical nerve stimulation and acupuncture may be helpful in some patients as well.

Acute symptomatic treatment of PTH pain is best treated with nonaddictive medication. Specific choices, including nonsteroidal anti-inflammatory drugs (NSAIDs), muscle relaxants, and others, are discussed below. Prophylactic pharmacological therapy for PTH should be considered when acute medications are ineffective, required frequently, or are not well tolerated. Doses should be low initially and advanced as necessary and as tolerated. Adverse-effect profiles should be tailored to the individual and carefully explained. Multiple symptoms should be targeted with the minimum of medications (e.g., the choice of tricyclic antidepressants for patients with concomitant depression and pain). Daily preventive medications should be challenged for effectiveness and discontinued when possible. The United States Headache Consortium has published evidence-based treatment guidelines that may be downloaded from the Internet (http://www.aan.com). These guidelines address both nonpharmacological and pharmacological options.

For TTHs that are intermittent, NSAIDs, including cyclooxygenase-2 inhibitors, can be useful. These may include over-the-counter or prescription drugs. Acetaminophen is also useful. Muscle relaxants may be used if there is significant neck discomfort. Frequent headaches may require prophylaxis, and amitriptyline or other tricyclic antidepressants in relatively small doses given at bedtime may be of great use.

Acute therapy of migraine has been revolutionized by the advent of the triptans. These serotonergic agents have possible therapeutic mechanisms, including vascular constriction and suppression of neurogenic inflammation (Moskowitz 1992). Currently, almotriptan, naratriptan, rizatriptan, sumatriptan, zolmitriptan, eletriptan, and frovatriptan are available. NSAIDs may be useful if given early in the attack and at high enough doses. A gastric motility–enhancing drug such as metoclopramide may improve absorption and increase efficacy. We have found hydroxyzine a useful adjunct for headache pain and associated nausea. Intranasal, subcutaneous, or intramuscular dihydroergotamine remains useful, although less convenient to use than the triptans. Selecting the correct route of drug administration is very important. It is important to consider nonoral routes for medication if there is prominent nausea or vomiting, or both. Injections, nasal sprays, and suppositories may be appropriate (Ward 1998). Troublesome attacks of TTH in patients with migraine may respond to triptan drugs, whereas TTH in nonmigraineurs usually does not (Lipton et al. 2000).

Numerous medications have been used for migraine prevention. Drug selection again is best made with consideration of comorbid and coexistent medical conditions (see Table 21–5). Choices with strong support in the literature include propranolol, valproic acid, amitriptyline, and methysergide. A useful strategy is to start with a low dose of medication, monitor progress with a headache calendar, and adjust the dose upward slowly every few weeks as tolerated and required. Occasional patients may require more than one preventive medication (Ward 2000).

Cluster headache is rarely triggered by trauma. The episodic form is characterized by bouts of headaches typically lasting weeks followed by remissions with no headaches for months or years. Individual attacks frequently respond to oxygen, subcutaneous sumatriptan, and transnasal butorphanol. When prevention is used, verapamil is usually the mainstay of therapy. Additional preventive drugs with efficacy include lithium, valproic acid, and methysergide (Ward 2000). An occipital nerve block performed ipsilateral to the pain may control the episodes until a remission occurs (Anthony 1987). Chronic cluster headache is the form that occurs essentially without a significant remission for longer than a year. Occasionally, inpatient therapy with repetitive dihydroergotamine is effective. Truly medically intractable cases may require neurosurgery.

Neuralgic syndromes can frequently co-occur with other headache types in patients with PTH. Local nerve infiltration with lidocaine or bupivacaine can be both diagnostic as well as palliative in patients with occipital neuralgia, supraorbital neuralgia, and Eagle's syndrome. In these neuralgias, percussion over the irritated nerve often provokes a Tinel's sign and reproduces the symptomatology. Trigger point injection, particularly in patients with cervicalgia, can be effective in selected cases.

Refractory daily or frequent severe headaches may require hospitalization. Repetitive intravenous dihydroergotamine as described by Raskin (1986) can be dramatically effective. Other intravenous protocols include chlorpromazine and valproic acid (Mathew et al. 1999). Appropriate selection and performance of these regimens often requires a high level of experience and knowledge. Referral of the patient to a knowledgeable headache expert or headache center may be the most efficient way to manage the patient, especially if more straightforward and simpler measures have failed to provide sufficient benefit. Such referrals are usually appropriate for those patients with unusual conditions, unclear diagnoses, poor response to therapies, or failure to improve over time.

Conclusion

The evaluation and management of patients with posttraumatic headache must be individualized and comprehensive. Attention to the fundamentals of thorough diagnosis and familiarity with all of the various therapeutic modalities available enables the initiation of a treatment plan that should alleviate symptoms and minimize disability. The majority of patients spontaneously improves within 6 months. The remainder can still be helped by a symptom-based approach that is both competently applied and compassionate. Because posttraumatic headache is often a component of postconcussion syndrome, awareness of that condition and the additional symptoms it causes allows the alleviation of suffering and benefit for the patient.

References

American Academy of Neurology: Assessment of brain SPECT: report of the Therapeutics and Technology Assessment Subcommittee of the American Academy of Neurology. Neurology 46:278–285, 1996

Anthony M: The role of the occipital nerve in unilateral headache, in Current Problems in Neurology: Advances in Headache Research. Edited by Rose FC. London, England, John Libbey, 1987, pp 257–262

Blumbergs PC, Jones NR, North JB: Diffuse axonal injury in head trauma. J Neurol Neurosurg Psychiatry 52:838–841, 1989

Dencker SJ, Lofving BA: A psychometric study of identical twins discordant for closed head injury. Acta Psychiatr Neurol Scand 122 (suppl):119–126, 1958

Gennarelli TA: Mechanisms of brain injury. J Emerg Med 1:5–11, 1993

Gfeller JD, Chibnall JT, Duckro PN: Postconcussion symptoms and cognitive functioning in posttraumatic headache patients. Headache 34:503–507, 1994

Gutkelch AN: Posttraumatic amnesia, post-concussional symptoms and accident. Eur Neurol 19:91–102, 1980

Guttman L: Post-contusional headache. Lancet 1:10–12, 1943

International Headache Society: Classification and diagnostic criteria for headache disorders, cranial neuralgias and facial pain. Cephalalgia 8 (suppl 7):1–96, 1988

Junger EC, Newell DW, Grant GA, et al: Cerebral autoregulation following minor head injury. J Neurosurg 86:425–432, 1997

Lipton RB, Stewart WF, Cady R, et al: Sumatriptan for the range of headaches in migraine sufferers: results of the Spectrum Study. Headache 40:783–791, 2000

Machado EB, Michet CJ, Ballard DJ, et al: Trends in incidence and clinical presentation of temporal arteritis in Olmsted County, Minnesota, 1958–1985. Arthritis Rheum 31:745–749, 1988

Mathew NT, Ravishankar K, Sanin LC: Coexistence of migraine and idiopathic intracranial hypertension without papilledema. Neurology 46:1226–1230, 1996

Mathew NT, Kailasam J, Meadors L, et al: Intravenous valproate sodium (Depacon) aborts migraine rapidly: a preliminary report (abstract). Cephalalgia 19:373, 1999

Moskowitz MA: Neurogenic versus vascular mechanisms of sumatriptan and ergot alkaloids in migraine. Trends Pharmacol Sci 13:307–311, 1992

Packard RC: Posttraumatic headache. Semin Neurol 14:40–45, 1994

Packard RC, Ham LP: Posttraumatic headache: determining chronicity. Headache 33:133–134, 1993

Packard RC, Ham LP: Pathogenesis of posttraumatic headaches and migraine: a common headache pathway? Headache 37:142–152, 1997

Pikus HJ, Phillips JM: Outcome of surgical decompression of the second cervical root for cervicogenic headache. Neurosurgery 39:63–71, 1996

Post RM, Silberstein SD: Shared mechanisms in affective illness, epilepsy, and migraine. Neurology 44:S37–S47, 1994

Raskin NH: Repetitive intravenous dihydroergotamine as therapy for intractable migraine. Neurology 36:995–997, 1986

Rimel RW, Giordani B, Barth JT: Disability caused by minor head injury. Neurosurgery 9:221–228, 1981

Rutherford WH, Merrett JD, McDonald JR: Symptoms of one year following concussion from minor head trauma. Injury 10:225–230, 1978

Taylor AB, Bell TK: Slowing of cerebral circulation after concussional head injury: a controlled trial. Lancet 2:178–180, 1996

Ward TN: Management of an acute primary headache. Clin Neurosci 5:50–54, 1998

Ward TN: Providing relief from headache pain: current options for acute and prophylactic therapy. Postgrad Med 108:121–127, 2000

Ward TN, Levin M, Phillips JM: Evaluation and management of headache in the emergency department. Med Clin North Am 85:971–985, 2001

Warner JS, Fenichel GM: Chronic post-traumatic headache often a myth? Neurology 46:915–916, 1996

Young WB, Packard RC, Ramadan N: Headaches associated with head trauma, in Wolff's Headache and Other Head Pain, 7th Edition. Edited by Silberstein SD, Lipton RB, Dalessio DJ. Oxford, England, Oxford University Press. 2001, pp 328–329

Zubkov AY, Pilkington AS, Bernanke DH, et al: Posttraumatic cerebral vasospasm: clinical and morphological presentations. J Neurotrauma 16:763–770, 1999

22 Balance Problems and Dizziness

Edwin F. Richter III, M.D.

DIZZINESS AND IMPAIRED balance are among the known consequences of traumatic brain injury (TBI). Dizziness may include sensations of unsteadiness, nausea, light-headedness, or other vague symptoms. Vertigo is a more specific sensation of the environment spinning around the patient. Because this is a more distinct phenomenon, some clinicians stress the term *true vertigo* in their assessments. Although the distinctions between vertigo and other forms of dizziness are of some importance, one should not conclude from the popular use of the term *true vertigo* that other complaints of dizziness are either false or unimportant.

Dizziness is a subjective symptom. It may be experienced at rest or when in motion. Objective examination findings may be associated with conditions known to cause dizziness. Even when such findings are present, patients express various levels of distress.

Impaired balance is an objective sign. Ability to maintain body position can be measured. Visual observation and other tests provide objective assessments of dysequilibrium. There may still be substantial differences in how individuals report their complaints for a given degree of impairment. Prior activity levels and current comorbidities influence perceptions of disability. Some patients with visible stigmata of recurrent falls, such as ecchymoses, may verbalize less distress than others who perceive themselves at risk for falls.

Various factors contribute to difficulty maintaining balance after TBI. Some are relatively easy to detect and understand. Patients with motor deficits may demonstrate difficulty controlling body position. Somatosensory deficits also cause balance deficits, especially if proprioception and kinesthesia are impaired. Cerebellar lesions may be associated with significant ataxia.

Vestibular deficits may cause functional impairments after head trauma. Gait may become less stable. Stabilizing gaze during head motions may become more difficult.

Balance deficits may be subtle. Some patients appear to ambulate normally under ordinary conditions but struggle with uneven terrain or moving surfaces. Environmental factors may trigger balance problems. A mismatch between subjective complaints and conventional examination findings may pose a management challenge.

Prevalence

The incidence of dizziness and balance problems after TBI varies with several factors. Dysfunction of the vestibular system can occur in approximately one-half of cases with skull fractures. If a temporal bone fracture is involved, incidence has been reported as great as 87%–100% (Toglia 1976; Tuohima 1978). Transverse fractures of the temporal bone are more likely to cause anatomical damage to the vestibular system. Unilateral injuries may include acute spontaneous nystagmus, provoked vertigo, and impaired balance. (Provoked vertigo is a spinning sensation elicited by various combinations of head turning, sudden eye movements, or other challenging stimuli.) Bilateral injuries may feature oscillopsia (to-and-fro eye motions) and profound balance disorders (Herdman 1990). Longitudinal temporal fractures more often cause anatomical injury to the middle ear, with prominent conductive hearing loss, but vestibular dysfunction may also be seen.

The overall incidence of balance problems or dizziness, or both, after TBI is difficult to determine accurately. Reports of vestibular symptoms ranging from 30% to 60% have been reported in various studies of TBI populations (Gibson 1984; Griffiths 1979; Healy 1982). Given varying access to services in populations at risk for brain injury and the potential for underreporting of mild TBI, a precise estimate may not be possible.

Physiology

To understand posttraumatic vestibulopathy, one must consider the structure of the vestibular apparatus (Hain and Hillman 2000; Shumway-Cook 2001). The peripheral sensory receptors are located within the membranous labyrinth of the inner ear. The structures include the semicircular canals, the utricle, and the saccule. These receptors and the vestibular fibers of cranial nerve VIII constitute the peripheral component of the vestibular system. Information from this system passes through the vestibular nuclei to ascending and descending tracts. The vestibular nuclei and the structures to which they connect constitute the central vestibular system.

Within each inner ear, the three semicircular canals are each oriented in a different plane. Each canal is paired with a symmetrical counterpart in the opposite ear. Each canal is filled with endolymphatic fluid and surrounded with perilymphatic fluid. If the head rotates in the plane of a canal, the endolymphatic fluid tends to stay at rest within the canal. Because the canal itself moves with the head, there is a relative motion of the fluid in the canal.

At the end of each canal is an enlarged area called the *ampulla*. Within each ampulla lie upward projections called *cupula*. They are deformed by motion of the canal because the endolymphatic fluid surrounding them does not initially move. The cupula contain projections from the hair cells. These tufts bend with the cupula during rotation within the plane of their canal.

The hair cells are connected to the vestibular nuclei via bipolar neurons. At rest, these neurons fire at a fixed rate. The firing frequency of these neurons changes with bending of the hair cells, increasing or decreasing depending on the direction of motion. Because the canals are paired, angular acceleration within the plane of a pair of canals results in activation of the receptors on both sides.

Hair cells within the vertical saccule and horizontal utricle project into masses called *otoliths*. These contain crystals called *otoconia*. Linear acceleration or lateral tilting of the head causes motion of the otoliths and bending of the hair cells. The presence of paired structures on opposite sides of the head allows concurrent input of data. Redundancy may allow for compensation for unilateral injuries.

Information from the hair cells travels along the vestibular nerve to the vestibular nuclei, located at the junction of the pons and medulla. There are also connections to the cerebellum, reticular formation, thalamus, and cerebral cortex. Proprioceptive, visual, and auditory information is also processed by the vestibular nuclei.

Information from the vestibular system drives the vestibuloocular reflex (VOR). This reflex rotates the eyes in the direction opposite to the direction of head rotation. A rapid resetting motion follows this eye rotation. This is called *nystagmus*. This system relies on the horizontal canals in particular to detect the direction and rate of acceleration of movement. Normally, each canal should generate signals of equal magnitude. (Unilateral injury may cause conflicting data to be presented to the central nervous system.)

Vestibular input also drives the vestibulospinal reflex. Rapid acceleration of head motion may excite the vestibulospinal tract, which activates antigravity muscles.

Reflex activation of cervical muscles to oppose detected motion also occurs. Vestibulocollic reflex head movement counters perceived head motion detected by the vestibular system.

The vestibular nuclei directly activate the reflexes, but the cerebellum plays a critical role in the central vestibular system. It regulates the sensitivity of the reflexes and probably plays a critical role in compensating for disorders.

Cortical interaction with the vestibular system is far from fully understood. Parietal processing of vestibular information occurs, but the exact process is not known. It is clear that the brain must somehow coordinate visual, vestibular, and proprioceptive information to facilitate gaze stability and postural stability.

Because multiple sites within the brain may be associated with modifying and perceiving input from the visual and vestibular systems, dysfunction may occur after even mild TBI. The sensory organs themselves may be either injured or intact in this scenario. If intact, they might be sending correct data that are not accurately processed. If sensory organs are injured, there might not be adequate ability to compensate in the central nervous system. Any resulting perceptions of dizziness or dysequilibrium would not help problems of irritability or distractibility.

Diagnostic Procedures

History

As with most clinical disorders, careful attention to the history is the most critical aspect of the diagnostic process. Many patients do not have a precise vocabulary for matters relating to dizziness and dysequilibrium (Table 22–1). Vague references to being "light-headed" or

---

TABLE 22–1.   Common somatic complaints associated with dysequilibrium after traumatic brain injury

Dizziness ("shaky," "light-headed," many other vague synonyms)

Vertigo (environment spins)

Imbalance (+/–falls), veering

Visual blurring and fatigue, difficulty reading (+/–headache)

Tinnitus (ringing or buzzing sensation in ears)

Difficulty distinguishing speech from background noise

Difficulty hearing

Sensitivity to noise

"floating" may be the first clues to the existence of a significant deficit. Other patients may have heard terms such as *vertigo* or *vestibular disorder* without accurately understanding them, and may then use them while relating their history.

Patients should be asked about the presence or absence of spinning sensations (vertigo), feeling off balance, vision problems, difficulty reading, hearing problems, or tendencies to veer to one side while walking. Exacerbating conditions should be noted if any of these problems are reported.

Patients should be asked about past history of inner ear disorders. Any premorbid visual or hearing impairment should be noted.

Academic and vocational history is sometimes used to infer levels of cognitive function before brain injury. Some patients may be able to recall their scores on the Scholastic Aptitude Test or their grades in school. A clinician may consider such information when neuropsychological testing reveals evidence of cognitive impairments. Few patients have had comparable formal balance testing before presenting with their complaints. One can sometimes infer from vocational or avocational histories how certain individuals previously functioned. A valid history of high-level athletic performance, prolonged work at elevated heights, or extensive exposure to extreme motion without prior difficulty can indicate good underlying vestibular system functioning. Individuals who always tended to develop motion sickness riding in conventional vehicles may have been living with less resilient vestibular systems. One may obtain a hint of past function by asking about prior experiences traveling by airplane or boat, past participation in relevant recreational sports, or even amusement park experiences.

In addition to eliciting a current list of symptoms, it is useful to inquire about performance of common func-

tional tasks. During reading, the eyes scan across pages in a manner that may challenge the compromised vestibular system. Shopping in a grocery store is potentially quite difficult. This activity requires scanning across both sides of an aisle, processing extensive visual information, while moving through the environment and avoiding both stationary and moving obstacles. The colorful packaging and ambient noise provide additional sensory stimuli.

Standard batteries have been developed. The Dizziness Handicap Inventory is a 25-item questionnaire with physical, emotional, and functional sets of questions (Jacobson and Newman 1990) (Figure 22–1). Correlation with balance platform testing has been shown (Robertson and Ireland 1995). A short form has recently been developed (Tesio et al. 1999). This 13-item version appears promising but has not been tested as widely as the original.

A detailed medication history should be taken, including any over-the-counter medications, vitamins, or herbal supplements. There is a trap to be avoided when reviewing medications of the patient with dizziness, because numerous medications are known to include dizziness as a potential side effect. One must always look carefully at the temporal relationship between the onset of dizziness and the initiation of any drug suspected of either causing or exacerbating the condition (Table 22–2). Stimulants, benzodiazepines, tricyclic antidepressants, tetracyclics, monoamine oxidase inhibitors, selective serotonin reuptake inhibitors, neuroleptics, anticonvulsants, selective serotonin agonists, and cholinesterase inhibitors are among the classes of drugs with multiple members reported to cause dizziness. There are also many medications that patients might be taking for conditions unrelated to brain injury that could cause dizziness.

Certain anticonvulsants, such as phenytoin, may cause nystagmus in the absence of any noxious symptoms. This is not so much an adverse reaction as a potential confounding factor for the physical examination.

Physical Examination

Observation of the patient begins before the formal parts of the physical examination. Grooming and attire may reflect how well an individual performs his or her morning routine of activities of daily living. Signs of recent minor injuries might indicate balance or coordination problems.

Ambulatory patients may be observed walking through a waiting area or within the examination room. One may note greater difficulty maneuvering through a busy environment than in a quiet area without distractions or hazards. Some patients with vestibular dysfunction after brain injury are very sensitive to visual or auditory distractions. (If a patient demonstrates much more

(E=emotional, F=functional, P=physical)
"Yes" 4 points, "Sometimes" 2 points, "No" 0 points.

P1.   Does looking up increase your problem?
E2.   Because of your problem do you feel frustrated?
F3.   Because of your problem do you restrict your travel for
        business or recreation?
P4.   Does walking down the aisle of a supermarket increase
        your problem?
F5.   Because of your problems do you have difficulty getting
        into or out of bed?
F6.   Does your problem significantly restrict your participation in
        social activities such as going out to dinner, movies,
        dancing, or parties?
F7.   Because of your problems do you have more difficulty
        reading?
P8.   Does performing more ambitious activities like sports,
        dancing, and household chores such as sweeping or
        putting away dishes increase your problem?
E9.   Because of your problem are you afraid to leave your home
        without having someone accompany you?
E10. Because of your problem have you been embarrassed in
        front of others?
P11. Do quick movements of your head increase your problem?
F12. Because of your problem do you avoid heights?
P13. Does turning over in bed increase your problem?
F14. Because of your problem is it difficult for you to do
        strenuous housework or yard work?
E15. Because of your problem are you afraid people may think
        you are intoxicated?
F16. Because of your problem is it difficult for you to go for a
        walk by yourself?
P17. Does walking down a sidewalk increase your problem?
E18. Because of your problem is it difficult for you to
        concentrate?
F19. Because of your problem is it difficult for you to walk
        around your house in the dark?
E20. Because of your problem are you afraid to stay home
        alone?
E21. Because of your problem do you feel handicapped?
E22. Has your problem placed stress on your relationships with
        members of your family or friends?
E23. Because of your problem are you depressed?
F24. Does your problem interfere with your job or household
        responsibilities?
P25. Does bending over increase your problem?

FIGURE 22–1.   Dizziness Handicap Inventory items.

Source.   Reprinted from Jacobson GP, Newman CW: "The Development of the Dizziness Handicap Inventory." *Archives of Otolaryngology—Head and Neck Surgery* 116:424–427, 1990. Used with permission.

difficulty with ambulation when formally asked to demonstrate walking than at other times, one may be concerned about an attempt at simulating pathology.)

Visual acuity screening is appropriate, but many visual impairments may be missed by use of an eye chart alone. A visual field cut, for example, might spare central vision, but loss of a peripheral visual field could create significant safety problems. Extraocular movements and pupillary responsiveness should be assessed. These evaluations may yield signs of cranial nerve injury. (Impaired eye movement may hinder efforts at teaching compensatory strategies. A therapist seek-

ing to teach a patient how to compensate for a field cut benefits from knowing how the eyes move during scanning.)

There are other components of the visual system examination that are of special interest when assessing patients with suspected vestibular disorders. *Nystagmus* describes involuntary rhythmic movements of the eye, with a rapid saccadic component followed by a slow return to the opposite direction. Spontaneous nystagmus is most often seen in acute settings. Gaze-induced nystagmus, noted during testing of smooth pursuit, is more common in subacute and chronic cases. A deviation of approxi-

---

---

mately 30 degrees is appropriate to test for this finding. At the extremes of eye movement, endpoint nystagmus may be seen in healthy individuals.

Other clinical visual tests include checking saccades (quick movements between targets), tracking a target while the head moves with it (vestibuloocular cancellation), and fixating on a target while the head is moved horizontally or vertically (vestibuloocular reflex; VOR). (Detailed reviews of vision tests and related issues are provided in Chapter 23, Vision Problems.) Clinicians who do not specialize in visual disorders may still incorporate brief screening in their own examination to guide a decision on referral to an appropriate eye specialist. Because many rehabilitation therapies present visual information to patients, visual impairments may impede progress.

Brief auditory screening can similarly be done in a bedside or office setting. Ability to hear a tuning fork vibrating at 512 Hz is one of the simplest parameters to test. Functional observation of how well a patient responds to auditory stimuli may also be useful. Audiometric testing is safe and painless but does require some basic ability to attend to a task and follow directions. Patients who are unlikely to do so may be referred instead for auditory evoked potentials. Auditory pathology may be present independent of vestibular pathology. Hearing problems may interfere with a patient's ability to process verbal instructions. There are data suggesting that impaired auditory sensory gating may produce attention and memory impairments (Arciniegas et al. 2000) after brain injury. One should look closely at auditory pathways in balance and dizziness evaluations given the close proximity of the systems.

Olfactory screening is rarely if ever performed by most clinicians (on the basis of personal observation after reviewing many hospital and office charts). The University of Pennsylvania Smell Identification Test (Doty et al. 1984) is a commercially available (Sensoronics, Haddon Heights, NJ) standardized test. Brain injury specialists are well aware of the risk of injury to olfactory nerves traversing the cribriform plate in frontal injuries. This can

cause hyposmia or anosmia. (A number of patients at our center have complained of somewhat disabling hyperacute olfactory function. There is no obvious mechanism by which brain injury would improve function of the nose, but these patients are easily distracted by odors in their environment.)

Somatosensory testing is undoubtedly critical when evaluating any patient with balance issues. Pinprick and light touch are most often documented in standard neurological examinations. Assessments of proprioception, kinesthesia, and vibration sense are also indicated in patients with balance issues.

Ataxia is not anticipated in patients with isolated vestibular deficits in the absence of cerebellar injury. (Both are common after TBI.) A patient with a remote history of head trauma is still at risk of developing a cerebellar or pontine tumor or stroke, multiple sclerosis, or other new disorder. Development of a new finding not explained by the known history would generate a legitimate need for further investigation.

Musculoskeletal factors should be evaluated carefully. Strength of postural muscles must be adequate for static and dynamic balance tasks before more subtle deficits can be addressed. Chronic problems such as leg-length discrepancies or skeletal deformities may no longer be compensated for adequately if balancing mechanisms sustain an injury. Patients who sustained musculoskeletal injuries in addition to brain injuries may have residual impairments limiting mobility. (Vestibular symptoms may not be noted if a patient is confined to a bed or wheelchair during acute care.)

Direct examination of balance can be performed in several ways. Severe deficits can be picked up on observation of poor sitting or standing balance or a markedly unsteady gait. Patients with mild to moderate brain injuries may look normal in this context or their deficits may only be evident when fatigued or otherwise stressed. (Variability that can be logically explained differs conceptually from "inconsistency," which raises concerns about efforts to simulate pathology.)

Romberg testing begins with a patient standing with feet apart and eyes open. The feet are placed directly together at the heels and toes. (Some patients need extensive prompting to do so and may "cheat" by moving the feet apart if not monitored.) If patients can maintain balance in this condition, then they are instructed to close their eyes. Ability to maintain balance and extent of sway are noted over at least 60 seconds if the patient is able to maintain for that long. The degree of difficulty can be increased by changing the positions of the feet. Standing with one foot directly in front of the other provides the sharpened Romberg position. Ability to stand on one leg is another test of standing balance, with a somewhat greater dependence on lower extremity motor power.

Office testing of static balance is usually performed on a conventional floor. Sensitivity can be increased by adding use of a foam mat. Lighting and background noise may also affect aspects of performance.

Dynamic testing attempts to simulate some of the challenges faced in the "real world," where the body's center of gravity moves during functional tasks. The Fukuda Stepping Test (Fukuda 1959) evaluates ability to march in place with eyes open and closed. Moving forward more than 50 cm or turning more than 30 degrees is abnormal.

Functional reach from a standing position is another readily measured dynamic assessment. It is easily measured with a measuring tape or ruler, correlates with center of pressure testing, and has some ability to predict falls (Duncan et al. 1992).

The Dynamic Gait Index is a low-tech quantitative measure using a shoe box, cones, and stairs (Shumway-Cook 1995). It consists of eight tasks related to gait. Patients can score up to 3 points on each task. Scores below 19 suggest an increased fall risk in elderly patients.

The Berg Balance Scale (Berg 1989; Thorbahn and Newton 1996) is a 14-item test of various balancing tasks. Up to 4 points are awarded on each task, for a maximum total of 56. Scores below 36 correlate with very significant fall risks in elderly patients. Although published studies have primarily looked at predicting falls in geriatric populations, it is reasonable to use this scale for evaluation of patients with TBIs.

For patients with TBI, it has been suggested that tests of balance should be combined with performance of cognitive tasks (Shumway-Cook 2000). This would reflect the reality that in normal life people do not concentrate on how they are maintaining their equilibrium while they move through their environment. A patient with marginal balance might be able to compensate when concentrating on a specific balancing task in a clinical setting. This does not necessarily mean that he or she could repeat the performance while multitasking in a community setting. One could observe performance while engaging a patient in conversation as a simple application of this concept. Therapists may take patients on community excursions such as a trip to a store.

Physical examinations should also include evaluation for medical disorders that might contribute to gait or balance disorders. Problems such as orthostatic hypotension should be addressed appropriately.

When evaluating older patients after brain injury, one may consider vascular pathology. Vertebrobasilar disease may mimic vestibular dysfunction. Screening for verte-

TABLE 22–3. Points to cover during physical examination after brain injury

Observation

Olfactory (optional)

Eyes: acuity, tracking, saccades, nystagmus

Ears: hearing screen (otoscopic examination and/or ear, nose, and throat referral if abnormal)

Sensation: sharp, light touch, proprioception, vibration

Motor: power, coordination

Balance: sitting, sit-to-stand transfer, standing (eyes open or closed, feet apart or together or in tandem stance, or on one leg)

Gait: walking, tandem walking, turning

brobasilar insufficiency carries potential pitfalls. Flow in the vertebral or basilar artery may be compromised by atherosclerotic disease or external masses, and when combined with the effects of certain neck positions, patients may experience dizziness or even syncope. Cervical rotation and extension performed in supine position may elicit symptoms of benign positional vertigo. Testing in a seated position avoids this potential confounding factor (Clendaniel 2000). Table 22–3 highlights points to cover during a physical examination.

Laboratory Tests

The diagnostic workup after head trauma routinely includes imaging by at least computed tomography scanning, and often may include magnetic resonance imaging (MRI). In patients with dizziness and balance problems, one might consider the value of MRI in evaluating the posterior fossa (Halmagyi and Cremer 2000). This helps exclude subtle infarctions, tumors, and demyelinating disorders. (One might therefore pursue such testing when the correlation between onset of dizziness and TBI is not clear.) Negative studies do not exclude either central or peripheral forms of vestibular dysfunction. Patients who cannot undergo MRI might benefit from computed tomography scanning, with particular attention to the posterior fossa.

Electronystagmography (ENG) is an electrodiagnostic test of eye movements. It relies on differences of potential between the cornea and the retina, which allow surface electrodes to detect eye rotation. Data can be recorded graphically and electronically. ENG is notably less sensitive than direct inspection by an examiner and is not able to quantify vertical movements because of the confounding effects of blinking (Honrubia 2000). Despite those limitations, ENG does allow reliable objective measurement of horizontal rotation. It can be combined with various provocative maneuvers to record physiological data.

One can elicit the VOR with caloric stimulation. Caloric testing requires irrigating the external auditory canals with water at 7°C higher or lower than body temperature. The patient is positioned supine with the head tilted back 60 degrees from the upright position. The resulting temperature gradients in the horizontal canals create currents within the endolymphatic fluid, triggering deformation of hair cells. With warm water, there is a slow deviation away from the site of irrigation followed by nystagmus toward that side. (The response is named by convention on the basis of the direction of the nystagmus.) Cold water elicits the opposite response. (Thus, the mnemonic *COWS* refers to the principle of *c*old *o*pposite, *w*arm *s*ame in this situation.)

There are limitations to this test. Anatomical variations may alter the process of heat transfer. Fixation allows some individuals to suppress nystagmus to varying degrees. Quantitative analysis can be performed with use of ENG. One can compare the maximum slow component velocity of nystagmus between left ear and right ear stimulation responses or measure the ability to suppress with fixation. There are many procedural variables to consider (Honrubia 2000). The test does have some ability to localize lesions. Unilateral response would indicate contralateral peripheral dysfunction. Bilateral normal responses would not rule out some central pathology.

Rotatory (Barany) chair testing can be performed in a simple manner by rapidly rotating a chair, with the backrest tilted back 60 degrees. One can then observe the duration of resulting nystagmus or record the severity of subjective complaints. More sophisticated testing uses ENG and automated programs of rotation (Honrubia 2000).

Quantitative balance testing can be performed in several ways. Force platforms can record the perturbations of the center of gravity in varying conditions. Removing visual input or providing visual inputs that contrast with actual conditions can pose added challenges.

One might seek information about how postural muscles respond to environmental challenges. Dynamic posturography can include electromyographic measurement of lower extremity muscle responses on a moving platform. Patients may rely on varying strategies to maintain balance, including use of motions about the ankle or hip. Muscles stabilizing the ankle respond to perturbations of smaller amplitude or velocity. Hip muscles are recruited in more severe challenges. The most severe perturbations require moving the feet (Pai and Patton 1997). Patients who lose their balance during testing before initiating typical strategies may be given exercises to address deficits in involved muscles or may be trained to recruit these muscles sooner with biofeedback.

Attention has been paid to indicators of psychogenic balance disorders (Goebel et al. 1997). Worse performances on easier conditions, unusually large variability within trials of the same test, and a regular frequency of sway all raise concerns. Krempl and Dobie (1998) reported that dynamic posturography was effective in distinguishing between malingering and best-effort performance in healthy subjects. Table 22–4 provides a summary of laboratory testing.

TABLE 22–4. **Laboratory test summary**

Test	Purpose	Indication
Magnetic resonance imaging/ computed tomography	Shows anatomy	To localize visible lesions; may lead to surgery
ENG	Records eye motion	To record/localize signs of oculomotor pathology; may guide therapy or document change on retesting
Caloric stimulation	Tests VOR	To provoke involuntary response, measurable with ENG (see above), not dependent on effort
Rotatory chair	Tests VOR	To provoke involuntary response, measurable with ENG (see above), not dependent on effort
Posturography: force plates	Tests balance	To record signs of balance pathology or potential simulation; may guide therapy or allow documentation of change on retesting
Posturography: surface electromyography	Tests balance	To add information on motor strategies to platform tests (see above)

Note. ENG=electronystagmography; VOR=vestibuloocular reflex.

Peripheral Vestibular Dysfunction

Benign Positional Paroxysmal Vertigo

The most commonly attributed cause of vertigo after TBI is benign positional paroxysmal vertigo (BPPV). It is also the most common cause of vertigo seen in outpatient populations in general. Vertigo and dysequilibrium are elicited by common motions or positions. The proposed etiology is a disturbance of semicircular canal function caused by debris from the otolithic organs. Provocative maneuvers can be used to elicit vertigo and nystagmus. The Hallpike-Dix (also referenced as Dix-Hallpike) maneuver (Dix and Hallpike 1952) involves rotating the head 45 degrees and quickly lying down with the head hanging 30 degrees below horizontal. Within 30 seconds, this maneuver will elicit nystagmus if the affected side is inferior.

Single-treatment interventions for BPPV have been developed on the basis of the underlying problem of debris that was displaced from otolithic organs into the canals (Epley 1992; Herdman et al. 1993). Simply put, these interventions all involve maneuvering the head to facilitate flow of the debris out of the canals. Habituation regimens teach patients to repeatedly position themselves several times a day in provoking positions (Brandt and Daroff 1980).

Developers of all of these techniques have reported high success rates. Although most reports lacked control groups, it does appear that the rapid remission of symptoms can often be attributed to the intervention. (A much-delayed response might reflect a spontaneous recovery.) One problem is that patients must tolerate the transient induction of symptoms that these procedures require. They must also comply with instructions regarding positioning over a 2- to 5-day period. Use of a cervical collar may be indicated during this period.

Patients who sustained TBIs may have cervical pathology. Cervicalgia in the absence of demonstrated orthopedic or neurological cervical pathology would not formally contraindicate these maneuvers, but patient response might be problematic.

Perilymphatic Fistula

Trauma to the round or oval windows may lead to a perilymphatic fistula, with communication between the middle and inner ears. A popping sensation may be noted at the time of onset. Symptoms include vertigo, tinnitus, and hearing loss. Valsalva maneuvers may exacerbate the symptoms.

Diagnosing this condition may be difficult because usually no single test is definitive. Application of pressure over the tympanic membrane may induce vertigo (Hen-nebert's sign) or nystagmus. Concurrent use of computerized balance platform testing allows quantitative measurement of increased sway during this maneuver. (This form of posturography uses force plates under the feet to detect displacement of the center of gravity.) Audiometric testing may show significant hearing loss, especially at higher frequencies. ENG may show dysfunction in the affected ear.

Bed rest with the head elevated may be of some help. Avoidance of constipation or other causes of straining is advisable. Persistent symptoms may be managed surgically, with exploration and repair of defects of the windows. Differing opinions about the success rate of surgical interventions have been offered (Fetter 2000; Fitzgerald 1995). It is reasonable to suppose that a number of patients with chronic dizziness have undiagnosed perilymphatic fistulas, but identifying this subset of patients can be difficult.

Ménière's Disease

Classically, Ménière's disease is regarded as an idiopathic disorder that typically begins in middle age. It begins with potentially severe bouts of vertigo accompanied by a sense of fullness in the affected ear, episodic hearing reduction, and tinnitus. The hearing loss does not always remit after each episode.

A syndrome such as Ménière's can be seen after head trauma (Healy 1982). Bleeding into the membranous labyrinth or altered bony anatomy after temporal fracture are two possible mechanisms.

The disorder is associated with endolymphatic hydrops (excessive accumulation of fluid). This is usually attributed to malabsorption of endolymph. Restriction of sodium, caffeine, nicotine, and alcohol intake has been recommended traditionally, whereas diuretics and fluid restrictions are also sometimes added. There is a lack of strong data to support these interventions. The relapsing and remitting nature of the disorder would make further investigation difficult.

The effectiveness of endolymphatic sac surgery is controversial, but such procedures are not expected to harm any existing function of the vestibular and auditory systems. Labyrinthectomy and vestibular nerve resections are both effective at stopping vertigo (Mattox 2000), but the latter is preferred if preserving hearing is a goal.

Central Vestibular Dysfunction

Although the reflex circuits from the vestibular sensory organs to oculomotor, cervical, and postural muscles are

TABLE 22–5. Medications for dizziness and vertigo

Medication	Dosage (typical ranges)	Precautions (common)	Reactions (partial list)
Meclizine (Antivert)	12.5–25.0 mg, bid–tid	Bladder obstruction, asthma, glaucoma	Sedation, confusion, dry mouth (common), ototoxicity, tachycardia hallucinations (serious)
Prochlorperazine (Compazine)	5–10 mg, tid–qid	Bladder obstruction, asthma, glaucoma, bone marrow depression, epilepsy, many others	Sedation, confusion, dry mouth (common), hematologic, hepatic, neuroleptic malignant syndrome (serious)
Promethazine (Phenergan)	12.5–25.0 mg, qid	Bladder obstruction, asthma, glaucoma, epilepsy, liver dysfunction	Sedation, confusion, dry mouth, tachycardia (common) hematologic, respiratory depression, bradycardia (serious)
Scopolamine (Transderm Scop)	1.5-mg patch, apply 4 hours before travel, lasts 72 hours	Bladder or intestinal obstruction, asthma, glaucoma, epilepsy, liver or kidney dysfunction	Sedation, confusion, dry mouth, respiratory depression, bronchospasm

the best-identified pathways, it is clear that data must also flow to other areas within the central nervous system. By convention, pathology involving this network is referred to as *central vestibular dysfunction* even if the sensory end organs are intact. The central vestibular system may be defined as the vestibular nuclei and their connections to other parts of the brain and spinal cord. A subset of brain-injured patients presents with complaints of dizziness and imbalance related to central dysfunction. It is to some extent a diagnosis of exclusion because imaging of the vestibular apparatus or testing of the reflex arcs (e.g., caloric stimulation) can help to uncover peripheral lesions. Patients who fit a profile of vestibular dysfunction after brain injury but who do not have evidence of a peripheral lesion or other etiologies are included in the central category.

An important role for the cerebellum in the vestibular system has been accepted. The cerebellar flocculus, in particular, seems to play a critical role in VOR adaptations. There is reason to believe that some forms of learning and adaptation take place in areas of the cerebellum and the brainstem (du Lac et al. 1995). Trauma affecting the cerebellum may therefore affect subjective sensations of dizziness or objective signs of balance problems even if gross ataxia is not present.

Brandt and Dieterich (1994, 1995) have made extensive reviews of central vestibular syndromes. Sites from the brainstem to the thalamus to sensory cortex have been implicated (including an area of the parietoinsular cortex in monkeys). Reviews of cases of individuals with well-circumscribed lesions are, of course, critical to the current understanding of brain pathology. Functional MRI studies are adding new dimensions to that knowledge. Opto-

kinetic stimulation has been noted to activate vestibular cortex on functional MRI (Dietrich et al. 1998).

Pharmacological Management

Medications for dizziness and vertigo may be referred to as *vestibular sedatives* (Table 22–5). They tend to have generally sedating properties. Their exact mode of action for dizziness reduction is not known. Meclizine, which has antihistaminic and anticholinergic properties, is a common choice. Promethazine and prochlorperazine also have properties of phenothiazines. Transdermal scopolamine is another anticholinergic option.

There are general precautions about use of vestibular sedatives in patients with asthma, glaucoma, or prostatic hypertrophy. More specifically, there is little basis for prolonged use of these medications for chronic dizziness (Zee 1985). They may be quite helpful for acute motion sickness or other acute disorders but have not been shown effective in chronic deficits after brain injury. Vestibular sedatives might actually slow the process of adaptation after injury. Sedating effects may negatively affect arousal. The potential for drug interactions in patients taking other medications should also be considered. Polypharmacy also poses additional problems for cognitively impaired patients who have difficulty keeping track of medications.

Benzodiazepines and other sedating drugs are sometimes prescribed for patients with dizziness. These may address associated anxiety but are not known to be of direct benefit. Prolonged use in patients with brain injury should be approached with great caution.

Vestibular Rehabilitation

Techniques of therapy have been developed for patients with various vestibular disorders. These have been used in brain-injury populations, although it is widely understood that patients with multiple areas of dysfunction face special challenges.

Vertiginous symptoms are addressed with habituation exercises (Brandt and Daroff 1980). Repetition of movements that provoke vertigo eventually reduces symptoms. Behavioral or cognitive problems are known to increase the difficulty in applying this approach to brain-injured patients (Shumway-Cook 2000).

Gaze stabilization exercises are used to improve the efficiency of vestibuloocular coordination. These exercises are initially performed with the head still and later are performed during movement.

Balance retraining may stress challenging vestibular function by minimizing availability of other sensory inputs. For patients who cannot progress with this approach, efforts at optimizing their use of visual or proprioceptive strategies for balance may be proposed.

To whatever extent normal function cannot be restored, adaptive techniques can be taught. Patients may need to modify how they perform routines for dressing and grooming. A shower bench may be needed if they cannot balance safely with eyes shut. These interventions may require collaboration between physical and occupational therapists. If patients or family members resist such recommendations, then psychologists or social workers on the rehabilitation team will need to understand the underlying rationale to intervene effectively.

Our center uses a separate team of physical therapists for vestibular therapy. Given the known emotional challenges of vestibular disorders, a pathway has been established to facilitate referral of patients without brain injury to psychologists with expertise in treating this population. For patients with brain injury, particularly mild TBI, we have found that an interdisciplinary team can provide a closer level of coordination and communication. Occupational therapists, speech pathologists, and neuropsychologists may need to modify their approaches to accommodate patients with limited tolerance of visual or auditory stimuli. Social workers and vocational counselors should understand these issues as they advise families or employers.

It is important for clinicians and patients to understand that aspects of a vestibular therapy program may make the patient feel worse acutely. The potential for facilitating habituation should be explained. As patients practice fixing gaze on a target while turning the head as quickly as possible or walking through a hallway while turning to look at targets on the walls, dizziness may be elicited. With further practice, however, the central vestibular system may adapt and no longer perceive discomfort. As patients practice maintaining balance on soft foam pads or moving platforms, their bodies may become more efficient at maintaining their center of gravity in a stable position.

Extra emotional support might be needed in the early stages of a program. As time passes, reviewing measurable clinical progress is a reasonable strategy to counteract discouragement over any persistent symptoms. One can review clinical measures such as the rate at which patients can turn their heads from side to side while keeping their eyes fixed on a target. The length of time that balance is maintained during Romberg testing is another easily measured parameter. Functional performance in daily life can also be reviewed, such as the length of time spent out of bed or distance ambulated daily.

Once progress is made, the reinforcement of compliance with home exercises may be necessary. If a plateau is reached after a prolonged course of therapy, counseling should focus on the need to move on with life rather than hope for a dramatic improvement with more of the same treatment.

Emotional Factors

Dizziness and nausea are noxious stimuli. Impaired balance carries a risk of injury that is readily understood by most patients. These problems can therefore have an adverse emotional effect on patients. There is also concern that expressions of vestibular symptoms might reflect a primary psychiatric disorder or pursuit of secondary gain.

Patients with dizziness have a significant risk of psychiatric dysfunction. Rates as high as 50% have been cited for either panic disorder or depression in patients with vestibular hypofunction (Eagger et al. 1992). (The subset of dizzy patients who present after head trauma was not studied separately.) Anxiety and dizziness overlap more than would be predicted by chance and carry a worse prognosis for resolution of dizziness and greater degree of reported handicap, but this does not mean that vestibular symptoms should be readily dismissed as not having a physiological basis. Jacob and Furman (2001) proposed a linkage via overlapping circuits, including the parabrachial nucleus network. A better understanding of the neurophysiology underlying anxiety and dizziness may reduce the temptation to dismiss "psychogenic dizziness" as strictly an emotional disorder.

Clinicians who do not have a mental health background, conversely, should be aware of the potential emotional effect of dizziness and impaired balance. Awareness of comorbidities can at least lower the threshold for appropriate consultations and referrals.

Patients may be asked to undertake various challenging forms of therapy, and one should remember that vestibular symptoms might escalate during rehabilitation activities. If this process also leads to more overt mood disturbances, it can be difficult to distinguish the basis for decreased compliance with various types of exercises. This need not be limited to the physical therapy regimen alone because activities in occupational or speech therapy or cognitive remediation may tax a patient's vestibular system capacity.

Beliefs should also be considered. Handicap levels at a 6-month follow-up were predicted by baseline beliefs about negative consequences of dizziness (Yardley et al. 2001). Negative beliefs were reduced in patients who underwent vestibular therapy.

Interactions with significant others may be problematic. As with many other effects of brain injury, the subjective symptoms of dizziness are not visible. Patients may limit their activities out of fear, or they might be advised by therapists to avoid certain exacerbating conditions. If the situation is not properly explained to their families or other caregivers, it may engender feelings of resentment. Kay (1992) has offered compelling explanations of how psychological overlay accumulates with time, causing increasing dysfunction. Patients who sense that their symptoms are not accepted may be inadvertently encouraged to exaggerate their problems.

Outcomes

Patients with vestibular dysfunction after TBI have been shown to recover more slowly and to a lesser degree than other populations (Pfaltz and Kamath 1983). There is certainly potential for injury to peripheral and central components of the vestibular system. Even when the peripheral system is intact (within the current ability to test it), central pathology is difficult to treat. One cannot achieve quick success with maneuvers for BPPV if a significant central deficit is present.

Coordinating interventions for these patients is often difficult. Medications that temporarily alleviate vestibular symptoms often have problematic risk–benefit ratios for long-term use. Rehabilitation techniques may exacerbate symptoms, after which team members may draw different conclusions about how to proceed. Mixed messages may

be sent. One physician may be encouraging a patient to increase use of sedating medication, while another advises avoiding use of the same medication. A vestibular therapist may advise some patients to limit their exposure to visual and auditory stimulation, while occupational and therapeutic recreation therapists may be offering treatments that are highly stimulating. A vision therapist may recommend limits on reading that conflict with a cognitive remediation treatment plan.

In the absence of rigorous evidence-based pathways, there may be differences in practice patterns. Interdisciplinary communication between professionals would at least allow discussion of potential areas of conflict. The patient might not have to choose between contradictory instructions if such conflicts could be resolved by the clinicians.

References

Arciniegas D, Oliney A, Topkoff J, et al: Impaired auditory gating and P50 non-suppression following traumatic brain injury. J Neuropsychiatry Clin Neurosci 12:77–85, 2000

Berg K: Balance and its measure in the elderly: a review. Physiother Can 41:304–311, 1989

Brandt T, Daroff RB: Physical therapy for benign positional vertigo. Arch Otolaryngol 106:484–485, 1980

Brandt T, Dieterich M: Vestibular syndromes in the roll plane: topographic diagnosis from brainstem to cortex. Ann Neurol 36:337–347, 1994

Brandt T, Dieterich M: Central vestibular syndromes in the roll, pitch, and yaw planes: topographic diagnosis of brainstem disorders. Neuro-ophthalmology 15:291–303, 1995

Clendaniel R: Cervical vertigo, in Vestibular Rehabilitation. Edited by Herdman S. Philadelphia, PA, FA Davis, 2000, pp 494–495

Dieterich M, Bucher SF, Seelos KC, et al: Horizontal or vertical optokinetic stimulation activates visual motion-sensitive, ocular motor, and vestibular cortex areas with right hemispheric dominance: an fMRI study. Brain 121:1479–1495, 1998

Dix MR, Hallpike CS: Pathology, symptomatology and diagnosis of certain disorders of the vestibular system. Proc R Soc Med 45:341–347, 1952

Doty RL, Shaman P, Kimmelman CP, et al: University of Pennsylvania Smell Identification Test: a rapid quantitative olfactory function test for the clinic. Laryngoscope 94:176–178, 1984

du Lac S, Raymond JL, Sejnowski TJ, et al: Learning and memory in the vestibulo-ocular reflex. Annu Rev Neurosci 18:409–441, 1995

Duncan PW, Studenski S, Chandler J, et al: Functional reach: predictive validity in a sample of elderly male veterans. J Gerontol 47:M93–M98, 1992

Eagger S, Luxon LM, Davies RA, et al: Psychiatric morbidity in patients with peripheral vestibular disorders: a clinical and neuro-otological study. J Neurol Neurosurg Psychiatry 55:383–387, 1992

Epley JM: The canalith repositioning procedure: for treatment of benign paroxysmal positional vertigo. Otolaryngol Head Neck Surg 107:399–404, 1992

Fetter M: Vestibular system disorders, in Vestibular Rehabilitation, 2nd Edition. Edited by Herdman SJ. Philadelphia, PA, FA Davis, 2000, pp 97–98

Fitzgerald DC: Persistent dizziness following head trauma and perilymphatic fistula. Arch Phys Med Rehabil 76:1017–1020, 1995

Fukuda T: The stepping test: two phases of the labyrinthine reflex. Acta Otolaryngol 50:95, 1959

Gibson W: Vertigo associated with trauma, in Vertigo. Edited by Dix R, Hood JD. New York, Wiley, 1984

Goebel JA, Sartaloff RT, Hanson JM, et al: Posturographic evidence of nonorganic sway patterns in normal subjects, patients and suspected malingerers. Otolaryngol Head Neck Surg 117:293–302, 1997

Griffiths MV: The incidence of auditory and vestibular concussion following minor head injury. J Laryngol Otol 93:253–265, 1979

Hain TC, Hillman MA: Physiology of the vestibular system, in Vestibular Rehabilitation. Edited by Herdman S. Philadelphia, PA, FA Davis, 2000, pp 3–24

Halmagyi DM, Cremer PD: Assessment and treatment of dizziness. J Neurol Neurosurg Psychiatry 68:129–134, 2000

Healy GB: Hearing loss and vertigo secondary to head injury. N Engl J Med 306:1029–1031, 1982

Herdman SJ: Treatment of vestibular disorders in traumatically brain-injured patients. J Head Trauma Rehabil 5:63, 1990

Herdman SJ, Tusa RJ, Zee DS, et al: Single treatment approaches to benign paroxysmal positional vertigo. Arch Otolaryngol Head Neck Surg 119:450–454, 1993

Honrubia V: Quantitative vestibular function tests and the clinical examination, in Vestibular Rehabilitation, 2nd Edition. Edited by Herdman SJ. Philadelphia, PA, FA Davis, 2000, pp 105–171

Jacob RG, Furman JM: Psychiatric consequences of vestibular dysfunction. Curr Opin Neurol 14:41–46, 2001

Jacobson GP, Newman CW: The development of the Dizziness Handicap Inventory. Arch Otolaryngol Head Neck Surg 116:424–427, 1990

Kay T: Neuropsychological diagnosis: disentangling the multiple determinants of functional disability after mild traumatic brain injury, in Rehabilitation of Post-Concussive Disorders: Physical Medicine and Rehabilitation: State of the Art Reviews. Edited by Horn L, Zasler N. Philadelphia, PA, Hanley & Belfus, 1992, pp 109–127

Krempl GA, Dobie RA: Evaluation of posturography in the detection of malingering subjects. Am J Otol 19:619–627, 1998

Mattox DE: Surgical management of vestibular disorders, in Vestibular Rehabilitation, 2nd Edition. Edited by Herdman SJ. Philadelphia, PA, FA Davis, 2000, pp 256–259

Pai YC, Patton J: Center of mass velocity-position predictions for balance control. J Biomech 30:347–354, 1997

Pfaltz CR, Kamath R: Central compensation of vestibular dysfunction. Adv Otorhinolaryngol 30:355–363, 1983

Robertson D, Ireland D: Dizziness Handicap Inventory correlates of computerized dynamic posturography. J Otolaryngol 24:118–124, 1995

Shumway-Cook A: Motor Control. Baltimore, MD, Williams & Wilkins, 1995, pp 323–324

Shumway-Cook A: Traumatic brain injury, in Vestibular Rehabilitation. Edited by Herdman S. Philadelphia, PA, FA Davis, 2000, pp 476–493

Shumway-Cook A: Motor Control Theory and Practical Applications. Baltimore, MD, Lippincott Williams & Wilkins, 2001, pp 74–77

Tesio L, Alpinia D, Cesarini A, et al: Short form of the Dizziness Handicap Inventory: construction and validation through Rasch analysis. Am J Phys Med Rehabil 78:233–241, 1999

Thorbahn LD, Newton RA: Use of the Berg Balance Test to predict falls in the elderly. Phys Ther 76:576–583, 1996

Toglia JU: Acute flexion extension injury of the neck. Neurology 26:808–814, 1976

Tuohima P: Vestibular disturbances after acute mild head injury. Acta Otolaryngol Suppl (Stockholm) 359:7–67, 1978

Yardley L, Bech S, Weinman J: Influence of beliefs about the consequences of dizziness on handicap in people with dizziness, and the effect of therapy on beliefs. J Psychosom Res 50:1–6, 2001

23 Vision Problems

Neera Kapoor, O.D., M.S.

Kenneth J. Ciuffreda, O.D., Ph.D.

VISION IS ONE of the primary sensory modalities involved in tasks such as stance, gait, reading, and other basic activities of daily living (ADLs). Furthermore, adequate vision is a requisite for evaluation and treatment performed during most types of rehabilitation, such as optometric, ophthalmological, neuropsychological, physical, vestibular, occupational, and speech and language therapies. Nonetheless, diagnosis and management of functional vision deficits have been frequently overlooked in textbooks and teaching curricula used by many rehabilitation professionals (Wainapel 1995). The recent increasing interest in functional vision and its integrative effect on rehabilitation in patients with traumatic brain injury (TBI) (Altner et al. 1980; Fisher 1987; Tinette et al. 1995; Wainapel et al. 1989) serves as the impetus for this chapter.

In this chapter, we discuss the prevalence and pathophysiology of vision problems and provide an overview of functional vision anomalies in patients with TBI. A glossary of ophthalmic terms used in the following text is found in the appendix at the end of the chapter.

Prevalence of Vision Problems in TBI

Vision problems have been reported in TBI patients with varying prevalence, depending on the source used and diagnostic criteria adopted (Al-Qurainy 1995; Baker and Epstein 1991; Gianutsos et al. 1988; Hellerstein et al. 1995; Lepore 1995; Sabates et al. 1991; Schlageter et al. 1993; Suchoff and Gianutsos 2000; Suchoff et al. 1999, 2000; Suter 1995; Zost 1995) (Table 23–1). The most common problems adversely affecting visual function directly are versional and vergence oculomotor anomalies, accommodative dysfunctions, dry eye, cataracts, and visual field defects. Other vision problems affecting function more indirectly include orbital fractures, lid anomalies, blepharitis, blepharoconjunctivitis, pupillary anomalies, optic nerve anomalies, and retinal defects (Suchoff et al. 1999).

Pathophysiology

The pathophysiology for all vision deficits in TBI has not been reported in the literature in detail, but it is more evident for some deficits than for others. Oculomotor deficits (Table 23–2) resulting in diplopia, loss of place while reading, nystagmus, and oscillopsia may occur because of sheared or severed cranial nerves (CNs) (i.e., CN III, CN IV, CN VI), mechanical restriction of an extraocular muscle, or damage at the level of the neuromuscular junction (Baker and Epstein 1991). Accommodative deficits resulting in blurred vision may occur as a result of damage to the oculomotor nerve (i.e., CN III), more central neurological anomalies, or a side effect of medications (Ciuffreda 1991; Cooper 1998; Suchoff et al. 2000).

With respect to ocular pathology, dry eye resulting in intermittent blurred vision and a gritty sensation is quite common in the TBI population. It is typically an ocular side effect of antidepressants, antihypertensives, and oral contraceptives (Bartlett and Jaanus 1995; Jaanus and Bartlett 1984). Blepharitis and blepharoconjunctivitis are also frequently found and typically occur because of poor lid hygiene (Catania 1988). Pupillary anomalies may result from damage along the pupillary pathway in association with a CN III palsy, asymmetrical optic nerve disease or anomaly, the presence of a space-occupying lesion, or disrupted autonomic innervation. Visual field defects such as noncongruous hemianopias and quadrantanopias may oc-

TABLE 23–1. Percentage of visual and ocular conditions in acquired brain-injured (ABI) sample with comparative values for a random adult population

Ocular/visual condition	Occurrence in an ABI sample (%)	Occurrence in a random adult population (%)	Occurrence in an ABI/random adult occurrence
Exophoric deviations	41.9	2.1	19.9
Esophoric deviations	1.6	1.3	1.3
Vertical deviations	9.7	1.6	6.1
Oculomotor dysfunctions	39.7	NA	NA
Accommodative dysfunctions	9.6	NA	NA
External eye pathologies: dry eye/blepharitis/keratitis/pterygium/corneal degeneration	22.6	11.2	2.0
Lid defects: ptosis/dermatochalasis/blepharochalasis	4.8	2.1	2.3
Aphakia/pseudophakia/cataracts	24.1	12.3	2.0
Optic nerve cupping/optic atrophy/glaucoma suspect/glaucoma	19.4	8	2.4
Color vision defect	0	8.3 (male); 0.5 (female)	0
Contrast sensitivity defect	0	NA	NA
Posterior pole anomalies: retinopathies (including diabetic retinopathy, hypertensive retinopathy, and maculopathy)	9.7	1.5	6.5
Retinal defects/detachments	1.6	0.1	20.0
Peripheral retinal degenerations/vitreoretinal degenerations	9.7	2.6	3.7
Blindness/enucleation	6.5	1.6	4.1
Pupillary anomaly	1.6	1	1.6
Visual field defects	32.5	NA	NA

Note. NA=normative data for a random adult population not available.
Source. Adapted from Suchoff IB, Kapoor N, Waxman R, et al: "The Occurrence of Ocular and Visual Dysfunctions in an Acquired Brain-Injured Patient Sample." *Journal of the American Optometric Association* 70:301–309, 1999. Used with permission.

cur with TBI depending on the nature and severity of the injury, but they are more typically associated with stroke. Clinical experience has demonstrated that TBI patients present with scattered visual field defects and no evidence of hemifield lateralization, as described in the section Visual Field Deficits. The etiology of this scattered visual field defect remains poorly understood.

There are other ocular sequelae that may occur with blunt trauma to the periorbital region but are not common in TBI. These sequelae are orbital fracture, lid anomaly, corneal abrasion, lens dislocation, angle recession, traumatic glaucoma, traumatic cataract, traumatic uveitis, and retinal or vitreal detachment (Vogel 1992). The pathophysiology of these conditions is not addressed further because it is beyond the scope and aim of this chapter.

However, in the TBI population, there is an increased frequency of some of the above conditions when compared with the non-brain-injured population (Suchoff et al. 1999; Vogel 1992), which may result in reduced visual acuity, reduced contrast sensitivity, and/or visual field defects. Orbital fractures and lid anomalies secondary to blunt and severe head trauma require immediate medical intervention because of the concern of additional inflammation or infection (e.g., orbital cellulitis). Inflammation, infection, shearing, or compression may occur at any point along the optic radiations in the primary visual pathway between the occipital cortex and retina as a result of trauma. Retinal defects and tears occur often with severe blunt trauma. Retinal vascular insufficiencies, which are often associated with hypertension and diabetes, are also possible sequelae. Such

TABLE 23–2.   Visual deficits after traumatic brain injury

Deficit	Possible underlying mechanism	Clinical manifestation
Blurred vision	Ocular injury to cornea, lens, and/or retina	Constant or intermittent blurred vision in one or both eyes
	Damage to the optic nerve or anywhere along the primary visual pathway	Fatigue or eyestrain with sustained visual tasks
	CN III damage	
	Midbrain injury	
	Refractive error	
	Amblyopia	
Binocular vision anomalies	Diminished oculomotor control (i.e., paresis or palsy of CN III, CN IV, or CN VI)	Constant or intermittent diplopia in some or all positions of gaze
	Midbrain injury affecting medial longitudinal fasciculus and/or the oculomotor nuclei	Reduced accuracy of depth perception
		Difficulty localizing objects in space
		Confusion with sustained visual activities
Nystagmus	Brainstem damage	Abnormal ocular oscillations resulting in oscillopsia, nausea, blurred vision, and visual confusion
	Cerebellar damage	
Deficits of pursuit	Lesion in either hemisphere with or without brainstem damage	Difficulty tracking in any plane
Deficits of saccades	Lesion in frontal eye field (area 8) or parietal area	Difficulty in rapid localization of objects in space
		Difficulty with reading

Note.   CN=cranial nerve.
Source.   Reprinted from Hellerstein LF: "Visual Problems Associated With Brain Injury," in *Understanding and Managing Vision Deficits: A Guide for Occupational Therapists.* Edited by Scheiman M. Thorofare, NJ, Slack, 1997, pp 233–247. Used with permission.

vascular compromise may occur at the level of the ophthalmic artery or at the level of the carotid arterial supply from which the ophthalmic artery arises. Additionally, there is an increased frequency of cataracts and glaucoma, but the pathophysiology remains unclear.

Vision Care Professionals

As with any health condition, appropriate diagnosis is required for the effective treatment and management of vision deficits. Diagnosis of vision problems in the TBI population is made appropriately through two professions involved in vision care: ophthalmology and optometry.

Ophthalmology is a medical specialty with several relevant subspecialties that relate to the treatment of individuals with TBI, such as neuro-ophthalmology, plastics, reconstructive, retina, strabismus, and low vision, to name a few. If vision anomalies are evident during the acute stage of TBI, the neuro-ophthalmologist is recruited for the patient's management. There are occasions on which retinal and plastics ophthalmologists may be called depending on the nature and severity of the physical insult to the globe and the associated periorbital region. However, ophthalmology does not maintain a dominant, long-term role in the rehabilitation of the TBI patient.

In contrast, *optometry* is a profession specializing in nonsurgical, noninvasive, and often rehabilitative primary eye care. Additionally, optometry's scope of practice has expanded significantly over the past 20 years to include the use of diagnostic and therapeutic pharmaceutical agents.

Optometry's rich history of treating patients by incorporating components of vision therapy, low vision, ophthalmic optics, refraction, and visual perception provides the basis for its ability to address functional vision problems in the TBI population. In addition, this background provides the basis for optometry's long-term involvement as a contributing and productive member of the TBI interdisciplinary rehabilitation team.

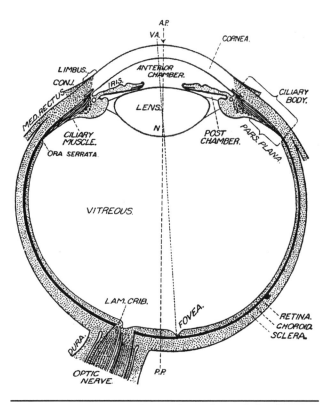

FIGURE 23–1. **Horizontal section of the human eye.**

PP = posterior pole; AP = anterior pole; VA = visual axis; CONJ = conjunctiva; MED = medial; N = nodal point; LAM CRIB = lamina cribrosa.

Source. Reprinted from Last RJ: *Wolff's Anatomy of the Eye and Orbit.* Philadelphia, PA, WB Saunders, 1968, pp 39–181. Used with permission of the publisher.

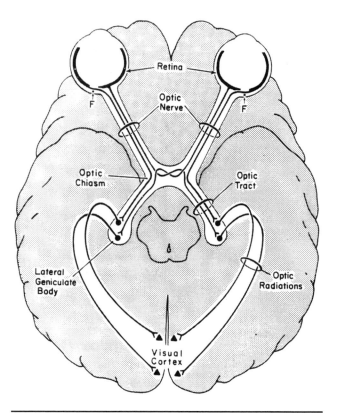

FIGURE 23–2. **Schematic representation of primary neural visual pathways.**

F = fovea.

Source. Reprinted from Trobe JD, Glaser JS: *The Visual Fields Manual: A Practical Guide to the Testing and Interpretation.* Gainesville, FL, Triad Publishing, 1983, pp 29–62. Used with permission of the publisher.

Ocular Anatomy and the Visual Pathways

The globe of the human eye, from anterior to posterior, consists of the following major structural anatomical components: cornea, conjunctiva, sclera, iris, aqueous humor, anterior and posterior chamber, crystalline lens, vitreous, retina, choroid, and sclera (Last 1968; Trobe and Glaser 1983) (Figure 23–1).

Primary Visual Pathway

The primary visual pathway commences at the level of the retina, where axons of the two types of ganglion cells (i.e., the *magnocellular* or *transient cells,* and the *parvocellular* or *sustained cells*) exit the retina as the *optic nerve* via the optic nerve head (Martin 1989; Solan 1994). The axons of the optic nerve proceed to the *optic chiasm,* where there is a *partial decussation* of the nerve fibers from each eye. This partial decussation ensures that visual information from the right and left sides of the visual field is separated and sub-

sequently corresponds to the left and right sides of this pathway, respectively.

From the optic chiasm, the fibers proceed via the *optic tract* to the *lateral geniculate body,* where the visual input is combined with nonvisual neural inputs (Martin 1989; Solan 1994). Some of these fibers then proceed to the following areas: 1) the primary visual cortex, or the *occipital cortex,* via the *optic radiations,* to perform the early stages of visual information processing; 2) the *tectum* to participate in pupillary function; or 3) the *superior colliculus,* to participate in eye movement and related multisensory integrative behaviors. The routes of these fibers constitute the *primary visual pathway* (Martin 1989; Solan 1994) (Figure 23–2).

Secondary Visual Pathway

There is a second level of visual information processing that begins at the *extrastriate portion of the visual cortex* and is referred to as the *secondary visual pathway* (Kaas 1989; Martin 1989; Solan 1994). From the extrastriate visual cortex, the parvocellular cells communicate with the *inferior temporal* area, which has been shown to be associated with visual identification and recognition of objects, or the "what" aspect of visual perception. However, the magnocellular cells proceed to the middle temporal area and eventually to the posterior parietal cortex, which is associated with motion and spatial vision, or the "where" aspect of visual perception (Kaas 1989; Martin 1989; Robertson and Halligan 1999; Solan 1994; Stein 1989).

Some cortical areas that are common to many of these oculomotor subsystems include the cerebellum, midbrain, frontal eye fields, superior colliculus, parietal cortex, and visual cortex. Therefore, damage to one or more of these areas might affect a range of ocular motility functions (Baker and Epstein 1991; Ciuffreda et al. 1991; Leigh and Zee 1991; Sabates et al. 1991; Suchoff et al. 2000) (Table 23–3).

TABLE 23–3. Clinical categories of traumatic brain injury

General category	Specific areas of vision difficulty
Soft-tissue injuries	Extraocular muscle avulsion
	Hemorrhage and edema
Orbital fractures	Floor
	Medial wall
	Lateral wall
	Roof
Cranial neuropathies	Oculomotor nerve
	Trochlear nerve
	Abducens nerve
	Sphenocavernous syndrome
	Orbital apex syndrome
Intraaxial brainstem damage	Internuclear ophthalmoplegia
	Horizontal gaze paresis
	Vertical gaze paresis
	Parinaud's syndrome
	Skew deviation
	Abnormalities of accommodation, convergence, and fusion
	Cerebellar lesions
	Vestibular system dysfunctions
Cerebral lesions	Saccade
	Pursuit

Source. Adapted from Baker RS, Epstein AD: "Ocular Motor Abnormalities from Head Trauma." *Survey of Ophthalmology* 35:245–267, 1991. Used with permission.

Standard Protocol for the Vision Examination

The initial stage of the vision examination of the TBI patient involves an extensive case history, as outlined below. Subsequent to the case history, the vision examination includes an assessment of the following major areas: refractive, sensorimotor, and ocular health status, including special testing as appropriate. Below is an overview of the testing involved for each of the four elements of the vision examination (Eskridge et al. 1991).

1. *Case history*, including specific queries regarding reading ability, eyestrain or fatigue, blurred vision, diplopia, visual field loss, light sensitivity, dizziness, loss of balance, vertigo, and motion sensitivity.
2. *Refractive assessment*, including visual acuity, keratometry, retinoscopy, and subjective refraction to determine the appropriate refractive correction at far and at near (i.e., emmetropia, myopia, hyperopia, astigmatism, and presbyopia).
3. *Sensorimotor assessment*, including the assessment of versional ocular motility, vergence ocular motility, stereopsis, and accommodation.
4. *Ocular health assessment and special testing*, including confrontation visual field, color vision, pupils, anterior segment evaluation, applanation tonometry, posterior segment evaluation, and automated perimetry. Special testing includes visual evoked potentials, contrast sensitivity testing, application of tinted lenses, and application of yoked prisms.

Functional Vision Anomalies After TBI

Functional vision anomalies may negatively affect the ability of the TBI patient to perform basic ADLs such as reading, writing, walking, shopping, driving, and navigating through crowded environments, to name a few (Hellerstein 1997; Suchoff and Gianutsos 2000; Suchoff et al. 2000; Suter 1995). Even simpler tasks such as reviewing mail, washing dishes, doing laundry, and dusting can be troublesome to the TBI patient with impaired functional vision. Several common functional vision anomalies, as well as their associated signs and symptoms, are described in the following sections (Al-Qurainy 1995; Ciuffreda et al. 2001a; Gianutsos et al. 1988; Hellerstein et al. 1995; Suchoff and Gianutsos 2000; Suchoff et al. 2000; Suter 1995).

Convergence Insufficiency

Convergence insufficiency (CI) is a binocular vision vergence anomaly in which the eyes cannot rotate inward and maintain single vision at close distances (Borish 1970; Griffin and Grisham 1995; Press 1997; Schieman and Wick 1994). This condition is quite common in TBI patients, varying in occurrence from approximately 41% to 65% (Ciuffreda et al. 2001a; Cohen et al. 1989; Gianutsos et al. 1988; Hellerstein et al. 1995; Suchoff and Gianutsos 2000; Suchoff et al. 1999, 2000; Suter 1995). Vision-related symptoms associated with nearwork include eyestrain (ocular "fatigue"), intermittent closing of one eye, diplopia, abnormal sensitivity to visual motion, and the perception that printed text is "floating above the page" or "shimmering." Patients with CI may also position themselves relatively far from or not be able to maintain eye contact with people during conversation to avoid diplopia. If the magnitude of the CI is sufficient to produce frequent diplopia at near, fusional prisms may be prescribed. CI is amenable to oculomotor rehabilitation (i.e., optometric vision therapy; Ciuffreda 2002) designed to increase the extent, stability, and sustainability of the vergence response (Freed and Hellerstein 1997; Han et al., in press; Kapoor and Ciuffreda 2002; Kapoor et al., in press; Kerkhoff and Stogerer 1994; Morton 1995).

Vertical Oculomotor Deviations

Vertical oculomotor deviations, including heterophorias and heterotropias, are more complex to manage because of the variability in magnitude of the deviation as a function of gaze position and time of day. In addition to the complaints outlined in the section above for CI, patients with vertical deviations may also report impaired binocular depth perception and headaches. The aim of oculomotor rehabilitation is to train sensory and motor fusion (i.e., single binocular vision) initially in primary gaze and then increase the field of fusion (Borish 1970; Caloroso and Rouse 1993; Griffin and Grisham 1995; Press 1997; Schieman and Wick 1994). Surgical intervention is also an option, depending on the status of the patient's overall health. If oculomotor rehabilitation is unsuccessful, and surgery is not an option, then occlusion of one eye as needed to eliminate diplopia may be recommended. Although neurological or mechanical restriction of the extraocular muscles does limit the benefit of oculomotor rehabilitation for increasing the range of horizontal and vertical fusion, it still should be attempted to improve vision function and overall visual efficiency (Caloroso and Rouse 1993; Han et al., in press; Kapoor and Ciuffreda 2002; Kapoor et al., in press; Suchoff et al. 2000; Suter 1995).

Versional Oculomotor Deficits

Versional oculomotor deficits, including those of pursuit, saccades, and fixation, affect the ability to track objects smoothly, track objects as they move rapidly from point A to point B, and maintain steady visual fixation on a target, respectively (Ciuffreda and Tannen 1995). Individuals with versional oculomotor deficits primarily complain of reading difficulties: reading slowly, loss of place while reading, misreading or rereading words and paragraphs, text that appears to "swim" and "shimmer," and, occasionally, apparent visual motion perhaps related to vergence misalignment and/or frank oscillopsia. Some of these symptoms may also be related to vestibular deficits (see the section Visual-Vestibular Disturbances). Oculomotor rehabilitation is also beneficial for versional deficits (Ciuffreda et al. 1996, 2001a; Freed and Hellerstein 1997; Griffin and Grisham 1995; Han et al., in press; Kapoor and Ciuffreda 2002; Kapoor et al., in press; Press 1997; Ron 1981, 1982; Schieman and Wick 1994).

Refractive Changes

Refractive changes may sometimes be the cause of blurred vision in the TBI population. Reduced best-corrected visual acuity may arise because of damage along the primary visual pathway anywhere from the optic nerve head to the occipital cortex via the optic radiations (Sabates et al. 1991; Suchoff et al. 2000). Because there is a visual basis for many of the evaluative and treatment strategies involving TBI rehabilitation, optimizing and stabilizing visual acuity by initially assessing the refractive status are of utmost importance.

For example, there are cases in the TBI population in which prepresbyopic patients may require a near-vision correction. Relatively small amounts of hyperopia in younger individuals without TBI can easily be typically overcome by their accommodative mechanism. However, if a 20-year-old hyperopic patient who did not previously wear a near-vision correction experiences damage to CN III as a result of a brain injury, this patient might experience blurred near vision and require a reading correction because of the newly developed accommodative dysfunction secondary to the brain injury.

Prescribing spectacles for TBI is important in terms of functional vision for prepresbyopic, nonemmetropic patients with accommodative deficits, as well as for presbyopic patients, because they require different spectacle corrections for distance and near vision. Despite optical and cosmetic advances, the progressive, or "invisible," bifocal lens is not appropriate for the TBI population because of its residual optical distortions as well as the requirement for precise and coordinated eye, head, and neck movement on the part of the patient (Han et al. 2003). These peripheral optical distortions also produce dizziness, nausea, and illusory motion in many TBI patients during ambulation and therefore adversely affect daily function. Often, the range of head and neck movement is limited in TBI patients because of the injuries incurred at the time of their initial trauma. For these reasons, *all* multifocal lenses are contraindicated for ambulation in the TBI population, especially in those with vestibular deficits and sensitivity to visual motion. To optimize vision function by allowing minimal head and neck movement and, hence, minimal adverse effects, one should prescribe separate distance and near single-vision spectacles.

Accommodative Dysfunctions

Accommodative dysfunctions in the prepresbyopic TBI population may impair a patient's ability to sustain near vision for prolonged time periods without ocular fatigue, thereby decreasing overall visual efficiency and reading ability. The most common accommodative dysfunction in the TBI population is accommodative insufficiency, for which the primary diagnostic criterion is reduced amplitude of accommodation. Symptoms of general accommodative dysfunctions include intermittent blurred vision, inability to sustain prolonged near vision, tearing, and occasionally headaches (Al-Qurainy 1995; Baker and Epstein 1991; Gianutsos et al. 1988; Hellerstein 1997; Hellerstein et al. 1995; Suchoff et al. 2000). Prescribing separate reading spectacles with or without concurrent oculomotor rehabilitation may benefit the patient by enhancing the amplitude, facility, and sustainability of accommodation (Borish 1970; Griffin and Grisham 1995; Press 1997; Schieman and Wick 1994).

Visual Field Defects

Visual field defects, such as homonymous hemianopias with or without visual inattention, are more common among the stroke population but do occur in the TBI population as well (Gianutsos and Suchoff 1997; Gianutsos et al. 1988; Hellerstein 1997; Hellerstein et al. 1995; Kapoor et al. 2001b; Suchoff and Ciuffreda 2004; Suchoff and Gianutsos 2000; Suchoff et al. 1999, 2000). Patients with hemianopia complain of either of the following: 1) "being told" that part of their visual field is missing, if they have visual inattention; or 2) being aware that part of their visual field is missing, if they do

not have visual inattention. They may have difficulty reading (e.g., finding the beginning of the next line of print because of a left hemianopia) or manifest slow and laborious reading as they saccade cautiously in small steps from left to right into their blind field (because of a right hemianopia) (Ciuffreda 1994). Hemianopic patients may also complain that they bump into objects on one side, miss food on one side of the plate, have trouble dressing one side of their body, and have problems navigating streets and buildings (Gianutsos et al. 1988; Halligan and Marshall 1993; Hellerstein 1997; Hellerstein et al. 1995; Gianutsos and Suchoff 1997; Robertson and Halligan 1999; Suchoff and Ciuffreda 2004; Suchoff and Gianutsos 2000; Suchoff et al. 2000). Hemianopia significantly and irreversibly alters numerous basic functional aspects of patients' lives. It often limits their independence through the restriction or even prevention of common tasks, such as driving and unaccompanied ambulation.

In some hemianopic patients, laterally displacing (i.e., yoked) prism spectacles, half-Fresnel prisms, and mirrors can be useful (Suchoff and Ciuffreda 2004; Suchoff and Gianutsos 2000; Suchoff et al. 2000). These optical devices are designed to increase the patient's awareness of the affected field. Scanning techniques, either alone or in conjunction with a field-enhancing optical device (Chedru et al. 1973; Diller and Weinberg 1977; Gur and Ron 1992; Kerkhoff et al. 1992; Ron 1981; Ron 1982; Webster et al. 1984), may also benefit the patient (Kapoor et al. 2001a, 2001b).

Another type of visual field defect that we typically find in the TBI population is a scattered visual field pattern (Figure 23–3). Patients presenting with this type of field loss do not report functional vision limitations. Such field defects should be monitored twice yearly for any variation over time. Optical devices have not been helpful in these cases.

Photosensitivity

Photosensitivity, even in the absence of ocular inflammation and pain, produces significant discomfort. In the literature, this increased light sensitivity is often referred to as *photophobia*, which really refers to elevated light sensitivity in conjunction with frank ocular pain because of contraction and relaxation of inflamed ocular tissue (Stedman's Medical Dictionary 1990). It is our opinion that, because TBI patients experience varying degrees of increased light sensitivity in the absence of any such ocular pain, this phenomenon should be referred to as *photosensitivity* rather than *photophobia*. The discomfort associated with photosensitivity can be alleviated considerably

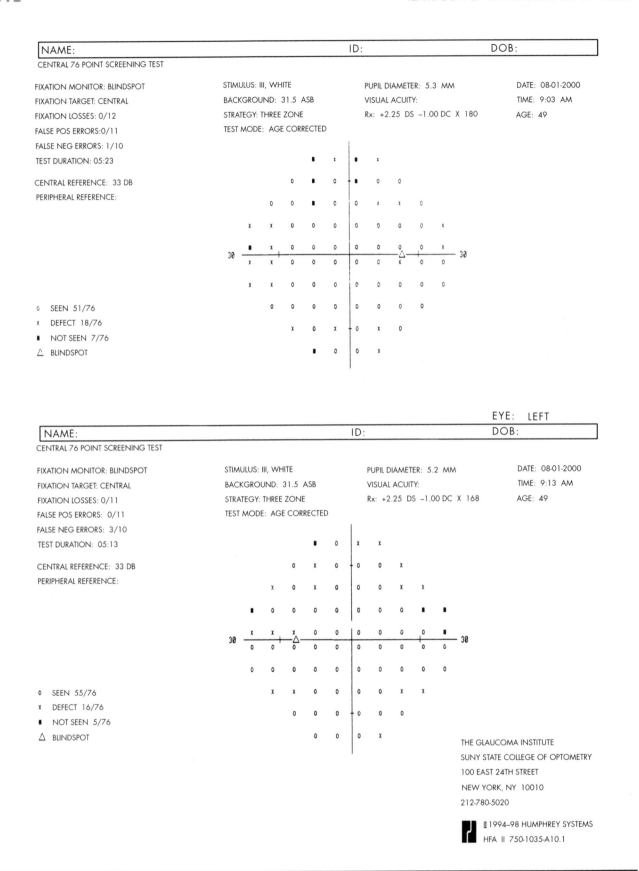

FIGURE 23–3. Typical scattered visual field defect pattern after traumatic brain injury.

with the application of specific tinted lenses (Jackowski 2001; Jackowski et al. 1996, 1998). Typically, a lighter tint is used indoors, and a darker tint is used outdoors.

Visual-Vestibular Disturbances

Visual-vestibular disturbances result in complaints of dizziness, loss of balance, vertigo, nausea, motion sensitivity, oscillopsia, and, frequently, photosensitivity. Patients with visual-vestibular disturbances report difficulty shopping in department stores with high shelving because of the sensation of visual motion in their periphery (Ciuffreda 1999), being in visually crowded environments such as busy restaurants, watching movies or television because of the rapid movement from scene to scene, reading because of the sensation of "shimmering" and "floating," and using the computer monitor because of screen flickering.

Patients with vestibularly based complaints are referred typically to neurology, neuro-otolaryngology, and, finally, vestibular rehabilitation, an area in which vision becomes especially important (Malamut 2001). One particular subset of vestibular exercises directly incorporates the vestibuloocular reflex (VOR) and is referred to as *gaze stability training* (Baloh and Honrubia 1990). To develop a functional VOR, stable fusion is required, especially under dynamic conditions. The dynamic VOR must rapidly adapt with changes in target distance involving complex vestibular-vergence interactions (Leigh and Zee 1991). Despite the fact that the patient and target are stationary during standard clinical binocular vision testing, unstable fusion in association with symptoms of nausea and dizziness during the actual binocular vision clinical testing is often evident in patients with vestibular dysfunction.

Oculomotor rehabilitation, with the incorporation of fusional prisms for diplopia and tinted lenses for photosensitivity, is designed to improve and stabilize fusional vergence under static and dynamic viewing conditions. Additionally, as stated in the section Refractive Changes, it is important to prescribe single-vision spectacles for patients requiring different corrections for far and near viewing for presbyopia and accommodative deficits. Oculomotor rehabilitation and spectacle correction have been shown to markedly enhance one's ability to perform gaze stabilizing techniques and other aspects of vestibular rehabilitation and to function in terms of basic ADLs (Malamut 2001).

Conclusion

The primary sensory input for most aspects of rehabilitation in the TBI patient is vision (Wainapel 1995). There-fore, increased awareness of the visual system's anatomy, physiology, neurology, clinical evaluative procedures, and key related anomalies is important for the physician who treats individuals with TBI (Ciuffreda et al. 2001b). Heightened awareness and recognition of these vision anomalies on the part of the physician lead to improvement in the patient's ability to function in terms of overall rehabilitation as well as in basic activities of daily living.

References

Al-Qurainy IA: Convergence insufficiency and failure of accommodation following midfacial trauma. Br J Oral Maxillofac Surg 33:71–75, 1995

Altner PE, Rusin JJ, DeBoer A: Rehabilitation of blind patients with lower extremity amputations. Arch Phys Med Rehabil 61:82–85, 1980

Baker RS, Epstein AD: Ocular motor abnormalities from head trauma. Surv Ophthalmol 35:245–267, 1991

Baloh RW, Honrubia V: Clinical Neurophysiology of the Vestibular System, 2nd Edition. Philadelphia, PA, FA Davis, 1990

Bartlett JD, Jaanus SD: Clinical Ocular Pharmacology, 3rd Edition. Boston, MA, Butterworth-Heinemann, 1995, pp 127–617

Borish IM: Clinical Refraction, 3rd Edition. New York, Professional Press, 1970, pp 189–256

Caloroso EE, Rouse MW: Clinical Management of Strabismus. Boston, MA, Butterworth-Heinemann, 1993

Catania LJ: Primary Care of the Anterior Segment. East Norwalk, CT, Appleton and Lange, 1988, pp 24–30

Chedru F, Leblanc M, Lhermitte F: Visual searching in normal and brain-damaged subjects (contribution to the study of unilateral inattention). Cortex 9:94–111, 1973

Ciuffreda KJ: Accommodation and its anomalies, in Vision and Visual Dysfunction, Vol. 1. Edited by Charman WN. London, Macmillan, 1991, pp 231–279

Ciuffreda KJ: Reading eye movements in patients with oculomotor disturbances, in Eye Movements in Reading. Edited by Ygge J, Lennerstrand G. New York, Pergamon, 1994, pp 163–188

Ciuffreda KJ: Visual vertigo syndrome: a clinical demonstration and diagnostic tool. Clin Eye Vis Care 11:41–42, 1999

Ciuffreda KJ: The efficacy of and scientific basis for optometric vision therapy in non-strabismic accommodative and vergence disorders. Optometry 73:735–762, 2002

Ciuffreda KJ, Tannen B: Eye movement basics for the clinician. St. Louis, MO, Mosby, 1995, pp 1–9

Ciuffreda KJ, Levi DM, Selenow A: Amblyopia: Basic and Clinical Aspects. Boston, MA, Butterworth-Heinemann, 1991, pp 165–241

Ciuffreda KJ, Suchoff IB, Marrone MA, et al: Oculomotor rehabilitation in traumatic brain-injured patients. J Behav Optom 7:31–38, 1996

Ciuffreda KJ, Ciuffreda YH, Kapoor N, et al: Oculomotor consequences of acquired brain injury, in Visual and Vestibular Consequences of Acquired Brain Injuries. Edited by Suchoff IB, Ciuffreda KJ, Kapoor N. Santa Ana, CA, Optometric Extension Program Foundation, 2001a, pp 77–88

Ciuffreda KJ, Suchoff IB, Kapoor N, et al: Normal vision function, in Downey and Darling's Physiological Basis of Rehabilitation Medicine, 3rd Edition. Edited by Gonzalez EG, Myers SJ, Edelstein JE, et al. Boston, MA, Butterworth-Heinemann, 2001b, pp 241–261

Cohen M, Groswasser Z, Barchadski R, et al: Convergence insufficiency in brain injured patients. Brain Inj 3:187–191, 1989

Cooper J: Accommodative dysfunction, in Diagnosis and Management in Vision Care. Edited by Amos J. Boston, Butterworth, MA, 1998, pp 431–459

Diller L, Weinberg J: Hemi-inattention and rehabilitation: the evolution of a rational treatment program, in Advances in Neurology, Vol. 18. Edited by Weinstein EA, Freidland RP. New York, Raven, 1977, pp 63–82

Eskridge JB, Amos J, Bartlett JD (eds): Clinical Procedures in Optometry. Philadelphia, PA, Lippincott, 1991

Fisher R: Rehabilitation of the blind amputee: a rewarding experience. Arch Phys Med Rehabil 68:382–383, 1987

Freed S, Hellerstein LF: Visual electrodiagnostic findings in mild traumatic brain injury. Brain Inj 11:25–36, 1997

Gianutsos R, Suchoff IB: Visual fields after brain injury: management issues for the occupational therapist, in Understanding and Managing Vision Deficits: A Guide for Occupational Therapists. Edited by Scheiman M. Thorofare, NJ, Slack, 1997, pp 333–358

Gianutsos R, Ramsey G, Perlin R: Rehabilitative optometric services for survivors of acquired brain injury. Arch Phys Med Rehabil 69:573–578, 1988

Griffin JR, Grisham JD: Binocular Anomalies: Diagnosis and Vision Therapy, 3rd Edition. Boston, MA, Butterworth-Heinemann, 1995

Gur S, Ron S: Training in oculomotor tracking: occupational health aspects. Israel J Med Sci 28:622–628, 1992

Halligan PW, Marshall JC: The history and clinical presentation of neglect, in Unilateral Neglect: Clinical and Experimental Studies. Edited by Robertson IH, Marshall JC. Hillsdale, NJ, Erlbaum, 1993, pp 3–19

Han Y, Ciuffreda KJ, Selenow A, et al: Dynamic interactions of eye and head movements during return-sweep saccades when reading with single vision and progressive lenses in a simulated computer-based environment. Invest Ophthal Vis Sci 44:1534–1545, 2003

Han Y, Ciuffreda KJ, Kapoor N: Reading-related oculomotor testing and training protocols for acquired brain injury. Brain Res Protocols (in press)

Hellerstein LF: Visual problems associated with brain injury, in Understanding and Managing Vision Deficits: A Guide for Occupational Therapists. Edited by Scheiman M. Thorofare, NJ, Slack, 1997, pp 233–247

Hellerstein LF, Freed S, Maples WC: Vision profile of patients with mild brain injury. J Am Optom Assoc 66:634–639, 1995

Jaanus SD, Bartlett JD: Adverse ocular effects of systemic drug therapy, in Clinical Ocular Pharmacology. Edited by Bartlett JD, Jaanus SD. Boston, MA, Butterworth, 1984, pp 917–939

Jackowski MM: Altered visual adaptation in patients with traumatic brain injury: photophobia, abnormal dark adaptation, and reduced peripheral visual field sensitivity, in Visual and Vestibular Consequences of Acquired Brain Injuries. Edited by Suchoff IB, Ciuffreda KJ, Kapoor N. Santa Ana, CA, Optometric Extension Program Foundation, 2001

Jackowski MM, Sturr JF, Taub HA, et al: Photophobia in patients with traumatic brain injury: uses of light-filtering lenses to enhance contrast sensitivity and reading rate. Neurorehabilitation 6:193–201, 1996

Jackowski MM, Sturr JF, Turk MA, et al: Altered dark adaptation in patients with traumatic brain injury. Invest Ophthalmol Vis Sci 39(suppl):401, 1998

Kaas JH: Changing concepts of visual cortex organization, in Neuropsychology of Visual Perception. Edited by Brown JW. Hillsdale, NJ, Erlbaum, 1989, pp 3–38

Kapoor N, Ciuffreda KJ: Vision disturbances following traumatic brain injury. Curr Treat Options Neurol 4:271–280, 2002

Kapoor N, Ciuffreda KJ, Harris G, et al: A new portable clinical device for measuring egocentric localization. J Behav Optom 12:115–118, 2001a

Kapoor N, Ciuffreda KJ, Suchoff IB: Egocentric localization in patients with visual neglect, in Visual and Vestibular Consequences of Acquired Brain Injuries. Edited by Suchoff IB, Ciuffreda KJ, Kapoor N. Santa Ana, CA, Optometric Extension Program Foundation, 2001b, pp 131–144

Kapoor N, Ciuffreda KJ, Han Y: Oculomotor rehabilitation in acquired brain injury: two case reports. Arch Phys Med Rehabil (in press)

Kerkhoff G, Stogerer E: Recovery of fusional convergence after systemic practice. Brain Inj 8:15–22, 1994

Kerkhoff G, MunBinger U, Haaf E, et al: Rehabilitation of homonymous scotomata in patients with postgeniculate damage of the visual system: saccadic compensation training. Restor Neurol Neurosci 4:245–254, 1992

Last RJ: Wolff's Anatomy of the Eye and Orbit. Philadelphia, PA, WB Saunders, 1968, pp 39–181

Leigh RJ, Zee DS: The Neurology of Eye Movements, 2nd Edition. Philadelphia, PA, FA Davis, 1991

Lepore FE: Disorders of ocular motility following head trauma. Arch Neurol 52:924–926, 1995

Malamut D: Vestibular therapy and ocular dysfunction in traumatic brain injury: a case study, in Visual and Vestibular Consequences of Acquired Brain Injuries. Edited by Suchoff IB, Ciuffreda KJ, Kapoor N. Santa Ana CA, Optometric Extension Program Foundation, 2001

Martin JH: The visual system, in Neuroanatomy: Text and Atlas. New York, Elsevier, 1989, pp 135–163

Morton RL: Visual dysfunctions following traumatic brain injury, in Traumatic Brain Injury Rehabilitation. Edited by Ashley MJ, Krych DK. Boca Raton, FL, CRC Press, 1995, pp 171–186

Press LJ: Accommodative and vergence therapy, in Applied Concepts in Vision Therapy. Edited by Press LJ. St. Louis, MO, Mosby, 1997, pp 222–245

Robertson IH, Halligan PW: Spatial Neglect: A Clinical Handbook for Diagnosis and Treatment. Hove, East Sussex, UK, Psychology Press, 1999

Ron S: Plastic changes in eye movements in patients with traumatic brain injury, in Progress in Oculomotor Research. Edited by Fuchs AF, Becker W. New York, Elsevier North-Holland, 1981, pp 237–251

Ron S: Can training be transferred from one oculomotor system to another?, in Physiological and Pathological Aspects of Eye Movements. Edited by Roucoux A, Crommelinck M. London, W. Junk, 1982, pp 83–88

Sabates NR, Gonce MA, Farris BK: Neuro-ophthalmological findings in closed head trauma. J Clin Neuroophthalmol 11:273–277, 1991

Schieman M, Wick B: Clinical Management of Binocular Vision: Heterophoric, Accommodative, and Eye Movement Disorders. Philadelphia, PA, JB Lippincott, 1994

Schlageter K, Gray K, Shaw R, et al: Incidence and treatment of visual dysfunction in traumatic brain injury. Brain Inj 7:439–448, 1993

Solan HA: Transient and sustained processing: dual subsystem theory of reading disability. J Behav Optom 5:149–154, 1994

Stedman's Medical Dictionary, 25th Edition. Baltimore, MD, Williams & Wilkins, 1990

Stein JF: Representation of egocentric space in the posterior parietal cortex. J Exper Physiol 74:583–606, 1989

Suchoff IB, Gianutsos R: Rehabilitative optometric interventions for the acquired brain injured adult, in Physical Medicine and Rehabilitation: The Complete Approach. Edited by Grabois M, Garrison SJ, Hart KA, et al. New York, Blackwell Scientific, 2000, pp 608–620

Suchoff IB, Ciuffreda KJ: A primer for the optometric management of unilateral spatial inattention. Optometry 75:305–318, 2004

Suchoff IB, Kapoor N, Waxman R, et al: The occurrence of ocular and visual dysfunctions in an acquired brain-injured patient sample. J Am Optom Assoc 70:301–309, 1999

Suchoff IB, Gianutsos R, Ciuffreda K, et al: Visual impairment related to acquired brain injury, in The Lighthouse Handbook on Vision Impairment. Edited by Silverstone B, Lang MA, Rosenthal B, et al. New York, Oxford University Press, 2000, pp 517–539

Suter PS: Rehabilitation and management of visual dysfunction following traumatic brain injury, in Traumatic Brain Injury Rehabilitation. Edited by Ashley MJ, Krych DK. Boca Raton, FL, CRC Press, 1995, pp 198–220

Tinette M, Inouye S, Gill T, et al: Shared risk factors for falls, incontinence, and functional dependence. JAMA 273:1348–1353, 1995

Trobe JD, Glaser JS: The Visual Fields Manual: A Practical Guide to Testing and Interpretation. Gainesville, FL, Triad Publishing, 1983, pp 29–62

Vogel MS: An overview of head trauma for the primary care practitioner, part II: ocular damage associated with head trauma. J Am Optom Assoc 8:542–546, 1992

Wainapel SF: Vision rehabilitation: an overlooked subject in physiatric training and practice. Am J Phys Med Rehabil 74:313–314, 1995

Wainapel SF, Kwon YS, Fazzari PJ: Severe visual impairment on a rehabilitation unit: incidence and implications. Arch Phys Med Rehabil 70:439–441, 1989

Webster JS, Jones S, Blanton P, et al: Visual scanning training with stroke patients. Behav Ther 15:129–143, 1984

Zost MG: Diagnosis and management of visual dysfunction in cerebral injury, in Diagnosis and Management of Special Populations. Edited by Maino DM. New York, Mosby, 1995, pp 75–134

Appendix 23–1

Glossary of Ophthalmic Terms

accommodation: the crystalline lens-based mechanism used to obtain and maintain a clear retinal image of an object of interest.

accommodative amplitude: the closest point of clear vision.

accommodative facility: the ability to change focus rapidly.

ametropia: uncorrected blurred distance vision.

astigmatism: uncorrected blurred distance vision in selected meridians.

diopter: the unit of lens power.

esophoria: inward turning of one eye when binocular vision is prevented.

exophoria: outward turning of one eye when binocular vision is prevented.

fusion: single vision under binocular viewing conditions.

heterophoria: the turning of one eye relative to the other when binocular vision is prevented.

hyperopia: far-sightedness.

myopia: near-sightedness.

near point of convergence: the closest point of binocular, single vision.

orthophoria: absence of the turning of one eye when binocular vision is prevented.

oscillopsia: the apparent sensation of movement of stationary targets.

prism diopter: the unit of prism power.

relative accommodative range: lens-mediated change in focus without a concurrent change in vergence.

relative fusional range: prism-mediated change in vergence without a concurrent change in focus.

strabismus (heterotropia): the turning of one eye relative to the other under binocular viewing conditions.

vergence: the coordinated inward/outward or upward/downward movement of the eyes when tracking objects moving in depth.

version: the coordinated movement of the eyes (laterally, vertically, or obliquely) when tracking objects at a fixed distance.

24 Chronic Pain

Nathan D. Zasler, M.D.

Michael F. Martelli, Ph.D.

Keith Nicholson, Ph.D.

A Brief Overview of Pain

Pain is defined by the International Association for the Study of Pain (Merskey and Bogduk 1994) as "an unpleasant sensory and emotional experience associated with actual or potential tissue damage, or described in terms of such damage." Acute pain, usually occurring in response to identifiable tissue damage or a noxious event, has a time-limited course during which treatment is aimed at correcting the underlying pathological process (if any such intervention is deemed necessary). Chronic pain (generally considered as pain persisting for longer than 6 months) may or may not be associated with any obvious tissue damage or pathological process. In the latter case, presentation may be characterized by maladaptive protective responses or pain behaviors, protracted courses of medication use and minimally effective medical services, and marked behavioral or emotional changes, including restrictions in daily activities. Pain-related avoidance behaviors and reduced activity are likely to result in a cyclic disability-enhancing pattern. The longer pain persists, the more recalcitrant it becomes and the more treatment goals focus on improved coping with pain and its concomitants (Kulich and Baker 1999; Martelli et al. 1999a). Finally, there is increasing evidence and growing acceptance that persistent pain may be associated with peripheral sensitization or central sensitization effects in which hyperresponsiveness or spontaneous discharge of components of the pain system develops (Lidbeck 2002; Nicholson 2000c, 2000d). In this regard, it has been noted that there is an association between posttraumatic stress reactions and the development of chronic pain (Bryant et al. 1999; Miller 2000; Sharp and Harvey 2001), with uncontrollable pain after physical injury potentially representing the core trauma, resulting in posttraumatic symptomatology (Schreiber and Galai-Gat 1993).

It is widely held that pain should be considered as a multidimensional, subjective experience mediated by emotion, attitudes, and other perceptual influences. Variability in pain responses is the rule rather than the exception and appears to reflect complex biopsychosocial interactions between genetic, developmental, cultural, environmental, and psychological factors (Hinnant 1994; Turk and Holzman 1986). Important distinctions between pain and suffering (Fordyce 1988) or impairment and disability (World Health Organization 1980) reflect the variability in response to pain problems. Although some pain patients appear to present with unusual and possibly exaggerated suffering or disability, others present with a "belle indifference" in which extremely high reported pain severity may produce no apparent affective distress, pain behavior, or interference in many life activities. In some cases, the onset, maintenance, severity, or exacerbation of pain is primarily associated with psychological factors and may warrant a DSM-IV-TR (American Psychiatric Association 2000) diagnosis of pain disorder associated with psychological factors. However, it is cautioned that one should avoid the pitfalls of mind–body dualism and always consider both psychological and organic factors in the presentation of any chronic pain patient (Nicholson et al. 2002).

Finally, it should be recognized that complexities in pain presentation warrant referral to pain management specialists or specialty interdisciplinary pain programs, or both. Referral is particularly warranted in cases of intractable pain and/or functionally disabling pain, regardless of whether the pain is considered chronic.

Neuroanatomy of Pain

The neuroanatomical pathways associated with pain perception are complex and not completely understood. Readers are referred to more in-depth sources for further detail (Bromm and Desmedt 1995; Vogt et al. 1993; Willis and Westlund 1997). Primary afferents are composed of A delta fibers and C fibers. A delta fibers are small, thin, myelinated neurons 1–5 μm in diameter with conduction velocities in the range of 5–30 m per second. Pain mediated by A delta fibers tends to be fast, sharp, localized, and well defined. These fibers have small receptive fields and tend to be modality specific. They are divided into thermoresponsive and mechanoresponsive subgroups. C fibers are small, unmyelinated afferent fibers with diameters of 0.25–1.5 μm and conduction velocities from 0.5 to 2.0 m per second. Pain mediated by C fibers tends to be slow, diffuse, poorly localized and of a burning, throbbing, or gnawing nature. These polymodal fibers subserve noxious nociceptive input from thermal, mechanical, and chemical stimuli, as well as non-noxious, low-intensity stimulation. Input to the primary afferents is provided through nociceptors that are the first step in the sensory pathway of transduction of a painful stimuli to a relevant neural signal. Nociceptors occur in cutaneous, muscular, and visceral structures.

Pain centers involve widely distributed neural networks. The distinction between the lateral and medial pain systems (Vogt et al. 1993) is considered to be of paramount importance. The former may mediate primarily the sensory-discriminative components of pain, whereas the latter may mediate primarily emotional-motivational components. However, these systems are heavily interconnected, reflecting the unitary experience of pain. There has also been the suggestion that the lateral and medial pain systems are mainly responsible for processing acute and chronic pain, respectively (Albe-Fessard et al. 1985). The lateral pain system involves inputs to the thalamus and somatosensory cortex from the lateral spinothalamic tract. The medial pain system involves projections of the medial thalamic nuclei to area 24 of the anterior cingulate cortex and other forebrain areas. The anterior cingulate cortex is an extensive area of the limbic cortex overlying the corpus callosum and is involved in the integration of cognition, affect, and response selection. The descending connections of the anterior cingulate cortex to the medial thalamic nuclei and to the peri-aqueductal gray in the brainstem suggest that this system may also be involved in the modulation of reflex responses to noxious stimuli.

Pain may be triggered by sensory inputs, especially when acute, but may also be generated independently, especially when chronic. Sensitization effects represent hyperresponsiveness in either the peripheral or central components of the nervous system. Supraspinal sensitization effects associated with the medial pain system (Vogt et al. 1993) and related limbic structures (Chapman 1996; Gabriel 1995) seem to mediate the pain response. Thus, pain could be produced by the output of a widely distributed neural network in the brain, rather than directly by peripheral nociceptive stimuli. Importantly, the central pain control processes seem to encompass the cognitive-evaluative, motivational-affective, and sensory-discriminative systems (Melzack 2001) that characterize the pain response. Finally, it should be noted that the pain system is intimately related to other systems in the brain (e.g., motor, mnemonic, and social systems).

Traumatic Brain Injury, Chronic Pain, and Cognitive Dysfunction

There is a high comorbidity of chronic pain problems with cranial trauma as well as traumatic brain injury (TBI). Indeed, headache is the primary complaint in virtually all surveys of postconcussion syndrome (e.g., Nicholson 2000d). The frequency of posttraumatic headache (PTH) in the immediate postaccident period has been estimated to be as high as 90%, with problems continuing beyond 6 months in as many as 44% of patients (Martelli et al. 1999a). In addition to headache, many other pain problems may follow trauma, including back pain, complex regional pain syndrome (CRPS), and fibromyalgia, among others. Curiously, most studies report that pain problems are much more common in less severe as compared with more severe TBI (Martelli et al. 1999d; Nicholson 2000d; Zasler and Martelli 2002), although pain problems may also be common in the latter (Lahz and Bryant 1996). Although more severe brain injuries may result in reduced sensitivity to pain because of lesions of the central nervous system (CNS) structures involved in processing pain (as observed in some dementias [Nicholson 2000c]) or may reflect optimal posttraumatic healing because of reduced activity, or both, it has also been suggested that there is increased likelihood for developing a central sensitization or neurosensitization effect (Miller 2000; Nicholson 2000b) after milder injuries.

There is increasing awareness of the role that pain may play in symptom presentation after TBI, especially with regard to cognitive complaints. Several recent reviews have addressed this issue, including Martelli et al. (1999a), Nicholson (2000b, 2000d), and Hart et al. (2000). In addition, Martelli et al. (2001a, 2001b) reviewed these reviews.

In summary, available evidence strongly supports the conclusion that pain and pain-related symptomatology, independent of TBI or neurological disorder, can and often do produce impairment of cognitive functioning as assessed on neuropsychological tests. Measures of attentional capacity, processing speed, memory, and executive functions are most likely to be affected. This pattern of impairment closely resembles that observed in mild or even more severe TBI. Clearly, chronic pain and associated problems can complicate the symptom picture in TBI (McCraken and Iverson 2001). Especially in cases of persistent sequelae after mild TBI, increasing evidence suggests that headache or other pain problems contribute to or maintain symptoms. This evidence provides strong support for the argument that resolution of postconcussion syndrome and successful adaptation to residual sequelae frequently rely on successful coping with PTH or other pain, or both, and associated symptomatology.

Pain Assessment

Because pain is a subjective experience, the patient's self-report of pain is the cornerstone of pain assessment. There are several important aspects of the experience of pain that should be assessed. Inquire about pain character, onset, location, duration, and factors that exacerbate or relieve. The clinician should also query about pain frequency and intensity and interference with everyday activities. A couple of useful methods of assessing pain intensity in adults are the Visual Analogue Scale (Galer and Jensen 1997) and the Verbal Analogue Scale. The visual scale is a 10-cm line with anchors of "no pain" and "the most pain imaginable," whereas the verbal scale solicits a rating of pain on a 0–10 scale with the same anchors. These scales are sensitive to treatment changes and are widely used in clinical settings.

Because pain is a complex perceptual process composed of behavioral, affective, cognitive, and sensory components, evaluation is conducted not only of a patient's medical findings, but also physiological, behavioral, and cognitive-affective functioning, including vulnerabilities and strengths. A comprehensive, biopsychosocial assessment becomes critical when pain is chronic, and should address beliefs about a patient's condition, coping strategies, psychological adjustment, and activity level and quality of life (Gatchel and Turk 1999). Psychological assessment is a required element of pain treatment programs accredited by the Commission on Accreditation of Rehabilitation Facilities (Gonzales et al. 2000) as well as several managed care companies. A brief survey of general classes and useful pain assessment instruments on the ba-

sis of previous work (Martelli and Zasler 2002) is included in Table 24–1.

Finally, chronic pain and associated symptoms are frequently accompanied by complaints of impairment in cognitive functioning. As noted in the section Traumatic Brain Injury, Chronic Pain, and Cognitive Dysfunction, the available evidence strongly supports the conclusion that pain and pain-related symptomatology can independently produce impairments in cognitive functioning, especially in attentional capacity, processing speed, memory, and executive functions. This pattern of impairment closely resembles that observed in TBI and can complicate the symptom picture, especially in cases of persistent postconcussion symptomatology. Some simple, basic recommendations to assess and minimize the confounding effects of chronic pain during neurocognitive examinations are presented in Table 24–2.

Pain Management

The goal of pain management is to modulate and, ideally, negate the associated physical and psychological symptoms of pain, prevent chronicity, and reduce functional disability. Realistic endpoints of pain relief consistent with the clinical situation should be established. Pain management methods include nonpharmacological or pharmacological methods, or both. Clinicians should strive to identify pain generators and treat them as directly as possible versus simply treating the symptom of pain. The simplest and least invasive pain management approach should be used whenever possible. When pharmacological agents are used, analgesia should be delivered with minimal adverse effects and inconvenience to the patient, both of which will optimize compliance.

Medical Management Issues

In the acute care setting, already compromised neurological status may limit the array of pharmacotherapeutic agents that might be appropriate to use in a patient in whom the neurosurgical and neurological status is either stabilized or static, or both. Medications that potentially alter any aspect of the neurological assessment should be used with caution if there is a more significant brain injury or neurological instability, or both. Additionally, consideration should be given to medications with reversible effects (e.g., narcotic reversal with naloxone) whenever there is a question of medication effect versus ongoing deterioration of neurological status.

During the acute care phase, the primary pain generators in trauma patients are fractures, intra-abdominal in-

TABLE 24–1.   A brief sample of general classes and common instruments for assessing psychological variables relevant to adjustment and coping with chronic pain

General and specific measures of behavioral, cognitive/attitudinal, and emotional coping

The Vanderbilt Pain Management Inventory (Brown and Nicassio 1987) measures chronic pain coping strategies (e.g., active, passive) and provides useful information for treatment planning and recommendations.

The Cognitive Coping Strategies Inventory (Butler et al. 1989) assesses the degree to which patients engage in adaptive and maladaptive cognitive coping strategies.

The Coping Strategies Questionnaire (Rosensteil and Keefe 1983) rates the frequency of engagement in 48 different behavioral and cognitive coping strategies in response to pain or physical symptom experience.

General health behavior inventories

The Sickness Impact Profile (Bergner et al. 1981) is a behaviorally based measure of health status designed to assess both psychosocial and physical dysfunction. It has sound psychometric properties, is used widely with chronic pain patients, and can provide relevant information regarding degree of functional limitation in daily activity.

The Millon Behavioral Health Inventory (Millon 1999), one of the most frequently used health inventories in the United States, provides information across four broad categories: basic coping styles, psychogenic attitudes, specific disease syndromes, and prognostic indices. It has good psychometric properties, a large normative database of representative medical patients, with specific disease scales developed for specific patient groups. It has recently been upgraded to the Millon Behavioral Medicine Diagnostic test. It assists with identification of significant psychiatric problems, making specific recommendations, pinpointing personal and social assets to facilitate adjustment, identifying medical regimen compliance problems, and structuring posttreatment plans and self-care responsibilities in the patient's social network.

The Illness Behavior Questionnaire (Pilowsky and Spence 1975, 1976), although not a pure behavioral measure, does provide useful information about attitudes, perceived reactions of others, and psychosocial variables. It delineates seven factors that include general hypochondriasis, disease conviction, psychological vs. somatic focusing, affective disturbance, affective inhibition, denial, and irritability. In addition, it has value in identifying patients who rely on illness behavior as a coping style for need procurement.

Specific pain domain inventories

The Multiaxial Pain Inventory uses a biopsychosocial conceptualization to assess relevant psychosocial, cognitive, and behavioral aspects of responses to pain and includes specific norms for different statistically derived chronic pain subtypes (Turk 1978): interpersonally distressed with inadequate social support, globally dysfunctional coping, and adaptive coping. An inexpensive software scoring program is available (Rosensteil and Keefe 1983). This multiaxial classification system appears a psychometrically sound and objective method of evaluating chronic pain patients, at least in terms of integrating useful psychological information with data from multiple other sources, and offers benefit for matching patients to types of pain management interventions.

The Hendler Chronic Pain Screening Test (Green and Shellenberger 1991) assesses contribution of physical vs. psychological variables to pain behavior expressions. It represents a composite predictor approach for which ratings are derived, with higher scores reflecting less "objective" and more psychologically influenced pain responses. Higher scores reflect strong psychologically influenced or motivated pain behavior and suggest recommendations for conservative treatments with multimodality treatment programs. Very high scores typically require psychiatric referral and intervention.

The Cogniphobia Scale (Todd 1998) is a quick screening measure of unreasonable or irrational fear of headache or painful reinjury on cognitive effort or exertion. The scale is adapted from the kinesiophobia instrument and designed to assess anxiety-based avoidant behavior with regard to cognitive exertion. Like the Tampa Scale of Kinesiophobia, this instrument offers information about need for combination therapies that include such anxiety-reduction procedures as graduated exposure, cognitive reinterpretation, and systematic desensitization.

The Headache Disability Rating procedure of Packard and Ham (Montgomery 1995) is a scale that estimates impairment from headache rated on frequency, severity, and duration of attacks and how activities affect functional skills and activities of daily living. Importantly, it includes a modifier variable for rating motivation (i.e., treatment motivation, exaggeration/over concern, and legal interest) that are used to adjust the total impairment rating.

TABLE 24–1. A brief sample of general classes and common instruments for assessing psychological variables relevant to adjustment and coping with chronic pain (continued)

General psychological measures: mood, anger, and anxiety

The Beck Depression Inventory-2 (Beck et al. 1961) is a common self-report measure that assesses depressive symptomatology. It has been reported to differentiate chronic pain patients with and without major depression (Fordyce 1979) (optimal cutoff score of 21) and has well-documented predictive validity.

The Zung Self-Rating Depression Scale (Zeigler and Paolo 1995) appears well suited for medical (vs. psychiatric) settings and has several advantages over other measures. It is shorter, simpler to administer and score, requires a lower reading level, fits well with medical and injury situations, and can be easily administered in an interview format (Rudy and Turk 1989). Items are self-ratings on a scale ranging from 1 to 4 ("Not at all" to "Most or all of the time") and are scored in the direction of increased depressive symptomatology, with a raw score cutoff for mild depression of approximately 40 points.

The State-Trait Anger Expression Inventory-2 (Skevington 1990) and its recent update is a reliable, well-normed instrument for assessing the experience, expression, and control of both current state and trait anger. Anger Expression and Anger Control scales assess four relatively independent anger-related traits: 1) expression of anger outward, 2) holding anger in, 3) controlling outward expression, and 4) controlling internal angry feelings. This instrument provides information regarding how experience, expression, and control of anger may contribute to psychophysiological arousal and symptoms and increase risk for developing somatic symptoms and medical problems. Indirectly, it offers suggestions for the direction of appropriate interventions.

The Beck Anxiety Inventory (BAI) (Spielberger 1999) is a screening measure of severity of patient anxiety. Specifically designed to reduce overlap with symptoms of depression, it assesses both physiological and cognitive components of anxiety in 21 items describing subjective, somatic, or panic-related symptoms. The BAI differentiates well between anxious and nonanxious groups in a variety of clinical settings.

The Perceived Stress Scale (PSS) (Cocchiarella and Andersson 2001) is a widely used instrument for measuring the degree to which situations in one's life are appraised as stressful. Items measure how unpredictable, uncontrollable, and overloaded respondents find their lives and directly queries current levels of experienced stress. Higher PSS scores have been associated with greater vulnerability to physical and psychological symptoms after stressful life events.

Comprehensive personality assessment

The Minnesota Multiphasic Personality Inventory (MMPI) (Dahlstrom et al. 1975) is the most widely used psychological assessment instrument in the United States. The MMPI is a 567-item (true/false), objective (i.e., 10 clinical and 3 [7 in revised version] validity scales are derived through empirical discrimination) measure of personality function and emotional status. Its predictive abilities are based on more than 50 years of actuarial data collection and analysis. It is a very sensitive measure of psychological states, traits, and styles (e.g., excessive anxiety, tension, hostility, somatization tendencies, sociopathy), as well as other traits (e.g., substance abuse, deviant thinking and experience, social withdrawal, problematic anger, and suicidal, homicidal, or other violent tendencies). Through configural interpretation of the relative scale elevations, tentative hypotheses regarding personality and coping style and relative degree of particular types of psychological disturbance can be gleaned. Importantly, although the MMPI can and is frequently misused and misinterpreted (e.g., application of psychiatric norms to medical patients tends to beg psychiatric interpretations), it represents one of the most useful adjuncts to personality assessment and treatment planning. Although efforts to distinguish organic vs. psychological causes for chronic pain and use of cookbook interpretations on the basis of psychiatric patient normative data (Pilowsky and Spence 1976; Schreiber and Galai-Gat 1993) represent failed applications, other significant information regarding emotional distress and coping styles can be derived.

juries, soft-tissue injuries, and pain associated with invasive procedures. Pain treatment should be tailored to the degree of pain assessed and reported via metric (e.g., Visual Analogue Scale) or qualitative (e.g., mild, moderate, severe, and excruciating) descriptors. For neurologically compromised patients with response limitations, prophylactic pain management should be practiced on the basis of injuries sustained and clinical presentation. Pharmacological pain prophylaxis should be considered in patients with low-level responses (e.g., vegetative or minimally conscious, or both) given 1) difficulty in assessment of

pain and controversies regarding pain appreciation and suffering in this patient group, and 2) the negative effect of pain (even in a vegetative state) related to subcortical physiological responses to nociceptive stimuli, including increased tone and posturing, tachycardia, tachypnea, and diaphoresis, in addition to other adverse effects.

In the subacute setting, many of the same issues present in the acute care setting continue to serve as pain generators. As patients are weaned from pain medication, pain experience can increase and acute pain generators can evolve into subacute pain generators. Ongoing atten-

TABLE 24-2. Recommendations for assessing and minimizing the confounding effects of pain during neurocognitive examination

Always assess pain when present, when posttraumatic adaptation seems compromised by pain and related symptomatology, or when limitations in daily functioning and decrements in test performance seem atypical. Clarify the frequency, intensity, and character of pain during the examination and, more generally, the characteristics of the chronic pain experience and related problems.

Assess problems that are commonly associated with chronic pain (e.g., sleep disturbance, fatigue, somatic preoccupation, anxiety, depression) because these all have the potential to markedly disrupt aspects of cognitive functioning.

Repeated administration of measures sensitive to the effects of pain-related fatigue (e.g., sustained, attention-demanding, timed tests) during examinations may help identify or corroborate fatigue-related deficits.

Motivation or effort level during examination and response bias to report problems should also always be assessed.

Consider postponing cognitive assessment in cases in which pain and related symptomatology have not been appropriately or aggressively treated.

Use accommodated procedures during examinations when possible [e.g., optimizing comfort, providing frequent breaks, allowing frequent position changes and use of personal orthotics (e.g., cushions or heating or ice pads), and modifying lighting and sound].

tion to pain management must be continued as patients are moved to neurosurgical step-down units or inpatient rehabilitation units, or both. Changes in patient status in the subacute setting may reflect underlying neural changes that are adaptive or maladaptive. Maladaptive changes can result in additional pain generators (e.g., progression or increase of tonal abnormalities, or both, resulting in hypertonicity and rigidity) as well as central pain phenomena. Pain often affects functional assessment in neurological patients with lower response levels, and the pain must be adequately assessed and treated. This includes pain associated with spasticity, posturing, fractures, pressure sores, peripheral nerve changes, CRPS, and postsurgical incisional pain.

Chronic pain has many elements of acute and subacute pain but is generally promulgated by additional factors, including psychological ones. Current evidence strongly supports mechanisms of central sensitization in chronic pain phenomena that are not present in the acute and subacute periods. Central sensitization is a phenomenon that has been demonstrated in both animal and human studies. Specifically, nociceptive input to the CNS may be increased because of activation or sensitization of peripheral sensory afferents. This barrage of nociceptive impulses may result in sensitization of second- and third-order neurons in the CNS. In this way, sensitization may play a role in initiation and maintenance of chronic pain (Bendtsen 2002; Bolay and Moskowitz 2002; Lidbeck 2002; Melzack 1999). It is likely that the effects of medication may be partly due to a reduction in sensitization. The patient experiencing chronic pain should be treated just as aggressively as a patient with acute or subacute pain but, because peripheral pain triggers are frequently less obvious, with different modalities. With chronic pain, biopsychosocial models for assessment and management are indicated, and inclusion and integration of behavioral and psychological interventions usually optimize treatment outcome.

It is critical in the context of assessment to take a thorough pain history for the clinician to provide an adequate foundation for identifying possible or probable pain generators. Clinicians are cautioned against assumptions that commonly reported pain symptoms are due to the brain injury itself (e.g., PTH) because pain and other symptoms are commonly produced by extracerebral injury (Martelli et al. 2004). Evaluating clinicians should be familiar with both the broad array of pain symptoms that may be reported by posttrauma patients and assessment methodologies for the various types of pain seen in this population. Clinicians are referred to various other sources for a more detailed description of patient assessment methodologies for persons with TBI or pain, or both (e.g., Turk and Melzack 1992).

Pharmacological Management

Mild pain medicines that should be considered typically include aspirin, acetaminophen, and nonsteroidal antiinflammatory drugs (NSAIDs). For moderate pain, the following may be considered: high-dose aspirin or acetaminophen, high-dose standard NSAIDs, newer generation NSAIDs such as cyclooxygenase-2 inhibitors, alternate NSAIDs, injectable NSAIDs, mixed narcotic analgesics with aspirin or acetaminophen (with or without caffeine), and tramadol. For severe pain, medications to consider would include parenteral narcotics (morphine sulfate is standard), mixed agonist antagonists (e.g., pentazocine, nalbuphine), partial agonist narcotics (e.g., buprenorphine), antidepressants, anticonvulsants, and/or atypical agents. Stimulants such as methylphenidate are used with opioid analgesics as adjuvant analgesics and to help manage opioid-induced sedation and cognitive impairment. Common medications used in pain management are included in Table 24–3.

TABLE 24–3. Medications for pain

Drug	Typical dose
Antidepressants (bedtime dose helps sleep and pain)	
Amitriptyline	75 mg qhs
Desipramine	75 mg qhs
Nortriptyline	75 mg qhs
Fluoxetine	20 mg qd
Venlafaxine	25 mg q8h
Paroxetine	20–40 mg qd
Analgesics	
Acetaminophen	650 mg q4–6h
Tramadol	100 mg q4–12h
Steroids	
Prednisone	20–80 mg qd
Dexamethasone	4–16 mg qd
Anticonvulsants (especially for lancinating pain)	
Carbamazepine	200 mg q8h
Valproic acid	250 mg q8h
Phenytoin	100 mg q8h
Clonazepam	0.5 mg q8h
Gabapentin	600 mg q8h
Levetiracetam	250–500 mg q12h
Lamotrigine	50–100 mg q12h
Oxcarbazepine	300–600 mg q12h
Local anesthetics	
Lidocaine	1.5 mg/kg iv
Mexiletine	225 mg q8h
Flecainide	150 mg q12h
Topical anesthetics	
Capsaicin	Topical qid
"Speed gel"	Topical tid–qid

Many posttrauma patients present with a number of different pain problems or pain processes, including 1) nociceptive pain associated with the normal operation of the pain system in response to a noxious peripheral stimulus or pathological process (e.g., mechanical pressure or inflammation), as well as 2) neuropathic or neurogenic pain resulting from the abnormal operation of the pain system associated with a primary lesion or dysfunction of the nervous system. Care should be taken to determine whether pain is idiopathic, given that such pain is often unresponsive to opioids or other pharmacological interventions.

Medications that have been used for opioid-insensitive pain include NSAIDs; tricyclic antidepressants (TCAs); newer generation antidepressants such as venlafaxine (Effexor); anticonvulsants, including carbamazepine-based derivatives, gabapentin, levetiracetam, and lamotrigine; as well as less commonly used agents such as mexiletine, among other drugs.

Adjuvant analgesics are drugs that are analgesic in specific circumstances but have primary indications other than for pain management. Adjuvant analgesics are usually combined with analgesics. Corticosteroids and anti-inflammatory medications, such as prednisone, are commonly used as short-term therapy to decrease pain and nausea and improve mood, appetite, and general sense of well-being. Adverse effects of short-term corticosteroid use include edema, dyspepsia, and neuropsychiatric changes. Patients with diabetes should be counseled about careful blood glucose monitoring while taking corticosteroids because of their hyperglycemic effect.

Antidepressants and anticonvulsants are used to manage a variety of neuropathic pain states that have not been responsive to opioid analgesics (Table 24–4). TCAs, particularly amitriptyline, have shown efficacy in the management of diabetic neuropathy and are used for other neuropathic states (Fishbain 2000a, 2000b, 2002; Lynch 2001; Mattia et al. 2002). TCAs can also manage underlying depression in pain states. Other TCAs such as nortriptyline, imipramine, and desipramine are also used. Agents such as venlafaxine, with mixed noradrenergic and serotonergic properties, have also been found effective in certain pain conditions (Fishbain 2000a, 2000b, 2002; Lynch 2001; Mattia et al. 2002). TCA adverse effects include anticholinergic effects (dry mouth, sedation), weight gain, orthostatic hypotension, and cardiac arrhythmias. Secondary amines such as nortriptyline and desipramine have fewer adverse effects and should be used in patients, such as the elderly, when there is concern for anticholinergic effects, sedation, and orthostatic hypotension. Antidepressants generally should be initiated at a low dosage and titrated up slowly on the basis of pain relief and patient tolerance.

Anticonvulsants, such as carbamazepine and gabapentin, can be effective for the management of neuropathic pain, particularly lancinating or paroxysmal pain. Because carbamazepine can decrease platelets, neutrophils, and red blood cells, patients who are taking carbamazepine should have complete blood cell counts performed routinely. Gabapentin has shown efficacy in diabetic neuropathy and postherpetic neuralgia and generally has a milder adverse effect profile, consisting of sedation and ataxia, and does not require routine laboratory work. As

TABLE 24–4.   **Opioids**

Short-acting			Long-acting[a]			Mixed short- and long-acting	
	Equivalent doses			Equivalent doses			
Drug	Oral	Parenteral	Drug	Oral	Parenteral	Drug	Oral
Morphine	30 mg q3–4h	10 mg q3–4h	MS-Contin	90–120 mg q12h	—	Avinza (morphine sulfate)	30–120 mg/ day as a single dose
Hydromorphone	7.5 mg q3–4h	1.5 mg q3–4h	Levorphanol	4 mg q6–8h	2 mg q6–8h		
Codeine	200 mg q3–4h	—	Methadone	20 mg q6–8h	10 mg q3–6h		
Hydrocodone	30 mg q3–4h	—	Oramorph SR	90–120 mg q12h	—		
Oxycodone	30 mg q3–4h	—	Oxymorphone	—	1 mg q3–4h		
Meperidine	300 mg q2–3h	100 mg q3h	Fentanyl	Transdermal: 25-g patch			
Fentanyl im or iv				45–135 mg			
				Morphine po over 24 hours			

[a]Opioid-naive adults and children ≥50 kg body weight.

with the antidepressants, begin at a low dosage and titrate slowly. Valproate, oxcarbazepine, lamotrigine, topiramate, phenytoin, and clonazepam are other anticonvulsants that also have been used for neuropathic pain.

Other agents that have more recently been recognized as adjuvants in the pharmacological management of pain include tizanidine and sodium amobarbital (Amytal). Mailis and Nicholson (2002) published an excellent review of the use of sodium Amytal infusion in the assessment and treatment of chronic pain (and functional disorders). Tizanidine, an α_2-adrenergic agonist, has also provided antinociception without producing pronounced hemodynamic changes. On the basis of experimental evidence, this drug depresses dorsal horn convergent neuronal activity, probably in part by a postsynaptic inhibitory action. Owing to the role of convergent neurons in pain processes, this could explain, at least partially, the analgesic action of this compound. It is thought to have several mechanisms of action resulting in a decrease in polysynaptic spinal cord reflex activity, including inhibition of the release of excitatory neurotransmitters from presynaptic sites and of substance P from nociceptive sensory afferents (Gray et al. 1999; Nance et al. 1994). Tizanidine has been shown to be effective in a variety of pain conditions, including fibromyalgia as well as tension-type headache.

Capsaicin can be used topically to help decrease pain associated with peripheral neuropathies. Capsaicin de-

pletes peptides such as substance P that mediate nociceptive transmission. Application of capsaicin is associated usually with a burning sensation, which may be severe enough to require premedication with either an oral analgesic or a topical lidocaine cream or ointment. Patients should be counseled not to touch mucous membranes after applying capsaicin. Compounded agents, typically formulated through "compounding pharmacies" may also play a role in pain management of the post-TBI patient. Such standard formulas as "speed gel" (contains amitriptyline, lidocaine, guaifenesin, and ketoprofen) can work quite well for neuropathic or neuralgic scalp pain. Similar compounded topicals with varying ingredients such as gabapentin, ketamine, and clonidine may be helpful as adjutants for CRPS-related pain.

Surgery produces pain by releasing pain and inflammatory mediators via damaged tissue. This pain is acute pain and improves as the wound heals and the patient convalesces. The goal of postoperative pain management is to provide continuous and effective analgesia with minimal adverse effects. NSAIDs such as parenteral ketorolac are used both intraoperatively and postoperatively to decrease the production of inflammatory prostaglandins released at the site of injury. The ketorolac dose is dependent on route, patient age, and weight and should only be continued at the appropriate dosage for 5 days because of the development of renal dysfunction and gastrointestinal toxicity. Opioid analgesics are the most commonly used medications for postoperative pain, usually administered intramuscularly or intravenously on an as-needed basis. This approach can lead to delays in the patient receiving adequate analgesia because of medication administration delays and intramuscular route absorption. Patients should be switched to oral opioid analgesics without diet restrictions when oral administration is tolerated. Patient-controlled analgesia (PCA) is a process in which the patient is allowed to self-administer low doses of intravenous opioid analgesics to maintain analgesia (Rudolf et al. 1999). To use PCA, a patient should be sufficiently cognizant to understand the goals of PCA and understand the use of the equipment. Patients who are confused or cognitively impaired are not good candidates for PCA. The number of injections and attempted injections can be monitored for efficacy and adverse effects in addition to the patient's report of pain. Opioid analgesics can also be administered into the epidural or intrathecal space combined with local anesthetics such as bupivacaine or ropivacaine for postoperative pain management. Patient-controlled epidural analgesia may be considered in specific circumstances. Current consensus among pain specialists dictates that concerns regarding addiction are generally not a contraindication to opioid treatment for otherwise intractable pain. We highly recommend that patients with prior drug abuse histories or addiction-prone personalities be carefully screened if being considered for chronic narcotic treatment for pain. Last, we always recommend the use of a "narcotics agreement" when using such agents for pain management (Fishman and Kreis 2001; see Appendix).

The physician should aim for drug prescriptions that optimize compliance and minimize potential side effects. Particularly in cognitively impaired patients, physicians should aim for once- to twice-a-day drug dosing. Patients should be counseled on the goals of treatment and what to expect regarding adverse effects, especially constipation with opioid analgesics or gastrointestinal side effects with NSAIDs. Fears regarding dependence should be openly discussed as should any sexual function side effects. Ideally, the clinician should aim for decreasing polypharmacy; however, when appropriate, combination drug regimens should be considered. It is critical to ascertain whether patients are taking their medicine correctly (e.g., taking scheduled medicine on an as-needed basis) and/or supplanting their prescribed medications with over-the-counter products.

Nonpharmacological Management

A wide variety of psychological, behavioral, physical (e.g., physiotherapy, exercise, chiropractic, and massage) or other medical interventions may be beneficial in the treatment of chronic pain. It is beyond the scope of this chapter to provide any comprehensive review. Rather, we focus on what we think are the most promising behavioral and medical treatments. Readers are referred to more comprehensive summaries such as the work of McQuay and Moore (1998), a recent review of evidence-based recommendations for management of chronic nonmalignant pain (College of Physicians and Surgeons of Ontario 2000), the reviews by Martelli et al. (1999a, 1999b), the work of Fishbain (2000a, 2000b; 2002), or the many systematic reviews prepared for the Cochrane Collaboration (e.g., Cochrane Library 2002).

Depending on the etiology of the pain generator in question, numerous nonpharmacological approaches may be considered in the management of pain conditions, including use of physical agents and modalities, injection therapies, exercise, biofeedback, adaptive equipment, and/or psychological interventions. These treatment modalities should all be given adequate consideration in conjunction with possible pharmacological alternatives if physicians are to develop adequate functionally oriented treatment regimens for addressing chronic pain issues in persons with TBI.

It should be emphasized that pain is a highly aversive condition. Mitigation of especially resistant and severe chronic pain can be extremely challenging to often unsatisfactory. Hence, search for pain relief can lead to both desperation on the part of persons with pain and premature claims of efficacy by practitioners and proponents of particular treatment modalities. Importantly, reviews of efficacy and evidence-based reviews, as well as clinical knowledge and common sense, should be relied on to guide the specific use of these interventions for specific diagnostic syndromes and conditions.

Physical Modalities

Physical agents used to modulate pain may include superficial heat and cold. The most common modalities used are hot/cold packs, heat lamps (incandescent or infrared), paraffin baths, and cryotherapy. Hydrotherapy interventions for pain management may involve prescription of whirlpool or contrast baths. Various diathermy techniques may also be used to facilitate pain control, including ultrasound, phonophoresis, as well as short-wave and microwave diathermy (Weber and Allen 2000). There are also a number of electrical stimulation techniques used in pain management such as transcutaneous electrical nerve stimulation and iontophoresis that are commonly employed as adjuvants for pain control (Mysiw and Jackson 2000).

Cranioelectrotherapy stimulation is a treatment for pain reduction that, unlike transcutaneous electrical nerve stimulation, targets CNS function. It involves attachment of electrodes carrying microcurrent across the scalp and induces an approximate 15-Hz cortical rhythm. A large number of studies, many well controlled, have examined cranioelectrotherapy stimulation since the 1970s. Findings from these studies, as well as experience of two of the authors (N.Z. and M.M), indicate that this relatively unknown intervention is a safe and surprisingly useful treatment for pain, especially chronic pain and its associated symptomatology of anxiety, depression, and insomnia (Kirsch 1999; Kirsch and Smith 2000).

Physical modalities tend to play a more predominant role in the treatment of pain complaints of musculoskeletal origin and may include traction, manual medicine techniques (e.g., joint manipulation, myofascial release techniques, and strain counter-strain), as well as massage (Atchinson et al. 2000). Injection techniques, including intra-articular, periarticular, peritendinous, ligamentous/fibrous tissue (i.e., prolotherapy), and trigger point, can all be used in various types of musculoskeletal pain disorders. Axial injections such as epidurals and zygapophyseal joint and sympathetic blocks may all be relevant considerations for pain treatment in this population, depending on the presumptive pain generators (Lennard 1994).

Exercise, in our experience, is an underappreciated and underprescribed treatment intervention (e.g., deLateur 2000; Philadelphia Panel Evidence Based Clinical Practice Guidelines on Selected Rehabilitation Interventions for Neck Pain 2001), especially in persons post-TBI with pain complaints. Exercise can play a significant role in controlling pain both on a central and peripheral basis and in commensurately improving weight control, affect, and general state of health and well-being. Adaptive equipment such as reachers, sock aides, long-handled scrubbers, and/or brushes as well as ergonomically modified work environments are a few of the many different interventions that may also facilitate greater pain modulation and tolerance (Trombly 1995).

Fear of pain and related pain and anxiety-based avoidant behaviors often represent significant impediments to recovery through decreased activity that can prevent normal restoration of function and perpetuate painful experience. Graduated activity programs that combine re-education; anxiety-reduction procedures such as graduated exposure, cognitive reinterpretation, and promotion of adaptive attitudes; and treatment participation and cooperation are especially helpful (Martelli et al. 1999b).

Behavioral–Psychological Management

Behavioral treatment interventions in persons with TBI and concomitant chronic pain typically begin with an assessment of relevant treatment issues (e.g., personality variables, social support) and facilitation of the patient–therapist relationship. A detailed clinical interview; personality, emotional status, and coping measures; and specific pain assessment instruments may be supplemented by psychophysiological assessment (e.g., examination of muscle tension or electromyography for different muscle groups). These results are integrated into a specifically tailored treatment plan that provides a framework for treatment, defines goals and patient/therapist expectations and sequences, and provides psychoeducational information about the particular type of chronic pain and rationale for treatment (Gonzales et al. 2000; Martelli et al. 1999a).

Although there is an abundance of available treatment outcome studies (e.g., van Tulder et al. 2001), relatively few specifically examine the behavioral treatment of pain after TBI. However, the available literature suggests that, with the exception of some reports of greater treatment resistance, there are mostly similarities in clinical presentations, pathophysiologies, and treatment responses for persons with chronic pain who do and do not have an associated TBI (Andrasik 1990). Especially in cases of posttraumatic pain, the severity and frequency of pain attacks and chronic pain-related sequelae such as coping abilities, depression, and anxiety may be significantly improved by combined psychological treatment protocols (Eccleston et al. 2003; Jenson et al. 1987; Lazarus and Folkman 1984; Martelli 1997; Rosensteil and Keefe 1983; van Tulder et al. 2001). Supportive counseling that begins early after trauma and is continuous results in better patient response (e.g., Rosensteil and Keefe 1983), and combination treatments appear to increase likelihood of benefit (e.g., Grayson 1997).

McQuay and Moore (1998) and Martelli et al. (1999a) reviewed various behaviorally based chronic pain treatment interventions for which efficacy data are available. Recent authors have more systematically reviewed the evidence supporting the utility of these behavioral interventions (e.g., Eccleston et al. 2003; van Tulder et al. 2001). Table 24–5 includes a summary of frequently used strategies for which there is empirical support.

Conclusion

Most current approaches to chronic pain assessment and management use a biopsychosocial perspective (Green and Shellenberger 1991; Martelli et al. 1999b). Biopsychosocial models conceptualize health and illness as occurring in a dynamic and interactive system of interdependent biological, psychological, and social subsystems. These subsystems each reflect individual differences and variabilities, and in this conceptualization, pain experi-

---

TABLE 24–5. Summary of useful behavioral treatments for chronic pain

Patient education: The most modifiable pain-contributing factor is the stress reaction component. The best treatment packages generally contain elements targeting numerous factors. Posture may be addressed by awareness training. Stress management can assist with reducing sympathetic arousal/discharge that exacerbates pain. Accurate information and expectancies help with this and also assist with coping with pain more adaptively. Education about expected symptoms and course after mild traumatic brain injury has been shown to reduce the anxiety and selective attention and misattribution that can unnecessarily prolong symptoms (Mittenberg et al. 1998).

Biofeedback: Abundant research supports the utility of EMG or thermal biofeedback for both headache pain and chronic musculoskeletal pain disorders more generally. The forehead, trapezii, frontal-posterior neck, and neck areas are frequent EMG feedback sites. Patterns of pathophysiological neuromuscular activity that underlie pain complaint and functional limitations, which can be remediated through feeding back physiological information to allow self-correction, include 1) stress-related hyperarousal in musculoskeletal or other physiological systems; 2) postural dysfunction; 3) hyper- or hypotonicity induced by reflex systems activated by inflammation, active trigger points, and cumulative strain or recurrent trauma; 4) learned guarding or bracing to mitigate anticipated pain or injury; 5) learned inhibition or avoidance of muscle activation/activity; 6) chronic compensation for joint hyper- or hypomobility (e.g., muscles taking over the role of damaged joint tissue); and 7) faulty motor schema and muscle imbalance, reflecting development of one or more of the preceding syndromes and resulting in the lack of coordination and stability between typically coordinated muscle groups. Finally, data are emerging that indicate that EEG biofeedback and associated EEG-driven stimulation offer efficacy in treatment of some persistent pain and persistent postconcussion symptoms (Arena et al. 1997; DeVore 2002).

Relaxation training: PMR is the most studied relaxation procedure (Blanchard 1994). PMR involves the systematic tensing and relaxing of various muscle groups to elicit a deepening relaxation response, usually with combination of muscle groups and addition of diaphragmatic breathing to shorten the protocol. Meta-analytic reviews generally conclude that relaxation training and biofeedback training are equally effective. Relaxation training presumably serves to 1) reduce proprioceptive input to the hypothalamus, thereby decreasing sympathetic nervous system activity, and 2) directly reduce muscle tension or pre-headache vasoconstriction. (e.g., Auerbach and Gramling 1998; Ham and Packard 1996).

Operant treatment: Treatment based on the operant model (e.g., Fordyce 1974, 1976) requires altering environmental contingencies to eliminate pain behaviors (e.g., verbal complaints, inactivity, and avoidance) and reward "well" behaviors (e.g., incrementally increased exercise and activity level).

Cognitive-behavioral treatments: Cognitive approaches typically involve instruction in identification and refutation of maladaptive beliefs concerning pain. Specific cognitive strategies and skills are taught to replace inappropriate negative expectations and beliefs that maintain physiological arousal and complicate symptom resolution (e.g., Holroyd and Andrasik 1978; Keefe 1996). Mittenberg et al. (1996) demonstrated successful treatment of postconcussion syndrome that included headache with a treatment package consisting of education about how expectations and misattributions can perpetuate symptoms, along with cognitive restructuring to shape more adaptive interpretations and expectancies.

Social and assertiveness skills training: Skills training may help some patients with more effective communication of needs. Increased need fulfillment decreases distressful emotions, reducing the physiological arousal that contributes to pain experience (Miller 1993).

Imagery and hypnosis: Using a combination of autohypnosis, suggestions of relaxation, and visual imagery, patients are generally instructed to visualize the pain (i.e., give it form) and focus on altering the image to reduce the pain. Imagery-based treatment is most effective after establishment of a good therapeutic alliance to facilitate compliance (Forsa et al. 2002; Martin 1993; Olness et al. 1999).

Habit reversal: These treatment packages teach pain patients to detect, interrupt, and reverse maladaptive habits (e.g., maladaptive head/jaw posture, jaw tension, and negative cognitions). Specific skills are taught to both reverse poor functional habits and stressful thoughts as well as feelings that precipitate or perpetuate them (Gramling et al. 1996).

Note. EEG=electroencephalography; EMG=electromyography; PMR=progressive muscle relaxation.

---

ence can have multiple expressions and causal pathways. From this perspective, the most suitable interventions are ones that are offered holistically, addressing function in somatic, psychological, and psychosocial domains.

There are a wide variety of pharmacological or other medical or physical interventions, and many of the more useful and promising ones were reviewed in this chapter. Currently, multicomponent treatment packages are the preferred treatment choice for chronic pain (Martelli et

al. 1999a; Miller 1993, 2000). The most promising current treatment interventions are combination treatments that are holistic in nature, that target not only the pain but also the patient's reaction to it within his or her daily life, and that emphasize self-control (vs. more narrowly focused treatments, such as medication management or nondrug therapies alone; Miller 1990).

Importantly, there is increasing evidence for an interactive biological and psychological conceptualization of chronic pain that represents a convergence of findings across multiple specialties. Most forms of chronic pain are now considered to include a hyperresponsiveness of the pain system involving "wind up" or sensitization in the CNS or brain (e.g., Jay et al. 2001; Nicholson 2000a, 2000b, 2000c, 2000d; Nicholson et al. 2002), along with dysregulation in pain inhibitory mechanisms. Conceptually, the thrust of current efforts in chronic pain management seem to be toward "desensitization" of the CNS through combination treatments. Using this conceptual model, we consider that currently available and potentially useful chronic pain treatment approaches can be categorized according to specific area and manner of desensitization targeted. Table 24–6 offers a preliminary classification model that has been found useful in our treatment planning, especially for more challenging chronic pain situations. Additionally, it fits nicely with the growing consensus regarding central and peripheral nervous system hyperarousal in chronic pain. Finally, it offers an intuitively appealing classification system for conceptually organizing the wide variety of available treatment interventions and in planning combination treatments.

TABLE 24–6. **A desensitization model for chronic pain treatment interventions**

Desensitizing peripheral CNS procedures

Electromyography biofeedback; various relaxation and imagery procedures; transcutaneous electrical nerve stimulation

Desensitizing CNS medications

Antiepileptic drugs, tizanidine HCL, sodium amobarbital (Amytal), neuroimmunomodulators, selective serotonin reuptake inhibitors, etc.

Desensitizing behavioral activity procedures

Operant behavioral activity programs; graduated exposure and graduated activity programs

Desensitizing psychotherapeutic procedures

Emotional desensitization of catastrophic reaction to injury and pain and other fears and trauma; splinting of emotional reactions and calming of catastrophic reactions and hypervigilance to pain; specific formal pain and fear desensitization procedures

Desensitizing neurophysiological procedures

Cranioelectrotherapy stimulation: consider electroencephalography biofeedback or adjunctive procedures such as sound and light (audiovisual stimulation), transcranial magnetic stimulation, and brain electrical stimulation.

Note. CNS=central nervous system.

References

Albe-Fessard D, Berkley KJ, Kruger L, et al: Diencephalic mechanisms of pain sensation. Brain Res 356:217–296, 1985

American Psychiatric Association: Diagnostic and Statistical Manual of Mental Disorders, 4th Edition, Text Revision. Washington, DC, American Psychiatric Association, 2000

Andrasik F: Psychologic and behavioral aspects of chronic headache. Neurol Clin 8:961–976, 1990

Arena JG, Bruno GM, Brucks AG: The use of EMG biofeedback for the treatment of chronic tension headache. Electromyography: Applications in Physical Therapy. Biofeedback Foundation of Europe. Available at: http://www.bfe.org/protocol/pro08eng.htm, 1997. Accessed June 18, 2004.

Atchinson JW, Stoll ST, Cotter AC: Manipulation, traction and massage, in Physical Medicine and Rehabilitation, 2nd Edition. Edited by Braddom RL. New York, WB Saunders, 2000

Auerbach SM, Gramling SE: Stress Management: Psychological Foundations. New York, Prentice-Hall, 1998

Beck AT, Ward CH, Mendelson M, et al: An inventory for measuring depression. Arch Gen Psychiatry 4:561–571, 1961

Bendtsen L: Sensitization: its role in primary headache. Curr Opin Investig Drugs 3:449–453, 2002

Bergner M, Bobbitt RA, Carter WB, et al: The Sickness Impact Profile: development and final revision of a health status measure. Med Care 19:787–805, 1981

Blanchard EB: Behavioral medicine and health psychology, in Handbook of Psychotherapy and Behavior Change. Edited by Bergin EA, Garfield W. New York, Wiley, 1994

Bolay H, Moskowitz MA: Mechanisms of pain modulation in chronic syndromes. Neurology 59 (suppl 2):S2–S7, 2002

Bromm B, Desmedt JE (eds): Pain and the Brain: From Nociception to Cognition. New York, Raven, 1995

Brown GK, Nicassio PM: The development of a questionnaire for the assessment of active and passive coping strategies in chronic pain patients. Pain 31:53–65, 1987

Bryant RA, Marosszeky JE, Crooks J, et al: Interaction of posttraumatic stress disorder and chronic pain following traumatic brain injury. J Head Trauma Rehabil 14:588–594, 1999

Butler R, Damarin F, Beaulieu C, et al: Assessing cognitive coping strategies for acute post-surgical pain: psychological assessment. J Consult Clin Psychol 1:41–45, 1989

Chapman CR: Limbic processes and the affective dimension of pain. Prog Brain Res 110:63–81, 1996

Cocchiarella L, Andersson GBJ (eds.): Guides to the Evaluation of Permanent Impairment, 5th Edition. Chicago, IL, AMA Press, 2001

Cochrane Library, Issue 2. Oxford, England, Update Software, Ltd. 2002. The Cochrane Collaboration available at: http://www.Cochrane.org/index0.htm. Accessed June 18, 2004

College of Physicians and Surgeons of Ontario: Evidence-based recommendations for medical management of chronic non-malignant pain. November, 2000 http://www.cpsbc.ca/physician/documents/pain.htm. Accessed August 13, 2004.

Dahlstrom WG, Welsh GS, Dahlstrom LE: An MMPI Handbook: Research Applications, Vol 2. Minneapolis, MN, University of Minnesota Press, 1975

deLateur BJ: Therapeutic exercise, in Physical Medicine and Rehabilitation, 2nd Edition. Edited by Braddom RL. New York, WB Saunders, 2000, pp 392–412

DeVore JR: Applied psychophysiology: state of the art, in Functional Medical Disorders, State of the Art Reviews in Physical Medicine and Rehabilitation. Edited by Zasler ND, Martelli MF. Philadelphia, PA, Hanley & Belfus, 2002, pp 21–36

Eccleston C, Yorke L, Morley S, et al: Psychological therapies for the management of chronic and recurrent pain in children and adolescents. Cochrane Database Syst Rev CD003968, 2003

Fishbain DA: Evidence-based data on pain relief with antidepressants. Ann Med 32:305–316, 2000a

Fishbain DA: Non-surgical chronic pain treatment outcome: a review. Int Rev Psychiatry 12:170–180, 2000b

Fishbain DA: Chronic nonmalignant pain. J Rheumatol 29:2243–2244, 2002

Fishman SM, Kreis PG: The opioid contract. Clin J Pain 18:S70–S75, 2001

Fordyce WE: Pain viewed as learned behavior. Adv Neurol 4:415–422, 1974

Fordyce WE: Behavioral Methods for Chronic Pain and Illness. St. Louis, MO: CV Mosby, 1976

Fordyce WE: Use of the MMPI in the assessment of chronic pain, in Clinical Notes on the MMPI. Edited by Butcher J, Gynther W, Schofield W. Nutley, NJ, Hoffman LaRoche, 1979

Fordyce WE: Pain and suffering: a reappraisal. Am Psychol 43:276–283, 1988

Forsa EA, Sexton H, Gottesman G: The effect of guided imagery and amitriptyline on daily fibromyalgia pain: a prospective, randomized, controlled trial. J Psychiatr Res 36:179–187, 2002

Gabriel M: The role of pain in cingulate cortical and limbic thalamic mediation or dance learning, in Forebrain Areas Involved in Pain Processing. Edited by Besson JM, Guilbaud G, Ollat H. Paris, France, John Libbey Eurotext, 1995, pp 197–211

Galer BS, Jensen MF: The development and preliminary validation of a pain measure specific to neuropathic pain: the Neuropathic Pain Scale. Neurology 48:332–338, 1997

Gatchel RJ, Turk DC (eds): Psychosocial Factors in Pain. New York, Guilford, 1999

Gonzales VA, Martelli MF, Baker JM: Psychological assessment of persons with chronic pain. NeuroRehabilitation 14:69–83, 2000

Gramling SE, Neblett J, Grayson RL, et al: Temporomandibular disorder: efficacy of an oral habit reversal treatment program. J Behav Ther Exp Psychiatry 27:212–218, 1996

Gray AM, Pache DM, Sewell RD: Do alpha 2 adrenoreceptors play an integral role in the antinociceptive mechanism of action of antidepressant compounds? Eur J Pharmacol 378:161–168, 1999

Grayson RL: EMG biofeedback as a therapeutic tool in the process of cognitive behavioral therapy: preliminary single case results. Poster presented at the Association for Advancement of Behavior Therapy (AABT), 31st annual convention, Miami, Florida, November, 1997

Ham LP, Packard RC: A retrospective, follow-up study of biofeedback-assisted relaxation therapy in patients with posttraumatic headache. Biofeedback Self Regul 21:93–104, 1996

Hart RP, Martelli MF, Zasler ND: Chronic pain and neuropsychological functioning. Neuropsychol Rev 10:131–149, 2000

Hinnant DW: Psychological evaluation and testing, in Handbook of Chronic Pain Management. Edited by Tollison DC, Satterwhite JR, Tollison JW. Baltimore, MD, Williams & Wilkins, 1994, pp 18–35

Holroyd KA, Andrasik F: Coping and the self-control of chronic tension headache. J Consult Clin Psychol 5:1036–1045, 1978

Jay GW, Krusz JC, Longmire DR, et al: Current Trend in the Diagnosis and Treatment of Chronic Neuromuscular Pain Syndromes: Myofascial Pain Syndrome, Chronic Tension-Type Headache, and Fibromyalgia. Sonora, CA, American Academy of Pain Management, 2001

Jenson MP, Turner JA, Romano JM: Self-efficacy and outcome expectancies: relationship to chronic pain coping strategies and adjustment. Pain 44:263–269, 1987

Keefe FJ: Cognitive behavioral therapy for managing pain. Clin Psychol 49:4–5, 1996

Kirsch DL: The Science Behind Cranial Electrotherapy Stimulation. Edmonton, Alberta, Canada, Medical Scope Publishing, 1999

Kirsch DL, Smith RB: The use of cranial electrotherapy in the management of chronic pain: a review. NeuroRehabilitation 14:85–94, 2000

Kulich RJ, Baker WB: A guide for psychological testing and evaluation for chronic pain, in Evaluation and Treatment of Chronic Pain. Edited by Aranoff GM. Baltimore, MD, Williams & Wilkins, 1999, pp 301–312

Lahz S, Bryant RA: Incidence of chronic pain following traumatic brain injury. Arch Phys Med Rehabil 77:889–891, 1996

Lazarus RS, Folkman S: Stress, Appraisal, and Coping. New York: Springer, 1984

Lennard TA (ed): Physiatric Procedures in Clinical Practice. Philadelphia, PA, Hanley & Belfus, 1994

Lidbeck J: Central hyperexcitability in chronic musculoskeletal pain: a conceptual breakthrough with multiple clinical implications. Pain Res Manage 7:81–92, 2002

Lynch ME: Antidepressants as analgesics: a review of randomized controlled trials. J Psychiatry Neurosci 26:30–36, 2001

Mailis A, Nicholson K: The use of sodium Amytal in the assessment and treatment of functional or other disorders, in Functional Medical Disorders, State of the Art Reviews in Physical Medicine and Rehabilitation. Edited by Zasler ND, Martelli MF. Philadelphia, PA, Hanley & Belfus, 2002, pp 131–146

Martelli MF: The Vulnerability to Disability Rating Scale (VDRS). Test in the public domain. Glen Allen, Virginia, Concussion Care Centre of Virginia, 1997

Martelli MF, Zasler ND: Useful psychological instruments for assessing persons with functional medical disorders, in Functional Medical Disorders, State of the Art Reviews in Physical Medicine and Rehabilitation. Edited by Zasler ND, Martelli MF. Philadelphia, PA, Hanley & Belfus, 2002, pp 147–162

Martelli MF, Grayson R, Zasler ND: Post traumatic headache: psychological and neuropsychological issues in assessment and treatment. J Head Trauma Rehabil 1:49–69, 1999a

Martelli MF, Zasler ND, Mancini AM, et al: Psychological assessment and applications in impairment and disability evaluations, in Guide to Functional Capacity Evaluation with Impairment Rating Applications. Edited by May RV, Martelli MF. Richmond, VA, NADEP Publications, 1999b, pp 1–84

Martelli MF, Zasler ND, Nicholson K, et al: Masquerades of brain injury, I: Chronic pain and traumatic brain injury. The Journal of Controversial Medical Claims 8:1–8, 2001a

Martelli MF, Zasler ND, Nicholson K, et al: Masquerades of brain injury, II: response bias in medicolegal examinees and examiners. The Journal of Controversial Medical Claims. 8:13–23, 2001b

Martelli MF, Zasler ND, Bender MC, et al: Psychological, neuropsychological, and medical considerations in assessment and management of pain. J Head Trauma Rehabil 19:10–28, 2004

Martin PR: Psychological Management of Chronic Headaches. New York, Guilford, 1993

Mattia C, Paoletti F, Coluzzi F, et al: New antidepressant in the treatment of neuropathic pain: a review. Minerva Anestesiol 68:105–114, 2002

McCraken LM, Iverson GL: Predicting complaints of impaired cognitive functioning in patients with chronic pain. J Pain Symptom Manage 21:392–396, 2001

McQuay H, Moore A: An Evidence Based Resource for Pain Relief. Oxford, England, Oxford University Press, 1998

Merskey H, Bogduk N (eds): Classification of Chronic Pain. 2nd Edition. Seattle, WA, IASP Press, 1994

Melzack R: Pain: an overview. Acta Anaesthesiol Scand 43:880–884, 1999

Melzack R: Pain and the neuromatrix in the brain. J Dent Educ 65:1378–1382, 2001

Miller L: Chronic pain complicating head injury recovery: recommendations for clinicians. Cognitive Rehabilitation 8:12–19, 1990

Miller L: Psychotherapy of the Brain Injured Patient. New York, WW Norton, 1993

Miller L: Neurosensitization: a model for persistent disability in chronic pain, depression, and posttraumatic stress disorder following injury. NeuroRehabilitation 14:25–32, 2000

Millon T: The MBHI and the MBMD, in Interpretive Strategies for the Millon Inventories. Edited by Strack S. New York, Wiley, 1999

Mittenberg W, Trement G, Zielinski RE, et al: Cognitive-behavioral prevention of postconcussion syndrome. Arch Clin Neuropsychol 11:139–145, 1996

Mittenberg W, Luis C, Essig S: Psychological treatment: mild head trauma. Recovery 9:26–27, 1998

Montgomery GK: A multi-factor account of disability after brain injury: implications for neuropsychological counseling. Brain Inj 9:453–469, 1995

Mysiw WJ, Jackson RD: Electrical stimulation, in Physical Medicine and Rehabilitation, 2nd Edition. Edited by Braddom RL. New York, WB Saunders, 2000, 464–474

Nance PW, Bugaresti J, Shellenberger K, et al: The North American Tizanidine Study Group. Efficacy and safety of tizanidine in the treatment of spasticity in patients with spinal cord injury. Neurology 44 (suppl 9):S44–S52, 1994

Nicholson K: At the crossroads: pain in the 21st century. NeuroRehabilitation 14:57–68, 2000a

Nicholson K: The neuropsychology of pain. Paper presented at the meeting of the National Academy of Neuropsychology, Washington, DC, November, 2000b

Nicholson K: Pain associated with lesion, disorder or dysfunction of the central nervous system. NeuroRehabilition 14:3–14, 2000c

Nicholson K: Pain, cognition and traumatic brain injury. NeuroRehabilitation 14:95–104, 2000d

Nicholson K, Martelli MF, Zasler ND: Myths and misconceptions about chronic pain: the problem of mind body dualism, in Pain Management: A Practical Guide for Clinicians, 6th Edition. Edited by Weiner RB. Boca Raton, FL, St. Lucie Press, 2002, pp 465–474

Olness K, Hall H, Rozniecki JJ, et al: Mast cell activation in children with migraine before and after training in self-regulation. Headache 39:101–107, 1999

Philadelphia Panel Evidence Based Clinical Practice Guidelines on Selected Rehabilitation Interventions for Neck Pain. Phys Ther 81:1701–1717, 2001

Pilowsky I, Spence ND: Patterns of illness behavior in patients with intractable pain. J Psychosom Res 19:279–287, 1975

Pilowsky I, Spence ND: Illness behavior syndromes associated with intractable pain. Pain 2:61–71, 1976

Rosensteil AK, Keefe FJ: The use of coping strategies in chronic low back pain patients: relationship to patient characteristics and current adjustment. Pain 17:33–44, 1983

Rudolph H, Packer JS, Cade JF, et al: Pain relief using smart technology: an overview of a new patient-controlled analgesia device. IEEE Trans Inf Technol Biomed 3:20–27, 1999

Rudy TE, Turk DC: Multiaxial Assessment of Pain: Multidimensional Pain Inventory Computer Program User Manual, Version 2.1. Pittsburgh, PA, University of Pittsburgh, 1989

Schreiber S, Galai-Gat T: Uncontrolled pain following physical injury as the core-trauma in post-traumatic stress disorder. Pain 54:107–110, 1993

Sharp TJ, Harvey AG: Chronic pain and posttraumatic stress disorder: mutual maintenance? Clin Psychol Rev 21:857–877, 2001

Skevington SM: A standardized scale to measure beliefs about controlling pain (BPCQ): a preliminary study. Psychol Health 4:221–232, 1990

Spielberger C: State-Trait Anger Expression Inventory, Research Edition. Professional Manual. Odessa, FL, Psychological Assessment Resources, 1999

Todd DD: Kinesiophobia: the relationship between chronic pain and fear-induced disability. The Forensic Examiner 7:14–20, 1998

Trombly CA: Retraining basic and instrumental activities of daily living, in Occupational Therapy for Physical Dysfunction, 4th Edition. Edited by Trombly CA. Baltimore, MD, Williams & Wilkins, 1995, pp 289–316

Turk DC: Cognitive behavioral techniques in the management of pain, in Cognitive Behavior Therapy: Research and Application. Edited by Foreyt JP, Rathjen RP. New York, Plenum, 1978, pp 119–130

Turk DC, Holzman AD: Chronic pain: interfaces among physical, psychological and social parameters, in Pain Management: A Handbook of Psychological Treatment Approaches. Edited by Holzman AD, Turk DC. New York, Pergamon, 1986, pp 1–9

Turk DC, Melzack R: The measurement of pain and the assessment of people experiencing pain, in Handbook of Pain Assessment. Edited by Turk DC, Melzack R. Guilford, New York, 1992, pp 3–14

van Tulder MW, Ostelo R, Vlaeyen JW, et al: Behavioral treatment for chronic low back pain: a systematic review within the framework of the Cochrane Back Review Group. Spine 26:270–281, 2001

Vogt BA, Sikes RW, Vogt LJ: Anterior cingulate cortex and the medial pain system, in Neurobiology of Cingulate Cortex and Limbic Thalamus: A Comprehensive Handbook. Edited by Vogt BA, Gabriel M. Cambridge, MA, Birkhäuser Boston, MA, 1993, pp 313–344

Weber DC, Allen WB: Physical agent modalities, in Physical Medicine and Rehabilitation, 2nd Edition. Edited by Braddom RL. New York, WB Saunders, 2000, pp 445–463

Willis WD, Westlund KN: Neuroanatomy of the pain system and of the pathways that modulate pain. J Clin Neurophysiol 14:2–31, 1997

World Health Organization: International Classification of Impairments, Disabilities and Handicaps. Geneva, World Health Organization, 1980

Zasler ND, Martelli MF: Post-traumatic headache: practical approaches to diagnosis and treatment, in Pain Management: A Practical Guide for Clinicians, 6th Edition. Edited by Weiner RB. Boca Raton, FL, St. Lucie Press, 2002, pp 313–344

Zeigler DK, Paolo AM: Headache symptoms and psychological profile of headache-prone individuals: a comparison of clinic patients and controls. Arch Neurol 52:602–606, 1995

Appendix 24–1

PATIENT AGREEMENT FOR
CONTROLLED SUBSTANCE PRESCRIPTIONS

Controlled substance medications (i.e., narcotics, tranquilizers, and barbiturates) are very useful but have a high potential for misuse and are, therefore, closely controlled by local, state, and federal governments. They are intended to relieve pain, thus improving function and/or ability to work. Because my physician is prescribing controlled substance medications to help manage my pain, I agree to the following conditions:

1.   **I am responsible for the controlled substance medications prescribed to me.** If my prescription is lost, misplaced, or stolen, or if I "run out early," I understand that **it will not be replaced.**

2.   **Refills of controlled substance medications:**

Will be made only during regular office hours Monday through Friday, in person, once a month, during a scheduled office visit. Refills will not be made at night, on weekends, or during holidays.

Will not be made if I "run out early," or "lose a prescription," or "spill or misplace my medication." I am responsible for taking the medication in the dose prescribed and for keeping track of the amount remaining.

Will not be made as an "emergency," such as on Friday afternoon because I suddenly realize I will "run out tomorrow." I will call at least twenty-four (24) hours ahead if I need assistance with a refill.

3.   It may be deemed necessary by my doctor that I see a medication-use specialist at any time while I am receiving controlled substance medications. I understand that if I do not attend such an appointment, my medications may be discontinued or may not be refilled beyond a tapering dose to completion. I understand that if the specialist feels that I am at risk for psychological dependence (addiction), my medications will no longer be refilled.

I agree to comply with random urine, blood, or breath testing, documenting the proper use of my medications as well as confirming compliance. I understand that driving a motor vehicle may not be allowed while taking the controlled substance medications and that it is my responsibility to comply with the laws of the state while taking the prescribed medications.

I understand that **if I violate any of the above conditions,** my prescription for controlled substance medications may be terminated **immediately.** If the violation involves obtaining controlled substance medications from another individual, or the concomitant use of nonprescribed illicit (illegal) drugs, it may also be reported to my physicians, medical facilities, and appropriate authorities. I understand that the **main treatment goal is to reduce pain and improve my ability to function and/or work.** In consideration of this goal, and the fact that I am being given a potent medication to help me reach my goal, I agree to help myself by the following better health habits: exercise, weight control, and avoidance of the use of tobacco and alcohol. I must also comply with the treatment plan as prescribed by my physician. I understand that a successful outcome to my treatment will only be achieved by following a healthy lifestyle.

I understand that the **long-term advantage and disadvantages of chronic opioid use have yet to be scientifically determined** and my treatment may change at any time. I understand, accept, and agree that there may be unknown risks associated with the long-term use of controlled substances and that my physician will advise me of any advances in this field and will make treatment changes as needed.

I have been fully informed by Dr. ---------- and his staff regarding psychological dependence (addiction) of controlled substance medications, which I understand is rare. I know that some individuals may develop a tolerance to the medications, necessitating a dose increase to achieve the desired effect, and that there is a risk of becoming physically dependent on the medication. This will occur if I am on the medication for several weeks. Therefore, when I need to stop taking the medication, I must do so slowly and under medical supervision or I may have withdrawal symptoms. I have read this contract and the same has been explained to me by Dr. ------------. In addition, I fully understand the consequences of violating this agreement.

Patient Signature: _____

Witness Signature: _____

Date: _____

25 Sexual Dysfunction

Nathan D. Zasler, M.D.

Michael F. Martelli, Ph.D.

TRAUMATIC BRAIN INJURY (TBI) may adversely affect the expression of sexuality because of a variety of different factors. Alterations in physical, cognitive, and behavioral status, as well as communication skills, can all adversely affect expression of sexuality. Brain injury may produce sexual dysfunction at the genital level as well as adversely affect expression of sexuality at the nongenital level. Ultimately, the mediating factors in these functional alterations include disruption of neuroanatomical pathways or aberrations in neurophysiological function, or both, as a result of the TBI. To better comprehend the effect of brain injury on sexuality, one must understand the basic neuroanatomical pathways and neurophysiological mechanisms involved in the mediation of sexual function.

Appropriate neuromedical, psychiatric, and rehabilitative intervention should be available to the TBI patient population to allow for maximal reintegration into preinjury sexual lifestyles at the personal, family, and community levels. Professionals must address the area of sexuality as they do other functional areas of human "performance," including mobility, activities of daily living, and bowel and bladder function, to provide a comprehensive approach to the problem and minimize any resultant functional impairment. By providing appropriate early intervention after trauma, the professional allows for a smoother transition and accommodation to potential postinjury sexuality issues.

Sexual Neuroanatomy and Neurophysiology

To understand how sexual function and sexuality may be adversely affected by TBI, an appreciation of neuroana-

tomical, neurophysiological, and neurochemical correlates of sexual function is critical. By gaining a sense of the myriad interactions required for "normal" sexual function, diagnosis and treatment can be improved when functional difficulties occur.

Sexual Neuroanatomy

Studies involving mapping of neuronal pathways in animal models have allowed scientists to develop a better understanding of the neuronal organization of central nervous system pathways involved in controlling various aspect of sexual functioning. Retrograde and anterograde tracing techniques have allowed the identification of many such pathways. Agents such as neurotropic viruses have been used as neuronal tracers to map entire networks of neurons in various animal models.

The multiplicity of neural networks involved are believed to include structures in the peripheral nervous system (both autonomic and somatic), brainstem, subcortex, and cortex (Table 25–1). Given the propensity for frontotemporal focal cortical contusion and diffuse axonal injury, it is not surprising that sexual dysfunction commonly occurs after any significant brain insult (Horn and Zasler 1990).

Cortical structures, including the paralimbic cortex, are involved in the mediation of sexual function. Stimulation of cortical structures has produced genital hallucinations and erections (MacLean 1975). Certain cortical structures, such as the piriform cortex, are in intimate connection with more primitive "sexual" systems, including the olfactory system. Animal studies have shown that lesions in these areas may produce hypersexuality (Mesulam 1985). The frontal lobes are intimately involved with limbic and paralimbic structures via numerous neural

TABLE 25–1.   Sexual neuroanatomy: substructures and theoretical behavioral correlates

Neuroanatomical structure	Neuroanatomical substructure	Theorized behavioral correlate
Cortical	Piriform cortex	Modulation of drive, initiation, and sexual activation
	Frontal lobes	
	Temporal lobes	
Subcortical	Hippocampus	Modulation of sexual behaviors and genital responses
	Amygdala	
	Septal complex	
	Hypothalamus	
Brainstem	Reticular activating system	Maintenance of arousal and alertness and conduit for information
	Afferent input	
	Efferent output	
Peripheral nervous system	Autonomic	Genital sexual function
	Sympathetic	
	Parasympathetic	
	Somatic	

connections. Frontal injury may result in various behavioral abnormalities. Inferomedial frontal injury may produce disinhibited and sexually inappropriate behavior, whereas dorsolateral frontal injury typically results in impaired sexual initiation (Walker 1976). Clinical experience has revealed that certain patients with frontal injury demonstrate a compromised ability to fantasize that may impede masturbation. Observations derived from patients who have had strokes suggest that right brain injury results in a greater degree of sexual impairment (Coslett and Heilman 1986). However, frontal involvement rather than laterality may be the more significant factor (Horn and Zasler 1990).

Research has demonstrated that lesions in the nondominant hemisphere may lead to a cornucopia of deficits that compromise expression of sexuality, including dysprosody, visuoperceptual problems, and anosognosia (Zasler 1991). Additionally, the nondominant temporal lobe has been theorized to be the sexual activation center for the brain (Cohen et al. 1976). Lesions in the dominant hemisphere may produce aphasias and apraxias, thereby compromising both communication and motor performance (Zasler 1991).

The midbrain central gray or periaqueductal gray has been shown to be involved with control of both male and female sexual function. Stimulation of this area can result in elicitation of sexual responses. These neurons have extensive connections with brainstem sites and also have significant projections to other subcortical structures (McKenna 2001).

Subcortical structures, including the hippocampus, amygdala, septal complex, and hypothalamic nuclei, play important roles in mediation of sexual function. MacLean (1975) hypothesized that penile tumescence is modulated by the hippocampus (Steers 2000). The septal complex has been theorized to be involved in erection as well as pleasurable sexual sensations similar to orgasm (Heath 1964; Penfield and Rasmussen 1950; Steers 2000). The amygdala has been studied quite extensively through ablation and stimulation studies. Among the classic studies were those involving removal of the anterior temporal lobes, resulting in so-called Klüver-Bucy syndrome, with hypersexuality as a behavioral hallmark; discrete lesions of the amygdala, however, do not seem to induce hypersexual behavior. The hypersexuality induced by large lesions of the temporal lobes is likely caused by loss of inhibitory control secondary to destruction of the pyriform cortex.

The anterior hypothalamus is involved in endocrine activity and associated copulatory behaviors. The posterior hypothalamus has been linked functionally to copulatory behaviors and precocious puberty (Bauer 1959; Boller and Frank 1982). The paraventricular nucleus of the hypothalamus contains multiple projections to the autonomic outflow as well as direct projections to pelvic autonomic and somatic efferents. The paraventricular nucleus receives extensive input from the medial preoptic area and may mediate genital as well as nongenital autonomic components of sexual arousal. Thalamic relays from sensory afferents in the ventrolateral and intralaminar nuclei have also been postulated to play important roles in normal sexual functioning (Horn and Zasler 1990). Stimulation of ascending thalamic sensory inputs has been shown to produce erection (MacLean 1975; Walker 1976). Hypersexuality has also been reported as a sequelae of thalamic lesion (Miller et al. 1986). Basal ganglia stimulation may produce complex forms of species-specific ritualistic sexual behaviors (MacLean 1975).

Brainstem structures such as the catecholaminergically "driven" pontine and mesencephalic reticular activating systems are responsible for maintaining arousal and alertness. These systems innervate limbic and frontal structures responsible for many sexually oriented behaviors. The brainstem also serves as the conduit for sexual information carried by afferent and efferent fibers (Horn and Zasler 1990). Injury to brainstem pathways can result in decreased ability to prepare the organism for processing incoming information. This fact takes on additional importance given the evidence supporting the need for activation within certain limbic and cortical structures for normal libido and potency (Coslett and Heilman 1986; Miller et al. 1986). On the basis of current theory, there is a discrete population of neurons in the rostral medulla that tonically inhibit spinal sexual reflexes through serotonergic mediation. Studies have demonstrated a role of the nucleus paragigantocellularis in the medulla in modulating normal sexual functioning (McKenna 2001).

The peripheral autonomic and somatic nervous systems comprise the remaining structures involved with sexual function. Penile and clitoral erection are influenced by sensory innervation through the pudendal nerve, proerectile parasympathetic innervation, antierectile sympathetic innervation, and somatic innervation that contributes to penile rigidity. Autonomic activity is mediated through the sympathetic and parasympathetic nervous systems. Sympathetic fibers emanate from the T10 to L2 level and from the inferior mesenteric ganglion and merge to form the hypogastric plexus and provide innervation to the testes, prostate, seminal vesicles, and vas deferens. Parasympathetic innervation occurs via the nervi erigentes formed by the preganglionic fibers that originate in the intermediolateral nuclei of the sacral spinal cord between S2 and S4. These fibers innervate the penis, prostate, seminal vesicles, and vas deferens. An afferent parasympathetic system also exists via the posterior roots at the S2 to S4 level. The pudendal nerve, which arises from S2 to S4, carries somatic innervation in both sexes and provides motor innervation to pelvic floor musculature with the sensory dermatomes being supplied by S2 to S5. The pudendal nerve becomes the dorsal nerve distally in both the female and the male (Goutier-Smith 1986). In females, the sympathetic nerve supply is mixed; however, the parasympathetic nerve supply is through the pelvic nerves via the uterine and hypogastric plexi. The uterus and ovaries receive only sympathetic innervation, whereas other genital structures receive mixed autonomic innervation (Horn and Zasler 1990; Zasler 1991).

Sexual Neurophysiology

The major pituitary hormones involved in the regulation of sexual function include follicle-stimulating hormone (FSH), luteinizing hormone (LH), and prolactin (PRL). These glycoproteins regulate levels of gonadal hormones; specifically, testosterone in males and estrogen in females. Testosterone secretion is stimulated by the effect of LH on the cells of Leydig in the testes. FSH acts on the seminiferous tubules complementing the effects of LH relative to spermatozoa maturation. FSH and LH in females

are mainly involved with the control of the menstrual cycle. PRL levels are suppressed in the presence of hypothalamic portal system dopamine. PRL secretion is increased secondary to stress, in association with certain types of seizure disorders, and as a consequence of certain medications (mainly antidopaminergic drugs such as neuroleptics). Normally, increases in PRL exert an inhibitory effect on the hypothalamic-pituitary-gonadal axis (Horn and Zasler 1990).

Cells in the arcuate nucleus of the hypothalamus secrete gonadotropin-releasing hormone into the portal circulation and subsequently stimulate the release of both LH and FSH from the anterior pituitary. Gonadotropin-releasing hormone release is regulated by feedback from gonadal hormone levels, PRL levels, and other extrahypothalamic structures in the brainstem and limbic system. Oxytocin levels are greatly increased by sexual arousal. It seems likely that oxytocin may activate penile erection at both hypothalamic and spinal sites.

Gonadal hormones play an integral role in normal sexual maturation and function. The principal male gonadal hormone is testosterone. Androgens, including testosterone, are secreted mainly by the cells of Leydig in the testes but also in smaller amounts by the ovary and adrenal glands. Testosterone is responsible for the development of the male sexual organs, secondary sexual characteristics, and behavioral patterns. Ovarian hormones consist principally of estrogens, progesterones, and small amounts of androgens, and are required for normal female sexual maturation, including sex organ development, secondary sexual characteristics, menstruation, and libido. Please refer to Table 25–2 for a summarization of sexual hormones and their origin and effect.

In addition to neuroendocrine dysfunction, there are multiple neuroactive substances that may affect sexual behavior. The relationship of neurotransmitters and neuromodulators to sexual function is important also because certain pharmacotherapeutic agents may adversely affect sexual function, whereas others may be therapeutically beneficial (Horn and Zasler 1990; Zasler 1991; Zasler and Horn 1990) (Table 25–3).

Review of Research Literature

There is a growing literature on sexual dysfunction in persons after TBI. Bond (1976), for example, examined issues of psychosocial changes arising from severe brain injury using interview assessments. He found that the level of sexual activity was not related to posttraumatic amnesia, level of physical disability, or level of cognitive impairment. Specific sexual function patterns were not examined. Rosenbaum

TABLE 25–2. Sexual neurophysiology: hormone source and effect

Hormone	Site of release	Physiological effect
Gonadotropin-releasing hormone	Hypothalamus	Stimulate release of LH/FSH
FSH	Pituitary	Sperm maturation
LH	Pituitary	Increase testosterone secretion
Prolactin	Pituitary	Inhibit hypothalamic-pituitary-gonadal axis
Testosterone	Testes	Primary and secondary male sexual characteristics and libido
Estrogen and progesterone	Ovaries	Primary and secondary female sexual characteristics and libido

Note. FSH=follicle-stimulating hormone; LH=luteinizing hormone.

TABLE 25–3. Sexual pharmacology: drug class and clinical effect

Drug class	Clinical effect
Anabolic steroid Methandrostenolone	(–) Decreased libido
Anorexiant Amphetamines	(–) Decreased libido, impotence, ejaculatory dysfunction, anorgasmia
Anticholinergic Oxybutynin Scopolamine	(–) Inhibited erection and ejaculation, decreased libido
Anticonvulsant Carbamazepine Phenytoin	(–) Impotence and decreased libido
Antidepressant Nortriptyline Doxepin	(–) Decreased libido, delayed orgasm in women, ejaculatory and erectile dysfunction
Antihypertensive β-Blockers Methyldopa Clonidine	(–) Impotence, decreased libido, and ejaculatory dysfunction
Antiparkinsonian Levodopa Bromocriptine	(+) Generally increased libido, may also improve erectile function
Antipsychotic Haloperidol Risperidone Olanzapine Quetiapine	(–) Impotence, decreased libido, ejaculatory dysfunction, hyperprolactinemia, and priapism
Antispasticity Baclofen	(–) Impotence, ejaculatory dysfunction, and menstrual irregularities
Diuretic Thiazides	(–) Decreased libido and impotence
Estrogens	(–) Decreased libido in both sexes
H2 antihistamine Ranitidine	(–) Decreased libido, erectile dysfunction
Nonsteroidal antiinflammatory Naproxen	(–) Erectile problems and anejaculation
Noradrenergic agonist Yohimbine	(+) Increased libido in both sexes

(continued)

and Najenson (1976) interviewed wives of wartime patients with either brain or spinal cord injuries (SCIs). Reduced sexual function and emotional distress were present more often in the brain injury group relative to a group of uninjured individuals. The greatest level of mood disturbance was found for the wives of men with brain injury when compared with the wives of the spinal cord–injured group and the control group. There was no significant relationship between the locus of injury and the specific area of sexual dysfunction. Oddy et al. (1978) studied 50 adults with TBI who were at least 6 months postinjury and had a minimum of 24 hours of posttraumatic amnesia. One-half of the 12 married patients reported an increase in sexual intercourse, and one-half reported a decrease. In a subsequent study, Oddy and Humphrey (1980) investigated alterations in sexual behavior 1 year after injury. Slightly less than 50% of spouses reported that they were significantly less affectionate toward their injured partners. Lezak (1978) reported that many patients demonstrated completely absent libido whereas others reported increases in sexual drive. Generally, altered sexual interest as well as other commonly seen posttraumatic cognitive-behavioral problems contributed to family and marital difficulties. Social adjustment 2 years after severe TBI was assessed by Weddell et al. (1980). They interviewed relatives of a group of patients after they completed a rehabilitation program. Although no direct inquiries were made regarding sexuality issues, personality changes were examined. Irritability was the most frequent behavioral alteration, followed by altered expression of affection. This study reinforced per-

TABLE 25–3. Sexual pharmacology: drug class and clinical effect *(continued)*

Drug class	Clinical effect
Phenoxybenzamine	(–) Ejaculatory dysfunction
Progestin	(–) Decreased libido, impotence
Medroxyprogesterone	
Serotonergic agonists and atypical/mixed antidepressants	(–)/(+) In general, decreased libido; however, reports of increased libido have occurred. Abnormal ejaculation/orgasm, dyspareunia, impotence, painful erection.
Trazodone	
Selective serotonin reuptake inhibitors	
Mirtazapine	
Venlafaxine	
Bupropion	

Note. +=positive; –=negative.

ceptions regarding the deleterious effects of poor interpersonal skills on community reentry and psychosocial reintegration commonly seen in survivors of significant TBI.

One of the best early studies on alterations in sexual function after brain injury was done by Kosteljanetz et al. (1981) of a group of 19 male patients who had experienced concussions. They found that a majority of patients (53%) reported reduced libido and that a lesser but still significant percentage (42%) reported erectile dysfunction (ED). A positive correlation was noted between reports of sexual dysfunction and intellectual impairment. A survey of 40 wives and mothers of male patients with brain injury (not necessarily after trauma) by Mauss-Clum and Ryan (1981) found that a large proportion (47%) of the respondents reported that the survivor was either disinterested in sex or preoccupied with it. Forty-two percent of wives also reported that they had no sexual outlet. Miller et al. (1986) suggested that sexual behavior changes were related to injury neuropathology; specifically, medial basal-frontal or diencephalic injury was more highly correlated with hypersexuality, whereas limbic injury was more likely to result in altered sexual preference. Kreutzer and Zasler (1989) developed the Psychosexual Assessment Questionnaire and administered it to 21 sexually active male patients after TBI. This 11-item questionnaire assesses changes in sexual behavior, affect, self-esteem, and heterosexual relationships. The majority of these patients reported negative changes in sexual behavior, including decreased libido, ED, and decreased frequency of intercourse. There was no relationship between the level of mood change and altered sexual

behavior. Despite negative changes, there was evidence that the quality of the marital relationships was preserved.

Garden et al. (1990) studied 11 men and 4 women who had sustained TBI at least 2 months before the evaluation. Both the spouses and the patients completed a sexual history and function questionnaire. A variety of factors were assessed. Only a few significant positive correlations were found. Intercourse frequency decreased for 75% of female patients, whereas 55% of the male patients reported a decline. Although male genital sexual dysfunction rarely was reported, female spouses reported a significant decline in their ability to achieve orgasm after their partner was injured. O'Carroll et al. (1991) examined the psychosexual and psychosocial sequelae of TBI in a series of 36 patients followed for up to 4 years after injury. Using several previously validated scales, they assessed both patients and partners. Approximately one-half of all male patients scored within the dysfunctional range on the psychosexual profiles. The major psychosexual complaint was decreased frequency of sexual intimacy, including intercourse. There was a clear relationship noted between advancing patient age and psychosexual dysfunction. Neurologic injury severity did not correlate highly with psychosexual complaint rate. Time since injury was positively correlated with the degree of sexual dissatisfaction among male survivors of TBI in this study.

An excellent study by Sandel et al. (1996) demonstrated that, in a group of 52 outpatients with a history of TBI, persons with frontal lobe lesions reported an overall higher level of sexual satisfaction and functioning than those individuals without such lesions. Overall, persons with TBI in this study reported lower orgasm and sexual drive than noninjured individuals on the Derogatis Interview of Sexual Function. Sexual arousal dropped off with time postinjury. Perhaps counterintuitively, persons with right hemispheric lesions reported higher sexual arousal and sexual experiences. Elliott and Biever (1996) reviewed the literature dealing with TBI and sexuality and mainly focused on the behavioral consequences of the injury. In particular, they discussed problems with impulsivity, sexual inappropriateness, libidinal alterations, and sexual dysfunction.

A number of studies dealing with sexuality and TBI have been published by the Israeli researcher Aloni and her group at Beit Loewenstein Hospital (Aloni and Katz 1998, 1999; Aloni et al. 1999). These authors have recognized the complex underpinnings of sexual dysfunction in persons with TBI relative to the contributions of primary versus secondary sexual problems. In their 1999 study, Aloni et al. concluded that in the early postinjury phase, most individuals after severe TBI had relatively high self-ratings of self-confidence, sex appeal, and mood levels. Only 7.7% reported sexual function difficulties. The authors concluded that, on the basis of their findings and the literature on the high incidence of sexual complaints in the more chronic phases post-TBI, sexual dysfunction seen in the later stages of recovery was most probably because of "reactive behavioral changes" and not underlying organic brain damage. They also went on to argue in their second article published that year in *Brain Injury* that it was difficult to accurately differentiate between primary and secondary sexual problems after TBI and the manner in which each problem might affect sexual function.

In a study examining partner relations and functioning after SCI as well as TBI, Kreuter et al. (1998b) found that the majority (55%) of relationships in persons with TBI were established after injury. Both SCI and TBI were associated with significantly more depressive feelings compared with a noninjured control group. Overall quality of life ratings were lowest in persons with SCI. Single persons rated themselves significantly lower on global quality of life measures than those with partners. Another study by the same first author (Kreuter et al. 1998a) looked at sexual adjustment after TBI and its predictors. Ninety-two persons were studied (65 men and 27 women). Median time postinjury was 9 years. Of note is that more than one-half of the participants had a stable partner relationship at the time of the investigation. A high degree of physical independence and maintained sexual ability were the most important predictors for sexual adjustment. Common complaints included decreased erectile ability, diminished orgasmic capability, and decreased frequency of sexual intercourse.

A long-term outcome study of a small male population of TBI survivors (*n*=14) with complaints of sexual dysfunction authored by Crowe and Ponsford (1999) found that those with TBI scored lower than non-brain-injured control subjects (*n*=14) on the Sexual Imagery subscale of the Imaginary Processes Inventory. It should be noted that the researchers corrected for the level of depression via analysis of covariance. Of note, was the fact that persons with TBI had lower levels of performance on the Sexual Imagery subscale of the Imaginary Processes Inventory than matched control subjects after correction for mood. The researchers concluded that sexual arousal disturbances might therefore exist above and beyond the disturbances to affect associated with the psychosocial effects of the TBI. That is, factors other than mood were likely mediating reported alterations in sexual function.

A long-term, retrospective outcome study examining sexual dysfunction after TBI was authored by Hibbard et al. in 2000 that examined a large group of TBI survivors (*n*=322), both men and women, as well as a control group of nondisabled individuals (*n*=264). They found that age was the only variable that related to reports of sexual dif-

ficulties in individuals with TBI and men without disability. Age at onset and severity of injury were negatively correlated to reports of sexual difficulties in persons with TBI. In men with TBI and without disability, the most sensitive predictor of sexual dysfunction was level of depression. For women without disability, an endocrine disorder was the most sensitive predictor of sexual dysfunction. For women with TBI, age at injury and milder injuries predicted greater difficulties, yet depression and an endocrine disorder combined were the most sensitive predictor of sexual dysfunction. The authors concluded by emphasizing the need for broader based assessment of sexual functioning in persons post-TBI in conjunction with implementation of treatment studies to enhance sexual functioning in persons after these types of injuries.

In a paper authored by Bell and Pepping (2001), the authors pointed out the lack of a more adequate research data on women and TBI. They noted that, although most of the effects of TBI are gender neutral, there are a plethora of issues unique to women relative to endocrine, reproduction, and sexual functioning. Additionally, they endorsed the view that TBI in women would affect family dynamics differently than in men because of female roles of wife, mother, and daughter.

There is a great deal of literature on temporal lobe epilepsy (TLE); however, the patient populations that formed the bases of these studies were typically quite heterogeneous and not necessarily posttraumatic. However, given the frequency of post-TBI TLE (more than 20% of all posttraumatic epilepsy), it is important to mention the effect of TLE on sexual behavior. Herzog (1984) found that 40%–58% of males with TLE were impotent or hyposexual, and up to 40% of women had menstrual irregularities. Blumer (1970a) reported that 70% of patients with TLE reported sexual problems. The most chronic alteration in sexual behavior was hyposexuality, indicative of a loss of libido. Anecdotal observations suggest that mesial temporal involvement may be correlated with libidinal alterations in TLE; however, no well-controlled studies have confirmed this finding (Blumer 1970b; Blumer and Walker 1967). Less commonly, hypersexuality (which may follow surgical intervention or be related to anticonvulsant medication), homosexual behavior, and ictal or postictal sexual arousal have been reported.

In summary, the literature in the area of sexuality and sexual dysfunction in patients with TBI is developing slowly, with a significant number of studies being published in the last 10 years or so. Few studies have focused specifically on sexual behavior, and many of these have disparate results. Many of the studies are anecdotal reports and do not provide empirical evidence to guide clinical decision making or relate information to patients and families. It is not surprising that alterations in sexuality as well as sexual function occur in patients with TBI. As of now, there is only a sense of the magnitude of this area of functional deficit, which is unfortunate given the importance of sexuality to most people, whether single or married.

Clinical Evaluation

Problems occurring after TBI can result from a number of factors, including nongenital and genital dysfunction. Genital dysfunction can include ED, ejaculatory problems, orgasmic dysfunction, vaginal lubrication problems, and vaginismus. Nongenital problems that may adversely affect sexual intimacy include sensorimotor deficits, communication deficits, perceptual deficits, limited joint range of motion, neurogenic bowel and bladder dysfunction, dysphagia with or without problems controlling secretions, motor dyspraxias, posttraumatic behavioral deficits, as well as alterations in self-image and self-esteem (Zasler and Horn 1990).

A decreased serum testosterone level, in an otherwise healthy male, often first manifests as a decrease in libido and later as impotence and infertility. There may also be loss of secondary sexual characteristics. Females with acquired hormonal dysregulation may present with oligomenorrhea or amenorrhea, infertility, and signs of relative androgen access, such as acne and hirsutism (Horn and Zasler 1990). It is critical that professionals treating patients after TBI recognize clinical presentations suggestive of neuroendocrine dysfunction.

Clinicians working with this patient population must have an appreciation for the appropriate assessment and management of this class of functional deficits. One protocol that has been proposed is the General Rehabilitation Assessment Sexuality Profile, which divides assessment into the sexual history, sexual physical examination, and clinical diagnostic testing (Zasler and Horn 1990) (Table 25–4).

Sexual History

A thorough sexual history defines needs, expectations, and behavior. Additionally, it identifies problems, misconceptions, and areas for education, counseling, and reassurance in relation to sexuality issues. When possible, interviews should be conducted with both the patient and the sexual partner. The assessment should include demographic and personal information as well as past medical history to identify medical disorders that potentially affect sexual function. Questions pertaining to premorbid sexual functioning, practices, and relationships should be

TABLE 25–4. General Rehabilitation Assessment Sexuality Profile

Sexual history

Interview both patient and partner if possible.

Obtain information about preinjury medical and sexual status and performance.

Delineate sexuality concerns.

Provide a private room and take your time.

Use appropriate vocabulary.

Clarify sexual preference.

Sexual physical examination

Assess general mobility and activities of daily living.

Assess general hygiene.

Inspection and palpation of genitalia.

Neurourological assessment: rectal examination, sensory testing, lumbosacral reflex arc testing.

Clinical sexual diagnostic testing

Urodynamics

Male: penile biothesiometry, dorsal nerve somatosensory-evoked potential, nocturnal penile tumescence, and response to intracavernosal pharmacotherapy

Female: photoplethysmography, thermal clearance, and heat electrode

Neuroendocrine evaluation: follicle-stimulating hormone, luteinizing hormone, prolactin with testosterone (male) and estradiol and dehydroepiandrosterone (female)

Source. Adapted from Zasler ND, Horn LJ: "Rehabilitative Management of Sexual Dysfunction." *The Journal of Head Trauma Rehabilitation* 5:14–24, 1990.

asked. Both partners should be questioned about genital function as well as sexuality concerns, including birth control, fertility, genital dysfunction, libidinal alterations, and others. Sexuality issues may not be important for all patients. This fact must be recognized by treating professionals. Key points when interviewing include provision of a private atmosphere, not rushing the interview, being frank yet empathic, and using nonconfrontational techniques and appropriate vocabulary relative to the patient's educational and cultural background (e.g., "do you suffer from premature ejaculation?" versus "do you cum too quickly?"). The clinician should avoid putting the patient in conflict with religious or moral beliefs by, for example, advocating that a practicing Catholic use birth control. Last, the status of an individual's sexual preference should be clarified and discussed. Ultimately, the interview can serve as a foundation for demonstrating to the patient that he or she has a right to be sexual and that sexual expression resulting in intimacy, not necessarily vaginal intercourse, is the goal of the process (Zasler 1991).

Sexual Physical Examination

The sexual physical examination begins when the clinician first sees the patient. Mobility deficits may provide clues as to physical limitations that may adversely affect sexuality and sexual function. Of particular importance are the flexibility of the hips and degree of adductor spasticity. The clinician should note the patient's general hygiene status and use of adaptive equipment. Obviously, ruling out other preexisting neurological or medical conditions that might contribute to sexual dysfunction is critical as well as assessing for posttraumatic neuromedical sequelae, including epilepsy, neuroendocrine dysfunction, and affective disorders.

The genitals should be examined from both a neurological and non-neurological standpoint by a physician comfortable in these examination procedures. In the female, direct visualization of the genitalia followed by a bimanual examination is critical. The vaginal walls must be evaluated for tone and mucosal alterations. In the male, the clinician must palpate the penis to assess for plaques as found in Peyronie's disease. Testicular presence in the scrotal sacs and size and consistency should all be evaluated. In both males and females, assessment of hair distribution in the genital region and in locations of secondary sexual hair growth is paramount to rule out possible endocrinopathies that could be either primary or secondary in nature. The neurological assessment of the genitalia includes a rectal examination, sensory testing, and assessment of lumbosacral reflex integrity. The skilled clinician can use the information from bedside testing to guide recommendations as well as prognosticate genital sexual function relative to the neurological insult in question (Zasler 1991; Zasler and Horn 1990).

Clinical Sexual Diagnostic Testing

Urodynamics can help obtain a better understanding of the integrity of genital innervation. Afferent neurological assessment can be performed with penile biothesiometry or dorsal nerve somatosensory-evoked potentials, or both. Penile biothesiometry, which measures the vibration perception threshold of the skin of the penis, is performed using a portable hand-held electromagnetic vibration device with a fixed frequency and variable amplitude. A dorsal nerve somatosensory-evoked potential provides an objective physiological assessment of the entire pudendal nerve afferent pathway. Efferent neurological assessment, whether motor or autonomic, can be performed in a gross manner via nocturnal penile tumescence or response to intracavernosal pharmacotherapy, or both (Padma-Nathan 1988).

Female sexual clinical assessment is less sophisticated and has been conducted with various techniques. Photoplethysmography, thermal clearance, and heat electrode techniques have been used to assess vaginal hemodynamics via indirect evaluation of vaginal wall blood flow parameters (Levin 1980). These techniques can be used to treat orgasmic and arousal deficits via biofeedback training (Levin 1980; Zasler 1991; Zasler and Horn 1990).

It is crucial to ascertain whether a patient is taking any prescribed drugs excessively or using illicit drugs in a way that may adversely affect sexual functioning. Alcohol, although often not seen as an agent of abuse or illicit substance, is the most widely used aphrodisiac in the United States. Acute and/or chronic substance misuse or abuse may affect sexual functioning in a variety of ways and therefore must be clarified as part of the relevant history. Other illicit drugs that must be inquired about include marijuana, cocaine, opiates, and amphetamines, among numerous others.

Initial laboratory evaluation should include assessment of FSH, LH, PRL, and free testosterone in males. Given the pulsatile cycle of the release of these hormones, it has been suggested that three samples be obtained approximately 20 minutes apart and then be combined for a single measurement. In females, the same hormones should be assessed in addition to estradiol and dehydroepiandrosterone. Because of normal menstrual variations, the best time for this assessment is during the early follicular phase. Provocative testing of pituitary function with such agents as thyrotropin-releasing hormone and gonadotropin-releasing hormone may be useful to assess for more subtle aspects of neuroendocrine dysfunction (Grossman and Sanfield 1994).

An awareness of appropriate neuroendocrine tests relative to specific clinical presentations is paramount for any practitioner working with patients with TBI (Table 25–5). Clinicians should keep in mind that other factors, such as medications or physiological stress in patients with acute TBI, may contribute to neuroendocrine abnormalities.

Clinical Management

The management of sexual dysfunction must take into consideration the many issues that may directly or indi-

TABLE 25–5. Posttraumatic neuroendocrine dysfunction: clinical presentation and appropriate laboratory evaluation

Clinical syndrome	Clinical presentation (possible symptoms)	Neuroendocrine evaluation
Male postpubertal sexual dysfunction	Decreased libido	FSH, LH, PRL, free testosterone
	Impotence	R/O associated medical condition
	Ejaculatory dysfunction	
	Infertility	
Female postpubertal sexual dysfunction	Oligomenorrhea	FSH, LH, PRL, estradiol, and dehydroepiandrosterone
	Amenorrhea	
	Virilization	R/O associated medical condition
	Galactorrhea	
	Decreased libido	
	Recurrent spontaneous abortions	
Male prepubertal sexual dysfunction	Delay in development of secondary sexual characteristics	FSH, LH, PRL, free testosterone
	Precocious puberty	
Female prepubertal sexual dysfunction	Delay in development of secondary sexual characteristics	FSH, LH, PRL, estradiol, and dehydroepiandrosterone
	Precocious puberty	
Sexual dysfunction associated with temporolimbic epilepsy	Male: impotence, decreased libido, and endocrine disturbances	Same as above
	Female: menstrual irregularities, endocrine disturbances, and polycystic ovarian syndrome	Same as above
		R/O drug side effect

Note. FSH=follicle-stimulating hormone; LH=luteinizing hormone; PRL=prolactin; R/O=rule out.

rectly contribute to alterations in sexual function after TBI, including neuroendocrine, nongenital, and genital dysfunction. Clinicians should be aware of how subjective complaints may provide clues to guiding treatment. Additionally, adequate knowledge of the potential benefits and side effects of pharmacological agents in this patient population is critical in optimizing outcome (see Table 25–3). There are also multiple issues related to sexuality after TBI that require management through counseling interventions, including matters of birth control, sex education, competency to engage in sexual activity, sexual abuse, and sexual "release."

Neuroendocrine Dysfunction

Neuroendocrine dysfunction may occur after TBI; however, the general clinical experience has been that this phenomenon is relatively rare in the TBI population. In

postpubertal females, cyclic administration of oral estrogen–progesterone preparations restores the menstrual cycle, maintains secondary sexual characteristics, and reduces the risk for osteoporosis. In the postpubertal male, hypogonadism may be treated with intramuscular testosterone (200–400 mg) replacement, typically given every 2–4 weeks. In cases of delayed puberty, treatment should begin during adolescence; males are typically treated with human chorionic gonadotropin (500–1,000 United States Pharmacopeia units three times per week for the first 3 weeks, followed by 500 United States Pharmacopeia units two times per week for 1–2 years) and subsequently followed by maintenance testosterone therapy. In females, cyclic estrogen and progesterone therapy should be instituted to establish menses and secondary sexual characteristics (Zasler and Horn 1990). Clinicians should be familiar with the myriad symptoms that may be indicators of underlying neuroendocrine dysfunction and the appropriate laboratory evaluation of those conditions (see Table 25–5).

Nongenital Dysfunction

Other areas of nongenital neurological impairment must also be assessed relative to treatment options, whether pharmacological, surgical, or compensatory. Sensorimotor deficits, cognitive and behavioral deficits, language-based alterations, changes in libido, as well as neurogenic bowel and bladder dysfunction can all be addressed by the clinician because they affect sexual expression (Zasler and Horn 1990). Libidinal changes can be treated behaviorally and pharmacologically. Hormonal treatment or serotonergic agents, or both, can be used for hypersexuality. Medroxyprogesterone acetate has been used in varying doses to suppress both aggressive behavior and sexual arousal (100–200 mg/week typically preceded by a loading dose of 400 mg/week over the first 2–3 weeks). There are numerous case reports in the literature regarding the use of "chemical castration" for hypersexuality after TBI. However, we are aware of no controlled, prospective studies (Britton 1998). There are also ethical, medicolegal, and patient rights issues that have been debated as related to the use of such agents as medroxyprogesterone that must be adequately discussed and considered by the treating clinician. We have had some success with serotonergic agents such as trazodone hydrochloride for suppression of libido in doses typically ranging from 3.0 to 5.0 mg/kg body weight. There has also been some recent literature on the use of selective serotonin reuptake inhibitors (SSRIs) in the treatment of sexual dysfunction, but none that we are aware of specific to post-TBI impairments. Clearly, there is a much larger literature on the adverse sexual side effects of this drug class than there is on the therapeutic use of such agents for treatment of sexual dysfunction (Montejo et al. 2001). SSRIs, however, tend to have a dose-dependent adverse effect on sexual functioning, including suppression of libido; however, other mechanisms, including reuptake mechanisms, anticholinergic side effects, inhibition of nitric oxide synthetase, and propensity for accumulation over time, must be considered (Rosen et al. 1999). LH-releasing hormone agonists have also been used for reducing sexual desire (Bradford 2001).

Noradrenergic agonists or hormonal supplementation, or both, have been used for hyposexuality, particularly in males (Blumer and Migeon 1975; Lehne 1986; McConaghy et al. 1988; Zasler and Horn 1990).

Clinicians should recall that patients with temporolimbic epilepsy may present with alterations in neuroendocrine status and sexual function. The presence of characteristic "temporal lobe personality" traits such as circumstantiality, viscosity, and obsessionalism in combination with altered sexuality, even in the absence of "clinical" seizures and/or electrographic seizures, suggests consideration for treatment with a psychoactive anticonvulsant such as carbamazepine or valproate (Gualtieri 1991). Patients with Klüver-Bucy syndrome have also shown hypersexual behaviors as part of this symptom complex that respond in a favorable fashion to treatment with psychotropic anticonvulsants such as carbamazepine (Stewart 1985).

Genital Dysfunction

Genital sexual dysfunction after TBI may take a number of potential forms. Males may present with erectile, ejaculatory, and/or orgasmic dysfunction. The present state of the art in neurological management of ED focuses on one of five main treatment categories: oral therapies such as phosphodiesterase type 5 inhibitors (e.g., sildenafil, tadalafil, and vardenafil) as well as the dopaminergic agonist apomorphine (Dinsmoor 2004), penile prostheses, intracavernosal pharmacotherapy, MUSE (medicated urethral system for erection), and external management (Meinhardt et al. 1999). Given the relative ease of use and good side-effect profile, agents like sildenafil (Jarrow et al. 1999) may become the mainstay of treatment for neurogenic ED after TBI; however, there are no studies that have looked specifically at this drug's application to ED in this population. Recently, some authors have found that tachyphylaxis effects may limit the long-term use of sildenafil (El-Galley et al. 2001). Enteral agents have been used, including noradrenergic agonists such as yohimbine (5.4–6.0 mg po tid) (Morales et al. 1982) as well as other drug classes such as dopamine agonists. Work is ongoing relative to the efficacy of enteral agents in patients with ED, including, but not limited to, sublingual apomorphine, oral phentolamine, and vardenafil (a phosphodiesterase type-5 inhibitor) (Rosen 2000). Problems with premature ejaculation should be first addressed behaviorally to assess how much of the problem is functionally based. Methods such as the "squeeze" technique, which involves application of pressure to the penile shaft just proximal to the glans penis when the male feels that he is about to ejaculate, can be taught to prolong the time until ejaculation. On occasion, medication could be considered for the male patient who complains of premature ejaculation; this could include topical anesthetics to the penile shaft (5%–10% lidocaine) or anticholinergic (imipramine, 100–200 mg/day) and sympatholytic medication (phenoxybenzamine, 10 mg bid to tid) administered orally. Recent literature and experience have also shown a role for SSRIs in the treatment of premature ejaculation (McMahon and Touma 1999). Orgasmic dysfunction is generally approached from a behavioral standpoint in both men and women. Females may complain of alterations in vaginal lubrication or orgasmic dysfunction, or both. Inadequate vaginal lubrication can generally be treated with artificial lubrication using water-soluble products. Behavioral therapy, including imagery and body exploration and sensitization training, may benefit some females who have arousal or orgasmic dysfunction (Halvorsen and Metz 1992; Sarwer and Durlak 1997; Zasler 1991).

Physicians should be aware of how certain medications may produce iatrogenic sexual dysfunction. Antipsychotic medications (both typical and atypical), antihypertensives, and anticholinergic medications are some of the more common "culprits" (Clayton and Shen 1998). Other drugs, including histamine-2 receptor blockers, may produce adverse effects through their antiandrogenic effect and increased central PRL. Anticonvulsant medication such as phenytoin may decrease circulating levels of sex hormone via induction of hepatic enzyme systems, resulting in a relative secondary hypogonadism. Assessment of medications and appropriate substitutions to optimize sexual functioning is critical in the physician's role in the management of sexuality issues in this population (Finger et al. 1997).

Counseling Issues

There are numerous controversial issues pertaining to sexuality in patients with TBI that affect medical, ethical, and legal fronts, thereby obliging clinicians to address them. Among these issues are matters pertaining to sex education, including birth control, sexually transmitted disease, sexual abuse, sexual release, and masturbation. Other issues that may arise include decisions regarding sterilization as well as more germane and "socially acceptable" issues such as dating, marriage, sexual preference issues, child-rearing matters, and psychosocial behavior.

Quite frequently, TBI patients assume that they will be unable to find a compatible sexual companion because they have had a brain injury. Various recommendations can be provided to maximize community reintegration, including attending church or synagogue functions, brain injury survivor meetings, local organization social gatherings, or participating in dating services for people with disabilities such as Handicapped Introductions and Date-Able (Garden 1988). Professionals also can assist clients by teaching or "reteaching" the psychosocial graces that

may many times be adversely affected by significant TBI before attempting more aggressive community reentry efforts. Responsible decisions regarding sexual relations are critical for both single and married people with brain injury, and ongoing follow-up is essential to ensure that there is compliance with the recommendations as well as sex life satisfaction.

Generally, patients who have been evaluated as competent and who have the capacity to understand and remember the ramifications of their actions are probably capable of being sexually active in a responsible fashion. Sexually active patients, whether male or female, should be instructed in the appropriate use of condoms given the ever-present fear of acquired immunodeficiency syndrome.

For patients demonstrating especially poor "sexual judgment" and/or uncontrollable sexual behaviors that are resistant to other treatments (e.g., indiscriminate masturbation or hypersexuality), the professional may need to consider either chemical or surgical sterilization. Given the variability in state laws regarding competency/capacity issues and decisions regarding sterilization, it is recommended that professionals consult legal counsel regarding each case in question.

Families and patients should be counseled regarding alternatives for sexual release, particularly for patients without active sexual partners. Masturbation should be discussed as one potential option as long as it is done in an appropriate social context. For those clients requiring external stimulation to aid in successful masturbation, sexual stimuli (e.g., erotic reading materials, pictures, videotapes, and telephone sex services) can be provided. Obviously, many of the aforementioned suggestions may not be acceptable to certain people because of their moral or religious beliefs, or both, but they should be discussed with all patients and families as appropriate.

Some health care professionals and family members have advocated, as well as condoned, the use of sexual surrogates and prostitutes in addressing the sexual frustrations of people after TBI who might otherwise never find sexual partners. Although there are differences between surrogates and prostitutes, many state laws do not make a legal distinction. In an era of high awareness regarding sexually transmitted diseases and legal liability, most professionals seem to be shying away from making use of this class of "community resources." Professionals should counsel patient and family alike regarding dealing with alterations in sexual preference, which are more commonly a result of lack of heterosexual partners (for heterosexual patients) than a result of organically based alterations in sexual orientation because of the TBI itself (Miller et al. 1986). Appropriate counseling for heterosexuals and homosexuals alike should be available. Counseling clinicians should always inquire about the patient's sexual orientation. All patients, regardless of sexual preference, should be counseled on high-risk sexual practices.

Sexual abuse of persons with TBI and/or by persons with TBI may be encountered on occasion. Although poorly documented because of a general trend toward not studying things that make people feel uncomfortable, clinicians must recognize abuse when they see it. Health care professionals are legally and morally obligated to ensure that the proper authorities are notified if a person with TBI, a family member, an attendant, or an acquaintance is engaged in sexual misconduct or abuse, or both. If sexual abuse is suspected, proper measures should be taken to either remove the patient from the environment in question or remove the suspected perpetrator from the patient's immediate milieu.

Family Issues

Sexuality is a classic example of an integrative function, requiring cognitive, physical, and psychobehavioral components. A double sensitivity often exists regarding sexuality and disability (Chigier 1980), which often prevents the person with a brain injury from being seen as a sexual being. All people, whether patient, family, or treating professionals, must learn to accept the fact that sexuality issues exist for most survivors, regardless of injury severity, and must be dealt with relative to sexual function issues, sexual rights, rehabilitation interventions, and family or attendant counseling. Family issues may arise in a variety of situations, including single individuals living with parents, married people living with spouses, and parents living with children with brain injuries (Zasler and Kreutzer 1991).

Sexual problems after TBI can occur in at least three different scenarios. First, people with brain injury (classically, adolescents or young adults) may be living with their parents. They commonly may be unable to maintain sexual relationships established before their injury or to establish new relationships after the injury, or both. Sexual problems for these individuals include finding a suitable partner as well as diminished physical capabilities.

Second, some TBI survivors are unable to maintain previously established relationships. These people may be married, living with a significant other, or single and dating. Diminished frequency of intercourse and physical dysfunction may stem from emotional or physical problems.

Third, sexual problems may arise between married relatives of the injured person and may be attributable to the negative consequences of brain injury in other family members (e.g., children, siblings, or parents). The stressors associated with alteration of preinjury roles related to caring for the injured person may cause a variety of psychological reactions, including burnout, feelings of guilt, and displacement, to name only a few, resulting in spousal alienation, sexual disinterest, and, potentially, sexual dysfunction.

Conclusion

Professionals are only beginning to examine the neurological and functional ramifications of TBI on sexual function. Presently, there is a relative dearth of information on which clinicians can base prognostication, assessment, or treatment; however, the knowledge base is expanding slowly but surely. Better acknowledgment of the importance of sexuality and sexual function to quality of life may stimulate researchers and clinicians alike to allocate more resources to answering many of the questions that remain. The treating physician must be able to address sexuality issues effectively by relying on an approach that holistically defines problematic areas, determines what changes can realistically be made, and works toward effecting those changes and accepting what cannot be changed. In the interim, clinicians and researchers alike should remain cognizant of the importance of sexual expression relative to other areas of human function after TBI. Awareness, in and of itself, will provide an impetus for further critical examination of this important area of psychophysiological function.

References

Aloni R, Katz S: Sexual function after traumatic brain injury. Harefuah 134:816–821, 1998

Aloni R, Katz S: A review of the effect of traumatic brain injury on the human sexual response. Brain Inj 13:269–280, 1999

Aloni A, Keren O, Cohen M, et al: Incidence of sexual dysfunction in TBI patients during the early post-traumatic inpatient rehabilitation phase. Brain Inj 13:89–97, 1999

Bauer HG: Endocrine and metabolic conditions related to pathology in the hypothalamus: a review. J Nerv Ment Dis 28:323–328, 1959

Bell KR, Pepping M: Women and traumatic brain injury. Phys Med Rehabil Clin N Am 12:169–182, 2001

Blumer D: Changes of sexual behavior related to temporal lobe disorders in man. J Sex Res 6:173–180, 1970a

Blumer D: Hypersexual episodes in temporal lobe epilepsy. Am J Psychiatry 126:1099–1106, 1970b

Blumer D, Migeon C: Hormone and hormonal agents in the treatment of aggression. J Nerv Ment Dis 160:127–137, 1975

Blumer D, Walker AE: Sexual behavior in temporal lobe epilepsy. Arch Neurol 16:31–43, 1967

Boller F, Frank E: Sexual Dysfunction in Neurological Disorders: Diagnosis, Management and Rehabilitation. New York, Raven, 1982

Bond MR: Assessment of psychosocial outcome of severe head injury. Acta Neurochir 34:57–70, 1976

Bradford JM: The neurobiology, neuropharmacology and pharmacological treatment of the paraphilias and compulsive sexual behavior. Can J Psychiatry. 46:24–25, 2001

Britton KR: Medroxyprogesterone in the treatment of aggressive hypersexual behavior in traumatic brain injury. Brain Inj 12:703–707, 1998

Chigier E: Sexuality of physically disabled people. Clin Obstet Gynaecol 7:325–343, 1980

Clayton DO, Shen WW: Psychotropic drug-induced sexual function disorders: diagnosis, incidence and management. Drug Saf 19:299–312, 1998

Cohen H, Rosen R, Goldstein L: Electroencephalographic laterality changes during human sexual orgasm. Arch Sex Behav 5:189–199, 1976

Coslett H, Heilman K: Male sexual function: impairment after right hemisphere stroke. Arch Neurol 43:1036–1039, 1986

Crowe SF, Ponsford J: The role of imagery in sexual arousal disturbances in the male traumatically brain injured individual. Brain Inj 13:347–354, 1999

Dinsmoor W: Treatment of erectile dysfunction. Int J STD AIDS 15:215–221, 2004

El-Galley R, Rutland H, Talic R, et al: Long-term efficacy of sildenafil and tachyphylaxis effect. J Urol 166:927–931, 2001

Elliott ML, Biever LS: Head injury and sexual function. Brain Inj 10:703–717, 1996

Finger WW, Lund M, Slagle MA: Medications that may contribute to sexual disorders: a guide to assessment and treatment in family practice. J Fam Pract 44:33–43, 1997

Garden FH: Dating services for the disabled: Sexuality Update Newsletter. American Congress of Rehabilitation Medicine 1:4, 1988

Garden FH, Bontke CF, Hoffman M: Sexual functioning and marital adjustment after traumatic brain injury. J Head Trauma Rehabil 5:52–59, 1990

Goutier-Smith PC: Sexual function and dysfunction. Clinical Neurobiology 1:634–642, 1986

Grossman WF, Sanfield JA: Hypothalamic atrophy presenting as amenorrhea and sexual infantilism in a female adolescent: a case report. J Reprod Med 39:738–740, 1994

Gualtieri CT: Neuropsychiatry and Behavioral Pharmacology. New York, Springer-Verlag, 1991

Halvorsen JG, Metz ME: Sexual dysfunction, II: diagnosis, management and prognosis. J Am Board Fam Pract 5:177–192, 1992

Heath RG: Pleasure response of human subjects to direct stimulation of the brain: physiologic and psychodynamic considerations, in The Role of Pleasure in Behavior. Edited by Heath RG. New York, Harper & Row, 1964, pp 219–243

Herzog A: Endocrinological aspects of epilepsy, in Neurology and Neurosurgery Update Series (5[11]). Princeton, NJ, Continuing Professional Education Center, 1984

Hibbard MR, Gordon WA, Flanagan S, et al: Sexual dysfunction after traumatic brain injury. NeuroRehabilitation 15:107–120, 2000

Horn LJ, Zasler ND: Neuroanatomy and neurophysiology of sexual function. J Head Trauma Rehabil 5:1–13, 1990

Jarrow JP, Burnett AL, Geringer AM: Clinical efficacy of sildenafil citrate based on etiology and response to prior treatment. J Urol 162:722–725, 1999

Kosteljanetz M, Jensen TS, Norgard B, et al: Sexual and hypothalamic dysfunction in post-concussional syndrome. Acta Neurol Scand 63:169–180, 1981

Kreuter M, Dahllof AG, Gudjonsson G, et al: Sexual adjustment and its predictors after traumatic brain injury. Brain Inj 12:349–368, 1998a

Kreuter M, Sullivan M, Dahllof AG, et al: Partner relationships, functioning, mood and global quality of life in persons with spinal cord injury and traumatic brain injury. Spinal Cord 36:252–261, 1998b

Kreutzer JS, Zasler ND: Psychosexual consequences of traumatic brain injury: methodology and preliminary findings. Brain Inj 3:177–186, 1989

Lehne GK: Brain damage and paraphilia: treatment with medroxyprogesterone acetate. Sex Disabil 7:145–157, 1986

Levin RJ: The physiology of sexual function in women. Clin Obstet Gynecol 7:213–252, 1980

Lezak MD: Living with the characterologically altered brain injured patient. J Clin Psychiatry 39:592–598, 1978

MacLean P: Brain mechanisms of primal sexual functions and related behavior, in Sexual Behavior: Pharmacology and Biochemistry. Edited by Sandler M, Gessa G. New York, Raven, 1975, pp 1–11

Mauss-Clum N, Ryan M: Brain injury and the family. J Neurosurg Nurs 13:165–169, 1981

McConaghy N, Balszczynski A, Kidson W: Treatment of sex offenders with imaginal desensitization and/or medroxyprogesterone. Acta Psychiatr Scand 77:199–206, 1988

McKenna KE: Neural circuitry involved in sexual function. J Spinal Cord Med 24:148–154, 2001

McMahon CG, Touma K: Treatment of premature ejaculation with paroxetine hydrochloride. Int J Impot Res 11:241–245, 1999

Meinhardt W, Kropman RF, Vermeij P: Comparative tolerability and efficacy of treatments for impotence. Drug Saf 20:133–146, 1999

Mesulam M: Principles of Behavioral Neurology. Philadelphia, PA, FA Davis, 1985

Miller BL, Cummings JL, McIntyre H, et al: Hypersexuality or altered sexual preference following brain injury. J Neurol Neurosurg Psychiatry 49:867–873, 1986

Montejo AL, Llorca G, Izquierdo JA, et al: Incidence of sexual dysfunction associated with antidepressant agents: a prospective multicenter study of 1022 outpatients. Spanish Working Group for the Study of Psychotropic-Related Sexual Dysfunction. J Clin Psychiatry 62:10–21, 2001

Morales A, Surridge DHC, Marshall PG, et al: Nonhormonal pharmacological treatment of organic impotence. J Urol 128:45–47, 1982

O'Carroll RE, Woodrow J, Maroun F: Psychosexual and psychosocial sequelae of closed head injury. Brain Inj 5:303–313, 1991

Oddy M, Humphrey M: Social recovery during the first year following severe head injury. J Neurol Neurosurg Psychiatry 43:798–802, 1980

Oddy M, Humphrey M, Uttley D: Subjective impairment and social recovery after closed head injury. J Neurol Neurosurg Psychiatry 41:611–616, 1978

Padma-Nathan H: Neurologic evaluation of erectile dysfunction. Urol Clin North Am 15:77–80, 1988

Penfield W, Rasmussen T: The Cerebral Cortex of Man. New York, Macmillan, 1950

Rosen RC: Sexual pharmacology in the 21st century. J Gend Specif Med 3:45–52, 2000

Rosen RC, Lane RM, Menza M: Effects of SSRIs on sexual function: a critical review. J Clin Psychopharmacol 19:67–85, 1999

Rosenbaum M, Najenson T: Changes in life patterns and symptoms of low mood as reported by wives of severely brain-injured soldiers. J Consult Clin Psychol 44:881–888, 1976

Sandel ME, Williams KS, Dellapietra L, et al: Sexual function following traumatic brain injury. Brain Inj 10:719–728, 1996

Sarwer DB, Durlak JA: A field trial of the effectiveness of behavioral treatment for sexual dysfunctions. J Sex Marital Ther 23:87–97, 1997

Steers WD: Neural pathways and central sites involved in penile erection: neuroanatomy and clinical implications. Neurosci Biobehav Rev 24:507–516, 2000

Stewart JT: Carbamazepine treatment of a patient with Klüver-Bucy syndrome. J Clin Psychiatry 46:496–497, 1985

Walker AE: The neurological basis of sex. Neurol India 24:1–13, 1976

Weddell R, Oddy M, Jenkins D: Social adjustment after rehabilitation: a two year follow-up of patients with severe head injury. Psychol Med 10:257–263, 1980

Zasler ND: Sexuality in neurologic disability: an overview. Sex Disabil 9:11–27, 1991

Zasler ND, Horn LJ: Rehabilitative management of sexual dysfunction. J Head Trauma Rehabil 5:14–24, 1990

Zasler ND, Kreutzer JS: Family and sexuality after traumatic brain injury, in Impact of Head Injury on the Family System: An Overview for Professionals. Edited by Williams J, Kay T. Baltimore, MD, Paul H Brookes, 1991, pp 253–270

PART IV

Special Populations and Issues

26 Sports Injuries

Jason R. Freeman, Ph.D.

Jeffrey T. Barth, Ph.D.

Donna K. Broshek, Ph.D.

Kirsten Plehn, Ph.D.

History

Mild traumatic brain injury (MTBI) has only recently come to be appreciated as a substantial interest and concern to medical science. It was the mid-1980s when it was first noted that MTBIs could result in serious and lasting consequences. With increasing awareness of the significance of MTBI has come an associated advancement in the study of sports-related brain injuries. Neuropsychology of sports-related brain injury is the study of cognitive and psychological consequences of sports-related central nervous system injury. Injuries are seen in athletic activities in which trauma to the head is common or in fact integral, such as in boxing, as well as in sports in which contact to the head is thought to be less common, such as basketball, cycling, and equestrian events.

Before the 1970s, research focused on moderate to severe brain injury and its sequelae. The lack of attention to MTBI was because of the belief that neurologic and neurocognitive changes as a result of MTBI were minor, transient, and of little consequence. In the 1970s and 1980s, three lines of research were pursued to further understand brain injury.

The first line of research examined human subjects through retrospective studies of MTBI (Barth et al. 1983; Gronwall and Wrightson 1974; Leininger et al. 1990; Rimel et al. 1981). These studies revealed evidence of neurocognitive deficits and delayed return to work in MTBI patients with postconcussive syndrome (PCS) symptoms. Neuropsychological impairments were documented in some MTBI patients 1 month postinjury, with resolution of symptoms commonly seen in 2–3 months (Dikmen et al. 1986; Levin et al. 1987a; 1987b). Although these studies augmented and improved the understanding of MTBI, they varied in many respects, such as inclusion and exclusion criteria, the use of different neuropsychological measures, variability in the type or a lack of controls, and failure to account for potential confounds, such as substance abuse or prior brain injuries.

The second line of research used animal models to examine the affect of forces on the brain (Gennarelli et al. 1981; Ommaya and Gennarelli 1974). In these original studies with primates, researchers demonstrated axonal tearing and shear strain as a result of linear acceleration-deceleration injuries. Although the research was highly fruitful, the ability to generalize animal findings to humans remains theoretical at best; yet, animal research offered the first clear evidence of potential neuropathological sequelae of MTBI.

A third course of research examined individuals' neuropsychological functioning pre- and post-MTBI. Beginning in the mid-1980s, a 4-year prospective study of MTBI in college athletics was initiated at the University of Virginia as part of the Sports Laboratory Assessment Model (SLAM) (Barth et al. 1989, 2002). This study involved 2,300 football players at 10 universities and used both pre- and post-MTBI neuropsychological assessment. Not only did this study use a matched control group, but it also used individuals as their own control subjects by collecting baseline preinjury data during the preseason. This study was the most comprehensive prospective examination of neurocognitive functioning after MTBI undertaken in the twentieth century.

The main goal of this large-scale football study was to determine the recovery curve for MTBI in young, healthy, well-motivated individuals. By-products included determining incidence estimates of football-related brain injuries, characterizing their cognitive effects, identifying projected recovery curves, distinguishing risk factors for injury, and examining the long-term effects of multiple MTBIs. Unlike other areas of research, research that uses athletes as participants has the advantage of a low incidence of complicating factors associated with cognitive decline such as poor health, advanced age, and substance abuse (Ruchinskas et al. 1997). Furthermore, issues of motivation or effort are uncommon with athletes insofar as there is less risk of secondary gain, as can be seen in litigation contexts. Athletes are usually highly motivated for recovery and return to play; in fact, they may hide deficits to avoid benching. In contrast to prior methods of research, this study verified the presence and course of recovery of significant acute deficits in healthy individuals with appropriate motivation and effort. Athletes demonstrated mild neurocognitive deficits and a 5–10 day natural recovery curve (when controlling for practice effects) after very mild brain injuries. Although primarily clinically motivated, this study provided the foundations for the study of the neurocognition of sports-related MTBIs, which are more broadly termed *concussions* in the sports arena.

Epidemiology

Ann Brown, Chairman of the U.S. Consumer Products Safety Commission, stated that reducing traumatic head injury is one of the commission's highest priorities (U.S. Consumer Products Safety Commission 1999). An estimated 1.5–2.0 million people, including athletes, sustain traumatic brain injuries each year, and in young adults and children, such injuries are the primary cause of long-term disability (Consensus Conference 1999). The prevalence rate of brain injury is estimated at 2.5–6.5 million individuals and therefore is "of major public health significance" (Consensus Conference 1999, p. 974). Because MTBI is so frequently underdiagnosed, the "likely societal burden is therefore even greater" (Consensus Conference 1999, p. 974). Persisting symptoms after brain injury include deficits in memory, attention, concentration, and frontal lobe functions (executive skills), as well as language and vision perception deficits that often go unrecognized (Consensus Conference 1999). Persisting neurologic symptoms also occur, such as headaches, seizures, sleep disorders, and vision deficits. In addition, there are multiple other sequelae, including behavioral

and mood disturbances, as well as social and economic consequences.

Determining the incidence of sports-related MTBI is further complicated by underreporting and unclear diagnostic criteria. Although only 3% of admissions to hospitals are for sports- or recreation-related traumatic brain injuries (TBIs), the majority (90%) of sports-related TBIs are mild and frequently unreported, resulting in a significant underestimate of the true incidence of such injuries (Consensus Conference 1999). Notably, MTBI is often not recognized or diagnosed when patients do not lose consciousness, and over 90% of cerebral concussions do not involve loss of consciousness (LOC) (Cantu 1998). Current methods of assessing concussion severity have been criticized for their reliance on LOC and length of posttraumatic amnesia (PTA). Recent research indicates that the former fails to correlate with outcome, and the latter is difficult to assess reliably (Forrester et al. 1994; Lovell et al. 1999; Paniak et al. 1998). Currently, there are "no objective neuroanatomic or physiologic measurements that can be used to determine if a patient has sustained a concussion or to assess the severity of insult" (Wojtys et al. 1999).

Sports-related TBI is a major public health concern because these injuries occur most frequently among children and young adults (ages 5–24 years), often resulting in lengthy periods of disability and interfering with patients' attainment of their full educational and occupational potential (Consensus Conference 1999). Approximately 300,000 people each year sustain a sports-related TBI, and this problem is compounded by the fact that athletes are at risk for multiple brain injuries (Thurman et al. 1998). Multiple brain injuries may increase the risk for poor outcome. Furthermore, a fatality has occurred in high school and college football every year between 1945 and 1999, excluding 1990, resulting in a total of 712 fatalities during that period (Mueller 2001). Sixty-nine percent of those deaths were because of brain injuries, with subdural hematoma being the cause of 74.5% of the fatal football-related brain injuries. During that same time period, 75% of the football-related fatalities that occurred because of brain injury occurred in high school athletes. Also of concern is the fact that 63 brain injuries sustained in high school football games resulted in permanent disability between 1984 and 1999 (Mueller 2001). Despite these poor outcomes, the National Institutes of Health Consensus Development Panel (Consensus Conference 1999, p. 976) noted that "there is great promise for prevention of sports-related TBI."

In an extraordinary 3-year study on the incidence of TBI in varsity athletics at 235 high schools, 1,219 MTBIs were recorded, constituting 5.5% of the total injuries

(Powell and Barber-Foss 1999). Football accounted for the largest number of concussions (63.4%), followed by wrestling (males, 10.5%), female soccer (6.2%), male soccer (5.7%), and female basketball (5.2%). Other sports accounted for less than 5% of injuries, including male basketball (4.2%), softball (females, 2.1%), baseball (males, 1.2%), field hockey (females, 1.1%), and volleyball (females, 0.5%). The majority of injuries resulted from tackles, takedowns, and/or collisions. In soccer, the majority of TBIs occurred during heading, but the data did not indicate whether the injuries resulted from head-to-ball, head-to-head, head-to-ground, or another type of collision that could create an acceleration-deceleration injury. Recent research on rugby suggests that despite this sport's high-impact image, rugby players sustain fewer concussions than football players and soccer players, possibly because of the mechanics of the rugby tackle (Farace and Alves 2000). On the basis of their sample, Powell and Barber-Foss (1999) estimate that the national incidence of MTBI across these 10 sports is 62,816 cases, with the majority occurring in football.

The annual survey of catastrophic football injuries that started in 1945 was expanded in 1982 with the establishment of the National Center for Catastrophic Sports Injury Research (Mueller 2001). The expansion involved collecting data on a wide range of high school and college sports in addition to football and was partially motivated by increasing participation by female athletes after the enactment of Title IX of the National Educational Assistance Act in 1972 and the lack of data on catastrophic injuries to female athletes. Data collected between 1982 and 1999 revealed that female athletes sustained fatalities or permanent disabilities in cheerleading, volleyball, softball, gymnastics, and field hockey. Notably, over 50% of the catastrophic injuries to female athletes during that period were due to cheerleading.

Although males have approximately twice the risk of females for sustaining a TBI in all age groups (Centers for Disease Control and Prevention 1997), few studies have examined the role of gender on outcome after TBI (Farace and Alves 2000; Kraus et al. 2000). A recent meta-analysis on gender differences found only nine studies that reported data by gender (Farace and Alves 2000). One study was excluded because of biased methodology, leaving eight studies reporting 20 outcome variables by gender. Females demonstrated poorer outcome in 17 of the 20 variables (85%), with an average effect size of –0.15. A recent prospective study of patients with moderate and severe TBI revealed that the female mortality rate was 1.28 times higher than that of males (Kraus et al. 2000). Additionally, the likelihood of poor outcome was 1.57 times higher for females. On the basis of a review of the

literature and their own prospective research, Kraus and colleagues (2000) suggest that future research in TBI should evaluate the effects of gender and examine any pathophysiological basis of differential outcome across gender. As increasing numbers of women participate in sports and other high-risk activities (e.g., rock climbing), a greater understanding of the role of gender on TBI outcome is needed (Farace and Alves 2000).

Animal research has revealed differential TBI outcomes on the basis of gender. In rats that underwent experimental TBI, estrogen had a protective effect for males, whereas it exacerbated injuries in females (Emerson et al. 1993). Using a fluid percussion-injury model, researchers have observed higher mortality rates in female rats (Emerson et al. 1993; Hovda 1996). The reported poorer outcome for women after TBI may have a hormone-based pathophysiological basis (i.e., a balanced hormonal system of testosterone and estrogen may have a positive effect on physical recovery) as suggested by these animal studies.

Although limited, the existing human research on MTBI also suggests a greater risk of poor outcome for females. Females have been noted to have a larger number of persisting symptoms 1 year after MTBI (Rutherford et al. 1979), a greater incidence of depression post-MTBI (Fenton et al. 1993), and a greater likelihood of PCS (Bazarian et al. 1999) than males. In contrast, other researchers have reported that females are more likely to return to school or work after TBI (Groswasser et al. 1998). Although cerebral glucose metabolic rates do not appear to vary by gender (Azari et al. 1992; Miura et al. 1990), healthy female control subjects have demonstrated higher mean cerebral blood flow (CBF) than healthy male control subjects (Gur and Gur 1990; Warkentin et al. 1992).

Brain Injury in Organized Sports

Boxing

Boxing is the sole competitive, organized, athletic endeavor in which injury—specifically, neurologic injury—is the goal. Inducing LOC via blows to the head is the objective of this sport rather than a competitive risk. Contrary to many other sports-related injuries, brain injury in boxing tends to be moderate to severe in nature and thus receives considerable attention. Accounts of associated neurological changes (so called punch-drunk syndrome) have been documented from as early as 1928 (Martland). Early accounts of neurological sequelae from boxing injuries described a progressive pattern of deficits, including initial confusion and loss of coordination followed by worsening latency of speech and motor functioning with associated upper-body tremors. Martland (1928) observed that the pattern of symptoms seen in punch-drunk boxers often resembled that of Parkinson's disease patients. It is estimated that 9%–25% of professional boxers ultimately develop punch-drunk syndrome (Ryan 1987). This neurological change has been referred to as "chronic boxer's encephalopathy" (Serel and Jaros 1962), "traumatic boxer's encephalopathy" (Mawdsley and Ferguson 1963), and "dementia pugilistica" (Lampert and Hardman 1984).

The greater degree of neurological damage observed in boxers versus other athletes is hypothesized to be because of the multiple mechanisms of possible damage in boxing. Injuries can occur as a result of direct blows to the head as well as from rotational torque, thereby creating the potential for focal and diffuse injury. Specifically, the means of injury in boxing and other contact sports are likely to include rotational acceleration (shearing), linear acceleration (resulting in compressive and tensile stress on axons), carotid injuries, and deceleration on impact (Cantu 1996; Lampert and Hardman 1984). Injury to carotid arteries may create reflexive hypotension, with resulting lightheadedness that increases the risk of further injury. Furthermore, boxers are subject to successive head trauma (concussive and subconcussive blows), resulting in a host of other neurological difficulties, including increased vulnerability for subsequent neurodegenerative conditions (Jordan 1987, 1993). Neuropathological changes observed in boxers include cerebral atrophy, cellular loss in the cerebellum, and cortical as well as subcortical neurofibrillary tangles (Corsellis et al. 1973). Jordan (1987) showed that the genetic protein apolipoprotein E (*apoE*) with the ε4 allele is a risk factor for the development of dementia pugilistica, just as it appears to be a risk factor for the development of Alzheimer's disease (AD) in the general population.

Research on the neurocognitive effects of sports-related injuries in boxers has revealed mixed findings. In his review of research on this subject, Mendez (1995) found that the status of the athlete (amateur vs. professional) accounted for the greatest variation in cognitive functioning. Excluding athletes who showed positive findings on neuroimaging, amateur boxers demonstrated neuropsychological functioning similar to that of other amateur athletes. In contrast, professional boxers with associated imaging evidence of neurological conditions, including subdural hematomas and perivascular hemorrhage, demonstrated a broad range of neuropsychological deficits. These findings were supported by a review of amateur boxers that found no consistent evidence of neuropsychological deficiency with the exception of decreased, but not impaired, non-

dominant-hand fine motor coordination (Butler 1994). This result was hypothesized to reflect mild peripheral nerve damage as a result of boxers' propensity to lead with their nondominant hand. Other findings have suggested little difference between the neurocognitive functioning of amateur boxers and matched soccer-player control subjects (Thomassen et al. 1979). In a study of amateur boxers in Ireland, concussion was found to be the most common injury (Porter and O'Brien 1996). Furthermore, such injuries occurred solely during matches, unlike peripheral injuries to the hands, wrists, or knees, which occurred in the course of training as well as competition.

In contrast to the above research, several studies have suggested that some boxers appear to have greater vulnerability to neuropsychological impairments. McLatchie and colleagues (1987) compared 20 amateur boxers with 20 matched control athletes who had orthopedic injuries. Authors found significant neuropsychological impairments in boxers relative to control subjects, as well as eight irregular electroencephalograms (EEGs), seven atypical clinical examinations, and one abnormal computed tomography (CT) scan. Of these findings, neuropsychological tests were believed to be the most sensitive measures of cerebral dysfunction. It was noted that only a few of the boxers demonstrated severe impairment; thus, neuropsychological and other measures were necessary to discern generally subtle differences between boxers and control subjects. Authors attributed this pattern of findings to specific vulnerability to neuropsychological deficits in the boxing population. Similar studies of boxers and matched control subjects have supported this assertion (N. Brooks 1987; Levin et al. 1987b).

Research on boxing-related injuries has suffered from methodological criticism regarding selection bias and lack of appropriate control groups. As recently as the mid-1980s, it was commonly believed that neurological and neuropsychological deficits observed in boxers were artifacts of prior substance abuse, poor education, and poor training (American Medical Association Council of Scientific Affairs 1983). In response to such criticism, Casson et al. (1984) selected 18 current and former professional boxers. The subjects had no history of neurological illness or substance abuse, and all had "responsible jobs, [and] secondary or college education" (p. 2663). Measures included EEG, CT, and neuropsychological testing. The authors found abnormalities on at least two of these assessments for the majority of boxers, and the remaining subjects showed deficiency on at least some neuropsychological measures (e.g., immediate and delayed verbal memory). These findings were not related to number of concussions or amnestic episodes. Notably, neuropsychological performance was found to be the most sensitive measure of cerebral dysfunction in this study.

Perhaps the most comprehensive study to date is the longitudinal study conducted by Stewart and colleagues (1994) of 484 amateur United States boxers. Between 1986 and 1990, neurological and neuropsychological data were gathered at baseline and subsequent 2-year follow-up. Although neither frequency of sparring nor bouts between evaluations was associated with cognitive deficits, the number of bouts before baseline was statistically significant. Specifically, the number of prebaseline bouts was associated with perceptual motor, visuoconstructional, and memory deficiency. The authors hypothesized that the number of bouts fought before the advent of increased safety measures in 1984 predicted cognitive deficiency. Decreased neurological and neuropsychological injury likely resulted from the implementation of new policies that paired boxers according to skill, prevented boxers with recent head injury from competing, and improved and mandated protective headgear (Stewart et al. 1994).

Other researchers have investigated the relationship between neuropsychological testing and functional neuroimaging in amateur boxers (Kemp et al. 1995). The number of bouts was positively correlated with poorer neuropsychological test performance. Deficits in neuropsychological testing for boxers occurred even in the absence of abnormalities on their cerebral single-photon emission computed tomography (SPECT) scans. In sum, research reveals significant risk for brain injury among boxers, with neuropsychological assessment being the most sensitive indicator of cerebral dysfunction.

Football

Because of the frequency of impact and the nature of the sport, United States football has long had a high incidence of significant brain injuries. In an epidemiological study of catastrophic football injuries (defined as "football injuries that result in death, brain, or spinal cord injury, or cranial and spinal fracture") from 1977 to 1998, researchers found 118 deaths attributed to central nervous system injuries, with an additional 200 neurological injuries with incomplete recovery (Cantu and Mueller 2000). Similar to results observed in boxing, the severity of neurocognitive deficiency after football-related head injuries is closely tied to the number and recency of prior head injuries. Numerous case studies have demonstrated the potentially fatal outcome of football injuries, particularly in the case of repeated injury in close proximity to prior brain trauma (Harbaugh and Saunders 1984; Schneider 1973).

Although serious injuries while playing football have drawn attention from researchers, it is only relatively recently that MTBI in football has received scientific investigation. Multiple studies have indicated that the rate of concussion in football is as high as 5% of all acquired injuries (DeLee and Farney 1992; Karpakka 1993). It is often the case that athletes receive "dings" or "see stars," but until recently these symptoms were largely ignored or minimized by players so that they might return to play (Magnes 1990). Some of the lack of cohesion regarding return to play is attributable to the lack of consensus in developing criteria for classification of MTBI (see the section Return-to-Play Criteria).

As described in the section History, a University of Virginia study (Barth et al. 1989) examined mild cognitive dysfunction with rapid recovery in a population of 2,300 football players with MTBI without LOC, yet with some level of confusion or alteration of consciousness. All participants received preseason baseline assessments. All concussed athletes, as well as matched control subjects, then received serial assessments at 24 hours, 5 days, and 10 days postinjury. The injured athletes and matched control subjects were also assessed at the end of the season. The results showed that concussed players had mild deficits or failed to show the expected practice effect on neuropsychological testing compared with the nonconcussed players. This trend was noted in the areas of sustained attention and visuomotor speed, with resolution of symptoms by the fifth to tenth day. The preseason assessment and the comparison with matched control subjects were critical in detecting and tracking subtle neurocognitive changes indicative of concussion. Subjective complaints of dizziness, headache, and memory dysfunction that largely resolved by the tenth day accompanied the neuropsychological dysfunction. This large-scale study demonstrated significant and measurable—but time-limited—neurocognitive deficits after concussion in a healthy, young, motivated sample of athletes (Macciocchi et al. 1996).

The findings of the University of Virginia study (Barth et al. 1989) were supported by Lovell and Collins (1998), who examined MTBI in 63 Division I college football players. Preseason neuropsychological assessment and subsequent evaluation postinjury of participants, including four players with documented concussion, revealed a lack of practice effects in players with head injury as well as performance below baseline levels, particularly in the areas of information processing speed and verbal fluency. As a result of this pioneering study, the use of preseason baseline neurocognitive screening as described by the SLAM model (Barth et al. 2001, 2002) is becoming the gold standard for concussion assessment and management.

Soccer

Soccer is a sport that enjoys worldwide popularity. Although contact between players is not fundamental to the sport as it is in American football, the aggressive nature of play makes the likelihood of brain injury high. Athletes risk potential injury from collision with the ground, the ball, the goalposts, and other players, with head injury estimated to account for 4%–20% of all soccer injuries (Roass and Nilsson 1979), although this figure includes all aspects of head injuries, such as lacerations, fractures, and eye injuries. In soccer players between the ages of 15 and 18 years, Powell and Barber-Foss (1999) reported an estimated 3.9 incidence of MTBI for boys and 4.3 incidence for girls. Study of the risk for brain injury in soccer has been complicated by the lack of clarity regarding the potential for head injury as a result of heading the ball. Although most of the potential causes of injury in soccer are incidental, heading the ball is an integral part of play. Estimates suggest that the average player has six or seven headers in each game (Tysvaer and Storli 1981). However, in their prospective study, Boden et al. (1998) found that head injuries were most frequently the result of head-to-head or head-to-ground contact rather than the result of head-to-ball contact. Head injuries resulting from contact with the ball were most often the result of accidental strikes rather than purposeful heading of the ball (Boden et al. 1998). Continued research exploring the direct mechanism of injury in soccer is warranted.

Early seminal research on brain injury in soccer was performed by Tysvaer and colleagues (Tysvaer and Storli 1981; Tysvaer et al. 1989), who conducted several studies examining the neurological and neuropsychological functioning of soccer players, both active and retired. Preliminary research consisted of data collected from a survey of 192 Norwegian professional soccer players, which revealed that half of this sample reported symptoms related to heading the ball (Tysvaer and Storli 1981). More comprehensive studies with both active and retired soccer players were conducted and published in subsequent years, showing mild EEG abnormalities as well as considerable subjective complaints of symptoms consistent with postconcussive syndrome in comparison with matched control subjects (Tysvaer et al. 1989). In a 1992 study, Tysvaer examined 69 active and 37 retired Norwegian soccer players and found significant differences in the retired population. Approximately 30% of the retired athletes reported postconcussive symptoms. Additionally, CT scans showed cerebral atrophy in one-third of the retired group, and approximately 80% of this group demonstrated deficiency on neuropsychological measures in the areas of attention, concentration, memory, and judgment in comparison to age-matched control subjects (Sortland and Tysvaer 1989).

These findings have not been consistently duplicated in subsequent research. Following on the work of Tysvaer

and colleagues, Haglund and Eriksson (1993) compared former and current professional soccer players to amateur boxers and track athletes. Neurological and neuropsychological studies failed to demonstrate evidence of neurocognitive deficits in the population of soccer players. Slight variability was seen in the finger-tapping speed of soccer players, but this finding was still within normal limits. Similarly, in a comparison of the 1994 United States World Cup soccer team with track athletes, there was no difference between the groups in terms of magnetic resonance imaging (MRI) findings, history of head injury, or alcohol abuse (Jordan et al. 1996). However, those soccer players who had experienced prior head injury did report a significantly higher number of subjective symptoms compared with soccer players without prior head injury. The authors suggest that history of concussion rather than exposure to heading increases the risk for reporting head injury symptoms. In a similar study, Pennsylvania State University conducted a prospective study that assessed college athletes at pre- and posttraining sessions, with one group participating in heading and the other group not participating in heading (Putukian et al. 2000). This investigation failed to show evidence of dysfunction, and the authors interpreted that there are no acute neuropsychological effects of heading in soccer.

In contrast, Matser and colleagues (1999) conducted a cross-sectional study of 33 amateur soccer players and 27 matched athlete control subjects in which participants were compared in terms of neuropsychological test performance. Researchers found that the amateur soccer players demonstrated deficits in planning and memory, and the number of concussions sustained by soccer players was inversely related to their performance on measures of simple auditory attention span, facial recognition, immediate recall of complex figures, rapid figural encoding, and verbal memory. These findings remained significant despite corrections for level of education, concussions unrelated to soccer, numbers of treatments with general anesthesia, and alcohol use. Notably, the sample of soccer players was found to have a statistically higher level of alcohol consumption than control subjects. This study suggests that amateur soccer play is associated with mild but enduring memory and planning deficiency.

There are several potential factors that may account for the variability of these findings. First, inclusion criteria vary widely from study to study. Changes in the composition and make of soccer balls have made them less water absorbent and therefore less heavy, thereby reducing the potential mass on impact (S.E. Jordan et al. 1996). Older and retired players likely used heavier and potentially more damaging balls, whereas younger players now benefit from technologically improved equipment. Furthermore, factors known to influence cognition, such as alcohol use and malnutrition, are often not considered in this research (Victor et al. 1989). Similarly, the presence of learning disorders is rarely accounted for, thus creating the potential for results to be skewed by preexisting factors. Last, early research often failed to accurately measure the history of concussion and brain injury outside of soccer play in athletes. Although players with brain injuries not incurred through soccer play were excluded, the impact of multiple concussions has not always been fully appreciated. Continued research with attention to these methodological issues will be beneficial.

Other Sports

Because of widespread enjoyment and media coverage of boxing, football, and soccer, brain injury in these well-known sports receives substantial attention. However, there are numerous less-publicized competitive and recreational sports that pose potential risks for brain injury that are often neglected. Heightened awareness regarding the potential risks for brain injury in these areas is warranted.

Skiing has a long history as a recreational sports activity, with an estimated 15 million participants (Hunter 1999). Although the overall incidence of skiing-related injuries has decreased in the recent past (Chissel et al. 1996) and the majority of injuries are minor, the number of brain injuries in skiing has remained stable. Head injury in fact now represents approximately 15% of all skiing-related injuries (U.S. Consumer Products Safety Commission 1999). As a result of the media coverage of the celebrity deaths of Sonny Bono and Michael Kennedy, the dangers of brain injury in winter recreational activities have gained increasing attention. In a review of the incidence, severity, and outcomes of skiing-related head injuries in Colorado between the years of 1994 and 1997, it was noted that a total of 118 skiers were hospitalized for head injuries (Diamond et al. 2001). Of those hospitalized, there was a preponderance of males (approximately a 2:1 ratio vs. females), although each gender appeared to have an equal risk for "serious" head trauma. Approximately one-fourth of the study sample received a skull fracture, and 29% continued to report difficulties on discharge from the hospital. These findings are similar to results from a study on a population of skiers in Switzerland (Furrer et al. 1995).

Snowboarding, a sport that is rapidly gaining popularity, is associated with unique risks for brain injury. In a 2-year study of snowboarding- and skiing-related head injuries in Nagano, Japan, researchers found a 6.5 per 100,000 incidence of head injury for snowboarders and a 3.8 per 100,000 incidence for skiers (Nakaguchi et al.

1999). Snowboarders who rated themselves as beginners were more likely to sustain head injuries than self-rated beginning skiers. The most frequent cause of injuries was falls sustained while jumping and falling backward, resulting in occipital impact. Although helmet use is gaining acceptance in winter sports, only a small proportion of individuals wear safety gear at present. The U.S. Consumer Products Safety Commission (1999) estimated that of those individuals sustaining head injuries in 1998, only 6% of them were wearing helmets.

Cycling is a widely enjoyed sport, with nearly 54 million people using a bike annually (U.S. Bureau of the Census 1993). Like other sports, however, it is not without risk. In the United States, bicycle-related accidents account for more than 500,000 annual emergency room visits (Sacks et al. 1988; Yelon et al. 1995). In a study of bicyclists in San Diego, California, 7% of brain injuries were bicycle related, indicative of an incidence rate of 13.5 injuries per 100,000 (Kraus et al. 1986). Similarly, the Royal Society for the Prevention of Accidents (1991) estimates that annual totals of cycling-related injuries in the United Kingdom are approximately 90,000. Furthermore, injuries in cycling occur across a wide range of ages. In 1993, it was determined that cycling-related injuries accounted for 15% of total trauma deaths to children in Ontario (Spence et al. 1993). Despite popular opinion to the contrary, off-road cycling does not appear to be associated with increased risk of brain injury compared with road cycling. In a review of injuries in a population of all-terrain cyclists in South Carolina, subjects were found to have had a high incidence of injury (lifetime rate of 84%, with 51% reporting injuries in the past year), but these injuries tended to be abrasions, lacerations, and contusions, and they were less severe than injuries seen in road cyclists (Chow et al. 1993). The high incidence of helmet use (88%) likely contributed to the low incidence of brain injury. In 1994, a poll of Pro/Elite competitors revealed an absence of catastrophic head injuries, with the majority of injuries occurring as wounds and contusions to the lower extremities and back (Pfeiffer 1994). As a result of the growing awareness of the potential dangers of bicycle use, potential protective factors in cycling are receiving increased public health attention.

Current research illustrates the significant impact of helmets in reducing the severity of brain injury in cycling (Bull 1988; Runyan et al. 1991; Wasserman and Buccini 1990). Most fatalities from bicycle accidents are caused by head and neck injuries (Ginsberg and Silverberg 1994; McCarthy 1991). It is estimated that helmet use can result in as much as a 50% reduction in the incidence of cycling-related head injuries (Sacks et al. 1988; Weiss 1991). Despite this knowledge, helmet use is quite low, and research has demonstrated that ownership of a helmet is not synonymous with use (Fullerton and Becker 1991). In a study of competitive cyclists, researchers found that despite a relatively high use of helmets (80%), cyclists complained of helmets being hot and heavy as well as "looking funny" (Runyan et al. 1991). Factors that contribute to increased helmet usage include use of helmets by companion cyclists as well as mandatory helmet laws (Dannenberg et al. 1993; Jaques 1994). Wearing helmets has also been associated with a sense of personal freedom because of feelings of increased safety and social responsibility (Everett et al. 1996).

Equestrian sports have been identified as the sports activity with perhaps the highest risk for brain injury. The United States hosts approximately 10,000 sanctioned equestrian events annually in addition to abundant unofficial events (W.H. Brooks and Bixby-Hammett 1998). Participants range from children to adults, with more than 12,000 active members of the United States Pony Clubs and nearly 25,000 children active in 4-H programs (W.H. Brooks and Bixby-Hammett 1998; Lamb 2000). Given the inherent difficulties of anticipating and directing the actions of such large animals, as well as factors such as the potential speed and force of horses and the height from which riders can fall when mounted, the potential for accidents is high (W.H. Brooks and Bixby-Hammett 1991). The predominance of equestrian-related injuries occurs as a rider makes impact with the ground, although acceleration-deceleration injuries may occur as a rider loses contact with the horse. In addition, equestrian events have the potential for "double impact" injuries, as a rider is injured when striking the ground or an obstacle and additional injury occurs as he or she is trampled or crushed by the horse (Whitlock 1999). These factors create the possibility for both focal and diffuse cerebral injury (W.H. Brooks and Bixby-Hammett 1998).

It is estimated that over 25,000 individuals required emergency room admission in 1997 as a result of equestrian-related injuries (Lamb 2000). Epidemiological studies indicate that head injuries are the most common causes for hospitalization in equestrian-related injuries (Frankel et al. 1998). For example, within a 4-year period in the 1990s, of the 30 patients admitted to the University of Kentucky Medical Center for equestrian-related injuries, 24 were admitted for treatment of a head injury (Kriss and Kriss 1997). Similarly, in a retrospective review of medical records at three University of Calgary hospitals, 91% of the 156 equestrian-related nervous system injuries recorded were head injuries (Hamilton and Tranmer 1993). The most common mechanism of injury was being thrown or otherwise falling from the horse, with associated secondary injuries. In Lexington, Kentucky, a neurosurgeon

gathered evidence on equestrian-related injuries seen in his practice (Brooks 2000). He found that of the 234 recorded injuries, the majority occurred during recreational riding. The most common form of head injury was concussion, followed by cerebral contusion, skull fracture, and intracranial hematoma. Skull fracture occurred most commonly in those not using protective headgear.

As with other sports, the use of helmets in equestrian events is inconsistent, although the issue is gaining greater attention. Recent attention to brain injury in equestrian events has resulted in focused efforts to improve the standards for equestrian helmets as well as to increase their use. Studies have addressed the ability of various helmets to withstand the impact of simulated injury as well as their ability to remain in proper position throughout the course of impact (Biokinetics & Associates Ltd. 2000). In some settings—namely the city of Plantation, Florida and the state of New York—proactive efforts by equestrian organizations have resulted in the passage of helmet-use laws (American Medical Equestrian Association 1999; Pinsky 2000). Despite such efforts, helmet use is estimated to be generally as low as 40%, with particularly poor use by Western riders (Condie et al. 1993; Lamb 2000). The commonly cited reasons for low levels of helmet use often mirror those given by cyclists, such as poor ventilation in heat and fears that one will look "silly" (Neal 1999). Many manufacturers of equestrian helmets, however, have put great effort into designing protective helmets that closely resemble traditional headgear, such as hunt caps and cowboy hats. As with all sporting activities discussed in this chapter, the value of education regarding the potential threat of brain injury, the use of safety gear, and factors related to compliance in the use of protective factors are important issues for future research and attention.

Neurophysiology of Concussion

MTBI is defined as the changes in consciousness, including potential LOC, and awareness as a result of head injury. As opposed to more severe brain trauma, MTBI is often subtle and can take several forms. Contusions are often present, usually in the frontal and temporal lobes. White matter may be affected by edema as well as by shearing (Bailes and Hudson 2001) as the brain receives compressive, tensile, and shearing forces. Furthermore, neurochemical changes such as functional changes in neurotransmitter release, receptor binding, and cholinergic functioning are seen as well (Dixon et al. 1993).

Initial injury commonly occurs as a blow to the head, and consequent acceleration results in axonal shearing as well as stretching and compression of long tract neurons (Gennarelli 1986). Such injuries may not be associated with significant neurological findings on examination; indeed, evidence of axonal injuries has been found in postmortem studies of individuals with only 1 minute of LOC (Blumbergs et al. 1994).

Understanding the Underpinnings of Mild Brain Injury: Animal Models

Physiological and metabolic disruption after cerebral concussion has been demonstrated using animal models (Hovda et al. 1999). Several researchers have consistently found reductions in CBF immediately after experimentally induced TBI (Dewitt et al. 1986; Goldman et al. 1991; Yamakami and McIntosh 1989; Yuan et al. 1988). Hovda et al. (1999) have speculated that the duration of reduced CBF after brain injury is likely to be the primary factor predictive of outcome. Cerebral concussion can be conceptualized as a posttraumatic neurological state clinically defined by altered consciousness, impaired cognition, and transient or lasting neuropsychological deficits (Hovda et al. 1999). To date, there are no objective neuroanatomical or physiological procedures or measures that absolutely confirm the presence of concussion or reliably assess the extent of any physical effects, but this is and will continue to be an important area of research.

Although the neurobiological understanding of concussion is preliminary, animal models have shown several neurobiological effects that follow concussion, including trauma-induced ionic flux, metabolic changes, and disruptions to CBF. When sufficient force is applied to the brain, either through a direct blow or an acceleration/deceleration injury, the intracellular concentration changes for several ions, including decreased potassim and magnesium and increased calcium (Hovda et al. 1999). Known as ionic flux, this state requires energy to restore the normal homeostatic functioning of the neuron; otherwise, the function of the cell can be drastically reduced, leading to cell death. It is believed that ionic flux triggers hyperglycolysis shortly after concussion, which provides the necessary energy for cell membrane pumps to restore cellular ionic homeostasis. Hyperglycolysis has been observed within minutes of injury in animal fluid percussion studies.

Hyperglycolysis does not persist, and in the most succinct terms, ionic flux and metabolic disruption can be conceptualized as an "energy crisis." This crisis must be ameliorated to restore the equilibrium and normal functioning of neurons. Research has shown (Giza and Hovda 2001; Hovda et al. 1999) that the crisis reflects an increased demand for energy that is initially accommodated via hyperglycolysis, but there is a subsequent decrease in

supply of glucose/blood. Animal models of TBI show reductions of CBF by as much as 50% shortly after the initiation of hyperglycolysis, thereby compromising the "supply" of glucose and other cellular nutrients necessary to restore cellular equilibrium. The imbalance of supply and demand can occur even in MTBI and is referred to as an "uncoupling" or disruption of CBF autoregulation (Hovda et al. 1999). In the normally functioning brain, autoregulation balances the cellular metabolic demands and the blood flow that provides the necessary nutrients to meet them. Disrupted autoregulation of the vascular supply therefore places brain-injured individuals at great risk for life-threatening consequences should a second such injury ensue (see Second Impact Syndrome).

Aspects of disrupted cellular metabolism last up to 10 days in mature animals. It is important to note that two pathophysiology studies (Hovda 1996; Hovda et al. 1999) showed increased morbidity as well as mortality in younger rodents relative to more mature mice, and return to physiological homeostasis was considerably longer in these immature rodents. These results seem to have implications for protecting younger athletes from the effects and vulnerabilities created by concussion.

Human Studies of TBI Pathophysiology

Although bench animal research yields a basic foundation for improving our understanding of concussion physiology, it may not generalize adequately to humans. Additionally, animal research cannot easily assess and track cognitive changes associated with TBI. Animal models do highlight temporal "windows" of altered ionic and metabolic function that mark vulnerability to a secondary insult and also indicate potential times for introducing pharmacological treatments to counter vulnerability (Hovda et al. 1999).

With respect to human pathophysiology research, impaired cerebral autoregulation after MTBI has been documented (Arvigo et al. 1985; Junger et al. 1997; Strebel et al. 1997). Additionally, hyperglycolysis has also been identified after human concussion with concomitant reductions in CBF (Shalmon et al. 1995). Hovda et al. (1999) assert that the duration of impaired autoregulation likely correlates strongly with brain injury outcome. From a neurochemical perspective, Wojtys and colleagues (1999) found that increased intracellular calcium is associated with a reduction in CBF in humans, and alterations in CBF have been observed in patients with MTBI (Arvigo et al. 1985; Junger et al. 1997; Strebel et al. 1997).

More research is still needed to verify the extent of neurochemical and metabolic disruption after brain injury, but there is an expanding literature showing the persisting effects of concussion in the absence of findings on traditional neuroimaging (e.g., MRI and CT). Using a xenon inhalation technique, Arvigo and colleagues (1985) compared 17 mildly brain-injured patients with matched control subjects. All of the patients with mild brain injury showed dramatically reduced CBF within 10 days of injury. At a follow-up measurement 1 week after the initial reading, six patients showed persisting CBF decline. All demonstrated normal CBF within 4 weeks of the initial reading, and CBF recovery correlated with improved Glasgow Coma Scale (GCS) and Galveston Orientation and Amnesia Test scores (Arvigo et al. 1985). Observed weaknesses of this study included the failure to investigate more complex neurocognitive functions and the lack of an age- and education-matched control population.

Neurometabolic functions have also been assessed noninvasively using fluorodeoxyglucose positron emission tomography for severely brain-injured patients (Bergsneider et al. 1997). Investigators found regional and global hyperglycolysis persisting up to 2 weeks posttrauma in all six patients with an initial GCS score between 3 and 8. This study was the first to extend and apply animal models of hyperglycolysis, which are reflective of ionic destabilization, after brain injury in humans. Bergsneider and colleagues noted that future treatment and management of concussion will depend on further elucidation of neurometabolism after brain injury.

Other noninvasive technological advances are being applied to the study of concussion as well. Junger and colleagues (1997) compared 29 MTBI patients (GCS score 13–15) with 29 matched control subjects using transcranial Doppler ultrasonography. This technique provides a measure of CBF and mean arterial blood pressure. Despite having equivalent mean arterial blood pressure at rest, MTBI patients experienced disrupted autoregulation after induced rapid and brief changes in arterial blood pressure. Decreased CBF in these situations may leave such patients vulnerable to ischemia, and increased mean arterial blood pressure to compensate for reductions in blood supply may place even MTBI patients at risk for secondary hemorrhage and/or edema (Junger et al. 1997). Clearly, these results demonstrate the vulnerability to drastic and potentially fatal effects as a result of second head traumas, even those mild in nature (see Second Impact Syndrome).

Much of the thinking regarding standard management of concussion/MTBI has been based on "traditional" symptoms or qualities. An abundance of literature has emphasized the use of these traditional hallmarks (i.e., LOC, significant retrograde or PTA, or evidence of pathology on standard neuroimaging) in determining the length of time for returning concussed athletes to competition (see Return-to-Play Criteria). Reliance on the presence or absence of these symptoms as well as their duration, particularly with respect to LOC, may be insufficient for predicting the extent and duration of functional changes after TBI (Lovell et al. 1999). Investigations of the neurocognitive, neurovascular, and neurochemical effects of MTBI in humans therefore represent a progressive area of research.

Although it is postulated that recovery of neurochemical and metabolic function will likely mirror the improvements in neuropsychological test performance seen in college football players within 5–10 days of injury (Barth et al. 1989), this concept has yet to be empirically demonstrated. Linking function and chemistry rather than form and function will yield the data necessary to better comprehend the length of vulnerability, how the vulnerability is manifested, and potentially how to evaluate the efficacy of various treatments. At a minimum, "treatment" should include abstinence from exertion and contact while recovering. We are clearly at a stage in our understanding of the physiology of concussion at which innovative extensions into human investigations are necessary. As our understanding grows, proactive mechanical (e.g., improved helmets) or even pharmacological interventions can be developed. Additionally, recovery-enhancing interventions can be validated.

Second Impact Syndrome

Compounding the potential dangers of managing concussion and making return-to-play decisions is the threat of "second impact syndrome" (SIS) (Cantu and Voy 1995; Schneider 1973). Diffuse cerebral swelling has been observed in numerous sports injuries, but at present the etiology of such injuries is somewhat unclear. One hypothesis is that this posttraumatic complication is the result of repeated mild injuries. Explicitly, Cantu and Voy (1995) defined *SIS* as an injury that results when "an athlete, who has sustained an initial head injury, most often a concussion, sustains a second head injury before symptoms associated with the first have fully cleared."

> What happens in the next 15 seconds to several minutes sets this syndrome apart from a concussion or even a subdural hematoma. Usually within seconds to minutes of the second impact, the athlete—conscious yet stunned—quite precipitously collapses to the ground, semicomatose with rapidly dilating pupils, loss of eye movement, and evidence of respiratory failure. (Cantu 1998, p. 38).

There appears to be a neurovascular mechanism behind this process, marked by the loss of cerebral vascular autoregulation that is different from that described in

Hovda et al.'s (1999) work after a singular TBI. The second injury is posited to result in vascular engorgement, with rapidly increasing intracranial pressure that leads to herniations in the uncus, the lobes below the tentorium, or the cerebellar tonsils through the foramen magnum (Cantu 1998). Often, the second injury is not severe, may not involve LOC, and may not even be noted by the individual or observers (Cantu and Voy 1995; Kelly et al. 1991). Within a short period of time, however, the athlete has a sudden decrease in functioning beginning with confusion and collapse, and often ending in death. The marked rapidity of the onset and changes associated with SIS has been documented in animal models as well as in humans (Bruce 1984; Bruce et al. 1981). As the literature on neurochemistry and neurometabolism suggests, the energy crisis and subsequent "vulnerability" that an initial, even mild, TBI creates is quite concerning, particularly given that the risk of a second concussion appears higher than likelihood of the first (Annegers et al. 1980; Salcido and Costich 1992).

Laurer et al. (2001) found that repeated MTBI resulted in intensified disruption of the blood-brain barrier in cortical regions, prolonged motor dysfunction, and increased axonal injury that appeared synergistic rather than simply additive from a previous MTBI 24 hours earlier. The investigators did not observe any cerebrovascular hypotension, an aforementioned proposed mechanism in SIS, after a repeated MTBI (Laurer et al. 2001). Although relatively rare in incidence, sports-related SIS has an extremely high mortality rate (McCrory and Berkovic 1998). In the literature, premature return to play after an initial concussion and SIS has been implicated, although incompletely substantiated, in at least 17 athlete deaths (Cantu and Voy 1995). The quickness of onset and the lethality of this syndrome make the prevention of SIS a high priority in the safety of athletes.

A recent article called the concept of SIS into question on the basis of a previous review of published cases (McCrory 2001; McCrory and Berkovic 1998). All published cases were reviewed for the following criteria: an observed first impact with subsequent medical review, documented ongoing symptoms between the first and second impacts, rapid cerebral deterioration after an observed second impact, and a neuroimaging or neuropathologic finding of cerebral edema without evidence of intracranial hematoma or other known cause (McCrory and Berkovic 1998). Of the 17 cases identified in the literature, none met these criteria for definite SIS and only five met the criteria for probable SIS. In addition, despite similar worldwide concussion rates across sports, virtually all of the SIS reports occurred in the United States. On the basis of these findings, McCrory (2001) argues that there

is insufficient evidence to name SIS as a clinical entity. He notes that there is a rare and catastrophic complication of head injury called "diffuse cerebral swelling," but that this condition is unrelated to whether a second impact occurs. Although McCrory argues that SIS is an unsubstantiated clinical entity, he notes that children and adolescents are at greater risk for diffuse cerebral swelling and that the etiology is often unknown. Therefore, he recommends that athletes who have sustained a concussion should not return to play until all symptoms have resolved and their neuropsychological functioning has returned to normal. In summary, McCrory urges that full neurological and neuropsychological symptom resolution should guide return to play rather than arbitrary guidelines based on fear of an unsubstantiated clinical condition (i.e., SIS).

Apolipoprotein E ε4 and Risk for Poor Outcome

Recent literature has implicated a particular form of apoE genotype as a marker for increased risk of negative consequences after brain injury. apoE is a plasma protein synthesized mainly in the liver that is implicated in encoding and transporting cholesterol. There are three major expressions of *apoE* that are the products of their respective alleles (*ε2*, *ε3*, and *ε4*). Whereas *apoE ε2* and *apoE ε3* have been shown to be involved in neuritic repair and expansion, *apoE ε4* appears to decrease growth and branching of neurites (Handelmann et al. 1992; Nathan et al. 1994; Sabo et al. 2000). Thus, it appears that apoE ε4 retards repair and therefore limits recuperation after brain injury. Evidence suggests that *apoE ε4* is a genetic risk factor in the development of AD (Strittmatter et al. 1993). Whereas 34%–65% of individuals with AD carry the *apoE ε4* allele, only 24%–31% of the nonaffected adult population possess this allele (Jarvik et al. 1995; Saunders et al. 1993). Furthermore, the presence of *apoE ε4* decreases the mean age at onset of AD from 84 to 68 years (Corder et al. 1993).

In addition to these findings, the presence of apoE has been linked to poorer outcomes from brain trauma (Mayeur et al. 1996). Individuals carrying the *apoE ε4* allele have demonstrated poorer recovery after intracerebral hemorrhage (Alberts et al. 1995). Other researchers have examined *apoE ε4* as a predictor of length of unconsciousness and recovery in individuals with TBI. In a prospective study, 69 consecutive inpatient and outpatient referrals were examined in a 6- to 8-month period (Friedman et al. 1999). Whereas 31% of participants without the *apoE ε4* allele had excellent functioning at follow-up, only 3.7% of the group with *apoE ε4* had the same results. Furthermore, participants with the *apoE ε4* allele had worse

GCS scores, and a greater percentage had LOC beyond 7 days. In sum, the presence of the *apoE ε4* allele predicted poorer short- and long-term functioning and recovery after TBI.

The association between the presence of the *apoE ε4* allele and poor outcome has significant implications for sports-related injuries. In his examination of 30 boxers, Jordan (1993) demonstrated that the combination of high exposure to risk of injury (as measured by participation in more than 11 bouts) and the presence of the *apoE ε4* allele accounted for significantly worse performance on a head injury scale. These findings were replicated in a study of cognitive status of younger versus older football players with and without the *apoE ε4* allele (Kutner et al. 2000). Kutner and colleagues conducted neuropsychological assessments and *apoE* genotyping of 53 active American professional football players, revealing lower-than-anticipated neuropsychological functioning in those players possessing the *apoE ε4* allele. In contrast, the Rotterdam study did not suggest that the presence of apoE is a potential risk factor for athletes at risk for head injury (Mehta et al. 1999). This study examined 6,645 subjects of the general population residing in a suburb of Rotterdam, Netherlands, age 55 years or older who were free from dementia at baseline assessment. The incidence of head trauma and LOC was measured at baseline and tracked over time, with genotype testing of 4,070 members of this sample. Subsequent analyses of individuals who had experienced a head injury in comparison with a cohort without head trauma revealed no increased risk for dementia on the basis of the incidence of mild head injury or the presence of *apoE ε4*. However, the length of the follow-up period was quite short (approximately 2.1 years), and the association was stronger for moderate and severe head injury versus mild. Clearly, the role and contribution of *apoE ε4* in recovery after head injury is a potentially fruitful area for future research, as is the potential contribution of *apoE ε4* to the development of degenerative neurological conditions.

Measuring the Severity of Injury

Sports brain injuries have inherent qualities that impede their identification and measurement. One is that athletes often deny or minimize symptoms in an effort to return to play. Another is that sequelae of MTBI may be subtle and not routinely reported by athletes. Finally, neuroimaging techniques typically do not identify evidence of MTBI. As a result, MTBIs in athletics are often overlooked or minimized.

Even when concussions are identified, a further complication is the determination of concussion severity. Classification is hindered by lack of clarity in the definition and description of different levels of injury. Because randomized prospective trials with human subjects are not feasible, researchers are limited in their ability to test hypotheses about gradations of MTBI. This results in significant variability in the classification systems for determining severity of injury, which were based on clinical consensus rather than an empirical basis.

In 1966, the Committee on Head Injury Nomenclature of the Congress of Neurological Surgeons defined *concussion* as "a clinical syndrome characterized by immediate and transient posttraumatic impairment of neural function, such as alteration of consciousness, disturbance of vision, equilibrium, etc., due to brainstem involvement" (p. 386). The broad nature of this description clearly limited classification. In an attempt to refine and clarify the variance in concussions, Maroon et al. (1980) proposed a graded system of classification of concussion on the basis of the length of unconsciousness. "Mild concussion" encompassed injuries with no LOC; "moderate concussion" included injuries with a brief LOC as well as retrograde amnesia; and "severe concussion" described injuries with a LOC of 5 minutes or more. Using his extensive experience as a team physician, Cantu (1986) combined these elements to create guidelines for determining severity of concussion using length of LOC and PTA. According to his grading system, Grade 1 concussion encompasses injuries with no LOC and less than 30 minutes of PTA, defined as any memory problems associated with brain trauma including retrograde amnesia and anterograde amnesia. Grade 2 includes injuries with LOC of less than 5 minutes in duration *or* PTA lasting longer than 30 minutes but less than 24 hours in duration. Grade 3 concussion refers to injuries with LOC of more than 5 minutes in duration *or* PTA lasting longer than 24 hours (Table 26–1).

TABLE 26–1.   Severity of concussion

Grade	Loss of consciousness		Duration of posttraumatic amnesia
1 (mild)	None		<30 minutes
2 (moderate)	<5 minutes	or	≥30 minutes but <24 hours
3 (severe)	≥5 minutes	or	≥24 hours

Source.   Reprinted with permission of WB Saunders Company. Originally printed in Cantu RC: "Return to Play Guidelines After a Head Injury," *Clinics in Sports Medicine* 17:52, 1998.

TABLE 26–2. American Academy of Neurology practice parameters for concussion severity

Grade	Symptoms	Loss of consciousness
1 (mild)	Transient confusion; symptoms or mental status abnormalities on examination resolve in <15 minutes	None
2 (moderate)	Transient confusion; symptoms or mental status abnormalities on examination last >15 minutes	None
3 (severe)	—	Any loss of consciousness, either brief (seconds) or prolonged (minutes)

Source. Adapted from Kelly JP, Rosenburg JH: "The Diagnosis and Management of Concussion in Sports." *Neurology* 48:575–580, 1997.

In contrast, the Colorado Medical Society (1991) guidelines propose a greater emphasis on LOC and confusion with amnesia. These guidelines were the precursors of the Practice Parameters established by the American Academy of Neurology (AAN; 1997). Unlike Cantu's system, these practice parameters consider any LOC a Grade 3 severe concussion, and they incorporate the concept of confusion as a hallmark of concussion. The AAN guidelines are organized as follows: Grade 1—Transient confusion, no LOC, concussion symptoms or mental status abnormalities on examination resolve in less than 15 minutes; Grade 2—Transient confusion, no LOC, concussion symptoms or mental status abnormalities on examination last more than 15 minutes; Grade 3—Any LOC, either brief (seconds) or prolonged (minutes) (Table 26–2).

A recent article by Cantu (2001) reproduced eight tables of concussion severity grading systems, but the most referenced methods are those of Cantu and the AAN Practice Parameters. In this same article, Cantu (2001) suggests some evidence-based modifications to his grading system on the basis of prospective studies of the connection between duration of PCS symptoms and PTA and results of neuropsychological assessment. This system introduces the consideration of PCS signs or symptoms that can be assessed on the sidelines using measures such as the Standardized Assessment of Concussion (SAC; McCrea et al. 1996) or other mental status or brief cognitive examinations/interviews. Cantu's new concussion severity rating system defines *Grade 1 concussion* as no

LOC with PTA or PCS symptoms less than 30 minutes. *Grade 2* is LOC less than 1 minute and PTA or PCS symptoms greater than 30 minutes and less than 24 hours. *Grade 3* is LOC greater than 1 minute or PTA greater than 24 hours, plus PCS symptoms longer than 7 days (Cantu 2000).

Each of the above grading systems has subtle distinctions, but each offers valuable guidelines for considering the seriousness of a concussion. The purpose of determining injury severity is to be sure to consider relevant neurologic and neurocognitive factors to help monitor recovery (or decline). Accurate assessment of these states has been the best effort to date in determining when full recovery has taken place and the brain is no longer vulnerable to the potential drastic effects of additional trauma (i.e., SIS). Determination of injury severity is a prerequisite for making return-to-play decisions, but clinical judgment is also necessary for dealing with these issues on a case-by-case basis.

In addition to concerns regarding the severity of single episodes of concussion, the cumulative aspects of multiple concussions must be considered as well. Although there is no general consensus and no data on the topic of how many concussions should result in termination of an athlete's career, Echemendia and Cantu (2004) suggest that two factors should be carefully considered. First, significant increases in the length of PCS symptoms—from days, to weeks, to months with each successive concussion—may indicate reduced resiliency. In other words, the athlete's capacity to recover from cumulative concussions has been depleted. Second, when lower levels of force and indirect blows (e.g., impact to the torso or legs) result in symptoms of concussion, it provides further indication that the athlete's "functional reserve" has been exhausted. Such indications that the athlete is at increasingly greater risk for additional concussions with more persisting symptoms should guide the decision to terminate an athlete's career.

Return-to-Play Criteria

Decisions about return to play are difficult to make because of the paucity of data regarding the effects of multiple concussions and the psychosocial pressures (i.e., coaches, family, players, and institutional needs) that are brought to bear on this question. Although there are no randomized, experimental studies assessing differences in long-term neurocognitive outcome as a function of different delays in return to play, there are data that provide some basis for specific return-to-play guidelines. For instance, the aforementioned University of Virginia foot-

TABLE 26–3. Guidelines for return to play after concussion

	First concussion	**Second concussion**	**Third concussion**
Grade 1 (mild)	May return to play if asymptomatic for 1 week	Return to play in 2 weeks if asymptomatic at that time for 1 week	Terminate season; may return to play next season if asymptomatic
Grade 2 (moderate)	Return to play after asymptomatic for 1 week	Minimum of 1 month; may return to play then if asymptomatic for 1 week; consider terminating the season	Terminate season; may return to play next season if asymptomatic
Grade 3 (severe)	Minimum of 1 month; may return to play if asymptomatic for 1 week	Terminate season; may return to play next season if asymptomatic	

Note.   *Asymptomatic* means no headache, dizziness, or impaired orientation, concentration, or memory during rest or exertion.
Source.   Reprinted with permission of WB Saunders Company. Originally printed in Cantu RC: "Return to Play Guidelines After a Head Injury," *Clinics in Sports Medicine* 17:56, 1998.

ball study (Barth et al. 1989; Macciocchi et al. 1996) offers clear indications of cognitive dysfunction after mild concussions, with a 5- to 10-day recovery cycle. The results of Hovda's (1996) mature rodent fluid percussion research, in which a "mild" concussion was induced, closely parallel this time line in terms of normalized glucose metabolism and CBF. At a minimum, common sense and medical concern regarding the vulnerability of the brain to more severe, catastrophic injury (i.e., SIS) dictate the need to hold players from contact situations until all neurologic/neuropsychological symptoms have subsided.

The Cantu and AAN concussion grading guidelines formed the basis of current return-to-play criteria (Table 26-3). These works extended and expanded Quigley's rule (Schneider 1973), which uniformly terminated an athlete's participation in contact sports after three concussions, regardless of severity. Cantu's guidelines for return to play recommend that an athlete be held from competition for 1 week if asymptomatic after sustaining his or her first Grade 1 concussion (Cantu 1998). In contrast, after the third Grade 1 concussion, the guidelines suggest that the athlete terminate play for the season. An athlete sustaining his or her first Grade 3 concussion would be held out of play for a minimum of 1 month and can then be returned to play after 1 week without symptoms during rest or exertion.

Echemendia and Cantu (2004) further advanced Quigley's rule by proposing a dynamic model of return-to-play decision making. They noted that most of the published return-to-play criteria are based on aspects of the concussion, such as LOC or PTA. They argued, however, that return-to-play decisions should involve consideration of multiple factors, including medical information, neuropsychological data, and player and team factors, in addition to severity of concussion and concussion history. Even extraneous factors, such as field condi-

tions and playing surface, should be considered. Echemendia and Cantu (2004) recommended that before an athlete is returned to play, all PCS symptoms must be absent while the athlete is at rest, the neurological examination must be normal, there should be no apparent structural lesions on CT or MRI, and the neuropsychological performance must return to or surpass the baseline performance. Once these criteria have been met, the athlete can slowly undergo exertional challenges, and as long as he or she remains symptom-free, the length and intensity of these challenges can be increased. The player factors to consider before returning an athlete to play include personality characteristics (e.g., his or her tendency to minimize or maximize symptoms), level of athletic skill, degree of investment in his or her sport, family issues, and attitude about return to play. Team factors include the level of competition (i.e., amateur vs. professional), the injured athlete's position on the team, and the likelihood of sustaining another concussion in that position, among other issues. Consideration of all these factors allows for making a return-to-play decision that is highly individualized and considers the athlete's best interests on multiple levels.

It is worth further comment to note how athlete personality factors may affect return-to-play decisions. Certainly, neuropsychiatric symptoms may emerge as a consequence of concussion, just as in more severe head injuries. Irritability, restlessness, depression, and fatigue may be experienced in the wake of MTBI, and these are important symptoms to identify and monitor during the recovery process. Because many athletes may be reluctant to acknowledge any symptoms, particularly psychiatric sequelae, careful assessment and observation are essential. Gathering corroborating data from coaches and teammates is often useful in determining if a concussed athlete's personality or behavior differs from the preinjury baseline. The physician should intervene, even if only by advising the patient to refrain from exertion, if the consensus is that the athlete's behavior is significantly different after injury. Just as neurocognitive symptoms need to resolve before returning to play, so, too, should emotional sequelae.

Sideline and Neuropsychological Assessment

To evaluate concussion severity accurately and objectively, preseason neurocognitive assessment is critical because it establishes a baseline to which one can compare an athlete's postconcussive performance. This is vitally important because there are many factors that would otherwise impede successful identification of mild concussion. First, the symptoms are often not immediately obvious. Furthermore, many athletes minimize their injuries to "play through the pain" and ensure playing time. In addition, comparing neurocognitive assessment findings to standard population normative data may underestimate concussion-related deficits, as performance in the "normal" range may still reflect significant decline for any given individual. Even comparing scores to sport-specific normative data would involve considerable risk for false negatives and false positives. Minimizing both is a priority in optimizing athlete health, and baseline testing permits an athlete to serve as his or her own control subject.

Once teammates, referees, athletic trainers, coaches, or team physicians have identified an athlete as having a possible concussion or the athlete self-reports symptoms, sideline assessment should be instituted. Such assessment should involve both neurocognitive screening and gross neurologic assessment to verify that a concussion indeed occurred, with resulting implications for removing the athlete from competition and eventual return to play. Most team physicians and athletic trainers agree with the AAN guidelines: persistence of any neurologic or cognitive symptoms for more than 15 minutes under conditions of rest and exertion precludes return to play during that event.

The most popular and well-studied brief sideline neurocognitive assessment measure is the SAC (McCrea et al. 1996). The SAC is a 5–10 minute evaluation of attention/concentration, memory, and rapid novel problem–solving typically administered after physical exertion. It is recognized as sensitive to mild cognitive and mental status impairment. When preseason baseline/number of errors is used, even one additional error suggests cognitive compromise. When coupled with a brief neurological examination, the SAC provides the minimum data for making immediate removal and return-to-play decisions.

To more completely evaluate severity of concussion and make eventual return-to-play decisions, the methodology used by SLAM (see History section above) (Barth et al. 1989, 2001) is the gold standard. This procedure uses preseason and extensive postconcussion neurocognitive assessment. A variety of assessment methods may be used, including traditional and standard paper-and-pencil neuropsychological tests, computerized assessment methods, and Web-based evaluative procedures. Many different neuropsychological tests, such as Trail Making Tests A and B from the Halstead-Reitan Neuropsychological Test Battery, the Paced Auditory Serial Addition Task, Rey Auditory Verbal Learning Test, the Hopkins Verbal Learning Test, the Digit Span subtest from the Wechsler Adult Intelligence Scale—III, and others, have been used with some success in sports concussion studies (Lezak 1995).

Ideally, all athletes at risk for concussion receive preseason screenings to determine each individual's baseline level of cognitive functioning (Barth et al. 2001; Lovell and Collins 1998). This is essential to control for any premorbid cognitive dysfunction, such as learning disabilities, attention-deficit/hyperactivity disorder (ADHD), history of concussion, or psychological factors (e.g., depression or anxiety), all of which have the potential to affect test results and mimic the neurocognitive effects of acute injury. Influences of learning disability and history of more than two concussions on testing have been found in some investigations (Collins et al. 1999; Matser et al. 1999). Other studies have found no effect of prior concussion on neurocognitive performance (Macciocchi et al. 2001). Neuropsychological screening of athletes usually takes 20–30 minutes and includes measures of cognition thought to be sensitive to the sequelae of concussion, including processing speed, attention/concentration, and memory (Lovell and Collins 1998). Any injured player should then receive a comprehensive evaluation, including repetition of baseline measures, within 24 hours of injury to detect any changes in performance. Neuropsychological assessment can thus serve as a sensitive tool in identifying any impairment that results from brain injury, even in the absence of radiographic or neurological findings (Broshek and Barth 2001). Repeated administrations of a test battery can then be used to track improved neurocognitive functioning over time to assist with the timing of return to play.

Computerized tests have been recently used. These procedures have numerous advantages, including less one-to-one test administration time, potential use of group-administered baseline measures, increased reliability of results, alternate forms, and ease and speed of statistical comparisons. Tests such as the Automated Neuropsychological Assessment Metric (ANAM) (Bleiberg et al. 2000; Reeves et al. 1995) and the more recently developed Immediate Post-Concussion Assessment and Cognitive Testing (ImPACT) (personal communication, M. Lovell, June 2001) provide the ease of automated assessment of the aforementioned cognitive/functional domains and rapidly available data for comparison with baseline scores.

Finally, the wave of the future will clearly involve brief computerized neurocognitive assessment that is easily accessible through the World Wide Web. Erlanger and colleagues at HeadMinder, Inc. have developed a system to deliver their Concussion Resolution Index (CRI), a set of neurocognitive tests of attention, reaction time, memory, and problem solving (Erlanger et al. 1999, 2001, 2002). With trainer supervision and use of a confidential, secure password, athletes may log into the system at any time and take the standard 20- to 30-minute neurocognitive battery. On completion, current test results are instantly compared with previous test results (e.g., baseline data) to determine whether there has been any decline or improvement. Medical and athletic personnel who are authorized to assist in making return-to-play decisions can then access these results. These tests have multiple forms, allowing testing each day if necessary to chart progress. Practice effects are controlled for by internal statistical analysis. Web-based assessment makes low-cost neurocognitive evaluation available to virtually everyone, but return-to-play decisions must be made on-site by medical, neuropsychological, and athletic trainer personnel.

Case Studies

The following case studies are included to demonstrate variability in clinical presentation among athletes who have sustained multiple concussions. Although not exhaustive, they are meant to exemplify the neurocognitive effects and decision-making process related to concussion.

Case Study 1

A 19-year-old female collegiate lacrosse player was referred for neuropsychological assessment after sustaining her eighth concussion, *none of which had resulted in LOC.* She was otherwise physically healthy, was not taking any medication, and reported that she had always excelled academically. The athlete sustained her first concussion while riding a skateboard in the second grade, sustaining a fractured jaw and several weeks of persisting headaches. In addition, her recall for that

accident was hazy. The second concussion occurred when she was in the eighth grade and was struck in the head with a lacrosse ball. She experienced approximately 2 days of confusion after that injury. Over the next few years, she sustained five more concussions during organized sports and, by self-report, generally fully recovered from each within 24–48 hours. When attempting to stand immediately after her fifth concussion, however, she collapsed to the ground. She was subsequently confused and dizzy for 2 days. She felt significantly better on the third day after injury and returned to practice.

Three weeks before the current evaluation, she sustained her eighth concussion while playing lacrosse when she collided with another player. Although the athlete did not feel that the impact was very hard, she felt very unsteady and dizzy and she had gaps in her memory for events that occurred after the impact. She was irritable and had difficulty concentrating for 2 days after the concussion, and her friends expressed concern that she was "not herself" during that time. She was held from practice for 1 week but had not yet returned to competition at the time of her evaluation.

Because of significant concerns about her history of multiple concussions, the athletic trainer referred her for a comprehensive neuropsychological evaluation. During the interview, the athlete reported that she never experienced persisting headaches, nausea, dizziness, irritability, or mood disturbance for more than 2 days after concussion. Academically, she felt that greater effort was required for her to achieve at her previous level, but she also acknowledged that her engineering courses had become significantly more difficult.

On the Wechsler Adult Intelligence Scale—III, the athlete's verbal and nonverbal intellectual ability fell within the superior range. Examination of her factor scores revealed that her working memory was high average and her processing speed was superior. On a novel problem-solving task that assesses nonverbal abstract reasoning, her performance was above average. On the Trail Making Test, which is very sensitive to cerebral dysfunction, her performance was superior. When compared with other individuals with superior intellect, her rapid serial addition ability was average. The athlete's performance on memory testing was average to superior. Her fine motor speed and dexterity were above average to superior, and she made no errors on sensory-perceptual testing. On the Personality Assessment Inventory, the athlete responded openly and candidly with no evidence of psychological distress.

Overall, the results of her neuropsychological evaluation revealed neurocognitive abilities that were not only intact but also exceptional when compared with her same age peers. Because she sustained two Grade II concussions during one season, it was recommended that she be held from competition for 1 month based on the Cantu guidelines. Although she did not appear to be experiencing any neurocognitive sequelae, it was concerning that she had a lifetime history of eight concussions. The athlete had a strong desire to return to play and was highly motivated to complete her collegiate athletic career. She was educated on the importance of avoiding future concussions, and it was suggested that she consider the use of protective headgear during practice to minimize her risk. The athlete was cleared for return to play by the team physician and athletic trainer after 1 month of rest. It was strongly recommended that she undergo another comprehensive neuropsychological assessment before return to practice or competitive play in the unfortunate event that she sustained another concussion.

Case Study 2

A neuropsychological screening was requested to evaluate a 19-year-old man who had suffered his sixth concussion during a college football scrimmage approximately 5 days before the appointment. The issue of multiple concussions and the persistence of subjective complaints led the neuropsychologist and head athletic trainer to expedite this referral. Prior concussions occurred after the age of 12, with some involving LOC and PTA. In one such instance, he recalled continuing to play in the contest despite having no memory of game events. For the most recent event, the athlete described having had a "ding" early in a scrimmage, but with no alterations in consciousness or neurological symptoms. A second head-to-ground contact later in that scrimmage resulted in immediate symptoms of confusion, headache, dizziness, and nausea, but he denied any LOC or true PTA. Nevertheless, he acknowledged persisting subjective short-term memory and attentional problems, as well as headaches that evolved during cognitive or academic challenges.

As part of his involvement in collegiate athletics, the athlete had participated in baseline neu-

TABLE 26–4. Results and interpretation for neuropsychological testing in Case Study 2

Test/subtest	Standard score	Interpretation
WAIS-III/Vocabulary	16	Very superior
WAIS-III/Block Design	15	Superior
Trail Making Test A	10	Average
Trail Making Test B	10	Average
Paced Auditory Serial Addition Task[a]	3	Moderately impaired
Rey Auditory Verbal Learning Test—Immediate/Delayed Recall	—	Average/average
Rey-Osterrieth Complex Figure Test Copy/Delayed Recall	—	Low average/ average

Note. WAIS-III=Wechsler Adult Intelligence Scale—III.
[a]During this measure, the athlete complained of developing a significant headache that had significantly disrupted his concentration skills.

rocognitive screening using the aforementioned CRI (Erlanger et al. 1999) (see Sideline and Neuropsychological Assessment section) to assess cognitive processing speed, reaction time, and visual memory. Two administrations subsequent to his most recent concussion showed performance between 1.5 and 3.0 standard deviations below his baseline CRI, as well as continued subjective reports of headaches, sleep disturbance, and diminished concentration and memory. These results suggested lingering neurocognitive sequelae from the injury. During the comprehensive assessment using standard paper-and-pencil neuropsychological tests, the athlete obtained the scores provided in Table 26–4.

Before clinically interpreting these results, other relevant contextual factors were also considered. First, the athlete had expressed ambivalence about his continued participation in his sport. He did not have career goals of playing at a higher level but instead indicated a desire to consider graduate training in education. Simultaneously, he reported long-standing pressures from parents and coaches to be a "star" athlete. Last, the athlete expressed significant emotional distress about how the cumulative effects of concussions might impact his cognition, as well as fear of having any further concussions. These concerns had not been previously discussed with the athletic training staff.

Straight interpretation of the data did not reveal concern that the athlete's history of concussions had caused any lasting neurocognitive effects, although the fact that he showed impaired performance on the Paced Auditory Serial Addition Task was of concern. Consistent with his self-report, sustained concentration efforts resulted in headache, which suggested that the measure was perhaps assessing the impact of his discomfort and not his true sustained attention skills. Nonetheless, development of symptoms during this "cognitive exertion" implied that return to physical exertion even without contact would be premature. As such, the primary decision was to hold the athlete from exertion, as well as contact, pending a neurosurgical consultation. When cleared by neurosurgery, the athlete was instructed to complete the CRI to determine whether he had returned to baseline. However, further contacts with this athlete during the intervening time allowed additional clinical context to enter the foreground. The neuropsychologist worked with the athlete to address his concerns with appropriate athletic staff, and in light of his career goals and personal concerns about how concussions might affect him in the future, the cooperative decision to retire the athlete was made.

These case studies emphasize concepts discussed in Echemendia and Cantu's (2004) previously cited dynamic model of return-to-play criteria. Although research will continue to illuminate the physiology of MTBI/concussion, there will always be individual differences among athletes. Each situation should be approached clinically from an idiographical perspective. Regardless of "hard" data, context from the athlete and collateral sources (e.g., parents, teams, and coaches) should play a prominent role in decisions regarding return to play and/or retirement from contact events. The perspective of the athlete and his or her concerns regarding the risks associated with concussion, career aspirations, investment in the sport or activity, and psychological adjustment are of considerable importance. In both of the above case studies, the athletes' wishes and fears played a dominant role in decisions regarding return to play and concussion management. These cases also demonstrate that there can be no predetermined or rigid cutoff for deciding how many concussions are too many. In some cases, one concussion may result in "retirement," whereas in other cases individuals show excellent neurocognitive functioning, little or no cognitive decline, and no elevated concern about additional injury despite having numerous prior concussions.

Although this is not to suggest that concussions occur without cost, the unique circumstances of each individual athlete must guide decision-making, and future research must account for these many complicated processes.

Prevention

According to the Centers for Disease Control and Prevention, the first step in preventing further cases of TBI is better data collection (Thurman et al. 1998). More information is needed on risk of injury by sport, typical causes of injury, and prevalence of injuries occurring at all levels of participation and competition (e.g., professional, community leagues, and youth sports). In addition to collecting injury data by sport, the collection of pooled data would provide common injury factors across sports, thereby suggesting global prevention strategies. Information should also be gathered on personal (e.g., appropriate use of protective equipment, substance abuse) and sports-specific risk (e.g., playing surface) factors to identify those risk factors that can be modified to prevent future injury.

Although education has not received sufficient emphasis to date, it clearly plays an important role in concussion prevention. Athletes should be instructed in the proper use and maintenance of protective headgear, the importance of inspecting their helmets daily, and techniques for reducing their risk of injury (Powell 1999). In addition, athletes should undergo conditioning and strengthening of the neck muscles as a means of reducing the transmission of impact forces to the brain (Johnston et al. 2001). The playing arena or surface should be inspected at each game to insure that there are no hazards that might increase the risk of injury (Powell 1999). Appropriate padding on goalposts and the corners of scorers' tables, as well as the removal of dangerous obstructions on the sidelines, may minimize injury.

For those athletes who have sustained a concussion, reviewing the film of the game or practice during which the injury occurred may provide additional information about the mechanism of injury (Oliaro et al. 2001). In addition to identifying the source of injury, such as head-to-ground or head-to-head contact, such reviews can identify improper or poor techniques that may be contributing to injury risk (Oliaro et al. 2001). Examples include spearing in football or incorrect heading style in soccer. Reviewing the athlete's technique and focusing on improving the athlete's playing style may prevent future concussions. Perhaps most importantly, athletes, coaches, and medical personnel should be educated about the seriousness of concussion so that athletes receive proper medical attention and are withheld from play until they have fully recovered.

Hard Science for Hard Questions

Laws of Motion and Mechanics of Injury

Varney and Roberts (1999) suggested that fundamental Newtonian formulas be used to describe linear and rotational vector forces on the head and brain as a model for understanding the role of acceleration and deceleration in clinical aspects of MTBI. Using these formulas, it is possible to estimate the g-forces applied to the brain, yielding models for comprehending the stresses and energy displacement on neural fibers in sport and nonathletic conditions (e.g., motor vehicle accidents). Determining g-forces (acceleration/deceleration) may make it possible to "calculate" an injury's severity. Use of these formulas would improve the empirical rating of brain injury severity and clarify the impact on neurocognitive functioning when used in conjunction with neuropsychological testing (Barth et al. 2001). Such research will improve our understanding of the mechanics of TBI and outcome, particularly when using the SLAM model (Barth et al. 1999, 2001).

Many sports-related brain injuries reflect sudden changes in velocity or generally rapid deceleration of the head and, consequently, the brain. Using the formula

$$a = (v^2 - v_o^2)/2sg$$

it is easy to compute the deceleration (a) using the observed initial speed (v_o) in a given direction before deceleration starts, the directional speed at the end of deceleration (v), and the distance traveled during the deceleration (s). The result is then obtained in terms of g, which is equivalent to 10.73 yards/sec^2 (Barth et al. 2001; Varney and Roberts 1999). In the majority of sports concussions, the player is often brought to a halt (v=0) by hitting another player, striking the ground, or hitting another immovable object such as a goalpost (Barth et al. 2001). For this common situation, the formula can be simplified as follows:

$$a = -v_o^2/2sg$$

After measuring the acceleration in sports-related injuries, estimates of the force applied to the individual athlete can then be calculated. This is achieved using Newton's second law of motion, in which force (F) equals mass (m) times acceleration (a):

$$F = ma$$

In the simplest case, if a player simply falls to the ground, *a* is solely the acceleration due to gravity, or 1 g, yielding the formula:

$$F = mg$$

It is easy to see that the forces applied to the body can quickly mount as the mass and the change in velocity increase. The amount of g-force necessary to induce clinically relevant functional and/or structural changes in the brain has yet to be empirically demonstrated, in part because it depends on numerous factors (e.g., direction of acceleration, state of preparedness for acceleration). These issues are the focus of "biomechanical studies" that investigate the physiological consequences in response to different injury situations. Some have suggested 200 g-force as the necessary threshold value for permanent damage to result from a single injury mechanism (Naunheim et al. 2000). These investigators used a triaxial accelerometer inserted in the helmets of four high school athletes during actual and simulated play. Naunheim and colleagues (2000) found "peak" g-forces during a simulated heading drill (54.7 g) were greater than "peak" values for two football linemen (29.2 g) and one ice hockey defenseman (35.0 g). No study to date has examined changes in cognition or other functional areas after measured forces applied to the brain. Hence, it is not clear "how much is too much" or what are the specific functional and structural effects of repeated concussive or subconcussive blows.

Numerous factors likely interact to determine the severity of injury. These include magnitude of acceleration and duration of acceleration, the number of directions in which acceleration occurs (i.e., rotational/angled vs. linear impacts) and the athlete's state of preparedness for acceleration. With respect to the latter, if an athlete is expecting an impact, and hence acceleration, he or she is more likely to protect the head by aligning the body or tensing the muscles in such a way that the g-force is distributed across a larger surface area (i.e., the upper body) rather than merely the head. Therefore, forces applied to the brain are likely reduced when athletes are prepared for contact, and more severe brain injuries may result from unanticipated impact (Barth et al. 2001). In sum, it is clear that measuring the forces actually applied to the brain presents a complex challenge. According to Newtonian laws, potential for more serious sports-related brain injury occurs when acceleration occurs over a short distance (i.e., full speed to a sudden stop), when an athlete is not prepared for acceleration, and when there are significant changes in velocity in several directions (e.g., rotational injuries such as those caused by clotheslining). These multiple acceleration vectors likely account for the greatest histokinetic changes, as evidenced by axonal injury, found in MTBI (Barth et al. 2001). As a result, such traumas may lead to the most dramatic changes in neurobehavioral outcome after sports-related concussion.

Use of Newtonian laws is essential in determining how to best protect athletes from sports-related brain injury.

Not only are they applied to the development of protective equipment but also in the development of training, techniques, and rules of various athletic endeavors. Unfortunately, although these Newtonian principles were well known before to the first football game in 1869, no padding of any kind was worn, no helmets at all were used in football before 1896, and there were no hard-shelled helmets used before the early 1950s (Mueller 1998). Despite the advent of shelled helmets, between 1945 and 1994 there were 684 deaths caused by head and cervical spine injuries in football, and even as recently 1971–1975 there were 59 deaths that were directly related to brain trauma. The majority of these deaths occurred at the high school level of competition (Mueller 1998). Thus, even though the surface area of head impact had been increased through the use of helmets, the laws of physics still needed further application. Recently, heightened emphasis of strength conditioning of the head and neck musculature has reduced the risk of injury. More importantly, the banning of head-first tackling (i.e., spearing) in 1976 and 51 other rule changes, as well as requiring college and high school athletes to wear helmets certified by the National Operating Committee on Standards for Athletic Equipment, have substantially reduced the fatality incidence in football (Mueller 1998). In the future, rule changes should be considered in various sports if particular aspects of play are identified that result in greater risk of brain injury (Johnston et al. 2001). Despite progress in the application of physics to protect athletes in all sports, there were 26 fatalities between the years of 1994 and 1999 because of football (Mueller 2001). There is clearly still work to be done.

Future Directions

As discussed throughout this chapter, understanding the phenomenon of MTBI is a complex task at best. MTBI has physiological, metabolic, cognitive, and psychological repercussions. Although consequence of multiple injuries is still a matter for further research, concerns about second impact syndrome and the possible synergistic adverse effects of cumulative concussive and subconcussive blows emphasize the need for future research in these realms. Because of the diversity of adverse effects on neurocognitive, sensorimotor, and neurochemical functioning, a multidisciplinary approach to evaluating and researching MTBI is essential. By blending the efforts and expertise of neuropsychology, neurology, neuropsychiatry, mechanical engineering, physiology, and pharmacology, more effective ways of evaluating, treating, and preventing MTBI in sports will be achieved. Larger-scale studies that incorporate the best of technology in these various fields will promote this goal.

Applying physics formulas and developing mathematical models for how various components (e.g., soft tissue, cerebrospinal fluid, skull, and protective equipment) respond to forces will enhance the mechanical understanding of such injury. Sensitive neuropsychological data, such as that provided by computerized testing, and neurophysiological measures of functioning, such as Doppler and other imaging, will aid in the translation of "hard data measurements" of applied forces. Establishing relationships among these variables and validating mathematical models of injury will facilitate a feedback loop for developing more effective protective equipment as well as enhancing the safety of techniques and rules. Use of the Newtonian formulas provides a good conceptual basis for understanding the mechanics of forces applied to the brain during sports-related concussion. With greater knowledge of the histokinetic, metabolic, and neurocognitive changes after TBI, specific chemical agents may be tested to improve the recovery curve or perhaps even protect against the ill effects of TBI.

References

Alberts MJ, Graffagnino C, McClenny C, et al: ApoE genotype and survival from intracerebral haemorrhage. Lancet 346:575, 1995

American Academy of Neurology: Practice parameter: the management of concussion in sports (summary statement). Neurology 48:581–585, 1997

American Medical Association Council on Scientific Affairs: Brain injury in boxing. JAMA 248:254–257, 1983

American Medical Equestrian Association: City of Plantation, Florida, requires ASTM SEI helmet when riding on public property. American Medical Equestrian Association News 10:6–8, 1999

Annegers JF, Grabow JD, Kurland LT, et al: The incidence, causes, and secular trends of head trauma in Ulmstead Count, MN. Neurology 30:912–919, 1980

Arvigo F, Cossu M, Fazio B, et al: Cerebral blood flow in minor cerebral contusion. Surg Neurol 24:211–217, 1985

Azari NP, Rapoport SI, Grady CL, et al: Gender differences in correlations of cerebral glucose metabolism rates in young normal adults. Brain Res 574:198–208, 1992

Bailes JE, Hudson V: Classification of sports-related head trauma: a spectrum of mild to severe head injury. J Athl Train 36:236–243, 2001

Barth JT, Macciocchi SN, Giordani G, et al: Neuropsychological sequelae of minor head injury. Neurosurgery 13:529–533, 1983

Barth JT, Alves WM, Ryan T, et al: Mild head injury in sports: neuropsychological sequelae and recovery of function, in Mild Head Injury. Edited by Levin HS, Eisenberg HM, Benton AL. New York, Oxford Press, 1989, pp 257–275

Barth JT, Varney RN, Ruchinskas RA, et al: Mild head injury: the new frontier in sports medicine, in The Evaluation and Treatment of Mild Traumatic Brain Injury. Edited by Varney RN, Roberts RJ. Mahwah, NJ, Lawrence Erlbaum Associates, 1999, pp 81–89

Barth JT, Freeman JR, Broshek DK, et al: Acceleration-deceleration sports-related head injury: the gravity of it all. J Athl Train 36:253–256, 2001

Barth JT, Freeman JR, Broshek DK: Mild head injury, in Encyclopedia of the Human Brain, Vol 3. Edited by Ramachandran VS. San Diego, CA, Academic Press, 2002, pp 81–92

Bazarian JJ, Wong T, Harris M, et al: Epidemiology and predictors of post-concussive syndrome after minor head injury in an emergency population. Brain Inj 13:173–189, 1999

Bergsneider M, Hovda DA, Shalmon E, et al: Cerebral hyperglycolysis following severe traumatic brain injury in humans: a positron emission tomography study. J Neurosurg 86:241–251, 1997

Biokinetics and Associates, Ltd.: Equestrian headgear standards. American Medical Equestrian Association News 11:1–3, 2000

Bleiberg J, Kane RL, Reeves DL, et al: Factors analysis of computerized and traditional tests used in mild brain injury research. Clin Neuropsychol 14:287–294, 2000

Blumbergs PC, Scott G, Manavis J, et al: Staining of amyloid precursor protein to study axonal damage in mild head injury. Lancet 34:1055–1056, 1994

Boden BP, Kirkendall DT, Garrett WE Jr.: Concussion incidence in elite soccer players. Am J Sports Med 26:238–241, 1998

Brooks N: Neurobehavioral effects of amateur boxing. Paper presented at the European International Neuropsychological Society Meeting, Barcelona, Spain, 1987

Brooks WH: Neurologic injuries in equestrian sport, in Neurologic Athletic Head and Spine Injuries. Edited by Cantu RC. Philadelphia, PA, WB Saunders, 2000, pp 305–316

Brooks WH, Bixby-Hammett DM: Head and spinal injuries associated with equestrian sports: mechanisms and prevention, in Athletic Injuries to the Head, Neck and Face. Edited by Torg JS. St. Louis, MO, Mosby, 1991, pp 133–141

Brooks WH, Bixby-Hammett DM: Equestrian Sports, in Sports Neurology, 2nd Edition. Edited by Jordan BD. Philadelphia, PA, Lippincott-Raven, 1998, pp 381–391

Broshek DK, Barth JT: Neuropsychological assessment of the amateur athlete, in Neurological Sports Medicine: A Guide for Physicians and Athletic Trainers. Edited by Bailes J, Day A. Rolling Meadows, IL, The American Association of Neurological Surgeons, 2001, pp 155–179

Bruce DA: Delayed deterioration of consciousness after trivial head injury in childhood. BMJ 289:715–716, 1984

Bruce DA, Alavi A, Bilaniuk L, et al: Diffuse cerebral swelling following head injuries in children: the syndrome of "malignant brain edema." J Neurosurg 54:170–178, 1981

Bull JP: Cyclists need helmets. BMJ 296:1144, 1988

Butler RJ: Neuropsychological investigation of amateur boxers. Br J Sports Med 28:187–190, 1994

Cantu RC: Guidelines for return to contact sports after a cerebral concussion. Physician Sports Med 14:75–83, 1986

Cantu RC: Head injuries in sport. Br J Sports Med 30:289–296, 1996

Cantu RC: Second-impact syndrome. Clin Sports Med 17:37–44, 1998

Cantu RC: Posttraumatic retrograde and anterograde amnesia: pathophysiology and implications in grading and safe return to play. J Athl Train 36:244–248, 2001

Cantu RC, Mueller FO: Catastrophic football injuries: 1977–1998. Neurosurgery 47:673–677, 2000

Cantu RC, Voy R: Second impact syndrome: a risk in any sport. Physician Sportsmed 23:27–36, 1995

Casson IR, Siegel O, Sham R, et al: Brain damage in modern boxers. JAMA 251:2663–2667, 1984

Centers for Disease Control and Prevention: Traumatic brain injury: Colorado, Missouri, Oklahoma, and Utah, 1990–1993. MMWR Morb Mortal Wkly Rep 46:8–11, 1997

Chissel HR, Feagin Jr. JA, Warme WJ, et al: Trends in ski and snowboard injuries. Sports Med 22:141–145, 1996

Chow TK, Bracker MD, Patrick K: Acute injuries in mountain biking. Western J Med 159:145–148, 1993

Collins MW, Grindel SH, Lovell MR, et al: Relationships between concussion and neuropsychological performance in college football players. JAMA 282: 964–970, 1999

Colorado Medical Society: Report of the sports medicine committee: guidelines for the management of concussion in sports. Denver, CO, Colorado Medical Society, 1991

Committee on Head Injury Nomenclature of the Congress of Neurological Surgeons: Glossary of head injury including some definitions of injury to the cervical spine. Clin Neurosurg 12:386–394, 1966

Condie C, Rivara RP, Bergman AB: Strategies of a successful campaign to promote the use of equestrian helmets. Public Health Rep 108:121–126, 1993

Consensus Conference: Rehabilitation of persons with traumatic brain injury. NIH Consensus Development Panel on Rehabilitation of Persons with Traumatic Brain Injury. JAMA 282:974–983, 1999

Corder EH, Saunders AM, Strittmatter WJ, et al: Gene dose of apolipoprotein E type 4 allele and the risk of Alzheimer's disease in late onset families. Science 261:921–923, 1993

Corsellis JA, Bruton CJ, Freeman-Browne D: The aftermath of boxing. JAMA 3:270–303, 1973

Dannenberg AL, Gielen AC, Beilsenson PL, et al: Bicycle helmet laws and educational campaigns: an evaluation of strategies to increase children's helmet use. Am J Pub Health 83:667–674, 1993

DeLee JC, Farney WC: Incidence of injury in Texas high school football. Am J Sports Med 20:575–580, 1992

Dewitt DS, Jenkins LW, Wei EP, et al: Effects of fluid-percussion brain injury on regional cerebral blood flow and pial arteriolar diameter. J Neurosurg 64:787–794, 1986

Diamond PT, Gale SD, Denkhaus HK: Head injury in skiers: an analysis of injury severity and outcome. Brain Inj 15:429–434, 2001

Dikmen S, McLean A, Temkin N: Neuropsychological and psychological consequences of minor head injury. Neurosurgery 48:1227–1232, 1986

Dixon C, Taft W, Hayes R: Mechanisms of mild traumatic brain injury (mTBI). J Head Trauma Rehabil 8:1–12, 1993

Echemendia RJ, Cantu R: Return to play following cerebral head injury, in Traumatic brain injury in sports: a neuropsychological and international perspective. Edited by Lovell MR, Echemendia RJ, Barth JT, et al. Netherlands, Swets & Zeitlinger, 2004, pp 479–498

Emerson CS, Headrick JP, Vink R: Estrogen improves biochemical and neurological outcome following brain injury in male rats, but not in females. Brain Res 608:95–100, 1993

Erlanger DM, Feldman DJ, Kutner K: Concussion Resolution Index. New York, HeadMinder, Inc., 1999

Erlanger D, Saliba E, Barth J, et al: Monitoring resolution of postconcussion symptoms in athletes: preliminary results of a Web-based neuropsychological test protocol. J Athl Train 36:280–287, 2001

Erlanger DM, Feldman D, Kutner K, et al: Development and validation of a Web-based neuropsychological test protocol for sports-related return-to-play decision making. Arch Clin Neuropsychol 18:293–316, 2003

Everett SA, Price JH, Bergin DA, et al: Personal goals as motivators: predicting bicycle helmet use in university students. J Safety Res 27:43–55, 1996

Farace E, Alves WM: Do women fare worse: a metaanalysis of gender differences in outcome after traumatic brain injury. J Neurosurg 93:539–545, 2000

Fenton G, McClelland R, Montgomery A, et al: The postconcussional syndrome: social antecedents and psychological sequelae. Br J Psychiatry 162:293–497, 1993

Forrester G, Encel J, Geffen G: Measuring post-traumatic amnesia (PTA): an historical review. Brain Inj 8:175–184, 1994

Frankel HL, Haskell R, Digiacomo JC, et al: Recidivism in equestrian trauma. Am Surg 64:151–154, 1998

Friedman G, Froom P, Sazbon L, et al: Apolipoprotein E-ε4 genotype predicts a poor outcome in survivors of traumatic brain injury. Neurology 52:244–248, 1999

Fullerton L, Becker T: Moving targets: bicycle-related injuries and helmet use among university students. J Am Coll Health 39:213–217, 1991

Furrer M, Erhart S, Frutiger A, et al: Severe skiing injuries: a retrospective analysis of 361 patients including mechanisms of trauma, severity of injury, and mortality. J Trauma 39:737–741, 1995

Gennarelli T: Mechanisms and pathophysiology of cerebral concussion. J Head Trauma Rehabil 2:23–29, 1986

Gennarelli TA, Adams GH, Graham DI: Acceleration induced head injury in the monkey: the model, its mechanisms and physiological correlate. Acta Neuropathol 7:23–25, 1981

Ginsberg GM, Silverberg DS: A cost-benefit analysis of legislation for bicycle helmets in Israel. Am J Public Health 84:653–656, 1994

Giza CC, Hovda DA: The neurometabolic cascade of concussion. J Athl Train 36:228–235, 2001

Goldman H, Hodgson V, Morehead M, et al: Cerebrovascular changes in a rat model of moderate closed-head injury. J Neurotrauma 8:129–144, 1991

Gronwall D, Wrightson P: Delayed recovery of intellectual function after minor head injury. Lancet 2:604–609, 1974

Groswasser Z, Cohen M, Keren O: Female TBI patients recover better than males. Brain Inj 12:805–808, 1998

Gur RE, Gur RC: Gender differences in regional cerebral blood flow. Schizophr Bull 16:247–254, 1990

Haglund Y, Eriksson E: Does amateur boxing lead to chronic brain damage? a review of recent investigations. Am J Sports Med 21:97–109, 1993

Hamilton MG, Trammer BI: Nervous system injuries in horseback-riding accidents. J Trauma 34:227–232, 1993

Handelmann GE, Boyles JL, Weisgraber KH, et al: Effects of apolipoprotein E, β-very low density lipoprotein, and cholesterol on the extension of neurites by rabbit dorsal root ganglion neurons in vitro. J Lipid Res 33:1677–1688, 1992

Harbaugh RE, Saunders RL: The second impact in catastrophic contact-sports head trauma. JAMA 252:538–539, 1984

Hovda DA: Metabolic dysfunction, in Neurotrauma. Edited by Narayan RK, Wilberger JE Jr., Povlishock JT. New York, McGraw-Hill, 1996, pp 1459–1478

Hovda DA, Prins M, Becker DP, et al: Neurobiology of concussion, in Sports Related Concussion. Edited by Bailes JE, Lovell MR, Maroon JC. St. Louis, MO, Quality Medical, 1999, pp 12–51

Hunter RE: Skiing injuries. Am J Sports Med 27:381–389, 1999

Jaques LB: Rates of bicycle helmet use in an affluent Michigan county. Public Health Rep 109:296–301, 1994

Jarvik GP, Wijsman EM, Kukull WA, et al: Interaction of apolipoprotein E genotype, total cholesterol level, and sex in prediction of Alzheimer disease in a case-control study. Neurology 45:1092–1096, 1995

Johnston KM, McCrory P, Mohtadi NG, et al: Evidence-based review of sport-related concussion: clinical science. Clin J Sport Med 11:150–159, 2001

Jordan BD: Neurological aspects of boxing. Arch Neurol 44:453–459, 1987

Jordan BD: Chronic neurological injuries in boxing, in Medical Aspects of Boxing. Edited by Jordan BD. Boca Raton, FL, CRC Press, 1993, pp 177–185

Jordan SE, Green GA, Galanty HL, et al: Acute and chronic brain injury in United States National Team soccer players. Am J Sports Med 24:205–210, 1996

Junger EC, Newell DW, Grant GA, et al: Cerebral autoregulation following minor head injury. J Neurosurg 86:425–432, 1997

Karpakka J: American football injuries in Finland. Br J Sports Med 27:135–137, 1993

Kelly JP, Nichols JS, Filley CM, et al: Concussion in sports: guidelines for the prevention of catastrophic outcome. JAMA 266:2867–2869, 1991

Kemp P, Houston A, Macleod M, et al: Cerebral perfusion and psychometric testing in military amateur boxers and controls. J Neurol Neurosurg Psychiatry 59:368–374, 1995

Kraus JF, Fife D, Ramstein K, et al: The relationship of family income to the incidence, external causes, and outcomes of serious brain injury, San Diego County, California. Am J Pub Health 76:1345–1347, 1986

Kraus JF, Peek-Asa C, McArthur D: The independent effect of gender on outcomes following traumatic brain injury. Neurosurg Focus 8:2000, 2000

Kriss TC, Kriss VM: Equine-related neurosurgical trauma: a prospective series of 30 patients. J Trauma 43:97–99, 1997

Kutner KC, Erlanger DM, Tsai J, et al: Lower cognitive performance of older football players possessing apolipoprotein E ε4. Neurosurgery 47:651–657, 2000

Lamb C: Equestrian helmet use in the National 4-H program. American Medical Equestrian Association News 11:12–17, 2000

Lampert PW, Hardman JM: Morphological changes in brains of boxers. JAMA 251:2676–2679, 1984

Laurer HL, Bareyre FM, Lee VM, et al: Mild head injury increasing the brain's vulnerability to a second concussive impact. J Neurosurg 95:859–870, 2001

Leininger BE, Gramling SE, Ferrel AD, et al: Neuropsychological deficits in symptomatic mild head injury patients after concussion and mild concussion. J Neurol Neurosurg Psychiatry 53:293–296, 1990

Levin HS, Lippold SC, Goldman A, et al: Neurobehavioral functioning and magnetic resonance imaging findings in young boxers. J Neurosurg 67:657–667, 1987a

Levin HS, Mattis S, Ruff RN, et al: Neurobehavioral outcome following minor head injury: a three-center study. J Neurosurg 66 :134–243, 1987b

Lezak MD: Neuropsychological Assessment. New York, Oxford University Press, 1995

Lovell MR, Collins MW: Neuropsychological assessment of the college football player. J Head Trauma Rehabil 13:9–26, 1998

Lovell MR, Iverson GL, Collins MW, et al: Does LOC predict neuropsychological decrements after concussion? Clin J Sport Med 9:193–198, 1999

Macciocchi SN, Barth JT, Alves W, et al: Multiple mild head injury in college athletes. Neurosurgery 10:510–514, 1996

Macciocchi SN, Barth JT, Littlefield L, et al: Multiple concussions and neuropsychological functioning in collegiate football players. J Athl Train 36:303–306, 2001

Magnes SA: When a knee injury becomes a head injury. Phys Sports Med 12:53–67, 1990

Maroon JC, Steele PB, Berlin R: Football head and neck injuries: an update. Clin Neurosurg 27:414–429, 1980

Martland HS: Punch-drunk. JAMA 19:1103–1107, 1928

Matser JT, Kessels AGH, Lezak MD, et al: Neuropsychological impairment in amateur soccer players. JAMA 282:971–973, 1999

Mawdlsey C, Ferguson FR: Neurological disease in boxers. Lancet 2:795–801, 1963

Mayeur R, Ottoman R, Maestre G, et al: Synergistic effects of head injury and apolipoprotein ε4 in patients with Alzheimer's disease. Neurology 45:555–557, 1996

McCarthy M: Pedal cyclists, crash helmets, and risk. Public Health 105:327–334, 1991

McCrea M, Kelly JP, Randolph C: Standardized Assessment of Concussion (SAC): Manual for Administration, Scoring, and Interpretation. Waukesha, WI, CNS, Inc., 1996

McCrory P: Does second impact syndrome exist? Clin J Sport Med 11:144–149, 2001

McCrory PR, Berkovic MD: Second impact syndrome. Neurology 50:677–683, 1998

McLatchie G, Brooks N, Galbraith S, et al: Clinical neurological examination, neuropsychology, electroencephalography and computed tomographic head scanning in active amateur boxers. J Neurol Neurosurg Psychiatry 50:96–99, 1987

Mehta KM, Ott A, Kalmijn S, et al: Head trauma and risk of dementia and Alzheimer's disease. Neurology 53:1959–1962, 1999

Mendez MF: The neuropsychiatric aspects of boxing. Int J Psychiatry Med 25:249–262, 1995

Miura SA, Schapiro MB, Grady CL, et al: Effect of gender on glucose utilization rates in healthy humans: a positron emission tomography study. J Neurosci Res 27:500–504, 1990

Mueller FO: Fatalities from head and cervical spine injuries occurring in tackle football: 50 years' experience. Clin Sports Med 17:169–182, 1998

Mueller FO: Catastrophic head injuries in high school and collegiate sports. J Athl Train 36:312–315, 2001

Nakaguchi H, Fujimaki T, Ueki K, et al: Snowboarding head injury: prospective study in Chino, Nagano, for two seasons from 1995 to 1997. J Trauma 46:1066–1069, 1999

Nathan BP, Bellosta S, Sanan DA, et al: Differential effects of apolipoprotein E3 and E4 on neuronal growth in vitro. Science 264:850–852, 1994

Naunheim RS, Standeven J, Richter C, et al: Comparison of impact data in hockey, football, and soccer. J Trauma 48:938–941, 2000

Neal S: Approved vs. non-approved riding helmets in competition disciplines. American Medical Equestrian Association News 10:13–17, 1999

Oliaro S, Anderson S, Hooker D: Management of cerebral concussion in sports: the athletic trainer's perspective. J Athl Train 36:257–262, 2001

Ommaya AK, Gennarelli TA: Cerebral concussion and traumatic unconsciousness: correlation of experimental and clinical observations on blunt head injuries. Brain 97:633–654, 1974

Paniak C, MacDonald J, Toller-Lobe G, et al: A preliminary normative profile of mild traumatic brain injury (mTBI) diagnostic criteria. J Clin Exp Neuropsychol 20:852–855, 1998

Pfeiffer RP: Off-road bicycle related injuries—the NORBA Pro/Elite category: Care and prevention. Clin Sports Med 13:207–218, 1994

Pinsky BM: New York equestrian helmet legislation. American Medical Equestrian Association News 11:1–3, 2001

Porter M, O'Brien M: Incidence and severity of injuries resulting from amateur boxing in Ireland. Clin J Sport Med 6:97–101, 1996

Powell JW: Injury patterns in selected high school sports, in Sports Related Concussion. Edited by Bailes JE, Lovell MR, Maroon JC. St. Louis, MO, Quality Medical, 1999, pp 75–90

Powell JW, Barber-Foss KD: Traumatic brain injury in high school athletes. JAMA 282:958–963, 1999

Putukian M, Echemendia R, Mackin S: Acute effects of heading in soccer: a prospective neuropsychological evaluation. Clin J Sport Med 10:104–109, 2000

Reeves D, Kane R, Winter K, et al: Automated Neuropsychological Assessment Metrics (ANAM): Test Administration Manual (Version 3.11). St. Louis, MO, Missouri Institute of Mental Health, 1995

Rimel RW, Giordani B, Barth JT, et al: Disability caused by minor head injury. Neurosurgery 9:221–228, 1981

Roass A, Nilsson S: Major injuries in Norwegian football. Br J Sports Med 13:3–5, 1979

Royal Society for the Prevention of Accidents: Information Sheet FS3: Cycling Facts. London, Royal Society for the Prevention of Accidents, 1991

Ruchinskas RA, Francis JP, Barth JT: Mild head injury in sports. Appl Neuropsychol 4:43–49, 1997

Runyan CW, Earp JA, Reese RP: Helmet use among competitive cyclists. Am J Prevent Med 7:232–236, 1991

Rutherford WH, Merrett JD, McDonald JR: Symptoms at one year following concussion from minor head injuries. Injury 10:225–230, 1979

Ryan AJ: Intracranial injuries resulting from boxing: a review (1918–1985). Clin Sports Med 6:31–40, 1987

Sabo T, Lomnitski L, Nyska A, et al: Susceptibility of transgenic mice expressing human apolipoprotein E to closed head injury: the allele E3 is neuroprotective while E4 increases fatalities. Neuroscience 101:879–884, 2000

Sacks JJ, Holmgreen P, Smith SM, et al: Bicycle-associated head injuries and deaths in the United States from 1984 through 1988. JAMA 266:3016–3018, 1988

Salcido R, Costich JF: Recurrent traumatic brain injury. Brain Inj 6:293–298, 1992

Saunders AM, Strittmatter WJ, Schmechel D, et al: Association of apolipoprotein E allele ε-4 with late-onset familial and sporadic Alzheimer's disease. Neurology 43:1467–1472, 1993

Schneider RC: Head and Neck Injuries in Football: Mechanisms, Treatment, and Prevention. Baltimore, MD, Williams & Wilkins, 1973

Serel M, Jaros O: The mechanisms of cerebral concussion in boxing and their consequences. World Neurol 3:351–358, 1962

Shalmon E, Bergsneider M, Kelly DF, et al: Existence of regional coupling between cerebral blood flow and glucose metabolism following brain injury [abstract]. J Neurotrauma 12:141, 1995

Sortland O, Tysvaer AT: Brain damage in former association football players: an evaluation by cerebral computed tomography. Neuroradiology 31:44–48, 1989

Spence LJ, Dykes EH, Bohn DJ, et al: Fatal bicycle accidents in children: a plea for prevention. J Pediatr Surg 28:214–216, 1993

Stewart WF, Gordon B, Selnes O, et al: Prospective study of central nervous system function in amateur boxers in the United States. Am J Epidemiol 139:573–588, 1994

Strebel S, Lam AM, Matta BF, et al: Impaired cerebral autoregulation after mild brain injury. Surg Neurol 47:128–131, 1997

Strittmatter WJ, Saunders AM, Schmechel D, et al: Apolipoprotein E: high avidity binding to β-amyloid and increased frequency of type 4 allele in late-onset familial Alzheimer disease. Proc Natl Acad Sci U S A 90:1977–1981, 1993

Thomassen A, Juul-Jensen P, de Fine OB, et al: Neurological, electroencephalographic and neuropsychological examination of 53 former amateur boxers. Acta Neurol Scand 60:352–362, 1979

Thurman DJ, Branche CM, Sniezek JE: The epidemiology of sports-related traumatic brain injuries in the United States: recent developments. J Head Trauma Rehabil 13:1–8, 1998

Tysvaer AT: Head and neck injuries in soccer: impact of minor trauma. Sports Med 14:200–213, 1992

Tysvaer AT, Storli OV: Association football injuries to the brain: a preliminary report. Br J Sports Med 15:163–166, 1981

Tysvaer AT, Storli OV, Bachen NI: Soccer injuries to the brain: a neurological and electroencephalographic study of former players. Acta Neurol Scand 80:151–156, 1989

U.S. Bureau of the Census: Statistical Abstract of the United States: 1993, 113th Edition. Washington, DC, U.S. Government Printing Office, 1993

U.S. Consumer Product Safety Commission: Skiing Helmets: An Evaluation of the Potential to Reduce Head Injury. Washington, DC, U.S. Government Printing Office, 1999

Varney NR, Roberts RJ: Forces and accelerations in car accidents and resultant brain injuries, in The Evaluation and Treatment of Mild Traumatic Brain Injury. Edited by Varney RN, Roberts RJ. Mahwah, NJ, Lawrence Erlbaum Associates, 1999, pp 39–48

Victor M, Adams R, Collins G: The Wernicke Korsakoff and Related Disorders due to Alcoholism and Malnutrition. Philadelphia, PA, FA Davis, 1989

Warkentin S, Passant U, Minthon L, et al: Redistribution of blood flow in the cerebral cortex of normal subjects during head-up postural change. Clin Autonom Res 2:9–24, 1992

Wasserman RC, Buccini RV: Helmet protection from head injuries among recreational bicyclists. Am J Sports Med 18:96–97, 1990

Weiss BD: Bicycle helmets: effective, but underused. JAMA 266:3032–3033, 1991

Whitlock MR: Injuries to riders in the cross country phase of eventing: the importance of protective equipment. Br J Sports Med 33:212–214, 1999

Wojtys EM, Hovda D, Landry G, et al: Concussion in sports. Am J Sports Med 27:676–687, 1999

Yamakami I, McIntosh TK: Effects of traumatic brain injury on regional cerebral blood flow in rats as measured with radiolabeled microspheres. J Cereb Blood Flow Metab 9:117–124, 1989

Yelon JA, Harrigan N, Evans JT: Bicycle trauma: a five-year experience. Am Surg 61:202–205, 1995

Yuan X, Prough DS, Smith TL, et al: The effects of traumatic brain injury on regional cerebral blood flow in rats. J Neurotrauma 5:289–301, 1988

27 Children and Adolescents

Jeffrey E. Max, M.B.B.Ch.

THIS CHAPTER FOCUSES on the relatively under-studied area of neuropsychiatric aspects of pediatric traumatic brain injury (TBI). There are brief sections that review neurological, neurocognitive, language, and educational aspects of pediatric TBI with specific relevance to child neuropsychiatry. Citations for review articles on these topics are provided for readers who desire more in-depth reviews of each of these areas.

Epidemiology

TBI in children and adolescents is a major public health problem. The average incidence rate of all levels of brain injury severity in children younger than age 15 years is approximately 180 per 100,000 children per year (Kraus 1995). The ratio of deaths to hospital discharges to reported medically attended instances is approximately 1:32:152. The male to female incidence rate ratio is approximately 1.8:1.0 and increases to 2.2:1.0 when children ages 5–14 years are considered. The incidence in males and females is similar in those ages 1–5 years (160 per 100,000 population), but then increases at a higher rate in males. In late childhood and adolescence, brain injury rates increase for males but decrease for females. Higher incidence rates have been found to be related to median family income even when age and/or race and ethnicity were controlled (Kraus et al. 1990). The proportion of brain injury caused by motor vehicle or motor vehicle–related accidents increases with age, from 20% in children 0–4 years to 66% in adolescents (Levin et al. 1992). Pedestrian or bicycle-related injuries more likely affect younger children, whereas adolescents are more often injured in motor vehicle accidents. The mechanism of injury in almost 50% of cases of infant, toddler, and young child brain injury is related to assaults or child abuse and falls (Adelson and Kochanek 1998). The distri-

bution of brain injury by severity ranges from 80% to 90% for mild, 7% to 8% for moderate, and 5% to 8% for severe brain injury. *Mild TBI* is generally defined by a lowest postresuscitation Glasgow Coma Scale (GCS) (Teasdale and Jennett 1974) score of 13–15 with no brain lesion documented by computed tomography (CT) scan or magnetic resonance imaging. *Moderate TBI* is defined by a lowest postresuscitation GCS score of 9–12, or 13–15 with a brain lesion on CT scan or magnetic resonance imaging or a depressed skull fracture. *Severe TBI* is defined by a lowest postresuscitation GCS score of 3–8 (Williams et al. 1990).

Etiology and Pathophysiology

Focal injuries, including subdural, epidural, and intracerebral hematomas, occur with a higher incidence in adults (30%–42%) versus children (15%–20%). There is an anterocaudal gradient in the frequency of focal lesions. There is a higher frequency of children with lesions in the dorsolateral frontal region (middle and superior frontal gyri), orbitofrontal region (orbital, rectal, and inferior frontal gyri), and frontal lobe white matter; a few areas of abnormal signal in the anterior temporal lobe; and isolated areas in more posterior areas (Levin et al. 1993). Skull fractures occur in approximately 5%–25% of children and are less commonly associated with epidural hematomas (40%) than in adults (61%). Children, more frequently than adults, present with diffuse injury and cerebral swelling (44%), resulting in intracranial hypertension. Diffuse axonal injury or vascular injury, or both, are the principal histopathologic findings of a diffuse injury in children. For a more complete review of advances in the understanding of the pathophysiology of pediatric brain injury (including blood flow changes and biochemical cascades) as well as initial assessment, management, and treatment of pediatric brain injury, see Adelson and Kochanek (1998) and Chapter 2, Neuropathology.

Sequelae

Neurological Sequelae

Acute management of children with TBI may involve the diagnosis and treatment of delirium. The pillars of management are the interruption of the normal secondary response of the brain to trauma and the avoidance and treatment of secondary insults such as systemic deterioration or hypotension, or both, prolonged hypoxemia, and uncontrolled intracranial hypertension (Adelson and Kochanek 1998).

There are many potential neurological sequelae of TBI, depending on the nature and location of brain damage. These include paresis and peripheral neuropathy, which may require occupational or physical therapy or both. Other sequelae include movement disorder, the residua of associated musculoskeletal injuries, endocrine disturbances, and seizures.

Posttraumatic seizures are of particular interest and relevance to psychiatrists who treat children with TBI. The incidence of early seizures (within the first week of TBI) is approximately 5% among all individuals with TBI and is higher in young children, among whom the incidence is approximately 10% (Yablon 1993). Immediate seizures (within the first 24 hours of TBI) constitute 50%–80% of early seizures and are particularly frequent among children with severe TBI. Late seizures (beyond the first week after TBI) occur in approximately 4%–7% of adults with TBI and occur less frequently in children. A psychiatric study of compound depressed skull fractures reported that psychiatric disorder was more frequent, but not at a statistically significant level, in children with late-onset epilepsy (Shaffer 1995). However, elevated rates of psychiatric disorder are consistently found in cohorts of individuals with epilepsy who have not experienced a TBI (Ott et al. 2001). Antiepileptic drugs may positively influence behavioral or psychiatric presentation in children by helping to achieve seizure control or may compound psychiatric problems through side effects (Ott et al. 2001).

School Sequelae

Academic functioning within the school environment is the childhood equivalent of occupational functioning for adults. Adults are not guaranteed reentry into the occupational arena after severe TBI, but educators are mandated to provide services to children under the Individuals with Disabilities Education Act. The challenge for schools is substantial because it has been estimated that as many as 20 school-aged children in a school district of 10,000 will sustain a TBI and will require specialized educational provisions (Arroyos-Jurado et al. 2000). The special education services required for these TBI survivors have to be tailored toward their particular needs, which are often different from those of children with developmental learning disabilities. Special education services are necessary for various problems, including poor academic function related to 1) skill deficits in major domains such as arithmetic, spelling, and reading; 2) behavioral and emotional disorders; or 3) a combination of the preceding with or without underlying complications of preinjury developmental learning disabilities in some children.

Special Education: Skill Deficits in Arithmetic, Spelling, and Reading

The use of appropriate control groups, a luxury not available to school psychologists, generally allows the detection of significant decrements in academic function in children after severe TBI, but not after mild TBI, once preinjury risk factors are controlled (Bijur et al. 1990; Fay et al. 1994). The younger children are at the point of injury, the more vulnerable they may be to persistent deficits in academic skills (Ewing-Cobbs et al. 2004). A study that used preinjury group testing data (state-mandated tests) revealed that the higher the child's ability before mild to severe TBI the higher his or her reading and spelling achievement and adaptive functioning were at 2 years postinjury (Arroyos-Jurado et al. 2000). When decrements are present, they are not uniform across individuals and can include permutations of academic functional deficits in mathematics, spelling, and reading domains (Barnes et al. 1999; Chadwick et al. 1981b; Ewing-Cobbs et al. 1998; Jaffe et al. 1992, 1993; Knights et al. 1991). In general, however, word recognition scores may be relatively spared, whereas arithmetic scores and reading comprehension may be more vulnerable to TBI (Barnes et al. 1999; Berger-Gross and Shackelford 1985; Ewing-Cobbs et al. 1998).

Even if scores on standardized academics tests recover to the average range, classroom performance and academic achievement may not. This may imply that the standardized tests are relatively insensitive. This insensitivity may be related to the broad average ranges on the tests, such that a very large decline is necessary for scores to enter a "below average" range. The insensitivity may also be related to the "sanitized" environment of the testing room. In contrast, the classroom milieu is embedded with numerous auditory, visual, and social distractions.

Function in the major academic domains (arithmetic, spelling, and reading) may depend on a number of more basic or core cognitive skills that are frequently impaired after severe TBI (see Fay et al. 1994). For example, arithmetic may require working memory, visual memory, and visual-spatial skills; spelling may require phonological processing, visual memory, and visual-motor integration; and reading may require phonological processing, fluency of retrieval of names for visual stimuli, word decoding skill, vocabulary knowledge, and auditory working memory (Ewing-Cobbs et al. 2004).

Special Education: Behavioral and Emotional Problems

Another category of specialized educational needs stems from behavioral and emotional disorders that limit functional academic achievement. Specific psychiatric syndromes that may interfere with function include personality change (PC) due to TBI, in which low frustration tolerance can lead the child to become overly distressed, avoid work, or be ejected from class for markedly inappropriate social behavior. Attention-deficit/hyperactivity disorder (ADHD) may similarly interfere because of inattentive, impulsive, and hyperactive behavior. Major depression may leave a child without the emotional resources, drive, and concentration to work efficiently. Children with oppositional defiant disorder (ODD) may refuse to work or be so disruptive that they, too, may be ejected from class or else learn less. These and other psychiatric disorders are discussed further in the section Psychiatric Sequelae.

Special Education: Service Delivery

A common scenario in the case of children who survive a severe brain injury is for the children to face significant challenges when they return to school. Armstrong et al. (2001) reported that many children with TBI do not receive special education despite impaired functioning. These investigators reported that rates of special education services were higher in a severe TBI group (50%) than a moderate TBI group (14%) or orthopedic group (10%) approximately 4 years postinjury. The most common special classifications for children with TBI were "traumatic brain injury" and "learning disability." Predictors of special education services included more severe TBI, lower socioeconomic status, more pre- and postinjury behavior problems, lower ratings of pre- and postinjury academic performance, and weaker postinjury neuropsychological and achievement skills (Armstrong et al. 2001).

One reason that some children do not receive special education services is that frequently school personnel are not aware that the student has had a TBI, especially with greater elapsed time since the injury. Another reason that some children do not receive services or receive limited services is because of financial constraints in school districts. The quality of services may be limited because of insufficient training with regard to the specific challenges of children with TBI.

Appropriate training of educators can clarify some of the following issues. Behavior problems, including disinhibited remarks, hyperactivity, poor attention, and disruptive behavior, may be seen as volitional. The student's presentation may be complex because some aspects of his or her behavioral difficulty may in fact be volitional to escape academic demands that may not have been tailored to his or her altered capacity for academic work. Children who were volitionally disruptive before the TBI may continue to be so after the injury. Clinical assessment may be required to discern whether there is a component of their postinjury disruptiveness that has a direct relationship to brain injury. The more remote the TBI, the less likely it is for the injury to be thought of as playing a relevant role in current difficulties. Parents face an annual challenge to educate and inform school personnel about their child's particular problems. School personnel are sometimes skeptical about the relevance of a remote TBI because usually children with even severe TBI have a relatively normal physical appearance and, as noted in the section Special Education: Skill Deficits in Arithmetic, Spelling, and Reading, have intellectual function and even academic achievement standardized scores within the normal range. Comprehensive school-based identification and intervention programs have been proposed to address these issues (e.g., Ylvisaker et al. 2001).

Psychiatric Sequelae

Psychiatric disorders that occur after child and adolescent TBI pose major challenges to community reentry and to quality of life.

Methodological Concerns

Study design is critical to the determination of the quality and generalizability of data generated. Many of the controversial issues in the child and adolescent TBI clinical outcome field have their basis in the overinterpretation of data from studies with major design flaws. This is especially true in the debate concerning outcome after mild TBI in children (Satz et al. 1997). Most studies, with rare exceptions (e.g., Ewing-Cobbs et al. 1999), exclude children with a history of physical abuse. Therefore, unless otherwise indicated, this review refers only to accidental injury.

In general, psychiatric aspects of child and adolescent TBI have received scant attention from researchers. In fact, there have only been two prospective studies of consecutive hospital admissions of children and adolescents with TBI in which standardized psychiatric interviews were used to assess psychopathology (Brown et al. 1981; Max et al. 1997b). Other data that have informed the understanding of this topic are essentially of lesser quality because of study design. Table 27–1 lists psychiatric studies of childhood TBI according to design characteristics such as consecutive hospital admissions, prospective and retrospective psychiatric assessment, standardized interview assessment, and use of a control group. There is also a large literature that addresses postinjury behavioral changes reported by parents and teachers—typically by questionnaires, which tend not to be specific for generating a psychiatric diagnosis or a psychiatric treatment plan (e.g., Fletcher et al. 1990; Rivara et al. 1994; Schwartz et al. 2003; Yeates et al. 1997).

Preinjury Psychiatric Status

Preinjury behavioral status in children who have a TBI is an area of some debate. The only prospective psychiatric studies that have used standardized psychiatric interviews found that between one-third and one-half of children had a preinjury lifetime psychiatric disorder (Brown et al. 1981; Max et al. 1997e). The investigation of preinjury psychopathology using behavior checklists soon after the child's TBI has produced conflicting data. One group (Pelco et al. 1992) studied a sample of consecutively admitted children with TBI and found no evidence of increased preinjury psychopathology when compared with population norms on the Child Behavior Checklist (Achenbach 1991). Another investigator (Donders 1992) found no evidence for an increased level of preinjury psychopathology in a referred sample of children with severe TBI admitted to a rehabilitation center. However, others reported on a large nonreferred sample of prospectively followed children with mild TBI, orthopedic-injured control subjects, and community control subjects and found that significant preinjury differences on the Child Behavior Checklist were evident between the TBI and community control subjects, and neither group differed from the orthopedic children (Light et al. 1998). The mean ratings were not elevated at clinically significant levels in any of the groups. Bijur et al. (1988) conducted a large epidemiological study involving a birth cohort studied at age 5 years and then again at age 10 years. They found that children who went on to sustain injuries (e.g., mild brain injury, burns, and lacerations) in the follow-up period were rated as having more behavioral problems, particularly aggression, before their injuries when compared with children who did not have injuries.

A unique contribution to this literature was provided by Bloom et al. (2001), who sampled 46 consecutively admitted children from a prospective study of TBI in which children were enrolled only if a developmental screen for psychiatric disorders, including ADHD, was negative. Despite the effort to exclude youth with a history of psychopathology, a standardized psychiatric interview assessment conducted at least 1 year postinjury concluded that the onset of any psychiatric disorder and onset of ADHD, specifically, occurred in 35% and 22% of children, respectively, before the injury. This finding suggests that the lack of evidence for preinjury psychopathology in children with TBI, as assessed primarily by behavioral checklists or developmental screens, may be related to insensitivity of the instruments.

Postinjury Psychiatric Status

The first stage in the evolution of research in child and adolescent psychiatric outcome after TBI has focused on the emergence of new or novel psychiatric disorders. The term *novel psychiatric disorders* has been coined to describe two possible scenarios (Max et al. 1997e). First, a child with TBI free of preinjury lifetime psychiatric disorders could manifest a psychiatric disorder post-TBI. Second, a child with a lifetime psychiatric disorder could manifest another psychiatric disorder that was not present before the TBI. These disorders are varied, thus demonstrating that behavioral outcome after brain injury is not a unitary construct. This categorical classification system of new, or novel, disorders has value because it reflects functional outcome in children and has information about risk factors for psychiatric disorder in this population. The second stage in this evolution is the examination of characteristics, including risk factors and phenomenology of specific clusters of psychiatric symptoms or specific psychiatric disorders, that emerge after TBI. Research on specific new psychiatric disorders is necessary because it is likely that different disorders will have different psychosocial and biological (including lesion) characteristics. The findings from this research may have relevance to the understanding of phenotypically similar disorders in children who have not experienced brain injury.

New Psychiatric Disorders

New psychiatric disorders have been noted in 54%–63% of children approximately 2 years after severe TBI, in 10%–21% of children after mild-moderate TBI, and in 4%–14% of children after orthopedic injury (Brown et al. 1981; Max et al. 1997b; Max et al. 1998h). As shown in Table 27–2, predictors of novel psychiatric disorders include severity of injury, preinjury psychiatric disorders,

TABLE 27–1. Psychiatric studies of pediatric traumatic brain injury (TBI)

Study	Consecutive admissions	Prospective vs. retrospective	Referred sample source	Standardized psychiatric interview	Control subjects
Brown et al. 1981	x	Prospective	—	x	x
Max et al. 1997b	x	Prospective	—	x	—
Black et al. 1969	x	Prospective	—	—	—
Hjern and Nylander 1964	x	Prospective	—	—	—
Luis and Mittenberg 2002	x	Retrospective	—	x	x
Bloom et al. 2001	x	Retrospective	—	x	—
Lemkuhl and Thoma 1990	x	Retrospective	—	x	—
Max et al. 1998h	x	Retrospective	—	x	x
Schachar et al. 2004	x	Retrospective	—	—	x
Shaffer et al. 1975	x	Retrospective	—	x	—
Rune 1970	x	Retrospective	—	—	—
Gerring et al. 1998	—	Prospective	Rehabilitation center	x	—
Konrad et al. 2000	—	Retrospective	Rehabilitation centers	—	x
Max et al. 1997a	—	Retrospective	Pediatric brain injury clinic	x; chart review	—
Bender 1956	—	Retrospective	Child psychiatry inpatients	—	—
Blau 1936	—	Retrospective	Child psychiatry inpatients	—	—
Strecker and Ebaugh 1924	—	Retrospective	Child psychiatry inpatients	—	—
Max et al. 1997c	—	Retrospective	Child psychiatry inpatients	—	x
Harrington and Letemendia 1958	—	Retrospective	Child psychiatry outpatients	—	—
Kasanin 1929	—	Retrospective	Child psychiatry outpatients	—	—
Max and Dunisch 1997	—	Retrospective	Child psychiatry outpatients	—	x
Otto 1960	—	Retrospective	Child psychiatry outpatients	—	—
Dillon and Leopold 1961	—	Retrospective	Litigants	—	—
Max et al. 1998b	—	Retrospective	Litigants	—	x
Ackerly and Benton 1947	—	Retrospective	Case report	—	—
Eslinger et al. 1992	—	Retrospective	Case report: adult with childhood TBI	—	—
Price et al. 1990	—	Retrospective	Case report: adult with childhood TBI	—	—
Marlowe 1992	—	Retrospective	Case report	—	—
Russell 1959	—	Retrospective	Case report	—	—
Williams and Mateer 1992	—	Retrospective	Case report	—	—

preinjury family function, family psychiatric history, socioeconomic status and preinjury intellectual function, and preinjury adaptive function (Brown et al. 1981; Max et al. 1997b). The most consistent predictor of novel psychiatric disorders in one study was preinjury family func-

tion (Max et al. 1997b). Because preinjury psychiatric disorders are predictors of novel psychiatric disorders, the importance of retrospectively assessing whether these disorders were present before the injury cannot be overstated. One prospective study (Max et al. 1997b) found

TABLE 27–2. Predictive variables of novel psychiatric disorders in the 2 years after childhood traumatic brain injury

Severity of injury

Lifetime preinjury psychiatric disorder

Preinjury teacher-rated behavior

Preinjury parent-rated adaptive function

Family psychiatric history

Preinjury family function

Socioeconomic status

Preinjury intellectual function

that there was no child with a mild-moderate TBI who was free of a preinjury lifetime psychiatric disorder who went on to manifest a novel psychiatric disorder in the second year after injury. All mild-moderate TBI children who exhibited a preinjury psychiatric disorder and then developed a novel disorder had either preinjury traits of what turned out to be the novel disorder, the disorder was transient, or the disorder was apparently unrelated to the brain injury itself (e.g., adjustment to an unrelated individual or family environmental stressor).

A large epidemiological study of a Finnish birth cohort reported that either inpatient- or outpatient-treated TBI before age 15 years in males was associated with a twofold increased risk of development of later inpatient-treated psychiatric disorder and a fourfold risk of later comorbid inpatient-treated psychiatric disorder and registry-classified criminality (Timonen et al. 2002). However, this finding does not necessarily confirm causality. Raw data revealed that 9% of children with TBI (vs. 2% of the noninjured group) developed a psychiatric disorder that was eventually treated with hospitalization, and 16% of children with TBI (vs. 10% of the noninjured group) developed registry-classified criminality. Furthermore, 5% of those individuals treated as inpatients for psychiatric disorder had a history of TBI, and 4% of classified criminals had a history of TBI.

Family Function and Psychiatric Disorder in Children With TBI

When children and adolescents have a TBI, the family is affected. Only one study has investigated the relationship of postinjury family function and psychiatric complications of TBI (Max et al. 1998f). This study shows that the strongest influences on family functioning after childhood TBI are preinjury family functioning and the devel-

opment of a novel psychiatric disorder. Preinjury family life events or stressors and immediate postinjury coping style emerge as significant variables later in the follow-up. The importance of novel psychiatric disorders for family functioning is evident at 6, 12, and 24 months postinjury. The direction of these effects are in the expected direction (worse outcome with poorer family function, presence of novel psychiatric disorder, more stressors, and use of fewer sources of support).

Other studies also show that family function (pre- and postinjury) and child behavior (pre- and postinjury) are closely related. Thus, pre- and postinjury family function predicted behavioral problems after TBI (Taylor et al. 1999; Yeates et al. 1997), and behavior problems developing shortly after TBI were associated with family burden, family distress, or poorer family function at follow-up (Barry et al. 1996; Rivara et al. 1992, 1993). Furthermore, Taylor et al. (2001) have demonstrated tentative support for bidirectional influences of child behavior and family function after TBI.

Specific Psychiatric Disorders and Symptom Clusters

Personality Change due to TBI

The most common novel disorder after severe TBI is PC due to brain injury (Max et al. 2000, 2001) or its approximations in other diagnostic nomenclatures. The Neuropsychiatric Rating Schedule (Max et al. 1998d) can be used to establish a diagnosis of PC. Approximately 40% of consecutively hospitalized children with severe TBI had ongoing persistent PC an average of 2 years postinjury (Max et al. 2000). Additionally, approximately 20% had a history of a remitted and more transient PC. PC occurred in 5% of mild-moderate TBI patients, but was always transient. Other studies of consecutive TBI admissions found that 5 of 31 (16%) (Brown et al. 1981) to 17 of 45 (38%) (Lehmkuhl and Thoma 1990) children with severe TBI developed a syndrome that resembled PC. The labile, aggressive, and disinhibited subtypes of this syndrome are common, whereas the apathetic and paranoid subtypes are uncommon (Max et al. 2000; 2001). Table 27–3 shows the items rated on the Neuropsychiatric Rating Schedule and the frequencies of PC symptoms after severe TBI. In children with severe TBI, persistent PC was significantly associated with severity of injury, particularly impaired consciousness longer than 100 hours and a concurrent diagnosis of secondary ADHD (SADHD) but was not significantly related to any psychosocial adversity variables. Persistent PC was also significantly associated with adaptive and intellectual function-

TABLE 27–3. Frequency of positively rated Neuropsychiatric Rating Schedule items among 37 consecutively admitted subjects with severe traumatic brain injury (TBI)

Subtype or symptom	Frequency	Percentage
(1) Personality change	21/37	57
(2) **Affective instability**	18/37	49
(3) Marked shifts from normal mood to depression	3/37	8
(4) Marked shifts from normal mood to irritability	15/37	41
(5) Marked shifts from normal mood to anxiety	2/37	5
(6) Rapid shifts between sadness and excitement	4/37	11
(7) Laughs inappropriately and/or excessively	9/37	24
(8) Sudden euphoria/elation	3/37	8
(9) Pathological crying	7/37	19
(10) **Recurrent outbursts of aggression or rage that are grossly out of proportion to any precipitating stressors**	14/37	38
(11) **Markedly impaired social judgment**	14/37	38
(12) Uninhibited/disinhibited (acts)	12/37	32
(13) Disinhibited vocalization/verbalization	15/37	41
(14) Lack of tact or concern for others; not sensitive to others' feelings/reactions	8/37	22
(15) Inability to plan ahead (lack of foresight, inability to judge consequences of actions)	10/37	27
(16) Sexually inappropriate (not part of a manic episode or delirium, dementia, or posttraumatic amnesia)	6/37	16
(17) **Marked apathy or indifference** (little interest or pleasure in activities, apathetic, does not care about anything, lack of initiative)	5/37	14
(18) **Suspiciousness or paranoid ideation**	2/37	5
(19) Explosive subtype predominates	12/37	32
(20) Perseveration	13/37	35
(21) Echolalia	1/37	3
(22) Immaturity	9/37	24

Note. The frequency of positively rated (occurring at least some point postinjury) Neuropsychiatric Rating Schedule items among 37 consecutively admitted severe-TBI subjects is shown. **Bold headings** correspond to subtypes of personality change because of TBI. Numbers in parentheses correspond to numbered items on the Neuropsychiatric Rating Schedule.

Source. Adapted from Max JE, Robertson BAM, Lansing AE: "The Phenomenology of Personality Change due to Traumatic Brain Injury in Children and Adolescents." *Journal of Neuropsychiatry and Clinical Neurosciences* 13:161–170, 2001. Used with permission.

ing decrements. Accurate diagnosis is especially important because recognition of PC may alert the clinician to certain pharmacological interventions.

When PC is present, it typically encompasses the most impairing symptoms in a particular child even if other syndromes may co-occur. Many of these children are slow to learn from their mistakes. One reason for poor learning in children with PC is that the children almost invariably have poor insight regarding their condition. That is, parents report believable affective instability, aggression, disinhibition, apathy, or paranoia, but children deny such behavior. When they do acknowledge the be-

haviors, most children do not appear to comprehend the grave implications of their behavior.

Secondary Attention-Deficit/ Hyperactivity Disorder

Secondary ADHD (SADHD) is the term used for ADHD that develops after TBI. SADHD is associated with increasing severity of injury and adaptive and intellectual function deficits as well as family dysfunction when children with mild to severe TBI are studied. When the samples are limited to severe or to severe-moderate TBI, adaptive deficits are still evident, but findings regarding intellectual function outcome are mixed (Gerring et al. 1998; Max et al. 2004). However, in these samples of constricted range of injury severity, the following variables are not associated with SADHD: injury severity, family function at the time of assessment, socioeconomic status, family stressors, family psychiatric history, gender, and lesion area. An overlapping study of attention-deficit/hyperactivity symptoms found a similar relationship with severity and also found that overall attention-deficit/hyperactivity symptoms were associated with poorer preinjury family functioning (Max et al. 1998a). A referred sample of children dominated by children with severe TBI had similar findings, and the SADHD children had greater premorbid psychosocial adversity (Gerring et al. 1998). An association of SADHD with lesions of the right putamen or thalamic lesions has been reported and awaits replication (Gerring et al. 2000; Herskovits et al. 1999).

There is no doubt that SADHD can follow severe TBI (Brown et al. 1981; Gerring et al. 1998; Max et al. 2004). It can follow moderate TBI, but, thus far, this has been convincingly demonstrated only in the presence of preinjury ADHD traits (Max et al. 2004). SADHD has also followed mild TBI and orthopedic injury (in the absence of brain injury) at similar rates (Max et al. 2004). The attribution of brain injury as the primary etiological factor for SADHD after mild TBI has been inconclusive.

Findings from a prospective study found that omission errors on a continuous performance test in the acute period after TBI predicted later SADHD (Wassenberg et al. 2004). A recent retrospective study (Schachar et al. 2004) provides some insight into the relationship of SADHD and inhibition deficit, as measured with the Stop Signal Reaction Time (Logan 1994), in nonconsecutively injured children with mild to severe TBI and uninjured control children. An inhibition deficit, similar to that usually seen in developmental ADHD, was found only in children with severe TBI who also had SADHD. SADHD was diagnosed by cut-off points on the Survey Diagnostic Instrument behavioral questionnaire (Boyle et al. 1996). An earlier study (Konrad et al. 2000) yielded similar findings. The neuropharmacology of SADHD was explored in a pioneering study of catecholamine function in children with TBI, noninjured children with ADHD, and control subjects (Konrad et al. 2003). Children with SADHD excreted significantly more normetanephrine in resting situations (possibly reflecting chronic overactivation of the noradrenergic system) and less epinephrine after cognitive stress, and they showed a decreased blink rate (possibly reflective of hypofunctioning of the dopamine system) compared with normal control subjects.

Oppositional Defiant Disorder

One study showed that ODD symptomatology in the first year after TBI was related to preinjury family function, social class, and preinjury ODD symptomatology (Max et al. 1998c). Increased severity of TBI predicted ODD symptomatology 2 years after injury. Change (from before TBI) in ODD symptomatology at 6, 12, and 24 months after TBI was influenced by socioeconomic status. Only at 2 years after injury was severity of injury a predictor of change in ODD symptomatology. The influence of psychosocial factors appears greater than severity of injury in accounting for ODD symptomatology and change in such symptomatology in the first but not the second year after TBI in children and adolescents. This appears related to persistence of new ODD symptomatology after more serious TBI. A study using a referred brain injury clinic sample found that children who developed ODD/conduct disorder after TBI, when compared with children without a lifetime history of the disorder, had significantly more impaired family functioning, showed a trend toward a greater family history of alcohol dependence and abuse, and had a milder TBI (Max et al. 1998i).

Posttraumatic Stress Disorder

It is apparent that posttraumatic stress disorder (PTSD) and subsyndromal posttraumatic stress disturbances occur despite neurogenic amnesia. In one study, only 2 of 46 children (4%) with at least one follow-up assessment developed PTSD (Max et al. 1998e). However, the frequency with which children experienced at least one PTSD symptom ranged from 68% in the first 3 months to 12% at 2 years in assessed children. The presence of an internalizing (mood or anxiety) disorder at time of injury followed by greater injury severity were the most consistent predictors of PTSD symptomatology. Another group of investigators (Levi et al. 1999) found a significant relationship between parent- and child-reported PTSD symptomatology with severe TBI versus moderate TBI and orthopedic injury even after controlling for ethnicity, social disadvantage, and age at injury. However, family socioeconomic disadvantage was associated with greater PTSD symptomatology across groups. A third study found similarly that PTSD occurred in 13% of children with severe TBI recruited from a rehabilitation center (Gerring et al. 2002). PTSD by 1 year postinjury was associated with female gender and early postinjury anxiety symptoms. Posttraumatic symptoms at 1 year postinjury were predicted by preinjury psychosocial adversity, preinjury anxiety symptoms, and injury severity, as well as early postinjury depression symptoms and nonanxiety psychiatric diagnoses. Patients who met the reexperiencing criterion for PTSD in this study had significantly fewer lesions in limbic system structures on the right than subjects who did not meet this criterion (Herskovits et al. 2002). Similarly, the presence of left temporal lesions and the absence of left orbitofrontal lesions were significantly related to PTSD symptoms and hyperarousal symptoms (Vasa et al. 2004).

Other Anxiety Disorders

Obsessive-compulsive disorder can occur after TBI in adolescence (Max et al. 1995b; Vasa et al. 2002). Frontal and temporal lobe lesions may be sufficient to precipitate the syndrome in the absence of clear striatal injury (Max et al. 1995b). A wide variety of other anxiety disorders have been documented after childhood TBI. These include overanxious disorder, specific phobia, separation anxiety disorder, and avoidant disorder (Max et al. 1997b, 1997d, 1998h, 1998j; Vasa et al. 2002). No statistically significant increase has been demonstrated in any single anxiety disorder compared with preinjury frequencies, but there was a trend in this regard for overanxious disorder (Vasa et al. 2002). However, a significant increase in anxiety symptoms after injury compared with before injury has been demonstrated. Preinjury anxiety symptoms and younger age at injury correlated positively with postinjury anxiety symptoms (Vasa et al. 2002). In this study, greater volume and number of orbitofrontal lesions correlated with decreased risk for anxiety disorder and anxiety symptoms (Vasa et al. 2004).

Mania or Hypomania

A number of case reports have been published on the development of mania or hypomania after childhood TBI (Cohn et al. 1977; Joshi et al. 1985; Khanna and Srinath 1985; Sayal et al. 2000). However, there is only one report of this disorder from a child TBI cohort. Four of 50 children (8%) from a prospective study of consecutive children hospitalized after TBI developed mania or hypomania (Max et al. 1997d). The phenomenology regarding the overlapping diagnoses of mania, ADHD, and PC, or the "frontal lobe syndrome," are important considerations in differential diagnosis (Max et al. 2000). Increased severity of injury, frontal and temporal lobe lesion location, and family history of major mood disorder may be implicated in the etiology of mania or hypomania secondary to TBI. Lengthy episodes and similar frequency of irritability and elation may be characteristic.

Depressive Disorders

One prospective study that used standardized psychiatric interviews found that 9 of 50 children had a preinjury lifetime history of major depressive disorder (MDD) or adjustment disorder with depressed mood or mixed mood. Follow-up for 2 years revealed that at some point 7 of these 9 children displayed clinically significant MDD, depressive disorder not otherwise specified, or adjustment disorder with depressed mood or mixed mood. In fact, of 5 children who developed a depressive mood disorder in the first month after TBI, 3 had preinjury depressive disorders, 1 had a first-degree relative with major depression, and another had a preinjury anxiety disorder (J.E. Max, "Depressive Disorders After Child and Adolescent Traumatic Brain Injury," Department of Psychiatry, University of California, San Diego, September 1998). These data imply that a substantial proportion of children who manifest depressed mood after TBI have a preinjury personal history of depressive disorders and that most of the remaining children have identifiable risk factors for a new-onset depressive disorder. A potentially related finding is that suicide attempts in adults with major depression and a remote history of TBI were related to a history of preinjury aggression in childhood (Oquendo et al. 2004). A retrospective psychiatric interview study (Max et al. 1998h) found that one-fourth of children with severe TBI had an ongoing depressive disorder and that one-third of the children had a depressive disorder at some point after the injury. A prospective recruitment study with retrospective psychiatric assessment 6 months after injury (Luis and Mittenberg 2002) found new mood disorders present in 16% of moderate-severe TBI patients, 21% of mild TBI patients, and 3% of orthopedic control subjects. Another group found that TBI increases the risk of depressive symptoms, especially among more socially disadvantaged children, and that depressive symptoms were not strongly related to postinjury neurocognitive scores (Kirkwood et al. 2000).

Psychosis

There have been only two cases of new-onset nonaffective psychosis reported in studies of consecutive admission of 224 children with TBI that used standardized psychiatric interviews (Brown et al. 1981; Lehmkuhl and Thoma 1990; Max et al. 1997b, 1998h). There has been interest in the possibility that early TBI increases the risk of psychosis in adult life (Wilcox and Nasrallah 1987). A more recent large study of the association of multiplex schizophrenia and multiplex bipolar pedigrees found that rates of TBI were significantly higher for those with a diagnosis of schizophrenia, bipolar disorder, and depression than for those with no mental illness (Malaspina et al. 2001). Members of the schizophrenia pedigrees, even those without a diagnosis of schizophrenia, had greater exposure to TBI compared with members of the bipolar disorder pedigrees. Furthermore, within the schizophrenia pedigrees, TBI was associated with a greater risk of schizophrenia consistent with synergistic effects between genetic vulnerability for schizophrenia and TBI. The study concluded, therefore, that post-TBI schizophrenia in multiplex schizophrenia pedigrees does not appear to be a phenocopy of the genetic disorder.

Autism

The absence of autism after childhood TBI is notable. However, other forms of brain injury have been implicated in the new onset of autism in childhood [e.g., brain tumors (Hoon and Reiss 1992) and "congenital hemiplegia" (Goodman and Graham 1996)].

Relationship of Psychiatric Disorder and Cognitive Function and Language Outcomes After TBI

There is an important relationship between psychiatric disorders and cognitive function after TBI (Brown et al. 1981; Max et al. 1999). The Max et al. study reported that severe TBI, when compared with mild TBI and orthopedic injury, was associated with significant decrements in intellectual and memory function. A principal components analysis of independent variables that showed significant ($P<0.05$) bivariate correlations with the outcome measures yielded a "neuropsychiatric factor" encompassing severity of TBI indices and postinjury psychiatric disorders and a "psychosocial disadvantage factor." Both factors were independently and significantly related to intellectual and memory function outcome. Postinjury psychiatric disorders added significantly to severity indices, and family functioning and family psychiatric history added significantly to socioeconomic status in explaining several specific cognitive outcomes. Similarly, Brown et al. (1981) found that new psychiatric disorders in children with severe TBI were most frequent when there was transient or persistent intellectual impairment versus no intellectual impairment. In most instances, this did not reach statistical significance. However, new psychiatric disorder was significantly more common in severe TBI patients than in control subjects even when there was no intellectual impairment. This suggests that the disorders were the result of brain injury rather than merely a reflection of intellectual impairment.

There is a great deal of evidence that cognitive outcome after TBI is related to severity of the injury (Barry et al. 1996; Chadwick et al. 1981a, 1981b; Fay et al. 1994; Fletcher et al. 1990; Jaffe et al. 1992, 1993; Knights et al. 1991; Levin et al. 1993, 1994; McDonald et al. 1994; Shaffer et al. 1975; Yeates et al. 1995, 1997), and there is some evidence that it is related to socioeconomic status

(Barry et al. 1996; Chadwick et al. 1981c; Rivara et al. 1994; Yeates et al. 1997). Less is known about other factors influencing cognitive outcome, including family functioning (Perrott et al. 1991; Rivara et al. 1994; Wade et al. 1996; Yeates et al. 1997).

There are potentially important relationships between executive function, discourse processing, and psychiatric disorders. However, with the exception of the studies of SADHD and inhibition noted above (Konrad et al. 2000; Schachar et al. 2004), these relationships have not been investigated. It is possible that more accurate classification of executive function or discourse deficits, or both, could lead to a better understanding of and potential interventions for psychiatric problems in children with TBI.

Relationship of Psychiatric Disorder and Adaptive Function After TBI

One group (Max et al. 1998g) described a relationship between psychiatric disorder and adaptive function after TBI. Family functioning, psychiatric disorder in the child, and IQ were significant variables that explained between 22% and 47% of the variance in adaptive functioning outcomes.

The literature on adaptive function after childhood TBI is burgeoning. Variables that have been linked to lower adaptive functioning outcome between 6 and 24 months after TBI include the following: 1) increasing severity of injury (Asarnow et al. 1991; Barry et al. 1996; Fay et al. 1994; Fletcher et al. 1990, 1996; Perrott et al. 1991; Rivara et al. 1993; Yeates et al. 1997), including one group's (Levin et al. 1997) finding that depth of brain lesion was directly related to severity of acute impairment of consciousness and inversely related to adaptive outcome; 2) poorer family functioning preinjury (Rivara et al. 1993; Yeates and Taylor 1997) and postinjury (Taylor et al. 1999); 3) poorer preinjury child functioning (Barry et al. 1996; Rivara et al. 1993); 4) new postinjury behavioral symptoms (Barry et al. 1996); and 5) younger age at injury, although the findings regarding the latter are mixed (Fletcher et al. 1996; Rivara et al. 1993; Yeates et al. 1997).

Clinical Decision Making

Investigators (Asarnow et al. 1991) have postulated at least six pathways to behavioral disturbance or psychiatric disorder:

   a) The behavior problem antedates the injury, and
   may actually contribute to the risk for incurring

the injury; b) the brain injury exacerbates a preexisting behavior problem; c) the behavior problem is a direct effect of a brain injury resulting from the accident; d) the behavior problem is an immediate secondary effect of the accident (e.g., an emotional response to the accident such as PTSD); e) the behavior problem is a long-term secondary effect of the accident (e.g., the conduct problems and decreased effectance motivation arising from frustration produced by the cognitive and other impairments caused by brain injury); f) the behavior problems are caused by factors other than head injury. (pp. 552–553)

As with any other clinical assessment, the development of a working biopsychosocial formulation is important in enriching one's approach to a case and in planning intervention. Key elements in such a formulation (Nurcombe and Gallagher 1986) are the pattern of symptomatology, precipitating events, under what circumstances the patient presented or was referred, predisposing factors, circumstances perpetuating the problem, and the prognosis with or without treatment. Research can guide the clinician in the determination of which one or combination of pathways may be most relevant in a particular case. Such postulated pathways can also guide research in examining behavior problems in children who have TBI.

The following vignettes illustrate some of the more common and important clinical differential diagnostic processes faced by clinicians working with children who have survived TBI. PC due to TBI is a disorder with which psychiatrists generally have least familiarity but is a disorder that should frequently enter the differential diagnosis.

Change of Personality Style Versus Personality Change

A 12-year-old girl experienced a mild brain injury in an accident in which her mother was killed. She had been wild and boisterous before the injury but had no definite psychiatric disorder. After the injury, she went through a period of appropriate mourning not complicated by depression. At assessments 6 and 12 months after TBI, she had been much more quiet, thoughtful, and responsible than she had been before the injury. She displayed no evidence of PTSD. Her friends and family noticed this difference and accepted that she had begun to take on more of a maternal role in the family. The girl said that she thought that accidents can happen easily, and this was why she developed a more cautious approach to life.

Comment: When personality styles change after a TBI, this need not necessarily be related to the direct effects of brain damage. Furthermore, PC is not a standard personality disorder with an organic etiology. Rather, it is a syndrome dominated by a new onset of potentially severe affective instability, aggression, or disinhibition or markedly impaired social judgment and, occasionally, by apathy or paranoia. These symptoms may be so severe and pervasive that observers may conclude that the child has undergone a change in personality. However, personality per se is not measured when making the diagnosis.

Attention-Deficit/Hyperactivity Disorder, Oppositional Defiant Disorder Versus Personality Change

PC overlaps symptomatically with other disorders, including most commonly with ADHD and ODD (Max et al. 2000). One should not make the diagnosis of PC if the symptomatology displayed can be sufficiently explained by ADHD or ODD. For example, children with comorbid ADHD and ODD have problematic hyperactivity, impulsivity, and/or inattention, as well as oppositional behavior, and may be easily angered. The diagnosis of PC is added in these children when poor anger control is more marked than oppositional behavior per se, when disinhibited behavior is a problem itself, and, of course, when these behaviors are a change from before a serious TBI.

A child with a mild TBI with preinjury ADHD and ODD had intense irritability (not caused by brain damage) before the injury. This was unchanged at an assessment 3 months after the injury. The child did not receive a diagnosis of PC.

Comment: If the child's irritability had increased only marginally or there was other psychosocial stress, or both, her affective instability would continue to be attributed to causes other than brain damage.

A child with a severe TBI with preinjury ADHD and ODD had clinically significant moderate irritability (not caused by brain damage) before the injury. After the injury and for 6 months, he experienced significant worsening of his irritability. There were no obvious major psychosocial stressors, and his school reentry program was well suited to his abilities. A significant component of his affective instability 6 months after injury was attributed to brain injury, and thus he received a diagnosis of PC, affective instability subtype.

Comment: If the clinician thinks that a particular symptom is significantly related to direct brain damage, the affective instability should be considered part of a PC syndrome.

Major Depression and Personality Change or Postconcussion Syndrome

A child with a mild TBI who was treated overnight at the hospital developed a month-long problem with intense irritability and anger, but no violent outbursts. This made home life miserable. He had headaches and attentional difficulties during most of this month. The syndrome had resolved after approximately 1 month postinjury. Before the injury, he had an easy-going temperament (according to an assessment immediately after the injury before problems developed). There were no significant psychosocial stressors in the first month after injury. He did meet criteria for an MDD during the first month. The syndrome did not depend on irritability for the diagnosis. He was sad and persistently drew pictures of graves and tombs, expressed hopelessness, and had vegetative signs of depression. He thus received a diagnosis of postconcussional syndrome as well as a diagnosis of MDD.

Comment: This is an example of the affective instability subtype of transient PC (i.e., without the duration criterion of 1 year) that can occur after mild TBI. It would be recognized as a postconcussional syndrome (i.e., related to brain injury) by clinicians treating individuals with TBI. A judgment call was made that the child's entire presentation could not be adequately explained by the diagnosis of MDD alone. The presence of headaches influenced this decision, as did the severity of attentional difficulties, even though decreased concentration is a symptom overlapping with MDD.

Adjustment Disorder Versus Personality Change

A child with a moderate TBI (i.e., depressed skull fracture that was elevated without complications) had mild attentional problems for 2 weeks after the injury. The next 8 months were uneventful. At that point, her parents began experiencing marital conflict. The child became irritable and angry and destroyed some property.

Comment: The child's affective change was not considered to be a direct consequence of brain injury because of the clear serious stressor and the relatively uncomplicated 7.5-month period before symptoms emerged. It is incumbent on the clinician to weigh the possibilities that symptoms di-

rectly related to brain damage may occur (most likely, soon after injury), although there is a possibility that children will "grow into their disability or syndrome" because a lesioned area may take over an important function later in development (Goldman 1974). Another organic-mediated, delayed-onset mechanism may involve the rare late onset of a seizure disorder in fewer than 5% of children with severe TBI. A history of seizures would clarify the clinical decision.

School Failure

A child with a severe TBI experienced new-onset ADHD and significant problems with pragmatics of communication, including narrative discourse. Regulation of mood states was unremarkable. Six months after injury, he began to be challenged more at school and could not keep up with his class. He became irritable, angry, and sad and was diagnosed with an adjustment disorder with mixed emotional features.

Comment: In the preceding case, the child's affective instability was thought to be an indirect result of his TBI (i.e., cognitive difficulties ultimately led to school failure, and he responded to this with irritability and sadness).

A child with a severe TBI experienced new-onset ADHD and significant problems with pragmatics of communication, including narrative discourse. Regulation of mood states was impaired in the hospital and remained so until an assessment 12 months after the TBI. Six months after injury, she began to be challenged more at school and could not keep up with her class. She became even more irritable, angry, and sad but did not meet criteria for a major depression.

Comment: In this case, the child's affective instability was thought to be a direct result of her TBI (i.e., poor affective regulation and cognitive difficulties led to school failure and complicated her teacher's efforts to work with her).

Treatment: Psychopharmacology

Personality Change due to TBI: Affective Instability and Rage Subtypes

There are no studies of treatment of children with PC; therefore the following guidelines are anecdotal. Clinically, it is important to differentiate the subtypes because the treatment approaches are different. The affective instability and aggressive types frequently co-occur (Max et al. 2001) and respond similarly to treatment. Mood-stabilizing medications such as carbamazepine and valproic acid can be particularly effective when combined with a behavior modification program targeting aggression. The substituted use of a mood stabilizer or the added use of a selective serotonin reuptake inhibitor (SSRI) to a mood stabilizer may be helpful as well. This may be counterintuitive for clinicians who work with children because of the well-known side effects of irritability and restlessness with SSRIs. Adults with affective instability (e.g., pathological laughter and pathological crying) have responded well to SSRIs (Robinson et al. 1993).

Personality Change due to TBI: Disinhibited, Paranoid, Apathetic Subtypes

The disinhibited subtype is particularly difficult to treat pharmacologically or behaviorally. School aides may be required to closely supervise the children. Parent education and support are particularly important to maximize overall family function. The paranoid subtype is rare. Careful assessment is necessary to determine whether a child with paranoid thoughts is truly impaired by these symptoms and whether they actually influence the child's behavior. Use of neuroleptic medication such as risperidone may be helpful in the acute hospitalization or rehabilitation unit if the child or adolescent is overtly paranoid and the symptoms are impeding compliance with treatment regimens. The potential risks regarding modification of neuronal recovery have been elucidated but not well demonstrated (Gaultieri 1988). The apathetic subtype is also rare and may respond to stimulant medication or SSRIs.

There may be periods when the child has intense affective instability, aggression, hyperactivity, and inattention and may meet criteria for overlapping syndromes of PC, ADHD, and mania or hypomania (Max et al. 1997d). Mood stabilizers may be helpful, and, if stimulants are being used, they should be reevaluated, although the mania or hypomania should not be considered a contraindication to stimulant use (Max et al. 1995a).

Attention-Deficit/Hyperactivity Disorder

Some reports of stimulants administered to children with TBI who have attention and concentration deficits have shown positive results (Gaultieri 1988; Hornyak et al. 1997; Mahalick et al. 1998), whereas another was negative (Williams et al. 1998). I have anecdotal evidence that children diagnosed with SADHD respond to stimulant medication. Popular belief that children with brain damage do not respond to this treatment is unfortunate and may impede the appropriate treatment of children who could

benefit from therapy. This belief may derive, in part, from the fact that even when SADHD has been treated with a stimulant, the child with a severe TBI may still have other psychiatric disorders that may require management and may have adaptive function and cognitive impairments that require other interventions. Methylphenidate is generally the first choice of clinicians, paralleling use in children with developmental ADHD. The literature on a decreased seizure threshold accompanying methylphenidate use in people with brain injury is extremely weak. In recent years, there have been a number of studies demonstrating the safety of methylphenidate in rehabilitation center–treated individuals with severe TBI (e.g., Wroblewski et al. 1992). The risk of seizures after closed head injury is small, and methylphenidate has been considered a safe choice of drug. It is prudent for the clinician to inform the parents and the child of the warnings in the *Physicians' Desk Reference* (1999) regarding the risk of seizures and interpret these before embarking on a trial of methylphenidate. Some families refuse a methylphenidate trial, or the trial may be unsuccessful. In this circumstance, a trial of D-amphetamine is safe and often effective. Families can be reassured that D-amphetamine was once considered a weak anticonvulsant (Weiner 1980) and therefore is not likely to be associated with decreasing seizure threshold. There have been no studies of tricyclic antidepressant medication, atomoxetine, or bupropion for SADHD. Caution should be observed when prescribing the former class of antidepressants, especially in terms of cardiac conduction side effects. Atomoxetine may be helpful, particularly in children who experience increased irritability while taking stimulant medication. The use of bupropion is generally avoided because of the risk of seizures. This may be an unnecessary precaution in this population, but there are no research data to guide usage in children with TBI.

Depression

There are no treatment studies of depressive disorders after childhood TBI. Clinical experience suggests that use of fluoxetine is effective, because it has been shown to be effective when used for childhood depression in the absence of TBI (Emslie et al. 2002). The author of this chapter has anecdotal evidence of effectiveness of amitriptyline in a child with comorbid posttraumatic migraines who could not tolerate an SSRI.

Treatment: Psychosocial

There are rare studies of psychosocial treatments for complications from childhood TBI (Singer et al. 1994).

Research findings are clear that preinjury family function is a significant predictor of child outcome as well as postinjury family function. Therefore, family needs should be assessed soon after injury and at various junctures thereafter. Education, clinical, and advocacy services should be offered to families who are in need. These services may improve child outcome by empowering the family to manage the child appropriately as well as limit secondary complications from delay in the diagnosis and treatment of medical, psychiatric, cognitive, and academic problems in the post-acute and chronic phases after TBI.

In the absence of studies to justify specific guidelines for treatment of emotional or behavioral problems (e.g., phobias, PTSD, ODD/conduct disorder) after TBI, general principles of psychosocial treatment should be applied. An important and specific psychoeducational preventive and/or treatment intervention is to warn about and modify some families' apparent overindulgence of their injured child after injury. When overindulgence occurs, it tends to be self-limiting unless complicated by a parent's excessive sense of guilt. Other families at the opposite extreme may insist on prematurely reexposing their children to the proximal hazard that resulted in the TBI (e.g., three-wheeler racing). These parents may be more likely to accept the recommendations of a neurosurgeon than a psychiatrist.

Prevention

The prevention of accidents should be the first objective in the battle to limit the societal and personal costs of pediatric TBI. Education regarding the use of bicycle helmets, improved motor vehicle safety, steps to decrease alcohol-related motor vehicle accidents, and programs to decrease the risk of child abuse and neglect are just some of the ways to prevent or limit the damage caused by pediatric TBI (Kraus 1995).

Summary and Conclusion

TBI in children and adolescents is a major public health problem. Particularly after severe TBI there may be neurological sequelae, including seizures, which can complicate behavioral outcome. Academic and cognitive function impairments make school reentry and long-term educational success a great challenge. When these impairments are associated with psychiatric problems, the challenge is magnified. Psychiatric disorders are common in children both before and after TBI. Postinjury psychiatric disorders are predicted by a variety of injury and psy-

chosocial variables that can be measured soon after injury. Therefore, children with TBI who are at high risk for impairing psychopathology are readily identifiable before the manifestations of the problems. The advantage of classification of psychiatric disorders into specific conditions (vs. T scores on domains of behavior such as internalizing or externalizing disorders) opens the possibility of specific and rational pharmacological and psychological treatment during the rehabilitative phase. Furthermore, the close relationship between family dysfunction and psychiatric disorders supports the case for family intervention research that may improve not only family function but the child's function as well. More research on biopsychosocial factor correlates of injury risk and psychiatric outcome should lead to more effective primary and secondary prevention efforts.

References

Achenbach T: Manual for the Child Behavior Checklist/4–18 and 1991 Profile. Burlington, VT, University of Vermont College of Medicine, 1991

Ackerly S, Benton AL: Report of a case of bilateral frontal lobe defect. Proceedings of the Association for Research in Nervous and Mental Disease 27:479–504, 1947

Adelson PD, Kochanek PM: Head injury in children. J Child Neurol 13:2–15, 1998

Armstrong K, Janusz J, Yeates KO, et al: Long-term attention problems in children with traumatic brain injuries. J Int Neuropsychol Soc 7:238, 2001

Arroyos-Jurado E, Paulsen JS, Merrell KW, et al: Traumatic brain injury in school-age children: academic and social outcome. J Sch Psychol 38:571–587, 2000

Asarnow RF, Satz P, Light R, et al: Behavior problems and adaptive functioning in children with mild and severe closed head injury. J Pediatr Psychol 16:543–555, 1991

Barnes MA, Dennis M, Wilkinson M: Reading after closed head injury in childhood: effects on accuracy, fluency, and comprehension. Dev Neuropsychol 15:1–24, 1999

Barry CT, Taylor HG, Klein S, et al: Validity of neurobehavioral symptoms reported in children with traumatic brain injury. Child Neuropsychol 2:213–226, 1996

Bender L: Personality problems of the child with a head injury, in Psychopathology of Children With Organic Brain Disorders. Springfield, IL, Charles C. Thomas, 1956, pp 66–96

Berger-Gross P, Shackelford M: Closed head injury in children: neuropsychological and scholastic outcomes. Percept Mot Skills 61:254, 1985

Bijur P, Golding J, Haslum M, et al: Behavioral predictors of injury in school-age children. Am J Dis Child 142:1307–1312, 1988

Bijur PE, Haslum M, Golding J: Cognitive and behavioral sequelae of mild head injury in children. Pediatrics 86:337–344, 1990

Black P, Jeffries JJ, Blumer D, et al: The posttraumatic syndrome in children: characteristics and incidence, in The Late Effects of Head Injury. Edited by Walker AE, Caveness WF, Critchley M, Research Group on Head Injuries, Springfield, IL, Charles C. Thomas, 1969, pp 142–149

Blau A: Mental changes following head trauma in children. Archives of Neurology and Psychiatry (Chicago) 35:723–769, 1936

Bloom DR, Levin HS, Ewing-Cobbs L, et al: Lifetime and novel psychiatric disorders after pediatric traumatic brain injury. J Am Acad Child Adolesc Psychiatry 40:572–579, 2001

Boyle MH, Offord DR, Racine Y, et al: Identifying thresholds for classifying childhood psychiatric disorder: issues and prospects. J Am Acad Child Adolesc Psychiatry 35:1440–1448, 1996

Brown G, Chadwick O, Shaffer D, et al: A prospective study of children with head injuries, III: psychiatric sequelae. Psychol Med 11:63–78, 1981

Chadwick O, Rutter M, Brown G, et al: A prospective study of children with head injuries, II: cognitive sequelae. Psychol Med 11:49–61, 1981a

Chadwick O, Rutter M, Shaffer D, et al: A prospective study of children with head injuries, IV: specific cognitive deficits. J Clin Neuropsychol 3:101–120, 1981b

Chadwick O, Rutter M, Thompson J, et al: Intellectual performance and reading skills after localized head injury in childhood. J Child Psychol Psychiatry 22:117–139, 1981c

Cohn CK, Wright JR, DeVaul RA: Post head trauma syndrome in an adolescent treated with lithium carbonate: case report. Dis Nerv Syst 38:630–631, 1977

Dillon H, Leopold R: Children and the post-concussion syndrome. JAMA 175:110–116, 1961

Donders J: Premorbid behavioral and psychosocial adjustment of children with traumatic brain injury. J Abnorm Child Psychol 20:233–246, 1992

Emslie GJ, Heiligenstein JH, Wagner KD, et al: Fluoxetine for acute treatment of depression in children and adolescents: a placebo-controlled, randomized clinical trial. J Am Acad Child Adolesc Psychiatry 41:1205–1215, 2002

Eslinger PJ, Grattan LM, Damasio H, et al: Developmental consequences of childhood frontal lobe damage. Arch Neurol 49:764–769, 1992

Ewing-Cobbs L, Fletcher JM, Levin HS, et al: Academic achievement and academic placement following traumatic brain injury in children and adolescents: a two-year longitudinal study. J Clin Exp Neuropsychol 29:769–781, 1998

Ewing-Cobbs L, Prasad M, Kramer L, et al: Inflicted traumatic brain injury: relationship of developmental outcome to severity of injury. Pediatr Neurosurg 31:251–258, 1999

Ewing-Cobbs L, Barnes M, Fletcher JM, et al: Modeling of longitudinal academic achievement scores after pediatric traumatic brain injury. Dev Neuropsychol 25:107–133, 2004

Fay GC, Jaffe KM, Polissar NL, et al: Outcome of pediatric traumatic brain injury at three years: a cohort study. Arch Phys Med Rehabil 75:733–741, 1994

Fletcher JM, Ewing-Cobbs L, Miner ME, et al: Behavioral changes after closed head injury in children. J Consult Clin Psychol 58:93–98, 1990

Fletcher JM, Levin HS, Lachar D, et al: Behavioral outcomes after pediatric closed head injury: relationships with age, severity, and lesion size. J Child Neurol 11:283–290, 1996

Gaultieri CT: Pharmacotherapy and the neurobehavioral sequelae of traumatic brain injury. Brain Inj 2:101–129, 1988

Gerring JP, Brady KD, Chen A, et al: Premorbid prevalence of ADHD and development of secondary ADHD after closed head injury. J Am Acad Child Adolesc Psychiatry 37:647–654, 1998

Gerring JP, Brady KD, Chen A, et al: Neuroimaging variables related to development of secondary attention deficit hyperactivity disorder after closed head injury in children and adolescents. Brain Inj 14:205–218, 2000

Gerring JP, Slomine B, Vasa RA, et al: Clinical predictors of posttraumatic stress disorder after closed head injury in children. J Am Acad Child Adolesc Psychiatry 41:157–165, 2002

Goldman PS: Functional development of the prefrontal cortex in early life and the problem of neuronal plasticity. Exp Neurol 32:366–387, 1974

Goodman R, Graham P: Psychiatric problems in children with hemiplegia: cross sectional epidemiological survey. BMJ 312:1065–1069, 1996

Harrington JA, Letemendia FJJ: Persistent psychiatric disorders after head injuries in children. J Ment Sci 104:1205–1218, 1958

Herskovits EH, Megalooikonomou V, Davatzikos C, et al: Is the spatial distribution of brain lesions associated with closed-head injury predictive of subsequent development of attention-deficit/hyperactivity disorder? Analysis with brain-image database. Radiology 213:389–394, 1999

Herskovits EH, Gerring JP, Davatzikos C, et al: Is the spatial distribution of brain lesions associated with closed-head injury in children predictive of subsequent development of posttraumatic stress disorder? Radiology 224:345–351, 2002

Hjern B, Nylander I: Acute Head Injuries in Children: Traumatology, Therapy and Prognosis, Vol 152. Stockholm, Sweden, Almqvist and Wiksells Boktryckeri AB, 1964

Hoon AH Jr, Reiss AL: The mesial-temporal lobe and autism: case report and review. Dev Med Child Neurol 34:252–259, 1992

Hornyak JE, Nelson VS, Hurvitz EA: The use of methylphenidate in paediatric traumatic brain injury. Paediatr Rehabil 1:15–17, 1997

Jaffe KM, Fay GC, Polissar NL, et al: Severity of pediatric traumatic brain injury and early neurobehavioral outcome: a cohort study. Arch Phys Med Rehabil 73:540–547, 1992

Jaffe KM, Fay GC, Polissar NL, et al: Severity of pediatric traumatic brain injury and neurobehavioral recovery at one year—a cohort study. Arch Phys Med Rehabil 74:587–595, 1993

Joshi P, Capozzoli JA, Coyle JT: Effective management with lithium of a persistent, post-traumatic hypomania in a 10-year-old child. J Dev Behav Pediatr 6:352–354, 1985

Kasanin J: Personality changes in children following cerebral trauma. J Nerv Ment Dis 69:385–406, 1929

Khanna S, Srinath S: Symptomatic mania after minor head injury (letter). Can J Psychiatry 30:236–237, 1985

Kirkwood M, Janusz J, Yeates KO, et al: Prevalence and correlates of depressive symptoms following traumatic brain injuries in children. Child Neuropsychol 6:195–208, 2000

Konrad K, Gauggel S, Manz A, et al: Inhibitory control in children with traumatic brain injury (TBI) and children with attention-deficit/hyperactivity disorder (ADHD). Brain Inj 14:859–875, 2000

Konrad K, Gauggel S, Schurek J: Catecholamine functioning in children with traumatic brain injuries and children with attention-deficit/hyperactivity disorder. Brain Res Cogn Brain Res 16:425–433, 2003

Knights RM, Ivan LP, Ventureyra EC, et al: The effects of head injury in children on neuropsychological and behavioural functioning. Brain Inj 5:339–351, 1991

Kraus JF: Epidemiological features of brain injury in children: occurrence, children at risk, causes and manner of injury, severity, and outcomes, in Traumatic Head Injury in Children. Edited by Broman SH, Michel ME. New York: Oxford University Press, 1995, pp 22–39

Kraus JF, Rock A, Hemyari P: Brain injuries among infants, children, adolescents, and young adults. Am J Dis Child 144:684–691, 1990

Lehmkuhl G, Thoma W: Development in children after severe head injury, in Brain and Behavior in Child Psychiatry. Edited by Rothenberger A. New York, Springer-Verlag, 1990, pp 267–282

Levi RB, Drotar D, Yeates KO, et al: Posttraumatic stress symptoms in children following orthopedic or traumatic brain injury. J Clin Child Psychol 28:232–243, 1999

Levin HS, Aldrich EF, Saydjari C, et al: Severe head injury in children: experience of the Traumatic Coma Data Bank. Neurosurgery 31:435–443; discussion 443–444, 1992

Levin HS, Culhane KA, Mendelsohn D, et al: Cognition in relation to magnetic resonance imaging in head-injured children and adolescents. Arch Neurol 50:897–905, 1993

Levin HS, Mendelsohn DB, Lilly MA, et al: Tower of London performance in relation to magnetic resonance imaging following closed head injury in children. Neuropsychology 8:171–179, 1994

Levin HS, Mendelsohn D, Lilly MA, et al: Magnetic resonance imaging in relation to functional outcome of pediatric closed head injury: a test of the Ommaya-Gennarelli model. Neurosurgery 40:432–440; discussion 440–441, 1997

Light R, Asarnow R, Satz P, et al: Mild closed-head injury in children and adolescents: behavior problems and academic outcomes. J Consult Clin Psychol 66:1023–1029, 1998

Logan GD: On the ability to inhibit thought and action: a users' guide to the stop signal paradigm, in Inhibitory Processes in Attention, Memory, and Language. Edited by Dagenbach D. San Diego, CA, Academic Press, 1994, pp 189–239

Luis CA, Mittenberg W: Mood and anxiety disorders following pediatric traumatic brain injury: a prospective study. J Clin Exp Neuropsychol 24:270–279, 2002

Mahalick DM, Carmel PW, Greenberg JP, et al: Psychopharmacologic treatment of acquired attention disorders in children with brain injury. Pediatr Neurosurg 29:121–126, 1998

Malaspina D, Goetz RR, Friedman JH, et al: Traumatic brain injury and schizophrenia in members of schizophrenia and bipolar disorder pedigrees. Am J Psychiatry 158:440–446, 2001

Marlowe WB: The impact of a right prefrontal lesion on the developing brain. Brain Cogn 20:205–213, 1992

Max JE, Dunisch DL: Traumatic brain injury in a child psychiatry outpatient clinic: a controlled study. J Am Acad Child Adolesc Psychiatry 36:404–411, 1997

Max JE, Richards L, Hamdan-Allen G: Case study: antimanic effectiveness of dextroamphetamine in a brain-injured adolescent. J Am Acad Child Adolesc Psychiatry 34:472–476, 1995a

Max JE, Smith WL, Lindgren SD, et al: Case study: Obsessive-compulsive disorder after severe traumatic brain injury in an adolescent. J Am Acad Child Adolesc Psychiatry 34:45–49, 1995b

Max JE, Lindgren SD, Knutson C, et al: Child and adolescent traumatic brain injury: psychiatric findings from a paediatric outpatient specialty clinic. Brain Inj 11:699–711, 1997a

Max JE, Robin DA, Lindgren SD, et al: Traumatic brain injury in children and adolescents: psychiatric disorders at two years. J Am Acad Child Adolesc Psychiatry 36:1278–1285, 1997b

Max JE, Sharma A, Qurashi MI: Traumatic brain injury in a child psychiatry inpatient population: a controlled study. J Am Acad Child Adolesc Psychiatry 36:1595–1601, 1997c

Max JE, Smith WL, Sato Y, et al: Mania and hypomania following traumatic brain injury in children and adolescents. Neurocase 3:119–126, 1997d

Max JE, Smith Jr WL, Sato Y, et al: Traumatic brain injury in children and adolescents: psychiatric disorders in the first three months. J Am Acad Child Adolesc Psychiatry 36:94–102, 1997e

Max JE, Arndt S, Castillo CS, et al: Attention-deficit hyperactivity symptomatology after traumatic brain injury: a prospective study. J Am Acad Child Adolesc Psychiatry 37:841–847, 1998a

Max JE, Bowers WA, Baldus D, et al: Pediatric traumatic brain injury and burn patients in the civil justice system: the prevalence and impact of psychiatric symptomatology. J Am Acad Psychiatry Law 26:247–258, 1998b

Max JE, Castillo CS, Bokura H, et al: Oppositional defiant disorder symptomatology after traumatic brain injury: a prospective study. J Nerv Ment Dis 186:325–332, 1998c

Max JE, Castillo CS, Lindgren, SD, et al: The Neuropsychiatric Rating Schedule: reliability and validity. J Am Acad Child Adolesc Psychiatry 37:297–304, 1998d

Max JE, Castillo CS, Robin DA, et al: Posttraumatic stress symptomology after childhood traumatic brain injury. J Nerv Ment Dis 186:589–596, 1998e

Max JE, Castillo CS, Robin DA, et al: Predictors of family functioning after traumatic brain injury in children and adolescents. J Am Acad Child Adolesc Psychiatry 37:83–90, 1998f

Max JE, Koele SL, Lindgren SD, et al: Adaptive functioning following brain injury and orthopedic injury: a controlled study. Arch Phys Med Rehabil 79:893–899, 1998g

Max JE, Koele SL, Smith WL Jr, et al: Psychiatric disorders in children and adolescents after severe traumatic brain injury: a controlled study. J Am Acad Child Adolesc Psychiatry 37:832–840, 1998h

Max JE, Lindgren SD, Knutson C, et al: Child and adolescent traumatic brain injury: correlates of disruptive behavior disorders. Brain Inj 12:41–52, 1998i

Max JE, Robin DA, Lindgren SD, et al: Traumatic brain injury in children and adolescents: psychiatric disorders at one year. J Neuropsychiatry Clin Neurosci 10:290–297, 1998j

Max JE, Roberts MA, Koele SL, et al: Cognitive outcome in children and adolescents following severe traumatic brain injury: influence of psychosocial, psychiatric, and injury-related variables. J Int Neuropsychol Soc 5:58–68, 1999

Max JE, Koele SL, Castillo CC, et al: Personality change disorder in children and adolescents following traumatic brain injury. J Int Neuropsychol Soc 6:279–289, 2000

Max JE, Robertson BAM, Lansing AE: The phenomenology of personality change due to traumatic brain injury in children and adolescents. J Neuropsychiatry Clin Neurosci 13:161–170, 2001

Max JE, Lansing AE, Koele SL, et al: Attention deficit hyperactivity disorder in children and adolescents following traumatic brain injury. Dev Neuropsychol 25:159–177, 2004

McDonald CM, Jaffe KM, Fay GC, et al: Comparison of indices of traumatic brain injury severity as predictors of neurobehavioral outcome in children. Arch Phys Med Rehabil 75:328–337, 1994

Nurcombe B, Gallagher RM: The Clinical Process in Psychiatry. Cambridge, England, Cambridge University Press, 1986

Oquendo MA, Friedman JH, Grunebaum MF, et al: Mild traumatic brain injury and suicidal behavior in major depression. J Nerv Ment Dis 192:430–434, 2004

Ott D, Caplan R, Guthrie D, et al: Measures of psychopathology in children with complex partial seizures and primary generalized epilepsy with absence. J Am Acad Child Adolesc Psychiatry 40:907–914, 2001

Otto U: The postconcussion syndrome in children. Acta Paedopsychiatrica: Int J Child Adolesc Psychiatry 27:6–20, 1960

Pelco L, Sawyer M, Duffield G, et al: Premorbid emotional and behavioural adjustment in children with mild head injuries. Brain Inj 6:29–37, 1992

Perrott SB, Taylor HG, Montes JL: Neuropsychological sequelae, familial stress, and environmental adaptation following pediatric head injury. Dev Neuropsychol 7:69–86, 1991

Physicians' Desk Reference. Montvale, NJ, Medical Economics Company, 1999

Price BH, Daffner KR, Stowe RM, et al: The compartmental learning disabilities of early frontal lobe damage. Brain 113:1383–1393, 1990

Rivara JB, Fay GC, Jaffe KM, et al: Predictors of family functioning one year following traumatic brain injury in children. Arch Phys Med Rehabil 73:899–910, 1992

Rivara JB, Jaffe KM, Fay GC, et al: Family functioning and injury severity as predictors of child functioning one year following traumatic brain injury. Arch Phys Med Rehabil 74:1047–1055, 1993

Rivara JB, Jaffe KM, Polissar NL, et al: Family functioning and children's academic performance and behavior problems in the year following traumatic brain injury. Arch Phys Med Rehabil 75:369–379, 1994

Robinson RG, Parikh RM, Lipsey JR, et al: Pathological laughing and crying following stroke: validation of a measurement scale and a double-blind treatment study. Am J Psychiatry 150:286–293, 1993

Rune V: Acute head injuries in children: a retrospective epidemiologic, child psychiatric and electroencephalographic study on primary school children in Umea. Acta Paediatr Scand Suppl 209:3–12, 1970

Russell WR: Brain Memory Learning. Oxford, England, Clarendon Press, 1959

Satz P, Zaucha K, McCleary C, et al: Mild head injury in children and adolescents: a review of studies (1970–1995). Psychol Bull 122:107–131, 1997

Sayal K, Ford T, Pipe R: Case study: bipolar disorder after head injury. J Am Acad Child Adolesc Psychiatry 39:525–528, 2000

Schachar R, Levin H, Max JE, et al: Attention deficit hyperactivity disorder symptoms and response inhibition after closed head injury in children: do preinjury behavior and injury severity predict outcome? Dev Neuropsychol 25:179–198, 2004

Schwartz L, Taylor HG, Drotar D, et al: Long-term behavior problems following pediatric traumatic brain injury: prevalence, predictors, and correlates. J Pediatr Psychol 28:251–263, 2003

Shaffer D: Behavioral sequelae of serious head injury in children and adolescents: the British studies, in Traumatic Head Injury in Children. Edited by Broman SH, Michel ME. New York, Oxford University Press, 1995, pp 55–69

Shaffer D, Chadwick O, Rutter M: Psychiatric outcome of localized head injury in children, in Outcome of Severe Damage to the Central Nervous System. Edited by Ciba F. Amsterdam, The Netherlands, New York, Elsevier, 1975, pp 191–213

Singer G, Glang A, Nixon C, et al: A comparison of two psychosocial interventions for parents of children with acquired brain injury: an exploratory study. J Head Trauma Rehabil 9:38–49, 1994

Strecker EA, Ebaugh FG: Neuropsychiatric sequelae of cerebral trauma in children. Arch Neurol Psychiatry 12:443–453, 1924

Taylor HG, Yeates KO, Wade SL, et al: Influences on first-year recovery from traumatic brain injury in children. Neuropsychology 13:76–89, 1999

Taylor HG, Yeates KO, Wade SL, et al: Bidirectional child-family influences on outcomes of traumatic brain injury in children. J Int Neuropsychol Soc 7:755–767, 2001

Teasdale G, Jennett B: Assessment of coma and impaired consciousness: a practical scale. Lancet 2:81–84, 1974

Timonen M, Miettunen J, Hakko H, et al: The association of preceding traumatic brain injury with mental disorders, alcoholism and criminality: the Northern Finland 1966 birth cohort study. Psychiatry Res 113:217–226, 2002

Vasa RA, Gerring JP, Grados M, et al: Anxiety after severe pediatric closed head injury. J Am Acad Child Adolesc Psychiatry 41:148–156, 2002

Vasa RA, Grados M, Slomine B et al: Neuroimaging correlates of anxiety after pediatric traumatic brain injury. Biol Psychiatry 55:208–216, 2004

Wade SL, Taylor HG, Drotar D, et al: Childhood traumatic brain injury: initial impact on the family. J Learn Disabil 29:652–661, 1996

Wassenberg R, Max JE, Lindgren SD, et al: Sustained attention in children and adolescents after traumatic brain injury: relation to severity of injury, adaptive functioning, ADHD and social background. Brain Inj 18:751–764, 2004

Weiner N: Norepinephrine, epinephrine, and the sympathomimetic amines, in The Pharmacologic Basis of Therapeutics, 6th Edition. Edited by Gilman AG, Goodman LS, Gilman A. New York, Macmillan, 1980, pp 138–175

Wilcox JA, Nasrallah HA: Childhood head trauma and psychosis. Psychiatry Res 21:303–306, 1987

Williams D, Mateer CA: Developmental impact of frontal lobe injury in middle childhood. Brain Cogn 20:196–204, 1992

Williams DH, Levin HS, Eisenberg HM: Mild head injury classification. Neurosurgery 27:422–428, 1990

Williams SE, Ris MD, Ayyangar R, et al: Recovery in pediatric brain injury: is psychostimulant medication beneficial? J Head Trauma Rehabil 13:73–81, 1998

Wroblewski BA, Leary JM, Phelan AM, et al: Methylphenidate and seizure frequency in brain injured patients with seizure disorders. J Clin Psychiatry 53:86–89, 1992

Yablon SA: Posttraumatic seizures. Arch Phys Med Rehabil 74:983–1001, 1993

Yeates KO, Taylor HG: Predicting premorbid neuropsychological functioning following pediatric traumatic brain injury. J Clin Exp Neuropsychol 19:825–837, 1997

Yeates KO, Blumenstein E, Patterson CM, et al: Verbal learning and memory following pediatric closed-head injury. J Int Neuropsychol Soc 1:78–87, 1995

Yeates KO, Taylor HG, Drotar D, et al: Preinjury family environment as a determinant of recovery from traumatic brain injuries in school-age children. J Int Neuropsychol Soc 3:617–630, 1997

Ylvisaker M, Todis B, Glang A, et al: Educating students with TBI: themes and recommendations. J Head Trauma Rehabil 16:76–93, 2001

28 Elderly

Edward Kim, M.D.

THE 65 YEARS and older age group accounts for nearly 13% of the United States population and will increase to 20% by 2030 (Malmgren 2000). Additionally, individuals ages 85 years and older represent the fastest growing segment of the United States population (Table 28–1). As a result, increasing attention must be paid to health care issues in the elderly. This chapter focuses on specific issues relevant to the older patient with traumatic brain injury (TBI).

Etiology and Risk Factors

Although motor vehicle accidents represent the most common cause of TBI in younger individuals, falls account for the highest proportion of TBIs in older individuals (Pennings 1993). This is largely because of the increased risk of falls in the aging population. Up to one-third of community-dwelling individuals older than age 65 years and up to 60% of nursing home residents fall each year (Fuller 2000). Falls cause 70% of accidental deaths in people older than age 75 years and represent the fifth leading cause of death in the elderly.

Additionally, certain age-related medical conditions may predispose individuals to falls (Table 28–2). These include orthopedic, neurological, and cardiac conditions (Tinetti 1997). Cognitive impairment is a significant risk factor for falls. This may be because of both decreased safety awareness and increased use of psychotropic medications in patients with dementia who develop psychiatric complications. Moreover, cognitive impairment is a risk factor for motor vehicle accidents, the second most common cause of TBI in this population (Dubinsky et al. 2000). Treatment with antipsychotic agents and benzodiazepines is associated with increased risk of falls in the elderly (Fuller 2000). Tricyclic antidepressants (TCAs), although highly effective in treating depression in late life,

may cause orthostatic hypotension and lead to falls. Selective serotonin reuptake inhibitors are known to have fewer cardiovascular and cognitive side effects than TCAs but may still be associated with falls (Thapa et al. 1998).

Influence of Age on TBI Outcome

Both animal and human studies provide substantial evidence that advanced age is associated with increased mortality and poorer outcomes after TBI. The greater plasticity of an immature brain leads to improved recovery from experimental injury in young animals (Finger 1978), whereas older rats experience increased mortality after experimental brain injury (Hamm et al. 1991). Additionally, older rats who survive experimental injuries demonstrate more motor and cognitive deficits than younger rats (Hamm et al. 1992). Despite the finding of poorer outcomes in numerous human studies of TBI involving older patients, numerous questions remain unanswered. In a critical review of the literature on outcomes after TBI in patients of advanced age, Rapaport and Feinstein (2000) noted methodological problems such as selection bias, small sample size, retrospective design, and the failure to control for preinjury functioning. They recommended larger prospective studies adjusted for premorbid cognitive and medical factors and using appropriate control groups. Such studies will help clarify the effect of aging on specific aspects of outcome after TBI as well as the interaction between aging and preinjury cognitive and physiological status.

Acute Outcome

The acute postinjury phase is characterized by an increased frequency of space-occupying lesions, secondary medical complications, and overall mortality. Com-

TABLE 28–1. Population ages 65 years and older: United States, 1950–2050

Population	1950	1995	2010	2030	2050
65+ (millions)	12.3	33.5	39.4	69.4	78.9
Percentage total population	8.1	12.8	13.2	20.0	20.0
85+ (millions)	0.6	3.6	5.7	8.5	18.2
Percentage total population	4.7	10.8	14.4	12.2	23.1

Source. Adapted from Malmgren R: "Epidemiology of Aging," in *Textbook of Geriatric Neuropsychiatry*, 2nd Edition. Edited by Coffey CE, Cummings JL. Washington, DC, American Psychiatric Press, 2000, pp 18–31.

TABLE 28–2. Factors associated with increased risk of falls

Sensory
  Impaired vision
  Impaired proprioception
  Impaired vestibular function
  Peripheral neuropathy
Musculoskeletal
  Muscle weakness, arthritis
Cardiovascular
  Postural hypotension
  Cardiac arrhythmias
Central nervous system
  Dementia
  Depression
  Movement disorders

Source. Adapted from Tinetti ME: "Falls," in *Geriatric Medicine*. Edited by Cassel CK, Cohen HJ, Larson EB, et al. New York, Springer-Verlag New York, 1997, pp 787–799.

paring patients older than and younger than 65 years old, Pentland et al. (1986) reported a threefold increase in intracranial hematomas in mild to moderate injuries; in severe injuries, there was no difference between age groups. However, another study comparing patients 60 years and older with patients ages 20–40 years with severe injuries [i.e., a Glasgow Coma Scale (GCS) score of 5 or less] noted a higher incidence of multiple brain lesions, hematoma, and contusions in the elderly patients (Pennings et al. 1993). Mortality in the older patient group was 79%, with one-third of these mortalities attributed to pulmonary, cardiac, or multisystem organ failure. By comparison, mortality in younger patients was 36%, all attributed to the primary brain injury. Comparing patients older than 70 years with TBIs of various severities, Kotwica and Jakubowski (1992) found that an initial GCS of less than 9 was associated with 85% mortality, whereas a GCS more than 12 was associated with 20% mortality, primarily from pneumonia. Ritchie et al. (2000) reviewed records of patients with TBI older than 65 years of age. There was a 33% mortality overall. An initial GCS score of less than 11 was associated with 78% mortality and poor outcomes necessitating discharge to nursing homes from the hospital. In patients older than 80 years, an initial GCS score of 13 was associated with poor outcomes. Rothweiler et al. (1998) followed 411 hospitalized patients with mild to severe TBI who were ages 18–89 years. Patients 60 years and older took longer than 7 days on average to become responsive to commands compared with less than 24 hours in younger patients. Additionally, the older patients were more likely to have complications such as cardiac arrest, ventriculitis, and sepsis. Thus, although mild injuries were associated with only slightly increased mortality and poorer outcomes in older versus younger patients, moderate and severe TBI were associated with substantially increased morbidity and mortality

in the elderly. This may be related to both physiological aspects of aging as well as limitations of the GCS in assessing severity of injury in older patients. These findings suggest that a GCS score alone may underestimate the severity of brain injury in patients with age-related cognitive and physiological changes.

Functional Outcome

There are conflicting data regarding the influence of age on functional outcome after TBI, with some investigators reporting no effect and others demonstrating substantially poorer functional outcomes in elderly patients (Carlsson et al. 1968; Jennett et al. 1976). Older patients may experience neurological deterioration after discharge, leading to nursing home placement, in contrast with the tendency of younger patients to improve neurologically after discharge (Pentland et al. 1986). Comparing patients older than and younger than 55 years matched for injury severity and gender, Cifu et al. (1996) observed that the older patient group had a significantly longer mean length of rehabilitation stay, higher total rehabilitation charges, and a slower rate of improvement on functional measures. Nonetheless, there was no difference between groups in discharge disposition (community vs. institutional setting). In this study, the mean GCS score was approximately 10 in both groups, suggesting a preponderance of moderate severity of injury. Therefore, although older patients required significantly longer and more costly inpatient rehabilitation stays, their dispositional outcomes were comparable to those of younger patients. Comparing psychosocial outcomes at 1 year postinjury in patients of various ages, Rothweiler et al. (1998) found that patients ages 60 years and older were significantly more disabled than those younger than 50 years of age, and those 50 years or older were significantly more disabled than those younger than 30 years. Significantly more patients older than 60 years required a change to a more supervised living situation than those younger than 50 years. Therefore, there is evidence that older patients may be able to achieve substantial gains, though at a much higher cost because of protracted inpatient rehabilitative treatments. These studies followed patients with a predominance of moderate to severe injuries. Rapaport and Feinstein (2001) compared subjects ages 60 years and older with those ages 18–59 years who had mild TBIs. Contrary to expectations, the older group had better functional and psychological outcomes at 1 month follow-up. Severity of injury is therefore an important factor to consider when predicting age-related variance of TBI outcomes (Table 28–3).

Cognitive Outcome

Cognitive functioning exerts a substantial influence on functional independence in all age groups. Older patients tend to have more cognitive impairment after TBI than younger patients, though the acute neuropsychological effects of mild TBI do not appear to be age-related (Fields 2000). Severity of injury generally influences the extent of resulting cognitive impairment, though at least one study found no such relationship (Mazzucchi et al. 1992). However, the use of a self-selected sample presenting to a neuropsychology clinic may have influenced this study's findings. Goldstein et al. (2001) compared elderly TBI patients with community-dwelling control subjects approximately 2 months after mild and moderate TBI. The TBI subjects had poorer performance on tests of language, memory, and executive functioning than the healthy control subjects. Aharon-Peretz et al. (1997) noted greater cognitive impairment in elderly TBI subjects compared with healthy control subjects. However, they also noted similar cognitive impairment in a comparison group of orthopedic inpatients. They hypothesized that preexisting cognitive impairment may have predisposed both TBI and orthopedic patients to falls that resulted in their hospitalization.

Another factor that is not directly related to aging is the role of medications, particularly polypharmacy, in the elderly. Age-related medical illnesses may necessitate the use

TABLE 28–3. Traumatic brain injury (TBI) outcome and advanced age

Author	Study group age (years)	Functional outcome
Pentland et al. 1986	65+ vs. <65	Older patients had more neurological deterioration, leading to nursing home placement.
Cifu et al. 1996	55+ vs. <55	Older patients had increased inpatient rehabilitation stay and charges, slower rate of improvement.
		No difference in discharge disposition.
Rothweiler et al. 1998	60+ vs. <50	Increased referral to supervised living.
Ritchie et al. 2000	>65	Ages 66–79 years: GCS <11=increased risk of nursing home placement.
		Age >79 years: GCS <13=increased risk of nursing home placement.
Rapaport and Feinstein 2001	>60 vs. 18–59 (mild TBI)	Older group had better functional and psychological outcomes at 1 month.

Note. GCS=Glasgow Coma Scale.

of multiple medications that may have adverse cognitive side effects, particularly medications with anticholinergic properties (Tune 2000). Advanced age is a risk factor for the inappropriate prescription of a variety of medications, particularly psychoactive drugs (Zhan et al. 2001). Diazepam, chlordiazepoxide, and amitriptyline are among the most commonly prescribed drugs deemed to be contraindicated by consensus panels (Aparasu and Sitzman 1999; Willcox et al. 1994). However, even appropriately prescribed nonpsychoactive medications such as antiparkinsonian, cardiac, antiinflammatory, and histamine 2 receptor antagonists can have substantial adverse effects on cognition (Moore and O'Keefe 1999). Thus, cognitive outcomes after TBI in advanced age are affected by factors not directly related to the neurobiology of aging.

Summary

Elderly patients who sustain TBIs are generally at risk for higher mortality as well as poorer cognitive and functional outcomes because of TBI. In particular, secondary organ failure is much more common and appears to contribute to increased mortality in older versus younger

TBI patients. In addition, older patients tend to require longer, more costly rehabilitative treatments, though they may benefit substantially from such interventions (Dobkin 2000). An additional concern is the concomitant use of psychoactive medications and other drugs that can have an adverse effect on cognition.

Pathophysiology of Aging and TBI

Age-related physiological changes contribute to the increased vulnerability of older patients to adverse consequences of TBI. These changes may involve brain structure and function that magnify the effects of head trauma and reductions in physiological reserve that predispose older patients to secondary organ failure.

Neurobiology of Aging

The human brain achieves full maturity in the second or third decade of life, and age-associated histological changes develop after age 40 years (Powers 2000). Studies in aging rodents show slowed protein synthesis and axonal transport, indicative of less active metabolism. Age-related cerebral atrophy in humans leads to a 0.4% decrease in brain volume per year after age 60 years (Akiyama et al. 1997). This atrophy may result from a loss of neurons, decrease in neuronal volume, and loss of synapses. Synaptic density declines with age, but the number of cortical neurons in many areas may remain stable through advanced age (Haug and Eggers 1991). In older rats, there is a decrease in the expression of neuronal growth-associated proteins. The expression of neuronal growth-associated proteins are considered to be an indication of neural plasticity, because they are necessary for the growth and synaptic proliferation of neurons. Nerve growth factor (NGF) administered to aging rodents reverses age-related atrophic changes in cortical pyramidal neurons (Mervis et al. 1991). Neurotrophic factors such as NGF are essential to the normal development and maintenance of cholinergic neurons (Powers 2000). In humans, there is evidence of decreased synthesis of NGF in the aging brain (Hefti et al. 1989). Thus, the aging brain may be less able to mount an effective regenerative response to brain trauma via neurotrophic factors. Age-related cerebrovascular changes also lead to a gradual reduction in cerebral perfusion (Choi et al. 1998). Finally, cerebral atrophy leads to brain shrinkage. This shrinkage increases the distance between the brain and skull, making dural vessels more vulnerable to shearing damage (Cummings and Benson 1992).

Neurochemical Changes

The neurochemical changes associated with TBI may represent protective reactions to trauma. Early after injury, there is a dramatic increase in cholinergic, serotonergic, and catecholaminergic turnover in the brain. Although cholinergic turnover may be involved in excitotoxic injury, increases in biogenic amines appear to reduce cerebral metabolism to counteract excitotoxic damage (Boyeson 1991; Pappius 1991). Subacutely, TBI appears to cause damage to cholinergic systems (Dewar and Graham 1996; Saija et al. 1988). Therefore, any age-related changes in these neurochemical states may render elderly patients more vulnerable to the neurochemical effects of TBI. These changes are summarized in Table 28–4.

Cholinergic Systems

Acetylcholine innervation is widely distributed throughout the brain. The majority of cholinergic fibers originate in the nucleus basalis of Meynert in the basal forebrain (Hedreen et al. 1984). No consistent loss of acetylcholine content is found in the brains of healthy elderly humans. In Alzheimer's disease (AD), choline acetyltransferase, the primary synthetic enzyme of acetylcholine, is reduced (Blennow and Cowburn 1996). However, the data in healthy aging humans indicates minimal reduction or no change at all (Muller et al. 1991). On the other hand, cerebrospinal fluid levels of the degradative enzyme acetylcholinesterase are increased in advanced age (Hartikainen et al. 1991; Muller et al. 1991), and the density of some cholinergic receptors decreases with advancing age. The nucleus basalis of Meynert begins to atrophy after age 60 years, with neuronal loss observed mainly in posterior regions (Finch 1993). Thus, there is a general age-related decrease in cholinergic activity that may render elderly patients more susceptible to cholinergic system dysfunction associated with TBI.

Aminergic Systems

The locus ceruleus is the primary source of noradrenergic fibers innervating the human forebrain (Powers 2000). Loss of noradrenergic neurons in the locus ceruleus begins in the fourth decade of life and progresses in a linear fashion (Mann et al. 1983, 1984). Decreased activity of the noradrenergic synthetic enzymes tyrosine hydroxylase and dopamine β-hydroxylase also occur in the aging brain (Powers 2000). Alterations in receptor densities vary depending on brain region, with no change in frontal

TABLE 28–4. Neurochemical changes associated with aging

Neurotransmitter	Location	Change	Receptor location	Receptor alterations
Acetylcholine	Nucleus basalis of Meynert	↓ or →	Neocortex	↓ M_1 and M_2
				↓ N
	Medial septal region	?	Hippocampus	↓ M_1, M_3, M_4
				↓ N
Serotonin	Raphe	?	Neocortex	↓ 5-HT_1, 5-HT_2
Norepinephrine	Locus ceruleus	↓	Neocortex	↓ α-adrenergic
				↓ β-adrenergic
Dopamine	Substantia nigra	↓	Basal ganglia	↑ Postsynaptic D_1
				↓ Postsynaptic D_2
				↓ Presynaptic D_1
				↓ Presynaptic D_2

Note. ↓=decreased; ↑=increased; →=no change; ?= unknown.
Source. Adapted from Powers RE: "Neurobiology of Aging," in *Textbook of Geriatric Neuropsychiatry*, 2nd Edition. Edited by Coffey CE, Cummings JL. Washington, DC, American Psychiatric Press, 2000, pp 33–79.

β-adrenergic receptors but decreased receptor densities in cingulate, precentral, temporal, and occipitotemporal cortices (Mendelsohn and Paxinos 1991). Thus, elderly patients may be at increased risk of depression.

Age-related loss of dopaminergic neurons in the nigrostriatal pathways begins in the fifth decade of life, leading to as much as 35% loss by age 65 years (Mann et al. 1984). Moreover, density of the D_1 and D_2 receptors declines after age 18 years (Antonio et al. 1993; Hubble 1998). In aging patients, decreased density of D_2 receptors is associated with cognitive dysfunction that is suggestive of frontal systems impairment (Volkow et al. 1998, 2000). Although dopaminergic agonists may be helpful to treat cognitive functioning secondary to TBI (Kraus and Maki 1997a; McDowell et al. 1998), older patients may potentially be less responsive to these treatments because of the reduced density of postsynaptic D_1 and D_2 receptors in elderly patients (Antonio et al. 1993; Hubble 1998). This age-related deterioration of pre- and postsynaptic dopaminergic functioning may also account for the heightened sensitivity of older patients to cognitive impairment secondary to dopamine antagonists such as antipsychotic medications (Byerly et al. 2001).

Densities of 5-HT_1 and 5-HT_2 receptors are decreased in elderly humans (see Table 28–4). Density of type 1 receptors is decreased by up to 70%, and type 2 receptor density is reduced by 20%–50% (Mendelsohn and Paxinos 1991). This reduction in central serotonergic functioning has been proposed as a potential contributor

to the development of disturbances of mood and behavior in elderly patients (Meltzer et al. 1998).

Other

Monoamine oxidase (MAO) activity is substantially altered in the aging human brain. MAO-A is not altered, but MAO-B activity increases with age (Fowler et al. 1997; Gottfries 1990). This increased activity may deplete dopamine and other catecholamines, increasing the risk of depression and attentional problems. The aging human brain also has diminished γ-aminobutyric acid content and glutamic acid decarboxylase activity (Powers 2000). Moreover, increased affinity of excitatory amino acid receptors occurs with age (Olney 1990). Experimental chemical injury to rat brains produces a more severe excitotoxic reaction in the mature animals compared with younger animals (Campochiaro and Coyle 1978). Excitotoxic damage has been implicated in the pathogenesis of AD (Drachman and Lippa 1992) and is also a factor in secondary brain injury after trauma (Faden et al. 1989).

Summary

Aging brain demonstrates mild to moderate neuronal loss, with much of the volume loss caused by neuronal and synaptic atrophy. Additionally, neural plasticity is greatly reduced in advanced age. These factors, in addition to reduced neuronal responsiveness to injury-induced neurotrophic factors, may contribute to less favorable outcomes from TBI in the elderly. Neurochemical changes in the aging brain may lead to increased vulnerability to excitotoxic effects of TBI as well as increased risk of post-TBI cognitive and affective disturbances.

TBI and Dementia

The high prevalence of dementia among former boxers with a history of multiple brain injuries even years after retirement has stimulated interest in the relationship between TBI and AD. Dementia pugilistica, or "punch drunk" syndrome, is associated with parkinsonian features such as dysarthria, tremor, ataxia, bradykinesia, and cognitive impairment (Roberts 1969). Histopathological findings include neurofibrillary tangles without the senile neuritic plaques seen in AD (Corsellis et al. 1973). Dementia pugilistica is associated with β-amyloid deposits similar to those seen in AD, suggesting a causative role of repetitive brain injuries in an AD-like dementia (Roberts et al. 1990). Postmortem studies of patients who died after TBI found β-amyloid deposits in 30% of patients (Roberts et al. 1991). Although β-amyloid deposition is relatively common in healthy elderly adults, this study included young adults and children. Roberts et al. (1994) hypothesized that increased expression of β-amyloid precursor protein may represent an early response to acute neuronal injury designed to facilitate repair.

Influence of Apolipoprotein E on Outcome

Apolipoprotein E (apoE) regulates lipid transport and metabolism in the liver and central nervous system, distributing cholesterol and phospholipids to neurons after injury. In this capacity, it may mediate neuronal repair, regeneration, and survival (Horsburgh et al. 2000). In humans, there are three common isoforms of apoE encoded by different alleles: ε2, ε3, and ε4 (apoE ε4). The apoE ε4 allele is a known risk factor for AD (Saunders et al. 1993) and also influences outcome after TBI through an unclear mechanism. Teasdale et al. (1997) prospectively followed 93 TBI patients. After adjustment for age, GCS, and computed tomography (CT) findings, 57% of patients with apoE ε4 had a poor outcome compared with 27% of patients without the apoE ε4 allele. Thus, the presence of the apoE ε4 allele was associated with a twofold increase in risk of a poor outcome (dead, vegetative state, or severe disability) when adjusted for age, severity of injury, and CT findings. Friedman et al. (1999) prospectively studied 69 survivors of TBI. Patients with the apoE ε4 allele were more than five times more likely to have prolonged coma (longer than 7

days) than those without the allele. Moreover, the odds ratio of a suboptimal outcome (fair or unfavorable) was 13.94 for patients with the apoE ε4 allele when adjusted for age and duration of coma. Lichtman et al. (2000) studied 31 patients who had completed an acute neurorehabilitation program after TBI. After controlling for coma duration, they found that patients with the apoE ε4 allele had significantly more functional impairment than those patients without the allele. No difference was found on cognitive measures. Kutner et al. (2000) studied 53 professional football players of various ages. They found that older players with the apoE ε4 allele performed more poorly on cognitive testing than players of all ages without the allele or younger players with the allele. This suggests that the apoE ε4 allele may interact with cumulative exposure to mild head trauma, leading to cognitive impairment. Nicoll et al. (1995) examined postmortem brains of 90 patients who died of TBI. Fifty-two percent of those with β-amyloid deposition had the apoE ε4 allele compared with only 16% of those without such deposition. Therefore, head trauma may trigger deposition of β-amyloid, particularly in patients with the apoE ε4 allele.

TBI and Alzheimer's Disease

The role of TBI as a risk factor for AD is contradictory. In studies comparing elderly patients with AD with elderly healthy control subjects, TBI was more than three times more common in patients with AD (Graves et al. 1990; Henderson et al. 1992; Mayeux et al. 1993; Mortimer et al. 1985). However, some studies have failed to find a significant association between TBI and AD (Amaducci et al. 1986; Broe et al. 1990; Chandra et al. 1987; Shalat et al. 1987; Williams et al. 1991). Mayeux et al. (1995) examined the risk of AD associated with TBI and apoE ε4 in 236 community-dwelling elderly persons. TBI alone was associated with no increased risk of AD. The apoE ε4 allele was associated with a twofold increase in risk of AD, and the presence of apoE ε4 as well as a history of TBI was associated with a 10-fold increase in risk of AD. Mehta et al. (1999) studied 6,645 subjects ages 55 years and older. A history of head trauma with loss of consciousness was not associated with an increased risk of AD in this population. Nemetz et al. (1999) reviewed medical records of 1,283 patients ages 40 years and older. A history of TBI was associated with no increased risk of developing AD, but in the TBI patients who developed AD, the median time between TBI and onset of AD was 10 years versus an age-adjusted median of 18 years. This suggests that TBI may reduce the time of onset of AD in vulnerable individuals.

Clinical Presentation

The clinical presentation of TBI in older patients differs from that of other populations because of age-related physiological changes and the different circumstances related to their injuries. Cognitive and neurological sequelae TBI in elderly patients may have a more insidious yet malignant onset and progression due to the high prevalence of subdural hematomas in even mild or moderate injuries. In this scenario, a patient may present with several weeks or months of progressive cognitive impairment. The patient may either have had a witnessed or unwitnessed fall or other head trauma that was not thought to warrant medical attention. The risk of social isolation in the elderly increases the likelihood that head trauma will either not be witnessed or the subacute evolution of signs and symptoms will not be observed.

Another presentation may involve the presence of orthopedic injuries resulting from a fall or cardiovascular pathology that precipitated a fall. These more emergent conditions may lead the primary treatment team to focus on acute stabilization, particularly in intensive care or surgical settings. Neuropsychiatric consultation may be requested later in the course of treatment as a result of emerging confusion or agitation that is attributed to complications of hospitalization rather than a pre-admission TBI. Careful history taking using collateral information sources may assist in the identification of an occult TBI.

Assessment

Clinical History

The GCS may be a less reliable measure of severity of injury in older individuals because of numerous factors, including sensory deterioration and preexisting dementia (Powers 2000). Moreover, because many fall-related TBIs may be unwitnessed, the duration of time before initial assessment may be more variable in this age group, further limiting the utility of the GCS. As a result, additional history must be obtained to clarify the extent of the insult and its effects on the patient. Particularly important is the establishment of a preinjury baseline. Age-related bias may lead clinicians to assume that post-TBI cognitive deficits are merely reflective of a preexisting dementia. In addition, previous brain injuries or cerebrovascular insults may have occurred over the course of the individual's lifetime. A detailed and accurate history of preinjury physical, cognitive, and psychological status is crucial. Frequently, such history must be obtained from relatives and friends. However, the protean

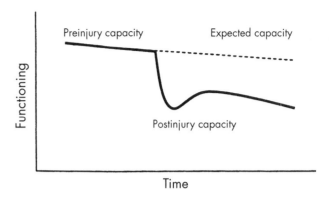

FIGURE 28–1. Alterations in functional capacity over time.

manifestations of TBI in the elderly are further complicated by the increased physiological variability between older individuals. Therefore, the clinician must use collateral information to develop an estimation of the patient's preinjury functioning as well as preinjury rate of functional decline (Figure 28–1). This process can help determine the influence of the injury on the patient's functional trajectory.

Neuroimaging

Given the high incidence of posttraumatic subdural hematomas in older patients, structural neuroimaging studies such as CT and magnetic resonance imaging may help identify such pathologies in verified or suspected TBI. Single-photon emission CT (SPECT) may also provide useful information regarding alterations in regional cerebral perfusion not detected by structural imaging (Masdeu et al. 1995). However, age-related changes in the brain may make interpretation of both structural and functional imaging results difficult. Global cerebral perfusion is diminished in normal aging (Choi et al. 1998), which may make interpretation of SPECT imaging difficult. Abnormalities in fronto-temporal perfusion are associated with behavioral disturbances in dementias (Hirano et al. 2000; Mychack et al. 2001). These findings suggest that SPECT imaging may be useful in confirming the presence of TBI when the presence of head trauma is not clear. However, nonspecific or dementia- and age-related changes may complicate interpretation of results.

Neuropsychological Assessment

Neuropsychological testing may help distinguish cognitive disturbances caused by TBI from age-related cognitive changes. Age-related decline in memory performance is characterized by a fairly narrow range of impaired performance in acquisition and retrieval of newly learned information (Peterson et al. 1992; Small et al. 1999). Moreover, decreased processing speed in healthy elderly subjects occurs only when multiple tasks are involved (Salthouse and Coon 1993). The cognitive deficits associated with TBI are more pervasive and may thus be distinguished from normal aging. Neuropsychological testing may also help distinguish cognitive effects of TBI from that of AD (Goldstein et al. 1996).

Summary

Assessment of the brain-injured older patient begins with maintaining a high index of suspicion for TBI even when the initial presentation or reason for consultation does not specify this history. Obtaining detailed collateral history of the presenting syndrome is critical, as is a history of prior injuries and cognitive functioning. Structural as well as functional neuroimaging provide important data regarding the effects of TBI on the brain, as does neuropsychological testing. Age-related alterations in brain structure and function require consideration of these changes when interpreting results. These factors that confound the use of formal testing and neuroimaging in the elderly accentuate the importance of a detailed pre- and postinjury history to determine the role of TBI in an older patient's functional problems.

Treatment

The necessity for a multidisciplinary biopsychosocial approach to management of TBI rehabilitation is present for all age groups. However, in older patients, even more attention must be paid to age-specific factors that affect the physiology, psychology, and social circumstances of brain-injured patients.

Pharmacological Treatment

Pharmacological interventions should take into consideration the increased sensitivity of elderly patients to medication side effects, particularly anticholinergic side effects. Additionally, attention must be paid to physiological changes that alter the pharmacokinetics of medications. Increases in body fat composition may increase elimination half-life of lipid-soluble medications, whereas decreased serum proteins may lead to increased bioavailability at equivalent serum levels. Additional factors include decreased gastric emptying and resulting slowed absorption and decreased renal and hepatic excretion (Table 28–5).

Environmental Interventions

Environmental interventions should address age-associated sensory decline. Areas should be well-lit and free from

excessive noise and other stimuli that may overwhelm and confuse the patient. Caregivers should be trained to approach the patient directly and speak clearly in brief, succinct sentences. Reinforcement of communication through repetition is vital. Management of older TBI patients may be similar to that of elderly patients with primary dementias. Neuropsychological testing may help identify areas of deficit and areas of preserved function. This may assist in the development of environmental and communication modifications to enhance function.

Psychotherapy

For the patient struggling with adaptation to new cognitive and functional impairments, supportive psychotherapy may be helpful in easing distress and obviating the need for psychotropic medications. This approach is addressed more completely in Chapter 35, Psychotherapy. Psychotherapy may be modified readily to accommodate the specific circumstances and needs of elderly patients and may prove quite effective for depressive disorders, particularly when combined with pharmacotherapy (Miller et al. 1997).

Family and Caregiver Work

The increased risk in older patients of functional impairment resulting from TBI may lead to drastic changes in role functioning in families that have often had stable roles for decades. Education of families and caregivers regarding the practical implications of these changes may reduce caregiver distress. In particular, engaging families with support groups that provide mentoring and education regarding the process of adjusting to TBI may reduce burnout. Caregivers and patients must be helped in the process of grieving lost functioning. As in the dementias, behavioral disturbances are a major cause of caregiver distress and an obstacle to successful community functioning. Likewise, such disturbances may accelerate the need for institutional placement (Dunkin and Anderson-Hanley 1998). In fact, caregiver distress exerts a major role independent of patient factors in predicting institutionalization in individuals with dementia (Cohen et al. 1993). Therefore, working with caregivers with supportive and educational interventions may improve functional outcomes.

Management of Neuropsychiatric Syndromes

Depression

Depression is an independent risk factor for mortality in advanced age and accounts for substantial functional

TABLE 28–5. Age-related physiological changes and pharmacokinetic implications

Function	Pharmacokinetic effect	Clinical implications in relevant drugs
Absorption	↓ Rate of absorption	Delayed onset, incomplete absorption, reduced effect
↑ Gastric pH		
↓ Gastric emptying		
↓ Mesenteric blood flow		
Distribution	↑ Volume of distribution for lipophilic drugs	↑ Time until steady-state plasma concentration
↓ Muscle mass	↑ Elimination half-life of lipophilic drugs	↓ Duration of effect of single doses
↓ Total body water		Slower titration
↑ Total body fat		
Plasma protein binding	↑ Free fraction of highly protein-bound drugs	↑ Potency and toxicity at lower doses
↓ Albumin		Reduced dosage
↓ γ_1-acid glycoprotein		
Hepatic metabolism	↑ Elimination half-life of hepatically metabolized drugs	↑ Time till steady-state plasma concentration
↓ Liver volume	↑ Ratio of parent drug to demethylated derivative	Reduced dosage
↓ Hepatic blood flow		Slower titration
↓ Oxidative metabolism		
↓ N-Demethylation		
→ Conjugation		
Renal clearance	↑ Elimination half-life of active hydrophilic drugs	↑ Time till steady-state plasma concentration
↓ Renal blood flow		Reduced dosage
↓ Glomerular filtration rate		Slower titration

Note. ↓=decreased; ↑=increased; →=no change.
Source. Adapted from Zubenko GS, Sunderland T: "Geriatric Neuropsychopharmacology: Why Does Age Matter?" In *Textbook of Geriatric Neuropsychiatry*, 2nd Edition. Edited by Coffey CE, Cummings JL, Lovell MR, et al. Washington, DC, American Psychiatric Press, 2000, pp 749–778.

impairment (Blazer et al. 2001). It may be characterized by more irritability and apathy, with less overt sadness. The changes in role functioning that often occur with aging may be exacerbated by the abrupt loss of functional capacity because of TBI. Greater dependence on others for cognitive and, at times, physical tasks may engender feelings of loss and helplessness. Antidepressant therapy may be extremely effective, particularly when depression is accompanied by vegetative or behavioral alterations from baseline. TCAs may cause orthostatic hypotension as well as lower seizure threshold (Wroblewski et al. 1990). By contrast, methylphenidate was not found to cause increased frequency of seizures

(Wroblewski et al. 1992). Therefore, stimulants or non-TCAs may be preferable.

Agitation and Psychosis

Agitation in the elderly TBI patient may represent an exacerbation of a preexisting dementia-related behavioral disorder. It may also be related to frontal disinhibition or dysphoric mania resulting from the injury itself. Mood stabilizers and atypical antipsychotics appear to be well tolerated in elderly dementia patients, though with appropriate decreases in dosage and rate of titration. Clarifying the symptom may be important to effective treatment. As mentioned in the section Depression, irritability and overt hostility may be a symptom of depression in the presence of advanced age and neurological disease. Another common occurrence in TBI is dysphoric mania, characterized by irritability, restless energy, and decreased need for sleep. Such patients respond well to mood stabilizers such as lithium, carbamazepine, and divalproex sodium (Kunik et al. 1994; Porsteinsson et al. 2001). Elderly patients may have altered metabolic clearance of drugs and different protein binding, necessitating careful dosing and titration of these medications. The therapeutic window may be exceedingly narrow. Increased sensitivity to side effects of sedation, tremor, and ataxia are common in older patients with any neurological disease. Atypical antipsychotic medications may reduce irritability and aggression in elderly patients with dementia. This is also true of elderly patients with behavioral complications of TBI. Care must be taken to provide the optimum degree of therapeutic benefit with a minimum of side effects. The atypical antipsychotic medications are well tolerated in the elderly and have varying side-effect profiles. Risperidone is less sedating but has greater potential for extrapyramidal side effects (EPSs). On April 16, 2003, the manufacturer of risperidone issued a letter warning of a small but statistically significant increase in cerebrovascular adverse events associated with treatment with risperidone compared with placebo, though the evidence does not point to a clear causal relationship (Smith and Beier 2004). Olanzapine may be more sedating at higher doses and has greater anticholinergic properties in vitro, but in clinical practice such side effects are reported less frequently than expected. Quetiapine is somewhat more sedating and carries a slightly increased risk for cataracts with chronic use. It is relatively free from anticholinergic side effects or EPSs. Ziprasidone is less sedating and less anticholinergic with minimal EPSs. In premarketing trials of ziprasidone, a slight increase in QT interval was found that was judged to be of subclinical significance in the general population. However, in elderly patients with known cardiac disease, particularly intraventricular conduction problems, ziprasidone should be used with caution (Glick et al. 2001).

Cognition

Acetylcholine has been recognized as a principal neurochemical mediator of cognition (Aigner 1995; Blokland 1995). However, dopaminergic functioning has also been identified as an important component to the neurochemistry of cognition (Kulisevsky 2000; Robbins 2000). Cholinergic therapies such as lecithin, physostigmine (Cardenas et al. 1994; Goldberg et al. 1982; Levin et al. 1986), and donepezil (Masanic et al. 2001; Morey et al. 2003; Taverni et al. 1998;

Walker et al. 2004; Whelan et al. 2000; Walker et al. 2004; Whitlock 1999; Zhang et al. 2004) may improve cognitive functioning in patients with TBI. These medications are well tolerated and therefore may be used to treat cognitive difficulties in elderly and younger TBI patients alike. Cholinergic dysfunction has been implicated in behavioral disturbances in dementia (Minger et al. 2000). Moreover, the psychotropic properties of cholinesterase inhibitors are being increasingly recognized in elderly patients with dementia (Cummings 2000). Therefore, these medications may demonstrate some behavioral benefits in elderly patients with TBI. There are currently no available data regarding behavioral improvements in this population.

Cognitive deficits may also respond to treatment with dopamine agonists. Both methylphenidate (Hornyak et al. 1997; Kaelin et al. 1996; Plenger et al. 1996; Whyte et al. 1997; Wroblewski et al. 1992) and amantadine (Kraus and Maki 1997b; Schneider et al. 1999) have been shown to improve attention, concentration, and processing speed in TBI patients. Amphetamine has been found to enhance functional recovery in a chart review study (Hornstein et al. 1996). In older patients who demonstrate reduced initiative and attention, these medications may be useful adjuncts to environmental stimulation.

Conclusion

The elderly represent a rapidly growing population with a specific set of risk factors for TBI that differ from that of the general population. Moreover, older patients are at high risk for less favorable outcomes and secondary complications. The thoughtful application of principles of geriatric medicine will improve the assessment and management of this complex patient group. Nevertheless, timely and appropriate rehabilitative and neuropsychiatric interventions may provide older patients with substantial functional and cognitive benefits.

References

Aharon-Peretz J, Kliot D, Amyel-Zvi E, et al: Neurobehavioral consequences of closed head injury in the elderly. Brain Inj 11:871–875, 1997
Aigner TG: Pharmacology of memory: cholinergic–glutamatergic interactions. Curr Opin Neurobiol 5:155–160, 1995
Akiyama H, Meyer JF, Mortel KF, et al: Normal human aging: factors contributing to cerebral atrophy. J Neurol Sci 152:39–49, 1997
Amaducci LA, Fratiglioni L, Rocca WA, et al: Risk factors for clinically diagnosed Alzheimer's disease: a case-control study of an Italian population. Neurology 36:922–931, 1986

Antonio A, Leender KL, Reist H, et al: Effect of age on D_2 dopamine receptors in normal human brain measured by positron emission tomography and ^{11}C-raclopride. Arch Neurol 50:474–480, 1993

Aparasu RR, Sitzman SJ: Inappropriate prescribing for elderly outpatients. Am J Health Syst Pharm 1:433–439, 1999

Blazer DG, Hybels CF, Pieper CF: The association of depression and mortality in elderly persons: a case for multiple, independent pathways. J Gerontol A Biol Sci Med Sci 56:M505–509, 2001

Blennow K, Cowburn RF: The neurochemistry of Alzheimer's disease. Acta Neurol Scand Suppl 168:77–86, 1996

Blokland A: Acetylcholine: a neurotransmitter for learning and memory? Brain Res Brain Res Rev 21:285–300, 1995

Boyeson MG: Neurochemical alterations after brain injury: clinical implications for pharmacologic rehabilitation. NeuroRehabilitation 1:33–43, 1991

Broe GA, Henderson AS, Creasey H, et al: A case-control study of Alzheimer's disease in Australia. Neurology 40:1698–1707, 1990

Byerly MJ, Weber MT, Brooks DL, et al: Antipsychotic medications and the elderly: effects on cognition and implications for use. Drugs Aging 18:45–61, 2001

Campochiaro P, Coyle JT: Ontogenetic development of kainate neurotoxicity; correlates with glutamatergic innervation. Proc Natl Acad Sci U S A 75:2025–2029, 1978

Cardenas DD, McLean A, Farrell-Roberts L, et al: Oral physostigmine and impaired memory in adults with brain injury. Brain Inj 8:579–587, 1994

Carlsson C-A, von Essen C, Losgren J: Clinical factors in severe head injuries. J Neurosurg 29:242–251, 1968

Chandra V, Philipose V, Bell PA, et al: Case-control study of late onset "probable Alzheimer's disease." Neurology 37:1295–1300, 1987

Choi JY, Morris JC, Hsu CY: Aging and cerebrovascular disease. Neurologic Clinics of North America 16:687–710, 1998

Cifu DX, Kreutzer JS, Marwitz JH, et al: Functional outcomes of older adults with traumatic brain injury: a prospective, multicenter analysis. Arch Phys Med Rehabil 77:883–888, 1996

Cohen CA, Gold DP, Shulman KI, et al: Factors determining the decision to institutionalize dementing individuals: a prospective study. Gerontologist 33:714–720, 1993

Corsellis JAN, Bruton CH, Freeman-Browne D: The aftermath of boxing. Psychol Med 3:270–273, 1973

Cummings JL: Cholinesterase inhibitors: a new class of psychotropic compounds. Am J Psychiatry 157: 4–15, 2000

Cummings JL, Benson DF: Dementia: A Clinical Approach, 2nd Edition. Boston, MA, Butterworths, 1992

Dewar D, Graham DI: Depletion of choline acetyltransferase activity but preservation of M_1 and M_2 muscarinic receptor binding sites in temporal cortex following head injury: a preliminary human postmortem study. J Neurotrauma 13:181–187, 1996

Dobkin BH: Rehabilitation, in Textbook of Geriatric Neuropsychiatry, 2nd Edition. Edited by Coffey CE, Cummings JL. Washington, DC, American Psychiatric Press, 2000

Drachman DA, Lippa CF: The etiology of Alzheimer's disease: the pathogenesis of dementia. The role of neurotoxins. Ann N Y Acad Sci 648:176–186, 1992

Dubinsky RM, Stein AC, Lyons K: Practice parameter: risk of driving and Alzheimer's disease (an evidence-based review): report of the Quality Standards Subcommittee of the American Academy of Neurology. Neurology 54:2205–2211, 2000

Dunkin JJ, Anderson-Hanley C: Dementia caregiver burden: a review of the literature and guidelines for assessment and intervention. Neurology 51 (suppl 1):S53–S60, 1998

Faden AI, Demediuk P, Panter SS, et al: The role of excitatory amino acids and NMDA receptors in traumatic brain injury. Science 244:798–800, 1989

Fields RB, Cisewski D, Coffey CE: Traumatic brain injury, in Textbook of Geriatric Neuropsychiatry, 2nd Edition. Edited by Coffey CE, Cummings JL. Washington, DC, American Psychiatric Press, 2000

Finch CE: Neuron atrophy during aging: programmed or sporadic? Trends Neurosci 16:104–110, 1993

Finger S: Recovery from Brain Damage. New York, Plenum, 1978

Fowler JS, Volkow N, Wang GJ: Age-related increases in brain monoamine oxidase B in living healthy human subjects. Neurobiol Aging 18:431–435, 1997

Friedman G, Froom P, Sazbon L, et al: Apolipoprotein E-ε4 genotype predicts a poor outcome in survivors of traumatic brain injury. Neurology 52:244–248, 1999

Fuller GF: Falls in the elderly. Am Fam Physician 61:2159–2168, 2000

Glick ID, Murray SR, Vasudevan P, et al: Treatment with atypical antipsychotics: new indications and new populations. J Psychiatr Res 35:187–191, 2001

Goldberg E, Gerstman LJ, Mattis S, et al: Selective effects of cholinergic treatment on verbal memory in posttraumatic amnesia. J Clin Neuropsychol 4:219–234, 1982

Goldstein FC, Levin HS, Roberts VJ, et al: Neuropsychological effects of closed head injury in older adults: a comparison with Alzheimer's disease. Neuropsychology 10:147–154, 1996

Goldstein FC, Levin HS, Goldman WP, et al: Cognitive and neurobehavioral functioning after mild versus moderate traumatic brain injury in older adults. J Int Neuropsychol Soc 7:373–383, 2001

Gottfries CG: Neurochemical aspects on aging and diseases with cognitive impairment. J Neurosci Res 27:541–547, 1990

Graves AB, White E, Koepsell TD, et al: The association between head trauma and Alzheimer's disease. Am J Epidemiol 131:491–501, 1990

Hamm RJ, Jenkins LW, Lyeth BG, et al: The effect of age on outcome following traumatic brain injury in rats. J Neurosurg 75:916–921, 1991

Hamm RJ, White-Gbadebo DM, Lyeth BG, et al: The effect of age on motor and cognitive deficits after traumatic brain injury in rats. Neurosurgery 31:1072–1077, 1992

Hartikainen P, Soininen H, Reinikainen KJ, et al: Neurotransmitter markers in the cerebrospinal fluid of normal subjects: effects of aging and other confounding factors. J Neural Transm (General Section) 84:103–117, 1991

Haug H, Eggers R: Morphometry of the human cortex cerebri and corpus striatum during aging. Neurobiol Aging 12:336–338, 1991

Hedreen JC, Struble RG, Whitehouse PJ, et al: Topography of the magnocellular basal forebrain system in human brain. J Neuropathol Exp Neurol 43:1–21, 1984

Hefti F, Hartikka J, Knusel B: Function of neurotrophic factors in the adult and aging brain and their possible use in the treatment of neurodegenerative disease. Neurobiol Aging 10:515–533, 1989

Henderson AS, Jorm AF, Korten AE, et al: Environmental risk factors for Alzheimer's disease: their relationship to age of onset and to familial or sporadic types. Psychol Med 22:429–436, 1992

Hirano N, Mega MS, Dinov I, et al: Left frontotemporal hypoperfusion is associated with aggression in patients with dementia. Arch Neurol 57:861–866, 2000

Hornstein A, Lennihan L, Seliger G, et al: Amphetamine in recovery from brain injury. Brain Inj 10:145–148, 1996

Hornyak JE, Nelson VS, Hurvitz EA: The use of methylphenidate in paediatric traumatic brain injury. Pediatr Rehabil 1:15–17, 1997

Horsburgh K, McCarron MO, White F, et al: The role of apolipoprotein E in Alzheimer's disease, acute brain injury and cerebrovascular disease: evidence of common mechanisms and utility of animal models. Neurobiol Aging 21:245–255, 2000

Hubble JP: Aging and the basal ganglia. Neurol Clin 16:649–657, 1998

Jennett B, Teasdale G, Braakmen R, et al: Predicting outcome in individual patients after severe head injury. Lancet 1:1031–1034, 1976

Kaelin DL, Cifu DX, Metthies B: Methylphenidate effect on attention deficit in the acutely brain-injured adult. Arch Phys Med Rehabil 77:6–9, 1996

Kotwica Z, Jakubowski JF: Acute head injuries in the elderly: an analysis of 136 consecutive patients. Acta Neurochir (Wien) 118:98–102, 1992

Kraus MF, Maki P: The combined use of amantadine and L-dopa/carbidopa in the treatment of chronic brain injury. Brain Inj 11:455–460, 1997a

Kraus MF, Maki PM: Effect of amantadine hydrochloride on symptoms of frontal lobe dysfunction in brain injury: case studies and review. J Neuropsychiatry Clin Neurosci 9:222–230, 1997b

Kulisevsky J: Role of dopamine in learning and memory: implications for the treatment of cognitive dysfunction in patients with Parkinson's disease. Drugs Aging 16:365–379, 2000

Kunik ME, Yudofsky SC, Silver JM, et al: Pharmacologic approach to management of agitation associated with dementia. J Clin Psychiatry 55 (suppl):13–17, 1994

Kutner KC, Erlanger DM, Tsai J, et al: Lower cognitive performance of older football players possessing apolipoprotein E ε4. Neurosurgery 47:651–657, 2000

Levin HS, Peters BH, Kalisky Z, et al: Effects of oral physostigmine and lecithin on memory and attention in closed head-injured patients. Cent Nerv Syst Trauma 3:333–342, 1986

Lichtman SW, Seliger G, Tycko B, et al: Apolipoprotein E and functional recovery from brain injury following postacute rehabilitation. Neurology 55:1536–1539, 2000

Malmgren R: Epidemiology of aging, in Textbook of Geriatric Neuropsychiatry, 2nd Edition. Edited by Coffey CE, Cummings JL. Washington, DC, American Psychiatric Press, 2000

Mann DMA, Yates PO, Hawkes J: The pathology of the human locus ceruleus. Clin Neuropathol 2:1–7, 1983

Mann DMA, Yates PO, Marcyniuk B: Monoaminergic neurotransmitter systems in presenile Alzheimer's disease and in senile dementia of Alzheimer type. Clin Neuropathol 3:199–205, 1984

Masanic CA, Bayley MT, Van Reekum R, et al: Open-label study of donepezil in traumatic brain injury. Arch Phys Med Rehabil 82:896–901, 2001

Masdeu JC, Abdel-Dayem H, Van Heertum RL: Head trauma: use of SPECT. J Neuroimag 5:S53–S57, 1995

Mayeux R, Ottman R, Tang MX, et al: Genetic susceptibility and head injury as risk factors for Alzheimer's disease among community-dwelling elderly persons and their first-degree relatives. Ann Neurol 33:494–501, 1993

Mayeux R, Ottman R, Maestre G, et al: Synergistic effects of traumatic head injury and apolipoprotein-ε4 in patients with Alzheimer's disease. Neurology 24:555–557, 1995

Mazzucchi A, Cattelani R, Missale G, et al: Head-injured subjects aged over 50 years: correlations between variables of trauma and neuropsychological follow-up. J Neurol 239:256–260, 1992

McDowell S, Whyte J, D'Esposito M: Differential effect of dopaminergic agonist on prefrontal function in traumatic brain injury patients. Brain 121:1155–1164, 1998

Mehta KM, Ott A, Kalmijn S, et al: Head trauma and risk of dementia and Alzheimer's disease: the Rotterdam Study. Neurology 53:1959–1962, 1999

Meltzer CC, Smith G, Price JC, et al: Reduced binding of [18F] altanserin to serotonin type 2A receptors in aging: persistence of effect after partial volume correction. Brain Res 813:167–171, 1998

Mendelsohn FAO, Paxinos G (eds): Receptors in the Human Nervous System. San Diego, CA, Academic Press, 1991

Mervis RF, Pope D, Lewis R, et al: Exogenous nerve growth factor reverses age-related structural changes in neocortical neurons in the aging rat: a quantitative Golgi study. Ann N Y Acad Sci 640:95–103, 1991

Miller MD, Wolfson L, Frank E, et al: Using interpersonal psychotherapy (IPT) in a combined psychotherapy/medication research protocol with depressed elders: a descriptive report with case vignettes. J Psychother Pract Res 7:47–55, 1997

Minger SL, Esiri MM, McDonald B, et al: Cholinergic deficits contribute to behavioral disturbance in patients with dementia. Neurology 55:1460–1467, 2000

Moore AR, O'Keefe ST: Drug-induced cognitive impairment in the elderly. Drugs Aging 15:15–28, 1999

Morey CE, Cilo M, Berry J, et al: The effect of Aricept in persons with persistent memory disorder following traumatic brain injury: a pilot study. Brain Inj 17:809–815, 2003

Mortimer JA, French LR, Hutton JT, et al: Head injury as a risk factor for Alzheimer's disease. Neurology 35:264–267, 1985

Muller WE, Stoll L, Schubert T, et al: Central cholinergic functioning and aging. Acta Psychiatr Scand 366 (suppl):34–39, 1991

Mychack P, Kramer JH, Boone KB, et al: The influence of right frontotemporal dysfunction on social behavior in frontotemporal dementia. Neurology 56:S11–S15, 2001

Nemetz PN, Leibson C, Naessens JM, et al: Traumatic brain injury and time to onset of Alzheimer's disease: a population-based study. Am J Epidemiol 149:32–40, 1999

Nicoll JA, Roberts GW, Graham DI: Apolipoprotein E4 allele is associated with deposition of amyloid beta-protein following head injury. Nat Med 1:135–137, 1995

Olney JW: Excitotoxin-mediated neuron death in youth and old age. Progr Brain Res 86:37–51, 1990

Pappius HM: Brain injury: new insights into neurotransmitter and receptor mechanisms. Neurochem Res 16:941–949, 1991

Pennings JL, Bachulis BL, Simous CT: Survival after severe traumatic brain injury in the aged. Arch Surg 128:787–793, 1993

Pentland B, Jones PA, Roy CW, et al: Head injury in the elderly. Age Ageing 15:193–202, 1986

Peterson RC, Smith G, Kokmen E, et al: Memory function in normal aging. Neurology 42:396–401, 1992

Plenger PM, Dixon CE, Castillo RM, et al: Subacute methylphenidate treatment for moderate to moderately severe traumatic brain injury: a preliminary double-blind placebo-controlled study. Arch Phys Med Rehabil 77:536–540, 1996

Porsteinsson AP, Tariot PN, Erb R, et al: Placebo-controlled study of divalproex sodium for agitation in dementia. Am J Geriatr Psychiatry 9:58–66, 2001

Powers RE: Neurobiology of aging, in Textbook of Geriatric Neuropsychiatry, 2nd Edition. Edited by Coffey CE, Cummings JL. Washington, DC, American Psychiatric Press, 2000

Rapaport MJ, Feinstein A: Outcome following traumatic brain injury in the elderly: a critical review. Brain Inj 14:749–761, 2000

Rapaport MJ, Feinstein A: Age and functioning after mild traumatic brain injury: the acute picture. Brain Inj 15:857–864, 2001

Ritchie PD, Cameron PA, Ugoni AM, et al: A study of the functional outcome and mortality in elderly patients with head injuries. J Clin Neurosci 7:301–304, 2000

Robbins TW: Chemical neuromodulation of frontal-executive functions in humans and other animals. Exp Brain Res 133:130–138, 2000

Roberts AJ: Brain Damage in Boxers. London, Pitman, 1969

Roberts GW, Allsop D, Bruton C: The occult aftermath of boxing. J Neurol Neurosurg Psychiatry 53:373–378, 1990

Roberts GW, Gentleman SM, Lynch A, et al: βA4 amyloid protein deposition in brain after head trauma. Lancet 338:1422–1423, 1991

Roberts GW, Gentleman SM, Lynch A, et al: Beta amyloid protein deposition in the brain after severe head injury: implications for the pathogenesis of Alzheimer's disease. J Neurol Neurosurg Psychiatry 57:419–425, 1994

Rothweiler B, Temkin NR, Dikmen SS: Aging effect on psychosocial outcome in traumatic brain injury. Arch Phys Med Rehabil 79:881–887, 1998

Saija A, Hayes RL, Lyeth BG, et al: The effect of concussive head injury on central cholinergic neurons. Brain Res 452:303–311, 1988

Salthouse TA, Coon VE: Influence of task-specific processing speed on age differences in memory. J Gerontol 48:P245–255, 1993

Saunders AM, Strittmatter WJ, Schmechel D, et al: Association of apolipoprotein E allele ε4 with late-onset familial and sporadic Alzheimer's disease. Neurology 43:1467–1472, 1993

Schneider WN, Drew-Cates J, Wong TM, et al: Cognitive and behavioural efficacy of amantadine in acute traumatic brain injury: an initial double-blind placebo-controlled study. Brain Inj 13:863–872, 1999

Shalat SL, Seltzer B, Pidcock, et al: Risk factors for Alzheimer's disease: a case-control study. Neurology 37:1630–1633, 1987

Small SA, Stern Y, Tang M, et al: Selective decline in memory function among healthy elderly. Neurology 52:1392–1396, 1999

Smith DA, Beier MT: Association between risperidone treatment and cerebrovascular adverse events: examining the evidence. J Am Med Dir Assoc 5:129–132. 2004

Taverni JP, Seliger G, Lichtman SW: Donepezil medicated memory improvement in traumatic brain injury during post-acute rehabilitation. Brain Inj 12:77–80, 1998

Teasdale GM, Nicoll JA, Murray G, et al: Association of apolipoprotein E polymorphism with outcome after head injury. Lancet 350:1069–1071, 1997

Thapa PB, Gideon P, Cost TW, et al: Antidepressants and the risk of falls among nursing home residents. N Engl J Med 339:875–882, 1998

Tinetti ME: Falls, in Geriatric Medicine. Edited by Cassel CK, Cohen HJ, Larson EB, et al. New York, Springer-Verlag New York, 1997

Tune LE: Serum anticholinergic activity levels and delirium in the elderly. Semin Clin Neuropsychiatry 5:149–153, 2000

Volkow ND, Gur RC, Wang G-J, et al: Association between decline in brain dopamine activity with age and cognitive and motor impairment in healthy individuals. Am J Psychiatry 155:344–349, 1998

Volkow ND, Logan J, Fowler JF, et al: Association between age-related decline in brain dopamine activity and impairment in frontal and cingulate metabolism. Am J Psychiatry 157:75–80, 2000

Walker W, Seel R, Gibellato M, et al: The effects of donepezil on traumatic brain injury acute rehabilitation outcomes. Brain Inj 18:739–750, 2004

Whelan FJ, Walker MS, Schultz SK: Donepezil in the treatment of cognitive dysfunction associated with traumatic brain injury. Ann Clin Psychiatry 12:131–135, 2000

Whitlock JA: Brain injury, cognitive impairment, and donepezil. J Head Trauma Rehabil 14:424–427, 1999

Whyte J, Hart T, Schuster K, et al: Effects of methylphenidate on attentional function after traumatic brain injury: a randomized, placebo-controlled trial. Am J Phys Med Rehabil 76:440–450, 1997

Willcox SM, Himmelstein DU, Woolhandler S: Inappropriate drug prescribing for the community-dwelling elderly. JAMA 272:292–296, 1994

Williams DB, Annegers JF, Kokmen E, et al: Brain injury and neurologic sequelae: a cohort study of dementia, parkinsonism, and amyotrophic lateral sclerosis. Neurology 41:1554–1557, 1991

Wroblewski BA, McColgan K, Smith K, et al: The incidence of seizures during tricyclic antidepressant drug treatment in a brain-injured population. J Clin Psychopharmacol 10:124–128, 1990

Wroblewski BA, Leary JM, Phelan AM, et al: Methylphenidate and seizure frequency in brain injured patients with seizure disorders. J Clin Psychiatry 53:86–89, 1992

Zhan C, Sangl J, Bierman AS, et al: Potentially inappropriate medication use in the community-dwelling elderly: findings from the 1996 Medical Expenditure Panel Survey. JAMA 286:2823–2829, 2001

Zhang L, Plotkin RC, Wang G, et al: Cholinergic augmentation with donepezil enhances recovery in short-term memory and sustained attention after traumatic brain injury. Arch Phys Med Rehabil 85:1050–1055, 2004

29 Alcohol and Drug Disorders

Norman S. Miller, M.D.

Jennifer Adams, B.S.

THE GREATEST RISK factors for traumatic brain injury (TBI) are alcohol/drug use and alcohol/drug disorder (A/DD). TBI is often an irreversible adverse consequence of the pharmacological effects and addictive use of alcohol and drugs. Of critical importance is that TBI is preventable. The prevention can include many aspects, but of primary importance is the treatment of A/DD before the onset of the TBI (Brismar et al. 1983; Brooks 1984; Field 1976; Sparadeo and Gill 1989).

The coexistence of TBI with A/DD requires concurrent treatment of both disorders. A/DD complicates the treatment of TBI and vice versa. Acceptance of both categories of disorders as independent and interactive enhances the total treatment of the patient (Alcohol and health, IV: treatment and rehabilitation 1981; Kreutzer 1996).

Clinicians working with individuals who have acute or chronic sequelae of TBI must be knowledgeable and skilled in the identification of A/DD whenever it exists in combination with TBI (Ksiazkiewicz 1998). If only one condition is the focus of the treatment, incomplete treatment and poor prognosis are likely to result for either condition. Because of the interplay between TBI and A/DD throughout the clinical course, treatment strategies must be developed that recognize the independence of and interaction between the two categories of disorders (Freund 1985). Research suggests that alcohol/drug dependence may play a mediating role in the outcomes of TBI (Bogner et al. 2001; Corrigan 1995). Proper treatment of both conditions may serve to lessen additive effects.

Treatment protocols can be implemented from the time of first contact during the acute intervention through chronic maintenance. Those who are actively involved in the treatment must be skilled in the intervention, referral, and, in some cases, the actual long-term management of both TBI and A/DD. Although a specialist may be employed for either category of disorder, he or she must know the ramifications of both disorders. For instance, the addiction specialist must know and work with the limitations of the alcohol- or drug-addicted patient with brain injury, and at the same time, the brain specialist must know the effect of both treated and untreated alcoholism and drug addiction on the patient with TBI. The two specialists, then, must work to coordinate the treatment of both disorders (Substance Abuse Task Force 1988).

Prevalence of the Problems

Between 29% and 52% of individuals admitted to a hospital with a TBI test positive for blood alcohol. Moreover, 58% of all surgical admissions and 72% of all hospital contacts, defined as visits to the hospital or emergency department, involve this same patient population. The reported prevalence of a history of alcohol dependence (addictive drinking) in patients with TBI ranges from 25% to 68%, which suggests that the majority of those involved in TBI at any time had a serious problem with alcohol use before the onset of the injury (Edna 1985; Elmer and Lim 1985). In an evaluation of substance use and dependence in TBI and spinal cord injury (SCI) patients, 81%–96% of individuals reported pretrauma drinking, whereas 42%–57% were heavy drinkers. This high degree of association strongly suggests that alcohol and TBI are causally related. Early identification of at-risk populations for TBI/SCI may be possible. If an A/DD is identified and treated in the early stages, TBI or SCI, or both, may be prevented (Kolakowsky-Hayner et al. 1999).

The role of drugs other than alcohol is not well documented because often specific testing and history taking for drugs are not part of either routine clinical practice or research studies. Many hospital records do not mention the implications of drug histories when clear evidence exists. The reasons for poor documentation are complex and include poor skills in assessing the importance of drugs and alcohol and ignorance that effective treatment for alcohol and drug disorders exists. Research protocols do not often include measurement of urine or blood for illicit or prescription medications. The common occurrence of multiple drug and alcohol use or addiction in high-risk populations for the development of TBI (namely, adolescents and young adults) makes routine assessment for alcohol and drug use mandatory in these populations when traumatic injury occurs. Conversely, it has been proposed that a major diagnostic error occurs in the presence of TBI veiled by the effects of alcohol. Many individuals are brought to the hospital by police after slight bodily injury. Physicians may miss the symptoms of a TBI or misattribute observed symptoms to the effects of alcohol in an intoxicated individual. It is essential that physicians look carefully for signs or symptoms of a TBI in an intoxicated individual.

The prevalence rate for alcoholism in the United States is approximately 15%. The long-term diagnosis of alcoholism can be made in 29% of men in the United States and 7% of women. The mean age at onset of alcoholism is 22 years in men and 25 in women, according to the Epidemiologic Catchment Area Study (Miller 1991b). The reported prevalence rate for drug addiction in the general population ranges from 9% to 20%. The majority of drug-addicted individuals are addicted to alcohol, and substantial numbers of alcoholic individuals are addicted to at least one other drug; namely, cannabis, cocaine, benzodiazepines, opiates, and/or hallucinogens, in decreasing order of frequency (Miller 1991b; Schuckit 1990). Despite these astonishing numbers, physicians often miss the diagnosis. In one evaluation of primary care physicians (Miller 2002), 94% were unable to identify a substance disorder as one of five diagnostic possibilities in case studies of patients with the early signs of an alcohol disorder. When case studies described early signs of a drug disorder in teenagers, 41% of pediatricians failed to provide substance disorder as one of five diagnostic possibilities. Also, nearly three-fourths of patients seeking treatment for a drug disorder did not receive guidance from their primary care physician. These results highlight the importance of physicians knowledgeable in addiction medicine to perform clinical examinations and assessments on drug use and history.

The prevalence rate for A/DD in psychiatric populations is 50%–75% and 25%–50% in medical populations. Treatment populations of addictive disorders show consistently high rates of multiple combinations of A/DD. The average age for men in treatment is 30–35 years, and the average age for women is 25–30 years. The proportion of men to women in typical treatment populations is 75% to 25% and 60% to 40% in membership surveys of Alcoholics Anonymous (AA) (Helzer and Pryzbeck 1988; Ries and Samson 1987).

Survey data provide evidence that alcohol and drugs are often involved with TBI. One hundred thousand people die annually in accidents in the United States. The leading cause of death for persons between the ages of 17 and 21 years is motor vehicle accidents. Fifty percent of all fatal accidents in the United States are motor vehicle accidents. Of these fatal motor vehicle accidents, 50% are associated with alcohol and drugs. Seventy percent of fatal injuries are from head trauma, and two-thirds of TBIs involve motor vehicle accidents. In fact, motor vehicle accidents appeared to be the most common cause of TBIs in a study of 322 patients at a rehabilitation center; however, violence-related injuries were found to occur most frequently in patients reporting substance dependence (Drubach et al. 1993). Similarly, 50% of all violent deaths from any cause are alcohol or drug related. However, the survival rate for people with severe TBI has increased to 60% since the 1980s. Most long-term survivors are young adult men (Sparadeo and Gill 1989; Sparadeo et al. 1990; Substance Abuse Task Force 1988).

The high degree of association of alcohol/drug use and addiction and TBI in young populations is clear. Despite what is known about the relationship between A/DD and TBI, there is much that is still unknown. Studies of prognosis and outcome after brain injury frequently exclude individuals who are addicted to drugs or alcohol, or both, before accidents, even though this practice produces significant and relevant distortions of data (Sparadeo and Gill 1989; Substance Abuse Task Force 1988).

Intervention in the Acute State

The first clinical caveat is that if alcohol or drug addiction, or both, is implicated in TBI, it is likely to have been a problem preceding and leading up to the injury. Precautions for the medical and psychiatric sequelae of acute and chronic drug and alcohol use should be undertaken. Frequent complications include drug–drug interactions, drug overdose, increased sensitivity to medication effects, and seizures either from drug intoxication or drug and alcohol withdrawal. Other possible complications include behavioral dyscontrol, hallucinations, delusions, anxiety, depression induced by intoxication and withdrawal from drugs and alcohol, and drug seeking because of the presence of an addictive disorder (Miller 1991b; Schuckit 1983) (Table 29–1).

TABLE 29–1. Psychiatric sequelae from drugs and alcohol

Drug–drug interactions

Drug overdose

Increased sensitivity to medication effects

Seizures either from drug intoxication or drug or alcohol withdrawal

Hallucinations

Delusions

Anxiety

Depression induced by intoxication and withdrawal from drugs

Alcohol and drug seeking from the presence of an addictive disorder

The second clinical caveat is that behaviors such as lethargy or agitation, confusion, disorientation, and respiratory depression after acute intoxication and overdose are similar to those following brain injury. Importantly, some intoxicated patients are discharged from the emergency department when in fact they have undiagnosed brain injuries. In a study of 167 patients (Gallagher and Browder 1968), alcohol obscured changes in consciousness, leading to misdiagnosis or delayed diagnosis of complications of brain trauma. In 21 patients, a subdural hematoma was diagnosed only at postmortem (Galbraith 1976), and others have reported similar results (Rumbaugh and Fang 1980).

Diagnosis of Alcohol and Drug Disorders

Once acute stabilization is achieved, the patient and family should be further evaluated for the presence and severity of an A/DD. Alcoholism and drug addiction are diagnosable according to established criteria in DSM-IV-TR (American Psychiatric Association 2000). Three of the seven criteria for the dependence syndrome reflect the behaviors of addiction; namely, 1) preoccupation with acquiring alcohol or drugs, 2) compulsive use of drugs despite adverse consequences, and 3) a pattern of relapse or inability to cut down on use despite adverse consequences. Two of the seven criteria reflect development of tolerance and dependence on alcohol and drugs. Any three of the nine criteria are required to make the diagnosis of alcohol or drug dependence, or both. Pervasive loss of control over use of alcohol and drugs sufficient to meet the criteria for the dependence syndrome in DSM-IV-TR

is often evident in the histories of patients with TBI. The manifest loss of control often is reflected by the circumstances surrounding and including the actual trauma that culminates in the brain injury (Table 29–2).

It has been well documented that the most effective clinical approach to both diagnosis and treatment of an alcohol or drug disorder involves the acknowledgment of substance dependence as a disease state rather than a moral or character problem. Twin and adoption studies provide adequate support for the powerful role of inheritance in alcohol or substance disorders. A parallel may be drawn between substance disorders and other inherited diseases such as hypertension, in which a person has little control over the development of the disorder but is solely responsible for treatment of the disorder. By using this approach in a clinical setting, patients often are able to overcome the common feelings of shame and blame associated with alcohol or drug dependence, accept responsibility for treatment, and adopt a commitment to long-term recovery. The use of medications for the treatment of withdrawal from alcohol or drugs and to assist patients with achieving abstinence may aid in the belief that alcohol or drug dependence is, in fact, a disease (Miller 2001).

Alcohol dependence and drug dependence are independent diagnoses. As independent disorders, each has a characteristic course and predictable consequences. The application of exclusionary criteria for A/DD is required before establishing other psychiatric disorders using DSM-IV-TR (Tamerin and Mendelson 1969).

There is little objective evidence that alcohol or drugs are used to "medicate" or ameliorate a mood state or an underlying or additional psychiatric disorder, including one caused by TBI (Miller and Goldsmith 2001). The preponderance of the studies show that alcohol and drugs cause psychiatric symptoms and worsen already existing symptoms from psychiatric disorders, especially those associated with TBI. Although alcoholic patients and those with drug addictions report drinking and using drugs because of anxiety and depression, objective and controlled studies fail to confirm the hypothesis that alcohol and drugs are used to improve mood and thinking. The conclusions from many studies are that continued alcohol and drug use results in the appearance and worsening of psychiatric symptoms in proportion to the amount and duration of alcohol and drug use (Mayfield and Allen 1967; Schuckit et al. 1990).

Family history is the best predictor for the onset of alcoholism and drug addiction in a given individual. A positive family history for alcohol and drug disorders can increase the index of suspicion for the presence of an A/DD in a TBI patient. Also family members may have A/DDs that require diagnosis, intervention, and treatment. Un-

---

TABLE 29–2.   **Criteria for substance dependence**

A maladaptive pattern of substance use, leading to clinically significant impairment or distress, as manifested by three (or more) of the following, occurring at any time in the same 12-month period:

(1) tolerance, as defined by either of the following:

    (a) a need for markedly increased amounts of the substance to achieve intoxication or desired effect

    (b) markedly diminished effect with continued use of the same amount of the substance

(2) withdrawal, as manifested by either of the following:

    (a) the characteristic withdrawal syndrome for the substance (refer to Criteria A and B of the criteria sets for withdrawal from the specific substances)

    (b) the same (or a closely related) substance is taken to relieve or avoid withdrawal symptoms

(3) the substance is often taken in larger amounts or over a longer period than was intended

(4) there is a persistent desire or unsuccessful efforts to cut down or control substance use

(5) a great deal of time is spent in activities necessary to obtain the substance (e.g., visiting multiple doctors or driving long distances), use the substance (e.g., chain-smoking), or recover from its effects

(6) important social, occupational, or recreational activities are given up or reduced because of substance use

(7) the substance use is continued despite knowledge of having a persistent or recurrent physical or psychological problem that is likely to have been caused or exacerbated by the substance (e.g., current cocaine use despite recognition of cocaine-induced depression, or continued drinking despite recognition that an ulcer was made worse by alcohol consumption)

Specify if:

With Physiological Dependence: evidence of tolerance or withdrawal (i.e., either Item 1 or 2 is present)

Without Physiological Dependence: no evidence of tolerance or withdrawal (i.e., neither Item 1 nor 2 is present)

Course specifiers:

Early Full Remission

Early Partial Remission

Sustained Full Remission

Sustained Partial Remission

On Agonist Therapy

In a Controlled Environment

Source.   Reprinted from American Psychiatric Association: *Diagnostic and Statistical Manual of Mental Disorders*, 4th Edition, Text Revision. Washington, DC, American Psychiatric Association, 2000. Used with permission.

---

treated family members with an addiction can have an adverse affect on the patient with A/DD and TBI that can interfere with the overall treatment (Cermak 1991; Miller et al. 1990).

Screening tests are available for alcohol disorders that can be modified for drugs by inserting drug for the word alcohol. The Brief Michigan Alcoholism Screening Test (a modified version of the Michigan Alcoholism Screening Test [Brief MAST]; Selzer et al. 1975; Figure 29–1) correlates with the clinical diagnosis of alcoholism. The CAGE questionnaire (Mayfield et al. 1974; Figure 29–2) is also a useful bedside screening test, which correlates well with a diagnosis of alcoholism (positive response to one question means probable alcohol dependence). The MAST and the CAGE can be self-administered and take

only a few minutes to complete. Both correlate highly with the DSM-III-R criteria (American Psychiatric Association 1987) for the substance use disorders, and they are commonly used and are well-established screening instruments. Fuller et al. (1994) recommend the CAGE or the Brief MAST be administered to any individual who has sustained a TBI.

In an effort to improve the diagnosis of alcohol and drug disorders within TBI populations, many studies have focused on tools that serve as valid A/DD identifiers in the traumatic, and often, disabled state of patients with brain injuries. Through the combination of blood alcohol levels (BALs), quantity and frequency of alcohol or drug consumption, or both, and the Short MAST, a comprehensive tool for recognizing substance disorders in TBI

Questions	Circle Correct Answer
1. Do you feel you are a normal drinker? (Normal means that you drink less than or as much as most other people.)	Yes (0) No (2)
2. Do friends or relatives think you are a normal drinker?	Yes (1) No (2)
3. Have you ever attended a meeting of Alcoholics Anonymous (AA)?	Yes (5) No (0)
4. Have you ever lost friends or girlfriends/boyfriends because of drinking?	Yes (2) No (0)
5. Have you ever gotten into trouble at work because of drinking?	Yes (2) No (0)
6. Have you ever neglected your obligations, your family, or your work for two or more days in a row because of drinking?	Yes (2) No (0)
7. Have you ever had delirium tremors (DTs) or severe shaking or heard voices or seen things that weren't there after heavy drinking?	Yes (2) No (0)
8. Have you ever gone to anyone for help about your drinking?	Yes (5) No (0)
9. Have you ever been in a hospital because of drinking?	Yes (5) No (0)
10. Have you ever been arrested for drunk driving or driving after drinking?	Yes (2) No (0)

FIGURE 29–1.   Brief Michigan Alcoholism Screening Test (MAST).

Note. If this is used as a self-administered written instrument, the scoring system should not be shown on the form. The scores on the Brief MAST correlate well with the full MAST. A score of 6 or above could identify an alcoholic patient.

Source. Reprinted from Selzer ML, Vinokur A, van Rooijen L: "A Self-Administered Short Michigan Alcoholism Screening Test (SMAST)." *Journal of Studies on Alcohol* 36:117–126, 1975. Copyright by Journal of Studies on Alcohol, Inc., Rutgers Center of Alcohol Studies, New Brunswick, NJ 08903. Used with permission.

patients can be shaped. The partnership of these assessment tools has been effective in a study by Cherner et al. (2001) who examined issues that obscured the measurement of the effects of alcohol in TBI populations. The Substance Abuse Subtle Screening Inventory (SASSI) and the Addiction Severity Index have also been recommended for the detection of an alcohol or drug disorder, or both, in individuals who have TBIs (Fuller et al. 1994). However, in an assessment of the utility of the SASSI-3 in individuals with TBIs, scores were most accurate when coupled with BALs. The SASSI-3 was found to be extremely sensitive to A/DD in TBI patients, whereas the BAL was more specific (Arenth et al. 2001).

1. Have you felt you ought to **C**ut down on your drinking?

2. Have people **A**nnoyed you by criticizing your drinking?

3. Have you ever felt bad or **G**uilty about your drinking?

4. Have you ever had a drink first thing in the morning to steady your nerves and get rid of a hangover? (**E**ye opener)

Scoring: Two or more positive responses suggest sufficient evidence of alcohol abuse at some point during lifetime to warrant further investigation

FIGURE 29–2.   CAGE questionnaire.

Source. Reprinted from Mayfield D, McLeod G, Hall P: "The CAGE Questionnaire: Validation of a New Alcoholism Screening Instrument." *American Journal of Psychiatry* 131:1121–1123. Used with permission.

Identification of the neural basis of pathological craving of alcohol and drugs may also serve as a vital tool for diagnosing patients with a substance dependency (Dackis and Miller 2003). Neuroimaging studies have identified limbic system pathways that are responsible for both normal and pathological cravings in human and animal studies. Changes in limbic system pathways have been identified in studies in which human and animal subjects have had chronic exposure to alcohol or drugs. It has been proposed that a change in homeostasis occurs. A new set point, or alleostasis, may be responsible for intense cravings that occur long after "liking" a drug. Structural neuroimaging studies have also revealed alcohol-induced brain atrophy, occurring in both limbic and frontal lobe structures. After a period of abstinence, the degree of atrophy in these regions tends to diminish, especially when abstinence occurs at a younger age. Further research on these issues may someday equip clinicians with an essential tool for the diagnosis and treatment of substance dependency (Netrakom and Krasuski 1999).

Treatment of Alcohol and Drug Withdrawal

The first step in treatment of A/DD is for the patient to discontinue the active use of alcohol and drugs. During this initial abstinence, the influence of alcohol and drugs on mood, cognition, and behavior, as well as the degree of drug-seeking behavior, can be assessed. A differential diagnosis for coexisting psychiatric disorders can also be assessed longitudinally apart from the effects of alcohol and drug intoxication and dependence (Blankfield 1986; Miller and Mahler 1991).

The principles used in the treatment of withdrawal from alcohol and drugs in addicted patients with TBI are similar to those used in patients without TBI, with some important exceptions. The identification of alcohol and drug intoxication and withdrawal follows the general principles of pharmacological dependence. The use of blood and urine toxicology is important to identify presence and levels of alcohol and drugs for assessment of intoxication and anticipation of withdrawal. The use of vital signs, particularly blood pressure, pulse, and temperature, is critical in determining the presence and severity of the withdrawal state (Miller 1991b).

The medications used in the treatment of withdrawal in TBI can be similar to those used in patients who have only drug or alcohol addiction, or both. However, the doses should be reduced to allow for the increased sensitivity of brain-injured patients to medication and drug effects. Individuals with TBI appear to have reduced tolerance to a wide variety of medications, particularly the sedatives used in treatment of withdrawal and agitation. The optimal level of medications for withdrawal can be assessed in an individual on an as-needed basis according to the clinical status of the patient. The patient's behavioral and vital signs can be assigned parameters for medication treatments (Miller 1991b).

For instance, for detoxification from alcohol, a dose of benzodiazepines can be given for systolic blood pressure greater than 150 mm Hg or diastolic pressure greater than 100 mm Hg, or both. For detoxification from benzodiazepines, a standing schedule can be designed for 2–3 weeks on the basis of estimates of doses taken during chronic use preceding withdrawal. For alcohol withdrawal, benzodiazepines should have a shorter-acting half-life (e.g., lorazepam) to avoid persistent sedation for patients with brain injury. However, for benzodiazepine withdrawal, the intermediate-acting preparations (e.g., diazepam) are preferred to avoid sharp peaks and troughs from short-acting preparations and persistent sedation from long-acting preparations that occur during the taper (Alexander and Perry 1991; Miller and Gold 1989; Miller et al. 1988). Previous research suggests that an important relationship may exist between prescription medications and outcomes for TBI patients with an A/DD. In a study by Chatham-Showalter et al. (1996), brain-injured patients with positive BALs tended to be on higher dosages of narcotic medications and benzodiazepines. These individuals were also given medications for longer periods when compared with individuals who did not have posi-

tive BALs. Further investigation on the effects of prescription medication on TBI patients with an A/DD is necessary because of the poorer prognosis often associated with individuals in this group.

In general, benzodiazepines are used to treat alcohol withdrawal (Table 29–3), and benzodiazepines or phenobarbital are used to treat sedative/hypnotic withdrawal (see Table 29–3), including withdrawal from benzodiazepines (Table 29–4). For cocaine, other stimulants, and cannabis withdrawal, medications usually are not required. For opiates, either clonidine or methadone can be used in 2-week or 4-week tapering schedules. As stated, other schemes for detoxification can be used, but only in lower doses for the drug-sensitive individual with TBI.

TABLE 29–3. Drug doses equivalent to 600 mg of secobarbital and 60 mg of diazepam

Drug (by class)	Dose (mg)
Benzodiazepines	
Alprazolam	6
Chlordiazepoxide	150
Clonazepam	24
Clorazepate	90
Flurazepam	90
Halazepam	240
Lorazepam	12
Oxazepam	60
Prazepam	60
Temazepam	90
Barbiturates	
Amobarbital	600
Butabarbital	600
Butalbital	600
Pentobarbital	600
Secobarbital	600
Phenobarbital	180
Glycerol	
Meprobamate	2,400
Piperidinedione	
Glutethimide	1,500
Quinazolines	
Methaqualone	1,800

Note. For patients receiving multiple drugs, each drug should be converted to its diazepam or secobarbital equivalent.

TABLE 29–4.   Signs and symptoms of benzodiazepine withdrawal

Symptoms of hyperexcitability

Agitation

Anxiety

Hyperactivity

Insomnia

Neuropsychiatric symptoms

Ataxia

Depersonalization

Depression

Fasciculation

Formication

Headache

Hyperventilation

Malaise

Myalgia

Paranoid delusions

Paresthesia

Pruritus

Tinnitus

Tremor

Visual hallucinations

Gastrointestinal symptoms

Abdominal pain

Constipation

Diarrhea

Nausea

Vomiting

Cardiovascular symptoms

Chest pain

Flushing

Palpitations

Genitourinary symptoms

Incontinence

Loss of libido

Urinary urgency, frequency

Assessment for other drug usage by a patient is indicated through history and clinical examination (Miller 1991b).

Pharmacological interventions must take into consideration possible drug–drug interactions with known and unknown drugs, both illicit and prescription medications. Persistent history taking from the patient and family and drug screens of urine and blood are essential in identifying the influence of alcohol and drugs in the precipitation of the brain injury and possible responses of the patient to pharmacological and behavioral managements. For instance, benzodiazepines may interact with alcohol or other sedatives, or both, acutely to further depress consciousness. On the other hand, acute withdrawal from alcohol that is not adequately treated with benzodiazepines may progress to agitation, delirium, and even death. The combination of clinical assessment and laboratory diagnosis is needed to manage these difficult clinical issues (Miller and Gold 1991).

Complications

Psychiatric Symptoms

The effects of alcohol and drugs on mood and behavior are numerous. In general, alcohol and other depressant drugs can cause depression, suicidal and homicidal thinking during intoxication, anxiety, hyperactivity, hallucinations, and/or delusions during withdrawal. Cocaine and other stimulant drugs can cause anxiety, hallucinations, and delusions during intoxication, and/or depression and suicidal thinking during withdrawal. As a consequence of addictive disorders, individuals can be withdrawn, asocial, antisocial (including violent behavior), hysterical, passive-aggressive, dependent, and/or narcissistic. Often, these personality features diminish after abstinence from alcohol and drugs and specific treatment of the addictive disorder. The aim of treatment of the addictive disorder is to alter attitudes and behaviors that are detrimental to personality (Blankfield 1986; Mayfield 1979; Miller and Mahler 1991; Schuckit 1983).

Length of Stay

The length of stay in the hospital for the individual with TBI is affected by the presence of alcohol or drugs. The TBI patients who are users of alcohol or drugs have a longer period of hospitalization. Sparadeo and Gill (1989) reported that patients with a negative BAL had an average stay of less than 3 weeks, with only 9.5% staying longer than 3 weeks and a maximum length of stay of 45 days. For patients with a positive BAL, twice as many patients (19.4%) stayed beyond 3 weeks, and the maximum length of stay was 102 days.

Agitation

The incidence of agitation is not significantly greater for patients with a positive BAL; however, the duration of agitation is significantly longer (Brismar 1983). Agitation is a serious complication for recovery from TBI in these patients because it interferes with nursing care, physical therapy, occupational therapy, speech therapy, and medical and surgical intervention. Importantly, families and staff are generally disturbed by agitated patients as well (Sparadeo and Gill 1989; Substance Abuse Task Force 1988).

Cognitive Status

Of considerable interest is that individuals who were intoxicated before brain injury have lower global cognitive scores at the time of discharge than do those who were not intoxicated. One could speculate that the trauma is more significant in those who are compromised by alcohol and drugs through a number of mechanisms. There is significantly and persistently reduced intellectual function in alcohol- and drug-addicted patients who use alcohol and drugs on a regular basis over time (Tarter and Edwards 1985).

Intellectual deficits in A/DD populations appear to be in large measure reversible in those patients without known brain trauma, and IQs improve with abstinence over time. The improvement in memory, abstraction, calculations, and other cognitive abilities occurs rapidly in the first 3–6 months of abstinence from alcohol and more gradually thereafter. Studies have shown improvement in intellect continuing at 2 years of abstinence, and clinical experience suggests that improvement continues beyond this initial period (Chelune and Parker 1981; Parsons and Leber 1981). There is usually some loss of intellectual functioning in TBI. Cognitive deficits are commonly seen in attention and concentration, short-term memory, and speed of processing information. There are often significant impediments to long-term recovery from TBI (Sparadeo and Gill 1989).

The effects of TBI and alcohol and drug abuse may be additive. Baguley et al. (1997) compared heavy social drinkers, individuals with a TBI who did not drink heavily, and a group with a history of both a TBI and heavy social drinking. Significantly more cognitive impairments were observed in those with a TBI who were also heavy social drinkers relative to the other two groups. Kelly et al. (1997) found that full-scale IQ and verbal IQ scores were significantly lower in participants who screened positive for alcohol consumption or dependence, or both, at the time of TBI compared with those injured who were negative for alcohol and to healthy control subjects.

Barnfield and Leathem (1998) studied New Zealand prison inmates and found high rates of substance disorders, TBIs, and recurrent TBIs. Furthermore, greater cognitive impairment was found in those individuals ex-periencing both an A/DD and a TBI. Similarly, individuals with a TBI who tested positive for cocaine on hospital admission showed significantly lower scores on the Rey Auditory Verbal Learning Test than those with TBI testing negative for cocaine (Barnfield and Leathem 1998).

Neuropathological Effects

The partnership of alcohol and TBI has been shown in numerous studies to cause measurable neuropathology in the brains of both human and animal models. In quantitative magnetic resonance imaging comparisons, patients experiencing a combination of both TBI and substance dependence exhibited greater atrophic changes when compared with individuals with either a TBI or an A/DD and healthy control subjects. TBI and alcohol/drug dependent groups also had significantly lower scores on the Glasgow Coma Scale when compared with TBI patients without A/DDs and healthy control subjects (Bigler et al. 1996). In animal studies, ethanol exposure at the time of brain injury has been shown to cause severe respiratory depression. This increase in postinjury apnea may lead to further injury or even death (Zink and Feustel 1995; Zink et al. 1993). The presence of ethanol intoxication at the time of brain trauma may potentiate responses both physiologically and metabolically that could play a causal role in secondary brain injury (Zink et al. 1998).

Hemodynamic depression, blood-brain barrier disruption, and derangements in homeostasis are some additional effects of intoxication at the time of brain injury. Upregulation of N-methyl-D-aspartate and downregulation of γ-aminobutyric acid receptor function may also arise because of chronic exposure to alcohol. Many factors, however, dictate the outcome of ethanol and brain trauma; proximity of intoxication to the time of injury, degree of use, and the affects of other injuries all may play a mediating role (Kelly 1995).

Economic Affect

A positive BAL is associated with higher costs for medical care. The longer length of stay, increased agitation, higher intensity and level of care, complications of treatment for TBI, and increased morbidity from alcohol and drug effects lead to greater expense in caring for alcohol- and drug-addicted or -using patients. Early identification and treatment of alcohol and drug problems can reduce expenses and allow greater numbers of patients to be treated (Miller and Ries 1991; Sparadeo and Gill 1989; Substance Abuse Task Force 1988).

TABLE 29–5. Resources for treatment of addictive disorders

Alcoholics Anonymous (AA) and Narcotics Anonymous (NA) and similar groups

Support groups patterned after AA and NA

Individual, group, and family alcohol and drug counseling

Outpatient and inpatient alcohol and drug treatment programs

Environmental control and behavior modification

Psychopharmacology

Intermediate and Long-Term Treatment

Principles

Generally, the most widely used treatment for A/DD uses the 12-step approach, which considers addiction as an independent disorder. This approach includes principles of recovery derived from AA, cognitive-behavioral therapies, group and individual modalities, and long-term management of the addictive disorders in AA or Narcotics Anonymous (NA; Table 29–5). The results of treatment outcome studies indicate that the 12-step method is an effective form of treatment for A/DD (Harrison et al. 1991). Overall abstinence rates for 1 year were 68% in 1,663 outpatients and 60% in 8,087 inpatients in a study derived from 35 different treatment sites (Hoffman and Miller 1992). The abstinence rates increased to 82% and 75%, respectively, with regular attendance at AA. Effective treatment strategies for chemical dependency in TBI populations should focus on behavioral, cognitive, and gestalt issues. The supportive network of AA and NA offer therapy on all of these levels (Kramer and Hoisington 1992).

In a study of 9,750 patients, motor vehicle accidents and moving traffic violations were significantly reduced in patients who received treatment for alcohol or drug addiction, or both, when rates before and after the treatment of the addictive disorder were compared. Of further interest is that the use of medical and psychiatric services dropped significantly and job performance improved significantly in those who received addiction treatment.

Experience in applying these treatment techniques to individuals with TBI is limited. Novel programs tailored to the needs of these individuals are being used, although clinical success awaits documentation in outcome studies. Attempts are under way to integrate standard care for TBI patients with standard treatment for addictive disorders (McLaughlin and Shaffer 1985; Miller and Mahler 1991; Substance Abuse Task Force 1988; Tobis et al. 1982) (Table 29–6).

TABLE 29–6. Techniques for therapy of traumatic brain injury (TBI) patients

People with TBI may digress or change course during conversation.

1. Redirect them using appropriate cues and reinforcers.
2. Teach prevention skills to the person with TBI that can be used in more than one life setting to maximize generalizability.
3. Focus on specific prevention goal.
4. Be redundant.
5. Never assume understanding or memory from previous session.
6. Always repeat the purpose, duration, and guidelines for each meeting.
7. Summarize previous progress and then restate where the previous meeting left off (Sparadeo et al. 1990).

Clinical experience suggests that individuals with TBI have specific persistent problems that may interfere with participating with other patients without TBI in mainstream programs (Jong et al. 1999). The major difference is that the pharmacological effects from alcohol and drugs are reversible, whereas those because of brain injury may not be totally reversible (Table 29–7).

It is imperative to achieve and maintain progress in addiction treatment to gauge any success in the treatment of the neuropsychiatric deficits from trauma. Basic principles used in working clinically with brain-injured individuals can be used in their addiction treatment as well. Individuals with TBI require concrete and structured programs tailored to their mental capacities. The addiction therapist must be knowledgeable in the assets and liabilities of individuals with brain injury, and skilled in applying traditional addiction treatment specifically to their

TABLE 29–7. Comparative effects of brain injury and drugs/alcohol

Possible effects of brain injury	Pharmacological effects of drugs/alcohol
Poor memory	Poor memory
Impaired judgment	Impaired judgment
Fine and gross motor impairments	Fine and gross motor impairments
Poor concentration	Poor concentration
Decreased impulse control	Decreased impulse control
Impaired language skills	Impaired language skills

needs. On the other hand, physicians, including psychiatrists and other therapists, must be knowledgeable in the priority of alcohol and drugs in the life of addicted patients and skilled in referring and collaborating with the addiction treatment team to provide a consistent, cogent, and effective treatment plan.

Research suggests that a window of opportunity for assisting those with a substance disorder to stop the abuse immediately after a TBI is usually present. Readiness to change in this time frame could prove useful if substance dependence is identified at the time of injury and treated appropriately (Bombardier et al. 1997). Another form of assistance for young adult men, the group displaying the highest risk for the duality of TBI and substance use disorders, has been proposed by Wehman et al. (2000). Because of high rates of unemployment in young adult men with both a history of TBI and A/DD, a supported employment approach has been suggested to assist these individuals on reentry into the workforce. This program may help alleviate frustrations in TBI/A/DD populations and assist in the transition toward a more normal lifestyle.

Treatment Strategy and Process

The following sections illustrate a program that provides a therapeutic milieu for the brain-injured patient to learn about and discuss his or her alcohol and drug problems.

Abstinence

The overall aim is for the individual with TBI to achieve and maintain abstinence from alcohol and drugs. The common denominator for recovery for alcohol- or drug-addicted individuals is loss of control over alcohol and drugs. The focus of treatment should be on abstaining from alcohol and drugs of addiction and what changes the patient must make to accomplish this goal. The process begins by admitting and optimally accepting that the use of alcohol and drugs results in adverse consequences to the individual. The success in maintaining abstinence by the addicted individual will be limited without the fundamental recognition by the therapist of the psychopathological processes in addictive use of drugs. The therapist must collaborate in the goals with the patient and be prepared to clarify for the patient the importance of abstinence from alcohol and drugs to recover from both addiction and TBI. At times, supportive confrontation may be necessary to dispel the denial inherent in the addictive process (Miller 1991a; Roman 1982; Vaillant 1983).

Confrontation of Denial

Denial is a major feature of the psychopathology of addictive disorders. Denial is both conscious and unconscious and appears to originate from multiple sources. The denial system stems in part from the pharmacological (organic) effects of alcohol and drugs and in many ways is indistinguishable from a dementia syndrome from other causes. The pharmacological effects of alcohol and drugs include impairment in judgment, insight, planning, and motivation, functions that are subserved by the frontal lobe. The result is a poorly motivated, addicted individual with little insight and judgment with regard to therapeutic intervention. The temporal lobes are also affected by alcohol and drugs such that short-term memory and the acquisition of memory for new events is impaired, resulting in faulty recall of associations between alcohol and drug use and the adverse consequences. Pharmacological disruption of the temporal lobe also leads to distortions in thinking and emotions that further augment the denial (Blanchard 1984).

The denial can be effectively confronted using the evidence of the adverse consequences from addictive use of alcohol and drugs. The associations can be made for the patient by the therapist in the concrete manner that is already used in the approach to the individual with TBI. The therapist is advised to remain in the "here and now" and concentrate on what must be done for the patient to abstain from alcohol and drugs. It is counterproductive to dwell on antecedent causes that are ultimately not directly related to the addictive use of alcohol and drugs. The addiction to alcohol and drugs is an independent and autonomous condition that is not generated by other causes. This is a crucial concept that must be incorporated into successful addiction treatment. Otherwise, distraction away from the central problem of addiction to other problems that are unrelated or secondary to the addiction will prevent the addicted patient from focusing on the addictive use of alcohol and drugs (Miller and Mahler 1991; Stead and Viders 1979).

The timing and method of confrontation about deficits, including alcohol and other drug problems, should be carefully coordinated with the interdisciplinary TBI treatment team. Educational points should be presented in the most effective cognitive and sensory mode. This information is best obtained from a TBI team member knowledgeable in cognitive deficits (Kreutzer et al. 1990).

Group Therapy

In group therapy, the primary treatment intervention is performed in a group setting where confrontation of denial and induction of acceptance of the individual's addiction are best accomplished. The group consists of peers who also have addiction(s) and brain injury and is led by professionals who are skilled in addiction therapy. The focus of the group is on the loss of control of alcohol and drug use and the attendant adverse consequences.

The group members share their experience, strength, and hope with each other in a supportively confrontational atmosphere (Langley 1991; Miller and Mahler 1991).

The group should have a prescribed structure and format that are facilitated by the therapist and actively used by the patients. Group members generally speak one at a time, with limited cross talk when patients "advise" other patients. Individuals are encouraged to speak from their own experiences and show how these may benefit others. The identification of one patient with another is central to the therapeutic process. The identification between individuals with both addiction and TBI is conducive to dissipating the destructive denial and to initiating constructive therapeutic changes. The shame, guilt, and hopelessness associated with addiction and TBI can be replaced through the mutual care and consideration of one individual toward another. There are no good studies illustrating the interactions between group members that produce the dramatic cohesion that can occur within the groups. Thus far, it has been impossible to explain how individuals with severe addiction and mental problems work together to produce this therapeutic milieu.

The clinical experience in this type of group process has been predominantly in addiction treatment. However, preliminary experience suggests that group therapy can be adapted to those who also have TBI. Special techniques that are commonly used in people with brain injury can be applied in addiction groups. The psychological approach to the person with brain injury shares commonalities with that used for the addiction patient. Techniques such as keeping it simple, focused, and concrete are useful in both populations. Being directive and supportive are also useful in treatment of individuals with addiction and TBI (Sparadeo et al. 1990).

Cost-effective treatment options for individuals with TBI and a substance use disorder have been proposed in a paper by Delmonico et al. (1998). The authors suggest group psychotherapy to help manage the frustration, poor impulse control, depression, anxiety, and many other common symptoms associated with TBI and A/DD. The average financial status of individuals with TBI and an A/DD requires a form of therapy that is affordable and long term. This psychotherapeutic group approach addresses preexisting coping skill deficits and psychological conditions while requiring minimal subsidy.

Community-based intervention for substance dependence in persons with TBI has been recommended in a paper by Corrigan et al. (1995). By combining a staff of individuals experienced in both TBI treatment and substance disorder therapy, a cost-effective program can be implemented. Community teams should treat patients on the basis of a theoretical model of changing addictive behaviors through community integration.

Treatment strategies that are both affordable and successful at bringing about recovery for substance dependents are imperative. Survival rates of persons with a substance dependency can be greatly improved through obtaining abstinence or complete recovery. Persons who do not achieve continual abstinence are at a much higher risk of mortality. Whether treatment is by means of group therapy, psychotherapy, community intervention, or some other form, all programs should focus on abstinence, which has been proven essential to the long-term health of those with a substance use disorder (Miller 1999).

Treatment Setting

The addiction-focused groups can be adjunctive in milieus that treat people with TBI. The addiction groups can be combined with the other therapies as an integral part of the overall therapy of those with TBI. Because more than 50% of individuals with TBI are likely to also have alcohol and drug addiction, the addiction groups can be incorporated as an essential therapeutic component for many patients in a given setting. Although it is not necessary for all members of the treatment staff to be skilled in addiction treatment, it is desirable that they have minimum knowledge regarding the nature of the illness and its effect on recovery from TBI. For instance, physicians and nurses must be able to identify drug seeking and differentiate it from other medical and psychiatric problems. In this way, addiction can be confronted and treated, and iatrogenic participation in addictive use of drugs can be minimized in the clinical care of these patients (Minkoff 1989).

All interventions should be directive in nature, short term, goal directed, and behaviorally anchored. The effects of severe brain injuries are typically so devastating to the family system that many family members "leave the field" when they come to appreciate what has occurred. Social isolation is common for people with TBI. The family system must be assessed and reassessed because it will fluctuate markedly in the first 4 years after TBI. The clinician should accentuate positive gains, using frequent social praise (Sparadeo et al. 1990).

Duration of Treatment

The duration of the addiction groups can be extended over time in a graduated fashion. The first month may have three 1-hour groups per week, on a Monday-Wednesday-Friday schedule. The remaining months may have one group per week in the setting, particularly if there is a prolonged stay. Also, it is important that the individuals attend meetings of AA or NA, either in the treatment setting or in the community. The service structure of AA offers assistance with holding meetings in institutions through the Cooperation with Professionals Committee. Also, some AA and NA meetings in the community are oriented toward having individuals attend on a regular basis (Chappel 1993; Appendices 1–3).

Generally, it is recommended that a patient with alcoholism and drug addiction undergo continuous treatment indefinitely. Both of these are chronic illnesses that can be characterized by a relapsing course in the untreated state. The relapse rate is highest in the first 3–6 months after cessation of alcohol and drug use, with up to 80% of individuals returning to alcohol and drug addiction in the untreated state. With treatment intervention, the abstinence rate can be increased to 70%–80% and higher with attendance at AA or NA meetings (Hoffman and Miller 1992). Abstinence rates are unknown for addicted individuals with TBI in long-term recovery.

The Hoffman and Miller (1992) treatment outcome study, as well as others in noninjured addicted individuals, further demonstrate improved cognition, emotional status, and attitudes toward self and others. The interpersonal relationships and responsibility toward self and others are improved in those with alcohol and drug addiction who continue in a sustained recovery program that includes attendance at aftercare for addiction treatment and AA. Personal responsibility is the cornerstone in recovery from addictive diseases (Alcoholics Anonymous 1976).

In a study by Miller et al. (1999), continuation in a sustained recovery program was a better predictor of posttreatment outcomes than lifetime depression or other pretreatment, clinical, or demographic variables. In fact, patients with a history of depression were more likely to be active in outpatient treatment and peer support groups when compared with substance dependents without a history of depression. One-year abstinence rates overall were 61% for patients taking part in outpatient treatment, 62% for patients without prior history of depression, and 60% for patients with a history of depression, thus indicating that abstinence rates were not significantly affected by depressive histories. Therapeutic interventions should focus on these findings when assessing plans for recovery.

Use of Medications in the Recovered Alcoholic or Addicted Patient With TBI

Studies do not find that standard psychiatric pharmacological and nonpharmacological treatments for depression and anxiety occurring in the setting of addiction are efficacious in reducing either the depression or the anxiety associated with addiction (Miller 2003). DSM-IV-TR (American Psychiatric Association 2000) requires exclusion of substance-induced disorders even before diagnosis or treatment. Anti-

depressants, antianxiety agents, and psychotherapy do not relieve the depression and anxiety induced by alcoholism or drug addiction or influence the overall course of the addictive use of alcohol and drugs. The same findings hold for other psychiatric disorders. Hallucinations and delusions induced by the addictive use of alcohol and drugs do not respond to conventional psychiatric pharmacological or nonpharmacological therapies, especially if the use of alcohol and drugs continues (Miller 1991b; Schuckit 1990).

Studies do confirm that specific treatment of the addictive disorders alleviates the addictive use of alcohol and drugs and the consequent psychiatric comorbidity. A period of observation of days to weeks may be necessary to examine important causal links in the genesis of psychiatric symptoms from addictive disorders and to establish independent psychiatric disorders (Miller 1991b; Tamerin and Mendelson 1969).

Most psychotropic medications can be used to treat independent psychiatric disorders in alcohol- and drug-addicted individuals with a TBI. Beyond the detoxifying period in the abstinent state, there is little evidence that the psychiatric disorders in those individuals with addictive disorders respond differently to most psychotropic medications. The caveat is that because of the addiction potential, alcoholic or addicted individuals are more likely to overuse and lose control of virtually any medications than individuals who are not addicted, particularly those medications with already established addictive potential (Miller 1991b).

The dose of psychotropic medications should be reduced because of the heightened sensitivity to both stimulants and depressants commonly seen in individuals with brain injury. The selection of medications can be similar to those for other psychiatric disorders, including diffuse brain damage from other causes. Miller (1991b) suggested the guiding principle of aiming for the lowest doses to reduce untoward effects while maximizing therapeutic efficacy.

The physician views medications as powerful and inherently good despite the potential for toxicity. Some psychiatrists do not view themselves as physicians or minimize their role as doctors if they do not prescribe medications for a clinical disorder. Moreover, clinicians skilled in the treatment of addictive disorders advocate that the patient who is addicted to alcohol or drugs needs a clear sensorium and access to feelings to make fundamental changes in attitudes and behaviors for continued abstinence. Medications may impair cognition and blunt feelings, albeit sometimes in a subtle way. A parallel illustration is the crucial point stressed by psychotherapists who advise judicious use of mood-altering chemicals that might interfere with the process of psychotherapy. This is a clinical caveat that pertains to the person with TBI as well (Miller 1991b).

The person with alcohol or drug addiction and TBI must take an active initiative in changing attitudes and feelings, and must abandon the long-held belief that alcohol or drugs, or both, can "fix" or "treat" life problems and uncomfortable psychological states during recovery. Clinically acknowledged, anxiety and depression can be motivating feelings to change without which the patient has little awareness of the need to change. A commonly used expression to explain this practice among recovering individuals is "no pain, no gain." The aim of pharmacotherapy to suppress symptoms such as anxiety and depression in the recovering addicted patient must take into consideration that these symptoms may be vital to the recovery and survival of the patient with alcohol or drug addiction. Enormous misunderstanding has arisen between physicians and patients with addiction and TBI because of a divergence in purpose and perspective toward medications and the lack of knowledge and skill in both (Miller 1991b).

The current standard of care for addictive disorders is nonpharmacological beyond the detoxification period. Several studies have shown that treatment of the addictive disorder with abstinence alone results in improvement in the psychiatric syndromes associated with alcohol and drug use or addiction. Severe depressive and anxiety syndromes induced by alcohol resolve within days to weeks after the onset of abstinence. Manic syndromes induced by cocaine resolve within hours to days, and schizophrenic syndromes with hallucinations and delusions resolve within days to weeks with abstinence as well (Mayfield and Allen 1967; Schuckit 1990).

Further studies are needed to confirm the clinical experience that psychiatric symptoms, including anxiety, depression, and personality disorders, respond to the specific treatment of addiction. The cognitive-behavioral techniques used in the 12-step–based treatment approach have been shown to be effective in the management of anxiety and depression associated with addiction (Miller 1991c).

Long-Term Recovery in Alcoholics Anonymous

Available data demonstrate abstinence rates from alcohol and other drugs, including cocaine, of 60%–80% after 2 years in both alcohol- and drug-addicted individuals who are in treatment programs on the basis of a 12-step approach with referrals to AA. Surveys also show recovery rates with continuous abstinence of 44% at 1 year, 83% between 1 and 5 years, and 90% at longer than 5 years with membership and attendance at meetings in AA (44% of alcoholic individuals in AA are also addicted to drugs; see Appendices 1 and 2). A recent controlled study revealed that the best treatment outcome is obtained when professional treatment and AA are combined (Keso and Salaspuro 1990). Studies are not yet available that examine the efficacy of psychiatric treatments in enhancing treatment outcome in addicted patients with psychiatric comorbidity, including TBI (Chappel 1993; Group for the Advancement of Psychiatry 1991; Schulz 1991; see Appendices 1–3).

Summary

Alcohol and drug use disorders are a major risk factor for TBI. The coexistence of TBI with A/DD requires concurrent treatment of both disorders. If only one condition is the focus of the treatment, incomplete treatment and poor prognosis are the likely outcomes for both conditions. A/DD complicates the treatment of TBI and vice versa. Clinicians working with individuals who have acute or chronic sequelae of TBI must be knowledgeable and skilled in the identification of A/DD whenever it exists in combination with TBI. Because of the interplay between TBI and A/DD throughout the clinical course, treatment strategies must be developed that recognize the independence of and interaction between the two categories of disorders. Such strategies must include early identification, family intervention, and the use of group, family, and individual therapies in combination with judicious psychopharmacological approaches.

References

Alcohol and health, IV: treatment and rehabilitation. Alcohol Health Res World 5:48–58, 1981

Alcoholics Anonymous: Alcoholics Anonymous, 3rd Edition. New York, AA World Services, 1976

Alexander B, Perry P: Detoxification from benzodiazepines: schedules and strategies. J Subst Abuse Treat 8:9–17, 1991

American Psychiatric Association: Diagnostic and Statistical Manual of Mental Disorders, 3rd Edition, Revised. Washington, DC, American Psychiatric Association, 1987

American Psychiatric Association: Diagnostic and Statistical Manual of Mental Disorders, 4th Edition, Text Revision. Washington, DC, American Psychiatric Association, 2000

Arenth PM, Bogner JA, Corrigan JD, et al: The utility of the Substance Abuse Subtle Screening Inventory-3 for use with individuals with brain injury. Brain Inj 15:499–510, 2001

Baguley IJ, Felmingham KL, Lahz S, et al: Alcohol abuse and traumatic brain injury: effect on event-related potentials. Arch Phys Med Rehabil 78:1248–1253, 1997

Barnfield TV, Leathem JM: Neuropsychological outcomes of traumatic brain injury and substance abuse in a New Zealand prison population. Brain Inj 12:951–962, 1998

Bigler Ed, Blatter DD, Johnson SC, et al: Traumatic brain injury, alcohol and quantitative neuroimaging: preliminary findings. Brain Inj 10:197–206, 1996

Blanchard MK: Counseling Head Injured Patients. Albany, NY, New York State Head Injury Association, 1984

Blankfield A: Psychiatric symptoms in alcohol dependence: diagnostic and treatment implications. J Subst Abuse Treat 3:275–278, 1986

Bogner JA, Corrigan JD, Mysiw WJ, et al: A comparison of substance abuse and violence in the prediction of long-term rehabilitation outcomes after traumatic brain injury. Arch Phys Med Rehabil 82:571–577, 2001

Bombardier CH, Ehde D, Kilmer J: Readiness to change alcohol drinking habits after traumatic brain injury. Arch Phys Med Rehabil 78:592–596, 1997

Brismar D, Engstrom A, Rydberg U: Head injury and intoxication: a diagnostic and therapeutic dilemma. Acta Chir Scand 149:11–14, 1983

Brooks N: Closed Head Injury. Oxford, England, Oxford University Press, 1984

Cermak TL: Co-addiction as a disease. Psychiatr Ann 21:266–272, 1991

Chappel J: Long term recovery in AA. Psychiatr Clin North Am 16:177–188, 1993

Chatham-Showalter PE, Dubov WE, Barr WE, et al: Alcohol level at head injury and subsequent psychotropic treatment during trauma critical care. Psychosomatics 37:285–288, 1996

Chelune JC, Parker JB: Neuropsychological deficits associated with chronic alcohol abuse. Clin Psychol Rev 1:181–195, 1981

Cherner M, Temkin NR, Machamer JE, et al: Utility of composite measure to detect problematic alcohol use in persons with traumatic brain injury. Arch Phys Med Rehabil 82:780–786, 2001

Corrigan JD: Substance abuse as a mediating factor in outcome from traumatic brain injury. Arch Phys Med Rehabil 76:302–309, 1995

Corrigan JD, Lamb-Hart GL, Rust E: A programme of intervention for substance abuse following traumatic brain injury. Brain Inj 9:221–236, 1995

Dackis C, Miller NS: Biology and behavior of cocaine dependence. Psychiatr Ann 33:584–592, 2003

Delmonico RL, Haneley-Peterson P, Englander J: Group psychotherapy for persons with traumatic brain injury: management of frustration with substance abuse. J Head Trauma Rehabil 13:10–22, 1998

Drubach DA, Kelly MP, Winslow MM, et al: Substance abuse as a factor in the causality, severity, and recurrence rate of traumatic brain injury. Md Med J 42:989–993, 1993

Edna T: Alcohol influence and head injury. Acta Chir Scand 148:209–212, 1985

Elmer O, Lim R: Influence of acute alcohol intoxication on the outcome of severe non-neurologic trauma. Acta Chir Scand 151:305–308, 1985

Field J: Epidemiology of Head Injury in England and Wales: With Particular Application to Rehabilitation. Leicester, England, Willsons, 1976

Freund G: Neuropathology of alcohol abuse, in Alcohol and the Brain: Chronic Effects. Edited by Tarter R, Van Thiel D. New York, Plenum, 1985, pp 3–17

Fuller MG, Fishman E, Taylor CA, et al: Screening patients with traumatic brain injuries for substance abuse. J Neuropsychiatry Clin Neurosci 6:143–146, 1994

Galbraith S: Misdiagnosis and delayed diagnosis in traumatic intercranial hematoma. BMJ 1:1438–1439, 1976

Gallagher JP, Browder J: Extradural hematoma experienced with 167 patients. J Neurosurg 29:1–22, 1968

Group for the Advancement of Psychiatry, Committee on Alcoholism and the Addictions: Substance abuse disorders: a psychiatric priority. Am J Psychiatry 148:1291–1300, 1991

Harrison PA, Hoffman NG, Streid SG: Drug and alcohol addiction treatment outcome, in Comprehensive Handbook of Drug and Alcohol Addiction. Edited by Miller NS. New York, Marcel Dekker, 1991, pp 1163–1700

Helzer JE, Pryzbeck TR: The co-occurrence of alcoholism with other psychiatric disorders in the general population and its impact in treatment. J Stud Alcohol 49:219–224, 1988

Hoffman NG, Miller NS: Effective treatment: abstinence based programs. Psychiatr Ann 22:1–5, 1992

Jong CN, Zafonte RD, Millis SR, et al: The effect of cocaine on traumatic brain injury outcome: a preliminary evaluation. Brain Inj 13:1017–1023, 1999

Kelly DF: Alcohol and head injury: an issue revisited. J Neurotrauma 12:883–890, 1995

Kelly MP, Johnson CT, Knoller N, et al: Substance abuse, traumatic brain injury and neuropsychological outcome. Brain Inj 11:391–402, 1997

Keso L, Salaspuro M: Inpatient treatment of employed alcoholics: a randomized clinical trial on Hazelden-type and traditional treatment. Alcohol Clin Exp Res 14:584–589, 1990

Kolakowsky-Hayner SA, Gourley EV 3rd, Kreutzer JS, et al: Pre-injury substance abuse among persons with brain injury and persons with spinal cord injury. Brain Inj 13:571–581, 1999

Kramer TH, Hoisington D: Use of AA and NA in the treatment of chemical dependencies of traumatic brain injury survivors. Brain Inj 6:81–88, 1992

Kreutzer J, Doherty K, Harris J, et al: Alcohol use among persons with TBI. J Head Trauma Rehabil 5:9–20, 1990

Kreutzer JS, Witol AD, Marwitz JH: Alcohol and drug use among persons with traumatic brain injury. J Learn Disabil 29:643–651, 1996

Ksiazkiewicz B, Bloch-Buguslawska E: [Diagnostic difficulties with skull and brain injury complications in alcoholic patients] (Polish). Pol Merkuriusz Lek 4:166–168, 1998

Langley MJ: Preventing post-injury alcohol-related problems: a behavioral approach, in Work Worth Doing: Advances in Brain Injury Rehabilitation. Edited by McMahon BT, Shaw LR. Orlando, FL, Paul M. Deutsch, 1991

Mayfield D: Alcohol and affect: experimental studies, in Alcoholism and Affective Disorders. Edited by Goodwin DW, Erickson CK. New York, SP Medical & Scientific Books, 1979

Mayfield D, Allen D: Alcohol and affect: a psychopharmacological study. Am J Psychiatry 123:1346–1351, 1967

Mayfield D, McLeod G, Hall P: The CAGE questionnaire: validation of a new alcoholism screening instrument. Am J Psychiatry 131:1121–1123, 1974

McLaughlin AM, Shaffer V: Rehabilitation or remold? family involvement in head trauma recovery. Cognitive Rehabilitation 3:1985

Miller NS: Drug and alcohol addiction as a disease, in Comprehensive Handbook of Drug and Alcohol Addiction. Edited by Miller NS. New York, Marcel Dekker, 1991a, pp 295–310

Miller NS: The Pharmacology of Alcohol and Drugs of Abuse and Addiction. New York, Springer-Verlag New York, 1991b

Miller NS: Special problems of the alcohol and multiple-drug dependent: clinical interactions, in Clinical Textbook of Addictive Disorders. Edited by Frances RJ, Miller SJ. New York, Guilford, 1991c, pp 194–218

Miller NS: Mortality risks in alcoholism and effects of abstinence and addiction treatment. J Addict Dis 22:371–383, 1999

Miller NS: Disease orientation: taking away blame and shame, in Addiction Recovery Tools: A Practical Handbook. Edited by Coombs RH. Thousand Oaks, CA, Sage, 2001, pp 99–110

Miller NS: Drug abuse, in Conn's Current Therapy. Edited by Rakel RE, Bope ET. 2002

Miller NS (ed): Treatment updates for pharmacotherapies for addictive disorders. Psychiatr Ann 33, 2003

Miller NS, Gold MS: Identification and treatment of benzodiazepine abuse. Am Fam Physician 40:175–183, 1989

Miller NS, Gold MS: Alcohol. New York, Plenum, 1991

Miller NS, Goldsmith RJ: Craving for alcohol and drugs in animals and humans: biology and behavior. J Addict Dis 20:87–104, 2001

Miller NS, Mahler JC: Alcoholics Anonymous and the "AA" model for treatment. Alcoholism Treatment Quarterly 8:39–51, 1991

Miller NS, Ries RK: Drug and alcohol dependence and psychiatric populations: the need for diagnosis, intervention, and training. Compr Psychiatry 32:268–276, 1991

Miller NS, Gold MS, Cocores JA, et al: Alcohol dependence and its medical consequences. N Y State J Med 88:476–481, 1988

Miller NS, Gold MS, Belkin B, et al: The diagnosis of alcohol and cannabis dependence in cocaine dependents and alcohol dependence in their families. Br J Addict 84:1491–1498, 1990

Miller NS, Ninonuevo F, Hoffmann NG, et al: Prediction of treatment outcomes: lifetime depression versus the continuum of care. Am J Addict 8:243–253, 1999

Minkoff K: An integrated treatment model for dual diagnosis of psychosis and addiction. Hosp Community Psychiatry 40:1031–1036, 1989

Netrakom P, Krasuski JS: Structural and functional neuroimaging findings in substance-related disorders. J Addict Dis 22: 1999

Parsons DA, Leber WR: The relationship between cognitive dysfunction and brain damage in alcoholics: causation or epiphenomenal? Clin Exp Res 5:326–343, 1981

Ries RK, Samson H: Substance abuse among inpatient psychiatric patients. Substance Abuse 8:28–34, 1987

Roman P: Barriers to the use of constructive confrontations with employed alcoholics. J Clin Psychiatry 43:53–57, 1982

Rumbaugh CL, Fang HEH: The effects of drug abuse on the brain. Med Times 3:37–52, 1980

Schuckit MA: Alcoholism and other psychiatric disorders. Hosp Community Psychiatry 34:1022–1027, 1983

Schuckit MA: Drug and Alcohol Abuse: A Clinical Guide to Diagnosis and Treatment. New York, Plenum, 1990

Schuckit MA, Irwin M, Brown SA: The history of anxiety symptoms among 171 primary alcoholics. J Stud Alcohol 51:34–41, 1990

Schulz JE: Long-term treatment in recovery from drug and alcohol addiction, in Comprehensive Handbook of Drug and Alcohol Addictions. Edited by Miller NS. New York, Marcel Dekker, 1991

Selzer ML, Vinokur A, van Rooijen L: A self-administered Short Michigan Alcoholism Screening Test (SMAST). J Stud Alcohol 36:117–126, 1975

Sparadeo FR, Gill D: Focus on clinical research: effect of prior alcohol use on head injury recovery. J Head Trauma Rehabil 4:75–82, 1989

Sparadeo FR, Strauss D, Barth JT: The incidence, impact, and treatment of substance abuse in head trauma rehabilitation. J Head Trauma Rehabil 5:1–8, 1990

Stead P, Viders J: A "SHARP" approach to treating alcoholism. Social Work 24:144–149, 1979

Substance Abuse Task Force: White Paper. Washington, DC, National Head Injury Foundation, 1988

Tamerin JS, Mendelson JH: The psychodynamics of chronic inebriation: observations of alcoholic during the process of drinking in an experimental group setting. Am J Psychiatry 125:886–899, 1969

Tarter R, Edwards K: Neuropsychology of alcoholism, in Alcohol and the Brain: Chronic Effects. Edited by Tarter R, Van Thiel D. New York, Plenum, 1985, pp 217–242

Tobis JS, Puri KB, Sheridan J: Rehabilitation of the severely brain-injured patient. Scand J Rehabil Med 14:83–88, 1982

Vaillant GE: The Natural History of Alcoholism. Cambridge, MA, Harvard University Press, 1983

Wehman P, Targett P, Yasuda S, et al: Return to work for individuals with TBI and a history of substance abuse. NeuroRehabilitation 15:71–77, 2000

Zink BJ, Feustel PJ: Effects of ethanol on respiratory function in traumatic brain injury. J Neurosurg 82:822–828, 1995

Zink BJ, Walsh RF, Feustel PJ: Effects of ethanol in traumatic brain injury. J Neurotrauma 10:275–286, 1993

Zink BJ, Sheinberg MA, Wang X, et al: Acute ethanol intoxication in a model of traumatic brain injury with hemorrhagic shock: effects on early physiological response. J Neurosurg 89:983–990, 1998

Appendix 29–1

Letter to Alcoholics Anonymous Sponsor of Member With Traumatic Brain Injury

The following is a letter to an Alcoholics Anonymous (AA) sponsor explaining the special characteristics of the alcohol- or drug-addicted individual with brain damage. A sponsor in AA (or Narcotics Anonymous [NA]) is someone who also is an alcoholic- or drug-addicted individual in recovery who assists the sponsoree in learning about the AA or NA program and "working" the steps of AA or NA (Henry 1988).

Dear Sponsor:

As a 12-stepper in AA or NA, you know fully well the horror chemical dependency thrusts into a person's life. Without concerted and persistent effort toward recovery, personal, family and social dimensions of life are deeply threatened and treacherously undermined. In the case of the person you are now sponsoring or are considering whether to sponsor, the addiction has been further compounded by a head injury that has, to some degree, caused damage to the brain. Because of this damage, the very physiological organ responsible for memory, language, reasoning, judgment, and behavior (among other skills and abilities) has been compromised. Consequently, problems have emerged that are a direct result of the trauma to the brain, and these problems now are inevitably overlapping and interacting with the individual's addictive nature.

At this stage in his or her recovery from the trauma, the individual with whom you are working has undoubt-edly regained many of those diminished abilities. However, in all probability, there are lasting effects ("seque-lae," in medical terminology) that remain and that you may now be witnessing. These residual problems may be manifested in obvious or subtle ways, and an explanation of their nature may be helpful.

The purpose of this letter is to acquaint you with some of the more common cognitive (i.e., having to do with perceiving, organizing, interpreting, and acting on information) and emotional problems that head-injured people face as a direct result of brain trauma. With a good medical recovery it is not at all unusual for these individuals to appear unimpaired unless one takes a close look, and your work as a sponsor certainly will require close interaction. These comments, then, are offered in a spirit of gratitude for your help to this person who must now come to grips with himself on several levels; who must now, en route to recovery from addiction, untangle a complex knot of problems, including the changing pretraumatic lifestyle, while dealing with the confusion and psychological pain that recently shattered cognition brings.

The human brain has specific sections that specialize in specific functions. If damage to any of these areas is severe enough, those functions—as well as higher level ones that they support—may be lastingly limited. Many of these regions of the brain interface to enable the performance of complex skills such as reading, or remembering and following through on lengthy directions. Because the brain's functioning is so dependent on the interrelationship of parts, and because any of those parts may be hurt in a trauma, many sorts of problems can result. The more prominent and frequently occurring ones, discussed in cognitive and emotional areas, are as follows:

Appendices reprinted courtesy of the National Head Injury Foundation (Substance Abuse Task Force: "White Paper." Washington, DC, National Head Injury Foundation, 1988, pp 53–59).

Cognitive

Attention

This includes maintaining attention for normal periods and the ability to shift attention to different areas after concentrating on one set of ideas. Also included here are difficulties screening out distractions (voices, noises, and visual things) in the environment, as well as suppressing one's own preoccupations while there is other work to be done.

Suggestions: Settle for smaller amounts of quality time rather than attempting longer amounts that may prove too fatiguing to the sponsoree. Cue him when he seems stuck in prior topics (e.g., "We're talking about now. . .") or when he seems to have drifted away ("Tune back in now, okay. . ."). Gradually lengthen the time of expected attention and concentration as increasing abilities permit.

Memory

The most common type of deficit resulting from brain injury is of short-term memory . This appears as difficulty holding onto several pieces of information while having also to think through each item (e.g., cooking while also staying mindful of the children's nearby play). Other common problems are in remembering to follow through on assigned tasks at specified times and in remembering recent experiences and conversations. Fortunately, memory for pretraumatic episodes are most often unimpaired by this time in the person's medical recovery.

Suggestions: Expect the person to use journals and date books—and to review them frequently and independently—to cue himself about past and future events. If such memory aids are necessary, consider this simply another component of the program to be worked; do not shy from expecting self responsibility. If the person is overloaded by doing two or more things simultaneously, encourage him to prioritize tasks and work out a time management schedule honoring that limitation.

Language

Both ability to understand others and to express one's own ideas clearly are often affected. In both cases, a slower speed of processing language is at play. Also, delays in recalling the words needed to articulate a thought are common. When speaking, the head-injured person may ramble and talk in a disorganized, circular kind of way, often failing to come to the point or himself losing it in the details of the conversation.

Suggestions: Encourage the person to ask questions and request clarification of information whenever needed to compensate for a slower rate of comprehension. For situations in which it is appropriate, encourage the head-injured person also to ask speakers to slow down, to repeat points, and to explain ideas in different words. Support may be required to downplay feelings of embarrassment to do these things. As a speaker, the sponsoree may need cues to see the need for making his point more clearly, simply, or briefly; working out a system for your providing such cues that you both feel comfortable with might be useful. As a general rule, encourage him to take time to think about what he wants to say, to plan how to say it, and to be unrushed in finding the words he needs.

Reasoning and Judgment

Basic skills such as cause-effect reasoning and/or the ability to make inferences are often reduced. Thinking may be excessively concrete, giving rise to confusion and misinterpretation of others' remarks (e.g., "Come off your high horse. . ."). Similarly, problem-solving skills are often marred by impulsive decision making, difficulty in considering several solutions to problems and in envisioning potential consequences of actions. Failure to note voice or facial cues of others that convey nonverbal messages also increases the chance of inappropriate remarks. Common, too, are related problems in inhibiting inappropriate behavior, determining what situations require which behaviors, and reflecting on the propriety of what he has just said or done.

Suggestions: As an overall rule, do not avoid openly addressing the issues raised by the above-mentioned behaviors or misunderstandings. Apply the very same gentle but firm advice-giving anyone working in a recovery program may require. It may be helpful to point out specific incidences as examples of behaviors that need to be avoided, or situations from which one can learn to "think first before saying or doing something." As you would with anyone looking to you for help, follow your good instincts to provide support in the amount, kind, and frequency that leads this particular person with this particular personality to the best levels of independence he can achieve.

Executive Functions

Executive functions refer to those abilities to initiate, organize, direct, monitor, and evaluate oneself. Self-insight is a crucial component. Owing to the very high level nature of these skills and to the vulnerability of the part of the brain responsible for their operation, they are frequently impaired in the person who has suffered a head trauma. As a result, even with other skills and abilities intact, the use of these executive functions in a directed, purposeful manner may be lacking, making the overall picture of brain operations rather like a full-member, competent orchestra without a conductor to organize and lead their many mixing harmonies; or, like a ready and able work crew without a foreman to coordinate and direct their labor.

Suggestions: If impairments in executive functions are apparent in the person you sponsor, it may well become especially important for you to assume a role of guiding some of these operations within the context in which you work together. To an extent, you would do this anyway; it is a large part of sponsorship. For a head-injured person, however, the need for such help may be deeper and more substantial. Your skills as a conductor, or foreman, may be particularly required. A little more firmly offered advice in decision making, for example—or better perhaps, encouragement to make one's own sound decisions with you available to monitor, affirm, give feedback, and gently correct when necessary. As noted earlier, in most cases it would be perfectly okay to talk openly about the need for your help in this regard because of the limitations imposed by the head injury. But be careful, of course, not to foster unnecessary dependence; increased well-being through healthy, clear-minded independence is always, as you know, the ultimate goal.

Emotional

There is an array of emotional problems typically related to head injury. These include irritability, poor frustration tolerance, dependence on others, insensitivity, lack of awareness of one's affect on others, and heightened emotionality. There may be tendencies toward overreaction to stressful situations, some paranoia, depression, withdrawal, or denial of problems. No single head-injured person evidences all of these problems, of course, and most would show only subtle signals of some of these psychosocial difficulties. They are mentioned, however, to familiarize you with some of the emotional problems that often accompany brain trauma, and to alert you to their similarity to those characteristics of many persons with histories of alcohol and drug addiction.

Suggestions: In your sponsoring of a head-injured person who may exhibit some of the above problems, the art of playing issues straight is recommended. Your sponsoree should know what problems you see impeding his

progress toward greater recovery. Because his well-being is the goal, your responsibility is as it would be with any other such partnership. Tactful but clear identification of problems, complete with acceptance of them as risks to continued sobriety or clean time that will necessitate work, is an appropriate attitude to adopt. Whether these sorts of problems are attributable to an addictive personality, or to the head injury, or to both, open, honest acknowledgment of the work to be done and the support needed to do it is what recovery is all about. The sponsorship concept, moreover, is a very plausible means of addressing those sorts of problems.

Please also be aware that there are three main avenues of assistance further available to you.

If the person with whom you work has received treatment from a rehabilitation center specializing in brain trauma, do not hesitate to contact the staff for advice They may be aware of approaches or strategies that work well with your individual.

For materials on brain injury and chemical dependency, contact the Brain Injury Association of America, 105 North Alfred Street, Alexandria, VA 22314. http://www.biausa.org/Pages/home.html

You are one of the main supports of the recovering chemically dependent, head-injured person. You deserve great thanks. The comments in this letter are not meant to frighten or dissuade you from sponsorship, but rather to provide you with basic information with which to enhance your preparedness and diffuse any unnecessary anxieties you may feel. Trust yourself in your work; your status as a 12-stepper well respected for your patience, intelligence, and straightforwardness. The recovering head-injured person receiving your help is fortunate to have you in his corner.

Kurt Vonnegut wrote that, "Detours are dancing lessons from God." You understand chemical dependency and recovery. Confronting a major life obstacle, you have learned to dance. Your sponsorship of the head-injured person with whom you are beginning involvement represents help for someone whose life has been shattered in a particularly devastating way, whose detour is indeed formidable. May your help in teaching that person to dance be gratifying, and blessed, and an occasion for joy and learning for you both.

Reference

Henry K: A letter to sponsors of chemically dependent head injured persons, in Task Force on Chemical Dependency. Southborough, MA, National Head Injury Foundation, 1988, pp 53–57

Appendix 29–2

Original Twelve Steps of Alcoholics Anonymous

1. We admitted we were powerless over alcohol; that our lives had become unmanageable.
2. Came to believe that a Power greater than ourselves could restore us to sanity.
3. Made a decision to turn our will and our lives over to the care of God as we understood Him.
4. Made a searching and fearless moral inventory of ourselves.
5. Admitted to God, to ourselves, and to another human being the exact nature of our wrongs.
6. Were entirely ready to have God remove all these defects of character.
7. Humbly asked Him to remove our shortcomings.
8. Made a list of all persons we had harmed and became willing to make amends to them all.
9. Made direct amends to such people wherever possible, except when to do so would injure them or others.
10. Continued to take personal inventory and when we were wrong, promptly admitted it.
11. Sought through prayer and meditation to improve our conscious contact with God as we understood Him, praying only for knowledge of His will for us and the power to carry that out.
12. Having had a spiritual awakening as the result of these steps, we tried to carry this message to alcoholics and to practice these principles in all our affairs.

Appendix 29–3

Traumatic Brain Injury
Explanation of the Twelve Steps

The following are the 12 steps of Alcoholics Anonymous that have been written for the traumatic brain injury (TBI) patient who has cognitive and mood disturbances. These steps can be understood by those who need concrete examples for understanding and using them in the recovery program for the TBI patient.

1. Admit that if you drink and/or use drugs your life will be out of control. Admit that the use of substances after having had a TBI will make your life unmanageable.
2. You start to believe that someone can help you put your life in order. This someone could be God, an Alcoholics Anonymous group, counselor, sponsor, etc.
3. You decide to get help from others or from God. You open yourself up.
4. You will make a complete list of the negative behaviors in your past and current behavior problems. You will also make a list of your positive behaviors.
5. Meet with someone you trust and discuss what you wrote in step 4.
6. Become ready to sincerely try to change your negative behaviors.
7. Ask God for the strength to be a responsible person with responsible behaviors.
8. Make a list of people your negative behaviors have affected. Be ready to apologize or make things right with them.
9. Contact these people. Apologize or make things right.
10. Continue to check yourself and your behaviors daily. Correct negative behaviors and improve them. If you hurt another person, apologize and make corrections.
11. Stop and think about how you are behaving several times each day. Are my behaviors positive? Am I being responsible? If not, ask for help. Reward yourself when you are able to behave in a positive and responsible fashion.
12. If you try to work these steps, you will start to feel much better about yourself. Now it's your turn to help others do the same. Helping others will make you feel even better. Continue to work these steps on a daily basis.

PART V

Social Issues

30 The Family System

Marie M. Cavallo, Ph.D.

Thomas Kay, Ph.D.

The Family System: Homeostasis and Involvement

Because hospitals and rehabilitation programs are under increasing pressure to become more efficient and generate more money at lower rates, and because managed care sets more limits on the nature, length, and coverage of "nonessential" services, non-reimbursed services and programs—such as family education and involvement of families in team meetings—of necessity decline. It can no longer be assumed that families of persons with traumatic brain injury (TBI) will be attended to and given what they need. It is our hope that this chapter will serve as an introduction to service providers across disciplines to sensitize them to the needs of families so that that the role of "family therapy" can be spread out and shared across the rehabilitation team and into the community.

The effect of TBI on the family system merits study for five important reasons.

1. TBI inevitably causes profound changes in every family system.
2. These changes dramatically influence the functional recovery of the person with brain injury.
3. The effect of TBI continues over the life cycle of the family, long after the initial adjustment to disability is made.
4. The lives of individual family members may be profoundly affected by a brain injury in another family member.
5. Family assessment and intervention are crucial at all stages of rehabilitation and adjustment after TBI, even when a pathological response is not present.

TBI is an event that affects and alters an entire family, not only the person with the injury. Families are systems with sets of relationships and roles that develop to maintain an effective balance in the day-to-day world. This homeostasis is broken at the moment one person in the family sustains a brain injury. The struggle of the family to "right itself" and reestablish a new homeostasis after TBI in one member is parallel to the process of rehabilitation and adjustment in the injured person. In the way that recovery is never complete for the individual after brain injury, the family as a unit can never return to its former "self." Assisting families in the process of reestablishing equilibrium, with new sets of roles, relationships, and goals, is the purpose of family assessment and intervention. Because of the range of physical, cognitive, and behavioral-affective changes that can result from TBI, the injured person is often more dependent on family members and therefore more intertwined in and affected by family dynamics. Consequently, the family's relative success or failure in establishing a functional equilibrium plays a significant role in determining the relative independence of the person with brain injury, making family interventions critical to the rehabilitation process.

Although it is generally agreed among professionals that families should be involved in the rehabilitation process, family involvement is often limited to keeping families informed of treatment plans and periodic appearances at team conferences, where families may be updated on progress and encouraged to participate in carrying out the team's care plan. This approach both lacks the active input of the family in defining the rehabilitation goals and process and fails to appreciate the needs of the recovering family system.

Equally unfortunate is the fact that psychiatric intervention is usually the consultation of last resort: when there is a crisis that no one else can manage, when medication is required, or (especially) when someone becomes suicidal. In our opinion, this is a serious underuse of potential psychiatric knowledge and skill in the area of family systems. The model developed in this chapter involves not primarily tertiary psychiatric intervention in the event of crisis, but instead a prospective, preventive, primary intervention model that calls for the psychodynamic and interpersonal expertise of the psychiatrist to be brought to bear in helping families cope from the moment of injury through long-term adjustment. In fact, this chapter is less concerned with delineating traditional psychiatric manifestations in the family and more concerned with articulating the effect of TBI on families, how they respond, what they need, and what psychiatric interventions are appropriate along the continuum of care.

Impact of TBI on the Family

The impact of TBI on the family can be conceptualized in three broad phases. In the acute phase, in which the primary issues are survival, medical stabilization, and minimization of permanent damage, the family coalesces and orients all of its energy toward the care of the injured person. In the rehabilitation phase, family roles are reorganized, and the goal is the restoration of as much physical and cognitive functioning as possible after brain injury. In the reintegration phase, the individual recovering from the injury attempts to return as much as possible to a level of maximum engagement and productivity in the community, while the family settles into longer-term patterns and equilibrium that allow them to resume their family life cycle with an altered identity. The primary issues the family faces during each of these phases are considered in the section A Model of Assessment and Intervention.

In the long run, however, TBI is distinguished from other catastrophic injuries in terms of effect on the family by the following facts: 1) cognitive, emotional, and behavioral sequelae, which alter the personality and capacities of the injured person, are constant (Kay and Lezak 1990); 2) the deficits are permanent, and the family must establish new patterns and goals to incorporate a member with brain damage; and 3) the demographics of TBI (primarily affecting young, adult men) dictate that, unlike strokes or dementing diseases affecting primarily the elderly, TBI affects families who are generally young and in the early stages of their development (Kalsbeek et al. 1980).

Research Literature on Families

The physical, emotional, psychosocial, and financial costs of TBI for the family of an injured person have been documented in a number of reviews (Bond 1983; Brooks 1991; Florian et al. 1989; Livingston 1990; Perlesz et al. 1999; Romano 1989). An overview of trends since the early 1970s distinguishes an evolution of TBI family research that includes four main phases (Kay and Cavallo 1991).

Phase I

In phase I, family members were studied as "windows" on the person with the brain injury (e.g., Bond 1976; Hpay 1970; Oddy et al. 1985). These studies were useful in documenting the cognitive, affective, and personality changes after brain injury and the persistence of symptoms over time.

Phase II

In phase II, studies that primarily documented the effects of brain injury on the patient also incidentally noted the effect of the injury on significant others. For example, Panting and Merry (1972) documented that 61% of wives and mothers required medication to help them cope with relatives with TBI, wives had more difficulty coping than mothers, and more than one-half of all relatives thought support services were inadequate. A series of studies by Oddy et al. (1978b) in London noted that increased dependence on families was associated with greater severity of injury, poorer family relationships at 1 year were associated with personality changes in the person with the brain injury (Oddy and Humphrey 1980), and personality changes were associated with greater family dependence (Weddell et al. 1980). These studies, however, did not have the family as their primary focus.

Phase III

In phase III, beginning in the late 1970s but peaking in the mid- to late 1980s, families—or at least individual family members—became a primary focus of research. By documenting the severity of injury, presence of a range of neurobehavioral symptoms, and the reactions of family members, these studies began to identify the factors that led to distress and burden on primary caregivers. For example, Oddy et al. (1978a) found that depression in family members correlated not primarily with severity of injury (as measured by coma or posttraumatic amnesia), but with the number and extent of cognitive symptoms, as well as with the failure to return to work and social isolation of the person with the injury. This theme—that the behavioral manifestations of the injury (both neuropsychological and functional), not the neurological severity of the TBI per se, affect family members—is a consistent one in this phase of family research.

In the 1980s, Brooks and colleagues in Glasgow published a series of papers articulating the nature and causes of subjective burden of family members after TBI (see Brooks [1991] and Livingston and Brooks [1988] for reviews). A number of themes can be considered established (summarized in Table 30–1). First, in the long run, behavioral, affective, and personality changes are most burdensome to families; physical deficits cause the least burden; and cognitive deficits cause intermediate burden (Brooks and McKinlay 1983; Brooks et al. 1987; McKinlay et al. 1981). Second, in a parallel finding, persons with brain injury and family members agree most when rating the nature and extent of physical problems, agree least about emotional-behavioral problems, and agree moderately on cognitive problems. Family members are most distressed by the changes persons with brain injury are least aware of: the impulsivity, disinhibition, irritability, anger outbursts, insensitivity, and changes in personality. Third, over the course of time, subjective family burden actually increases (Brooks et al. 1987). Subjective family burden becomes more strongly linked to personality changes (Brooks and McKinlay 1983) and less strongly linked to neurological severity (McKinlay et al. 1981). Fourth, there is no one-to-one correspondence between the degree of deficit and the degree of burden; personality characteristics of the family member appear to be a factor in how much burden that family member experiences. Although all family members experiencing high levels of burden report personality changes in the person with brain injury, it is not conversely true that whenever personality changes occur the result is high burden on the family (Brooks and McKinlay 1983). Similarly, although low levels of burden are associated with low levels of deficit, high levels of burden may be associated with either low or high levels of deficit (Brooks et al. 1987). However, relatives who rated the patient's emotional-behavioral problems as high also tended to have high neuroticism scores on the Eysenck Personality Questionnaire (Eysenck and Eysenck 1975). Because the Eysenck score represents a presumably durable personality trait involving maladaptive and anxiety-laden responses in stressful situations, it may be that family members with poorer ego integration experience more affective and behavioral distress from the person with the injury and therefore feel more burden. This suggestion was reinforced by Livingston (1987) who found that the preinjury psychiatric and health history of the relative accounted for 30% of the variance in the relative's rating of subjective burden.

TABLE 30–1. Glasgow research on subjective burden after traumatic brain injury

Behavioral, affective, and personality changes cause the most burden; cognitive changes cause intermediate burden; and physical changes cause the least burden.

Patients and family members agree most when rating physical problems, agree in an intermediate way about cognitive problems, and agree least about emotional-behavioral problems.

Over time, family burden increases, becoming more linked to personality changes and less to neurological severity.

No one-to-one correspondence between degree of deficits and degree of burden.

Note. For more information on subjective burden, see Brooks and McKinlay 1983; Brooks et al. 1987; Livingston 1987; McKinlay et al. 1981.

Although the bulk of work on caregiver burden took place in the mid- to late 1980s by Brooks and colleagues, other researchers continue to explore this area (e.g., Cavallo 1997; Cavallo et al. 1992; Groom et al. 1998; Koskinen 1998; Marsh et al. 1998).

In summary, subjective burden of family members tends to increase, not decrease, over time; it is most related to changes in personality, emotions, and behavior, of which the person with brain injury is least aware; it is the neurobehavioral manifestations of TBI and not the neurological severity per se that affect family members; and the adjustment of family members plays a large role in determining the subjective burden they experience. For overviews of burden issues, see Chwalisz (1992) and Cavallo (1997).

Phase IV

In phase IV of the research literature, predominantly from the late 1980s, the focus shifted from individual family members to families as systems and the effect of TBI on roles, relationships, and the family's status in society. For example, Kozloff (1987) used network analysis to document that the size of the social network of the person with the brain injury decreases, multiplex relationships increase (i.e., family members serve more and more functions as nonrelatives drop out), and families with higher socioeconomic status are more able to maintain existing relationships. Maitz (1989) compared families with a member with TBI to a group of families who did not have a person with TBI living with them but in which one of the members either had a sibling with TBI or a sibling married to a person with TBI. He found, using formal measures of family functioning, that families with a member with TBI had less (and more variable) cohesiveness and more variability in conflict resolution than those families who did not have a person with TBI living with them and showed a correlation between marital conflict and decreased cohesiveness. Peters et al. (1990) found that good dyadic adjustment (between person with TBI and spouse) was associated with less financial strain, low spousal ratings of patient psychopathology, and less severe injuries. Lifestyle changes in families with TBI were documented by Jacobs (1988), who found that families tend to be primarily responsible for providing support, socialization, and assistance to persons with brain injury, with two-thirds of such families experiencing financial adversity.

Moore et al. (1993) approached long-term outcome after TBI from a family life cycle model. They looked at a variety of family stressors in relation to distress in families. Perceived financial strain and age of the oldest child were found to be the factors most significantly related to an increase in distress in families. In an investigation of family response to injury in the acute stage of recovery, Curtiss et al. (2000) used Olson's Circumplex Model (Olson 1993; Olson et al. 1982) to examine changes in family response structure and coping responses pre- and post-TBI. Curtiss et al.'s results were consistent with Olson's Circumplex Model: significant changes in family structure and coping styles post-TBI were found, with differential changes on the basis of preinjury family structure.

Koscuilek and his colleagues (1994, 1996, 1997a, 1997b, 1998) found positive appraisal and family tension management ability to be predictive of successful family functioning and identified factors that enabled families to successfully adapt, such as support from friends. Minnes et al. (2000) found that "reframing" and "seeking spiritual support" as coping mechanisms after TBI were significantly related to more positive outcomes in family members. Douglas and Spellacy (1996) also found that the adequacy of social support for caregivers as well as length of PTA and current neurobehavioral functioning were predictive of long-term family functioning after TBI. However, Leach et al. (1994) found that perceived social support was not predictive of depression in individuals with TBI, though effective use of problem-solving and behavioral coping strategies by families was related to lower levels of depression for individuals with TBI.

Junque et al. (1997) concluded that residual affective-behavioral problems had the greatest effect on family functioning and that the presence of these symptoms was closely related to a need expressed by families for information concerning TBI. In fact, in a 1997 study assessing knowledge about TBI, Springer et al. found that, whereas families of individuals with TBI had a better understanding of the immediate significance of brain injury and its

negative effect on cognition, they had more misconceptions about potential long-term functioning, and they endorsed common misconceptions about TBI in the areas of unconsciousness, amnesia, and recovery.

There are a number of studies that focus on differing perceptions within families with a member with TBI on the basis of a variety of factors, including kinship, role, and gender. A group of researchers (Gervasio and Kreutzer 1997; Kreutzer et al. 1994a, 1994b; Serio et al. 1995) examined a variety of these factors potentially related to family functioning after TBI. Major findings included that outcome predictors, and perceived unmet needs of family members, differed for spouses and parents of individuals with TBI. Cavallo (1997), in comparing wives and mothers of individuals with TBI, found that although mothers were caring for more severely injured individuals with TBI, wives were reporting significantly more subjective burden related specifically to affective-behavioral and cognitive functioning of the individual with TBI. No differences were found between the two groups related to residual physical problems. However, Allen et al. (1994) suggest that there is little difference between parents and spouses in reported stress.

In a small number of studies (Cavallo 1997; Perlesz et al. 2000), it has been noted that men rarely identify as primary caregivers in families after a TBI. Perlesz et al. (2000) describe men as secondary or tertiary caregivers and further report that male caregivers may report their distress differently from female caregivers, perhaps as anger and fatigue, rather than depression and anxiety.

In studies of differing perceptions of residual problems and family functioning when comparing individuals with TBI to family members and/or professional staff working with them (Cavallo et al. 1992; Fordyce and Roueche 1986; Lanham et al. 2000; Malec et al. 1997; McKinlay and Brooks 1984), some basic concurrence of findings emerge. First, there tend to be differing amounts of agreement between individuals with TBI and their families or staff, or both, on the basis of the types of problems they are being asked to endorse. Second, there are differing amounts of agreement between individuals with TBI and their families or staff, or both, overall. Some have high agreement; some have low agreement, with families or staff, or both, endorsing more problem areas; and some have low agreement, with the individuals with TBI endorsing more problem areas. Third, in general, when family members are endorsing more problems than the individual with TBI, they tend to be in the affective-behavioral realm. Most significantly for this review, however, these studies generally represent a shift from generalizing about how all families respond to investigating differential responses within and among families.

In a study focusing on children with TBI and their families, Barry and Clark (1992) found that, regardless of severity of injury, children with TBI from nonintact families remained as inpatients in rehabilitation significantly longer than children from intact families. In a study of children of brain-injured parents, Pessar et al. (1993) found that, subsequent to the parent's brain injury, most of the children displayed increased negative behaviors, and correlates of poor outcome for these children included the injured parent's gender and level of depression. In an interesting study of children with TBI, Yeates et al. (1997) investigated the preinjury family environment as a predictor of outcome in children with TBI. They found that preinjury family functioning had a significant effect on 1-year outcome, even after accounting for injury-related variables. In 1998, another study of children with TBI by Max et al. confirmed this finding. They looked at preinjury psychosocial factors, injury factors, and postinjury factors (such as coping of family members and the development of psychiatric disorders in the child with TBI) as they related to family functioning in the first 2 years after TBI in children. The major findings were that the best predictor of family functioning after an injury was the preinjury family functioning as well as whether the child developed a psychiatric disorder. These findings of the effect of preinjury family functioning and chronic life stressors are consistent with earlier work with children by the Taylor group (Barry et al. 1996; Taylor et al. 1995; Wade et al. 1995, 1996) and the Rivara group (Rivara et al. 1992, 1993, 1994). A more recent study from the Taylor group (Wade et al. 2002) found that, although overall family stress and caregiver burden declined over time after both pediatric brain injuries and orthopedic injuries, families of children with severe brain injuries continued to experience high levels of stress and burden years after injury, especially when compared with families of individuals with orthopedic injuries.

It may be that elements in family situations that are beyond the influence of professionals (e.g., financial means and a network of family support) are the potent factors in family adaptation after TBI. Credence is lent to this hypothesis by the results of a recent study by Ergh et al. (2002). The authors found social support to be a significant factor moderating family functioning and caregiver burden after TBI. The more social support a family reported, the more functional the family was. Social support also moderated caregiver distress: in the absence of social support, caretakers were more vulnerable to the effects of time since injury, level of impairment, and lack of awareness on the part of the injured person.

One study that demonstrates the potential value of professionally based support is that of Albert et al. (2002). They studied the effects of offering an experimental social work liaison program for families of discharged rehabilitation inpatients with brain injuries of mixed types. In addition to offering education and emotional support, social workers offered practical advice about services and financial matters, and families were free to call at any time. Six months after patient discharge, caretakers who participated in the program showed decreased burden on six of nine scales when compared with caregivers who were tracked and interviewed but did not have access to the liaison program.

From a different perspective, Uysal et al. (1998) investigated the parenting skills of individuals with TBI and their spouses as well as the effects on children, specifically related to depression. They found that parents with TBI and their children experienced more symptoms of depression than their comparison groups, although the children did not have any greater frequency of behavior problems. They also found that there were specific areas of parenting in which individuals with TBI and their spouses differed from parents in the comparison group.

Finally, the diversity of styles of family adaptation has begun to be acknowledged in recent research. Our own work at New York University (NYU) Medical Center emphasizes the individuality of families and the influences of relationship, ethnicity, and culture and attempts to identify subgroups of family responses to TBI (Cavallo 1997; Cavallo and Saucedo 1995; Cavallo et al. 1992).

This recent phase of the research literature, the study of the family unit, depends on increasingly sophisticated and valid instruments and techniques for assessing family system functioning (see Bishop and Miller 1988 for a review of existing approaches). Most family assessment instruments are inadequately sensitive to particular issues specific to TBI. The NYU Head Injury Family Interview is one attempt to systematically survey family members about the effect of TBI on the person with the injury and on the family system (Kay et al. 1988, 1995).

The Head Injury Family Interview is a five-part structured interview designed for both research and clinical uses. It includes five sections covering premorbid, accident, rehabilitation, and community resource utilization (Table 30–2). It gathers information from both the person with the brain injury and significant others and provides a method for documenting the effect of the brain injury not only on the injured person, but on other family members as well. Most questions are hierarchically organized, beginning with open-ended questions (e.g., "What changes have you noticed since the injury?"), proceeding through structured areas (e.g., "Have you noticed any physical changes?"), and ending with focused questions (e.g., "Do you have problems with balance?"). Many of the main areas

TABLE 30–2.   New York University Head Injury Family Interview

Demographic and preinjury form

Demographic information

Accident/medical information

Preaccident history

Psychiatric history

Neurological history

Follow-up interview •

Routine medical care

Rehabilitation services

Psychotherapy

Living arrangements

Legal/insurance

Community service use

Significant other interview

Problems and changes

Problem checklist

Activities of daily living

Socialization and home activities

Patient competency rating

Interview for person with the brain injury

Problems and changes

Friendship and intimacy

Employment status

Homemaker status

Educational status

Problem checklist

Patient competency rating

Impact on the family

General

Questions for spouse

Questions for parents

Questions for adult siblings

Questions for younger siblings

Questions for adult children

Questions for younger children

of inquiry are asked both of the person with the injury and a significant other. Specific sections are provided for impact on parents, spouses, siblings, and children. The interview was developed over 9 years at the NYU Research and

Training Center on Head Trauma and Stroke out of a need for an instrument to gather detailed clinical and codable information specific to issues in TBI.

The research literature on the success of family intervention is small and relatively recent. Singer et al. (1994) compared two types of support groups for parents of individuals with TBI. They found that a stress management or coping skills approach was much more effective in reducing symptoms of anxiety and depression in families than an information and sharing approach. Carnevale (1996) outlined an approach called the *Natural-Setting Behavior Management Program* that trained individuals with TBI and their families to implement home-based behavior management programs. The results of the study support the success of this approach in managing behavioral issues after TBI. However, in a sobering follow-up article, Carnavale et al. (2002) found that neither education alone nor education combined with the Natural-Setting Behavior Management Program was effective in relieving caregiver burden.

There is also a small literature addressing family interventions that is more clinical and nonresearch based. DePompei and Williams (1994) describe a family-centered approach to rehabilitation and provide an excellent discussion of family life-cycle issues and episodic loss. Blosser and DePompei (1995) outline a family mentoring approach that can be used by professionals to help develop coping skills in family members and increase family involvement in planning and treatment. Maitz and Sachs (1995) provide an overview of treating families with TBI from a family systems perspective, specifically as it relates to family therapy and issues of power and authority. Kreutzer et al. (1997) outline case analyses and professionals' issues that contribute to the ability to successfully work with families after TBI. MacFarlane (1999) reviews the family therapy and rehabilitation literature on TBI treatment issues and discusses grief and loss reactions and stage theories of family adjustment.

Finally, four additional articles provide unique perspectives on family issues. Williams (1993) outlines how to train staff to provide family-centered rehabilitation; Rosen and Reynolds (1994) view services to individuals with TBI and their families from a public policy perspective; Hosack and Rocchio (1995) discuss the influence of managed care on the provision of services to families after TBI; and Cavallo and Saucedo (1995) discuss working with families from a variety of ethnic and cultural backgrounds after TBI.

Clinical Observations

In her classic article, Lezak (1978) provides observations on what it is like for family members living with the "characterologically altered" person with brain injury. She describes the personality changes that have primary impact on the family: 1) an impaired capacity for social perceptiveness, 2) stimulus-bound behavior (i.e., a concreteness, a failure to generalize), 3) impaired capacity for control and self-regulation, 4) emotional alterations (including apathy, irritability, and sexual changes), and 5) an inability to profit from experience (i.e., a tendency to repeat maladaptive patterns and not benefit from corrective strategies). As a result, family members may feel trapped, isolated, abandoned by outside relatives, and even abused, which often results in chronic or periodic depression among primary caregivers. Lezak's emphasis on the effect of characterological changes after brain injury (especially involving frontal systems) anticipated the later research documenting that personality and affective and behavioral changes in individuals with brain injury result in the greatest family burden.

Clinical experience bears out the research and descriptive literature cited in the preceding sections. Physical problems, although at times quite severe and necessitating specific family routines or limitations, are usually dealt with most successfully by the family in the long run, in large part because these problems are predictable, can be planned for, are within the awareness of the person with the brain injury, and are visible to and acknowledged by others. Cognitive problems, such as impaired attention, concentration, and memory, are more troublesome because they are less predictable and can invade all spheres of interaction and because their functional implications often are beyond the anticipation of the person with the brain injury. On the other hand, families often can be extremely creative in providing the external structures to minimize the effect of such deficits on everyday life. Emotional, behavioral, and personality changes, however, such as anger outbursts, self-centeredness, impulsivity, disinhibition, and social insensitivity, are extremely difficult to cope with because they can appear suddenly and unpredictably, have (even if not intended) a direct emotional impact on the recipient, are often embarrassing to others, and are extremely difficult to control. Not only do these characterological problems increase stress in internal family life, they also lead to family isolation as fewer friends visit, social outings decrease, and the immediate family bears increasing responsibility for the social network of the person with brain injury.

For example, a young father with brainstem and frontal lobe injuries after a high-speed motor vehicle accident and extended coma will typically have physical, cognitive, and behavioral changes. He may learn to compensate for an ataxic gait by walking slower, using a cane on uneven surfaces, and avoiding activities requiring speed and agil-

ity. He may learn to compensate in part for severe memory deficits by keeping a detailed memory book, writing down all telephone messages, keeping lists and checking things off as he does them, and posting visual cues around the house for things he needs to do. Adaptations to these physical and cognitive deficits may enable him to be a semiproductive and reliable helper at home. However, if he is behaviorally disinhibited, his outbursts of rage at his wife and children may make him difficult to be around, and his unpredictable and embarrassing disparagement of guests may make it impossible to have friends over, essentially isolating the family and leading to severe emotional and interpersonal problems within it.

These generalizations tend to apply to all "families" in which two or more persons are living together. Specific variations occur, however, depending on whether the person with TBI is a parent or a child, and brain injury in the family affects spouses, parents, siblings, and children in different ways. These variable effects on family roles are considered in the following section.

Family Structure and Role Changes

The impact of TBI on various members of the family system has been documented in the literature; for example, Williams and Kay (1991) included a number of first-person accounts from family members, and Lezak (1978, 1988) provided clinical commentary on various family roles.

Impact on Spouses

In many ways, the spouse, usually the wife, bears the greatest burden when the partner sustains a brain injury. An equal adult partnership has been broken, and the uninjured spouse is often thrust into the role of caregiver—both for the injured partner and for the family when there are children. The result is often financial burden, loss of support, and isolation. Younger spouses may become more dependent on their families of origin, especially if the injured partner is unable to independently carry out household responsibilities. In-law conflicts may erupt between the parents of the injured person and his or her spouse over care issues. In premarital, committed relationships, boyfriends or girlfriends may be excluded and shut out from contact by protective family members who "circle the wagons" against someone not perceived as being part of the family; this can have poisonous effects for years. In traditional families in which the husband was the "family executive," the wife may be thrust into managing and decision-making roles for which she is not prepared. (Increasingly, it is common for the wife to play this executive role.) Spouses often express the feeling of being "single parents": "My husband and I used to have two children; now I feel like I have three." Even in situations in which the injury is less severe and the injured partner is able to return to some type of work, it often is far below preaccident levels, and major lifestyle changes are required of the family. With social sympathy and concern flowing mainly toward the injured partner, the caretaking spouse often feels his or her needs go totally neglected, and this can lead to bitterness, despair, or burnout. When there are children, the spouse may be without an equal parenting partner, and in fact competition may develop between the children and the injured partner for the spouse's attention.

Especially in more severe injuries, spouses may feel married to a different person—one they no longer love or feel attracted to. Spouses face an enormous conflict between commitment and guilt if they consider leaving the relationship. This is particularly the case when the couple is young and have either no or young children. The spouse often realistically faces the choice of "sacrificing" his or her life to the injured partner or leaving the relationship to develop a new family. These are difficult moral and personal choices, and the professional is best advised to help the spouse sort out the options rather than imposing his or her own value system. In less tragic cases, enough of the personality and competence of the injured person remain on which to build a mutually satisfying commitment.

The situation in which the uninjured partner is considering divorce poses ethical and treatment dilemmas for the clinician. When the identified patient is clearly the person with TBI, it may be appropriate to find another therapist to help the partner, or the couple, deal with the divorce issues. When the identified "patient" is the family, however, it is appropriate for the clinician to work with the whole system—or the parental subsystem—to help the family face these issues. Unlike many mutually agreed-on divorces, however, divorces after TBI are often more unilaterally sought (by the uninjured partner), and the process of negotiating this transition is a combination of supporting the uninjured spouse (who is often ridden with guilt) and negotiating new support systems for the reluctant, angry, and frightened person with TBI—tasks usually more comfortably handled by two persons.

Countertransference issues often arise in working with young families of individuals with severe injuries if the personal value system of the clinician is at odds with the decisions of the uninjured partner, or the therapist's fantasies of improvement and happiness collide with the realities of the marital relationship. These feelings can arise in either direction: the therapist may unconsciously encourage the partner perceived as "trapped" to find a way out or unconsciously discourage a desperate spouse from "abandoning" the injured partner. Awareness of his or her personal feelings is crucial for the therapist, and transfer of the case is appropriate if the decisions of the uninjured partner make it impossible for the clinician to be fully supportive. Sorting out these countertransference issues, from realistically helping the partner to think through the consequences of his or her choices to knowing when to turn the case over to a colleague, is a crucial but tricky process, requiring self-searching by the therapist and, often, consultation with a colleague.

Even when marriages do survive, sexuality and intimacy are often difficult (see Chapter 25, Sexual Dysfunction). Persons with brain injury may have decreased capacity for intimacy and either heightened or lowered sexual drive and may be impaired in their ability to perform sexually (for physiological or psychological reasons). Wives in particular may be pressed to meet the sexual demands of the injured spouse, with little satisfaction for themselves. It is not uncommon for sexual relationships to stop entirely; when the spouse chooses to stay in the marriage, he or she may seek out (with much guilt and need for support) sexual relationships outside the marriage.

Impact on Parents

When a child is injured, special burdens and pressures exist for the parents. When a young child living at home is injured, the mother usually takes on the role of primary nurturer and caregiver. This may create tension within the marital relationship, and underlying cracks or strains in the relationship may become manifest. Husbands may unconsciously compete with the injured child for the mother's limited resources. When couples are composed of persons with complementary coping styles, the stress of caring for a severely injured child may drive them to opposite extremes of reaction and threaten the relationship; for example, the father may bury himself in his work while the mother drops everything (including any attention to her husband) and devotes all her energy to the injured child. Parents may also find it difficult to apportion their time and energy to other children or to elderly parents whom they may care for. Even when they work well together around the crisis, parents may find their lives dominated by the needs of the injured child and may be in jeopardy of neglecting their own marital relationship (e.g., no longer spending time together separate from their children) or may be cut off from adult social activities with friends.

When the injured child is an adult who had been living independently, parents often are thrown back into an earlier developmental phase of caring for a dependent child, with the complication that the grown child resents and resists the dependency. This is an extremely difficult position for both parents and child, especially when the child is male, recently past adolescence, and striving for autonomy. Driving, independent living, dating, and establishing friends and intimate relationships become volatile family issues. Parents often have great difficulty accepting the permanent changes in their children and in fact may complicate the rehabilitation process by refusing to give up unrealistic expectations ("My son *will* become a lawyer!"). Conflicts may develop between the parents over what is reasonable to expect of their adult child with brain injury. When adult children move back in with their parents for a period after a brain injury, it is not uncommon for old psychological terrain of the struggle for independence to be traversed again. How this was negotiated the first time around in adolescence is often predictive of how things will go the second time around. Sensitive clinicians can be extremely helpful to families during this period by normalizing the conflicts around independence and individuation and helping negotiate a series of compromises that respect both the needs of the parents to be protective and the needs of the adult child to start regaining independence.

Special issues attend the parent–school relationship for younger children through adolescents. These issues are addressed in the section Special Issues later in this chapter.

Impact on Children

Children of parents with brain injury face special problems over which they have little control. Younger children may suddenly find that they have lost the nurturance and guidance of a formerly loving and competent parent. The injured parent may be unpredictable, irritable, or even in competition with them for the uninjured parent's attention. Older children at home usually have increased responsibilities, less attention from the other parent, and an awkward home situation into which they are uncomfortable bringing their peers. Depending on the preexisting relationship, the child may be drawn emotionally closer to or driven farther away from and resent the injured parent. Older children may have more capacity to understand what has happened but also more freedom to create distance. It is not uncommon for school or behavioral problems to surface in children who are depressed, angry, or guilty about their new family situation.

When an older parent incurs a brain injury, adult children who are out of the house are inevitably faced with the issue of taking on increased responsibility. Because of

their own adult responsibilities, children are often limited in how much assistance they can actually contribute, with inevitable feelings of guilt. Adult children are often torn between the needs of their partners and children and those of their parents. Conflicts often develop between the caregiving adult child and his or her spouse, with resulting imbalance and conflict within the family. Conflicts can also erupt among siblings with an injured parent over perceptions of uneven participation in caregiving. Interventions with spouses of adult children with parents with TBI are often the most effective way to stabilize the support system for the injured parent. Therapists need to be realistic, however, in assessing how much any one child is willing and able to give and help other siblings deal emotionally with perceived inequalities.

Impact on Siblings

With most attention being paid to the child with the injury, uninjured siblings often become unrecognized "victims" of shifts in the family system after TBI. When the siblings are young and living at home with the injured child, the parents characteristically reorient all of their attention and energy toward the child with the brain injury. Children who suddenly feel lack of attention from their parents often act out their needs in ways not initially seen as related to their sibling's injury. This acting out may take the form of failing grades or getting into trouble at school. Parents need support in finding a balance in allocating limited resources among their children. Older children at home may, like children of injured parents, have more domestic responsibilities and perhaps also a socially awkward situation into which they are embarrassed to bring friends. Siblings of different personality styles and relationships with the injured child may also respond in different ways; one sibling may become closer to the injured child while another moves away in anger.

Older siblings who are not living at home experience stresses similar to those of adult children of injured parents. The demands of their own lives, perhaps including a spouse and children, compete against the need and desire to help their sibling. Typically, one adult sibling is designated as the primary caregiver, especially if the injured sibling is unmarried and the parents are distant or too old to take on a primary caregiving role. Support from the sibling's family is essential for him or her to play an effective role.

Impact on Extended Family

The impact of TBI on extended family networks is seldom discussed. The reality is that, especially in a mobile, urban society, kinship bonds often are more tenuous than they used to be, and aunts, uncles, and cousins seldom play a significant role in the primary care of any person with brain injury. (This does not hold in cultural groups in which a high value is placed on networks of extended families.) From our perspective, it is helpful for the nuclear family, whenever possible, to involve the extended family as early as possible in learning about the injury, the recovery process, and how to normalize the new person who emerges. Nuclear families who are able to tap into the support systems of extended families, even once or twice a year for respite, have a great advantage. Families often are unable to elicit the active support of relatives, however, because extended family members who do not live with the injured person often do not understand, are less sympathetic toward the family stresses, or are simply more wary of becoming involved. It is extremely useful for professionals working with families to include extended families in family meetings, especially early on, to establish a basis for a wider support network.

Family Responses to TBI: Stage Theories

The family's process of adjusting to TBI evolves over time; it involves becoming aware of the nature, extent, and permanence of neurobehavioral deficits and reestablishing a new set of family roles, structure, and routines to adapt to these changes. Successful clinical intervention with families requires the professional to be aware of where in this process of adjustment the family is; this determines what the family is able to hear and what kind of support is needed.

There are a number of useful ways to conceptualize the continuum of changes that families pass through. These are expressed as various stages, although it is clear that there is no objectively and universally true sequence. In discussing the effect of TBI on the family in the section Family Structure and Role Changes, we made reference to three main stages: the acute phase, the rehabilitation phase, and the integration phase. These stages are tied to a medically defined system of rehabilitation.

In the acute phase, the family is dealing with issues of survival and minimizing the extent of physical and neurological damage. The family generally is suspending normal routines and orienting all resources toward the injured person.

In the rehabilitation phase, the medically stable person enters a phase of intensive treatment aimed at restoration of functioning at the highest level possible. This is a time when high expectations for recovery pre-

TABLE 30–3. Stages of family adjustment
Initial shock
Emotional relief, denial, and unrealistic expectation
Acknowledgment of permanent deficits and emotional turmoil
Bargaining
Mourning or working through
Acceptance and restructuring

Source. Based on Rape RN, Busch JP, Slavin LA: "Toward a Conceptualization of the Family's Adaptation to a Member's Head Injury: A Critique of Developmental Stage Models." *Rehabilitation Psychology* 37:3–22, 1992.

dominate, and the family begins the task of receiving the injured person back into the family system and making the necessary structural adjustments. The rehabilitation may be on an inpatient or outpatient basis, but active treatment keeps open the possibility of unlimited improvement.

The integration phase is the lengthiest and most difficult and involves integration in two senses. First, the injured person is completing formal treatment and is, as much as possible, becoming gradually reintegrated into the community (e.g., socially and vocationally). Second, this is a time of reintegration for the family system. Expectations for complete recovery begin to recede as the reality of permanent neurobehavioral impairment in the injured person becomes apparent, and the family system attempts to strike a new, more permanent balance to allow its various members to proceed with their own lives. There is enormous variability during this final phase, which itself is composed of a series of stages of internal adjustment.

A number of other authors proposed stage theories of family adjustment after TBI. Rape et al. (1992) described and analyzed a number of these. These authors identified six major stages incorporated in most (but not all) of the stage theories they analyzed. (These stages are listed in Table 30–3.) Rape et al. noted that the hypothesized stages lacked empirical validation, often failed to meet the criteria for defining explanatory epigenetic stages, and contained conceptual problems (e.g., why some families adapt whereas others become stuck at one of the stages). They proposed integrating a family systems perspective into stage theories to solve some of these problems, and they advocated longitudinal research.

Prominent among the stage theories specific to TBI is Lezak's (1986) six-stage model of family adjustment after TBI, which introduces subphases into the integration phase. After the injured person returns home, the family passes through a series of perceptions, expectations, and reactions, beginning with minimizing problems and expecting full recovery and happiness about survival (I), through bewilderment and anxiety (II), discouragement and guilt (III), and depression, despair, and feeling trapped (IV). Families who ultimately move beyond their sorrow go through two final stages of grieving (V) and reorganization-emotional disengagement (VI). Lezak emphasized that many families are unable to move beyond chronic depression and despair. In our experience, it is often 2 years or more posttrauma before family members begin the true process of mourning that propels them to resume healthier life cycles for the rest of the family. Even then, some families seem better adapted than others to accepting the new realities and limits and are able to let go of old goals and hopes for complete recovery and find dignity in a new family constellation. Other families remain angry, bitter, and unaccepting, often blaming professionals for lack of recovery and constantly seeking the "right" rehabilitation program. Rape et al. (1992) provided some initial integration of systems theory and stage theory to account for these individual differences.

Kübler-Ross (1969) proposed an intrapsychic model of an individual's response to the prospect of death and dying, which is often applied to TBI, and described the process of the family as a system, or each individual family member, proceeding through the stages of denial, anger, bargaining, depression, and acceptance. Although it is absolutely true that each family member goes through some or all of these feelings in coping with TBI, we believe that there are some problems, indeed some dangers, in applying this model too simplistically to a family's response to TBI. First, the fact that the mourned person still lives and is present interferes with the normal grieving process in and of itself. Second, the denial so often noted in families of persons with brain injury (Romano 1974) often is treated as something to be dislodged by therapists if families do not heed therapists' prognostications early in the rehabilitation process about the permanence of deficits. The reality is that early denial—especially continuing to believe in the possibility of significant recovery—is an effective buffer against depression (Ridley 1989), may be necessary for the family to regroup, and should be respected by professionals. Third, the notion of a steady final stage of acceptance—in the sense of an emotionally peaceful embracing of the way things are—is neither realistic nor, perhaps, desirable to expect. Transitions in the family's life cycle bring episodic loss and rekindle the mourning process. It is also adaptive for families to keep their level of dissatisfaction alive because it can fuel needed periods of advocacy at different points of the injured person's life. Most important, harm has been done to families in turmoil years after an injury by professionals

who expect that because families are not demonstrating "acceptance" after so much time, a psychopathological process must be occurring. The reality is that living with an adult with brain injury brings cycles of adjustment, disequilibrium, and reestablishment of a new balance on a periodic basis, and this recycling never ends. The Kübler-Ross stages are best seen as an individual's internal responses that are likely to be replayed numerous times over the course of the life cycle. The family system's process of adjustment is too complex to reduce to such a set of stages.

That the grieving process after disability does not simply reach a steady state of acceptance has been recognized by a number of persons working outside the area of TBI. Olshansky (1962), for example, introduced the notion of "chronic sorrow" to describe the continued experience of sadness and ongoing adjustment that parents of mentally retarded children feel. Wikler (1981), working within the same framework, recognized that such chronic sorrow is punctuated by periods of more intense grieving at critical developmental junctures. Other formulations emphasized normal family life cycles (Carter and McGoldrick 1980) or life "spirals"—recurrent patterns of events that cycle through family systems across generations (Combrinck-Graham 1985). These are periods of normal transition (e.g., births, graduations, new jobs, marriages, and retirements) separating broader bands of life commitments (e.g., childhood, studenthood, and parenthood). Williams (1991a) applied these concepts to TBI and developed the notion of "episodic loss," in which the initial grieving process over the changed person is revisited at critical points in the family life cycle. The son with brain injury who does not begin to date normally, does not enter college, remains unmarried through early adulthood, and does not present grandchildren to his aging parents represents a situation in which the initial family adjustment to permanent disability must be emotionally recreated at critical times in the family's life cycle. Adjustment to loss is reexperienced episodically both by the injured person and by emotionally linked family members. Finally, Rolland (1987a, 1987b, 1990) developed a model that categorizes chronic illness according to its onset, course, outcome, and degree of incapacitation, describes its unfolding over time, and integrates concepts of family individuality and family life cycles.

A Model of Assessment and Intervention

Families are thrown into crisis at the moment a person is injured. Psychiatric intervention should not be reserved

---

TABLE 30–4.   A model of family assessment and intervention after traumatic brain injury

Concentric circles of intervention

    Individual family members

    The family as a system

    Relationship of family to community

Levels of intervention

    Information and education

    Support, problem solving, and restructuring

    Formal therapy

Stages of intervention

    Acute care

    Rehabilitation

    Community reintegration

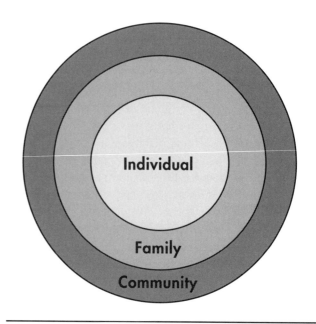

FIGURE 30–1.   Concentric circles of intervention.

for severe management problems or dysfunctional families. Family intervention should be proactive, flexible, health and prevention oriented, and responsive to the needs of families within the context of a progressive reestablishment of family equilibrium after brain injury.

The quality of family functioning has direct impact on the process of rehabilitation. "Dysfunctional" families may fail to join forces with the rehabilitation team, deliver conflicting messages, or respond to behaviors in ways that undercut the team's approach, all of which result in the patient's being caught between the family and treating professionals in a way that undermines the rehabilitation process. However, much of what professionals perceive as "dysfunctional" in families is the result of families being uninformed, underinvolved, and not having basic needs met, all of which may be preventable with appropriate interventions.

We propose a three-dimensional model of intervention (Table 30–4): *where* the intervention is aimed (concentric circles of intervention), *what* the intervention is (levels of intervention), and *when* it occurs (stages of intervention). Each of these dimensions itself contains three progressive levels.

Concentric Circles of Intervention

In evaluating the family of a person with brain injury, our model suggests thinking of that family as composed of three sets, or units, nested within each other (Figure 30–1): 1) the *individual family members*, 2) the *family as a system*, and 3) the *relationship of the family to the community*. Each of these systems must be assessed independently, and different interventions can be made at each level depending

on what stage the family is in. (The concept of concentric circles, as an alternative to the more traditional "unstable triad" of person, family, and society as bearing responsibility for the long-term care needs of persons with TBI, was first proposed by DeJong et al. in 1990.)

The clinician should evaluate individual family members in terms of their personality structure, their expectations for the injured person and the family, the individual strengths and weaknesses they bring to the family, and how they respond both to the person with the injury and to the current family situation. Individual family members may have particular attitudes, limitations, or strengths that become crucial in the rehabilitation process (e.g., a mother's need for her son not to hold a menial job, a father's need to not let others make decisions for his family, or a sibling's commitment to support an injured child). Individual family members may be at risk or in crisis, or may simply need support because they are shouldering a large share of the family's responsibilities. At times, the most effective family intervention is a targeted intervention with an individual family member.

The family system must be considered as a unit above and beyond its individual members. What are the structures and roles in this family, and how have they shifted as a result of the injury? What are the patterns of relationship and communication, and how are problems solved? How cohesive is the family unit, and what is the degree of enmeshment or disengagement? How flexible is the family in responding to challenges? What specific cultural norms do the family hold that may be different from the rehabilitation team's and that will color expectations of what is important in outcome, and how it is achieved? (See Williams and Savage 1991, for examples of cultural values applied to TBI rehabilitation.) What values do the family hold that will influence goals and expectations? (Strong cultural differences may exist among families, especially recent immigrant families.) Often, the failure of the rehabilitation team to appreciate strongly held family norms, values, or needs leads to conflict and an impasse in the rehabilitation process. Assessing the family system is crucial, and often strategic interventions within the family structure are critical to enabling a family to move on and cope more effectively.

The family's relationship to the community also must be assessed, and, often, crucial interventions need to be made not within the family system itself, but at the interface of the family and its community. The community is both the professional community of services that needs to be accessed and the psychosocial community of friends, recreation, and extended family. The history of a family's relationships to these communities is the best predictor of how they will respond in the crisis situation of TBI. In the early stages, intervention at this level almost always involves negotiating a good working relationship between the family (often as represented by one or two key members) and the rehabilitation team. Forging a strong working alliance is crucial for successful rehabilitation. In later stages, families must learn to deal with the world of multiple, often bureaucratic, community services, and if they are to overcome the natural tendency toward isolation, they must reestablish functional social and recreational opportunities. One often overlooked community relationship in the early stages is the family's need to establish quick communication with the world of insurance and legal matters. For families with injured children, the educational world is the major community relationship. Effective family intervention pays attention not only to the internal matters of the family, but to the family's relationship to various aspects of the community as well.

Special issues exist for recent immigrant families, often in large urban centers, who are locked into enclaves of culturally homogeneous families. Mainstream services often do not extend into such communities or are unknown or rejected. Language barriers often limit how effective outside professionals can be. In these situations, it is extremely helpful to identify a bilingual person within the family's community who can act as a translator throughout the process of community integration. Many large cities fund agencies to provide bilingual social workers or case managers for families from ethnic subcultures with special needs.

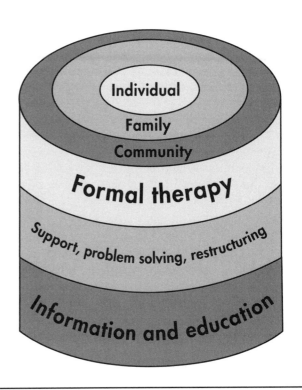

FIGURE 30–2. Levels of intervention.

Levels of Intervention

A second principle of our model is that family intervention need not equal family therapy. Effective family intervention requires that the clinician think in terms of levels of intervention that are appropriate to the situation (Muir et al. 1990; Rosenthal and Muir 1983). Our model defines three levels of intervention: 1) information and education; 2) support, problem solving, and restructuring; and 3) formal therapy. Figure 30–2 illustrates how these three levels of intervention—in ascending order from the most basic to the most complex—cut across the dimensions of individual, family, and community described in the section Concentric Circles of Intervention.

At the most basic level, families in which a brain injury has occurred need information and education at all stages of intervention (see next section), from acute care to community reentry. In the earliest acute phase, education is the most crucial intervention, although long-term prognostication is impossible. Families need to know what has physically happened to the person and his or her brain, what treatments are being given and why, what can be expected over the next few days and weeks, how to understand unusual behavior (e.g., confusion, agitation, and disinhibition) and how to respond to it, how to anticipate and respond to cognitive deficits (e.g., disorientation, severe memory problems, and lack of language), what treatment options should be considered, and what their insurance and legal options are.

The timing of providing information is also crucial, as is judging how much information the family is able to take in. In early stages of recovery, families need to sustain hope and cannot be overwhelmed with dire warnings and pessimistic projections. The seeds of long-term limitations are quietly planted early, but the skilled clinician will know when the family is ready to have them nurtured. Likewise, it is unethical to steer families toward program decisions without making them aware of the full range of options. Since the 1980s, an enormous amount of informational material (of variable quality) has been developed for families, and the Brain Injury Association of America is an excellent resource for such materials (see contact information in the section Brain Injury Association of America and Other Support Organizations). Most good rehabilitation facilities develop specific educational programs for families to inform them about TBI in a systematic way (Klonoff and Prigatano 1987; Rosenthal and Hutchins 1991). Educational programs that include open discussions also can be an excellent indirect and nonthreatening way to enable families to face their own emotional reactions in a way they would not if offered the more direct opportunity of group sessions run by psychologists or psychiatrists.

Support, problem solving, and restructuring can be effective family intervention at individual, system, or community-relations levels. For example, the overwhelmed wife of a husband with a brain injury may need structure and guided problem solving in deciding how to manage a family on limited resources. A large family whose mother returns home after a brain injury may need to sit down as a group and negotiate how family responsibilities should be reapportioned and deal with the inevitable feelings and conflicts generated by that process. The family who feels "trapped" at home with an impulsive and aggressive teenage son may need help in finding creative ways to maintain social relationships in the community or even how to take vacations. This level of intervention requires an active therapist who knows the realities of adjusting to brain injury and builds on the strengths and problem-solving capacities of the family and its individual members. As noted above in the section on review of research, there is increasing evidence that social support moderates how families function and how much burden caregivers experience. Sometimes, helping families negotiate transportation, figure out a way to pay for a piece of equipment, or find a weekend social program for their child is a more needed and effective intervention than ideas and psychological discussion.

Formal therapy becomes appropriate when severe problems are rendering the family system, or some part of it, dysfunctional. The stress and family changes inherent in TBI may cause family members to need individual therapy (often because the injured person is a family member previously seen as strong, such as a sibling or child). Individual family members who benefit from psychotherapy usually begin with issues related to brain injury, but often end up dealing with longer-standing personal or family of origin issues. This is what distinguishes this level of intervention from the previous two: all families benefit from education and problem solving; some family members require longer-term formal treatment because of issues outside the event of TBI. The same holds true for the family as a system. Families that were dysfunctional before the injury may require formal family therapy after the injury, with the added complication of learning to adjust their family structure. Decisions about the nature of this family therapy, and the extent to which the person with brain injury will be able to fully participate, should be on the basis of individual circumstances and the injured person's neurobehavioral competence.

Stages of Intervention

We have broadly divided the effect of TBI on the family into three main stages: 1) acute care, 2) rehabilitation, and 3) community reintegration, being fully aware that the third stage is open-ended and itself contains numerous subphases. This broad division, however, is useful in conceptualizing the nature of interventions that must be made during each stage. Figure 30–3 illustrates the concept that, at each of these temporal stages, interventions can be conceptualized at the three levels (information and education; support, problem solving, and restructuring; formal therapy) and within the three concentric domains (individual, family, community) described in the preceding sections.

In *acute care*, families gather their resources and organize around the injured person. This is a period of crisis intervention when education and information are crucial. Emotional support and permission to break standard family routines also are important. Later within this stage, when survival is assured, the family must quickly evaluate treatment options and insurance realities. Family intervention should be aimed at helping the family to cope effectively on numerous fronts while still in shock, including practical daily realities, emotional distress, and major decision making.

Rehabilitation is defined as the intermediate stage during which formal restorative treatment, inpatient or outpatient, is the primary family focus. During this stage, there is initially relief at survival and great hope for recovery, which the therapist should support, while gradually tempering hope with cautious reality. Even when therapists realistically assess severe limits of long-term func-

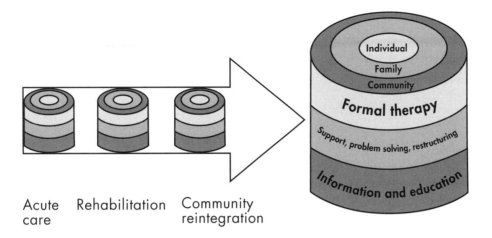

FIGURE 30–3. **Stages of intervention.**

tioning, families may be angered and alienated if this message is presented prematurely or too starkly. It is much better to help families gradually realize (rather than be told) emerging limitations through experience. It is during this stage when major family role restructuring often takes place, and individuals may need help in adjusting to their new roles. Toward the end of the rehabilitation stage, it will begin to become apparent that even though formal treatment is ending, complete recovery has not occurred, and the family faces the prospect of living with a permanently disabled person. This is a crucial time for intervention, when the therapist begins to deal with the anxieties and fears of the family.

Community reintegration, as noted in the section Concentric Circles of Intervention, refers both to the person with brain injury and to the family system as they struggle to reenter community life under drastically changed circumstances. This is when discouragement, depression, despair, and mourning begin to occur, often over the first few years after the end of rehabilitation. Family interventions usually become more needed, more intense, and longer term. The crucial turning point occurs when, after all formal rehabilitation ends, the family as a system faces the challenge of being able to reconstitute as an effective and functional system with a new balance and identity. Not all families are able to do so. In families who cannot, the life cycle is seriously disrupted, and individual members may be blocked from making natural life transitions in a healthy way. For example, a busy professional couple may be unable to reorganize their time and finances to care for a severely injured son who lives at home, and that role may fall to a teenage daughter. If she becomes trapped in that role, she may stay home after high school and devote herself to caring for her brother, with the result that her own development (college, career, boyfriends, marriage) may be seri-

ously blocked. Depending on her nature, she may either become seriously depressed or sacrifice herself for the sake of the family to her long-term "detriment." In working with such families, clinicians must be careful to sort out what is detrimental in their eyes from what is detrimental in the eyes of different family members. The decision to intervene when the self-sacrifice is in the service of homeostasis raises difficult countertransference and ethical issues, which must be dealt with honestly both by the therapist and directly with the family. Often, it is when a family member reaches a developmental transition (e.g., when the caregiving daughter's friends begin to marry) that the family becomes destabilized and productive intervention can begin.

Even when families do make the transition and their life cycle resumes, transitional points can bring episodic loss and mourning (see Family Responses to TBI: Stage Theories). For example, a family may adapt quite well to a severe TBI in a young child, but when his or her peers begin Little League and he or she does not, or when dating, high school graduation, college, and marriage do not occur as they naturally would, there is sadness for the family and a retouching of old hurts and losses. It is crucial during this period to help families build on their strength and dignity, and especially important to enable the person with the brain injury to find a productive and meaningful place in the family, with peers, and in the community.

The relationship of the family to the community is particularly important during this stage. Families need to learn to draw comfortably on the existing resources of extended family, friends, employers, churches, and other community organizations and to resist the tendency to become isolated, ashamed, and self-conscious or to shield the community from the injured person (although the conscious motive is usually the opposite). Family interventions should include a circle of support that is often wider than would initially be comfortable for the family. Family-to-family programs, self-help groups, family outreach and advocacy, and community networking are all concepts that the savvy family therapist uses (Williams 1991b). Family intervention at this final stage of reintegration should move beyond the confines of the office into the community.

Long-Term Issues

In the acute care and rehabilitation phases, as well as early in the community reintegration phase, most professional intervention provided to the family takes place within a "medical model" of service provision. As noted in the preceding section, once the family moves into the community reintegration phase, medical model supports become less available and, possibly, less useful, and the family's relationship to the community and community-based supports becomes more salient. In the past, community-based supports after TBI took the form of either informal family and community organizations (e.g., churches) or TBI-specific self-help groups that provide services such as educational materials, support groups, and mentoring or family-to-family programs, all of which are useful and important. However, in recent years, a variety of professional long-term community-based supports have become available. In fact, as funding for short-term medical model rehabilitation services has become more restricted (because of the influence of the managed care environment), funding streams, usually in the form of Medicaid Waivers or Trust Funds supported by fees on (for example) drunk drivers, have allowed for the proliferation of a variety of previously unavailable long-term community-based support systems (Digre et al. 1994; Rosen and Reynolds 1994; Spearman et al. 2001). Such supports—which are not equally available throughout the country—may include long-term service coordination ("case management"), in-home supervision and skill training, substance abuse services, and day programs.

Regarding community-based day programs (as opposed to medical model day treatment programs), probably the most widely known model is that of the Clubhouse, but in recent years other excellent models specific to the needs of individuals with TBI have developed. The Community-Based Day Rehabilitation model developed through the TBI Services Department of the Association for the Help of Retarded Children in New York City serves as an example of an approach to providing long-term (life-long if necessary) services to individuals with TBI within a day program environment. In this model, individuals attend a 6-hour-per-day program for as many days as they choose (Monday through Friday). The indi-

vidual sets the goals he or she has for him- or herself with the assistance and guidance of staff and family members. These goals may change as the needs of the individual change across his or her life span. The individual may attend the program as long as needed. For some, it is an excellent stepping stone for vocational advancement; for others, it may potentially provide a life-long learning and socialization environment. The program provides a variety of in-house cognitive, psychosocial, and skill groups and activities, but the primary work and socialization activities take place outside of the program site at a wide variety of settings within the community. Individuals choose the community activities they wish to be involved in and may go on a daily basis to community activities of their choice. They are accompanied into the community by a small group of peers (usually three other participants) and a staff person. Activities vary but are always associated with skill development. The overall goals of the program are the development and enhancement of skills, use of compensatory strategies in an increased variety of settings, increased awareness, increased socialization opportunities, and community inclusion.

The key points are that these community-based supports are long term (life-long, if necessary), supportive, person centered, and consumer driven. These types of supports are extremely helpful to families in the long run. The service coordination aspect alone relieves families of much of the logistical and practical, if not emotional, burdens. They also provide for ongoing interventions as needed. Some may even provide community living opportunities for individuals with an injury, which may help normalize as much as possible the family role and life cycle issues.

Over the long term, the issues families deal with tend to become more focused on quality of life rather than on the restoration of specific functions and abilities. Issues such as employment or productivity, intimacy, sexuality, and community inclusion become primary. In our experience, there is an ongoing sense of loss and visible grieving, not just by family members, but by the individuals themselves about their "lost self"; who they used to be, who they thought they were going to become, and their lost abilities and plans for the future. This may become less prominent with increased socialization opportunities and increased success in the community but rarely entirely disappears. In working with families whose member was injured 10, 15, or even 20 years earlier, we still see grief, anger, guilt, and even denial. The usual pattern is that these emotions "erupt" periodically and present in "waves" and appear to be the clinical manifestations of what we have described as episodic loss reactions or chronic sorrow (see Family Responses to TBI: Stage Theories).

Another interesting clinical observation is how family members will sometimes actively resist even positive change in the individual with TBI if it involves increased autonomy within the family and/or community or self-advocacy. Sometimes, what staff may see as progress in individuals with TBI in self-care, autonomy, or the ability to make decisions for themselves, the family sees as increased noncompliance with the newly established family routines, roles, and rules or as potentially dangerous situations. This may stem from fear for and protectiveness of the injured individual and from the many years of struggling to establish a new family homeostasis. Family members may have been forced to take on a greater role in the supervision and care of the injured individual. This may have become the new and accepted dynamic in the family, and disrupting it, even by positive change or opportunities, may lead to a need for further family restructuring and education. Families need support and guidance through this process.

Special Issues

Family Issues in Mild TBI

A special set of dynamics applies to mild TBI (see Chapter 15, Mild Brain Injury and the Postconcussion Syndrome), which deviates somewhat from some of the principles outlined in this chapter. *Mild TBI* refers to injuries with brief or no loss of consciousness, no long-term focal neurological abnormalities, usually normal computed tomography scans and magnetic resonance imaging studies, and a constellation of symptoms, including headache; irritability; fatigue; sleep disturbance; poor attention, concentration, and memory; depression; anxiety; poor self-esteem; and general inability to function (Kay 1986). Psychological overlay can accumulate with time and increases dysfunction, which usually reflects a complex interaction among organic, personality, and environmental factors. In many cases, a legitimate, if subtle, brain injury underlies and drives the dysfunction, which is layered over with maladaptive psychological reactions, many of which result from inappropriate environmental responses (Kay 1992).

Although in moderate to severe brain injury the family tends to rally around, support, and advocate for the injured person, one often sees a picture of initial concern followed by increasing alienation in families after mild TBI. This is the result of the injured person's apparent normalcy in the presence of his or her anxiety, depression, loss of self-esteem, and increasing dysfunction over time.

An essential part of any neuropsychiatric treatment of such complex and difficult cases is immediate family in-volvement. Family responses and reactions to the apparent discrepancy between severity of injury and severity of symptoms can either induce or exacerbate a dysfunctional postconcussional syndrome. The family needs information and education about the nature and consequences of concussion and how to understand and help the patient manage his or her symptoms. Also, any alienation that develops between the injured person and the family should be healed. Often, this involves addressing old issues, either intrapersonal or within the family system, which are in fact contributing to the excessive level of dysfunction. It is a mistake to see the obvious emotional overlay in such cases and dismiss the injured person as malingering or the problems as purely psychosomatic ones. The individual cannot be helped back to a level of productive functioning without addressing what is often a deteriorated family situation.

Parents and the School System

The normal relationship of parent to school is dramatically altered when a child has a TBI. The keys to successful adjustment for a student with TBI—from prekindergarten through high school—are contact, communication, consistency, and flexibility.

Contact

Unless the school is familiar with students with TBI and has special procedures in place—which is unusual and unlikely—the parents will need to be the ones to initiate contact with the school around the special needs of their child. This needs to start long before the child is ready to return to school—soon after the accident has occurred while the child is still in the acute or rehabilitation stage. The school should be apprised of the child's injury and school materials made available to rehabilitation professionals at the appropriate time. When the child is nearing discharge home, the parents need to make sure the rehabilitation team is putting together recommendations for school needs and help the team contact the appropriate school personnel. The parents should ask to sit down and meet with school staff in advance of the child's return and not be afraid to bring with them a member of the rehabilitation team or other expert in the community on TBI and education. Depending on the severity of the injury, the time since injury, and the student's stamina, the return to school may need to be gradual. Again, the parents should take the lead in contacting the school to work out these decisions. As the child's school career progresses, there may be needs for special evaluations or special services. Parents should be assertive in contacting the school about such special needs. They should not be afraid to identify advocates within the community and include them in school meetings. This does not mean there needs to be an adversarial relationship between the parents and the school. Quite the opposite: the goal is to establish a collaborative working relationship in which both school staff and parents are focusing on what is in the child's best interest. The message, however, is that the parents should be prepared to initiate contacts with the school around the child's needs.

Communication

Three levels of communication are critical when a child returns to school after a TBI: between parents and school, among those persons working with the child within the school, and between professionals working with the child outside the school and the school. First, parents need to take the initiative to meet on a regular basis with the teacher(s) and service providers within the school. This is particularly true on school reentry and at the beginning of each school year or semester, or both (when teachers and classes may be changing). Periodic team meetings with all involved persons should be the goal. More frequent face-to-face or telephone contact with the classroom or research room or homeroom teacher is appropriate. For younger children, a communications book in which the teachers, parents, and therapists write notes, requests, and concerns is often extremely helpful. Assignments should be checked for clarity so parents can monitor homework when necessary. Second, it is equally important that the child's school program be integrated— that is, that all the teachers and therapists are communicating with each other about their goals and the strategies they are using. When parents sense communication is not happening internally and services are becoming fragmented, it is appropriate for them to request that the school arrange time for the persons involved with the child to meet on a regular basis. Third, it is also important that there be communication between the school and those professionals treating the child outside the school setting. For example, physical therapists and occupational therapists (OTs) within and outside the school should communicate about their goals and strategies to learn from each other. It is also important that there be an open line of communication between the school and physicians, especially around behavioral issues, when seizures are suspected, or when medication is an issue. Physicians need input from the school on the child's behavior, and the school needs to know when medical changes have been made. It is the parents' responsibility to allow and foster such open communication.

Consistency

A child with TBI thrives most when there is consistency of approach between school and home. This is true in both cognitive and behavioral domains. When parents are involved in helping with homework, which they often are, they should discuss with teachers and therapists which compensatory strategies work best, and there should be consistency of implementation of these strategies across home and school settings as well as consistency across internal school settings. (For example, the history teacher, the science teacher, and the parents all should be using the same approach in helping a child with executive deficits develop a topic and outline for a paper.) Behaviorally, it is even more critical that difficult behaviors be dealt with in consistent ways at home and at school. This requires communication and problem solving on the part of parents, teachers, and school professionals. In the absence of such communication and consistency, behavioral problems are likely to become worse.

Flexibility

It is critical that parents and school personnel be flexible in their approaches to children with TBI. Children are developing rapidly, especially in their earlier years, even as they undergo recovery from the injury and the changing demands of new teachers, classes, routines, and schools. What is needed and working one semester may change the following semester or next school year. The child with TBI is especially at risk for breakdown at major transition points, including new teachers, moving from one classroom to multiple classes, and changing schools. As children grow older and the demands for more abstract and integrative thinking as well as for more independent and self-generated work increase, the need for academic assistance may increase. Individualized education programs may need to be revised on a more frequent basis than for other children. Teachers and parents should remain flexible in the approach they are taking with the child and communicate regularly to maintain consistency.

Dealing With "Unrealistic" Family Expectations

It is not uncommon for families to express goals, hopes, and expectations for the person with the brain injury that, in the judgment of the clinician, are simply not possible. When families react to such feedback with resistance, skepticism, or even anger, clinicians often see the family as being unaware, or in denial, and in need of education. Such scenarios often generate significant negative feelings and even outright conflict. How much is this the family's problem or the clinician's problem in knowing how to deal with the family?

Often, the clinician can diffuse such potential conflict and find a way of working with the family around the goals in question without placing the family in a position of giving up hope. Doing so requires a good bit of clinical savvy and use of language that permits the clinician to participate in exploration of certain goals and their feasibility without abandoning his or her clinical point of view.

The following principles are meant as possible tools for the clinician to use to work his or her way through difficult situations in which the family is expressing expectations and goals that appear unrealistic from the clinician's point of view.

Principle #1: Realities Are Subjective, and They Differ

Remember what any good marital therapist knows: each person's set of perceptions is absolutely real for them. To forcefully challenge the person's perceptions is tantamount to invalidating the person. Perceptions are driven not by cold, clear observation of obvious facts but by interpretations of cues that pass through a series of emotional filters. Families who express goals for the person with TBI that seem wildly unrealistic to a clinician are expressing hopes that may be coming from sacred places. These hopes must be dealt with gently and with respect. At the very least, do not immediately and offhandedly dismiss these hopes as unrealistic; it will be experienced as a crushing blow by the family, and you may lose them to work with. Show an interest in the goals and a willingness to discuss them.

Principle #2: We Do Not Know

Many families present having experienced professionals who made pronouncements that turned out to be false (e.g., "Your loved one will not survive"; "He survived, but he will not come out of the coma"; "He came out of the coma, but he will not communicate meaningfully"; "He communicates, but he will not walk"; "He walks, but he will not be independent"). Even in less severe cases, we really do not know what any given individual will be capable of—in both directions. Patients who look like they will make good recoveries languish; persons with severe impairments make achievements never dreamed possible. Clinicians develop a set of expectations on the basis of probabilities derived from experience. However, if it is true that 95% of persons with a given level of deficit will not go back to work, then 5% will. How does one know if this family represents the exception, not the rule? Clinicians owe it to the family to keep their minds open.

Principle #3: Never Underestimate Motivation

We have seen persons with severe brain injury being told in no uncertain terms they will never be able to teach again—only to do so—and injured students told that college would be impossible—who earned their degrees. In these cases, the professionals did not so much misjudge the severity of the injury as underestimate the motivation of the injured person and the family. This does not mean that all families will succeed at what they put their minds to; it does mean that clinicians should not short circuit the power of families who have a strong need to achieve a goal until they have given themselves a chance to try. Just as it is impossible to force a person with brain injury or his or her family to move in a direction they do not want to go, so, too, it is wise to see what motivates a patient or family and ride it as far as possible. The following principles are ways of encouraging a family's motivation, by endorsing the *spirit* of their goal, without necessarily endorsing the ultimate goal itself.

Principle #4: Elaborate and Collaborate: Find a Way of Endorsing the Spirit of the Goal

Elaboration and collaboration can be done in two major ways: 1) break the goal down into steps and take one at a time, and 2) find the spirit of the goal and substitute reasonable alternatives.

Break the goal down into steps and take one at a time. In practice, because families are often unrealistic about future goals soon after brain injury, it is most often the case that the "spirit of the goal" is identified first and then broken down into transitional steps that can be taken one at a time, as illustrated by the following example. A bright young woman in college had the (realistic) goal of becoming a doctor. After a TBI, she has significant memory and executive deficits. Her parents believe it is still possible for her to succeed and want her to resume college and take the Medical College Admission Test. The clinicians are absolutely convinced this is not possible. What options do the clinicians have?

One option is to confront the parents, saying that the goal is unrealistic. This is likely to provoke resistance and conflict. If the implications of their daughter's deficits were obvious, the parents would not be taking this stance in the first place. They are not likely to meekly respond by saying, "Oh, you're right, we never noticed that." Their expectations express deep-seated needs and hopes on their part, coupled with a willingness to believe that recovery, therapy, and determination will enable her to achieve her goal.

A smarter, more complex response is to first talk about what is required in medical school and in the practice of medicine and to relate those requirements to the changes in the young woman because of the injury that can be observed by the parents and clinicians. This is engaging the parents in a collaborative process of discovery to see how they respond to the explicit consideration of demands and capacities. Some families, in the face of such explicit comparison (which they probably have never done), begin on their own to modify their expectations. Other families admit skepticism, but are clear about wanting to move forward. Other families may in fact be in full blown denial—but again, contradicting them only fuels the denial (because it is acting as a defense mechanism).

When families remain determined to pursue goals professionals view as unrealistic, the best course of action is to break that goal down into component parts, and say "OK, let's take it one step at a time, and see how far we can go." It is perfectly fine for the clinician to express concerns that certain aspects of the demands may become too difficult for the injured person to handle. The process is then to implement the first step with support, see how it goes, and keep implementing steps as long as the person is succeeding. Ongoing monitoring and discussion are essential to evaluate progress and potential.

The medically aspiring young woman might enroll for a single course in a local community college. (A far cry from applying to medical school, but that goal is not being explicitly rejected.) Can she manage course reading? Can she take notes? What assistance does she need on examinations and papers? After taking one or two courses, the decision may be made for her to return to her college—or perhaps transfer to one with better support for students with disabilities. There she can take a science course or two and see how it goes.

The progression is obvious. By breaking the "unrealistic" goal down into steps, the professional can support each individual step and let the decision about how realistic medical school is emerge from the process itself, rather than being mandated a priori. When it is in fact unrealistic, both the injured person and his or her family will gradually realize that and be more at peace with letting go of the goal because they gave it their best shot.

Find the spirit of the goal and substitute reasonable alternatives. Many times, it is possible to discover the motivation behind a particular goal that may be unrealistic and satisfy the underlying need by substituting another, more reasonable goal. Most commonly, this process begins when an original goal has been broken down into steps and it becomes clear that the original goal is not achievable.

Many young persons with TBI become attached to and want to model themselves after therapists in their rehabilitation. One particular girl, a high school sophomore, loved her OT and on returning to school announced that becoming an OT was her career goal. The girl had severe visual problems, severe motor integration problems, and poor short-term memory. Her family was, at least superficially, supportive of her goals and told others of her plans.

There are two mistakes the professional can make in this scenario, at both extremes. The first is telling the girl and her family, point blank, that becoming an OT is an impossible goal. (This does not preclude serious discussions with the parents about what the obstacles would be.) This would prematurely deprive the girl of a much-needed aspiration and the reconstruction of her self-esteem by denying her a model with whom to identify. It could do significant harm. The other mistake is the opposite: to fully endorse the goal and reassure the girl that everyone will do everything possible to help her achieve that goal. That would feed into her unawareness or denial of the implications of her deficits, or both, and set her up for a particularly devastating failure.

The best path is the process of discovery (e.g., "OK, what do you need to do to go to OT school?" "What kinds of classes do you need to be able to pass? Let's give one a try"). When students return to school after severe brain injury, there is a benign tendency to grade them by their effort, not their achievement. In this example, it is important that the grade given the girl be a realistic one on the basis of the course expectations. It will probably become clear over the course of a semester that a diet of science is not realistic.

It is at this point that one is ready to explore the spirit of why the girl wanted to be an OT. Helping others, making suffering go away, or enabling a person to learn and succeed may emerge as the driving forces. It is then possible to explore other career or volunteer options that can meet those needs and give the girl an experience doing them in a supervised setting. But exploring the spirit of the goal in search of an alternative cannot take place until the injured person—and his or her family—is ready to let go of the original goal.

Principle #5: Use Controlled Failure (the Dignity of Risk)

As much as clinicians would like to save clients and their families additional pain, that is not always possible. There are times when all else fails and the injured person and family insist on embarking on a path that the clinician deems unrealistic. This may range from applying to college to returning to a job. Often, the reality is that the only way a family will confront the impossibility of a goal is to try it and fail. The key is to set up a safety net in the event the person fails. The wrong thing to do is simply say, "OK, give it a try," then shrug your shoulders and walk away. Setting up support services for the person, keeping clinical contact as he or she starts the process, identifying in advance what the difficult areas will be, and having a contingency plan if all comes crashing down are the responsible clinical approaches. That way, the injured person is protected as he or she comes to terms with what you knew: that the goal was unrealistic. Then again—the patient might fool you and succeed.

The one exception to allowing controlled failure is when the cost of failure could be catastrophic in terms of human or financial well-being. A trader responsible for millions of dollars a day—or an air traffic controller or a surgeon—should not be let loose to "see what happens," no matter how reliable the safety net. However, even in high-risk situations, it is often possible to create a supervised, less risky, job. Doctors, for example, can perform limited parts of examinations under supervision. But when the cost of failure is potentially too high, the risk of uncontrolled experimentation simply cannot be taken.

Principle #6: Ask the Person With the Injury What He or She Wants

Sometimes, clinicians become so caught up dealing with family expectations and demands that they fight the battle of what is realistic without ever inquiring what the injured person wants. Even though Dad and Mom are insisting their injured son will go back to law school, the eager-to-please son may be harboring his own doubts about whether he still wants to do that. Sometimes, it takes a number of sessions privately with the injured adolescent or young adult to help the person sort out what his or her goals are and how they may be different from the goals of the rest of the family.

Principle #7: Be Prepared to Challenge Overprotective Families That Are Negatively Unrealistic

A separate problem, but one that falls under the category of "unrealistic families," is the overprotective family that underestimates the capacities of the injured person. Most often, this occurs with persons with more severe injuries who have realistically significant limitations. However, the family, in the desire to protect the vulnerable family member, fails to appreciate capacities that the person has or risks that are reasonable to take. Often, this occurs with persons with frontal lobe injuries whose judgment may be compromised or persons with unstable medical conditions such as partially controlled seizures. The unpredictability of the injured person's behavior triggers an overprotective fear response on the part of the family. Such families may block efforts at continuing education, job trials, dating, or independent travel or living.

A number of strategies may be helpful to the clinician in this case. First and foremost is turning attention away from the person with the TBI to the fears of the family members in a position of decision making. An honest discussion of (usually parental) fears, coupled with a practical discussion of the risks involved (how realistic the risks are and what steps could be taken to minimize them) is often helpful. Second, it is often productive to sit down together with the person with TBI and the family to discuss goals and see if it is possible to set up a series of compromise steps that will allow a discovery of what is realistically possible.

For example, a young woman with a severe brain injury may be interested in learning to travel independently between her home and a job trial site. Her family, which may be all in favor of her having a job, may veto the goal of independent travel on the grounds that it is unsafe. To discuss this decision in the abstract may be unproductive. More helpful might be the approach taken in principle 4 as outlined in the preceding section: elaborate and collaborate. A multistep approach to travel training might be put forth explicitly as a compromise measure: it satisfies the injured person's desire to see how independent she can become in travel while satisfying the family's need to maintain a level of protection. Thus, the client might be guided to the work site, then develop a map and set of steps to follow, then accompanied one more time but encouraged to make her own decisions, then accompanied but tailed only, and so forth. Between each step, family members could be told how things went, and their consent could be sought for taking the next step.

As with any program of deconditioning, the idea is to introduce at each step a goal that has a high probability of success and that arouses a minimum amount of anxiety. Such an approach sidesteps the major conflict of whether the family will allow the injured person to travel alone, and introduces a stepwise process of gradual challenge in which the family is never asked to lose control of the process. Allowing families to retain a sense of control and safety in decisions about the injured person is a key concept in dealing with unrealistic expectations.

The preceding principles are not all inclusive. They are meant to represent some of the guidelines professionals can use when confronted with families whose goals are thought to be unrealistic. The key is to join with the family to develop a process of moving toward a goal to discover how realistic it is or to see if it can be reshaped in some way that works for the injured person. Simply telling the family that goals are unrealistic almost never works. It does not deter family members, and you lose your ability to work with them.

Legal Issues

Legal issues are touchy, and most professionals are wary of addressing them with families. Although it is certainly inappropriate for medical professionals to become involved in personal family matters regarding suing for damages and choosing lawyers, there are also ethical responsibilities about informing families about long-term care needs of the injured person and helping families avoid critical mistakes early on that will permanently prevent the injured person from receiving the resources he or she deserves. In our opinion, there are two circumstances in which medical professionals are justified in counseling families about legal issues.

First, not all personal injury lawyers are sophisticated in bringing injury cases to settlement or trial. They may terribly underestimate the long-term disability of the person and simply not be aware of what the long-term costs will be in terms of lost wages and care needs. This is especially true in severe injuries in which executive dysfunction may not be apparent in protected environments (including the lawyer's office) and in cases of mild brain injury. We have seen many families who were counseled by lawyers to settle early for sums of money grossly inadequate to care for the person in the long term and who bitterly look back on their legal advice wishing they knew then what they know now. When a clinician senses this is happening, we believe there are ethical grounds for discussing the situation with the family and urging them to seek consultation from a law firm more savvy and experienced in handling TBI cases.

Second, special situations exist with children who sustain TBIs at an early age. Many children "grow into" their deficits as the demands of school become greater and more complex and require more frontal lobe processing. Often, it is difficult to assess the long-term effect of a TBI on a child until he or she has worked his or her way through the school system. Many lawyers familiar with TBI in children prefer to wait years to try the case, except when the damages are immediately catastrophic and apparent. The failure to wait may mean families will accept a small settlement and then have an adolescent who is unable to support him- or herself and is genuinely in need of longer-term support. However, the risk of waiting to try the case is that other intervening events or variables over the years may cloud the picture and make it much more difficult in later years to tease out the impact of an early injury. In our opinion, in cases in which the child is too young for the true effect of the injury to be determined, and if the family is being pressured to accept a small, immediate settlement, there are ethical grounds for the clinician to discuss the legal issues with the family and to urge discussion of the issues with a lawyer as well.

Cultural Diversity

No discussion of family intervention after TBI is complete without the inclusion of the role of cultural back-

ground, which in the broadest sense includes race, religion, ethnicity, language, socioeconomic status, and even sexual orientation. Any or all of these factors may influence etiology, symptom manifestation, beliefs about the causation of disability, expectations regarding recovery and rehabilitation, participation in the rehabilitation process, and more (Chavira 1988; Fitzgerald 1992).

Consideration of cultural background is especially important as the United States increasingly becomes a multicultural nation. Early 2000 census data, for example, revealed that 18% of the United States population speaks a language other than English at home (in states such as California, New Mexico, Texas, New York, and Hawaii, it is approximately one-third of the population) (Schmitt 2001). In the 1990 census data, that figure was 14%, which was a 38% increase over the 1980 census figures (Barringer 1993). Despite this, there is little information in the TBI literature regarding the impact of language and culture on families after TBI or how to address the needs of these families in clinical situations.

The most comprehensive review and discussion of these issues in the TBI literature appears in Cavallo and Saucedo (1995). This article provides information regarding the epidemiology of TBI in culturally diverse populations and includes discussions of assessment, treatment, and factors that must be considered during service provision. Williams and Savage (1991) include ethnicity in a discussion of working with families of children with TBI. They make the important point that, in their clinical experience, families may identify more with their cultural heritage after an injury has occurred within their family. Horan (1987) describes working with families of children with TBI in the Native American community.

Rosenthal et al. (1996) looked specifically at how racial and ethnic status affects functional outcome and community integration after a TBI using data from the TBI Model Systems National Data Base. They found no significant differences between minorities and whites at time of admission to and discharge from inpatient rehabilitation and at 1 year postinjury for basic functional skills. However, at 1 year postinjury, they did find worse outcomes for minorities in return to work or school, in addition to decreased social contacts. They postulate that these differences may relate to the socioeconomic and social status of minorities in the United States, which is consistent with the discussion of socioeconomic, disability, and minority status in Cavallo and Saucedo (1995).

Orlandi et al. (1992) have defined cultural sensitivity as "an awareness of the nuances of one's own and other cultures." Cultural competency is defined as a "set of academic and interpersonal skills that allow individuals to increase their understanding and appreciation of cultural differences and similarities within, among, and between groups." It is imperative that professionals working with families after TBI actively seek to increase their level of cultural competency and sensitivity and to use this knowledge and understanding to enhance their ability to provide effective interventions. It would be difficult for any clinician to become an expert and have an in-depth understanding of all potential cultural differences he or she may encounter in the families he or she may work with. However, all clinicians should have a heightened awareness of the role that language, culture, race, and ethnicity may play in families' perceptions of and reactions to disability and rehabilitation.

Brain Injury Association of America and Other Support Organizations

The National Head Injury Foundation was founded in 1980 by Marilyn Price Spivack and Martin Spivack and a small group of families and professionals in Framingham, Massachusetts, because of the unmet needs of their brain-injured daughter. Today known as the Brain Injury Association of America, it has grown into a national advocacy organization centered in Arlington, Virginia, with affiliated chapters in most states. The Brain Injury Association encourages active participation of persons with brain injury, family members, and professionals; provides educational materials to families and professionals; organizes support groups at the local level; and acts as an advocacy organization at the state and national level for public policies and laws that support persons with brain injury and their families. At the professional level, the Brain Injury Association provides numerous opportunities for involvement through committees, task forces, and an annual national professional convention.

The Brain Injury Association of America is most easily reached via its Web site at http://www.biausa.org or by calling 703–761–0750. There is a toll-free hotline at 800–444–6443. The mailing address is Brain Injury Association of America, 8201 Greensboro Drive, Suite 611, McLean, VA, 22102. All of the associated state chapters can also be found through the Web site or by contacting the Brain Injury Association of America directly.

In local areas, other support and advocacy organizations, which may not be associated with the Brain Injury Association of America, have also evolved.

Family Individuality and Coping

Chapters such as this one can be written only by generalizing about families. A fitting way to end is with the caveat that all families are different. The effective clinician responds to the conscious and unconscious needs of an individual family and does not project onto the family his or her value system of what healthy adjustment is. Precisely because the person with brain injury is dependent on a network of significant others for his or her successful adaptation to disability, successful family intervention must proceed from within the framework of the unique family system. The rehabilitation team will not successfully impose goals, limits, or routines that are alien to the family. It is the role of the family therapist to help families meet needs, establish a new balance and identity that works for them, and negotiate a productive alliance between the rehabilitation team and the family. This can be done only by starting—and ending—with a healthy respect for the family's individuality.

References

Albert SM, Im A, Brenner L, et al: Effect of a social worker liaison program on family caregivers to people with brain injury. J Head Trauma Rehabil 17:175–189, 2002

Allen K, Linn RT, Gutierrez H, et al: Family burden following traumatic brain injury. Rehabil Psychol 39:29–48, 1994

Barringer F: For 32 million Americans, English is a second language. New York Times, April 28, 1993, p A18

Barry CT, Taylor HG, Klein S, et al: Validity of neurobehavioral symptoms reported in children with traumatic brain injury. Child Neuropsychology 2:213–226, 1996

Barry P, Clark D: Effects of intact versus non-intact families on adolescent head injury rehabilitation. Brain Inj 6:229–232, 1992

Bishop SD, Miller IW: Traumatic brain injury: empirical family assessment techniques. J Head Trauma Rehabil 3:31–41, 1988

Blosser J, DePompei R: Fostering effective family involvement through mentoring. J Head Trauma Rehabil 10:46–56, 1995

Bond MR: Assessment of psychosocial outcome of severe head injury. Acta Neurochir 34:57–70, 1976

Bond MR: Effects on the family system, in Rehabilitation of the Head Injured Adult. Edited by Rosenthal M, Griffith E, Bond M, Miller JD. Philadelphia, PA, FA Davis, 1983, pp 209–217

Brooks N: The head-injured family. J Clin Exp Neuropsychol 13:155–188, 1991

Brooks N, McKinlay W: Personality and behavioural change after severe blunt head injury—a relative's view. J Neurol Neurosurg Psychiatry 46:336–344, 1983

Brooks N, Campsie L, Symington C, et al: The effects of severe head injury upon patient and relative within several years of injury. J Head Trauma Rehabil 2:1–13, 1987

Carnevale GJ: Natural-setting behavior management for individuals with traumatic brain injury: results of a three-year caregiver training program. J Head Trauma Rehabil 11:27–38, 1996

Carnevale GJ, Anselmi V, Busichio K, et al: Changes in ratings of caregiver burden following a community-based behavior management program for persons with traumatic brain injury. J Head Trauma Rehabil 17:83–95, 2002

Carter EA, McGoldrick M (eds): The Family Lifecycle: A Framework for Family Therapy. New York, Gardner, 1980

Cavallo MM: Subjective burden in caregivers of persons with traumatic brain injury: the influence of family relationship. Unpublished doctoral dissertation, New York University, 1997

Cavallo MM, Saucedo C: Traumatic brain injury in families from culturally diverse populations. J Head Trauma Rehabil 10:66–77, 1995

Cavallo MM, Kay T, Ezrachi O: Problems and changes after traumatic brain injury: differing perceptions between and within families. Brain Inj 6:327–335, 1992

Chavira JA: Family, culture and decision making in the Mexican American population, in Disability, Rehabilitation and the Mexican American. Edited by Arnold BR. Edinburg, Texas, Pan American University; 1988, pp 91–97

Chwalisz K: Perceived stress and caregiver burden after brain injury: a theoretical integration. Rehabil Psychol 37:189–203, 1992

Combrinck-Graham L: A developmental model for family systems. Fam Process 24:139–150, 1985

Curtiss G, Klemz S, Vanderploeg RD: Acute impact of severe traumatic brain injury on family structure and coping responses. J Head Trauma Rehabil 15:1113–1122, 2000

DePompei R, Williams J: Working with families after TBI: a family centered approach. Topics in Language Disorders 15:68–81, 1994

DeJong G, Batavia AI, Williams JW: Who is responsible for the lifelong well-being of a person with a head injury? J Head Trauma Rehabil 5:9–22, 1990

Digre PG, Kamen D, Vaughn S, et al: Selected states' public policy responses to traumatic brain injury. J Head Trauma Rehabil 9:12–26, 1994

Douglas JM, Spellacy FJ: Indicators of long-term family functioning following severe traumatic brain injury in adults. Brain Inj 10:819–839, 1996

Ergh TC, Rapport LJ, Coleman RD, et al: Predictors of caregiver and family functioning following traumatic brain injury: social support moderates caregiver distress. J Head Trauma Rehabil 17:155–174, 2002

Eysenck HJ, Eysenck SBG: Eysenck Personality Questionnaire. London, England, Hodder and Stoughton, 1975

Fitzgerald MH: Multicultural clinical interactions. J Rehabil 58:388–342, 1992

Florian V, Katz S, Lahav V: Impact of traumatic brain damage on family dynamics and functioning: a review. Brain Inj 3:219–233, 1989

Fordyce DJ, Roueche JR: Changes in perspectives of disability among patients, staff and relatives during rehabilitation of brain injury. Rehabil Psychol 31:217–229, 1986

Gervasio AH, Kreutzer JS: Kinship and family members' psychological distress after traumatic brain injury: a large sample study. J Head Trauma Rehabil 12:14–26, 1997

Groom KN, Shaw TG, O'Connor ME, et al: Neurobehavioral symptoms and family functioning in traumatically brain-injured adults. Arch Clin Neuropsychol 13:695–711, 1998

Horan KT: Effects of head injury on the educational and vocational potential of American Indians. Rural Special Education Quarterly 8:19–22, 1987

Hosack KR, Rocchio CA: Serving families of persons with severe brain injury in an era of managed care. J Head Trauma Rehabil 10:57–65, 1995

Hpay H: Psycho-social effects of severe head injury, in International Symposium on Head Injuries, Edinburg and Madrid. New York, Churchill Livingstone, 1970, pp 110–119

Jacobs HE: The Los Angeles head injury survey: procedures and initial findings. Arch Phys Med Rehabil 69:425–431, 1988

Junque C, Bruna O, Mataro M: Information needs of the traumatic brain injury patient's family members regarding the consequences of the injury and associated perception of physical, cognitive, emotional and quality of life changes. Brain Inj 11:251–258, 1997

Kalsbeek WD, McLauren RL, Harris BSH, et al: The National Head and Spinal Cord Injury Survey: major findings. J Neurosurg 53:S19–S31, 1980

Kay T: The Unseen Injury: Minor Head Trauma. Framingham, MA, National Head Injury Foundation, 1986

Kay T: Neuropsychological diagnosis: disentangling the multiple determinants of functional disability after mild traumatic brain injury, in Rehabilitation of Post-Concussive Disorders: Physical Medicine and Rehabilitation: State of the Art Reviews. Edited by Horn L, Zassler N. Philadelphia, PA, Hanley & Belfus, 1992, pp 109–127

Kay T, Cavallo MM: Evolutions: research and clinical perspectives on families, in Head Injury: A Family Matter. Edited by Williams JM, Kay T. Baltimore, MD, Paul H Brookes, 1991, pp 121–150

Kay T, Lezak M: The nature of head injury, in Traumatic Brain Injury and Vocational Rehabilitation. Edited by Corthell D. Menomonie, WI, University of Wisconsin-Stout, 1990, pp 21–65

Kay T, Cavallo MM, Ezrachi O: Administration Manual, New York University Head Injury Family Interview (Version 1.2). New York, New York University Medical Center, Research and Training Center on Head Trauma and Stroke, 1988

Kay T, Cavallo MM, Ezrachi O, et al: The head injury family interview: a clinical and research tool. J Head Trauma Rehabil 10:12–31, 1995

Klonoff P, Prigatano GP: Reactions of family members and clinical intervention after traumatic brain injury, in Community Re-Entry for Head Injured Adults. Edited by Ylvisaker M, Gobble EMR. Boston, MA, College Hill, 1987, pp 381–402

Kosciulek JF: Relationship of family coping with head injury to family adaptation. Rehabil Psychol 39:215–230, 1994

Kosciulek JF: Dimensions of family coping with head injury: a replication and extension. Rehabil Couns Bull 41:43–53, 1997a

Kosciulek JF: Relationship of family schema to family adaptation to brain injury. Brain Inj 11:821–830, 1997b

Kosciulek JF, Lustig DC: Predicting family adaptation from brain injury-related family stress. Journal of Applied Rehabilitation Counseling 29:8–12, 1998

Kosciulek JF, Pichette EF: Adaptation concerns of families of people with head injuries. Journal of Applied Rehabilitation Counseling 27:8–13, 1996

Koskinen S: Quality of life 10 years after a very severe traumatic brain injury (TBI): the perspective of the injured and the closest relative. Brain Inj 12:631–648, 1998

Kozloff R: Networks of social support and the outcome from severe head injury. J Head Trauma Rehabil 2:14–23, 1987

Kreutzer JS, Gervasio AH, Camplair PS: Patient correlates of caregivers' distress and family functioning after traumatic brain injury. Brain Inj 8:211–230, 1994a

Kreutzer JS, Gervasio AH, Camplair PS: Primary caregiver's psychological status and family functioning after traumatic brain injury. Brain Inj 8:197–210, 1994b

Kreutzer JS, Sander AM, Fernandez CC: Misperceptions, mishaps, and pitfalls in working with families after traumatic brain injury. J Head Trauma Rehabil 12:63–73, 1997

Kübler-Ross E: On Death and Dying. New York, Macmillan, 1969

Lanham RA Jr, Weissenburger JE, Schwab KA, et al: A longitudinal investigation of the concordance between individuals with traumatic brain injury and family or friend ratings on the Katz Adjustment Scale. J Head Trauma Rehabil 15:1123–1138, 2000

Leach LR, Frank RG, Bouman DE, et al: Family functioning, social support and depression after traumatic brain injury. Brain Inj 8:599–606, 1994

Lezak MD: Living with the characterologically altered brain injured patient. J Clin Psychiatry 39:592–598, 1978

Lezak MD: Psychological implications of traumatic brain damage for the patient's family. Rehabil Psychol 31:241–250, 1986

Lezak MD: Brain damage is a family affair. J Clin Exp Neuropsychol 10:111–123, 1988

Livingston MG: Head injury: the relative's response. Brain Inj 1:33–39, 1987

Livingston MG: Effects on the family system, in Rehabilitation of the Adult and Child with Traumatic Brain Injury. Edited by Rosenthal M, Griffith ER, Bond MR, et al. Philadelphia, PA, FA Davis, 1990, pp 225–235

Livingston MG, Brooks DN: The burden on families of the brain injured: a review. J Head Trauma Rehabil 4:6–15, 1988

MacFarlane MM: Treating brain-injured clients and their families. Fam Ther 26:13–29, 1999

Maitz EA: The psychological sequelae of a severe closed head injury and their impact upon family systems. Unpublished doctoral dissertation, Temple University, 1989

Maitz EA, Sachs PR: Treating families of individuals with traumatic brain injury from a family systems perspective. J Head Trauma Rehabil 10:1–11, 1995

Malec JF, Machulda MM, Moessner AM: Differing problem perceptions of staff, survivors, and significant others after brain injury. J Head Trauma Rehabil 12:1–13, 1997

Marsh NV, Kersel DA, Havill JH, et al: Caregiver burden at 1 year following severe traumatic brain injury. Brain Inj 12:1045–1059, 1998

Max JE, Castillo CS, Robin DA, et al: Predictors of family functioning after traumatic brain injury in children and adolescents. Journal of the American Academy of Child Adolescent Psychiatry 37:83–90, 1998

McKinlay WW, Brooks DN: Methodological problems in assessing psychosocial recovery following severe head injury. J Clin Neuropsychol 6:87–99, 1984

McKinlay WW, Brooks DN, Bond MR, et al: The short-term outcome of severe blunt head injury as reported by relatives of the injured person. J Neurol Neurosurg Psychiatry 44:527–533, 1981

Minnes P, Graffi S, Nolte ML, et al: Coping and stress in Canadian family caregivers of persons with traumatic brain injury. Brain Inj 14:737–748, 2000

Moore A, Stambrooke M, Peters L: Centripetal and centrifugal family life cycle factors in long-term outcome following traumatic brain injury. Brain Inj 7:247–255, 1993

Muir CA, Rosenthal M, Diehl LN: Methods of family intervention, in Rehabilitation of the Adult and Child with Traumatic Brain Injury. Edited by Rosenthal M, Griffith ER, Bond MR, et al. Philadelphia, PA, FA Davis, 1990, pp 433–448

Oddy M, Humphrey M: Social recovery during the year following severe head injury. J Neurol Neurosurg Psychiatry 43:798–802, 1980

Oddy M, Humphrey M, Uttley D: Stresses upon the relatives of head-injured patients. Br J Psychiatry 133:507–513, 1978a

Oddy M, Humphrey M, Uttley D: Subjective impairment and social recovery after closed head injury. J Neurol Neurosurg Psychiatry 41:611–616, 1978b

Oddy M, Coughlan T, Tyerman A, et al: Social adjustment after closed head injury: a further follow-up seven years after injury. J Neurol Neurosurg Psychiatry 48:564–568, 1985

Olshansky S: Chronic sorrow: a response to having a mentally defective child. Soc Casework 43:190–193, 1962

Olson DH: Circumplex model of marital and family services, in Normal Family Processes. Edited by Walsh F. New York, Guilford, 1993, pp 104–137

Olson DH, Portner J, Bell RQ: FACES-II: Family Adaptation and Cohesion Evaluation Scales. St. Paul, MN, Family Social Science, University of Minnesota, 1982

Orlandi MA, Wesin R, Epstein LG: Cultural Competence for Evaluators. Washington, DC: US Department of Health and Human Services, 1992

Panting A, Merry PH: The long-term rehabilitation of severe head injuries with particular reference to the need for social and medical support for the patient's family. Rehabilitation 38:33–37, 1972

Perlesz A, Kinsella G, Crowe S: Impact of traumatic brain injury on the family: a critical review. Rehabil Psychol 44:6–35, 1999

Perlesz A, Kinsella G, Crowe S: Psychological distress and family satisfaction following traumatic brain injury: injured individuals and their primary, secondary, and tertiary carers. J Head Trauma Rehabil 15:909–929, 2000

Pessar LF, Coad ML, Linn RT, et al: The effects of parental traumatic brain injury on the behaviour of parents and children. Brain Inj 7:231–240, 1993

Peters LC, Stambrook M, Moore AD, et al: Psychosocial sequelae of closed head injury: effects on the marital relationship.
Brain Inj 4:39–47, 1990

Rape RN, Busch JP, Slavin LA: Toward a conceptualization of the
family's adaptation to a member's head injury: a critique of
developmental stage models. Rehabil Psychol 37:3–22, 1992

Ridley B: Family response in head injury: denial or hope for the
future? Soc Sci Med 29:555–561, 1989

Rivara JB, Fay GC, Jaffe KM, et al: Predictors of family functioning one year following traumatic brain injury in children, Arch Phys Med Rehabil 73:899–910, 1992

Rivara JB, Jaffe KM, Fay GC, et al: Family functioning and injury severity as predictors of child functioning one year following traumatic brain injury. Arch Phys Med Rehabil
74:1047–1055, 1993

Rivara JB, Jaffe KM, Polissar NL, et al: Family functioning and
children's academic performance and behavior problems in
the year following traumatic brain injury. Arch Phys Med
Rehabil 75:369–379, 1994

Rolland JS: Chronic illness and the life cycle: a conceptual
framework. Fam Process 26:203–221, 1987a

Rolland JS: Family illness paradigms: evolution and significance.
Fam Syst Med 5:482–503, 1987b

Rolland JS: Anticipatory loss: a family systems framework. Fam
Process 29:229–244, 1990

Romano MD: Family response to traumatic head injury. Scand
J Rehabil Med 6:1–4, 1974

Romano MD: Family issues in head trauma, in Traumatic Brain
Injury: Physical Medicine and Rehabilitation: State of the
Art Reviews. Edited by Horn L, Copi DN. Philadelphia,
PA, Hanley & Belfus, 1989, pp 157–168

Rosen B, Reynolds WE: The impact of public policy on persons
with traumatic brain injury and their families. J Head
Trauma Rehabil 9:1–11, 1994

Rosenthal M, Hutchins B: Interdisciplinary family education in
head injury rehabilitation, in Head Injury: A Family Matter. Edited by Williams JM, Kay T. Baltimore, MD, Paul H
Brookes, 1991, pp 273–282

Rosenthal M, Muir CA: Methods of family intervention, in Re-
habilitation of the Head Injured Adult. Edited by
Rosenthal M, Griffith ER, Bond MR, et al. Philadelphia,
PA, FA Davis, 1983, pp 407–419

Rosenthal M, Dijkers M, Harrison-Felix C, et al: Impact of minority status on functional outcome and community integration following traumatic brain injury. J Head Trauma
Rehabil 11:40–57, 1996

Schmitt E: Census data show a sharp increase in living standard.
New York Times, August 6, 2001, pp A1 and A10

Serio CD, Kreutzer JS, Gervasio AH: Predicting family needs
after brain injury: implications for intervention. J Head
Trauma Rehabil 10:32–45, 1995

Singer GHS, Glang A, Nixon C, et al: A comparison of two psychosocial interventions for parents of children with acquired brain injury: an exploratory study. J Head Trauma
Rehabil 9:38–49, 1994

Spearman RC, Stamm BH, Rosen BH, et al: The use of Medicaid waivers and their impact on services. J Head Trauma
Rehabil 16:47–60, 2001

Springer JA, Farmer JE, Bouman DE: Common misconceptions
about traumatic brain injury among family members of rehabilitation patients. J Head Trauma Rehabil 12:41–50, 1997

Taylor HG, Drotar D, Wade S, et al: Recovery from traumatic
brain injury in children: the importance of the family, in
Traumatic Brain Injury in Children. Edited by Broman SH,
Michel ME. New York, Oxford Press, 1995, pp 188–216

Uysal S, Hibbard MR, Robillard D, et al: The effect of parental
traumatic brain injury on parenting and child behavior.
J Head Trauma Rehabil 13:57–71, 1998

Wade SL, Drotar D, Taylor HG, et al: Assessing the effects of
traumatic brain injury on family functioning: conceptual and
methodological issues. J Pediatr Psychol 20:737–752, 1995

Wade SL, Taylor HG, Drotar D, et al: Childhood traumatic
brain injury: initial impact on the family. J Learn Disabil
29:652–661, 1996

Wade SL, Taylor G, Drotar D, et al: A prospective study of
long-term caregiver and family adaptation following brain
injury in children. J Head Trauma Rehabil 17:96–111, 2002

Weddell R, Oddy M, Jenkins D: Social adjustment after rehabilitation: a two-year follow-up of patients with severe head
injury. Psychol Med 10:257–263, 1980

Wikler L: Chronic stresses of families of mentally retarded children. Fam Relat 30:281–288, 1981

Williams JM: Family reaction to head injury, in Head Injury: A
Family Matter. Edited by Williams JM, Kay T. Baltimore,
MD, Paul H Brookes, 1991a, pp 81–99

Williams JM: Family support, in Head Injury: A Family Matter.
Edited by Williams JM, Kay T. Baltimore, MD, Paul H
Brookes, 1991b, pp 299–312

Williams JM: Training staff for family centered rehabilitation:
future directions in program planning, in Staff Development and Clinical Intervention in Brain Injury Rehabilitation. Edited by Durgin CJ, Schmidt ND, Fryer LJ. Gaith-
ersburg, MD, Aspen, 1993, pp 45–56

Williams JM, Kay T: Head Injury: A Family Matter. Baltimore,
MD, Paul H Brookes, 1991

Williams JM, Savage RC: Family culture and child development, in
Head Injury: A Family Matter. Edited by Williams JM, Kay T.
Baltimore, MD, Paul H Brookes, 1991, pp 219–238

Yeates KO, Taylor HG, Drotar D, et al: Preinjury family environment as a determinant of recovery from traumatic brain
injuries in school-age children. Journal of the International
Neuropsychology Society 3:617–630, 1997

31 Systems of Care

D. Nathan Cope, M.D.

William E. Reynolds, D.D.S., M.P.H.

System Concept

With the possible exception of some mild injuries, current thinking requires that traumatic brain injury (TBI), with its multiple and varied impairments, be managed by a diverse group of clinicians and other professionals in a variety of settings to achieve optimum results. This array of services is referred to by the term *comprehensive rehabilitation*. The clinician who undertakes to provide psychiatric care to the TBI population should have a basic understanding of this range and sequence of services and supports. Psychiatric interventions can thus be integrated into this broader context, and the clinician, when primary in the coordination of care, can efficiently and appropriately refer to these services for his or her patients with TBI.

The genesis of the system concept of care for TBI, to the extent that it can be delineated, lies with two seminal grants in 1977 by the Federal Rehabilitation Services Administration to New York University and Stanford University. These centers were the first to systematically investigate the long-term treatment and support needs and outcomes of survivors of severe TBI. The investigators concluded that the treatment of TBI required a multidisciplinary approach, applied both longitudinally over the course of recovery as well as in multiple settings beyond the traditional hospital-based care delivery sites previously extant (Berrol et al. 1982). Since that time, the experience and reports of these model system centers has stimulated an enormous growth of multiple treatment options and approaches for TBI. This federal support of the systematic processes of care requirements, outcomes, and other treatment and needs research has continued to this day and has expanded to the current 17 grant-supported model system research centers across the United States. These centers, supported by the National Institute on Disability and Rehabilitation Research (2004), continue to contribute to the scientific and clinical foundation of TBI care.

Patients with TBI have a broad array of physiologic deficits and functional impairments, each of which may require treatment by specific specialists. Some of these specialists are discussed in the section Professionals who Treat Individuals with TBI; however, beyond the individual treatment goals of a particular clinician, it is imperative that an overarching schema of care be developed and implemented that comprehensively addresses all significant deficits to ensure efficient and optimum recovery. This schema should not only encompass the 12–36 months postinjury during which "active" recovery is generally thought to proceed but should also end with implementation and maintenance of an appropriate life management plan for those persons with TBI who require it.

Over the past 20–30 years, as experience with the varying requirements of survivors with TBI has grown, a more or less standard array and sequence of services has evolved. (Although general patterns are evident in acquired brain injury service delivery, great individual differences obviously exist from patient to patient in specific composition, severity, and timing for such services.) The entirety of this deliberate interaction among many clinicians and sites of services has come to be referred to as the *system of coordinated supports and services*. Supports and services include any and all of the medical, therapeutic, rehabilitative, community-based, psychosocial, economic, educational, vocational, and other services necessary to enable the person with TBI to function in the community independently and productively (Bureau of Maternal and Child Health 2001).

In response to this growing awareness of the need to address the multifaceted issues facing many persons with TBI in a comprehensive way, Congress enacted the Traumatic Brain Injury Act of 1996 (Traumatic Brain Injury Technical Assistance Center 2004). The intentions of this act included supporting the conducting of expanded studies and the establishment of innovative programs with respect to TBI. Under the law, the U.S. Department of Health and Human Service's Health Resources and Services Administration has implemented a program to provide grants to states to improve access to health and other services for individuals with TBI and their families. The National Institutes of Health and the Centers for Disease Control and Prevention were assigned responsibilities in the areas of research, prevention, and surveillance.

In pursuance of this legislation, the National Institutes of Health convened a consensus conference on TBI rehabilitation methods in 1998. The panel concluded that "rehabilitation services, matched to the needs of persons with TBI, and community-based non-medical services are required [in addition to strictly medical services] to optimize outcomes over the course of recovery. Public and private funding for rehabilitation of persons with TBI should also be adequate to meet these acute and long-term needs, especially in consideration of the current health care environment where access to these treatments may be jeopardized by changes in payment methods for private insurance and public programs" (National Institutes of Health 1998, under "Abstract").

After initial trauma and neurosurgical management of the acute TBI and associated injuries, *early comprehensive rehabilitation* is perhaps the most important aspect of the care continuum for recently injured individuals with TBI. Numerous studies have linked early rehabilitation intervention after stabilization with greater functional recovery after TBI (Aronow 1987; Cope and Hall 1982; Mackay et al. 1992), including links between intervention directly after medical stabilization and shorter lengths of stay (Finset et al. 1995), higher functional levels at discharge (Bureau of Maternal and Child Health 2001; National Institutes of Health 1998), lower disability levels at discharge (Rappaport et al. 1989), and higher likelihood of discharge to the home (National Institutes of Health 1998). Similar studies suggest that benefits are derived from postacute services and other later services (Cope 1995; Cope et al. 1996).

A critical challenge for any clinician managing the care of a patient with TBI relates to the identification and appropriate application of an appropriate amalgam of these treatments for any individual case. This full array of treatment is often unavailable for many patients because of lack of the specific clinical services in the geographical area where the patient resides or, too often, because of lack of financial support (i.e., insurance and public reimbursement) for certain indicated elements or indicated duration of care. Similar to the circumstances surrounding mental health services, rehabilitation and other affiliated services (e.g., vocational and avocational services) are paid for via specific (and typically more limited) benefit structures by almost all payers. In addition, these service-delivery systems are almost universally fragmented and lack coordination, and points of entry into publicly funded systems are neither readily identified nor accessible. Thus, access by patients to a fully comprehensive system of care over the extended continuum of their recovery and postinjury life is a relatively rare event. Although acute medical and surgical care is typically comprehensively covered, there is incremental difficulty in obtaining funding and access for inpatient, outpatient, residential, cognitive, and behavioral rehabilitation as well as mental health services. The best results for individual patients are obtained when physicians and families understand and plan for these limitations and plan appropriate treatment allocations.

Clinicians who undertake the treatment of patients with TBI should develop familiarity with both the total conceptual array of indicated services and the particular availability and capabilities of such services in their communities. They should also become knowledgeable about the various funding options for patients with TBI, in particular the reimbursement practices that prevail in their communities.

Professionals Who Treat Individuals With TBI

A large variety of professionals in both private and public service-delivery systems are involved in the comprehensive treatment of TBI, including physicians, rehabilitation providers, and community-based providers, including school educators. Children with TBI have their own unique set of consequences of TBI. Interactions of physical, cognitive, and behavioral sequelae interfere with the major childhood task of new learning. The effect of early TBI may not become apparent until later in a child's development, although there is little explicit literature on the developmental consequences for infants who survive TBI. There may be a poor fit between the needs of children with TBI and the typical school educational programs. Children with TBI also may have difficulties with peers because of impaired cognitive processing, behavioral problems, or difficulty comprehending social cues. As noted in a National Institutes of Health Consensus Statement (1998), "Parents are faced with significant parenting challenges, including coping with changed academic aspirations and family goals."

Virtually the entire spectrum of medical specialties may be called on in various cases. Obviously, neurosurgeons are the primary physicians managing the acute component of care for patients with severe TBI, although for patients with mild TBI, the generalist, emergency department physician, or neurologist may often take primary accountability. Because many cases of severe TBI are caused by high-energy impacts (e.g., falls, motor vehicle accidents), general trauma surgeons and orthopedists are often also involved in the care and—from case to case—may have primary responsibility. Psychiatry is generally not involved in the immediate trauma management period, but many medical issues persist into the postacute period and thus have interplay with psychiatric and rehabilitation concerns. Medical conditions that may require the care of more acutely focused specialists for months and even years postinjury include—but are not limited to—delayed or recurrent subdural collections, hydrocephalus, posttraumatic epilepsy, fracture malunion or delayed healing, and infections. Thorough reviews of these issues are available and should be referenced for details on this portion of the care process (Feliciano et al. 1996; Horn and Zasler 1996; Jennet and Teasdale 1981).

After the immediate medical/surgical phase of care, for those with significant residual deficits from TBI, an array of rehabilitation professionals is required. This includes the physiatrist (a specialist in physical medicine and rehabilitation); rehabilitation nurse; speech and language pathologist; physical, occupational, and recreational therapists; clinical psychologist and neuropsychologist; orthotist and prosthetist (for occasional associated amputations); rehabilitation engineer; social worker; vocational counselor; special education teacher; often attorney; and others. Although it may seem unusual to include attorneys in this list, often the issues of third-party liability, workers' compensation regulations, governmental program eligibility, competency, and in some cases divorce and child custody and child protective services all lead to a very high rate of attorney involvement. It is in the patient's best interest to understand the important role that attorneys can play in facilitating (or impeding) treatment and recovery.

Each of these caregivers addresses a specific spectrum of deficits, disabilities, or needs as indicated for each patient with TBI, although there may be significant overlap in effort, such as physical and occupational therapy's shared ability to address upper extremity function or community ambulation, for example. Because of the vagaries of payer coverage, it may be necessary for the physician in charge of coordination and prescription of care to make

flexible use of whatever clinical professional is considered a covered benefit or available service. (One author of this chapter [N.C.] has had success integrating physical therapists into sophisticated behavioral contingency management programs when payers have denied "mental health coverage.") In its most comprehensive form, this care is typically delivered initially in a formalized coordinated inpatient treatment setting—the acute rehabilitation hospital (see Acute Inpatient Rehabilitation section)—under the direction of a rehabilitation physician, but as recovery proceeds and patients move to outpatient settings, individual clinicians may evolve to providing care in a more or less autonomous manner. It is unnecessary to elaborate on the particular expertise and focus of each of these clinical specialties; it is important, however, to discuss a number of general aspects of these clinicians' care delivery.

First, it should be recognized that the treatment of patients with TBI is a specific area of clinical expertise for each of these disciplines. Just as the expertise of neuropsychiatry is a subspecialty of general psychiatry, so must each of these professionals have the necessary experience and training to adequately provide care to TBI patients. One should exercise caution in assuming that a generalist clinician of any specialty or discipline can adequately assess or treat the patient with TBI; effort should be made to identify appropriately qualified providers. In particular, psychiatrists should be aware of the training and experience of the clinical and neuropsychologists involved. Erroneous diagnostic and treatment approaches are common if standard psychological methods and assessments are used with patients with TBI. As an obvious example, dynamic or insight-directed psychotherapy can be totally misdirected and ineffectual if the patient has deficient memory and frontal executive function (as is typical with TBI), which may preclude benefit from such approaches.

It is also critical to realize that each of these acutely focused professionals is highly likely to interact with the patient and his or her family in an intensely personal and educational manner. Virtually all of these clinicians have had at least some training in basic psychology/counseling processes and actively participate in the education and counseling of the patient and family. Many of the attitudes and beliefs that patients develop about their injury and condition are derived in large part from the prolonged input of these multiple participants in the care process. Thus, it is important both to be aware of this process and to understand what messages are being communicated. For example, it is not uncommon for many rehabilitation professionals (particularly those early in their careers with limited experience) to promote unrealistic expectations of recovery to both patients and family members. Doing so has the potential to create a destructive dynamic. One of

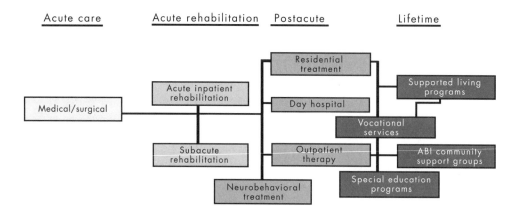

FIGURE 31–1. **Simplified schematic of treatment flow for the patient with traumatic brain injury: acute care, rehabilitation, and lifetime.**

ABI=acquired brain injury.

the authors of this chapter has seen numerous examples of entire families "held hostage" for years to unremitting 24 hour/day treatment programs by brain-injured children's parents who believe in unattainable recovery goals. These situations can result in sibling and spouse depression and anxiety, as well as divorce or broken families.

It is also critical, however, to appreciate the powerful opportunity such acutely focused clinicians bring to a comprehensive psychiatric management plan for a patient and family. Although not as psychiatrically sophisticated as many mental health professionals, these clinicians typically have an adequate foundation in basic psychology, psychopathology, and behavioral principles sufficient to allow their productive participation in general supportive psychological counseling, particularly behavioral management programs, if properly advised and supported by the neuropsychiatrist.

It is also often useful to utilize these professionals as sophisticated observers of patient and family behaviors. Doing so is critical to both gaining accurate diagnostic information and monitoring treatment responses to counseling, behavioral, or psychopharmacological interventions. All of these professionals generally perceive these behavioral and psychological monitoring functions to be appropriate aspects of their more specialized clinical roles in the care of the patient with TBI.

Finally, as implied in the above paragraphs, it is critical to consider the inputs, interfaces, and contributions of this array of professionals of differing backgrounds in considering the neuropsychiatric assessment and treatment planning for each case of TBI. Although doing so may initially require more time by the clinician devoted to gathering background information and to developing working relationships with the total treatment team, the

reward of more comprehensive and effective treatment more than compensates for this effort.

Settings of Care

As noted, the treatment of the patient with TBI typically takes place in a variety of settings designed to address the particular needs of each patient at specific points in the recovery process (Figure 31–1).

The flow diagram provided in Figure 31–1 is a simplification of the many variations of treatment programs that exist in various communities. The Brain Injury Association of America publishes a national directory of brain injury treatment programs, which is a valuable aid in locating appropriate local and regional treatment sites for individuals with TBI (Brain Injury Association of America 2004). Most state chapters of the Brain Injury Association of America have compiled supplemental information in state- and regional-level resource directories. Some have staff devoted to information and referral functions. These staff may be of great assistance to providers and persons with TBI and their families in locating appropriate services.

The Commission on Accreditation of Rehabilitation Facilities (CARF) is the accepted accrediting body for the various forms of brain injury rehabilitation programs. It accredits programs under six general categories (Table 31–1).

An annual printed directory of CARF-accredited programs has been published until recently; it has been replaced with an Internet-based directory available at http://www.CARF.org. CARF's accreditation requirements for inpatient units as well as for specialized downstream TBI

TABLE 31–1. Categories of Commission on Accreditation of Rehabilitation Facilities–certified rehabilitation programs

Inpatient

Outpatient

Home and community based

Residential

Long-term residential

Vocational

programs mandate an array of required therapy services as well as physician direction by a qualified specialist. A specific set of program evaluations is also mandated.

In addition, a number of states operate programs that include service coordination as well as a point of entry to the service system. In reference to Figure 31–1, it is important to appreciate that each patient will follow his or her own appropriate sequence of programs, and this progression need not be linear. Many patients skip components of care; some proceed at times from right to left in the diagram instead of conversely. Some patients need to have multiple opportunities for certain types of treatments. It is important to recognize the general indications for each type of care manifested by each patient. These indications must be matched against the array of services available in that patient's given locale. For certain types of care, consideration should be given to referral out of the patient's area for specialized expertise (e.g., specialized behavioral management or prosthetic services).

Acute Care

Since the 1980s, trauma systems have been increasingly formally developed to expedite the immediate evacuation of the injured patient to tertiary level facilities with comprehensive trauma-focused medical and surgical capabilities. These trauma systems—with level I and II centers being the appropriate triage destination for severe injury—have 24 hour/day surgical, intensive care unit, and imaging capabilities, and they have virtually immediate availability of the subspecialties required for trauma care—neurosurgical services in particular for patients with TBI. These systems have been demonstrated to improve survival and recovery from severe trauma. Evidence-based guidelines for acute neurosurgical and medical care have been developed that delineate those immediate-care procedures shown to improve clinical outcomes (Brain Trauma Foundation 1996). In addition to acute medical and surgical care, rehabilitation evaluation and preliminary interven-

tions should take place within a short time after injury in these settings as well; ideally, these steps should occur within the neurological intensive care unit setting during the first several days after injury.

From this point, determination of subsequent rehabilitation pathways is provisionally made on the basis of extent of injury and nature of recovery. Most commonly, for severe TBI survivors, the next treatment site is the acute inpatient rehabilitation facility. The full array of in- and outpatient programs is typically required only in severe cases of TBI. Mild and moderate cases typically do not require the inpatient components of this care spectrum but may require significant outpatient physical, occupational, psychological therapies; vocational and educational programs; and significant neuropsychiatric assistance.

Acute Inpatient Rehabilitation

As noted, inpatient, hospital-based rehabilitation is the usual next site of care after the acute hospital for severe TBI patients. The general conditions that lead to admission to these units are patients' specific patterns of significant medical and nursing care needs as well as self-care and functional deficits; however, patients should have the residual ability to participate in and benefit from intensive therapies. Inpatient acute rehabilitation programs offer medical monitoring and care from 24 hour/day nursing staff who have specialized expertise in issues relevant to severely disabled patients (e.g., pulmonary, skin, bowel, bladder, and nutritional management; skin and wound care management). Patients in this setting may require both management of residual medical/surgical issues and engagement in a full array of rehabilitation activities (e.g., physical therapy, occupational therapy, speech and language therapy, psychology). Typically, a variety of medical and surgical subspecialists also are routinely available as consultants in these settings. Because of the relative high cost of these programs, patients are typically dispatched to less acute levels of rehabilitation as soon as their medical and nursing care requirements are sufficiently resolved.

Subacute Rehabilitation

Subacute programs for survivors of TBI are designed for the very severely impaired patients who—because of the extent of injury, slowness of recovery, or other medical reasons—are unable to participate in full therapy programs. These programs are appropriate for patients who are in a "minimally responsive state" in which further arousal has not yet occurred but may be anticipated, leading to subsequent entry into acute rehabilitation. Patients in these programs are characterized by relative medical stability but high levels of nursing care needs. Therapies are provided at a lower level of intensity than in acute rehabilitation units, and often the focus is on relatively passive preservation of function via skin and joint maintenance programs, development of appropriate nutrition (e.g., gastrostomy tube feeding protocols), bowel and bladder management programs, and so forth. These subacute units or programs are typically distinct wards within acute hospitals or specialized programs within extended care or skilled nursing facilities.

Neurobehavioral Treatment

For the patient with TBI who develops significant agitation and/or aggressive behavior during recovery or at any extended point in time later, there are specialized programs in which focused neurobehavioral and psychopharmacological interventions can be provided while protecting the patient and others from his or her behavior. On occasion, this intervention is done on a formal neuropsychiatric unit, although more typically it is done in programs specifically designed for survivors of TBI. These programs may be subunits within inpatient units in rehabilitation hospitals, in skilled nursing facilities, or even in residential-type programs. They are characterized by relatively high levels of staff-to-patient ratios, with staff that have specific expertise in neurobehavioral management. The programs also are conducted in physically or architecturally designed "secure" physical plants, which prevent patient elopement or self-injury. Patients with TBI typically require these programs for a limited period during recovery while transiting Rancho Los Amigos Level of Cognitive Function Scale IV (i.e., while passing through the "confused, agitated" phase to more controlled levels of neural function; Hagen 1982). There is, however, also a small subset of patients who have persistent and severe behavioral disturbance that may last for many years after injury and are among the most distressing and difficult of patients with TBI to manage. Occasionally, a patient with TBI symptoms may require neurobehavioral intervention some time (occasionally years) after onset of injury.

Residential Treatment

For a number of patients without extensive medical or nursing care needs, treatment in an acute rehabilitation program is unnecessary, but for those with sufficient functional deficits, group residence programs exist that take place on "campuses" of various sorts, including rural "ranches," urban or suburban residential settings, dormi-

tories, and apartments. These programs have therapy areas as well as facilities such as kitchens and workshops to provide avocational/vocational training opportunities. These programs are staffed by professional clinicians of various disciplines as well as by laypersons who are provided in-program training in essentials of TBI rehabilitation management. Nursing services are typically provided (although usually not on a 24 hour/day basis) so that medical monitoring and dispensing of medications can take place. There is no onsite physician involvement, although typically there is a medical director (consultant) who sees the patients on a regular basis (usually weekly to monthly). These programs provide a safe and structured environment (often with graduated levels of autonomy through which patients move during recovery) to prepare patients for return to home or other long-term living arrangements.

Outpatient Day Hospital or Program

For many reasonably medically stable patients, it is possible to return home but still receive a full array of multidisciplinary therapy via a TBI day hospital or program. Such programs may or may not be attached to a hospital-based acute rehabilitation program within the outpatient department. At their best, these programs have specifically designed comprehensive activities and services for patients with TBI. These programs should have an identified medical director and regular team staffing to set and review treatment goals and progress for each patient with TBI. Not infrequently, however, what is termed a *day program* is simply an aggregation of individual therapies without an overall coordinating structure or TBI focus. Again, CARF accreditation standards delineate the minimum programmatic requirements indicated.

Outpatient Therapy

Very commonly, after more comprehensive treatment programs, patients with TBI require one or more individual therapy services for isolated residual functional deficits. More mildly to moderately injured patients with TBI also may require only one or a few isolated therapy services. For these cases, individual physical, occupational, speech, and psychological services are provided in a traditional manner within a hospital outpatient department or via individual office-based or home-health treatments.

Vocational Services

States receive federal funds through the Rehabilitation Act of 1973 (29 U.S.C. 723) to operate vocational programs for adults with TBI when return to work is a feasible rehabilitation goal. Current law mandates that even severely injured persons are assumed to have an ability to work and are therefore eligible for services. Vocational programs can include reeducation as well as worksite-related support and training. It is important to coordinate these services with traditional rehabilitation care so that the special needs of the TBI survivor can be incorporated into realistic vocational goals and training.

Special Educational Services

The Individuals With Disabilities Education Act (formerly called P.L. 94-142) mandates that the special educational needs of disabled children (up to age 18 years or until graduation from high school) be met within the public educational system. This law also requires the provision of related services (e.g., transportation, speech therapy, occupational therapy) that could assist the child's benefiting from the educational program. For school-age patients, often the fullest treatment programs can be obtained via establishment of a well-designed individualized educational program that can provide occupational and speech therapies, counseling, and specialized educational classes and tutoring. In the past, and to a significant extent still, students with TBI have been inappropriately classified (e.g., as mentally deficient) if they were identified at all. Placements made and services rendered have often been inappropriate to students with TBI. In the past decade, an increasing number of states have responded by developing guidelines and specialized training and technical assistance for the service of students with TBI (Goodall et al. 1994; Ylvisaker et al. 2001).

Lifetime Supported Living Services

Many persons with TBI are in need of long-term care and support services. These services include social, personal care, and supportive services. Often, the payment for rehabilitation ends within a few months after the injury although the period of recovery may extend to years. In addition, ongoing rehabilitation is often needed to maintain function. Such "maintenance" rehabilitation is often not reimbursed by insurers because it is beyond the scope of their benefits. Nearly 100 million Americans have a chronic illness or disability, yet the current health system is ill suited to provide the care that they need (LaForce and Wussow 2001). Twelve million people are unable to live independently, and six million of these are younger than age 65 years (Feder et al. 2000). However, the United States currently has no universal public or private mechanisms to pay for long-term care services (O'Keefe 1994).

Many seriously injured persons with TBI who are unable to return to an independent-living environment depend on informal supports provided by family and friends. When informal supports and personal finances are not available or have been exhausted, there is a patchwork of federal, state, and local programs that provides some home- and community-based services; however, these are limited and fragmented. The major source of public financing for long-term care services is Medicaid, the federal-state health program for individuals and families with low income, which funds primarily institutional services (Goodall et al. 1994). For persons with TBI, this circumstance often means inappropriate placement in nursing homes rather than living in the community with the aid of appropriate support services. These living arrangements are manifestly unsuitable for most persons with TBI, many of whom are young adults. However, in the 35 years since its enactment, Medicaid's "institutional bias" has been reduced through amendments to federal laws and policies (Office of the Assistant Secretary for Planning and Evaluation 2000). Recently, over one-half of states had used some type of Medicaid home and community-based (HCBS) waiver to provide services to persons with TBI (Spearman et al. 2001). In addition, many states have passed legislation creating programs and services specifically for individuals with TBI and their families. In general, these programs have been designed to fill in gaps in services by offering assistance not otherwise available through state and federal programs. Some states have entered into interagency agreements to coordinate systems so that they are better able to serve persons with TBI with limited resources (Vaughn and King 2001). Types of services provided through these state programs may include residential services provided in a self-contained setting by a single provider, but since the early 1990s, the trend has been toward increased use of community-based providers who emphasize natural and integrated settings to the extent possible. A diverse set of models of services continues to evolve.

Mental Health Services

Many people make a good recovery after suffering a severe TBI. However, a number of individuals have considerable difficulty with community integration after their rehabilitation and may need further services and supports (Feeney et al. 2001). In addition, many persons with TBI are not provided appropriate rehabilitation after the injury and later present with behavioral and cognitive problems that may lead to referral to the mental health system. Mental health services may be provided as a short-term benefit available through health insurance or another funding stream. Under such circumstances, the person with TBI can receive services from any appropriate provider. However, finding an appropriate provider often is a challenge because comprehensive education and training about TBI has not been routinely included in medical school or specialized training of psychiatrists and other mental health professionals. In addition, one of the key problems for persons with TBI who are attempting to access available services has been establishing that they are appropriate recipients of such services—this has often been true for mental health services. Insurance coverage has restrictions on benefits that may rule out its use as a source of payment for mental health benefits even when a provider is located.

Similar problems apply to the publicly funded mental health services available through state and local mental health programs designed to meet the needs of persons with chronic mental illness. As public mental health systems have reduced or nearly eliminated the use of large, state-operated psychiatric institutions, admissions have been restricted to those who are defined as appropriately matched to the services available within the institution and the community-based after-care system. Many states have determined that persons with TBI have needs that cannot be met within their psychiatric facilities. Advocates for persons with TBI have agreed because they wish to avoid the perceived stigma associated with mental illness. Such advocates supported the development of specialized programs for persons with TBI who have behavioral problems that jeopardize their ability to live successfully in the community rather than advocate for access to an apparently inappropriate mental health system. These programs have been described earlier in this chapter in the section Neurobehavioral Treatment.

Additionally, neurobehavioral programs for persons with TBI have been developed in a number of nursing homes (O'Keefe 1994). As previously stated, nursing homes are generally inappropriate for meeting the needs of persons with TBI, but they have been used for both rehabilitation and behavioral interventions for lack of more appropriate alternatives. The nursing home has become the default site for care and services for adults with a variety of chronic conditions because states can more readily use their Medicaid funds to pay for this type of care than for other alternatives. A small number of providers have responded to the opportunity to develop behavioral services in nursing homes and other residential settings because of the evident need and lack of alternatives. A few states use funds earmarked for services for persons with TBI to pay for other types of residential neurobehavioral programs that are not nursing homes. Such programs generally fall within the residential treatment or lifelong

supported living services described in the sections above by those names, depending on their specific goals.

In recent years, more states have developed appropriate services as part of their HCBS Medicaid waivers to address mental health and behavioral needs of persons with TBI. Among the few states that have comprehensively addressed the needs of persons with TBI who exhibit challenging behaviors, Massachusetts and Minnesota have developed specialized neurobehavioral units within hospitals operated directly by the state or under contracts with the state. New York has put a major emphasis on the development of statewide neurobehavioral resources within the structure of its community-based TBI program supported through its HCBS TBI waiver. New York has successfully transitioned hundreds of persons with TBI who were living in specialized nursing home units to community living. Full descriptions of New York's efforts have been provided elsewhere (LaForce and Wussow 2001; O'Keefe 1994).

Sources of Funding and Public Policy Aspects

Public and private funding for the rehabilitation of persons with TBI is needed to meet acute and long-term needs. Access to initial care and subsequent rehabilitation for persons with TBI varies depending on insurance coverage, treatment personnel, family and community characteristics, geographical location, knowledge of available resources, and the ability to navigate the medical care and rehabilitation system successfully. The outcome of injury depends not only on its severity but also on the speed and appropriateness of treatment.

Workers' Compensation

Some individuals with TBI who were injured on the job are eligible for worker's compensation. Workers' compensation legislation was initially enacted by most state legislatures in the first part of the 20th century. Its purposes included the provision of adequate benefits to injured workers in addition to limiting employers' liabilities. The system was designed to make prompt payments at predetermined levels to relieve employees and employers of uncertainty and to eliminate wasteful litigation (U.S. General Accounting Office 1996). The benefits are among the most comprehensive of all insurance coverage. They include medical care, extended rehabilitation, and partial wage replacement. Some states provide retraining and job placement services to assist the injured worker in returning to work, when feasible. Although this coverage provides a good opportunity for a person with TBI to resume his or her prior lifestyle, not many cases of TBI occur on the job, so few persons with TBI benefit from this coverage (Cavallo and Reynolds 1999; Wright 1993).

Automobile Liability Insurance

Automobile accidents are a frequent cause of TBI, especially in teenagers and young adults; therefore, automobile liability is an important source of payment for rehabilitation for such TBI survivors. Traditional automobile liability insurance is based on the concept that the party at fault for an accident is financially responsible for damage and injuries resulting from the accident. The owner of a car purchases insurance as protection from lawsuits. However, for the driver at fault and his or her passengers, automobile insurance does not cover the driver and passengers in the car driven by the party at fault. The party at fault and his or her passengers must seek reimbursement through their private health insurance or through Medicaid. Long delays associated with establishment of fault and obtaining settlements from the insurance companies are another problem. Such delays can adversely affect access to necessary rehabilitation (Spearman et al. 2001).

No-Fault Automobile Insurance

No-fault automobile insurance is an alternative to traditional liability insurance. The no-fault concept is designed to provide prompt payment for lost wages and medical expenses. Benefits are paid through one's own insurance company without the long delays associated with litigation (Spearman et al. 2001). Although the first state to enact a no-fault law did so in 1970, as of 2004 only 12 states had a no-fault law (Insurance Information Institute 2004; National Association of Insurance Commissioners 1999). Most no-fault states place a fairly low cap on the amount paid for medical care and rehabilitation (Michigan is the single exception). This amount typically may be $50,000, an amount totally inadequate to meet the needs of many persons with TBI. Active lobbying by trial lawyers' associations has contributed to weak no-fault laws (Spearman et al. 2001). Additional costs must be met by obtaining a settlement from the insurance company of the driver who was at fault. The person with TBI can also obtain reimbursement from his or her health insurance when no-fault means are exhausted (A.T. Doolittle, personal communication, October 2001).

Health Insurance

Health insurance often provides very few of the benefits beyond acute medical care needed by a person with a serious TBI. Private insurance pays primarily for acute care, and coverage decisions are generally made according to a narrow definition of *medical necessity* (Goodall et al. 1994). Limits typically are applied to the number of hospital days, skilled nursing facility days, and therapy sessions. Additional exclusions may exist for home health care, outpatient services, and all forms of long-term care. Health insurance policies rarely specify benefits for rehabilitation. Companies may negotiate an "extra contractual agreement" to cover such services (Spearman et al. 2001). As the majority of Americans participating in employer- and Medicaid-sponsored health plans have become enrolled in managed care plans, these preexisting limitations in health insurance coverage typically have continued, if not increased (DeJong and Sutton 1998).

Medicare

Medicare is a federal health insurance program covering services for persons ages 65 years and older as well as for 6.1 million persons younger than age 65 years with disabilities (data from 2003; Centers for Medicare and Medicaid Services 2004). Medicare pays primarily for acute care and a limited amount of postacute rehabilitation, nursing home, and home care. Medicare typically does not benefit many persons with TBI for two reasons. The first reason relates to the average age of persons with TBI. To be eligible for Social Security Disability Insurance (SSDI) and therefore eligible for Medicare, one must have a sufficient number of quarters of earnings, and many persons who sustain a TBI do not meet this qualification. Second, those who become eligible for SSDI must wait 2 years to become eligible for Medicare. Medicare eligibility therefore is not determined until after the postacute stage of injury, the period when TBI patients have the greatest need for rehabilitation services (Goodall et al. 1994).

Medicaid

The program known as *Medicaid* became law in 1965 as a jointly funded cooperative venture between federal and state governments to assist states in the provision of adequate medical care to eligible persons in need of it. One category of persons eligible for Medicaid that is of particular interest in regard to TBI is beneficiaries of the Supplemental Security Income program, which provides cash benefits to low-income disabled persons younger than the age of 65 years and to elderly persons with low income. Medicaid is the largest program providing medical and health-related services to America's lowest-income people. Within broad national guidelines, which the federal government provides, each of the states establishes its own eligibility standards; determines the type, amount, duration, and scope of services; sets the rate of payment for services; and administers its own program. Just as coverage for rehabilitation is often limited in health insurance plans and other private insurance, the Medicaid program benefits may or may not be adequate to meet the needs of persons with a recent TBI. This shortcoming may result from a state's failure to cover specific needed services that are not mandated by federal law or are not attainable because of the state's limitations on amount, duration, and scope of covered benefits.

Despite Medicaid's limitations in coverage of many people with low income, Medicaid provides a more comprehensive array of benefits than Medicare. Medicaid coverage can include rehabilitative services in addition to acute services. Medicaid covers long-term care services that are not covered by Medicare. In addition, some states provide an array of services appropriate to meet the needs of persons with TBI through optional Medicaid services including case management, personal assistance services, and HCBS waivers (Digre et al. 1994; Goodall et al. 1994; LaForce and Wussow 2001; Spearman et al. 2001).

For the clinician managing cases of TBI, in light of this daunting array of (typically inadequate) potential funding resources, the services of an experienced social worker or other reimbursement specialist are of critical importance in ensuring that survivors of TBI receive the optimum care possible.

Conclusion

In terms of sheer numbers of cases, patients with mild and moderate TBI far outnumber severely injured patients, and frequently the former are essentially physically independent individuals struggling with isolated psychiatric problems including depression, posttraumatic stress disorder, anxiety reactions, and less severe cognitive and behavioral disturbances. Appropriate psychological and psychiatric care is essential. For the more severely injured patient with TBI, however, a more complex pattern of care is typical. This chapter gives a general overview of the treatment context into which most neuropsychiatric care is placed. It has been a source of long-lasting surprise to the authors to see the degree to which the psychiatric "mental health" care for the patient with TBI has been provided in isolation from and disregard for the well-developed rehabilitation system developed over the past 25–30 years. This disconnection has frequently led to reduplication of care as well as each system's failure to garner the full value of the expertise in the other. It is hoped that as more awareness of these parallel resources emerges, better integration between them will occur, to the benefit of patients and families experiencing the consequences of TBI.

References

Aronow HU: Rehabilitation effectiveness with severe brain injury: translating research into policy. J Head Trauma Rehabil 2:24–36, 1987

Berroll S, Rappaport M, Cope DN, et al: Severe Head Trauma: A Comprehensive Medical Approach. Project 13-P-59156/9, Vols I and II. San Jose, CA, National Institute for Handicapped Research, 1982

Brain Injury Association of America: The 2003–2004 National Directory of Brain Injury Rehabilitation Services. McLean, VA, Brain Injury Association of America, 2004

Brain Trauma Foundation, American Association of Neurological Surgeons, Joint Section on Neurotrauma and Critical Care: Guidelines for the management of severe head injury. J Neurotrauma 13:641–734, 1996

Bureau of Maternal and Child Health, Health Services and Resources Administration, U.S. Department of Health and Human Services: Promising practices for state system of coordinated supports and services for people with brain injury and their families. Washington, DC, U.S. Government Printing Office, 2001

Cavallo M, Reynolds WE: TBI Act implementation project: a strategic process to refine a regional integrated system of services for persons with traumatic brain injury. Poster presented at Traumatic Brain Injury in the 21st Century: Learning from Models of Research and Service Delivery, Bethesda, MD, December 1999

Cope DN: The effectiveness of traumatic brain injury rehabilitation: a review. Brain Inj 9:649–670, 1995

Cope DN: Brain injury rehabilitation, in The State of the Science in Medical Rehabilitation, Vol 2. Edited by Sutton JP, Lehmkuhl DL, DeJong G, et al. Falls Church, VA, Birch and Davis Associates, 1996, pp 1–20

Cope DN, Hall K: Head injury rehabilitation: benefits of early rehabilitation. Arch Phys Med Rehabil 63:433–437, 1982

DeJong G, Sutton J: Managed care and catastrophic injury: the case of spinal cord injury. Topics in Spinal Cord Injury Rehabilitation 3:1–16, 1998

Digre PG, et al: Selected states' public policy responses to traumatic brain injury. J Head Trauma Rehabil 9:12–26, 1994

Feder J, Komisar H, Niefeld M: Long-term care in the United States: an overview. Health Aff (Millwood) 19:40–56, 2000

Feeney TJ, Ylvisaker M, Rosen BH, et al: Community supports for individuals with challenging behavior after brain injury: an analysis of the New York State behavioral resource project. J Head Trauma Rehabil 16:61–75, 2001

Feliciano DV, Moore EE, Mattox DL (eds): Trauma, 3rd Edition. Stamford, CT, Appleton and Lange, 1996

Finset A, Berstad J, Dyrnes S, et al: Regaining function following severe head injury: from primary rehabilitation to two years after the injury. Tidsskr Nor Laegeforen 115:210–213, 1995

Goodall P, Layer H, Wehman P: Vocational rehabilitation and traumatic brain injury: a legislative and policy perspective. J Head Trauma Rehabil 9:61–81, 1994

Hagen C: Language cognitive disorganization following closed head injury: a conceptualization, in Cognitive Rehabilitation: Conceptualization and Intervention. Edited by Trexler LE. New York, Plenum, 1982, pp 131–151

Centers for Medicare and Medicaid Services: Medicare Enrollment Trends 1966–2003. Available at: http://www.cms.hhs.gov/statistics/enrollment/natltrends/hi_smi.asp. Accessed August 5, 2004.

Horn LJ, Zasler ND (eds): Medical Rehabilitation of Traumatic Brain Injury. Philadelphia, PA, Hanley & Belfus, 1996

Insurance Information Institute: No-fault auto insurance. Available at: http://www.iii.org/media/hottopics/insurance/nofault. Accessed August 5, 2004.

Jennet B, Teasdale G: Management of Head Injuries. Philadelphia, PA, FA Davis, 1981

LaForce FM, Wussow J: Chronic Illness in America: Overcoming Barriers to Building Systems of Care. Lawrenceville, NJ, Center for Health Strategies, 2001

Mackay LE, Bernstein BA, Capman PE, et al: Early intervention in severe head injury: long-term benefits of a formalized program. Arch Phys Med Rehabil 73:635–641, 1992

National Association of Insurance Commissioners: No-Fault Auto Insurance. Kansas City, MO, National Association of Insurance Commissioners, 1999

National Institute on Disability and Rehabilitation Research: NIDDR Programs & Projects. Available at: http://www.ed.gov/rschstat/research/pubs/programs.html. Accessed June 29, 2004.

National Institutes of Health: Rehabilitation of Persons with Traumatic Brain Injury, Consensus Statement, October 26–28, 16:1–41, 1998

O'Keefe J: Long-term care and support services for persons with traumatic brain injury. J Head Trauma Rehabil 9:49–60, 1994

Office of the Assistant Secretary for Planning and Evaluation, U.S. Department of Health and Human Services: Understanding Medicaid home and community services: a primer. Washington, DC, U.S. Government Printing Office, 2000

Rappaport M, Herrero-Backe C, Rappaport ML, et al: Head injury outcome up to ten years later. Arch Phys Med Rehabil 70:885–892, 1989

Rehabilitation Act of 1973, Title 29, sec. 723. Available at http://www.ed.gov/policy/speced/teg/narrative.html. Accessed September 6, 2004.

Spearman RC, Stamm BH, Rosen BH, et al: The use of Medicaid waivers and their impact on services. J Head Trauma Rehabil 16:47–60, 2001

Traumatic Brain Injury Technical Assistance Center: About TBI State Grant Program. Available at http://www.tbitac.org/site/AboutTBI.cfm?page=aboutTBI. Accessed July 14, 2004.

U.S. General Accounting Office: Workers' Compensation. Selected Comparisons of Federal and State Laws. Washington, DC, U.S. General Accounting Office. GAO/GGD-96–76, 1996

Vaughn S, King A: A survey of state programs to finance rehabilitation and community services for individuals with brain injury. J Head Trauma Rehabil 16:290–233, 2001

Wright B: What Legislators Need to Know About Traumatic Brain Injury. Denver, CO, National Conference of State Legislatures, 1993

Ylvisaker M, Todis B, Glang A, et al: Educating students with TBI: themes and recommendations. J Head Trauma Rehabil 16:76–93, 2001

32 Social Issues

Andrew Hornstein, M.D.

FIFTY THOUSAND PEOPLE die of traumatic brain injury (TBI) every year in the United States, and more than 5 million TBI survivors are left with permanent disabilities. The economic burden of TBI approaches $40 billion annually. Most TBI victims are young, and many survivors need lifelong services (Centers for Disease Control and Prevention 1999). These facts highlight a major public health issue that has broad social as well as clinical implications. This chapter reviews some of these social implications. Areas to be covered are legislation affecting TBI patients, advocacy issues, insurance coverage, employment and vocational rehabilitation (VR) services, and litigation. Other important social aspects of TBI, prevention and broader legal issues, are covered in depth in Chapter 33, Ethical and Clinical Legal Issues, and Chapter 40, Prevention.

Public Policy and Legislation

Clinicians are often only vaguely aware of how public policy affects their work. However, the care of patients with TBI exemplifies the profound effect that government actions can have on the kind of care available to patients. As Rosen and Reynolds (1994) point out, "public policy decisions have an impact on every aspect of an individual's life following a traumatic brain injury...(affecting), for example, the training and skill level of emergency medical technicians, the configuration of the trauma system, the type and amount of rehabilitation services allowable through insurance, and the services available for long-term supports" (p. 1).

Before 1980, there was essentially no public policy specific to TBI (Spivack 1994). This began to change with the improvement in rates of survival from TBI as a result of better emergency care at accident sites, improved access to specialized trauma centers, and technological ad-

vances such as intracranial pressure monitors and magnetic resonance imaging scanning (Department of Health and Human Services 1989). There was a growing population of TBI survivors with a broad array of neurological deficits; some deficits subtle but devastating to vocational or social functioning, and some profound and necessitating institutional care. Few people other than TBI specialists understood the needs of these patients, and few resources were available to meet these needs. The American health care system is weighted overwhelmingly toward the provision of curative interventions for clearly defined, usually acute, conditions. The needs of the chronically disabled, such as TBI survivors, have been relegated by public and private insurers to the category of "maintenance," for which limited, if any, funds are available.

The burden of managing the daily needs of TBI survivors fell primarily on their families, who were further burdened by a paucity of information on TBI. The National Head Injury Foundation was founded in 1980 by family members of TBI survivors "to provide support, gather and disseminate information, and encourage program development" (Spivack 1994, p. 83). This organization evolved into the Brain Injury Association of America, which with its local and state chapters has been in the forefront of advocating for TBI survivors and their families. The Brain Injury Association has also become a vital source of information to TBI survivors and their families. It publishes an annual National Directory of Brain Injury Rehabilitation Services, periodicals for both the lay public and TBI professionals, and a series of resource guides on available public benefits.

The lobbying efforts of the Head Injury Foundation succeeded in a number of states, leading to legislation and executive orders addressing specific needs of TBI patients. Among the first was the Statewide Head Injury Program of Massachusetts, established in 1985, which provided case coordination and training on TBI issues to

TABLE 32–1. Spending by states for traumatic brain injury services

	AL	AZ	CA	FL	GA	KY	LA	MA	MN	MS	MO	NV	NM	NY	NC	PA	SC	TN	TX	VA
Health				X					X		X		X							
Rehabilitation services	X	X				X	X		X		X				X				X	X
Disability services			X			X									X		X			
Other					X															

Source. Reprinted from Vaughn SL, King A: "A Survey of State Programs to Finance Rehabilitation and Community Services for Individuals With Brain Injury." *The Journal of Head Trauma Rehabilitation* 16:23, 2001. Copyright 2001 Aspen Publishers, Inc. Used with permission.

schools, professionals, and the public. It also assisted with program development and direct funding of nonresidential services (Digre et al. 1994). Also in 1985, in conjunction with legislation mandating the use of seat belts, the State of Missouri established the Head Injury Advisory Council, which included members from the state legislature; administrators of state health, insurance, education, and VR agencies; and representatives from the local academic medical community. This Council has been instrumental in establishing numerous programs throughout the state to meet the needs of postacute TBI patients. In Florida, a more conservative fiscal climate precluded the use of existing public funds for expanding health care services to TBI patients. In 1987, a unique Impaired Driver's and Speeder's Trust Fund was legislated that charged an additional fine to those convicted of speeding or driving under the influence. The monies collected funded a statewide system of case managers and other services (Digre et al. 1994; Vaughn and King 2001). Table 32–1, from the review article of Vaughn and King (2001), illustrates the source and amount of funding provided by those states that have dedicated TBI programs. In their review, Vaughn and King note that in all these states, TBI programs are meagerly funded, are payers of last resort, and usually are staffed by fewer than six professionals.

At the federal level, active lobbying by the members of the National Head Injury Foundation led to increasing interest by members of Congress in the plight of TBI survivors and their families. In 1984, both the House of Representatives and the Senate passed resolutions directing various federal agencies dealing with the disabled to begin collecting data on the incidence of TBI as well as to assess the status of services, research, and unmet needs. In addition to increased recognition of TBI as a growing public health crisis, there were administrative initiatives that led to productive cooperation between federal and state officials involved with TBI issues (Spivack 1994). In 1987, at the direction of Congress, a Federal Interagency Head Injury Task Force issued a report that recommended,

among other things, consistent case definition and reporting of TBI, which had been lacking up until that time (Department of Health and Human Services 1989). Comprehensive regional brain injury centers were also established, but funding constraints limited full implementation of the report's recommendations.

Recognizing the large and growing public health problem that TBI survival represented, Congress passed the Traumatic Brain Injury Act in July 1996 (P.L. 104–166). The act directed the federal Centers for Disease Control and Prevention to carry out intra- and extramural projects to reduce the incidence of TBI by conducting research on strategies for prevention of TBI and by implementing public information and education programs on such prevention. The act also directed the National Institutes of Health to conduct research on

(A)...development of new methods and modalities for the more effective diagnosis, measurement of degree of injury, post-injury monitoring and prognostic assessment of brain injury for acute, subacute, and later phases of care; (B) the development, modification, and evaluation of therapies that retard, prevent, or reverse brain damage after acute brain injury, that arrest further deterioration following injury and that provide the restitution of function for individuals with long-term injuries; (C) the development of research on the continuum of care from acute care through rehabilitation, designed, to the extent predictable, to integrate rehabilitation and long-term outcome evaluation with acute care research; and (D) the development of programs that increase the participation of academic centers of excellence in brain injury treatment and rehabilitation research and training. (p. 5)

In addition, the Act provided matching funds for state demonstration projects designed to improve access to "health and other services regarding traumatic brain injury." The act called for the development of a uniform reporting system for TBI and for a consensus conference on TBI. Three million dollars per year for 3 years were allocated for these activities.

The National Institutes of Health held a Consensus Development Conference on Rehabilitation of Persons With Traumatic Brain Injury in October of 1998. The panel, whose 16 members represented multiple disciplines involved with TBI and public health, elicited expert and consumer opinion, with a focus on the following questions:

1. What is the epidemiology of TBI in the United States and what are its implications for rehabilitation?
2. What are the consequences of TBI in terms of pathophysiology, impairments, functional limitations, disabilities, societal limitations, and economic impact?
3. What is known about mechanisms underlying functional recovery after TBI, and what are the implications for rehabilitation?
4. What are the common therapeutic interventions for the cognitive and behavioral sequelae of TBI, what is their scientific basis, and how effective are they?
5. What are common models of comprehensive, coordinated, multidisciplinary rehabilitation for people with TBI, what is their scientific basis, and what is known about their short- and long-term outcomes?
6. On the basis of the answers to these questions, what can be recommended regarding rehabilitation practices for people with TBI?
7. What research is needed to guide the rehabilitation of people with TBI (National Institutes of Health Consensus Development Panel on Rehabilitation of Persons With Traumatic Brain Injury 1999)?

The panel's conclusions are listed in Table 32–2. The published report contains a detailed bibliography well worth the attention of the interested reader.

The Traumatic Brain Injury Act of 1996 also mandated that the Centers for Disease Control and Prevention publish a study of the national incidence and impact of TBI (Centers for Disease Control and Prevention 1999). The report presented available epidemiological data and concluded that TBI is a clearly important public health problem. The importance of primary prevention of the three main causes of TBI—transportation crashes, violence, and falls—was reiterated. Improved acute care and rehabilitation of TBI were called for, with specific focus on cognitive and emotional impairments. The need for improved data systems was also emphasized. The report described the decrease in TBI-related hospitaliza-

TABLE 32–2. Conclusions of the National Institutes of Health consensus conference on traumatic brain injury (TBI)

TBI is a heterogeneous disorder of major public health significance.

Consequences of TBI can be lifelong.

Given the large toll of TBI and absence of cure, prevention is of paramount importance.

Identification, intervention, and prevention of alcohol abuse and violence provide an important opportunity to reduce TBI and its effects.

Rehabilitation services, matched to the needs of persons with TBI, and community-based nonmedical services are required to optimize outcomes over the course of recovery.

Mild TBI is significantly underdiagnosed, and early intervention is often neglected.

Persons with TBI, their families, and significant others are integral to the design and implementation of the rehabilitation process and research.

Public and private funding for rehabilitation of persons with TBI should be adequate to meet acute and long-term needs.

Access to needed long-term rehabilitation may be jeopardized by changes in payment methods for private insurance and public programs.

Increased understanding of the mechanisms of TBI and recovery holds promise for new treatments.

Well-designed and controlled studies are needed to evaluate benefits of different rehabilitation interventions.

Basic and common classification systems of TBI are needed.

The evaluation of TBI interventions will require innovative research methods.

Funding for research on TBI should be increased.

Source. Reprinted from National Institutes of Health Consensus Development Panel on Rehabilitation of Persons With Traumatic Brain Injury: "Rehabilitation of Persons With Traumatic Brain Injury." *Journal of the American Medical Association* 282:981, 1999. Used with permission.

tion rates over the preceding 20 years and suggested that this decrease reflected fiscally driven restrictions in hospital admissions, leaving larger numbers of patients with less severe TBI with only emergency care. Uniform state-based surveillance systems of emergency department visits were recommended to determine the true frequency of different types of TBI (Centers for Disease Control and Prevention 1999) and to better determine the relationship between the initial severity of injury and long-term outcome. In October of 2000, a set of amendments to the Traumatic Brain Injury Act was passed, continuing funding for another 2 years and expanding the range of state rehabilitation and research programs that were eligible for federal grants. There was also continued explicit direction to the Centers for Disease Control and Prevention to study and clarify the epidemiology of TBI by developing consistent state registries.

Medicaid

The major sources of public funding for TBI services are Medicaid, VR, and independent living services (U.S. General Accounting Office 1998). Medicaid was established by the federal government in 1965 to provide health care for low-income and disabled adults and children. It provides health insurance for nearly 40 million Americans. Medicaid is a federally mandated program that is administered and partially funded by the individual states, with required services that all states must provide, such as inpatient and outpatient hospital care, physician services, and nursing facility care, and optional programs such as rehabilitation services and prescriptions.

Standard Medicaid programs do not provide funding for long-term community-based support services. In 1981, Congress passed the Home and Community Based Waiver, allowing states to waive certain Medicaid regulations to provide long-term services in the community, so long as these services cost less than institutional care (Goodall and Ghiloni 2001). These waiver programs now number 200 nationally and serve more than 250,000 individuals with such services as homemakers, personal care, and nonmedical transportation (U.S General Accounting Office 1998). Administrators of state programs for TBI patients were initially slow to invest the significant resources required to apply to the Health Care Financing Agency for waivers, especially because these services were designed primarily for individuals with physical rather than cognitive or emotional disabilities. However, regulatory changes in 1990 specifically eased the application process for TBI programs, and at this time more than one-half of the states use some type of Medicaid waiver to provide services for those with TBI (Spearman et al. 2001). Given the decentralized nature of the Medicaid program, every state TBI waiver program is unique. Table 32–3 illustrates some of the services various states provide.

However, the benefits of these waiver programs are limited to only a small fraction of TBI patients. Even in those states providing waiver services, the number of beneficiaries rarely exceeds 1,000 (U.S. General Accounting Office 1998). The General Accounting Office report cites the following barriers to TBI patients, using waivers: 1) many state programs are still weighted in favor of those with physical disabilities and are not equipped to

TABLE 32–3. Types of traumatic brain injury waiver services available

Case management

Residential rehabilitation

Transitional living

Independent living skills training and development

Adult day care and/or day treatment

Home and community support services (e.g., chores, supervision, companionship)

Substance abuse or mental health counseling

Psychological or behavioral counseling

Employment rehabilitation

Intensive behavioral support/crisis support

Home modifications

Specialized medical equipment and supplies/assistive technology

Nonmedical transportation

Respite care

Personal care/attendant services

Skilled nursing

Home-delivered meals

Expanded availability of physical, occupational, speech, and cognitive therapies

Source. Reprinted from Spearman RC, Stamm BH, Rosen BH, et al: "The Use of Medicaid Waivers and Their Impact on Services." *The Journal of Head Trauma Rehabilitation* 16:52, 2001, Aspen Publishers, Inc. Used with permission.

recognize or deal with individuals with, for example, subtle but incapacitating executive dysfunctions; 2) effective advocates are often needed to negotiate social service systems, especially for those TBI survivors with cognitive impairments; and 3) programs tend to exclude patients with problematic or aggressive behaviors; funding is only rarely available to provide the structured settings and professional supports necessary to properly manage TBI patients with behavioral problems. TBI waiver programs are expanding, however, and it is hoped that this trend will continue as policy makers are made more aware of the utility and cost-effectiveness of long-term community-based care for TBI.

Employment

A series of studies in the 1980s documented the fact that severe TBI precluded return to competitive employment for

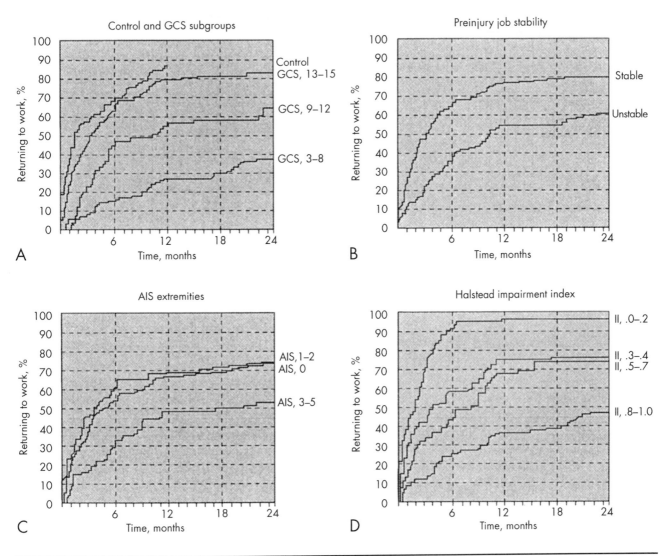

FIGURE 32–1.   **Return-to-work percentage by severity of traumatic brain injury, preinjury stability, physical disability, and neuropsychological status.**

Estimated percentage of patients first returning to work by subgroups defined on the basis of (A) initial Glasgow Coma Scale (GCS) score, (B) job stability, (C) Abbreviated Injury Scale (AIS) score for the extremities, and (D) neuropsychological performance at 1 month after injury using the Halstead Impairment Index (II).

Source.   Reprinted from Dikmen SS, Temkin NR, Machamer JE, et al: "Employment Following Traumatic Head Injuries." *Archives of Neurology* 51:182, 1994, American Medical Association. Used with permission.

the majority of survivors (Ben-Yishay et al. 1987; Brooks et al. 1987; Levin et al. 1979; McMordie et al. 1990; Rao et al. 1990). Despite methodological differences, the studies found the unemployment rate among survivors of severe TBI was generally in the range of 60%–80%. Factors correlated with poor employment outcome included severity of injury; degree of cognitive, physical, and psychosocial impairments; and vaguely defined "preinjury variables."

To clarify the impact of various risk factors on return to work, Dikmen et al. (1994) conducted a prospective study of 366 TBI patients and 95 control subjects with somatic trauma. Their results are illustrated in Figure 32–1.

The data show that 1 year after injury, 80% of TBI patients with Glasgow Coma Scale (GCS) scores of 13–15 returned to work, a level almost equal to that of control subjects. For patients with GCS scores of 9–12, less than 60% returned to work, and less than 30% of those with GCS scores of 8 or less were employed 1 year postinjury. Those with more severe injuries tended to show some improvement up to 2 years postinjury, whereas those with less severe injuries reached the asymptote by 1 year. The authors emphasize the importance of severity of injury, especially length of coma, as having a reliable and powerful predictive effect. Of those patients in their cohort who were not following commands 29 days after injury, only 8% were working 2 years after injury. They found that subjects older than age 50 years, those with less than a high school education, and those with unstable premorbid work histories were significantly less likely to be employed after TBI. In their group, moderate injury to other body systems did not lead to significant unemployment by 6 months after injury. A limitation of the Dikmen study is the restriction of study subjects to those fully employed at the time of injury, presumably a healthier group than the population at large, and their partial exclusion of patients with prior neurological, psychiatric, or substance abuse histories. An additional limitation of the Dikmen study is the fact that the outcome measure is time to return to work; employment retention, shown to be highly problematic for TBI survivors (Wehman et al. 1995), is not addressed.

Later studies have replicated and expanded these data (Gollaher et al. 1998; Hawkins et al. 1996). A study by Thornhill et al. (2000a) prospectively examined patients admitted to hospitals in Glasgow, Scotland, with a diagnosis of TBI. Although employment after brain injury was not a specific outcome measure of this study, the authors found an unexpectedly high incidence of disability after even mild TBI. Using the Glasgow Outcome Scale, which defines "good outcome" as resumption of premorbid lifestyle, the authors found that 55% of patients with mild TBI and 68% of patients with moderate TBI were at least moderately impaired 1 year after injury. Their data indicated that increased age, preexisting physical limitations, and a prior history of brain illness or injury were significant predictors of poor outcome. Sherer et al. (1999) found that a premorbid history of substance abuse resulted in an eightfold increase in post-TBI unemployment rates, all else being equal. Limited insight into deficits (anosognosia) has been shown to impede return to work (Sherer et al. 1998), as has depression (Satz et al. 1998). Fraser and Wehman (2001), among many others, found "cognitive barriers" to be the major difficulty in returning to work. Although no specific neuropsychological test or variable has been shown to be clearly predictive of real-life employability, impairments of so-called higher-level cognitive skills, such as the ability to screen out distracting or irrelevant stimuli, the ability to shift attention at will, the ability to plan and maintain a strategic sequence of activities, and the ability to inhibit responses, profoundly affect success in nearly every vocational setting (LeBlanc et al. 2000). Fraser and Wehman (2001) presented data, consistent with prior studies such as that of Eames (1988), showing that in their cohort, "diverse emotional concerns" and "preexisting characterological or behavioral difficulties" were each found to seriously adversely affect one-third of their patients. They cited the critical need for neuropsychiatric interventions (e.g., pharmacotherapy and/or behavioral and cognitive strategies) for population-wide improvements in the employment of TBI survivors.

Most of the literature on TBI and return to work focuses on competitive employment. Uysal et al. (1998) examined the effects of TBI on one's ability to function as a parent. In a group of parents 9 years postinjury, on average, they found more impairment in goal setting, skill development, nurturing, and involvement with children than in matched control subjects. Although the children of the families they examined were no more objectively dysfunctional than control subjects' families, TBI appeared to impair parenting ability.

Return to work has been used as a convenient endpoint for measuring recovery from TBI. It is clearly more than just a statistical tool, however. For many, if not most, TBI survivors, the inability to work epitomizes their sense of loss and diminishment. The inability to resume their accustomed social role, and their inability to support themselves and their families, exerts a highly corrosive effect on self-esteem. O'Neill et al. (1998) found employment status to be well correlated with perceived quality of life, social integration, and avocational activities. The workplace is also, in most cases, a major focus of one's social network. However, many TBI survivors face the loss of medical or disability benefits if they do return to work, a major difficulty especially if they cannot work full time or work at their premorbid levels. Recent changes in Social Security statutes, outlined in the following section, address this issue.

Disability Insurance

TBI survivors unable to work competitively must rely on disability insurance for maintenance of some income. The Social Security Administration is the largest disability insurance program in the country, providing benefits for up to 50% of those qualified as disabled (Ranavaya and Rondinelli 2000). It funds two distinct programs. Social Security Disability Insurance (SSD) was established in 1956 to provide pensions for workers older than the age of 50 years who are totally and permanently disabled. Benefits are available to workers who have contributed to the program through payroll and employer-paid taxes over a designated period of years, usually 5 of the preceding 10. More than 96% of jobs in the United States are covered by SSD (Robinson and Wolfe 2000). The Supplemental Security Income (SSI) program was established by Congress in 1972 to provide income support to the indigent disabled. It is a combined state and federal program that differs in its details and benefits from state to state. Eligibility for SSI benefits does not depend on work history; all those below designated levels of income and assets are eligible if they meet disability criteria. Congress mandated that recipients of either program undergo periodic continuing disability reviews to certify ongoing disability and, thus, eligibility for benefits. In 1995, approximately 13% of reviews led to termination of benefits (Robinson and Wolfe 2000). The benefits provided by these government programs are rather austere, with SSD replacing less than one-half the income of a person earning $25,000 annually and one-fourth the income of one earning $60,000. SSI payments average only 60% of SSD (Robinson and Wolfe 2000). Also, SSI is an asset-dependent benefit program; recipients lose benefits if they obtain money from other sources (e.g., successful litigation).

Approximately 40 million Americans have some sort of private long-term disability insurance, either purchased privately or acquired through the workplace (Ranavaya and Rondinelli 2000). Private disability insurance usually replaces 60% of an individual's usual income. However, these private policies are unique contracts between individuals (or groups) and the insurance company, thus making generalizations difficult. Increasing numbers of insurance companies are also issuing policies for long-term care providing reimbursement for institutional or home care in case of incapacity as demonstrated by inability to perform a predetermined set of activities of daily living. Such insurance can be helpful in the face of catastrophic incapacity, as with a severe TBI.

Vocational Rehabilitation

The history of federal legislative efforts on behalf of the disabled well illustrates the interacting themes of advocacy, public policy, and clinical impact. The federal government has promoted efforts to reemploy the disabled since 1918 when the Soldiers Rehabilitation Act authorized VR programs for injured veterans of World War I. This effort was expanded in 1920 with the Civilian Rehabilitation Act and set up as a permanent part of the Department of Labor with the Social Security Act of 1935 (Tate et al. 1998). Some of the more recent legislative efforts are discussed in the following paragraphs, but a brief description of VR is in order.

Vocational rehabilitation has been defined as any goods or services required to make the handicapped employable. As a government program that evolved piecemeal over decades, VR has no intrinsic definition, especially as it is (like Medicaid) a federal grant-in-aid program to the states, which authorize and define services as they see fit. Depending on the jurisdiction and the political climate, VR services can include the following: medical services (e.g., surgery or prostheses); tuition reimbursement for formal or vocational education; testing, including neuropsychological testing; assistive devices and technological aids; counseling and on-site job coaching; modification of the work environment; and cultivation of potential employers. The ways in which such services are provided has evolved since the 1970s.

Under the growing influence of the National Rehabilitation Association and other advocacy groups for the disabled, government attitudes toward the provision of vocational and other services began to shift in the 1960s from "top down" bureaucracies aiding those it labels as "handicapped" to a more "consumer oriented" approach. The Rehabilitation Act of 1973 (H.R. 8070) mandated that VR processes begin with the formulation of an Individualized Written Rehabilitation Plan, with active participation of the client. Subsequent amendments to the Rehabilitation Act have mandated greater consumer control over the types of employment and employment services available, as well as supporting the use of assistive technologies and supported or part-time employment. The Ticket to Work and Work Incentive Improvement Act of 1999 (P.L. 106-170) attempts to remove serious disincentives to returning to work experienced by SSD and SSI recipients (Golden 2001). Beneficiaries who return to work can now retain Medicare part A health insurance for up to 7.5 years. The availability of health insurance has been found to be a significant factor for successful return to work of TBI survivors (West 1995). Those who try returning to work but fail can have an expedited reinstatement of benefits without reapplication or a waiting period. Disability benefits continue for the first 9 months of work, considered a "trial work period." The act also partially "privatizes" VR services, allowing consumers to use approved private agencies whose reimbursement is in part tied to their success in helping people to no longer need disability program support (Golden 2001).

TBI patients have benefitted from such services, with studies showing the specific usefulness of supported employment—the presence on the job site itself of an employment specialist to provide training, counseling, and support on an ideally long-term basis, with subsequent skills generalization and increased productivity by the patient (Wehman et al. 1990, 1995). In their 1990 article, Wehman et al. cite the cost of such services as $8,700 per placement. Although this is an admittedly expensive investment of taxpayer dollars, alternatives such as chronic unemployment, dependence, and depression are far more expensive (Abrams et al. 1993).

The Rehabilitation Act of 1973 also guaranteed non-discrimination against persons with disabilities in any federally assisted program or activity. This guarantee was expanded by the Americans With Disabilities Act of 1990 to include all employment, public services, public transportation, places of accommodation such as hotels, and telecommunications. All firms with 15 or more employees had to accommodate their disabled employees unless this would impose "undue hardship."

Since the early 1970s, Congress has been funding Centers for Independent Living, autonomous, community-based agencies that provide peer counseling, information and referral, training in independent living skills, and advocacy to the disabled (Tate et al. 1998). Depending on available funding, some centers provide housing assistance and other concrete services. These Centers for Independent Living are unique in that they are managed and often staffed by the "handicapped" themselves, on the theory that they know better than bureaucrats (or physicians) what concrete services are needed. These centers, and groups modeled on them, teach TBI patients, among others, to be self-advocates—a role that can be deeply meaningful to people abruptly deprived by TBI of former capacities and often compelled to be dependent both on other individuals and on obtuse bureaucracies (Wehman 2001).

Litigation

The costs of care and rehabilitation for TBI are beyond the means of most people if they have to be paid for out of pocket (Sherer et al. 2000). As outlined in the section Disability Insurance, TBI patients and their families, to gain funding for treatment, typically have to deal with many insurance and governmental agencies, each with its own complicated sets of rules, requirements, and exclusions. The advocacy and clerical work that this requires (e.g., the establishment of contact with all available sources of funding, the verification of eligibility for benefits, and the collection of necessary data to justify services) is vitally important for most TBI patients but can easily consume much of a caregiver's time and energy. Psychiatrists working at TBI centers are often called to consult with distraught family members who are overwhelmed by the abrupt and horrifying impairment of a loved one and who, in the midst of their shock and grief, have to become highly effective advocates.

The challenges faced by patients and their caregivers become even more complicated when the TBI patient's injuries lead to litigation. It is estimated that most TBI patients become involved in litigation at some point, most

often as plaintiffs suing for damages or for wrongful denial of benefits (Miller 2000; Taylor 1997). Patients and their families then face the additional task of finding a lawyer who is competent and experienced in dealing with the multiple clinical and legal aspects of brain injury. Cases involving brain injury are considered among the most complex and "expert-intensive" areas of civil law practice (Taylor 2000). Increasing numbers of personal injury lawyers are specializing in what is called "neurolaw," a subdiscipline of attorneys with special competence in understanding the complex clinical issues involved in TBI (Taylor 1997). The legal literature has a number of recent articles and texts in the field of neurolaw (Miller 1998; Roberts 1996; Taylor 1997). Some of them (e.g., Miller 1998) can stand as thorough and sophisticated clinical reviews. The Brain Injury Association of America maintains a list of attorneys practicing neurolaw (http://www.biausa.org).

Litigation is often the only way TBI survivors can obtain even basic financial security. For those whose lives have been permanently impaired by the negligence of others, there are few ways other than litigation to obtain any sense of justice or closure. However, it is important for clinicians working with TBI survivors to realize that litigation can have serious adverse effects for the survivor. Strasburger (1999) points out that "few litigants are truly prepared for the forces of aggression that are released and sanctioned by our legal system." Ideally, seeking and obtaining compensation for multiple losses should be an empowering experience, especially for those who are powerless to fully restore their premorbid lives. However, even with successful outcomes, litigation can be deleterious to plaintiffs as well as defendants (Halleck 1997).

The goal of the legal system is to reduce all uncertain issues to clearly discernible dichotomies—guilty or innocent, for plaintiff or for defendant. A TBI survivor struggling with having to adapt to a life quite different from anything he or she could have imagined, whose life has become a series of novel and mostly unpleasant experiences, may have trouble conforming to forensic certainties. Patients experiencing the sequelae of TBI often feel damaged, helpless, and victimized. The incidence of posttraumatic stress disorder among TBI survivors is difficult to estimate, given the great variety of clinical and cognitive pictures presented. One may assume, however, that the typical avoidant defenses seen in general trauma survivors are used. The injury may evoke emotional memories of prior instances of victimization (e.g., childhood abuse), leading to a complex posttraumatic stress disorder (Raskin 1997). Judicial procedures can exacerbate these feelings and memories. Acute and chronic posttraumatic stress disorder symptoms can be sharply exacerbated by the unraveling of avoidant defenses resulting from the survivor having to repeatedly recount his or her history in law offices and in court (Pitman et al. 1996). A patient struggling to accept disability may find the articulate skepticism of opposing attorneys difficult and may feel compelled to prove to others and to themselves that the symptoms with which they are struggling are indeed real. This can cause an increased focus on symptoms and a tendency to overstate disability. In other words, survivors may feel compelled to assume a sick role that interferes with recovery (Bellamy 1997; Halleck 1997). In my experience, patients who are depressed and have self-doubt and who self-criticize are the most vulnerable to this process of having to "prove" symptoms. Narcissistic patients who need to minimize and deny any disability, lest they appear "defective," are also vulnerable to preoccupation with their symptoms. This process of symptom preoccupation can be conscious or unconscious and can lead to a preservation of self-esteem at the expense of worsening symptoms (Strasburger 1999). It should be stressed that these patients are not malingering—that is, deliberately exaggerating symptoms for financial gain—but are rather trying to adapt as best they can to a stressful and, at times, inquisitorial process.

The survivor may well have cognitive symptoms that impair the ability to competently participate in his or her case. For example, posttraumatic amnesia may interfere with both the ability to recall events after the injury and the ability to recall appointments, names of witnesses, and documents needed. Difficulty with organizing thoughts makes preparation for depositions and meetings with attorneys difficult. Increased distractibility may make the coherent presentation of information problematic, especially in the face of skeptical cross-examination. Symptoms of TBI, like all symptoms, can be exacerbated by stress (Feinstein et al. 2001; Finset et al. 1999). The TBI survivor can thus be caught in a vicious cycle, with cognitive symptoms worsening the ability to deal with litigation, and the consequent stress worsening cognitive symptoms.

Some authors conclude that the legal process itself is thus nociceptive, perpetuating pathology and disability in litigants (Bellamy 1997). In a meta-analysis of studies comparing litigating and nonlitigating TBI survivors, Binder and Rohling (1996) found that patients seeking compensation for injuries were more likely to show behavioral abnormalities and functional disability than control subjects, despite the fact that the litigating group had fewer neurological findings within 24 hours of injury and had a shorter period of posttraumatic amnesia. Time since lawsuit, rather than time since injury, has been found to be correlated with recovery, again implying that

litigation itself is toxic (Binder et al. 1991). In a prospective study of 100 patients with mild TBI, no demographic, neurological, or premorbid differences were found between litigating and nonlitigating patients; the litigants were significantly more anxious, depressed, dysfunctional, and likely to have a poor outcome than nonlitigants (Feinstein et al. 2001). These conclusions remain controversial, however. Authors such as Thornhill et al. (2000b) point out that TBI survivors with poor outcomes are more likely to seek damages than those who recover, accounting for the higher incidence of disability among litigants. They noted that among the patients in their prospective study who had impairments after mild brain injury, 80% were not involved in any litigation, implying that litigation is not a significant factor in poor outcome after TBI.

This controversy has a long and venerable history. Evans (1994), in his review article, details some of this history. The terms *railway spine* and *compensation neurosis* both date from the late nineteenth century, arising soon after the invention of both mechanized forms of transportation and of insurance awards for accident victims. The determination of feigned or exaggerated symptoms after TBI remains difficult and controversial, even with the current availability of both structural and functional scanning techniques (Alexander 1998; Ricker and Zafonte 2000). The importance of differentiating between frank malingering, posttraumatic stress disorder, somatoform disorders, and the often subtle neuropsychiatric symptoms of TBI has led to the evolution of forensic neuropsychology. Many graduate and postdoctoral programs in neuropsychology offer courses in the use of the tests that have been developed to try to clarify the etiology of posttraumatic symptoms. This challenging subject is beyond the scope of this chapter, and the interested reader is referred to recent review articles and books such as those of Iverson and Binder (2000), Reynolds (1998), and Rogers (1997).

Summary

TBIs have left ever-increasing numbers of survivors with serious disabilities. The cost of caring for these survivors is prohibitive for most families and has led to increasing numbers of government initiatives to provide assistance. After lobbying efforts by consumer groups such as the Brain Injury Association, the federal government passed legislation specifically to study the epidemiology of TBI and interventions to minimize morbidity and mortality. Medicaid waiver programs dedicated to TBI survivors, though of limited availability, provide extended rehabilitation and care. Social Security disability benefits provide a major source of income for TBI survivors. Vocational rehabilitation services, along with recent incentive programs in the Social Security system, are designed to help those disabled by TBI become self-supporting. TBI survivors are often involved in litigation that can be difficult and painful but that can also partially redress loss of income and perhaps even feelings of injustice.

The resources TBI survivors need to survive and to obtain clinical services are mostly funneled through major social institutions such as government bodies, insurance companies, and the judiciary. Social policy and effective advocacy profoundly affect the quantity and quality of resources available.

References

Abrams D, Barker LT, Haffney W, et al: The economics of return to work for survivors of traumatic brain injury: vocational services are worth the investment. J Head Trauma Rehabil 8:59–76, 1993

Alexander M: In pursuit of proof of brain damage after whiplash injury. Neurology 51:336–340, 1998

Bellamy R: Compensation neurosis: financial reward for illness as nocebo. Clin Orthop 336:94–106, 1997

Ben-Yishay Y, Silver SM, Piasetsky E, et al: Relationship between employability and vocational outcome after intensive holistic cognitive rehabilitation. J Head Trauma Rehabil 2:35–48, 1987

Binder LM, Rohling ML: Money matters: a meta-analytic review of the effects of financial incentives on recovery after closed-head injury. Am J Psychiatry 153:7–10, 1996

Binder RL, Trimble MR, McNeil DE: The course of psychological symptoms after resolution of lawsuits. Am J Psychiatry 148:1073–1075, 1991

Brooks N, McKinley W, Symington C, et al: Return to work within the first seven years of head injury. J Head Trauma Rehabil 1:5–19, 1987

Centers for Disease Control and Prevention: Traumatic Brain Injury in the United States: A Report to Congress. Washington, DC, 1999. Available at http://www.cdc.gov/doc.do?id=0900f3ec8001011c.

Department of Health and Human Services: Federal Interagency Head Injury Task Force Report. Washington, DC, Department of Health and Human Services, 1989

Digre PG, Kamen D, Vaughn S, et al: Selected states' public policy responses to traumatic brain injury. J Head Trauma Rehabil 9:12–26, 1994

Dikmen SS, Temkin NR, Machamer JE, et al: Employment following traumatic head injuries. Arch Neurol 51:177–186, 1994

Eames P: Behavior disorders after severe head injury: their nature, causes, and strategies for management. J Head Trauma Rehabil 3:1–6, 1988

Evans RW: The post-concussion syndrome: 130 years of controversy. Semin Neurol 14:32–39, 1994

Feinstein A, Ouchterlony D, Somerville J, et al: The effects of litigation on symptom expression: a prospective study following mild traumatic brain injury. Med Sci Law 41:116–121, 2001

Finset A, Anke AW, Hofft E, et al: Cognitive performance in multiple trauma patients 3 years after injury. Psychosom Med 61:576–583, 1999

Fraser RT, Wehman PH: Vocational rehabilitation status in traumatic brain injury: the need for revitalizing energies and cohesive direction. Brain Injury Source 5:22–47, 2001

Golden TP: Enhancing supports for career development and employment: the Ticket to Work and Work Incentives Improvement Act. Brain Injury Source 5:12–15, 2001

Gollaher K, High W, Sherer M, et al: Prediction of employment outcome one to three years following traumatic brain injury (TBI). Brain Inj 12:255–263, 1998

Goodall P, Ghiloni CT: The Changing Face of Publicly Funded Employment Services. J Head Trauma Rehabil 16:94–106, 2001

Halleck SL: Perils of being a plaintiff: impressions of a forensic psychiatrist. Clin Orthop Relat Res 336:72–78, 1997

Hawkins ML, Lewis FD, Medeiros RS: Serious traumatic brain injury: an evaluation of functional outcomes. J Trauma 41:257–263, 1996

Iverson GL, Binder LM: Detecting exaggeration and malingering in neuropsychological assessment. J Head Trauma Rehabil 15:829–858, 2000

LeBlanc JM, Hayden ME, Paulman RG: A comparison of neuropsychological and situational assessment for predicting employability after closed head injury. J Head Trauma Rehabil 15:1022–1040, 2000

Levin HS, Grossman RG, Rose JE, et al: Long-term neuropsychological outcome of closed head injury. J Neurosurg 50:412–422, 1979

McMordie WR, Barker SL, Paolo TM: Return to work (RTW) after head injury. Brain Inj 4:57–69, 1990

Miller L: Malingering in brain injury and toxic tort cases, in New Developments in Personal Injury Litigation. Edited by Wiley Law Editorial Staff. New York, Aspen, 1998, pp 225–289

Miller L: Psychological syndromes in traumatic brain injury litigation: personality, psychopathology, and disability. Brain Injury Source 4:18–43, 2000

National Institutes of Health Consensus Development Panel on Rehabilitation of Persons With Traumatic Brain Injury: Rehabilitation of Persons With Traumatic Brain Injury. JAMA 282:974–983, 1999

O'Neill J, Hibbard MR, Brown M, et al: The effect of employment on quality of life and community integration after traumatic brain injury. J Head Trauma Rehabil 13:68–79, 1998

Pitman RK, Sparr LF, Saunders LS, et al: Legal issues in PTSD, in Traumatic Stress. Edited by van der Kolk BA, McFarlane AC, Weisaeth L. New York, Guilford, 1996, pp 382–383

Ranavaya MI, Rondinelli RD: The major U.S. disability and compensation systems: origins and historical overview, in Impairment Rating and Disability Evaluation. Edited by Rondinelli RD, Katz RT. Philadelphia, PA, WB Saunders, 2000, pp 3–16

Rao N, Rosenthal M, Cronin-Stubbs D, et al: Return to work after rehabilitation following traumatic brain injury. Brain Inj 4:49–56, 1990

Raskin SA: The relationship between sexual abuse and mild traumatic brain injury. Brain Inj 11:587–603, 1997

Rehabilitation Act of 1973, H.R. 8070.

Reynolds CR: Detection of Malingering During Head Injury Litigation. New York, Plenum, 1998

Ricker JH, Zafonte RD: Functional neuroimaging and quantitative electroencephalography in adult traumatic brain injury: clinical applications and interpretive cautions. J Head Trauma Rehabil 15:859–868, 2000

Roberts AC: Head Trauma Cases—Law and Medicine, 2nd Edition. New York, Wiley, 1996

Robinson JP, Wolfe CV: Social Security Disability Insurance and Supplemental Security Income, in Impairment Rating and Disability Evaluation. Edited by Rondinelli RD, Katz RT. Philadelphia, PA, WB Saunders, 2000, pp 159–176

Rogers R: Clinical Assessment of Malingering and Deception, 2nd Edition. New York, Guilford, 1997

Rosen B, Reynolds WE: The impact of public policy on persons with traumatic brain injury and their families. J Head Trauma Rehabil 9:1–11, 1994

Satz P, Zaucha K, Forney DL, et al: Neuropsychological, psychosocial and vocational correlates of the Glasgow Outcome Scale at 6 months post-injury: a study of moderate to severe traumatic brain injury patients. Brain Inj 12:555–567, 1998

Sherer M, Bergloff P, Levin E, et al: Impaired awareness and employment outcome after traumatic brain injury. J Head Trauma Rehabil 13:52–61, 1998

Sherer M, Bergloff P, High W Jr, et al: Contribution of functional ratings to prediction of long term employment outcome after traumatic brain injury. Brain Inj 13:973–981, 1999

Sherer M, Madison CF, Hannay HJ: A review of outcome after moderate and severe closed head injury with an introduction to life care planning. J Head Trauma Rehabil 15:767–782, 2000

Spearman RC, Stamm BH, Rosen BH, et al: The use of Medicaid waivers and their impact on services. J Head Trauma Rehabil 16:47–60, 2001

Spivack MP: Pathways to policy: a personal perspective. J Head Trauma Rehabil 9:82–93, 1994

Strasburger LH: The litigant-patient: mental health consequences of civil litigation. J Am Acad Psychiatry Law 27:203–211, 1999

Tate DG, Heinrich RK, Paasuke L, et al: Vocational rehabilitation, independent living, and consumerism, in Rehabilitation Medicine, Principles and Practice, 3rd Edition. Edited by DeLisa JA, Gans BM. Philadelphia, PA, Lippincott–Raven, 1998, pp 1151–1162

Taylor JS: Neurolaw: Brain and Spinal Cord. Washington, DC, ATLA Press, 1997

Taylor JS: Introduction to neurolaw. Brain Injury Source 4:10–11, 2000

Thornhill S, Teasdale GM, Murray GD, et al: Disability in young people and adults one year after head injury: prospective cohort study. BMJ 320:1631–1635, 2000a

Thornhill S, Teasdale GM, Murray GD, et al: Disability in young people and adults one year after head injury: prospective cohort study. BMJ Electronic Letters. Available at http://www.bmj.com, 29 June 2000b

Ticket to Work and Work Incentive Improvement Act of 1999, Pub. L. 106-170.

Traumatic Brain Injury Act of 1996, Pub. L. No. 104-166, Stat. 110.1445

U.S. General Accounting Office: Traumatic Brain Injury Programs Supporting Long-Term Services in Selected States. GAO/HEHS-98-55, 1998

Uysal S, Hibbard MR, Robillard D, et al: The effect of parental traumatic brain injury on parenting and child behavior. J Head Trauma Rehabil 13:57–71, 1998

Vaughn SL, King A: A survey of state programs to finance rehabilitation and community services for individuals with brain injury. J Head Trauma Rehabil 16:20–33, 2001

Wehman P: People with traumatic brain injury helping themselves. Brain Injury Source 5:6, 2001

Wehman PH, Kreutzer JS, West MD, et al: Return to work for persons with traumatic brain injury: a supported employment approach. Arch Phys Med Rehabil 71:1047–1052, 1990

Wehman PH, West MD, Kregel J, et al: Return to work for people with severe traumatic brain injury: a data based approach to program development. J Head Trauma Rehabil 10:27–39, 1995

West MD: Aspects of the workplace and return to work for persons with brain injury in supported employment. Brain Inj 9:301–313, 1995

33 Ethical and Clinical Legal Issues

Robert I. Simon, M.D.

TRAUMATIC BRAIN INJURY (TBI) patients, especially those who manifest difficulties in judgment, mood regulation, memory, orientation, insight, and impulse control, often present complex ethical and clinical legal problems. In addition, they are likely to have a plethora of psychiatric symptoms. In litigation, brain injuries can result in large monetary awards if the patient becomes unemployable. In combination with current and future medical expenses, compensable damages from head trauma can be substantial. Depending on the extent of functional impairment, even "mild" brain injuries can result in seven-figure verdicts.

Ethical Considerations

During the first half of the twentieth century, the principle of patient autonomy was clearly recognized in the medical malpractice case *Schloendorff v. Society of New York Hospital (1914)*. Justice Cardozo enunciated the principle of patient self-determination by stating that "every human being of adult years and sound mind has a right to determine what shall be done with his own body, and a surgeon who performs an operation without his patient's consent commits an assault, for which he is liable in damages" (Schloendorff 1914).

Since the late 1950s and early 1960s, the medical profession has moved away from an authoritarian, physician-oriented model toward a more collaborative relationship with patients concerning their health care decisions. This is reflected in contemporary ethical principles (American Psychiatric Association 2001). Psychiatry, on ethical grounds, endorses granting competent patients the legal right to autonomy in determining their medical care. Without legal compulsion, most psychiatrists disclose pertinent medical information to their patients to enhance the therapeutic alliance (Simon 1992a).

The ethical principles of beneficence, nonmaleficence, and respect for the dignity and autonomy of the patient compose the moral–ethical foundation for the doctor-patient relationship. In preserving patient dignity and autonomy, a brain injury that interferes with a patient's decision-making capacity requires the psychiatrist to obtain informed consent from substitute decision makers. The rights of all patients are the same—only how these rights are exercised is different (Parry and Beck 1990).

The ethics of social justice calls for the fair allocation of medical resources in accord with medical need (Ruchs 1984). Although seemingly a new development, the ethical concerns about equitable health care distribution are found in the Hippocratic oath and in the tradition of medicine and psychiatry (Dyer 1988). For example, it would be unethical to discriminate against an individual who receives a TBI during the course of committing a felony by not providing adequate treatment and management resources.

Ethical issues arise daily for psychiatrists who treat TBI patients. Medical decision making, informed consent, resuscitation, "brain death," organ transplantation, the withholding and withdrawing of life support, and the allocation of medical resources all give rise to complex ethical and clinical legal problems (Luce 1990). Moreover, that which is considered ethical in clinical practice today may become a legal requirement tomorrow.

Competency: The Basic Concept

A 36-year-old man with traumatic dementia inherits $5 million. His physician becomes concerned when the patient proposes to pay for a 90-day around-the-world trip for himself and three of his longtime friends. A psychiatric consultation is requested. The mental status evaluation reveals adequate judgment and insight. Short-term memory is moderately disturbed. Sensorium and orientation are intact. Affective lability is present, particularly when frustration is experienced. The patient's brother requests a competency hearing and an appointment of a guardian for financial matters. After hearing testimony, the court finds that the patient has the minimal mental capacity to manage his financial matters. The court notes that decisions that seem idiosyncratic or even foolish do not necessarily denote mental incompetence.

Nearly every area of human endeavor is affected by the law and, as a fundamental condition, requires one to be mentally competent. *Competency* is defined as "having sufficient capacity, ability…[or] possessing the requisite physical, mental, natural, or legal qualifications…" (Black 1990, p. 284). This definition is deliberately vague and ambiguous because competency is a broad concept encompassing many different legal issues and contexts. As a result, competency requirements and application can vary widely depending on the circumstances in which it is measured (e.g., health care decisions, executing a will, or confessing to a crime).

As noted in the preceding example, *competency* refers to some *minimal* mental, cognitive, or behavioral ability, trait, or capability required to perform a particular legally recognized act or to assume some legal role. The term *incapacity*, which is often interchanged with *incompetency*, refers to an individual's functional inability to understand or to form an intention with regard to some act, as determined by a health care provider (Mishkin 1989). In TBI patients, fluctuations in mental capacity are common, particularly in the days and even months after injury.

The legal designation of *incompetent* is applied to an individual who fails one of the mental tests of capacity and is therefore considered *by law* not to be mentally capable of performing a particular act or assuming a particular role. The adjudication of incompetence by a court is subject or issue specific. For example, the fact that a TBI patient is adjudicated incompetent to execute a will may not automatically render that patient incompetent to do other things such as consenting to treatment, testifying as a witness, marrying, driving, or making a legally binding contract.

Generally, the law recognizes only those decisions or choices that have been made by a competent individual. The law seeks to protect incompetent individuals from the harmful effects of their acts. People older than the age of majority, which is now 18 years, are presumed to be com-

petent (*Meek v. City of Loveland 1929*; The Legal Status of Adolescents 1980, published in 1981). This presumption, however, is rebuttable by evidence of an individual's incapacity (*Scaria v. St. Paul Fire and Marine Ins Co 1975*). For the TBI patient, perception, short- and long-term memory, judgment, language comprehension, verbal fluency, and reality orientation are mental functions that courts scrutinize regarding capacity and competency.

The issue of competency, whether in a civil or criminal context, is commonly raised when the person is a minor or is mentally disabled. In many situations, minors are not considered legally competent and therefore require the consent of a parent or designated guardian. There are exceptions to this general rule, however, such as minors who are considered emancipated (Smith 1986), mature (*Gulf S I R Co v. Sullivan 1928*), or competent to consent in some cases of medical need (*Planned Parenthood v. Danforth 1976*) or emergency (*Jehovah's Witnesses v. King County Hospital 1967*, published in 1968).

The mentally disabled, which often include TBI patients, present complex problems in evaluating competency. Lack of capacity or competency cannot be presumed either from treatment for mental disorders (*Wilson v. Lehman 1964*) or from institutionalization of such persons (*Rennie v. Klein 1978*). Mental disability or disorder does not automatically render a person incompetent or incompetent in all areas of functioning. Neither do idiosyncratic or foolish decisions, by themselves, denote mental incompetence. Making foolish decisions is part of the human condition. Instead, scrutiny should be given to determine whether there are specific functional incapacities that render a person incapable of making a particular kind of decision or performing a particular type of task.

Respect for individual autonomy (Schloendorff 1914) demands that individuals be allowed to make decisions of which they are capable, even if they are seriously mentally ill, developmentally arrested, or organically impaired. As a rule, a patient with a TBI that causes mental incapacity generally must be judicially declared incompetent before that patient's exercise of his or her legal rights can be abridged. The person's current physical and mental illness is but one factor to be weighed in determining whether a particular test of competency is met.

Health Care Decision Making

Informed Consent

A 43-year-old man with a traumatic amnestic syndrome develops major depression. To obtain informed consent for treatment, the psychiatrist describes the risks and benefits of antidepressant medications to the patient. The psychiatrist quickly realizes that the patient lacks the mental capacity to retain this information long enough to consider it. In frustration and embarrassment, the patient consents to take any medication. The psychiatrist obtains proxy consent from the patient's wife after explaining the diagnosis, risks and benefits of treatment, alternative treatments with their risks and benefits, and the prognosis with and without treatment. Proxy consent by next of kin is permitted by statute in the state where the patient lives.

Patients with TBI frequently demonstrate impaired mental capacity. Obtaining a competent informed consent to proposed diagnostic procedures and treatments can be both challenging and frustrating. The capacity to consent, particularly after brain injury, may be present one moment and gone the next. Lucid intervals may permit the obtaining of competent consent for health care decisions.

The need to obtain competent, informed consent is not negated simply because it appears that the patient is in need of medical intervention or would likely benefit from it. Instead, clinicians must assure themselves that the patient or an appropriate substitute decision maker has given a competent consent before proceeding with treatment. In the preceding example, the psychiatrist realized that the patient was giving an incompetent consent to treatment and obtained proxy consent. In a number of states, proxy consent by next of kin may not be available for psychiatric patients. When patients agree to treatment, their competency to assent is often not questioned. An increasing number of states require a judicial determination of incompetence and the court's substituted consent before the administration of neuroleptic treatment to a patient who is deemed by a health care provider to lack functional mental capacity (Simon 1992a).

Under the doctrine of informed consent, health care providers have a legal duty to abide by the treatment decisions made by competent patients unless a compelling state interest exists. The term *informed consent* is a legal principle in medical jurisprudence, which holds that a physician must disclose to a patient sufficient information to enable the patient to make an informed decision about a proposed treatment or procedure (Black 1990, p. 779). For a patient's consent to be considered informed, it must adequately address three essential elements: competency, information, and voluntariness. In general, the patient must be given enough information to make a truly knowledgeable decision. The decision (consent) must be made voluntarily by a person who is legally competent. Each of these elements must be met or any consent given will not be considered informed and legally valid (Table 33–1).

TABLE 33–1.   Informed consent: reasonable information to be disclosed

Although there exists no consistently accepted set of information to be disclosed for any given medical or psychiatric situation, as a rule of thumb, five areas of information are generally provided:

1. Diagnosis—description of the condition or problem

2. Treatment—nature and purpose of proposed treatment

3. Consequences—risks and benefits of the proposed treatment

4. Alternatives—viable alternatives to the proposed treatment, including risks and benefits

5. Prognosis—projected outcome with and without treatment

Source.   Reprinted from Simon RI: *Clinical Psychiatry and the Law,* 2nd Edition. Washington, DC, American Psychiatric Press, 1992, p. 128. Used with permission.

The law recognizes several circumscribed exceptions to the requirement of informed consent (Rozovsky 1984). The most notable is the "emergency exception," which states that consent is implied in circumstances in which the patient is unable to give consent (e.g., unconsciousness) and has an acute, life-threatening crisis that requires immediate medical attention. Frequently, the TBI patient is initially brought for emergency care. Because the patient may be unconscious or manifest significant impairment in consciousness, treatment may be initiated under implied emergency consent. Another common clinical situation in which this exception might arise is in the treatment of the violent TBI patient. For example, patients diagnosed with frontal lobe or temporal lobe damage are known to have sudden, violent outbursts that may require immediate intervention to prevent serious injury to the patient or to third parties (Devinsky and Bear 1984).

Legally, the term *competency* is narrowly defined and equated with cognitive capacity. There are no established criteria for determining a patient's competence. A basic level of decision-making capacity exists when the patient is able to understand the particular treatment choice proposed, make a treatment choice, and communicate that decision.

The problem with the preceding standard of decision-making capacity is that it obtains a simple consent from the patient rather than an informed consent, because alternative treatment choices are not provided. A review of case law and scholarly literature reveals four general standards for determining incompetency in decision making (Appelbaum et al. 1987). By ascending levels of mental capacity required, these standards include 1) communication of choice, 2) understanding of information provided, 3) appreciation of one's situation and the risks and benefits of options available, and 4) rational decision making. *Task-specific competence* has been defined as the individual's ability to make a choice, to have a factual understanding of the information provided, to rationally manipulate the information, and to have a realistic appreciation of his or her situation (Pinals and Appelbaum 2000). For example, a TBI patient with frontal lobe damage may have difficulty with a realistic appreciation of his or her situation because of diminished insight and denial of the illness. Psychiatrists generally feel most comfortable with a rational decision-making standard in determining incompetency.

Most courts prefer the first two standards: communication of choice and understanding the information provided. An informed consent reflecting the patient's autonomy, personal needs, and values occurs when rational decision making is applied to the risks and benefits of appropriate treatment options provided to the patient by the clinician. When the patient seems competent, a decision that appears irrational is not, by itself, a basis for a determination of incompetence (Benesch 1989). Persons who are fully competent may make foolish decisions. Legal advice may be needed if the competency issue cannot be resolved by additional medical and psychiatric consultation.

The psychiatrist who treats a patient with TBI suspected of having neuropsychiatric deficits should conduct a thorough assessment of cognitive functioning. The sole objective of such an evaluation should be the determination of the TBI patient's ability to meet the minimal requirements for consent. At the very least, a mental status assessment of the patient's language comprehension, memory, judgment, insight, affect, orientation, and attention span should be performed (Folstein et al. 1975). Some TBI patients may be cognitively intact but manifest such severe affective lability that they are rendered mentally incompetent.

Except in an emergency, an authorized representative or appointed guardian must make health care decisions on behalf of patients with TBI who lack health care decision-making capacity (*Aponte v. United States 1984*; Frasier v. Department of Health and Human Resources 1986). Table 33–2 lists a number of consent options that may be available for such patients, depending on the jurisdiction.

Incompetent Patients

In what was hoped to be the "final word" on the difficult and personal question of patient autonomy, the U.S. Supreme Court ruled in *Cruzan v. Director, Missouri Department of Health (1990)* that the state of Missouri could refuse to remove a food and water tube surgically

TABLE 33–2. Common consent options for patients lacking the mental capacity for health care decisions

Proxy consent of next of kin

Adjudication of incompetence; appointment of a guardian

Institutional administrators or committees

Treatment review panels

Substituted consent of the court

Advance directives (living will, durable power of attorney, and health care proxy)

Statutory surrogates (spouse or court-appointed guardian)[a]

[a]These laws authorize certain persons, such as a spouse or court-appointed guardian, to make health care decisions when the patient has not stated his or her wishes in writing.
Source. Reprinted from Simon RI: *Clinical Psychiatry and the Law,* 2nd Edition. Washington, DC, American Psychiatric Press, 1992, p. 109. Used with permission.

implanted in the stomach of Nancy Cruzan without clear and convincing evidence of her wishes. She had been in a persistent vegetative state for 7 years. In other words, without clear and convincing evidence of a patient's decision to have life-sustaining measures withheld in a particular circumstance, the state has the right to maintain that individual's life, even against the family's wishes.

Although this decision seems to leave unanswered more questions than it answers, the court's decision does buttress the position of "right to refuse" treatment advocates in the following three significant ways:

1. The court seemed to give constitutional status to a competent person's right to refuse treatment. Furthermore, if individuals appoint relatives or friends to make decisions about medical treatment should they become incompetent, states "may well be constitutionally required" to defer to the wishes of such "surrogate decision makers."
2. The court did not distinguish between artificially administered food and water and other life-sustaining measures, such as respirators. This distinction has been a hotly contested sticking point in some previous, lower court decisions.
3. An incompetent person who makes his or her wishes known in advance, such as through a living will, may have a constitutional right to halt life-sustaining intervention, depending on the proof of those wishes.

The *Cruzan* decision is important for clinicians who treat severely or terminally impaired TBI patients because it requires that they seek clear and competent instructions regarding foreseeable treatment decisions. This information is best provided in the form of a living will, durable power of attorney agreement, or health care proxy. Any written document that clearly and convincingly sets forth the patient's wishes would serve the same purpose. Although physicians have historically feared civil or criminal liability for stopping life-sustaining treatment, liability may now arise from overtreating critically or terminally ill patients (Weir and Gostin 1990).

Do-Not-Resuscitate Orders

A 53-year-old woman with TBI has a cardiac arrest and is resuscitated. A psychiatric consult determines that the patient retains sufficient mental capacity to make health care decisions. The patient instructs her physician not to resuscitate her if another cardiac arrest occurs. The family disagrees. They want the patient to be resuscitated because they think the do-not-resuscitate (DNR) decision is based on impaired judgment caused by the brain injury. Nevertheless, the primary physician determines that the patient is competent when she makes the request. The physician writes the DNR order.

Cardiopulmonary resuscitation (CPR) is a medical life-saving technology. To be effective, it must be applied immediately, leaving no time to think about the consequences of reviving a patient. Ordinarily, patients requiring CPR have not thought about or expressed a preference for or against its use.

In the critically ill TBI patient, the psychiatrist and the substitute medical decision maker may have time to consider whether CPR should be offered on the basis of the patient's earlier expressed wishes. The ethical principle of patient autonomy justifies the position that the patient or substitute decision maker should make the final decision regarding the use of CPR. In the case example, the patient's direction concerning DNR should be followed, if made competently. Malpractice liability for not offering or providing futile care is unlikely, and the psychiatrist is exposed to greater liability exposure if such care is provided (March and Staver 1991). Schwartz (1987) noted that two key principles have emerged concerning DNR decisions:

1. In accordance with the ethical principle of autonomy and with the legal doctrine of informed consent, DNR decisions should be reached consensually by the attending physician and the patient or substitute decision maker.
2. DNR orders should be written and the reasoning for the DNR order documented in the chart.

Hospital CPR policies make DNR decisions discretionary (Luce 1990). However, psychiatrists should be familiar with the specific hospital policy whenever a DNR order is written. Medicolegal-ethical principles have been promulgated concerning CPR and emergency cardiac care (American Medical Association 1991, 1992).

Advance Directives

The use of advance directives such as a living will, health care proxy, or a durable medical power of attorney is recommended to avoid ethical and legal complications associated with requests to withhold life-sustaining treatment measures (Simon 1992a; Solnick 1985). The Patient Self-Determination Act, which took effect on December 1, 1991, requires hospitals, nursing homes, hospices, managed care organizations, and home health care agencies to advise patients or family members of their right to accept or refuse medical care and to execute an advance directive (LaPuma et al. 1991). These advance directives provide a method for individuals, while competent, to choose proxy health care decision makers in the event of future incompetency. A living will can be contained as a subsection of a durable power of attorney agreement. In the ordinary power of attorney created for the management of business and financial matters, the power of attorney generally becomes null and void if the person creating it becomes incompetent.

Federal law does not specify the right to formulate advance directives; therefore, state law applies. State legislators have recognized that individuals may want to indicate who should make important health care decisions in case they become incapacitated and unable to act in their own behalf. All 50 states and the District of Columbia permit individuals to create a durable power of attorney (i.e., one that endures even if the competence of the creator does not) (*Cruzan v. Director, Missouri Department of Health 1990*, n 3). A number of states and the District of Columbia have durable power of attorney statutes expressly authorizing the appointment of proxies for making health care decisions (*Cruzan v. Director, Missouri Department of Health 1990*, n 2).

Generally, durable power of attorney has been construed to empower an agent to make health care decisions. Such a document is much broader and more flexible than a living will, which covers only the period of a diagnosed terminal illness, specifying only that no "extraordinary treatments" may be used that would prolong the act of dying (Mishkin 1985). To rectify the sometimes uncertain status of the durable power of attorney as applied to health care decisions, a number of states have passed or are considering passing health care proxy laws. The health care proxy is a legal instrument akin to the durable power of attorney but specifically created for health care decision making (Appendix 33–1). Despite the growing use of advance directives, there is increasing evidence that physician values rather than patient values are more critical in end-of-life decisions (Orentlicher 1992).

In a durable power of attorney or health care proxy, general or specific directions are set forth about how future decisions should be made in the event one becomes unable to make these decisions. The determination of a patient's competence is not specified in most durable power of attorney and health care proxy statutes. Because this is a medical or psychiatric question, the examination by two physicians to determine the patient's ability to understand the nature and consequences of the proposed treatment or procedure, the ability to make a choice, and the ability to communicate that choice are minimally sufficient. This information, like all significant medical observations, should be documented in the patient's file.

Because of the frequent absence of advance directives, statutory surrogate laws have been enacted in some states. These laws authorize certain persons, such as a spouse or court-appointed guardian, to make health care decisions when the patient has not stated his or her wishes in writing. A number of states have enacted statutory surrogate laws.

The application of advance directives to neuropsychiatric patients poses some difficulties. The classic example arises when a currently stable TBI patient with organic personality syndrome and occasional bouts of severe affective instability draws up a durable power of attorney agreement or health care proxy directing that "If I become mentally unstable again, administer medications even if I strenuously object or resist." This has been described as the "Ulysses Contract" (T. Gutheil, personal communication, September 1985). In Greek mythology, Ulysses was bound to the mast of his ship so he could hear the beautiful, although lethal, sirens' song. All the other sailors covered their ears. When he heard the irresistible song of the sirens, Ulysses tried to struggle loose to go to them. When that failed, he demanded to be untied. Similarly, when mood instability recurs, the TBI patient may strenuously object to treatment.

Because durable power of attorney agreements or health care proxies can be easily revoked, the treating psychiatrist or institution has no choice but to honor the patient's refusal, even if there is reasonable evidence that the patient is incompetent. Legal consultation should be considered at this point. If the patient is grossly disordered and is an immediate danger to self and others, the physician or hospital is on firm ground medically and legally to temporarily override the patient's treatment refusal. Otherwise, it is generally better to seek a court order for treatment than to risk legal entanglement with the patient by attempting to enforce the original terms of the advance directive. Unless there are compelling medical reasons to do otherwise, courts will honor the patient's original treatment directions given while competent.

Guardianship

A guardianship is a method of substitute decision making for individuals who have been judicially determined as unable to act for themselves (Brakel et al. 1985). Historically, the state or sovereign possessed the power and authority to safeguard the estates of incompetent persons.

This traditional role still reflects the purpose of guardianship today. In some states, there are separate provisions for the appointment of a "guardian of one's person" (e.g., health care decision making) and for a "guardian of one's estate" (e.g., authority to make contracts to sell one's property) (Sale et al. 1982, p. 461). This latter guardian is frequently referred to as a *conservator*, although this designation is not used uniformly throughout the United States. A further distinction, also found in some jurisdictions, is general (plenary) versus specific guardianship (Sale et al. 1982, p. 462). As the name implies, the latter guardian is restricted to exercising decisions about a particular subject area. For instance, the specific guardian may be authorized to make decisions about major or emergency medical procedures, with the disabled person retaining the freedom to make decisions about all other medical matters. General guardians, by contrast, have total control over the disabled individual's person, estate, or both (Sale et al. 1982, pp. 461–462).

Guardianship arrangements, which are increasingly used for patients who demonstrate dementia, particularly acquired immunodeficiency syndrome–related dementia and Alzheimer's disease, can also be of use for TBI patients (Overman and Stoudemire 1988). Under the Anglo-American system of law, an individual is presumed to be competent unless adjudicated incompetent. Incompetence is a legal determination made by a court of law on the basis of evidence, provided by health care providers and others, that the individual's functional mental capacity is significantly impaired. Laws governing competency in many states are based on the Uniform Guardianship and Protective Proceeding Act or the Uniform Probate Code (Mishkin 1989). Drafted by legal scholars and practicing attorneys, uniform acts serve as models whose purpose is to achieve consistency among the state laws by enactment of model laws.

General incompetency is defined by the Uniform Guardianship and Protective Proceeding Act as "impaired by reason of mental illness, mental deficiency, physical illness or disability, advanced age, chronic use of drugs, chronic intoxication, or other cause (except minority) to the extent of lacking sufficient understanding or capacity to make or communicate reasonable decisions."

Some TBI patients may meet the preceding definition. Generally, the appointment of a guardian is limited to situations in which the individual's decision-making capacity is so impaired that he or she is unable to care for personal safety or provide such necessities as food, shelter, clothing, and medical care, likely resulting in physical injury or illness (In re Boyer 1981). The standard of proof required for a judicial determination of incompetency is clear and convincing evidence. Although the law does not assign percentages to proof, clear and convincing evidence is in the range of 75% certainty (Simon 1992b).

States vary concerning the extent of their reliance on psychiatric assessments. Nonmedical personnel such as social workers, psychologists, family members, friends, colleagues, and even the individual who is the subject of the proceeding may testify.

Substituted Judgment

Psychiatrists usually find that the time required to obtain an adjudication of incompetence is unduly burdensome and frequently interferes with the provision of quality treatment. Moreover, families often are reluctant to face the formal court proceedings necessary to declare their family member incompetent, particularly when sensitive family matters are disclosed. A common solution to both of these problems is to seek the legally authorized proxy consent of a spouse or relative serving as guardian when the refusing TBI patient is believed to be incompetent. Proxy consent, however, is not available in every state (Simon 1992a). A number of states exclude surrogate authorizations for the treatment of mental disorders.

Some states permit proxy decision making by statute, mainly through their informed consent statute (Solnick 1985). A few state statutes specify that another person may authorize consent on behalf of the incompetent patient; others mention specific relatives. Unless proxy consent by a relative is provided by statute or by case law authority in the state where the psychiatrist practices, it is not recommended that the good-faith consent of next of kin be relied on in treating a TBI patient believed to be incompetent (Klein et al. 1983). The legally appropriate procedure is to seek judicial recognition of the family member as the substitute decision maker.

There are clear advantages associated with having the family serve as decision maker (Perr 1984). First, the use of responsible family members as surrogate decision makers maintains the integrity of the family unit and relies on the sources that are most likely to know the patient's wishes. Second, it is more efficient and less costly than adjudication. Nonetheless, there are some disadvantages. Proxy decision making requires synthesizing the diverse values, beliefs, practices, and prior statements of the patient for a given specific circumstance (Emanuel and Emanuel 1992). As one judge characterized the problem, any proxy decision making in the absence of specific directions is "at best only an optimistic approximation" (In re Jobes 1987). Ambivalent feelings, conflicts within the family and with the patient, and conflicting economic interest may make certain family members suspect as guardians (Gutheil and Appelbaum 1980). Also, relatives may be unavailable or unwilling to become involved.

The President's Commission for the Study of Ethical Problems in Medicine and Biomedical and Behavioral Research (1982) recommended that the relatives of incompetent patients be selected as proxy decision makers for the following reasons:

- The family is generally most concerned about the good of the patient.
- The family will also usually be most knowledgeable about the patient's goals, preferences, and values.
- The family deserves recognition as an important social unit to be treated, within limits, as a single decision maker in matters that intimately affect its members.

Some TBI patients treated in an emergency may be expected to recover competency during lucid intervals or within a few days. As soon as the patient is able to competently consent to further treatment, such consent should be obtained directly from the patient. For the patient who continues to lack mental capacity for health care decisions, an increasing number of states provide administrative procedures authorized by statute that permit involuntary treatment of the incompetent and refusing mentally ill patients who do not meet current standards for involuntary civil commitment (Hassenfeld and Grumet 1984; Zito et al. 1984). In most jurisdictions, a durable power of attorney agreement permits the next of kin to consent through durable power of attorney statutes (Solnick 1985). In some instances, however, this procedure may not meet judicial challenge. To avoid this problem, a number of states have created health care proxies specifically for advance health care decision making.

A debate continues about the theory of substitute decision making. Should the substitute decision maker act in the patient's best interest (the "objective test"), or should he or she rely on what the patient would have decided if competent (the "subjective" or "substituted judgment" approach)? The increasingly used subjective test is difficult to implement for patients who have never been competent, who have made improvident or less than competent past decisions, or who have never openly stated choices to be implemented by others. Also, the values of substitute decision makers can be easily substituted for the patient's regardless of which test is used (Roth 1985). Both the best interest and the substituted judgment standards lead to predictable biases by those who implement them. Use of the best interest standard leads to treatment of patients and sustaining life. Application of the substituted judgment standard favors treatment refusal and the upholding of civil liberties (Robertson 1989).

The substituted judgment standard has found considerable judicial favor. Courts find authority and inspiration from J.S. Mill:

> The only purpose for which power can be rightfully exercised over any member of a civilized community against his will, is to prevent harm to others. His own good, either physical or moral, is not a sufficient warrant. He cannot rightfully be compelled to do or forebear because it will be better for him to do so, because it will make him happier, because in the opinion of others, to do so would be wise, or even right. (Mill 1951, pp. 316–333).

Criminal Proceedings

Among criminal defendants, a history of severe brain injury is often present. The possibility of TBI should be thoroughly investigated in criminal defendants. For example, Lewis et al. (1986) studied 15 death row inmates who were chosen for examination because of imminent execution rather than evidence of neuropathology. In each case, evidence of severe brain injury and neurological impairment was found.

The causal connection between brain damage and violence, however, remains frustratingly obscure. Violent behavior spans a wide spectrum, from a normal response to a threatening situation to violence emanating directly from an organic brain disorder such as Klüver-Bucy syndrome, hypothalamic tumors, or temporal lobe epilepsy (Strub and Black 1988). Moreover, violent behavior is the result of the interaction between an individual and a specific situation. Brain damage or mental illness may or may not play a significant role in this equation. Psychiatrists should acknowledge limitations in their expertise concerning the possible connection between brain damage and violence.

Criminal Intent (*Mens Rea*)

Under the common law, the basic elements of a crime are 1) the mental state or level of intent to commit the act (known as the *mens rea* or "guilty mind"), 2) the act itself or conduct associated with committing the crime (known as *actus reus* or "guilty act"), and 3) a concurrence in time between the guilty act and the guilty mental state (*Bethea v. United States 1977*). To convict a person of a particular crime, the state must prove beyond a reasonable doubt that the defendant committed the criminal act with the requisite intent. All three elements are necessary to satisfy the threshold requirements for the imposition of criminal sanctions.

The question of intent is a particularly vexing problem for the courts. Under most circumstances, everyone would agree that killing another person is deplorable conduct. But should the accidental death of a child in a car accident, the heat-of-passion shooting by a husband of his wife's lover, and the cold-blooded murder of a bank teller by a robber all result in the same punishment? The determination of the defendant's intent, or *mens rea*, at the time of the offense is the law's "equalizer" and trigger mechanism for deciding criminal culpability and the appropriate division of retribution. For instance, a person who deliberately plans to commit a crime is more culpable than the person who accidentally commits one.

There are two classes of intent used to categorize *mens rea*: specific and general. Specific intent refers to the *mens rea* in those crimes in which a further intention is present beyond that which is identified with the physical act associated with an offense. For instance, the courts frequently state that the intent necessary for first-degree murder includes a "specific intent to kill" or a person might commit an assault "with the intent to rape" (Melton et al. 1997). Unlike general criminal intent, specific criminal intent cannot be presumed from the unlawful criminal act but must be proven independently.

General criminal intent is more elusive. General criminal intent may be presumed from commission of the criminal act. It usually is used by the law to explain criminal liability in which a defendant was merely conscious or should have been conscious of his or her physical actions at the time of the offense (Melton et al. 1997). Because of the imprecision of these categories, modern statutory codes have created more precise criteria for defining mental states (Melton et al 1997).

Persons with certain mental handicaps or impairments, such as the TBI patient, represent a challenge for prosecutors, defense counsel, and judges in determining what, if any, retribution is justifiable. Mental impairment often raises serious questions about the intent to commit a crime and the appreciation of its consequences.

In addition to *mens rea*, a defendant's mental status can play a deciding role in whether he or she will be ordered to stand trial to face the criminal charges (*Dusky v. United States 1960*), be acquitted of the alleged crime (*M'Naghten's Case 1843*), be sent to prison, be hospitalized (Mental Aberration and Post Conviction Sanctions 1981), or, in some extreme cases, be sentenced to death (*Ford v. Wainright 1986*). Before any defendant can be criminally prosecuted, the court must be satisfied that the accused is competent to stand trial—that is, he or she understands the charges and is capable of rationally assisting counsel with the defense.

Competency to Stand Trial

In every situation in which competency is a question, the law seeks to reiterate a common theme: that only the acts of a rational individual are to be given recognition by society (*Neely v. United States 1945*). In doing so, the law attempts to reaffirm the integrity of the individual and of society in general.

The legal standard for assessing pretrial competency was established by the U.S. Supreme Court in *Dusky v. United States (1960)*. Throughout involvement with the trial process, the defendant must have "sufficient present ability to consult with his lawyer with a reasonable degree of rational understanding and … a rational as well as factual understanding of the proceedings against him" (*Dusky v. United States 1960*).

Typically, the impairment that raises the question of the defendant's competence is associated with a mental disease or defect. A person may be held to be incompetent to stand trial even if there is no mental disease or defect as defined by DSM-IV-TR (American Psychiatric Association 2000). For example, children who are younger than a certain age ordinarily are deemed incompetent to stand trial.

Although the majority of impairments implicated in competency examinations are functional, rather than organic (Reich and Wels 1985), neuropsychiatric impairments frequently raise questions about a defendant's competency to stand trial. For example, in *Wilson v. United States (1968)* the defendant had no memory regarding the time of the alleged robbery because of permanent retrograde amnesia. The amnesia was caused by injuries he sustained in an automobile accident that occurred as he was being pursued by the police after the offense. Of the various criteria the court established in determining the defendant's competence to stand trial for the robbery, the following are directly relevant to the issue of neuropsychiatric impairment:

- The extent to which the amnesia affected the defendant's ability to consult with and assist his lawyer
- The extent to which the amnesia affected the defendant's ability to testify in his own behalf

Amnesia by itself is insufficient to support a finding of incompetency to stand trial or of not guilty by reason of insanity (Rubinsky and Brandt 1986). Significant impairment of cognitive and communicative abilities, however, is likely to affect the decision regarding a defendant's competency. Nevertheless, it is the actual functional mental capability to meet the minimal standard of trial competency and not the severity of the deficits that determines whether an individual is cognitively capable of being tried.

For example, Slovenko (1995) questioned whether psychiatric diagnosis is relevant to competency to stand trial. The presence or absence of a mental illness is irrelevant if the defendant is capable of meeting competency requirements. It is legal criteria, not medical or psychiatric diagnosis, that governs competency. Diagnosis is relevant only to the question of restoring the defendant's competency to stand trial with treatment.

Checklists and structured interviews have been developed to assess specific psychological factors applicable to the competency standards established in *Dusky* (McGarry 1973). The Interdisciplinary Fitness Interview, for use by lawyers and mental health professionals (Schreiber et al. 1987), provides for a detailed examination of psychopathology and legal knowledge, using explicit scales for rating each response to the competency evaluation. *Evaluating Competencies: Forensic Assessments and Instruments*, by Grisso (1986), is a standard reference in the field.

A defendant's impairment in one particular function, however, does not automatically render the accused incompetent. For example, the fact that the defendant is manifesting certain deficits because of damage to the parietal lobe does not necessarily mean that he or she lacks the requisite cognitive ability to aid in his or her own defense at trial (Tranel 1992). The ultimate determination of incompetency is solely for the court to decide (*United States v. David 1975*). Moreover, the impairment must be considered in the context of the particular case or proceeding. Mental impairment may render an individual incompetent to stand trial in a complicated tax fraud case but not incompetent for a misdemeanor trial.

Psychiatrists and psychologists who testify as expert witnesses on a defendant's competency to stand trial are most effective if their findings are framed according to the degree to which the defendant is cognitively capable of meeting the standards enunciated in *Dusky*.

Insanity Defense

In American jurisprudence, one of the most controversial issues is the insanity defense. Defendants with TBI who are found competent to stand trial may seek acquittal on the basis that they were not criminally responsible for their actions because of insanity at the time the offense was committed.

Criminals commit crimes for a variety of reasons, but the law presumes that all of them do so rationally and of their own free will. As a result, the law concludes that they are deserving of some form of punishment. However, some offenders are so mentally disturbed in their thinking and behavior that they are thought to be incapable of acting rationally. Under these circumstances, civilized societies have deemed it unjust to punish a "crazy" or insane person (Blackstone 1769). This is in part because of fundamental principles of fairness and morality. Additionally, the punishment of a person who cannot rationally appreciate the consequences of his or her actions thwarts the two major tenets of punishment—retribution and deterrence. Although the insanity defense is rarely used, a successful insanity defense is even rarer.

A generally accepted, precise definition of legal insanity does not exist. Over the years, tests of insanity have been subject to much controversy, modification, and refinement (Brakel et al. 1985, p. 707). The development of the insanity defense standard in the United States has had the following four basic elements:

- Presence of a mental disorder
- Presence of a defect of reason
- A lack of knowledge of the nature or wrongfulness of the act
- An incapacity to refrain from the act

The existence of a mental disorder has remained a consistent core of the insanity defense, whereas the other elements have varied over time (Brakel et al. 1985, p. 709). Thus, there is variability in the insanity defense standard in the United States, depending on which state or jurisdiction has control over the defendant raising the defense.

After the acquittal by reason of insanity of John Hinckley, Jr., on charges of attempting to assassinate President Reagan and murder others, an outraged public demanded changes in the insanity defense. Federal and state legislation to accomplish that result ensued. Between 1978 and 1985, approximately 75% of all states made some sort of substantive change in their insanity defense standards (Perlin 1989). A number of states continued to adhere to the American Law Institute insanity de-

fense standard or a version of it. The American Law Institute test provides that

> A person is not responsible for criminal conduct if at the time of such conduct as a result of mental disease or defect he lacks substantial capacity either to appreciate the criminality [wrongfulness] of his conduct or to conform his conduct to the requirements of law.
>
> As used in this Article, the terms *mental disease* or *mental defect* do not include an abnormality manifested only by repeated criminal or otherwise antisocial conduct (Model Penal Code §4.01 [1962], 10 U.L.A. 490–91 [1974]).

This standard contains both a cognitive and a volitional prong. The cognitive prong derives from the M'Naghten rule, pronounced in England in 1843, exculpating the defendant who does not know the nature and quality of the alleged act or does not know the act was wrong. The volitional prong is a vestige of the irresistible-impulse rule, which states that the defendant who is overcome by an irresistible impulse that leads to an alleged act is not responsible for that act. It is on the volitional prong that experts disagree the most in individual criminal cases.

By contrast, defendants tried in a federal court are governed by the insanity defense standard enunciated in the Comprehensive Crime Control Act of 1984 (P.L. 98-473). The act provides that insanity is an affirmative defense to all federal crimes in which, at the time of the offense, "the defendant, as a result of a severe mental disease or defect, was unable to appreciate the nature and quality or the wrongfulness of his acts. Mental disease or defect does not otherwise constitute a defense" (Id 402, 98 Stat at 2057). This codification eliminates the volitional or irresistible impulse portion of the insanity defense. That is, it does not allow an insanity defense on the basis of a defendant's inability to conform his or her conduct to the requirements of the law. The defense is now limited to only those defendants who are unable to appreciate the wrongfulness of their acts (i.e., the *cognitive portion* of the defense).

The federal courts require the defendant to prove insanity by clear and convincing evidence. The burden of proof varies among the states. In a minority of states, the prosecution has the burden of proving beyond a reasonable doubt that the defendant was sane. In a majority of states, the defendant must bear the burden of proving by a preponderance of the evidence that she or he was insane (Melton et al. 1997, pp. 201–202). A few states have abolished the special plea of insanity. At the same time, evidence of insanity is admissible to negate *mens rea*.

A 29-year-old woman sustains a TBI in an automobile accident. She is subsequently diagnosed as having an organic personality syndrome secondary to frontal lobe damage. The patient is taking carbamazepine to control severe affective lability and poor impulse control. During an argument with her boyfriend, she impulsively pulls out a loaded gun from a drawer and kills him. She is charged with second-degree murder. She pleads not guilty by reason of insanity. Experts on both sides agree on the diagnosis. The defense forensic psychiatric expert testifies that the defendant was unable to form any intent to commit murder. Although she knew what was happening, it was like a bystander watching a murder take place. Rather, the shooting was a momentary impulsive act arising from her TBI. The prosecution expert testifies that the defendant has little cognitive impairment. Furthermore, she kept a loaded gun readily available, despite the knowledge of her own poor impulse control. At the moment of the murder, the defendant knew that she was killing her boyfriend. Because the case is heard in federal court, the insanity defense standard enunciated in the Comprehensive Crime Control Act of 1984 is applied. The court finds the defendant guilty of second-degree murder because she was "able to appreciate the nature and quality or the wrongness of her act."

The preceding case example illustrates that the threshold issue in making an insanity determination is not the existence of a mental disease or defect per se, but the lack of substantial mental capacity because of it. Therefore, the lack of capacity from causes other than TBI may be sufficient. For instance, mental retardation may represent an adequate basis for the insanity defense under certain circumstances.

Impulse disorders that allegedly arise secondary to TBI, such as intermittent explosive disorder, kleptomania, pathological gambling, and pyromania, generally have not fared much better under an insanity defense than the "purely" psychological impulse disorders. Persons with these conditions do not meet the criteria for the cognitive prong of an insanity defense. Presumably, the volitional prong would be applicable, but it is usually insufficient by itself. Moreover, courts and juries tend to view criminal acts arising from impulse disorders as impulses not resisted rather than irresistible impulses.

Diminished Capacity

It is possible for a person to have the required *mens rea* and yet still not be found criminally responsible. For instance, a defendant's actions may be considered so bizarre that a jury finds the defendant criminally insane and therefore not legally responsible, even though the defendant's knowledge of the criminal act (e.g., committing a murder) is relatively intact. The law recognizes that there are "shades" of mental impairment that obviously can affect *mens rea* but not necessarily to the extent of completely nullifying it. In recognition of this fact, the concept of "diminished capacity" was developed (Melton et al. 1997, pp. 204–208).

Diminished capacity permits the defendant to introduce medical and psychological evidence that relates directly to the *mens rea* for the alleged crime, without the necessity of pleading insanity (Melton et al. 1997, pp. 204–208). For example, in a case of assault with the intent to kill, psychiatric testimony would be permitted to address whether the offender acted with the purpose of committing homicide. When a defendant's *mens rea* for the criminal charge is nullified by psychiatric evidence, the defendant is acquitted only of that charge (Melton et al. 1997, pp. 204–208). In the preceding example, the prosecutor may still try to convict the defendant of an offense requiring a lesser *mens rea*, such as manslaughter. TBI patients who commit criminal acts may be eligible for a diminished capacity defense.

The diminished capacity concept has been gradually losing ground, largely because of the unevenness of its application by the courts (Brakel et al. 1985, p. 711). In California, where it originated, the use of diminished capacity has been abolished by state statute, largely in response to a public outcry against the court's ruling in the notorious "Twinkie defense" of Dan White (Cal Penal Code 28[b] [West 1981]). White was charged with killing the mayor of San Francisco and a county supervisor. He was found guilty by a jury of voluntary manslaughter rather than first-degree murder. A diminished capacity defense was used on the basis of testimony that mental distress was aggravated by chemical imbalances caused by the ingestion of large quantities of refined sugar (*People v. White 1981*, 117 Cal App 3d 270, 172 Cal Rptr 612 [1981]).

Guilty but Mentally Ill

In a number of states, an alternative verdict of guilty but mentally ill (GBMI) has been established. Under GBMI statutes, if the defendant pleads not guilty by reason of insanity, this alternative verdict is available to the jury (Slovenko 1982). Under an insanity plea, the verdict may be

- Not guilty
- Not guilty by reason of insanity
- Guilty but mentally ill
- Guilty

The problem with GBMI is that it is an alternative verdict without a difference from finding the defendant simply guilty. The court must still impose a sentence on the convicted person. Although the convicted person will receive psychiatric treatment if necessary, this treatment provision is also available to any other prisoner. Moreover, the frequent unavailability of appropriate psychiatric treatment for prisoners adds an additional element of spuriousness to the GBMI verdict.

Exculpatory and Mitigating Disorders

Psychotic disorders of differing etiologies form the most common basis for an insanity defense. In addition to the major psychiatric and organic brain disorders, a number of other conditions may provide a foundation for an insanity or diminished capacity defense.

Automatisms

For conviction of a crime, not only must there be a criminal state of mind (*mens rea*) but also the commission of a prohibited act (*actus reus*). The physical movement necessary to satisfy the *actus reus* requirement must be conscious and volitional. In addition to statutory and common law in many jurisdictions, Section 2.01(2) of the Model Penal Code (1962) specifically excludes from the *actus reus* the following:

> (a) a reflex or convulsion; (b) a bodily movement during unconsciousness or sleep; (c) conduct during hypnosis or resulting from hypnotic suggestion; [and] (d) a bodily movement that otherwise is not the product of the effort or determination of the actor....

A defense claiming that the commission of a crime was an involuntary act usually is referred to as an *automatism defense*. The classic, although rare, example is the person who commits an offense while "sleepwalking." Courts have held that such an individual does not have conscious control of his or her physical actions and therefore acts involuntarily (*Fain v. Commonwealth 1879*; *H.M. Advocate v. Fraser 1878*). A conscious, reflexive action carried out under stressful circumstances may qualify for an automatism defense. For example, during a domestic dispute, the husband points a gun at his wife's head. Instinctively, she raises her hands to protect herself. The gun is knocked from his hand by her reflexive reaction. The gun hits the floor and discharges, killing the husband. Other situations relevant to psychiatry in which the defense might be used arise when a crime is committed during a state of altered consciousness caused by a concussion after a brain injury,

involuntary ingestion of drugs or alcohol, hypoxia, metabolic disorders such as hypoglycemia, or epileptic seizures (Low et al. 1982).

There are, however, limitations to the automatism defense. Most notably, some courts hold that if the person asserting the automatism defense was aware of the condition before the offense and failed to take reasonable steps to prevent the criminal occurrence, then the defense is not available. For example, if a defendant with a known history of uncontrolled epileptic seizures loses control of a car during a seizure and kills another, that defendant will not be permitted to assert the defense of automatism.

Intoxication

Ordinarily, intoxication is not a defense to a criminal charge. Because intoxication, unlike mental illness, mental retardation, and most neuropsychiatric conditions, is usually the product of a person's own actions, the law is cautious about viewing it as a complete defense or mitigating factor. Most states view voluntary alcoholism as relevant to the issue of whether the defendant possessed the *mens rea* necessary to commit a specific crime or whether there was premeditation in a crime of murder. The mere fact that the defendant was voluntarily intoxicated will not justify a finding of automatism or insanity. A distinct difference does arise when, because of chronic, heavy use of alcohol, the defendant demonstrates an alcohol-induced organic mental disorder such as alcohol hallucinosis, withdrawal delirium, amnestic disorder, or dementia associated with alcoholism. If clinical evidence is presented that an alcohol-related neuropsychiatric disorder caused significant cognitive or volitional impairment, a defense of insanity or diminished capacity could be upheld.

Temporal Lobe Seizures

Another "mental state" defense occasionally raised by defendants regarding assault-related crimes is that the assaultive behavior was involuntarily precipitated by abnormal electrical patterns in the brain. This condition is frequently diagnosed as temporal lobe epilepsy (Devinsky and Bear 1984). Episodic dyscontrol syndrome (Elliot 1978; Monroe 1978) has also been advanced as a neuropsychiatric condition causing involuntary aggression. Studies have hypothesized that there are "centers of aggression" in the temporal lobe or limbic system—primarily the amygdala. This hypothesis has promoted the idea that sustained aggressive behavior by these persons may be primarily the product of an uncontrollable, randomly occurring, abnormal brain dysrhythmia. Hence, the legal argument is raised that these individuals should not be held accountable for their actions. Despite its simplicity and occasional success in the courts, there are few empirically significant data to support this theory at this time (Blumer 1984).

Metabolic Disorders

Defenses based on metabolic disorders have also been tried. The so-called Twinkie defense was used as part of a successful diminished capacity defense of Dan White in the murders of San Francisco Mayor George Mosconi and Supervisor Harvey Milk. This defense was based on the theory that the ingestion of large amounts of sugar contributed to a state of temporary insanity (*People v. White 1981*). The forensic psychiatric report stated that the defendant had been "filling himself up with Twinkies and Coca-Cola" (Blinder 1981–1982, p. 16). After specifying a number of factors that contributed to the murders, the forensic examiner concluded with the following opinion concerning Dan White's ingestion of certain food:

> Finally, there is much evidence to suggest recently recognized physiological aberrations consequent to consumption of noxious edibles by susceptibles. There are cases in the literature challenged with large quantities of refined sugar. Furthermore, there are studies of cerebral allergic reactions to the chemicals in highly processed foods; some studies have documented a marked reduction in violent and antisocial behavior in "career criminals" upon the elimination of these substances from their diet, as well as the production of rage reactions in susceptible individuals when challenged by the offending food substances. For these reasons, I would suggest a repeat electroencephalogram preceded by a glucose-tolerance test, as well as a clinical challenge of Mr. White's mental functions with known food antigens, in a controlled setting. (Blinder 1981–1982, pp. 21–22)

Hypoglycemic states also may be associated with significant psychiatric impairment (Kaplan and Sadock 1989). The brain is dependent on a steady supply of glucose through the bloodstream. When the glucose level drops significantly, the brain has no backup energy source to compensate. Metabolism naturally slows down, and cerebral function is impaired. Because the cerebral cortex and parts of the cerebellum metabolize glucose at the highest rate, they are the first to show impairment when there is an energy depletion (Wilson et al. 1991). When a substantial depletion occurs, a wide variety of responses may occur, including episodic and repetitive dyscontrol, temporary amnesia, depression, and hostility, with spontaneous recovery (quick recovery after the consumption of appropriate nu-

trients). The degree of mental abnormality associated with hypoglycemic states varies from mild to severe according to the blood glucose level. It is the degree of disturbance, not the mere presence of an etiologic metabolic component, that determines a mental state defense. This principle also applies to mental dysfunctions produced by disorders originating in the hepatic, renal, and adrenal systems, as well as the neuroendocrine system (premenstrual syndrome) (Parry and Berga 1991).

Civil Litigation

Expert Testimony

The ensuing civil litigation in brain injury cases generally requires the evaluation and testimony of psychiatrists (neuropsychiatrists) as well as neurologists, psychologists, neuropsychologists, and other mental health professionals. Psychiatrists can become involved in litigation as witnesses in one of two ways: as treaters or as forensic experts. An increasing number of psychiatrists are practicing the subspecialty of forensic psychiatry, which is defined as "a subspecialty of psychiatry in which scientific and clinical expertise is applied to legal issues in legal contexts embracing civil, criminal, correctional or legislative matters" (American Academy of Psychiatry and the Law 1987, p. 1).

Treating Clinician

Psychiatrists who venture into the legal arena must be aware of the fundamental difference in role that exists between a treating psychiatrist and the forensic psychiatric expert. Treatment and expert roles do not mix (Greenberg and Shuman 1997; Strasburger et al. 1997). For example, unlike the orthopedist who possesses objective data such as the X ray of a broken limb to demonstrate orthopedic damages in court, the treating psychiatrist must rely heavily on the subjective reporting of the patient. In the treatment context, psychiatrists are interested primarily in the patient's perception of his or her difficulties, not necessarily the objective reality. As a consequence, many treating psychiatrists do not speak to third parties or check pertinent nonmedical records to gain additional information about patients or to corroborate their statements. The law, however, is interested only in that which can reasonably be established by facts. Uncorroborated, subjective patient reporting is frequently attacked in court as speculative, self-serving, and unreliable. The treating psychiatrist usually is not well equipped to counter these charges.

Credibility issues also abound. The treating psychiatrist is, and must be, a total ally of the patient. This bias in favor of the patient is a proper treatment stance that fosters the therapeutic alliance. Furthermore, to be an effective therapist, no practitioner can treat a patient for very long whom he or she dislikes. The psychiatrist is the ally of the patient. Moreover, the psychiatrist looks for mental disorders to treat. This is the appropriate clinical role for the treating psychiatrist.

When a treating psychiatrist testifies in court, his or her credibility may be attacked. Opposing counsel will take every opportunity to portray the treating psychiatrist as a subjective mouthpiece for the patient-litigant—which may or may not be true. Also court testimony by the treating psychiatrist may compel the disclosure of information that may not be legally privileged, but nonetheless is viewed as intimate and confidential by the patient. This disclosure by a previously trusted therapist is bound to cause psychological damage to the therapeutic relationship (Strasburger 1987). In addition, psychiatrists must be careful to inform patients about the consequences of releasing treatment information, particularly in legal matters. Section 4, Annotation 2 of the Principles of Medical Ethics with Annotations Especially Applicable to Psychiatry (American Psychiatric Association 2001) states:

> The continuing duty of the psychiatrist to protect the patient includes fully apprising him/her of the connotations of waiving the privilege of privacy. This may become an issue when the patient is being investigated by a government agency, is applying for a position, or is involved in legal action.

Finally, when the treating psychiatrist testifies concerning the patient's need for further treatment, a conflict of interest is readily apparent. In making such treatment prognostications, the psychiatrist stands to benefit economically from the recommendation of further treatment. Although this may not be the intention of the psychiatrist at all, opposing counsel is sure to point out that the psychiatrist has a financial interest in the case.

The American Academy of Psychiatry and the Law (1987), in its ethics statement, advises that "a treating psychiatrist should generally avoid agreeing to be an expert witness or to perform an evaluation of his patient for legal purposes because a forensic evaluation usually requires that other people be interviewed and testimony may adversely affect the therapeutic relationship" (p. 4).

The treating psychiatrist should attempt to remain solely in a treatment role. If it becomes necessary to testify on behalf of the patient, the treating psychiatrist should testify only as a fact witness, not as an expert witness. As a fact witness, the psychiatrist will be asked to describe the number and length of visits, diagnosis, and treatment. Generally, no opinion evidence will be requested concerning causation of the injury or extent of damages. However, in some jurisdictions, the court may convert a fact witness into an expert at the time of trial. Many double agent roles that can develop when mixing psychiatry and litigation (Simon 1992a).

Forensic Expert

The forensic expert, on the other hand, is usually free from the encumbrances of the treating psychiatrist. During forensic evaluation, no doctor-patient relationship is created with a treatment bias toward the patient. The expert can review a variety of records and usually be able to speak to a number of people who know the litigant. Furthermore, the forensic expert, because of a clear appreciation of the litigation context and the absence of treatment bias, is not easily distracted from considering exaggeration or malingering. Finally, the forensic psychiatrist is not placed in a conflict-of-interest position of recommending treatment from which he or she would personally benefit. The forensic expert, however, is frequently viewed by opposing counsel as a "hired gun."

In evaluating the TBI patient, both the treating psychiatrist and the expert psychiatric witness will need to coordinate their efforts with other medical and nonmedical professionals. Obtaining additional information from others who are also assisting the patient fosters both good treatment and credible testimony.

Forensic Psychiatric Evaluation of the TBI Claimant

The forensic psychiatric evaluation of the TBI claimant differs in a number of significant ways from the traditional psychiatric evaluation of the TBI patient. As noted in the preceding sections, the distinction between the role of treating psychiatrist and that of forensic evaluator should be maintained in the litigation context. Problems in treatment and testimony invariably arise for clinicians when these roles are confused.

Most psychiatrists who enter the legal arena understand that equities usually exist on both sides of a case; otherwise, it would probably not have been brought to litigation in the first place. The fact that opposing experts disagree does not necessarily mean that one side or the other is wrong. The opinions of opposing experts should be carefully considered.

Team Approach

The comprehensive forensic psychiatric evaluation requires cooperation with a number of other practitioners and specialists. Usually, the forensic psychiatrist who is evaluating the TBI claimant will require the input of a neurologist, a neuropsychologist, and an internist or general practitioner. Depending on the complexities of the case, a number of other disciplines may need to be consulted. The forensic evaluator also should consider the findings of other examinations performed at the request of opposing counsel. The burgeoning number of complicated brain studies becoming available makes consultation with a qualified neurologist virtually a necessity in cases involving claims of brain injury.

No Doctor-Patient Relationship

The psychiatrist should inform the claimant at the time of the examination that no doctor-patient relationship will be formed. That is, the psychiatrist will not treat the claimant. The psychiatrist should explain that he or she has been retained by (name the specific party) to perform an independent psychiatric examination. The sole purpose of the examination is to provide information to the party retaining the psychiatrist.

No Confidentiality

The claimant should be informed that, unlike the usual doctor-patient relationship, confidentiality surrounding the forensic evaluation may not exist. Once the retaining attorney decides to disclose the findings of the evaluation in litigation, the information will be available to both sides and may become a public record.

Standard Diagnostic Schema

The diagnostic evaluation of TBI claimants should be made according to the multiaxial classification system contained in DSM-IV-TR. All five axes should be used. Axis I permits the clinician to consider the major clinical psychiatric syndromes, either single or multiple. TBI claimants often have concurrent Axis I diagnoses. For example, the presence of alcohol or drug abuse may directly contribute to the brain injury. Concurrent Axis I disorders may preexist or may be exacerbated by the brain injury.

Axis II requires the clinician to consider personality disorders that are often overlooked or ignored in the forensic evaluation of a claimant. The occurrence of significant brain injuries is high among the violent criminal population in whom a higher incidence of antisocial personality disorders exists (Lewis et al. 1986; Petursson and Gudjonsson 1981).

On Axis III, the relationship of medical disorders and their treatments to the patient's clinical presentation on Axis I should be carefully evaluated. TBI claimants may have a number of injuries requiring extensive pharmacotherapy that further complicates the patient's clinical picture. Moreover, a host of medical disorders may present or have associated symptoms of cerebral dysfunction. Prior brain injuries or preexisting central nervous system disorders should be considered. For example, young adults who have a history of learning disabilities or attention-deficit disorder are likely to develop serious incapacity when they sustain a TBI.

Axis IV permits the evaluation of psychosocial and environmental problems occurring usually within the year preceding the current evaluation that may have contributed to the development of a new mental disorder or recurrence of a prior mental disorder or may have become a focus of treatment. The search for multiple psychosocial stressors must be carefully conducted. It is the rare claimant who has only one psychosocial stressor affecting his or her life. A brain injury often occurs in the context of other preexisting psychosocial stressors such as sustained interpersonal difficulties, financial problems, occupational distress, or other personal losses.

Finally, functional impairment should be assessed on Axis V according to the DSM-IV-TR Global Assessment of Functioning Scale in combination with other standard methods of evaluation of psychiatric impairment discussed in the following sections.

DSM-IV-TR contains a cautionary statement about its use in litigation. Lawyers and courts refer to DSM-IV-TR extensively. Psychiatrists perform an important service to the judicial system by appropriately applying DSM-IV-TR in litigation. Lawyers and courts have a tendency to cloak clinical guidelines and diagnostic manuals with a certainty more properly given to the reading of statutes and codes.

Collateral Sources of Information

In the treatment situation, the psychiatrist relies almost exclusively on the subjective reporting of the patient. The patient is presumed to be candid and without conscious hidden agendas. In litigation, however, the claimant must naturally be expected to favor his or her own legal case. The possibility of malingering should be kept in mind (Table 33–3). Malingering is not limited to the fabrication of symptoms. Most often, malingering is manifested by the exaggeration of symptoms. Litigants also may consciously deny or minimize a significant past

TABLE 33–3. Increased index of suspicion for malingering

Litigation context (e.g., financial compensation, evading criminal prosecution)

Marked discrepancy between clinical findings and subjective complaints

Lack of cooperation with evaluation and treatment

Antisocial personality traits or disorder

Overdramatization of complaints

History of recurrent accidents or injuries

Evidence of self-induced injuries

Vaguely defined symptoms

Poor work history

Unable to work but retains capacity for pleasurable activities

history of mental illness. Thus, the psychiatrist should consider a broad array of information.

During the course of legal discovery by both parties to the suit, a great deal of information is developed. The forensic examiner should request that the retaining lawyer provide all relevant information. Incomplete information will likely be exposed by opposing counsel in court, undercutting the psychiatrist's testimony and possibly damaging the claimant's case. The forensic psychiatrist should review all data carefully before reaching a conclusion. The collateral source information list in Table 33–4, although not exhaustive, indicates major areas for inquiry.

TABLE 33–4. Collateral information sources

Other physicians and health care providers (e.g., reports, direct discussions)

Hospital records

Family

Other third parties

Military records

Educational records

Police records

Witness information

Work records

Work products (e.g., letters, work projects)

Legal discovery (e.g., depositions, legal documents)

Prior medical and psychiatric records

Prior psychological and neuropsychological evaluations

Mental Status Examination

In evaluating the mental status of the claimant, the psychiatrist must conduct a thorough mental status examination. If possible, it may be better to conduct the examination in divided sessions over the course of 2 days because of possible fluctuations in the mental status of the TBI claimant. The practice of performing a perfunctory mental status examination or relying solely on the assessment of the neuropsychologist is unwarranted. Neuropsychological assessment can be a valuable adjunct to the neuropsychiatric assessment of the TBI claimant (Becker and Kay 1986). Nevertheless, the psychiatrist will have little basis for critically reviewing the neuropsychological findings unless he or she can perform a competent mental status examination. Moreover, the mental status assessment is an integral part of the psychiatric examination that cannot be delegated to others. The mental status examination as described by Strub and Black (1988) provides a scored, comprehensive, reliable format for mental status evaluation.

The role of neuropsychological testing must be critically evaluated in each case. Neuropsychological tests are not totally objective. The qualifications and experience of the neuropsychologist are important variables. Tests of behavior in neuropsychological testing are subject to the control of the person performing the task. Thus, the consideration of motivation is critical. Also, low test scores may be caused by factors other than brain damage (Table 33–5). For example, the impact of somatic therapies and psychopathology as confounding factors in neuropsychological testing has been noted (Cullum et al. 1991; Finlayson and Bird 1991). Doctors, not tests, make diagnoses. A neuropsychological test score, by itself, cannot point to a specific cause of the litigant's injury. In litigation, whether legal causation exists between an injury and alleged incapacity (harm) is a matter for the finder of fact to determine.

Base rate neuropsychological deficits typically exist in the normal population. If impairments are noted without evaluation of the claimant's prior history and level of neuropsychological functioning, overinterpretation of the test data is likely. The critical review of educational and work records to determine the prior level of intellectual functioning is important in establishing baseline performance. Neuropsychological impairments observed among a healthy population increase with the age of the population. Lower IQ score and slower responses are also associated with normal aging.

Brain Injury Mimics

A number of psychiatric disorders may mimic TBI. Some of the more common TBI mimics include conversion, factitious, somatization, and depressive disorders presenting with

---

TABLE 33–5.   Major factors affecting neuropsychological test findings

Original endowment

Environment (e.g., education, occupation, and life experiences)

Motivation (e.g., effort)

Physical health

Age

Psychological distress

Psychiatric disorders (e.g., affective and somatoform disorders)

Medications (e.g., anticonvulsants and psychotropics)

Qualifications and experience of neuropsychologist

Errors in scoring

Errors in interpretation

---

symptoms of neurological and cerebral dysfunction. Conversion disorder symptoms classically mimic neurological disease. Dissociative symptoms may present with amnesia or atypical memory loss. Depressive pseudodementia is a commonly recognized clinical disorder in the elderly. Posttraumatic stress disorder manifesting symptoms of difficulty in concentration and psychogenic amnesia can also mimic brain injury. Similarly, anxiety disorders may be associated with memory complaints secondary to the inability to concentrate. On the other hand, TBI can cause anxiety and depression, so these symptoms may occur together with TBI.

To complicate matters, TBI litigants may be prescribed psychoactive substances, either for their symptoms of brain injury or for concurrent psychiatric and medical disorders. Antipsychotics, antidepressants, lithium, and, particularly, benzodiazepines can produce side effects that mimic neurological and brain disorders. Psychoactive substances may produce serious memory difficulties, either directly on brain chemistry or indirectly through sedation. It is common for practitioners to prescribe two or more drugs concurrently, particularly when the claimant appears refractory to treatment during the course of litigation. Various combinations of medications may interact to produce a host of side effects that involve the central nervous system. Psychoactive drug abuse is distressingly common in these cases, especially when the TBI litigant complains of persistent pain. Narcotics and barbiturates, especially in combination with nonnarcotic pain medications, are commonly abused.

Comorbidity and drug effects also should be considered when evaluating the results of neuropsychological test assessments. Questionable results will be obtained in the neuropsychological testing if the effects of concurrent psychiatric disorders and medications are not considered.

Disability Determinations

In addition to the psychiatric diagnosis, an assessment of functional impairment and disability must be made. In litigation, it is the degree of functional impairment, not the psychiatric diagnosis per se, that determines the amount of the monetary awards for damages. The psychiatrist also must understand the difference between impairment and disability. An impaired individual may not necessarily be disabled. Psychiatric impairment is considered disabling only when a psychiatric disorder limits a person's capacity to meet the demands of living. A traumatic blow to the eye of a company president that causes visual impairment may not significantly impair occupational functioning. The same injury to a major league baseball player would likely be totally disabling and end his career.

Similarly, a TBI patient may have moderate impairment but only mild disability in social or occupational functioning because of the development of compensatory coping mechanisms. Most psychiatric clinicians have seen TBI patients who have mild impairments but who are seriously disabled. This situation commonly occurs in litigation. For claimants presenting the latter clinical picture, the psychiatrist should pay particular attention to the possible presence of concurrent Axis IV psychosocial and environmental problems, comorbidity, substance abuse, medication effects, and litigation issues on the clinical presentation of the TBI claimant.

Standard impairment assessment methods should be used in combination with the DSM-IV-TR Axis V global assessment of functioning. The credible psychiatric assessment of functional impairment will avoid strictly subjective, conclusory pronouncements about the claimant's impairment and the need for future treatment. Instead, whenever possible, the TBI claimant's functional impairment and future treatment needs should be evaluated according to standard impairment measures such as the American Medical Association's Guide to the Evaluation of Permanent Impairment (American Medical Association 2000). The guide closely follows the Social Security Administration's guidelines for the assessment of disability. Assessment of permanent impairment should not be made until maximum medical improvement has been achieved.

Conclusion

The ethical and legal issues in the treatment and management of the TBI patient are challenging and complex. The legally informed psychiatrist is in a stronger position to provide good clinical care to the TBI patient within the context of burgeoning regulation of psychiatry by the courts and through legislation. Moreover, psychiatrists are increasingly required to testify in court concerning TBI patients. Familiarity and comfort with the role of fact or expert witness will facilitate competent psychiatric testimony.

References

American Academy of Psychiatry and the Law: Ethical Guidelines for the Practice of Forensic Psychiatry. Baltimore, MD, American Academy of Psychiatry and the Law, adopted May 1987 (revised October 1989 and 1991)

American Medical Association: Guidelines for the appropriate use of do-not-resuscitate orders (Council on Ethical and Judicial Affairs). JAMA 265:1868–1871, 1991

American Medical Association: Guidelines on cardiopulmonary resuscitation and emergency cardiac care, part VIII: ethical considerations in resuscitation. JAMA 268:2282–2288, 1992

American Medical Association: Guides to the Evaluation of Permanent Impairment, 5th Edition. Chicago, IL, American Medical Association, 2000

American Psychiatric Association: Diagnostic and Statistical Manual of Mental Disorders, 4th Edition, Text Revision. Washington, DC, American Psychiatric Association, 2000

American Psychiatric Association: Opinions of the Ethics Committee on the Principles of Medical Ethics with Annotations Especially Applicable to Psychiatry. Washington, DC, American Psychiatric Press, 2001

Aponte v United States, 582 FSupp 555, 566–69 (D PR 1984)

Appelbaum PS, Lidz CW, Meisel A: Informed Consent: Legal Theory and Clinical Practice. New York, Oxford University Press, 1987, p 84

Becker B, Kay GC: Neuropsychological consultation in psychiatric practice. Psychiatr Clin North Am 9:255–265, 1986

Benesch K: Legal issues in determining competence to make treatment decisions, in Legal Implications of Hospital Policies and Practices. Edited by Miller RD. San Francisco, CA, Jossey-Bass, 1989, pp 97–105

Bethea v United States, 365 A2d 64, (DC 1976) cert denied, 433 US 911 (1977)

Black HC: Black's Law Dictionary, 6th Edition. St. Paul, MN, West Publishing, 1990, p 284

Blackstone W: Commentaries vol. 4, 24–25 (1769); Coke E: Third Institute 6 (1680)

Blinder M: My examination of Dan White. Am J Forensic Psychiatry 2:12–22, 1981–1982

Blumer D: Psychiatric Aspects of Epilepsy. Washington, DC, American Psychiatric Press, 1984

Brakel SJ, Parry J, Weiner BA: The Mentally Disabled and the Law, 3rd Edition. Chicago, IL, American Bar Foundation, 1985, p 370

Comprehensive Crime Control Act of 1984, Pub. L. No. 98-473, 98 Stat. 1837

Cruzan v Director, Missouri Department of Health, 110 S Ct 284 (1990)

Cullum CM, Heaton RK, Grant I: Psychogenic factors influencing neuropsychological performance: Somatoform disorders, factitious disorders and malingering, in Forensic Neuropsychology: Legal and Scientific Bases. Edited by Doerr HO, Carlin AS. New York, Guilford, 1991, pp 141–171

Devinsky P, Bear DM: Varieties of aggressive behavior in patients with temporal lobe epilepsy. Am J Psychiatry 141:651–655, 1984

Dusky v United States, 362 U.S. 402 (1960)

Dyer AR: Ethics and Psychiatry: Toward Professional Definition. Washington, DC, American Psychiatric Press, 1988

Elliot FA: Neurological aspects of antisocial behavior, in The Psychopath. Edited by Reid WH. New York, Brunner/Mazel, 1978, pp 146–149

Emanuel EJ, Emanuel LL: Proxy decision making for incompetent patients—an ethical and empirical analysis. JAMA 267:2067–2071, 1992

Fain v Commonwealth, 78 Ky 183 (1879)

Finlayson MAJ, Bird DR: Psychopathology and neuropsychological deficit, in Forensic Neuropsychology: Legal and Scientific Bases. Edited by Doerr HO, Carlin AS. New York, Guilford, 1991

Folstein MF, Folstein SE, McHugh PR: "Mini-Mental State": a practical method of grading the cognitive state of patients for the clinician. J Psychiatr Res 12:189–198, 1975

Ford v Wainwright, 477 US 399 (1986); Note, The Eighth Amendment and the Execution of the Presently Incompetent, 32 Stan L Rev:765 (1980)

Frasier v Department of Health and Human Resources, 500 So2d 858, 864 (La Ct App 1986)

Greenberg SA, Shuman DW: Irreconcilable conflict between therapeutic and forensic roles. Journal of Professional Psychology: Research and Practice 28:50–56, 1997

Grisso T: Evaluating Competencies: Forensic Assessments and Instruments. New York, Plenum, 1986

Gulf S I R Co v Sullivan, 155 Miss 1, 119 So 501 (1928)

Gutheil TG, Appelbaum PS: Substituted judgment and the physician's ethical dilemma: with special reference to the problem of the psychiatric patient. J Clin Psychiatry 41:303–305, 1980

Hassenfeld IN, Grumet B: A study of the right to refuse treatment. Bull Am Acad Psychiatry Law 12:65–74, 1984

H.M. Advocate v Fraser, 4 Couper 70 (1878)

In re Boyer, 636 P2d 1085 1089 (Utah 1981)

In re Jobes, 108 NJ 394 (1987)

Jehovah's Witnesses v King County Hospital, 278 FSupp 488 (WD Wash 1967), affd, 390 US 598 (1968)

Kaplan HI, Sadock BJ: Comprehensive Textbook of Psychiatry, 5th Edition, Vol 2. Baltimore, MD, Williams and Wilkins, 1989, pp 1219–1220

Klein J, Onek J, Macbeth J: Seminar on Law in the Practice of Psychiatry. Washington, DC, Klein and Farr, 1983, p 28

LaPuma J, Orentlicher D, Moss RJ: Advance directives on admission: clinical implications and analysis of the Patient Self-Determination Act of 1990. JAMA 266:402–405, 1991

Lewis DO, Pincus JH, Feldman M, et al: Psychiatric, neurological and psychoeducational characteristics of 15 death row inmates in the United States. Am J Psychiatry 143:838–845, 1986

Low P, Jeffries J, Bonnie R: Criminal Law: Cases and Materials. Mineola, NY, The Foundation Press, 1982, pp 152–154

Luce JM: Ethical principles in critical care. JAMA 263:696–700, 1990

March FH, Staver A: Physician authority for unilateral DNR orders. J Leg Med 12:115–165, 1991

McGarry AL: Competency to Stand Trial and Mental Illness, a monograph sponsored by the Center for Studies of Crime and Delinquency, National Institute of Mental Health, DHEW Pub. No. (HSM) 73–9105, Rockville, MD, 1973

Meek v City of Loveland, 85 Colo 346, 276 P 30 (1929)

Melton GB, Petrila J, Poythress NG, et al: Psychological evaluation for the courts. New York, Guilford, 1987, p 128

Melton GB, Petrila J, Poythress NG, et al: Psychological Evaluations for the Courts: A Handbook for Mental Health Professionals and Lawyers, 2nd Edition. New York, Guilford, 1997, pp 204–205

Mental Aberration and Post Conviction Sanctions, 15 Suffolk UL Rev:1219 (1981); State v Hehman, 110 Ariz 459, 520 P2d 507 (1974); Commonwealth v Robinson, 494 Pa 372, 431 A2d 901 (1981)

Mill JS: On liberty, in The World Literature, Vol 2. Edited by Anderson GK, Warnock R. Chicago, IL, Scott, Foresman and Company, 1951, pp 316–336

Mishkin B: Decisions in Hospice. Arlington, VA, The National Hospice Organization, 1985

Mishkin B: Determining the capacity for making health care decisions, in Issues in Geriatric Psychiatry (Advances in Psychosomatic Medicine Series, Vol 19). Edited by Billig N, Rabins PV. Basel, Switzerland, Karger, 1989, pp 151–166

M'Naghten's Case, 10 Cl. F. 200, 8 Eng. Rep. 718 (H.L. 1943); United States v. Brawner, 471 F2d 969 (DC Cir 1972)

Monroe RR: Brain Dysfunction in Aggressive Criminals. Lexington, MA, Lexington Books, 1978

Neely v United States, 150 F2d 977 (DC Cir), cert denied 326 US 768 (1945)

Orentlicher D: The illusion of patient choice in end-of-life decisions. JAMA 267:2101–2104, 1992

Overman W, Stoudemire A: Guidelines for legal and financial counseling of Alzheimer's disease patients and their families. Am J Psychiatry 145:1495–1500, 1988

Parry BL, Berga SL: Neuroendocrine correlates of behavior during the menstrual cycle, in Psychiatry, Vol 3. Edited by Cavenar JO. Philadelphia, PA, JB Lippincott, 1991, pp 1–22

Parry JW, Beck JC: Revisiting the civil commitment/involuntary treatment stalemate using limited guardianship, substituted judgment and different due process considerations: a work in progress. Medical and Physical Disability Law Reporter 14:102–114, 1990

People v White, 117 Cal App 3d 270, 172 Cal Rptr 612 (1981)

Perlin MJ: Mental Disability Law: Civil and Criminal, Vol 3. Charlottesville, VA, Michie, 1989, p 404

Perr IN: The clinical considerations of medication refusal. Legal Aspects of Psychiatric Practice 1:5–8, 1984

Petursson H, Gudjonsson GH: Psychiatric aspects of homicide. Acta Psychiatr Scand 64:363–372, 1981

Pinals DA, Appelbaum PS: The history and current status of competence and informed consent in psychiatric research. Isr J Psychiatry Relat Sci 37:82–94, 2000

Planned Parenthood v Danforth, 428 US 52, 74 (1976) (abortion); Ill Ann Stat ch. 91 1/2, para 3–501(a) (Smith-Hurd Supp 1990) (mental health counseling)

President's Commission for the Study of Ethical Problems in Medicine and Biomedical and Behavioral Research: Making Health Care Decisions, Vol 1. (A report on the ethical and legal implications of informed consent in the patient-practitioner relationship.) Washington, DC, Superintendent of Documents, October 1982

Reich J, Wels J: Psychiatric diagnosis and competency to stand trial. Compr Psychiatry 26:421–432, 1985

Rennie v Klein, 462 FSupp 1131 (DNJ 1978), modified, 653 F2d 836 (3d cir 1981), vacated, 458 US 1119 (1982), on remand, 720 F2d 266 (3d Cir 1983)

Robertson ED: Is "substituted judgment" a valid legal concept? Issues Law Medicine 5:197–214, 1989

Roth LH: Informed consent and its applicability for psychiatry, in Psychiatry, Vol 3. Edited by Cavenar JO. Philadelphia, PA, JB Lippincott, 1985, pp 1–17

Rozovsky FA: Consent to Treatment: A Practical Guide. Boston, MA, Little, Brown, 1984, pp 87–122

Rubinsky EW, Brandt J: Amnesia and criminal law: a clinical overview. Behavioral Sciences and the Law 4:27–46, 1986

Ruchs VR: The "rationing" of medical care. N Engl J Med 311:1572–1573, 1984

Sale B, Powell DM, Van Duizend R: Disabled Persons and the Law: State Legislative Issues, 1982, p 461

Scaria v St. Paul Fire and Marine Ins Co, 68 Wis2d 1, 227 NW2d 647 (1975)

Schloendorff v Society of New York Hospital, 211 NY 125, 105 NE 92 (1914), overruled, Bing v Thunig, 2 NY2d 656, 143 NE2d 3, 163 NYS2d 3 (1957)

Schreiber J, Roesch R, Golding S: An evaluation of procedures for assessing competency to stand trial. Bull Am Acad Psychiatry Law 155:187–203, 1987

Schwartz HR: Do not resuscitate orders: the impact of guidelines on clinical practice, in Geriatric Psychiatry and the Law. Edited by Rosner R, Schwartz HR. New York, Plenum, 1987, p 91

Simon RI: Clinical Psychiatry and the Law, 2nd Edition. Washington, DC, American Psychiatric Press, 1992a

Simon RI: Clinical Psychiatry and the Law, 2nd Edition. Washington, DC, American Psychiatric Press, 1992b; citing, Addington v Texas, 441 US 418 (1979)

Slovenko R: Commentaries on psychiatry and the law: "Guilty but Mentally Ill." J Psychiatry Law 10:541–555, 1982

Slovenko R: Assessing competency to stand trial. Psychiatr Ann 26:392–393, 397, 1995

Smith JT: Medical Malpractice: Psychiatric Care. Colorado Springs, CO, Shephards McGraw-Hill, 1986, pp 178–179

Solnick PB: Proxy consent for incompetent nonterminally ill adult patients. J Leg Med 6:1–49, 1985

Strasburger LH: "Crudely, without any finesse": the defendant hears his psychiatric evaluation. Bull Am Acad Psychiatry Law 15:229–233, 1987

Strasburger LH, Gutheil TG, Brodsky A: On wearing two hats: role conflict in serving as both psychotherapist and expert witness. Am J Psychiatry 154:448–456, 1997

Strub RL, Black FW: Neurobehavioral Disorders: A Clinical Approach. Philadelphia, PA, FA Davis, 1988

The Legal Status of Adolescents 1980, U.S. Department of Health and Human Services, 41 (1981)

Tranel D: Functional neuroanatomy: neuropsychological correlates of cortical and subcortical damage, in American Psychiatric Press Textbook of Neuropsychiatry, 2nd Edition. Edited by Hales RE, Yudofsky SC. Washington, DC, American Psychiatric Press, 1992, pp 70–75

Uniform Guardianship and Protective Proceeding Act, sec. 5–101

United States v David, 511 F2d 355 (DC Cir 1975)

Weir RF, Gostin L: Decisions to abate life-sustaining treatment for nonautonomous patients: ethical standards and legal liability for physicians after Cruzan. JAMA 264:1846–1853, 1990

Wilson v Lehman, 379 SW2d 478, 479 (Ky 1964)

Wilson v United States, 391 F2d 460, 463 (DC Cir 1968)

Wilson JD, Braunwald E, Isselbacher KJ: Harrison's Principles of Internal Medicine, 12th Edition, Vol 2. New York, McGraw-Hill, 1991, p 1759

Zito JM, Lentz SL, Routt WW, et al: The treatment review panel: a solution to treatment refusal? Bull Am Acad Psychiatry Law 12:349–358, 1984

Appendix 33–1

Health Care Proxy

(1) I, _____ hereby appoint _____ (name, home address, and telephone number) as my health care agent to make any and all health care decisions for me, except to the extent that I state otherwise. This proxy shall take effect when and if I become unable to make my own health care decisions.

(2) Optional instructions: I direct my agent to make health care decisions in accord with my wishes and limitations as stated below, or as he or she otherwise knows. [Attach additional pages if necessary.]

_____

_____

(Unless your agent knows your wishes about artificial nutrition and hydration [feeding tubes], your agent will not be allowed to make decisions about artificial nutrition and hydration. See instructions below for samples of language you could use.)

(3) Name of substitute or fill-in agent if the person I appoint above is unable, unwilling, or unavailable to act as my health care agent.

_____ (name, home address, and telephone number)

(4).Unless I revoke it, this proxy shall remain in effect indefinitely, or until the date or conditions stated below. This proxy shall expire (specific date or conditions, if desired):

_____

(5) Signature _____

Address _____

Date _____

Statement by Witnesses (must be 18 or older)

I declare that the person who signed this document is personally known to me and appears to be of sound mind and acting of his or her own free will. He or she signed (or asked another to sign for him or her) this document in my presence.

Witness 1 _____

Address _____

Witness 2 _____

Address _____

Source.　From Simon RI: *Clinical Psychiatry and the Law,* 2nd Edition. Washington, DC, American Psychiatric Press, 1992, pp 614–617. Used with permission.

About the Health Care Proxy

This is an important legal form. Before signing this form, you should understand the following facts:

1. This form gives the person you choose as your agent the authority to make all health care decisions for you, except to the extent you say otherwise in this form. "Health care" means any treatment, service, or procedure to diagnose or treat your physical or mental condition.

2. Unless you say otherwise, your agent will be allowed to make all health care decisions for you, including decisions to remove or provide life-sustaining treatment.

3. Unless your agent knows your wishes about artificial nutrition and hydration (nourishment and water provided by a feeding tube), he or she will not be allowed to refuse or consent to those measures for you.

4. Your agent will start making decisions for you when doctors decide you are not able to make health care decisions for yourself.

You may write on this form any information about treatment that you do not desire and/or those treatments that you want to make sure you receive. Your agent must follow your instructions (oral and written) when making decisions for you.

If you want to give your agent written instructions, do so right on the form. For example, you could say:

If I become terminally ill, I do/don't want to receive the following treatments: . . .

If I am in a coma or unconscious, with no hope of recovery, then I do/don't want . . .

If I have brain damage or a brain disease that makes me unable to recognize people or speak and there is no hope that my condition will improve, I do/don't want . . .

I have discussed with my agent my wishes about _____ and I want my agent to make all decisions about these measures.

Examples of medical treatments about which you may wish to give your agent special instructions are listed below. This is not a complete list of the treatments about which you may leave instructions.

Artificial respiration

Artificial nutrition and hydration (nourishment and water provided by feeding tube)

Cardiopulmonary resuscitation (CPR)

Antipsychotic medication

Electroconvulsive therapy

Antibiotics

Psychosurgery

Dialysis

Transplantation

Blood transfusions

Abortion

Sterilization

Talk about choosing an agent with your family and/or close friends. You should discuss this form with a doctor or another health care professional, such as a nurse or social worker, before you sign it to make sure that you understand the types of decisions that may be made for you. You may also wish to give your doctor a signed copy. **You do not need a lawyer to fill out this form.**

You can choose any adult (older than 18), including a family member, or close friend, to be your agent. If you select a doctor as your agent, he or she may have to choose between acting as your agent or as your attending doctor; a physician cannot do both at the same time. Also, if you are a patient or resident of a hospital, nursing home, or mental hygiene facility, there are special restrictions about naming someone who works for that facility as your agent. You should ask staff at the facility to explain those restrictions.

You should tell the person you choose that he or she will be your health care agent. You should discuss your health care wishes and this form with your agent. Be sure to give him or her a signed copy. Your agent cannot be sued for health care decisions made in good faith.

Even after you have signed this form, you have the right to make health care decisions for yourself as long as you are able to do so, and treatment cannot be given to you or stopped if you object. You can cancel the control given to your agent by telling him or her or your health care provider orally or in writing.

Filling Out the Proxy Form

Item (1) Write your name and the name, home address, and telephone number of the person you are selecting as your agent.

Item (2) If you have special instructions for your agent, you should write them here. Also, if you wish to limit your agent's authority in any way, you should say so here. If you do not state any limitations, your agent will be allowed to make all health care decisions that you could have made, including the decision to consent to or refuse life-sustaining treatment.

Item (3) You may write the name, home address, and telephone number of an alternate agent.

Item (4) This form will remain valid indefinitely unless you set an expiration date or condition for its expiration. This section is optional and should be filled in only if you want the health care proxy to expire.

Item (5) You must date and sign the proxy. If you are unable to sign yourself, you may direct someone else to sign in your presence. Be sure to include your address.

Two witnesses at least 18 years of age must sign your proxy. The person who is appointed agent or alternate agent cannot sign as a witness.

PART VI

Treatment

34 Psychopharmacology

Jonathan M. Silver, M.D.

David B. Arciniegas, M.D.

Stuart C. Yudofsky, M.D.

MANY USEFUL THERAPEUTIC approaches are available for those who have experienced brain injury. As has been found with treatment of psychiatric disorders such as depression, panic disorder, and obsessive-compulsive disorder, a combination of therapeutic interventions administered simultaneously often provides more effective treatment than using a single modality. Individual, cognitive, behavioral, and family therapy, as well as environmental manipulation, all may affect symptoms and the patient's ability to cope with them (see Chapters 30 and 35–37). For many patients, the appropriate use of medications can be beneficial in the treatment of neuropsychiatric symptoms. In this chapter, we review the psychopharmacologic treatment of these symptoms when they occur after traumatic brain injury (TBI).

Evaluation

It is critical to conduct a thorough assessment of the patient before any intervention is initiated. For purposes of discussion, we assume that a complete psychiatric, developmental, and neurological history has been obtained, as presented in Chapter 4, Neuropsychiatric Assessment. Two issues require particular attention in the evaluation of the potential use of medication. First, the presenting complaints must be carefully assessed, defined, and operationalized, preferably through the use of objective rating scales such as the Overt Aggression Scale (Silver and Yudofsky 1991) (see Chapter 14, Aggressive Disorders), the Neurobehavioral Rating Scale—Revised (Levin et al. 1987; McCauley et al. 2001) (see Chapter 4), or the Neuropsychiatric Inventory (Cummings et al. 1994). In addition to clarifying the type, frequency, and severity of symptoms before treatment, repeated use of such scales during treatment improves the accuracy and objectivity of symptom monitoring. Second, the use and effectiveness of all ongoing treatments must be reevaluated, including pharmacological and nonpharmacological therapies as well as prescribed and self-administered agents. Although consultation may be requested to decide whether a new medication would be helpful, it is often the case that 1) other treatment modalities have not been properly applied, 2) there has been misdiagnosis of the problem, or 3) there has been poor communication among treating professionals. On occasion, a potentially effective medication has not been beneficial because it has been prescribed in a dose that is too low or for a period of time that is too brief. In other instances, the most appropriate pharmacological recommendation is that no medication is required and that other therapeutic modalities should be reassessed.

Portions of this chapter were previously published in Silver JM, Hales RE, Yudofsky SC: "Neuropsychiatric Aspects of Traumatic Brain Injury," in *The American Psychiatric Publishing Textbook of Neuropsychiatry*, 4th Edition. Edited by Yudofsky SC, Hales RE. Washington, DC, American Psychiatric Publishing, 2002, pp 363–395. Used with permission.

When reviewing the patient's current medication regimen, three key issues should be addressed: 1) the indications for all drugs prescribed, 2) whether currently the prescribed medications are still necessary, and 3) the potential side effects of these medications. Patients who have had severe brain trauma may be receiving many medications that result in psychiatric symptoms such as depression, mania, hallucinations, insomnia, nightmares, cognitive impairments, restlessness, paranoia, or aggression (Table 34–1). Specific issues with the use of anticonvulsant medications are discussed in the section Concerns Regarding Pharmacotherapy.

General Principles

There have been few controlled clinical trials to assess the effects of medication in patients with brain injury. Therefore, the decision regarding which medication (if any) to prescribe is based on 1) current knowledge of the efficacy of these medications in other psychiatric disorders, 2) side-effect profiles of the medications, 3) the increased sensitivity to side effects shown by patients with brain injury, 4) analogies from the brain injury symptoms to the recognized psychiatric syndromes (i.e., amotivational syndrome after TBI may be analogous to the deficit syndrome in schizophrenia), and 5) hypotheses regarding how the neurochemical changes after TBI may affect the proposed mechanisms of action of psychotropic medications.

There are several general guidelines that should be followed in the pharmacological treatment of the psychiatric syndromes that occur after TBI (see Table 34–2 for a summary of these treatment principles). They are

1. Start low, go slow
2. Therapeutic trial of all medications
3. Continuous reassessment of clinical condition
4. Monitor drug–drug interactions
5. Augment partial response
6. Discontinue or lower the dose of the most recently prescribed medication if there is a worsening of the treated symptom soon after the medication has been initiated (or increased)

In our experience, patients with brain injury of any type are far more sensitive to the side effects of medications than are patients who do not have brain injury. Doses of psychotropic medications must be raised and lowered in small increments over protracted periods, although patients with TBI ultimately may require the same doses and serum levels that are therapeutically effective for patients without brain injury.

When medications are prescribed, it is important that they be given in a manner that will enhance the probability of benefit and reduce the possibility of adverse reactions. Medications often should be initiated at dosages that are lower than those usually administered to patients without brain injury. However, comparable doses to those used to treat primary psychiatric disorders may be necessary to treat TBI-related neuropsychiatric conditions effectively. Dose increments should be made gradually to minimize side effects and enable the clinician to observe adverse consequences. It is important that such medications be given sufficient time to impart their full effects. Thus, when a decision is made to administer a medication, the patient must receive an adequate therapeutic trial of that medication in terms of dosage and duration of treatment.

Because of frequent changes in the clinical status of patients after TBI, continuous reassessment is necessary to determine whether each prescribed medication is still required. For depression after TBI, the standard guidelines for the treatment of major depression offered by the American Psychiatric Association (2000b) may offer a reasonable framework within which to develop a working treatment plan, including continuation of medication for a minimum of 16–20 weeks after complete remission of depressive symptoms. For this and all other neuropsychiatric sequelae of TBI, however, no formal treatment guidelines specific to this population are available. Although there is increasingly useful literature regarding the types and doses of medications useful for the treatment of such problems, there are few if any studies regarding the optimal duration of treatment and/or the issues pertaining to treatment discontinuation and relapse risk. In general, if the patient has responded favorably to initial medication treatment for one or another neuropsychiatric problem after TBI, the clinician must use sound judgment and apply risk: benefit determinations to each specific case in deciding whether and/or when to taper and attempt to discontinue the medication after TBI. Continuous reassessment is necessary because spontaneous remission of some symptoms may occur, in which case the medication can be permanently discontinued, or a carryover effect of the medication may occur (i.e., its effects may persist after the duration of treatment), in which case a reinstatement of the medication may not be required.

When a new medication is initiated in combination with medications previously prescribed, the clinician must be vigilant for the development of drug–drug interactions. These interactions may include alteration of pharmacokinetics that result in increased half-lives and serum levels of medications, as can occur with the use of

TABLE 34–1. Psychiatric side effects of neurological drugs

Symptom	Medications	Comments
Depression	Amantadine	Common at usual doses
	Anticonvulsants	Usually at higher blood levels
	Corticosteroids, ACTH	More common with high doses; may occur on withdrawal
	Benzodiazepines	Depression may also decrease in anxious, depressed patients
	Barbiturates	Common side effect
	Narcotics	—
	Levodopa	Greater risk with prolonged use
	Antihypertensives	Has been reported with many preparations
	Propranolol	Can occur at usual doses
	Vinblastine	Rare
	Asparaginase	Common side effect with higher doses
	Cimetidine	—
	Oral contraceptives	In as many as 15% of all cases
	Ibuprofen	Rare
	Metoclopramide	Usual doses
Mania	Baclofen	Usually appears after sudden withdrawal
	Bromocriptine	Symptoms may continue after drug is withdrawn
	Captopril	Symptoms may continue after drug is withdrawn
	Corticosteroids, ACTH	Usually at higher doses
	Dextromethorphan	—
	Levodopa	More frequent in elderly patients; risk increases with prolonged use
	Antidepressants	In bipolar and some patients with chronic depression
	Digitalis	In bipolar patients with higher doses
	Cyclobenzaprine	Reported in one patient
Hallucinations	Amantadine	Rare; more common in elderly patients
	Anticonvulsants	Visual and auditory
	Antihistamines	Especially with higher doses
	Anticholinergics	Usually with delirium
	Corticosteroids, ACTH	See above[a]
	Digitalis	Usually at higher blood levels
	Indomethacin	Especially in elderly patients
	Methysergide	Occasional
	Propranolol	At usual or increased doses
	Methylphenidate	More likely in children
	Levodopa	See above[a]
	Ketamine	Common
	Cimetidine	Usually in higher doses and in elderly patients
Nightmares	Antidepressants	When entire dose is taken at night
	Amantadine	Especially in elderly patients

(*continued*)

TABLE 34–1.   Psychiatric side effects of neurological drugs *(continued)*

Symptom	Medications	Comments
	Baclofen	Usually after sudden withdrawal
	Ketamine	Also produces hallucinations, crying, changes in body image, and delirium
	Levodopa	Often after dosage increase
	Pentazocine	During treatment
	Propranolol	See above[a]
	Digitalis	See above[a]
Paranoia	Asparaginase	May be common
	Bromocriptine	Not dose related
	Corticosteroids, ACTH	See above[a]
	Amphetamines	Even at low doses
	Indomethacin	Especially in elderly patients
	Propranolol	At any dose
	Sulindac	Reported in a few patients
Aggression	Bromocriptine	Not dose related; may persist
	Tranquilizers and hypnotics	A release phenomenon
	Levodopa	See above[a]
	Phenelzine	May be separate from mania
	Digitalis	See above[a]
	Carbamazepine	In children and adolescents

Note.   ACTH=adrenocorticotropic hormone.
[a]Same comments apply as for previous reactions on this drug.
Source.   Reprinted from Dubovsky SL: "Psychopharmacological Treatment in Neuropsychiatry," in *The American Psychiatric Press Textbook of Neuropsychiatry*, 2nd Edition. Washington, DC, American Psychiatric Press, 1991, pp 694–695. Used with permission.

TABLE 34–2.   General principles of pharmacotherapy for patients with traumatic brain injuries

Start low, go slow	Initiate treatment at doses lower than those used in patients without brain injuries, and raise doses more slowly than in patients without brain injuries.
Adequate therapeutic trial	Although patients with brain injuries may be more sensitive to the side effects of many medications, standard doses of such medication may be needed to treat adequately the neuropsychiatric problems of these patients.
Continuous reassessment	The need for continued treatment should be reassessed in an ongoing fashion, and dose reduction or medication discontinuation should be attempted after achieving remission of target symptoms. Spontaneous recovery occurs, and in such circumstances continued pharmacotherapy is unnecessary.
Monitor drug–drug interactions	Because patients with brain injuries are often sensitive to medication side effects and because they may require treatment with several medications, it is essential to be aware of and to monitor these patients for possible drug–drug interactions.
Augmentation	A patient experiencing a partial response to treatment with a single agent may benefit from augmentation of that treatment with a second agent that has a different mechanism of action. Augmentation of partial responses is preferable to switching to an agent with the same pharmacological profile as that producing the partial response.
Symptom intensification	If targeted psychiatric symptoms worsen soon after initiation of pharmacotherapy, lower the dose of the medication; if symptom intensification persists, discontinue the medication entirely.

multiple anticonvulsants. Additionally, alterations of pharmacodynamics may develop during the administration of medications with additive or synergistic clinical effects (i.e., increased sedative effects when several sedating medications are administered simultaneously).

If a patient does not respond favorably to the initial medication prescribed, several alternatives are available. If there has been no response, changing to a medication with a different mechanism of action is suggested, much as is done in the treatment of depressed patients without brain injury. If there has been a partial response to the initial medication, addition of another medication may be useful. The selection of a second supplementary or augmenting medication should be based on consideration of the possible complementary or contrary mechanisms of action of such agents, the individual and combined side-effect profiles of the initial and secondary agents, and their potential pharmacokinetic and pharmacodynamic interactions.

Although individuals after TBI may experience multiple concurrent neuropsychiatric symptoms (i.e., depressed mood, irritability, poor attention, fatigue, and sleep disturbances), suggesting a single psychiatric diagnosis such as major depression, we have found that some of these symptoms often persist despite treatment of the apparent "diagnosis." In other words, diagnostic parsimony should be sought but may not always be the best or most accurate diagnostic approach in this population. For this reason, the neuropsychiatric approach of evaluating and monitoring individual symptoms is necessary and differs from the usual syndromal approach of the present conventional psychiatric paradigm. Several medications may be required to alleviate several distinct symptoms after TBI, although it is prudent to initiate such treatments one at a time to determine the efficacy and side effects of each prescribed drug.

Studies of the effects of psychotropic medications in patients with TBI are few, and rigorous double-blind placebo-controlled studies are rare (see Arciniegas et al. 2000b). The recommendations contained in this chapter represent a synthesis of the available treatment literature in TBI, extensions of the known uses of these medications in phenotypically similar non–brain-injured psychiatric populations of patients with other types of brain injuries (e.g., stroke and multiple sclerosis), and the opinion of the authors of this chapter. We recognize that the pathophysiology of these symptoms may differ in patients with TBI, and, thus, generalization of response to treatment seen in the context of other forms of brain dysfunction (e.g., stroke and Alzheimer's disease) to TBI may not always be valid. Where there are treatment studies in the TBI population to offer guidance regarding medication treatments, these are noted and referenced for further consideration by interested readers.

Neurotransmitter Changes After TBI

Neuropsychiatric symptoms arising from penetrating or focal trauma, or both, are often understandable given the functions known to be subserved by the site of injury (e.g., behavioral disinhibition and aggression after bilateral orbitofrontal contusion), but the etiology of cognitive impairments after nonpenetrating (or "nonfocal") injuries is relatively less well understood. Cytotoxic processes such as calcium and magnesium dysregulation, free radical–induced injury, neurotransmitter (especially glutamate and cholinergic) excitotoxicity, and diffuse axonal injury because of straining and shearing biomechanical forces may be produced by nonpenetrating injuries (see Chapter 2, Neuropathology, and Chapter 39, Pharmacotherapy of Prevention, as well as McIntosh et al. 1999 and Halliday 1999 for review). These processes functionally and structurally disrupt the neural networks, subserving many critical neuropsychiatric functions (i.e., cognition, emotion, and behavior). Although TBI-induced glutamatergic disturbances are almost certainly important in the genesis of injury to areas critical to neuropsychiatric function (see Obrenovitch and Urenjak 1997 for review), there are at present no therapies available to directly ameliorate neuropsychiatric problems predicated on disturbances in this system. Several studies of neurochemical changes subsequent to TBI suggest that alterations in neurotransmitter production or delivery, or both, occur within these networks both acutely and chronically and may therefore play a role in the development of neuropsychiatric problems after TBI. These studies have shown that neurotransmitter systems, including norepinephrine, serotonin, dopamine, and acetylcholine, are altered by TBI, although the timing of such effects after TBI is important to consider. Multiple pharmacotherapies are available to modify the function of these neurotransmitter systems and the neuropsychiatric problems arising from disturbances within them.

In this chapter, we focus on TBI-induced neurotransmitter disturbances that are both related to neuropsychiatric functioning and amenable to modification using agents presently available. These two limits focus this portion of the discussion on disturbances in dopamine, norepinephrine, serotonin, and acetylcholine.

Catecholamines

Discrete lesions to ascending monoaminergic projections may interfere with the function of systems dependent on such afferent pathways (Morrison et al. 1979). Monoaminergic afferents course from the brainstem anteriorly, curving around the hypothalamus, the basal ganglia, and the frontal cortex, placing them in anatomical areas that are especially vulnerable to the effects of TBI.

Two studies found markedly elevated plasma norepinephrine levels after acute brain injury (Clifton et al. 1981; Hamill et al. 1987). However, most of the studies in this area suggest only that acute elevations of striatal dopamine are predictive of poor recovery from TBI (Donnemiller et al. 2000; Hamill et al. 1987; Woolf et al. 1987). Only the study of Tang et al. (1997) related alterations in dopamine function to cognitive performance, and their findings suggest that dopamine antagonism, but not agonism, may improve performance speed on the water maze task in experimentally injured mice. The observed pairing of striatal hyperdopaminergia with post-TBI memory deficits in mice is puzzling in light of the long-standing inference of reduced dopamine function after TBI in humans. It is noteworthy that this inference is drawn from the observation of cognitive benefits after augmentation of dopaminergic function in persons with TBI, an observation for which several hypotheses (e.g., correction of primary dopamine deficiency or correction of secondary dopamine dysfunction because of dysregulation in complementary neurotransmitter systems) may be generated. Few other experimental injury studies (Eghwrudjakpor et al. 1991; Kmeciak-Kolada et al. 1987; Tang et al. 1997) offer support for the hypothesis that cerebral catecholamine levels are chronically altered by TBI. No human studies have demonstrated a clear relationship between in vivo markers of dopaminergic function and long-term cognitive deficits in traumatically brain-injured humans. Thus, the extent of dopaminergic and noradrenergic dysfunction in the late period after TBI remains uncertain, and the implications of such findings with respect to long-term neuropsychiatric disturbances require further study. Nonetheless, the observation of cognitive improvements (e.g., arousal, speed of processing, attention, and, perhaps, memory) among some persons with TBIs during treatment with agents that increase dopaminergic neurotransmission suggests that dopamine dysfunction (primary, secondary, or both) may play an important role in the genesis of cognitive impairment after TBI.

Serotonin

Serotonergic projections to the frontal cortical areas are susceptible to biomechanical injury, and both diffuse axonal injury and contusions may produce dysfunction in this neurotransmitter system. Secondary neurotoxicity that is caused by excitotoxins and lipid peroxidation may also damage the neuronal systems that mediate serotonin

(Karakucuk et al. 1997) and perhaps also norepinephrine. Studies of serotonin activity after TBI are somewhat variable in their findings, although differences in the methodology (especially location of cerebrospinal fluid [CSF] sampling) appear to account for many of the differences in study findings. Pappius (1989) demonstrated widespread increases in hemispheric serotonin levels after experimentally induced brain injury in rats and noted that increases in serotonin appeared to produce decreases in cerebral glucose utilization. Busto et al. (1997) found a prompt increase in the extracellular levels of serotonin in cortical regions adjacent to the impact site in an experimental injury study in rats. Tsuiki et al. (1995) demonstrated in an experimental injury paradigm that serotonin synthesis was significantly increased in cortical areas throughout the injured hemisphere, and particularly in the dorsal hippocampus and area CA3, the medial geniculate, and the dorsal raphe, concurrent to a depression in cortical glucose use. Eghwrudjakpor et al. (1991) demonstrated a rapid increase in hemispheric concentration of serotonin, dopamine, and norepinephrine shortly after experimentally induced TBI in rats, with continued increases to three to four times control levels by 24–48 hours postinjury. These authors also reported significant regional differences in serotonin levels after experimental TBI, with increases in the hemispheres but decreases in the spinal cord.

This may offer some explanation for the discrepancy of findings related to CSF serotonin, norepinephrine, and dopamine metabolites after TBI in humans; namely, that the site from which samples are obtained may yield substantially different findings. Consistent with this experimental observation, Vecht et al. (1975) and Bareggi et al. (1975) found that lumbar CSF 5-hydroxyindoleacetic acid (5-HIAA) was below normal in conscious patients and normal in patients who were unconscious. Decreased CSF levels of serotonin were reported by Karakucuk et al. (1997) in 45 adults undergoing minor surgery with spinal anesthesia within 24 hours of TBI. However, Porta et al. (1975) demonstrated elevated ventricular CSF 5-HIAA levels in patients within days of severe TBI. Additionally, focal and diffuse lesions may result in differences with respect to monoaminergic alterations after TBI. For example, Van Woerkom et al. (1977) investigated patients with frontotemporal contusions and those with diffuse contusions. They documented decreased levels of 5-HIAA in patients with frontotemporal contusions but increased 5-HIAA levels in those with more diffuse contusions. In summary, the animal and human studies suggest acute increases in hemispheric serotonin levels after TBI and suggest that such increases are associated with decreased glucose utilization. Whether or to what extent similar changes persist into the late period after TBI remains uncertain, as does the role of such changes in the genesis of neuropsychiatric symptoms after TBI.

Acetylcholine

Findings from both basic and clinical neuroscience suggest both acute and long-term alterations in cortical cholinergic function develop after TBI. Multiple animal studies (Ciallella et al. 1998; DeAngelis et al. 1994; Dixon et al. 1994a, 1994b, 1997a, 1997b; Saija et al. 1988) demonstrate both acute and chronic alterations in hippocampal cholinergic function after experimentally induced TBI as well as a robust relationship between such alterations in cholinergic function and persistent cognitive impairments, including memory dysfunction. One of the most compelling demonstrations of relatively selective cholinergic injury after TBI is the report of Schmidt and Grady (1995). They induced a fluid-percussion brain injury sufficient to cause a 13- to 14-minute loss of righting reflex in rats anesthetized with halothane. Rats with experimentally induced midline injury had significant bilateral reductions in cholinergic neurons, including reductions in area Ch1 (medial septal nucleus; 36%), Ch2 (nucleus of the diagonal band of Broca; 44%), and Ch4 (nucleus basalis of Meynert; 41%). In animals with lateralized injuries, similarly severe losses of cholinergic neurons were observed ipsilaterally and lesser (11%–28%) losses were observed contralateral to the injury site. The authors noted that these losses did not extend to brainstem cholinergic nuclei (Ch5 and Ch6), and there were no observable effects on forebrain dopaminergic or noradrenergic innervation. These findings suggest that cholinergic losses may exceed those of other neurotransmitter afferents.

TBI appears to produce an acute increase in cholinergic neurotransmission followed by chronic reductions in neurotransmitter function and cholinergic afferents. Consistent with observations in experimental injury studies, Grossman et al. (1975) demonstrated that patients with TBI had elevated acetylcholine levels in fluid obtained from intraventricular catheters or lumbar puncture in the acute period after TBI. Dewar and Graham (1996) and Murdoch et al. (1998) demonstrated cortical cholinergic dysfunction (loss of cortical cholinergic afferents with concurrent preservation of postsynaptic muscarinic and nicotinic receptors) weeks after severe TBI. Arciniegas et al. (1999, 2000a, 2001), using the hippocampally mediated cholinergically dependent P50-evoked waveform response to paired auditory stimuli, demonstrated electrophysiological abnormalities consistent with reduced hippocampal cholinergic function in patients with

chronic symptoms of impaired auditory gating, attention, and memory in the late (longer than 1 year) period after TBI (see Chapter 7, Electrophysiological Techniques).

Pharmacological Treatment of Specific Neuropsychiatric Syndromes

Neuropsychiatric symptoms resulting from the neurotransmitter disturbances produced by TBI are amenable to treatment with a variety of medications. Where possible, selection of these medications should be guided by an understanding of the relationship between the neurochemistry most likely related to the symptom, the injury location in the patient with that symptom, or (preferably) both. In this section, we review the major neuropsychiatric symptoms and syndromes after TBI that may respond to medications. We also present recommendations for the use of psychotropic medications to treat these syndromes as well as review their significant side effects.

Emotional Disturbances

Emotional disturbances, including mood disorders and disorders of affect regulation, are common consequences of TBI and may be detrimental to a patient's rehabilitation and socialization (for reviews on these issues, see Arciniegas and Topkoff 2000; Arciniegas et al. 2000b; Hurley and Taber 2002; Silver et al. 1990, 1991). The literature regarding treatment of these conditions after TBI is limited when compared with that for phenotypically similar primary psychiatric disorders but is actively developing.

Depression

Depression after TBI can be responsive to psychopharmacologic treatment. Because of the safety profile, selective serotonin reuptake inhibitors (SSRIs) are the preferred medications. Cassidy (1989) conducted an open trial using fluoxetine for eight patients with severe TBI and associated depression. He found that two had marked improvement and three had moderate improvement. One-half of the patients experienced sedative side effects, and three out of the eight patients reported an increase in anxiety. Bessette and Peterson (1992) reported the case of a 41-year-old woman who experienced an episode of major depression after a mild brain injury and responded favorably to treatment with fluoxetine, 20 mg/day. Wroblewski et al. (1992a) reported a case in which improvement in depression after treatment with fluoxetine, 20 mg/day, after treatment with desipramine alleviated depressive symptoms but also precipitated posttraumatic seizures; however, this patient developed seizures while on fluoxetine as well, prompting the addition of phenytoin. It is difficult to reach conclusions regarding the safety (or efficacy) of a medication based on single case reports. Thus, we remain circumspect with regard to the potential for fluoxetine to lower significantly the seizure threshold among patients with posttraumatic epilepsy. Nonetheless, the published observation of precipitation of posttraumatic seizures with both of these generally well-tolerated agents suggests that the possibility of altering seizure threshold by their administration should not be dismissed offhandedly. Additionally, the observation supports the suggestion that this possibility should be discussed during the process of providing informed consent to treatment with these (or almost any) antidepressant agents in this population.

Fann et al. (2000) described improvement in depression secondary to mild TBI using sertraline (dose range, 25–200 mg by end of study) in an 8-week, nonrandomized, single-blind, placebo run-in trial conducted on 15 patients diagnosed with major depression between 3 and 24 months after a mild TBI. Thirteen (87%) had a decrease in Hamilton Rating Scale for Depression score of 50% or more ("response"), and 10 (67%) achieved a score of 7 ("remission") or less by treatment week 8. Significant improvements were also observed in ratings of psychological distress, anger and aggression, functioning, and postconcussive symptoms during treatment, and only one patient discontinued treatment because of side effects. In a subsequent report, Fann et al. (2001) described improvements in psychomotor speed, recent verbal memory, recent visual memory, and general cognitive efficiency as well as improvements in patient perception of cognitive symptoms as an effect of treatment of post-TBI depression with sertraline.

Turner-Stokes et al. (2002) performed an open-label trial of sertraline for depression after brain injuries, including TBI, in 21 adult patients. They reported clinical improvement as assessed by DSM-IV (American Psychiatric Association 1994) criteria in all of these patients. Among the 17 patients able to complete the Beck Depression Inventory before and after treatment, significant decreases in depressive symptoms were associated with treatment in this group. Of these, 11 had failed previous treatment with a different selective serotonin reuptake inhibitor.

However, Meythaler et al. (2001) performed a placebo-controlled trial of sertraline for arousal and attentional impairments in 11 subjects with severe TBI in the acute rehabilitation setting and failed to find a statistically significant treatment effect on these cognitive functions.

Horsfield et al. (2002) performed an 8-month open-label study of the effects of fluoxetine, 20–60 mg/day in five patients with TBI and varying levels of depression to determine whether this medication conferred mood and/or cognitive benefits. They observed improvements in mood as well as improvement on several measures of attention, processing speed, and working memory in this small group of patients. They suggested that fluoxetine's ability to stimulate expression of brain-derived neurotrophic factor and its specific tyrosine kinase receptor, which has in rodents been demonstrated to produce neuritic elongation and increased dendritic branching density of some hippocampal neurons, may explain the apparent benefits of this agent on posttraumatic cognitive impairments. Although their suggestion is intriguing, support for it in experimental injury models is lacking. For the present, it is simpler to interpret their findings as reflecting the well-known activating effects of fluoxetine.

Kant et al. (1998) reported that sertraline may also reduce irritability and aggression (as assessed using the Overt Aggression Scale—Modified for outpatients) and depressive symptoms (as assessed using the Beck Depression Inventory) after TBI at doses of 50 mg or greater. Notably, in this study, sertraline appeared to have a more robust effect on irritability and aggression than on depressive symptoms.

Although Khouzam and Donnelly (1998) reported a reduction in TBI-induced compulsive behavior in response to treatment with venlafaxine, there are at the time of this writing no reports offering support for the use of newer antidepressants such as venlafaxine or mirtazapine in the treatment of depression after TBI. Common clinical experience suggests that many of these agents may be useful in the treatment of depression after TBI, but their use must be undertaken knowing that there has been no published information in this population to assist clinicians in ascertaining the likelihood of benefit and the risk of adverse consequences. Because of the concern about hepatotoxicity with nefazodone, we would consider this medication only for individuals who have not been responsive or tolerant to other antidepressants.

When using the SSRIs, we would start at equivalent dosages of sertraline, 25 mg, or citalopram, 10 mg, and gradually increase the dose on a weekly basis (i.e., sertraline, 50 mg for 1 week, then 100 mg, or increase citalopram to 20 mg after 1 week). Usual antidepressant dosages may be required.

Tricyclic antidepressants (TCAs) may not be as effective a treatment for depression after TBI as for primary major depressive episodes, and they are associated with increased risks of adverse events in patients with TBI. Saran (1985) conducted a crossover study of phenelzine and amitriptyline administered at therapeutic doses to 10 patients with "minor brain injury" and 12 patients with major depression without TBI. All of the patients with major depression improved after 4 weeks of amitriptyline, but none of the TBI patients improved. Of note, however, the patients were reported to be the "melancholic" subtype, but they did not have significant weight loss or difficulty sleeping, which are typical symptoms of melancholic depression; therefore, the diagnostic categorization of these patients must be questioned. A subsequent study by Varney et al. (1987) found that 82% of 51 patients with major depressive disorder and TBI who received treatment with either TCAs or carbamazepine reported at least moderate relief of depressive symptoms. However, Dinan and Mobayed (1992) subsequently reported 85% of patients with major depressive disorder responded to amitriptyline, whereas only 31% of similarly depressed TBI patients responded to this treatment.

Nortriptyline and desipramine are used commonly in clinical practice, but there remains less evidence to guide their use and with which to assess the risks entailed by their use in persons with TBI than in other populations. Wroblewski et al. (1996) performed a modified, blinded, placebo lead-in treatment study of 10 patients with depression after severe TBI using desipramine and demonstrated improvement in six of seven patients (86%) able to complete the study. However, three patients (30%) discontinued the study, including one who developed seizures and one who developed mania during treatment. An additional patient experienced a seizure during treatment with desipramine but continued treatment with this medication nonetheless. In a study comparing nortriptyline versus fluoxetine in poststroke depression, nortriptyline was superior in efficacy to fluoxetine, and fluoxetine demonstrated no benefit above placebo (Robinson et al. 2000). Stroke is not pathophysiologically equivalent to TBI, and the studies comparing antidepressant efficacy may not be equally applicable to both populations. Both stroke and TBI may produce discrete white matter lesions that interrupt catecholaminergic or serotonergic pathways (source, projection, or target), and mood disorders after such injuries may result from dysfunction in these neurotransmitter systems. Many persons with TBI may not have discrete lesions to these systems but may instead experience diffuse axonal injuries; such injuries may modestly affect ascending catecholaminergic or serotonergic pathways and also glutmatergically dependent systems, cholinergic projections, and a host of other cortico-cortico or cortico-subcortical pathways and cortical and/or subcortical structures. Additionally, TBI, but not stroke, produces bihemispheric injury in this manner. Therefore, the neuroanatomical and neurochemical consequences of TBI may not be the same as those resulting from stroke. That being so, there is reason to predict and also to explain observed differences in treatment effects and side effects in these two populations. The published treatment data for these two populations suggest the possibility that there are differences in TCA efficacy in these two populations (more effective in stroke than in TBI) and also that there may be a greater risk of adverse effect in TBI patients.

If a heterocyclic antidepressant is chosen, we suggest nortriptyline (initial doses of 10 mg/day), or desipramine (initial doses of 25 mg/day), and a careful plasma monitoring to achieve plasma levels in the therapeutic range for the parent compound and its major metabolites (e.g., nortriptyline levels 50–150 ng/mL; desipramine levels greater than 125 ng/mL). Should the patient become sedated, confused, or severely hypotensive, the dosage of these drugs should be reduced.

Depressed mood because of TBI may respond to treatment with methylphenidate. Gualtieri and Evans (1988) reported significant improvement on ratings of mood and cognitive performance among 15 patients with TBI after treatment with methylphenidate using a double-blind, placebo-controlled crossover design study. Although these results were modest and suggestive of a possible role for methylphenidate in the treatment of the mood and cognitive disturbances after TBI, they have often been interpreted as strong evidence of a role for this medication in the treatment of neuropsychiatric sequelae of TBI. Although other studies offer support for the role of methylphenidate in the treatment of cognitive impairment after TBI (discussed in the section Cognitive Impairment), it is not clear if or for how long such benefits on either mood or cognition might be sustained by this treatment. Common clinical experience suggests that dextroamphetamine may be similar in its effects on mood and cognition after TBI, but no reports document a clear role for this medication in the treatment of depression after TBI.

Monoamine oxidase inhibitors (MAOIs) are not often used in persons with depression after TBI. This may reflect the high likelihood of difficulties with compliance to the complex dietary restrictions required during use of these medications given the cognitive impairments experienced by many TBI patients. Additionally, the literature offers little support for the effectiveness of these medications in the TBI population. In the studies by Saran (1985) and Dinan and Mobayed (1992) noted above, phenelzine was tried unsuccessfully in patients who had depression after TBI, even among those failing to respond to amitriptyline. Moclobemide, a selective MAO-A inhibitor, afforded improvement in 23 of 26 patients (88%) with depression after TBI (Newburn et al. 1999).

Because moclobemide does not affect the isoenzyme MAO-B, its use does not entail the dietary restrictions associated with other MAOIs. However, moclobemide is not available in the United States.

Electroconvulsive therapy (ECT) remains a highly effective and underused modality for the treatment of depression in general, and it appears to be an effective treatment of depression after acute TBI (Crow et al. 1996; Ruedrich et al. 1983; Zwil et al. 1992). Kant et al. (1999) reported on the safety and efficacy of ECT in patients with brain injury in a retrospective review of 11 patients hospitalized as a result of neuropsychiatric problems after TBI. Of these subjects, 9 experienced a major depression or other mood disorder because of TBI. All of the patients with neuropsychiatric problems because of TBI responded favorably to ECT, as assessed by the Montgomery-Åsberg Rating Scale for Depression and Global Assessment Scale, and did so without significant adverse cognitive or physical sequelae. Functional improvement occurred irrespective of baseline cognitive functioning or severity of injury. These studies suggest that ECT may be a safe treatment for chronic and severe neuropsychiatric disorders because of TBI. When ECT is used, we recommend treatment with the lowest possible energy levels that will generate a seizure of adequate duration (longer than 20 seconds), using pulsatile currents, increased spacing of treatments (2–5 days between treatments), and fewer treatments in an entire course (four to six). If the patient also has significant cognitive (especially memory) impairments because of TBI, nondominant unilateral ECT may be the preferable technique if this treatment is used in this population.

Adverse effects of antidepressants. The most common and disabling side effects of antidepressants in patients with neurological disorders are those associated with the anticholinergic properties of these medications, which can impair attention, concentration, and memory. For example, patients with Parkinson's disease have shown increased confusion when treated with anticholinergic medications (De Smet et al. 1982; Dubois et al. 1990). Experimental evidence in traumatically brain-injured rats supports this observation (Dixon et al. 1994b, 1995), as does common clinical experience in the treatment of patients with TBI. Such observations are consistent with the observed effects of both experimental and human TBI on cortical cholinergic function noted in the section Acetylcholine. The antidepressants amitriptyline, trimipramine, doxepin, and protriptyline have high affinities for the muscarinic receptors; given their strong anticholinergic properties, these medications should be prescribed only after careful consideration of alternative medications.

The choice of SSRI may require similar consideration; Schmitt et al. (2001) demonstrated that healthy middle-aged adults experienced significantly greater impairments of delayed recall in a word learning test during treatment with paroxetine, 20–40 mg/day, than during treatment with placebo, an effect attributed to paroxetine's nontrivial antimuscarinic properties. This study also demonstrated significant improvements in verbal fluency among healthy middle-aged adults treated with sertraline, 50–100 mg, when compared with treatment with placebo, an effect attributed to sertraline's dopamine reuptake inhibition. Whether similar differences in cognitive profiles distinguish between these and other SSRIs in the TBI population is not yet clear. Nonetheless, observations of distinct cognitive profiles among these agents may merit consideration when selecting an agent in this population.

Additionally, many antidepressants (e.g., doxepin, amitriptyline, trimipramine, imipramine, maprotiline, and trazodone) are highly sedating, resulting in significant problems of arousal in the TBI patient. Again, these medications should be prescribed only after careful consideration of other therapies.

TCAs may be associated with nontrivial rates of adverse events, particularly seizures. Wroblewski et al. (1990) reviewed the records of 68 patients with TBI who received antidepressant and, predominantly, TCA treatment for at least 3 months. The frequency of seizures was compared for the 3 months before treatment, during treatment, and after treatment. Seizures occurred among 6 patients during the baseline period, 16 during antidepressant treatment, and 4 after treatment was discontinued. Fourteen patients (20%) had seizures shortly after the initiation of treatment. For 12 of these patients, no seizures occurred after treatment with the antidepressant was discontinued. Importantly, 7 of these patients were receiving anticonvulsant medication before and during antidepressant treatment. Also, the occurrence of seizures was related to greater severity of brain injury. Wroblewski et al. (1992a) also observed seizures in a patient receiving fluoxetine for depression after TBI, suggesting that this medication, and perhaps other SSRIs, may be associated with an increased risk of seizures during antidepressant therapy after TBI. In addition to the TCAs, maprotiline and bupropion are often suggested to be associated with a higher incidence of seizures in otherwise healthy psychiatric patients (Davidson 1989; Pinder et al. 1977). Such suggestions prompt caution before prescribing these agents in patients with depression after TBI. However, Johnston et al. (1991), in a 102-site study of 1,986 patients treated with bupropion for depression, reported seizure rates of 0.24%–0.40%, and, among those receiving 300–450 mg/day, the cumulative rate of seizure was 0.36%.

This large data set suggests that bupropion may not be more likely to reduce seizure threshold than other antidepressants. Whether the same is true of bupropion's effects on seizure threshold after TBI is not clear at present, nor are there any data with which to assess the likelihood of similar problems during treatment with maprotiline in this population.

Among patients with established epilepsy, Ojemann et al. (1987) found that seizure control does not appear to worsen if psychotropic medication is introduced cautiously and if the patient is on an effective anticonvulsant regimen. There are, at present, no indications that treatment of depression in patients with posttraumatic epilepsy differs from that in patients with epilepsy of other etiologies. Although we conclude that antidepressants can be used safely and effectively in patients with TBI, including patients with posttraumatic epilepsy, we recommend that these agents be prescribed with caution and that treatment with them should include assiduous monitoring for adverse effects, including change in seizure frequency.

There are several important drug interactions that may occur among antidepressants and other drugs commonly prescribed for neurological conditions (Dubovsky 1992). Many antiparkinsonian drugs and neuroleptics have anticholinergic effects that are additive to those of the antidepressants. Antidepressant levels are likely to be decreased—often below therapeutic range—by the anticonvulsants phenytoin, carbamazepine, and phenobarbital. Similarly, antidepressants such as fluoxetine may raise the plasma levels of the anticonvulsants phenytoin (Jalil 1992), valproate (Sovner and Davis 1991), and carbamazepine (Grimsley et al. 1991). Carbamazepine induces the metabolism of sertraline. Therefore, patients receiving treatment with medications that require therapeutic blood level monitoring should have more frequent monitoring when antidepressants are administered. Although they may be highly efficacious drugs in patients with primary major depression, MAOIs should be less frequently prescribed for the treatment of depression in patients with TBI and particularly among those who are also taking other drugs that affect the central nervous system (CNS). For example, interactions with stimulants such as dextroamphetamine and with levodopa may result in lethal hypertensive reactions. (For a review of the safe use of MAOIs, see Marangell et al. 2003.)

Mania

Mania and bipolar disorder are less common consequences of TBI, although we believe they have been underdiagnosed in these individuals (see Chapter 10, Mood Disorders, and Hurley and Taber 2002 for review).

Several small case series suggest that lithium carbonate may be useful for the treatment of mania after TBI, although partial response, relapse of symptoms, or need for a second mood stabilizer is often observed (Bamrah and Johnson 1991; Parmalee and O'Shanick 1988; Starkstein et al. 1988, 1990; Stewart and Hemsath 1988; Zwil et al. 1993). Lithium has been reported to aggravate confusion in patients with brain damage (Schiff et al. 1982) and may relatively easily produce nausea, tremor, ataxia, and lethargy in persons with neurological disorders. In addition, lithium may lower seizure threshold (Massey and Folger 1984). Hornstein and Seliger (1989) reported a patient with preexisting bipolar disorder who experienced a recurrence of mania after closed head injury. This patient's mania, before injury, was controlled with lithium carbonate without side effects. However, subsequent to brain injury, dysfunctions of attention and concentration emerged that reversed when the lithium dosage was lowered. Because lithium carbonate may exacerbate cognitive impairments or cause confusion, especially in combination antidepressants, anticonvulsants, and antipsychotic medications, we suggest limiting the use of lithium in patients with TBI to those with mania or recurrent depressive illness that preceded their brain damage and who previously responded well to this treatment. Furthermore, and to minimize lithium-related side effects, we begin with low doses (300 mg/day). Patients with mania after TBI may respond to treatment with lithium despite relatively low blood levels (e.g., 0.2–0.5 mEq/L), highlighting the need for a "start low, go slow" approach to the care of these patients.

Manic episodes occurring after TBI may also respond to carbamazepine (Nizamie et al. 1988; Stewart and Hemsath 1988), although often only after addition of lithium (Stewart and Hemsath 1988) or antipsychotics (Sayal et al. 2000; Starkstein et al. 1988). For patients with mania subsequent to TBI, carbamazepine should be initiated at a dosage of 200 mg bid and adjusted to obtain plasma levels of 8–12 μg/mL. Because carbamazepine may produce or exacerbate cognitive impairments (Massagli 1991), monitoring for this effect when using this agent in patients with TBI is suggested. Brain damage appears to increase susceptibility to neurotoxicity induced by combination therapy with carbamazepine and lithium (Parmelee and O'Shanick 1988). As is true for patients without histories of TBI, clinicians should be aware of the potential risks associated with carbamazepine treatment, particularly bone marrow suppression (including aplastic anemia) and hepatotoxicity. Complete blood cell counts and liver function tests should be regularly monitored (Marangell et al. 1999). The most common signs of carbamazepine-induced neurotoxicity include lethargy, confusion, drowsiness, weakness, ataxia, nystagmus, and increased seizures. Pleak et al. (1988) described the development of mania, irritability, and aggression with carbamazepine treatment; however, in our experience, this reaction is unusual.

Pope et al. (1988) suggested that sodium valproate may be a useful mood stabilizer for patients with symptoms of bipolar disorder after TBI, and Monji et al. (1999) suggested that this benefit may extend to patients with rapid cycling mood disorders after TBI. In Monji et al.'s retrospective report, patients with such symptoms after TBI appeared to respond more robustly than those with similar symptoms in the absence of TBI (88% vs. 46%). The small sample sizes in this study do not permit extrapolation of this observation to TBI patients more generally, but are nonetheless encouraging of the use of this medication in the TBI population. As with carbamazepine, valproate may exacerbate cognitive impairments (Massagli 1991), and its use should include ongoing assessment of cognition in persons with TBI. Valproate is begun at a dosage of 250 mg bid and gradually increased to obtain plasma levels of 50–100 μg/mL. Tremor and weight gain are common side effects. Hepatotoxicity is rare and usually occurs in children who are treated with multiple anticonvulsants (Dreifuss et al. 1987).

For mania or manic-like syndromes after TBI that do not respond to conventional mood-stabilizing therapies, relatively more novel approaches may be useful to consider. Bakchine et al. (1989) described a manic-like state in a 44-year-old right-handed woman with bilateral orbitofrontal and right temporoparietal traumatic contusions that responded to clonidine after her behavior failed to respond to carbamazepine and worsened with levodopa. Dubovsky et al. (1987), Levy and Janicak (2000), and others have suggested that verapamil may be a useful agent for the treatment of mania alone or in combination with other mood stabilizers. To date, there are no studies of verapamil for the treatment of mania after TBI, but this agent might be worth considering when other conventional treatments fail or produce intolerable side effects. Clark and Davison (1987) also reported that ECT effected improvement in manic symptoms after nonpenetrating trauma, and the authors suggested that this therapy may be valuable to consider in such cases. Lamotrigine, oxcarbazepine, and gabapentin are other options, although evidence as to efficacy in individuals with TBI is not presently available.

Affective Dysregulation (Affective Lability and Pathological Crying/Laughing)

In contrast to mood disorders, conditions in which the baseline emotional state is pervasively disturbed over a relatively long period (i.e., weeks), disorders of affect denote conditions in which the more moment-to-moment variation and regulation of emotion is disturbed. The classic disorder of affective dysregulation is pathological laughing and/or crying (PLC), also sometimes referred to as *emotional incontinence* or *pseudobulbar affect*. Patients with this condition experience episodes of involuntary crying and/or laughing that may occur many times per day, often provoked by trivial (i.e., not sentimental) stimuli, are quite stereotyped in their presentation, are uncontrollable, do not evoke a concordant subjective affective experience, and do not produce a persistent change in the prevailing mood (Poeck 1985). In this classic presentation, PLC appears to be a relatively infrequent (5.3%) consequence of TBI (Zeilig et al. 1996). Affective lability differs from PLC in that both affective expression and experience are episodically dysregulated, the inciting stimulus may be relatively minor but is often somewhat sentimental, and the episodes are somewhat more amenable to voluntary control and are less stereotyped. However, these episodes do not produce a persistent change in mood and are often sources of significant distress and embarrassment to patients who otherwise (quite correctly) report their mood as "fine" (euthymic). The prevalence of affective lability after TBI is not clear, although Jorge and Robinson (2003) suggested a 1-year prevalence of approximately 12% among persons with TBI.

Although the neurobiology of mood and affect regulation overlap, the treatment of affective dysregulation in patients with brain injury overlaps but is not identical with the treatment of "uncomplicated" depression after TBI (Lauterbach and Schweri 1991; Panzer and Mellow 1992; Schiffer et al. 1985; Seliger et al. 1992; Sloan et al. 1992). The treatment literature overwhelmingly supports the use and effectiveness of relatively low doses (below typical antidepressant doses) of serotonergically and noradrenergically active antidepressants (Andersen et al. 1993; Lawson et al. 1969; Robinson et al. 1993; Schiffer et al. 1985) and to a lesser extent dopaminergic (Udaka et al. 1984) and noradrenergic (Evans et al. 1987; Sandyk and Gillman 1985) agents for the treatment of PLC and affective lability. Whether the lack of distinct therapies for these two disorders of affect reflects inseparable commonalities in their neurobiology or is instead an artifact of the diagnostic heterogeneity of patients included in the available treatment reports is unclear (Arciniegas and Topkoff 2000). It is noteworthy that the majority of treatment studies of these problems derives from the stroke, and not TBI, literature. Nonetheless, similar findings in multiple case series support the benefit of these agents for affective lability and PLC after TBI.

There are multiple reports of the beneficial effects of fluoxetine for "emotional incontinence" secondary to neurological disorders (Panzer and Mellow 1992; Seliger et al.

1992), including TBI (Nahas et al. 1998; Sloan et al. 1992). Brown et al. (1998) treated 20 patients with poststroke "emotionalism" (either PLC or affective lability) with fluoxetine in a double-blind placebo-controlled study. Those individuals receiving fluoxetine exhibited statistically and clinically significant improvement. In general, these investigators began treatment with 20 mg/day of fluoxetine, and patients often exhibited response within 5 days. We have had similar success with fluoxetine raised to higher doses (40–80 mg/day) and with sertraline, often starting and remaining at 25 mg/day and occasionally increasing gradually to 100 mg/day. A single-case report (Breen and Goldman 1997) and a small open-label trial (Muller et al. 1999) demonstrated reductions in affective lability during treatment with paroxetine; the latter of these two reports also compared the effectiveness of paroxetine and citalopram for the treatment of affective lability after brain injury and found both medications effective and citalopram somewhat better tolerated. Although only 2 of 26 patients included in the series described by Muller et al. (1999) were patients with TBI (the remainder being patients with strokes), both remained successfully treated for 1 year with paroxetine and relapsed after drug discontinuation. Andersen et al. (1999) also describe improvement in episodic crying after TBI in a 6-year-old child with citalopram, 2.5 mg daily. As is often seen in the treatment of affective lability, treatment response occurred within 2 days of beginning treatment, a response more rapid than that usually encountered in the treatment of depressed mood or major depressive episode.

TCAs may also be effective for affective lability and PLC. Allman (1992) described a marked decrease in pathological laughter in a patient treated with imipramine, 150 mg/day, with improvement occurring by the second week of treatment. Common clinical practice using TCA for PLC and affective lability after stroke (Robinson et al. 1993) suggests that nortriptyline may be of considerable benefit to patients with these conditions, and often at doses lower than those generally used to treat major depressive episodes. However, we emphasize that for many patients it may be necessary to administer these medications at standard antidepressant dosages to obtain full therapeutic effects, even when patients begin responding within days of initiating treatment at relatively low doses.

Although psychostimulants and dopaminergic agents are used most often for the treatment of cognitive impairments or diminished motivation, or both, after TBI, they may also offer some relief from affective lability during treatment of these other problems as well. Evans et al. (1987) reported reduced affective lability as well as cognitive improvements in a young man treated with methylphenidate or dextroamphetamine during a single-case, double-blind, placebo-controlled, dose-response study.

Gualtieri et al. (1989) described a sustained reduction of agitation and aggression, decreased distractibility, and improvement in affective stability among 19 of 30 TBI patients taking amantadine, 50 to 400 mg/day (average dose of 290 mg/day). Udaka et al. (1984) also reported reductions of PLC in response to amantadine or levodopa in approximately 50% of stroke or TBI patients. When patients present with affective lability or PLC in addition to cognitive and/or motivational impairments, methylphenidate, dextroamphetamine, amantadine, or levodopa may offer some relief from both sets of problems.

In the event that the first-line therapies (i.e., serotonergically and/or dopaminergically active agents) do not provide adequate relief from affective lability after TBI, particularly if affective lability is comorbid with posttraumatic aggression, treatment with mood-stabilizing agents may be necessary and of some benefit. Glenn et al. (1989) described an open-label trial of lithium carbonate for the treatment of affective instability and aggressive behavior in 10 patients (8 TBI and 2 stroke). The patients' symptoms included episodic aggressive or self-destructive behavior, "mood swings," tearfulness, and euphoria. Six of these patients demonstrated marked or moderate improvement in these target symptoms, one improved transiently, one failed to respond, and two patients worsened with this treatment. Three patients were on concomitant neuroleptic therapy and experienced neurotoxic side effects that prompted discontinuation of the lithium. Additionally, one patient experienced decreased attentiveness, and one patient experienced a seizure during this treatment. Lithium levels associated with clinical improvement ranged between 0.5 and 1.4 mEq/L.

Lewin and Sumners (1992) described a single case report of carbamazepine treatment of posttraumatic "episodic dyscontrol," a term used in their report to denote uncontrolled disproportionate episodic violence, depression, tearfulness, and irritability toward and intolerance of others. Treatment with carbamazepine, 200 mg/day, produced a good response, with no violent outbursts over the 12-month period of observation.

Both of these reports suggest possible benefit of mood-stabilizing agents for the treatment of some forms of affective lability after TBI, especially when mixed with irritability, aggression, or both. However, and as noted before, a cautious approach to dosing and continuous reassessment of benefit and adverse effects is needed in this population when using such agents.

Cognitive Impairment

Medication treatments for cognitive impairments after TBI follow one or both of two major neuropharmacolog-

TABLE 34–3. **Medications to treat impaired cognition and arousal**

Drug	Initial dose	Maximum dose
Methylphenidate	2.5 mg bid	20 mg tid
Dextroamphetamine	2.5 mg bid	20 mg tid
Amantadine	100 mg qam	200 mg bid
Bromocriptine	2.5 mg qam	20 mg tid
Sinemet (levodopa/carbidopa)	10/100 tid	25/250 qid
Modafinil	100 mg qam	200 mg bid
Donepezil	5 mg qd	10 mg qd

ical themes: dopaminergic augmentation or cholinergic augmentation. Because agents augmenting either of these neurotransmitter systems may improve several types of cognitive impairments (e.g., impaired attention, speed of processing, memory, and executive function), this section is organized by medication type rather than by type of cognitive impairment. The types of cognitive impairments responsive to each medication are discussed within these sections accordingly.

Methylphenidate and Related Psychostimulants

Psychostimulants, such as dextroamphetamine and methylphenidate, and dopaminergically active agents, such as amantadine and bromocriptine, may be useful for the treatment of diminished arousal, slowed speed of cognitive processing, attentional impairments, apathy, irritability, impulsivity, and fatigue after TBI (Table 34–3) (Evans et al. 1987; Glenn 1998; Kraus 1995; Lipper and Tuchman 1976; Marin et al. 1995; Weinstein and Wells 1981) and may afford such benefits in both the acute inpatient rehabilitation and also outpatient settings. Stimulants may also increase neuronal recovery after brain injury by a variety of dopaminergically mediated mechanisms (Crisostomo et al. 1988).

Stimulant medications act on central monoaminergic systems in a variety of complex and often reciprocally interactive ways. Methylphenidate and dextroamphetamine increase the release of dopamine and norepinephrine and, at higher doses, block the reuptake of these monoamines. These agents also appear to inhibit monoamine oxidase, which, in combination with these other effects, facilitates increased monoaminergic neurotransmission. The effect of such increases in the ascending reticular activating system, the striatum, and the several cortical-subcortical circuits in which these areas are involved appears to be an increase in arousal, speed of processing, and attention.

Kaelin et al. (1996) described the effect of methylphenidate, 15 mg twice daily, on the course of recovery in 11 patients with TBI during an acute inpatient rehabilitation setting. Using an A-A-B-A design, they demonstrated that methylphenidate significantly improved attention as measured by performance on digit span and symbol search tasks and was associated with improved Disability Rating Scale scores. Although one subject was withdrawn from the study because of tachycardia, methylphenidate was generally well tolerated. Plenger et al. (1996) demonstrated a significant effect of methylphenidate on attention, Disability Rating Scale scores, and motor performance during subacute recovery from TBI in a randomized, double-blind, placebo-controlled study. They found that attention and performance were significantly improved by treatment with methylphenidate at day 30, but were not different from placebo treatment at day 90. In this study, although methylphenidate treatment did not affect the ultimate level of recovery on these measures, it did improve the rate of recovery. Both studies suggest that methylphenidate may be used during the postacute recovery period after TBI to increase the rate of recovery, an effect that may facilitate increased involvement and compliance with acute rehabilitation and perhaps also permit earlier hospital discharge.

Similarly, Gualtieri and Evans (1988) reported significant improvement on ratings of mood and performance among 15 patients with TBI after treatment with methylphenidate using a double-blind, placebo-controlled, crossover design study. Although these results were modest and suggestive of a possible role for methylphenidate in the treatment of the neurobehavioral sequelae of TBI, they have often been interpreted as strong evidence for a role for this medication. However, in a similarly designed study performed several years later, Speech et al. (1993) found no effect of methylphenidate on attention, learning, processing speed, or social interaction in a group of 12 brain-injured patients treated a year or more after their injuries. More recently, Whyte et al. (1997) performed a randomized, double-blind, placebo-controlled, repeated crossover design study to assess the effect of methylphenidate on attention in TBI patients referred for treatment of attentional impairment. In this study, methylphenidate had no significant effect on any aspect of attention but did significantly improve speed of processing.

Dextroamphetamine is frequently used in the treatment of attention and memory impairment after TBI and is thought to have additional beneficial effects on depression, anergia, and impaired motivation. However, a thorough *MEDLINE*-based literature search undertaken at the time of this writing yielded only two reports to support its use in this population. The first report (Evans and Gualtieri 1987) described improvement in verbal memory and learning skills in response to treatment with either this agent or methylphenidate in a single adult male treated in the late postinjury period. The second report (Hornstein et al. 1996) reviewed the use of dextroamphetamine in the treatment of individuals during acute rehabilitation after TBI. Of the 27 patients so treated, 15 appeared to benefit from treatment with dextroamphetamine as measured by the Glasgow Outcome Scale.

Protriptyline, a secondary amine tricyclic agent, has also been suggested to have sufficient psychostimulant properties to permit its use for anergia and diminished motivation in TBI patients (Wroblewski et al. 1993). Reinhard et al. (1996) administered amitriptyline (one patient) and desipramine (two patients) and found improvement in arousal and initiation after TBI. They hypothesized that this effect resulted from the noradrenergic effects of the TCA. Showalter and Kimmel (2000) reported better-than-expected improvements in level of arousal in 9 of 13 severe (Rancho Los Amigos Scale I–III) TBI patients taking lamotrigine during the postacute recovery period (up to 10 months). They suggested that lamotrigine's ability to block sodium channels and inhibit glutamate release may prevent or facilitate recovery from injury; although not directly activating, lamotrigine may permit more rapid emergence from deeper stages of diminished arousal after TBI than might occur spontaneously. Pachet et al. (2003) also reported improvements in cognition and other neurobehavioral functions (as assessed by the Functional Independence Measure) in a single case study in a 40-year-old man with severe TBI treated with lamotrigine for approximately 4 months in the late (1.0–1.5 years) period after his injury. Additional studies are needed to ascertain the validity of this suggestion.

The published literature is quite variable with regard to the beneficial effects of psychostimulants on cognitive impairments after TBI. In light of the lack of in vivo evidence of long-term dopaminergic or noradrenergic dysfunction after TBI, the variability of benefit in the published reports is not surprising. At present, it appears that some patients may experience cognitive improvements during treatment with psychostimulants. To the extent that improved arousal or speed and efficiency of information processing can improve attention and memory, methylphenidate and related psychostimulants may be of benefit to some cognitively impaired TBI patients. However, additional studies are needed to clarify the role of these agents in the treatment of cognitive impairment after TBI before formal guidelines can be offered regarding their use.

Unlike most other medications, stimulants begin to take effect within a relatively short time (0.5–1.0 hour) and lose effect after a few hours. Thus, the goal is to first determine the effective dosage and then determine the frequency of dosing. Many individuals need repeat dosing every 3–4 hours. We suggest using an initial dosage of methylphenidate, 5 mg, or dextroamphetamine, 5 mg. There are now available multiple formulations of longer acting methylphenidate or dextroamphetamine preparations (such as Adderall, Concerta, and Metadate). Although no studies have been conducted on these formulations, some individuals may experience longer duration of response.

In clinical practice, careful assessment of arousal, speed of processing, and attention should be undertaken before and serially during treatment with these agents. Although such assessments may be difficult (Whyte 1992), they are important to perform to determine whether these medications impart sufficient benefit to merit their continued use in a given patient. Assessment with appropriate neuropsychological tests may be particularly helpful in determining response to treatment with these agents.

Other Dopaminergically Active Agents

Lal et al. (1988) reported on the use of levodopa/carbidopa (Sinemet) in the treatment of 12 patients with brain injury (including anoxic damage). Levodopa is a dopamine precursor that, when coupled with carbidopa to decrease the extent of its metabolism in the periphery, increases dopamine levels in the CNS. With treatment, patients exhibited 1) improved alertness and concentration; 2) decreased fatigue, hypomania, and sialorrhea; and 3) improved memory, mobility, posture, and speech. Dosage administered was 10/100 mg to 25/250 mg qid.

Bromocriptine is sometimes used as a psychostimulant in light of its effects on dopamine function when used at higher doses. At such doses, it appears to act directly on postsynaptic dopamine receptors—particularly dopamine type 2 (D_2) receptors—and serves as an agonist in dopaminergically mediated systems. At low doses, bromocriptine acts as a presynaptic D_2 agonist and thereby reduces dopaminergic release and function in dopaminergically mediated systems. Its net effect at midrange doses appears to be that of dopamine agonism (Berg et al. 1987). Eames (1989) suggested that bromocriptine may be useful in treating cognitive initiation problems of brain injury patients who are at least 1 year subsequent to injury. He recommended starting at 2.5 mg/day with treatment for at least 2 months at the highest dose tolerated (up to 100 mg/day). Other investigators found that patients with nonfluent aphasia (Gupta and Mlcoch 1992), akinetic mutism (Echiverri et al. 1988), and apathy (Catsman-Berrevoets and Harskamp 1988) improved after treatment with bromocriptine. Parks et al. (1992) suggested that bromocriptine exerts specific effects on the frontal lobe, thus increasing goal-directed behaviors. In the largest study of bromocriptine in this population, McDowell et al. (1998) studied 24 subjects using a counterbalanced, double-blind, placebo-controlled crossover design. Bromocriptine improved performance on some frontally mediated tasks such as executive function and dual-task performance but did not improve working memory. No other effects on cognition were demonstrated. Unlike the other psychostimulants, bromocriptine has not been demonstrated to have a consistent effect on affective lability or mood disorders because of TBI.

Amantadine may be beneficial in the treatment of anergia, abulia, mutism, and anhedonia subsequent to brain injury (Chandler et al. 1988; Gualtieri et al. 1989; Nickels et al. 1994; Van Reekum et al. 1995). Kraus and Maki (1997) administered amantadine, 400 mg/day, to six patients with TBI. Improvement was found in motivation, attention and alertness, as well as executive function. These authors also reported that amantadine reduced impulsivity and emotional (affective) lability. The mechanism of action of amantadine is not entirely clear but may involve increased dopamine release, decreased presynaptic dopamine reuptake, stimulation of the dopamine receptors, and/or enhancement of postsynaptic dopamine receptor sensitivity. In addition, amantadine is an *N*-methyl-D-aspartate glutamate receptor antagonist (Weller and Kornhuber 1992). As such, amantadine may inhibit *N*-methyl-D-aspartate receptor–mediated stimulation of striatal acetylcholine release. Although amantadine does not possess direct anticholinergic activity per se at conventional therapeutic doses, it is not uncommon for patients treated with this agent to develop anticholinergic-like symptoms. Amantadine is often started at a dose of 50 mg bid and increased every week by 100 mg/day to either symptomatic improvement or medication intolerance. In our experience, amantadine, 100 mg twice daily, is often sufficient to impart maximal benefit without undue side effects. When higher doses are necessary, the maximum dosage of amantadine should not exceed 400 mg/day.

Adverse effects of psychostimulants and dopaminergic agents. Adverse reactions to psychostimulants and dopaminergic agents are most often related to increases in dopamine activity. Dextroamphetamine and methylphenidate have the potential to produce paranoia, dysphoria, agitation, and irritability, although these adverse effects are in practice uncommon at the doses typically used to treat cognitive impairment after TBI. Side effects of bromocriptine include sedation, nausea, psychosis, headaches, and delirium. Amantadine may cause confusion, hallucinations, edema, and hypotension; these reactions occur more often in elderly patients than in younger patients. Because depressed mood and increased fatigue may develop after dis-

continuation of psychostimulants and other activating agents, these medications should be discontinued gradually.

Clinicians are sometimes reluctant to make use of psychostimulants out of concern that they might lower seizure threshold in patients with TBI, because at least a subgroup of this population appears to be at increased risk for posttraumatic seizures (see Chapter 16, Seizures). Wroblewski et al. (1992b) examined changes in seizure frequency after initiation of methylphenidate among 30 patients with both severe brain injury and posttraumatic seizures. The seizure frequency was monitored for 3 months before treatment with methylphenidate, 3 months during treatment, and 3 months after treatment was discontinued. They found that whereas only 4 patients experienced more seizures during methylphenidate treatment, 26 had either fewer or the same number of seizures during treatment. Although many patients in this study were treated concomitantly with anticonvulsant medications that may have conferred some protection against the development of seizures, 13 patients nonetheless experienced fewer seizures when treated with methylphenidate. The authors of this study concluded that there was no increased risk of lowering seizure threshold during methylphenidate treatment even in this group of TBI patients at high risk for seizures.

Similarly, in a double-blind, placebo-controlled study of the effects of methylphenidate (0.3 mg/kg body weight bid) in 10 children with well-controlled seizures and attention-deficit disorder, no seizures occurred during the 4 weeks of treatment with either active drug or placebo (Feldman et al. 1989). Dextroamphetamine has been used adjunctively in the treatment of refractory seizures (Livingston and Pauli 1975), and bromocriptine may also have some anticonvulsant properties (Rothman et al. 1990). It seems, therefore, that this class of medications is generally well tolerated with respect to its effects on seizure frequency and may in some patients be associated with reduced seizure frequency. One exception to this generality is amantadine, which may lower seizure threshold (Gualtieri et al. 1989); we also have observed several patients who had not experienced seizures for months before the administration of amantadine but who had a seizure within weeks after its prescription. Although amantadine may be of benefit for diminished arousal, attention, and executive function for some TBI patients, caution is indicated in patients with a history of pre- or posttraumatic epilepsy or among patients at high risk for this latter condition (see Chapter 16, Seizures, for a discussion of risk factors for posttraumatic epilepsy).

Cholinesterase Inhibitors

Cognitive impairments after TBI may, at least in part, result from disruption of cholinergic function (Arciniegas et al. 1999; Whitlock 1999). As noted in the section Acetylcholine, both animal and human studies support this suggestion. Additionally, the susceptibility of TBI patients to exacerbation of cognitive impairments during treatment with anticholinergic medications also suggests that these patients may have a relatively reduced reserve of cholinergic function. Several reports describe cognitive improvements after administration of physostigmine, both in the acute (Bogndanovitch et al. 1975) and post-acute (Eames and Sutton 1995; Goldberg et al. 1982) injury period. Levin et al. (1986) performed a double-blind, placebo-controlled study of combined oral physostigmine and lecithin in 16 patients with cognitive impairment after moderate to severe TBI. Sustained attention on the continuous performance test was more efficient under physostigmine than placebo, and lecithin did not appear to increase this effect. Cardenas et al. (1994), in a double-blind, placebo-controlled, crossover design study of physostigmine, placebo, and scopolamine (a cholinergic antagonist) in 36 males with memory impairment of at least 3 months' duration after TBI demonstrated improved memory scores on the long-term storage component of the Selective Reminding Test in 44% of subjects during treatment with oral physostigmine but not placebo or scopolamine. Although physostigmine may be of benefit to cognitively impaired TBI survivors, the systemic toxicity associated with this medication limits its acceptability as a treatment in this population; we do not recommend using physostigmine for the treatment of cognitive impairment after TBI.

The second-generation cholinesterase inhibitors (e.g., tacrine, donepezil, rivastigmine, and galantamine) may be similarly useful, but donepezil is the only agent for which there are published reports supporting use in the TBI population. Taverni et al. (1998) described improvements in refractory memory impairments on the Rivermead Behavioral Memory Test and Ross Immediate Processing Assessment in the late postinjury period in two traumatically brain-injured patients; these benefits were apparent after approximately 3 weeks of treatment with donepezil, 5 mg/day. Whelan et al. (2000) performed an open-label study of donepezil in 53 outpatients receiving care for long-term cognitive and neuropsychiatric problems after TBI. Patients treated with donepezil, 5–10 mg daily, for an average of 12 months were rated by clinicians as improved. A subset (22) of these patients were assessed with the Wechsler Adult Intelligence Scale—Revised and demonstrated improvements in full-scale IQ. Although these improvements occurred well after the period during which spontaneous recovery and "practice effects" might offer better explanations for them, the design of the study offers only suggestion of benefit with this treatment. Masanic et al. (2001) described significant improvements

in learning and short- and long-term recall on the Rey Auditory Verbal Learning Test and the complex figure test, and a trend toward improvements in behavior as assessed using the Neuropsychiatric Inventory, in four patients treated with donepezil, 5–10 mg daily.

Kaye et al. (2003) performed an 8-week, open-label study of 10 persons with remote (1–5 years; mean=1.2 years) TBI in an outpatient setting using a forced titration protocol of donepezil (5 mg/day for 4 weeks followed by 10 mg/day for 4 weeks). Subjects ranged in age from 26 to 60 years (mean age=41 years), and included six with mild, one with moderate, and three with severe TBI. Eight subjects completed the study; one subject was dropped from the study due to treatment noncompliance, and one subject discontinued treatment due to intolerable gastrointestinal side effects. Among those completing the study, ratings of Clinical Global Impression improved, although not necessarily as a function of improvements in memory. The authors reported that Clinical Global Impression improvements instead appeared to reflect the subject reports of improvements in "focus, attention, and clarity of thought." They noted that several subjects reported being better able "to keep multiple ideas in mind simultaneously," and that subjects' family members frequently described "improved socialization."

Morey et al. (2003) studied the effectiveness of donepezil for the treatment of chronic memory impairments in a group of seven patients with TBI. Subjects were on average 33 months postinjury (range=20–65 months) and mean age was 31 years (range=19–51 years). All subjects were without other medical, psychiatric, or physical problems that could have interfered with ability to participate in neuropsychological assessment, and none was taking medications with anticholinergic properties. Measures of cognitive function included the Brief Visual Memory Test—Revised, Hopkins Verbal Learning Test, Digit Span, and Letter-Number Sequence subtests of the Wechsler Adult Intelligence Scale—Revised, Controlled Oral Word Association Test, and the Memory Functioning Questionnaire, all of which were administered pre- and posttreatment during the two treatment phases of the study. These phases included donepezil, 5 mg daily for 1 month, followed by donepezil, 10 mg daily for an additional 5 months; after a 6-week washout period, patients were treated for an additional 6 months with donepezil, 5 mg daily. Treatment-emergent side effects (lethargy and somnolence) were observed in two subjects, prompting their removal from the study. Improvements in immediate and delayed memory as assessed by the Brief Visual Memory Test—Revised were reported as a function of treatment with donepezil, 10 mg/day, but not 5 mg/day. No other significant effects on cognition were observed during treatment with donepezil at either dose.

More recently, Zhang et al. (2004) reported findings from a 24-week, randomized, placebo-controlled, double-blind crossover trial of donepezil, 10 mg daily, in 18 subjects with TBI seen in two university-based hospitals. They had impairment on tests of attention or short-term memory and could not have a number of co-occurring conditions, including depression and epilepsy, or be treated with psychotropic medications. Donepezil and placebo were given in a randomized, double-blind, placebo-controlled crossover study, with 10 weeks on one treatment, a 4-week washout, and crossover to 10 weeks on the second treatment phase. When compared with baseline scores on the Wechsler Memory Scale Auditory and Visual Immediate Indices and the Paced Auditory Serial Addition Task, significant improvement was seen after treatment with donepezil. For those individuals who received donepezil first, no deterioration was seen after the 4-week washout and 10 weeks of placebo. This controlled trial in a subacute TBI population (average, 4–5 months post-TBI), demonstrated efficacy of donepezil. Limitations impair generalization to broader clinical populations because these individuals did not have co-occurring psychiatric disorders (which are very common) or were receiving other psychotropic medications. Whether this improvement would apply for those with a more remote history of TBI was not studied. The presence of a possible carryover effect is intriguing. Certainly, this at least is a caution for crossover studies and suggests that short-term treatment may have prolonged effects. Nonetheless, this study offers reasonably strong evidence that donepezil improves attention and memory impairments in the postacute injury period.

Although individuals with TBI may have difficulty maintaining attention on single tasks, many also experience difficulty mounting robust selective attention in the face of multiple competing stimuli (Arciniegas et al. 1999). This latter problem is referred to as *impaired sensory gating*, and it is experienced by so-affected individuals as difficulty focusing on any of several competing stimuli such that the stimuli become "blurred together" and "overwhelming." Many of these patients endorse the experience of impaired sensory gating as analogous to listening to a radio receiving two stations on the same frequency such that one is aware that there are two sources of information but is unable to clearly discern the content of one from the other. Impaired auditory gating can be distinguished clinically from distractibility, which refers to difficulty with sustained (but not selective) attention that results in brief but robust shifting of attention between competing stimuli. Impaired auditory gating is associated with abnormal middle latency (50 milliseconds) electrophysiological responses to closely paired (500-millisecond interstimulus interval) auditory stimuli, and this abnormal response is referred to as *P50*

nonsuppression (Arciniegas et al. 1999, 2000a; see Chapter 4). Importantly, distractibility (as may be seen in adults with attention-deficit/hyperactivity disorder) is associated with normal P50 suppression (Olincy et al. 2000), suggesting that the experience of impaired sensory gating reflects a physiological process distinct from that underlying distractibility. Arciniegas et al. (2002) reported normalization of P50 physiology during treatment with donepezil, 5 mg/day, in 10 patients with impaired auditory sensory gating in the late period after TBI in a randomized, double-blind, placebo-controlled, crossover design study. Notably, subjects in this study did not maintain normalized P50 physiology during treatment with donepezil, 10 mg/day, or either placebo condition, suggesting that there may be a therapeutic window for response of impaired sensory gating using cholinesterase inhibitors. This and the previously noted studies suggest that there may be a role for cholinesterase inhibitors in the treatment of impaired memory and impaired sensory gating after TBI.

Cytidine 5'-Diphosphocholine

Cytidine 5'-diphosphocholine (CDP-choline or citicoline) is an essential intermediate in the biosynthetic pathway of phospholipids incorporated into cell membranes that appears to activate the biosynthesis of structural phospholipids in neuronal membranes, increase cerebral metabolism, and enhance activity of dopamine, norepinephrine, and acetylcholine (Dixon et al. 1997a; Secades and Frontera 1995). A single-blind, randomized study of 216 patients with severe or moderate TBI demonstrated improved motor, cognitive, and psychiatric function during treatment with CDP-choline, and this treatment decreased length of stay in the hospital (Calatayud et al. 1991). Levin (1991) performed a double-blind, placebo-controlled study of 14 patients to evaluate the efficacy of CDP-choline (1 g/day) for the treatment of postconcussional symptoms in the first month after mild to moderate TBI. This treatment reduced the severity of postconcussional symptoms and improved recognition memory for designs but did not influence other aspects of neuropsychological performance. CDP-choline is available only as an over-the-counter agent; because content, purity, and effective dose may be difficult to predict in present formulations, patients electing to undertake treatment with CDP-choline should be cautioned about these potential problems and monitored carefully for both benefit and adverse reactions during its use.

Apathy

States of diminished motivation, or apathy, are common consequences of TBI (see Chapter 18, Disorders of Diminished Motivation). Diminished motivation or apathy denotes a neuropsychiatric syndrome in which there is a clinically significant decrease in goal-directed cognition, emotion, and/or behavior. Apathetic states occur on a continuum of severity, with states of mildly diminished motivation at one end of that continuum and akinetic mutism at the other end. Determining whether an individual patient's apathy is a symptom of another neuropsychiatric condition such as depression or is instead an independent syndrome is imperative before undertaking treatment. When apathy is a feature of depression, treatment of the underlying depression with agents such as the SSRIs may relieve both mood and apathy symptoms. However, when apathy occurs as an independent problem, the SSRIs are unlikely to improve the apathy and may actually worsen this problem. Complicating matters, apathy not uncommonly co-occurs with behavioral dyscontrol (i.e., disinhibition, impulsivity, and aggression). This seemingly odd combination of behavioral problems may occur in the setting of injury to both the anterior cingulate-subcortical circuits (resulting in apathy) and lateral orbitofrontal-subcortical circuits (resulting in a behavioral dyscontrol syndrome). In such circumstances, patients appear apathetic at baseline and demonstrate episodic behavioral dyscontrol when an environmental or somatic stimulus produces automatic (and often aggressive or appetitive) behaviors. This combination of apathy and behavioral dyscontrol presents substantial challenges to clinicians attempting to treat such problems because the therapies to improve apathy may worsen behavioral dyscontrol and the therapies for behavioral dyscontrol may worsen apathy. If clinicians select apathy as the target of treatment, psychostimulants and other dopaminergically active medications are the principal pharmacotherapies. Because these drugs are also used for the treatment of cognitive dysfunction, the reader is referred to the section Cognitive Impairment for guidelines on use.

Fatigue

Stimulants (methylphenidate and dextroamphetamine) and amantadine can diminish the profound daytime fatigue experienced by patients with TBI. Dosages utilized would be similar to those used for treatment of diminished arousal and concentration. These medications may be of particular benefit in patients with apparent depression after TBI in whom fatigue persists despite improvement in mood during treatment with antidepressants.

Modafinil, a medication recently approved for the treatment of excessive daytime somnolence in patients with narcolepsy, also may have a role in treatment of post-TBI fatigue. Although the exact mechanism of action of modafinil is not known, animal studies suggest that its promotion of wakefulness may result from an indirect, dose-dependent reduction of the release of γ-aminobutyric acid (GABA) in the cerebral cortex, medial preoptic area, and posterior hypothalamus (Ferraro et al. 1996, 1997b); activation of hypocretin (Orexin) neurons in the lateral hypothalamus (Chemelli et al. 1999); and dose-dependent increases in glutamate release in the ventrolateral and the ventromedial thalamus (Ferraro et al. 1997a). Some combination of these mechanisms in humans may increase arousal via activation in regions critical to this purpose, either directly via glutamatergic thalamic activation, indirectly via reduction of GABA function, or through the secondary effects of lateral hypothalamic projections to regions involved in control of arousal and the sleep-wake cycle (the tuberomammillary nucleus and the locus ceruleus) (Lin et al. 1999).

Studies of the effect of modafinil on fatigue and excessive sleepiness in patients with multiple sclerosis (Rammohan et al. 2002; Zifko et al. 2002) and Parkinson's disease (Nieves and Lang 2002) suggest benefit. Elovic (2000) has suggested that modafinil may be of similar benefit in patients with TBI. Teitelman (2001) described his use of modafinil among 10 outpatients with nonpenetrating TBI and functionally significant excessive daytime sleepiness and in two patients with somnolence because of sedating psychiatric medications. The patients included in his report were between the ages of 42 and 72 years, all were outpatients, and were treated in an open-label fashion. Doses of modafinil ranged between 100 mg and 400 mg taken once each morning. Nine of these patients reported marked improvements in excessive daytime sleepiness, and three reported moderate improvements. Some patients reported subjective improvements in attention as well as other cognitive benefits. Although this medication was generally well tolerated, Teitelman also described treatment intolerance because of increased "emotional instability" in two women with brain injury complicated by multiple other medical conditions and receiving multiple additional medications. At the time of this writing, there are no published clinical studies with which to evaluate the effectiveness or tolerability of modafinil for posttraumatic hypersomnolence or fatigue. If modafinil is used in this population, dosages should start with 100 mg in the morning and can be increased to up to 400 mg/day administered in either a single daily dose or two divided doses (i.e., 200 mg in the morning and 200 mg in the afternoon). Higher doses (up to 600 mg/day) are sometimes used, but there is no evidence in any patient population that such doses offer benefit beyond that achieved with 400 mg/day.

Coldness

Complaints of feeling cold, without actual alteration in body temperature, are occasionally seen in patients who have experienced brain injury. This feeling can be distressing to those who experience it. Patients may wear excessive amounts of clothing and adjust the thermostat so that other members of the family are uncomfortable. Although this is not a commonly reported symptom of TBI, Hibbard et al. (1998) have found that in a sample of 331 individuals with TBI, 27.9% complained of changes in body temperature and 13% persistently felt cold. Eames (1997), while conducting a study of the cognitive effects of vasopressin (DDAVP) nasal spray in patients with TBI, reported incidentally that 13 patients had the persistent feeling of coldness, despite normal sublingual temperature. All were treated with nasal DDAVP spray for 1 month. Eleven of these patients stopped complaining of feeling cold after 1 month of treatment, and one other patient had improvement in the symptom, without complete relief.

Silver and Anderson (1999) performed a pilot study of the effects of intranasal DDAVP twice daily for 1 month among six patients who complained of persisting coldness after brain injury. Five of the six patients had a dramatic response to DDAVP—some as soon as 1 week after initiating treatment—and no longer complained of feeling cold. This response persisted even after discontinuation of treatment. Patients denied any side effects from treatment with this agent. The authors of this study suggested that DDAVP may reverse physiological effects of a relative deficit in DDAVP in the hypothalamus caused by injury to the DDAVP precursor, producing cells in the anterior hypothalamus, and may thereby correct an internal temperature set-point disrupted by the brain injury.

Psychosis

Antipsychotic and Neuroleptic Medications

Typical antipsychotic medications are used commonly to control agitation and psychosis after TBI but are not benign treatments in this population. Side effects such as hypotension, sedation, and confusion are common. Patients with brain injury are particularly subject to dystonias, akathisias, and other parkinsonian side effects—even when relatively low doses of antipsychotic medications are prescribed (Wolf et al. 1989). Stanislav (1997) demonstrated improvement in cognitive performance in brain-injured patients after discontinuation of antipsychotic medications, the magnitude of which appeared to be greater after discontinuation of thioridazine (Mellaril) than of haloperidol (Haldol). Although both medications appeared to negatively affect cognitive performance, Stanislav suggested that the greater improvement observed after discontinuation of thioridazine is attributable to the brain-injured patients' reduced tolerance to the anticholinergic properties of this agent. Similarly, Sandel et al. (1993) observed new-onset delusions in a TBI patient receiving chlorpromazine for the treatment of agitation after

TBI, an effect that may also be attributable to the significant anticholinergic properties of this agent. Antipsychotic medications have also been reported to delay neuronal recovery after brain injury (Feeney et al. 1982). Consistent with this observation, Rao et al. (1985) found that patients treated with haloperidol in the acute period after TBI experienced significantly longer periods of posttraumatic amnesia, although the acute rehabilitation outcome did not differ from those not treated with this medication. Consistent with their greater sensitivity to medications affecting the CNS, patients with brain injury are more sensitive to the development of extrapyramidal side effects during treatment with typical antipsychotic medications (Rosebush and Stewart 1989; Vincent et al. 1986; Wolf et al. 1989; Yassa et al. 1984a, 1984b).

Given this literature and the availability of several atypical antipsychotic medications, we strongly discourage the use of typical and, particularly, the low-potency typical antipsychotic medications among persons with TBI. However, there is at present a dearth of reports to guide selection among the atypical antipsychotic agents in this population. Michals et al. (1993) used clozapine (Clozaril) to treat nine brain-injured patients with psychotic symptoms or outbursts of rage and aggression that had failed to respond to other medications. Three of these patients demonstrated marked improvements in aggression and/or psychosis, three demonstrated decreased agitation and auditory hallucinations, and an adequate duration of treatment was not achieved in three patients. Two of the nine patients experienced seizures during treatment. Burke et al. (1999) also reported improvement in refractory psychotic symptoms after TBI during treatment with clozapine. These reports suggest that clozapine may be useful in the treatment of psychosis and aggressive behavior after brain injury, but this treatment carries a relatively high risk of adverse effects, including seizures. Whether clozapine may also exacerbate cognitive impairments given its substantial anticholinergic properties is not clear but seems likely in light of the effects of other low-potency antipsychotic agents.

Schreiber et al. (1998) reported a case in which risperidone (Risperdal) treated delusions and sleep disturbance after TBI effectively. One of us (D.A.) has used this medication in two patients who developed psychosis (paranoid delusions, auditory hallucinations) after TBI in the acute rehabilitation setting. Each patient responded with decreasing psychotic symptoms with risperidone, 4 mg/day, and without significant adverse effect. The second of these patients was treated in an A-B-A-B fashion, and psychosis recurred during each reduction of risperidone below 3 mg/day. There are, to date, no studies reporting improvement in psychosis after TBI during treatment with olanzapine, quetiapine, aripiprazole (Abilify), or ziprasidone.

Each of these medications may be of benefit in this population, but specific benefits and side-effect profiles relevant to their use in TBI remain to be determined.

Special Consideration in the Use of Antipsychotic Agents

Neuroleptic malignant syndrome is a potentially life-threatening disorder that may emerge after the use of any antipsychotic agent and has been reported among patients receiving haloperidol after TBI (Vincent et al. 1986; Wilkinson et al. 1999). Patients experiencing neuroleptic malignant syndrome become severely rigid and occasionally catatonic. Fever, elevated white blood cell count, tachycardia, abnormal blood pressure fluctuations, tachypnea, and diaphoresis occur. Although medications such as bromocriptine and dantrolene sodium have been suggested to treat neuroleptic malignant syndrome, the most important therapeutic interventions are discontinuation of antipsychotic medications, treatment of any underlying infections or other concurrent medical illnesses, and symptomatic treatment of fever and hypertension (Rosebush et al. 1991).

Many psychotropic medications affect seizure threshold. This is of particular concern in this population given the risk of posttraumatic seizures after TBI. Among all the first-generation antipsychotic drugs, molindone and fluphenazine have consistently demonstrated the lowest potential for lowering the seizure threshold (Marangell et al. 1999; Oliver et al. 1982). Clozapine treatment is associated with a significant dose-related incidence of seizures (ranging from 1% to 2% of patients who receive doses below 300 mg/day, and 5% of patients who receive 600–900 mg/day) (Lieberman et al. 1989). The observations of Michals et al. (1993) suggest that this risk may be increased in patients with TBI; if this agent is prescribed at all in these patients, its use should be undertaken with extreme caution and only for the relief of refractory psychotic symptoms.

Anxiety Disorders and Posttraumatic Stress Disorder

Because of the side effects and danger of dependence associated with benzodiazepine use, we generally prefer to treat complaints of anxiety in brain injury patients with supportive psychotherapy and social interventions. TBI is highly associated with alcoholism and drug dependency (see Chapter 29, Alcohol and Drug Disorders), which further increases our caution in prescribing benzodiazepines for these patients. However, when the symptoms are so severe that they require pharmacological intervention, treatment with SSRIs, buspirone, or benzodiazepines may be considered.

Benzodiazepines may produce sedation and impair memory and motor function. In some instances, sedation may be the desired effect of benzodiazepines, but this side effect poses risk for further impairing the patient's cognitive and physical functioning. These drugs can produce amnesia (Angus and Romney 1984; Lucki et al. 1986; Roth et al. 1980) and will worsen preexisting memory difficulties. Problems with balance, ataxia, and coordination that occur subsequent to brain injury are likely to be exacerbated by benzodiazepines. Walburga et al. (1992) examined the effects of anxiolytic medications (buspirone and diazepam) on driving performance of outpatients with generalized anxiety disorder who had no neurological impairment. Each week, the subjects were tested for driving ability by a 100-kilometer on-the-road driving test. The diazepam-treated group showed significantly impaired performance in the first, second, and third weeks. No impairment was detected in the subjects who received buspirone. Importantly, these effects were demonstrated in subjects without neuropsychiatric impairments before the study. The likelihood of similar or worse effects among TBI patients is not trivial and poses serious concerns with respect to the effect of benzodiazepines on both everyday function and potentially risky endeavors such as driving or operating heavy machinery. This constellation of adverse effects make the use of benzodiazepines for the treatment of anxiety in patients with brain injury undesirable, and their use as first-line treatments for anxiety after TBI is not encouraged.

Buspirone may be less deleterious with respect to cognitive functioning in patients with TBI than benzodiazepines, and the former is not associated with dependency. Buspirone's therapeutic effects may occur after a latency of several weeks. Gualtieri (1991a, 1991b) found that four out of seven patients with "postconcussion syndrome" experienced "decreased anxiety, depression, irritability, somatic preoccupation, inattention, and distractibility" after treatment with buspirone. Side effects from buspirone are dizziness, lightheadedness, and, paradoxically, increased anxiety.

Patients with brain injury also may develop other anxiety disorders, such as panic disorder, obsessive-compulsive disorder, posttraumatic stress disorder (PTSD), and phobias. The most important step in the treatment of the patient with PTSD is the careful assessment and diagnosis of comorbid DSM-IV-TR Axis I or II conditions (American Psychiatric Association 2000a). When no pervasive comorbid condition is diagnosed, antidepressant medications should be the initial pharmacological treatment. Serotonergically active antidepressants are the medications initially indicated for the treatment of PTSD and other posttraumatic anxiety disorders.

The positive symptoms of PTSD, including reexperiencing of the event and increased arousal, often improve with medication. The negative symptoms of avoidance

TABLE 34–4.   Psychopharmacological treatment of chronic aggression

Agent	Indications	Special clinical considerations
Antipsychotics	Psychotic symptoms	Oversedation and multiple side effects
Benzodiazepines	Anxiety symptoms	Paradoxical rage
Anticonvulsants: carbamazepine (CBZ), valproic acid (VPA)	Seizure disorder	Bone marrow suppression (CBZ) and hepatotoxicity (CBZ and VPA)
Lithium	Manic excitement or bipolar disorder	Neurotoxicity and confusion
Buspirone	Persistent, underlying anxiety and/or depression	Delayed onset of action
Propranolol and other β-blockers	Chronic or recurrent aggression	Latency of 4–6 weeks
Antidepressants	Depression or mood lability with irritability	May need usual clinical doses

and withdrawal usually respond poorly to pharmacotherapy and may require additional treatment with psychotherapy targeting reductions of these symptoms.

Sleep

Sleep patterns of patients with brain damage are often disordered (see Chapter 20, Fatigue and Sleep Problems), with impaired rapid eye movement recovery and multiple nocturnal awakenings (Prigatano et al. 1982). Hypersomnia that occurs after severe penetrating brain injury most often resolves within the first year after injury, whereas insomnia that occurs in patients with long periods of coma and diffuse injury has a more chronic course (Askenasy et al. 1989). Barbiturates and long-acting benzodiazepines should probably be avoided in this population, and if prescribed at all, they should be used with great caution. These drugs interfere with rapid eye movement and stage 4 sleep patterns and may contribute to persistent insomnia (Buysse and Reynolds 1990). Clinicians should warn patients of the dangers of using over-the-counter preparations for sleeping and for colds because of the prominent anticholinergic side effects of these agents.

Trazodone, a sedating antidepressant medication that is devoid of anticholinergic side effects, may be used for nighttime sedation. A dose of 50 mg should be administered initially; if ineffective, doses up to 150 mg may be prescribed. Nonpharmacological approaches should be considered, including minimizing daytime naps, maintaining regular sleep onset times, and engaging in regular physical activity during the day.

Aggression and Agitation

We suggest using the framework provided by the Expert Consensus Panel for Agitation in Dementia (1998) when addressing aggression and agitation in persons with TBI. After appropriate assessment of possible etiologies of these behaviors, treatment is focused on the occurrence of comorbid neuropsychiatric conditions (e.g., depression, psychosis, insomnia, anxiety, and delirium), whether the treatment is being undertaken in the acute phase (hours to days) or the chronic phase (weeks to months), and the severity of the behavior (mild to severe). The pharmacotherapy of aggression and agitation is summarized in Table 34–4 and reviewed in detail in Chapter 14, Aggressive Disorders.

Concerns Regarding Pharmacotherapy

There has been a bias held by patients, families, and, often, treatment centers against the use of medications for the treatment of neuropsychiatric disorders in patients with brain injury. The issue is important, because the neuropsychiatrist is often faced with resistance from patients, families, and staff about the use of medications. The bias against the use of psychiatric medications may have several sources, including the stigma associated with mental illness and psychiatric treatment and, in some cases, the patient's previous suboptimal experience with psychotropic medications. Stigma may relate to the view that psychiatric symptoms are signs of weakness, indolence, or even moral decline. We have suggested that the neuropsychiatric paradigm—one that rejects the misleading demarcation between "brain" and "mind" and emphasizes the neurobiological bases of all cognitive, emotional, and behavioral problems regardless of the relationship of such problems to brain injury—as our strongest weapon against stigma (Arciniegas and Beresford 2001; Yudofsky and Hales 1989). Patients struggling to accept treatment in the face of old stigmas may benefit from an explanation of symptoms as the products of alterations in neurotransmitters, brain structures, brain networks, or some combination of these and presentation of treatments as designed to alleviate or compensate for such brain dysfunctions.

However, particularly for patients with TBI, the use of psychotropic medications indeed has often been a negative one. Antipsychotic medications, and particularly typical antipsychotics, are widely misused as a general "tranquilizer" to sedate patients agitated after TBI, with resulting impairment in alertness, cognition, and initiation, and the production, over time, of severe extrapyramidal side effects. For example, we evaluated in consultation one patient who had been treated with low-dose fluphenazine to control agitated behavior. One month later, the staff and family complained that she was "underaroused." On our examination, the patient had severe cogwheel rigidity that had not been diagnosed previously. One hour after administration of benztropine, 1 mg, she was "active" again.

Another fear about medication is that it will interfere with a "natural healing process" that occurs after TBI. Evidence obtained from animal models suggests that certain drugs, particularly agents that potently antagonize D_2 receptors, may interfere with recovery after neuronal injury. Feeney et al. (1982) studied the effect of D-amphetamine on recovery from hemiplegia after ablation of the sensorimotor cortex in rats. They found that D-amphetamine accelerated the rate of recovery and that this effect was blocked by haloperidol. In addition, haloperidol, when administered alone, resulted in delayed recovery. Importantly, recovery was affected only when the animal was allowed to move during drug administration. This implies that haloperidol delays the recovery process during active rehabilitation rather than interfering with spontaneous recovery per se. In another model, Hovda et al. (1985) found that haloperidol blocked the positive effect of D-amphetamine on recovery of depth perception after visual cortex injury.

It has been suggested that the mechanism of action of haloperidol in delaying recovery also operates through its effects as an α-adrenergic antagonist (Sutton et al. 1987). Clonidine, an α_2-adrenergic agonist, and prazosin, an α_1-adrenergic antagonist, reinstate deficits after sensorimotor cortex ablation (Sutton and Feeney 1987), an effect not seen with propranolol (Boyeson and Feeney 1984). Other studies have demonstrated that clonidine has deleterious effects on recovery (Feeney and Westerberg 1990; Goldstein and Davis 1990). It should be noted that these experimental methods in animals do not produce the same neuropathological findings as contusions or diffuse axonal injury in humans, and, therefore, may not apply fully to many patients with TBI.

In animal studies involving the neurotransmitter GABA, increased GABA function has been associated with greater neuromotor deficits and poorer recovery (Boyeson 1991). Increased production of GABA associated with benzodiazepine administration may result in greater glutamate neurotoxicity (Simantov 1990). Diazepam has been found to block recovery of sensory deficits after rat neocortex ablation (Schallert et al. 1986).

The preceding studies relating psychotropic use to impaired neuronal recovery after laboratory-induced brain injury have all used animal models. The study by Rao et al. (1985) appears to offer support for the notion of delayed recovery after administration of haloperidol by virtue of its demonstration of increased duration of posttraumatic amnesia among patients receiving this medication. However, there have been no carefully controlled clinical trials of this important relationship in humans. When the medical records of recovering stroke patients were reviewed, the use of antihypertensive medications or haloperidol was associated with poorer recovery (Porch et al. 1985). Goldstein and Davis (1990) found that when patients who had had ischemic strokes were administered phenytoin, benzodiazepines, dopamine receptor antagonists, clonidine, or prazosin, they showed poorer sensorimotor function and lower activities of daily living than stroke patients who did not receive those drugs.

Many patients are prescribed anticonvulsant drugs (ACDs) after TBI and may still be receiving them at the time of neuropsychiatric consultation in the period after acute rehabilitation. It is important, as discussed in Chapter 16, to ascertain whether such agents were prescribed for the treatment of active seizures, for seizure prophylaxis, or for the treatment of another neuropsychiatric problem.

ACDs can result in cognitive and emotional symptoms (Reynolds and Trimble 1985; Rivinus 1982; Smith 1991). Phenytoin has more profound effects on cognition than does carbamazepine (Gallassi et al. 1988). Dikmen et al. (1991) described greater cognitive impairment during treatment with phenytoin for prophylaxis of posttraumatic seizures when compared with placebo in a study of 244 patients with TBI. Intellectual deterioration in children on chronic treatment with phenytoin or phenobarbital also has been documented (Corbett et al. 1985). Dikmen et al. (2000) found no adverse cognitive effects of valproate when administered for 12 months after TBI. In a double-blind, placebo-controlled study of the cognitive and emotional effects of phenytoin (40 patients) and carbamazepine (42 patients) in TBI patients being treated with these medications for seizure prophylaxis, Smith et al. (1994) noted that both of these medications (but particularly carbamazepine) produced significantly more cognitive and motor slowing than did placebo. They found that both phenytoin and carbamazepine had negative effects on cognitive performance, especially those that involved motor and speed performance. Although in the patient group as a whole the effects were of questionable clinical significance, some patients experienced clinically significant negative cognitive effects during treatment with either of these agents. This is concordant with other observations of carbamazepine's potential to significantly impair cognition in neurologically vulnerable patients when cognition is properly assessed (Meador et al. 1999).

However, some patients do tolerate the cognitive effects of valproate or carbamazepine, or both, relatively well. Minimal impairment in cognition was found with both valproate and carbamazepine in a group of patients with epilepsy (Prevey et al. 1996); although those included in this study were not TBI patients, this observation suggests that at least some neurologically vulnerable patients may not experience significant cognitive impairment during treatment with this agent. Similarly, Persinger (2000) reported that 12 of 14 patients treated with carbamazepine in the late period after TBI retrospectively reported improvements in episodes of confusion and depression, increases in attention and focus, and reduction or elimination of subtle psychotic-like experiences ("aversive sensed presence"). Persinger suggested that this finding indicates an electrical (although not epileptic) nature for such symptoms that may be amenable to treatment with carbamazepine or other anticonvulsants.

Among the newer anticonvulsant medications, topiramate, but not gabapentin or lamotrigine, has been demonstrated to adversely affect cognition in healthy young adults (Martin et al. 1999). Treatment with more than one anticonvulsant (polytherapy) has been associated with increased adverse neuropsychiatric reactions (Reynolds and Trimble 1985). Hoare (1984) found that the use of multiple ACDs to control seizures resulted in an increase in disturbed behavior in children.

Patients who have a seizure immediately after brain injury often are placed on an ACD for seizure prophylaxis. Temkin et al. (1990) showed that the administration of phenytoin acutely after traumatic injury had no prophylactic effect on seizures that occurred subsequent to the first week after injury. Similarly, valproate did not demonstrate any efficacy in preventing late posttraumatic seizures (Temkin et al. 1999). It should be noted that there was a nonsignificant trend toward a higher mortality during treatment with valproate in this context. Anticonvulsant medications are not recommended after 1 week of injury for prevention (prophylaxis) of posttraumatic seizures (Brain Injury Special Interest Group of the American Academy of Physical Medicine and Rehabilitation 1998). Any patient with TBI who is treated with anticonvulsant medication requires regular reevaluations to substantiate continued clinical necessity for such treatment.

These studies suggest that careful monitoring of cognition during treatment with anticonvulsants in brain-injured patients is warranted. In general, treatment with these medications should be reserved for patients with established seizure disorders, mania, or severe aggression. These agents may also be useful for the treatment of affective lability that does not respond to more conventional antidepressant or dopaminergic agents.

Conclusion

It would be ideal if cognitive impairments, psychosis, depression, anxiety, aggression, and agitation after TBI could be controlled without medications. However, these neuropsychiatric problems are associated with significant distress and considerable functional disability; without treatment, some of these problems may also endanger the patient and others. In many cases, behavioral treatment and cognitive rehabilitation cannot be effective until psychopharmacological interventions are initiated. In other psychiatric conditions such as major depression, there is evidence that delay of effective treatment may result in refractoriness of the condition. Post (1992) reported that recurrent affective disorder becomes more difficult to treat the longer the condition persists. Thus, there are theoretical reasons for prompt initiation of pharmacological treatment of psychiatric syndromes in patients with TBI.

In this chapter, we reviewed the role of medication in the treatment of the most frequently occurring neuropsychiatric symptomatologies that are associated with TBI. When appropriately administered, medications may significantly alleviate these symptoms and improve rehabilitation efforts.

References

Allman P: Drug treatment of emotionalism following brain damage. J R Soc Med 85:423–424, 1992

American Psychiatric Association: Diagnostic and Statistical Manual of Mental Disorders, 4th Edition, Text Revision. Washington, DC, American Psychiatric Association, 2000a

American Psychiatric Association: Diagnostic and Statistical Manual of Mental Disorders, 4th Edition. Washington, DC, American Psychiatric Association, 1994

American Psychiatric Association: Practice Guideline for the Treatment of Patients With Major Depressive Disorder, 2nd Edition. Washington, DC, American Psychiatric Press, 2000b

Andersen G, Vestergaard K, Riis JO: Citalopram for post-stroke pathological crying. Lancet 342:837–839, 1993

Andersen G, Stylsvig M, Sunde N: Citalopram treatment of traumatic brain damage in a 6-year-old boy. J Neurotrauma 16:341–344, 1999

Angus WR, Romney DM: The effect of diazepam on patients' memory. J Clin Psychopharmacol 4:203–206, 1984

Arciniegas DB, Beresford TP: Neuropsychiatry: An Introductory Approach. Cambridge, England, Cambridge University Press, 2001

Arciniegas DB, Topkoff J: The neuropsychiatry of pathological affect: an approach to evaluation and treatment. Semin Clin Neuropsychiatry 5:290–306, 2000

Arciniegas D, Adler L, Topkoff J, et al: Attention and memory dysfunction after traumatic brain injury: cholinergic mechanisms, sensory gating, and a hypothesis for further investigation. Brain Inj 13:1–13, 1999

Arciniegas D, Olincy A, Topkoff J, et al: Impaired auditory gating and P50 nonsuppression following traumatic brain injury. J Neuropsychiatry Clin Neurosci 12:77–85, 2000a

Arciniegas DB, Topkoff J, Silver JM: Neuropsychiatric aspects of traumatic brain injury. Curr Treat Options Neurol 2:169–186, 2000b

Arciniegas DB, Topkoff J, Anderson CA, et al: Low-dose donepezil normalizes 50 physiology in traumatic brain injury patients. J Neuropsychiatry Clin Neurosci 14:115, 2002

Askenasy JJM, Winkler I, Grushkiewicz J, et al: The natural history of sleep disturbances in severe missile head injury. Journal of Neurological Rehabilitation 3:93–96, 1989

Bakchine S, Lacomblez L, Benoit N, et al: Manic-like state after bilateral orbitofrontal and right temporoparietal injury: efficacy of clonidine. Neurology 39:777–781, 1989

Bamrah JS, Johnson J: Bipolar affective disorder following head injury. Br J Psychiatry 158:117–119, 1991

Bareggi SR, Porta M, Selenati A, et al: Homovanillic acid and 5-hydroxyindole-acetic acid in the CSF of patients after a severe head injury, I: lumbar CSF concentration in chronic brain post-traumatic syndromes. Eur Neurol 13:528–544, 1975

Berg MJ, Ebert B, Willis DK, et al: Parkinsonism: drug treatment, part I. Drug Intelligence and Clinical Pharmacy 13:10–21, 1987

Bessette RF, Peterson LG: Fluoxetine and organic mood syndrome. Psychosomatics 33:224–226, 1992

Bogdanovitch UJ, Bazarevitch GJ, Kirillov AL: The use of cholinesterase in severe head injury. Resuscitation 4:139–141, 1975

Boyeson MG: Neurochemical alterations after brain injury: clinical implications for pharmacologic rehabilitation. Neurorehabilitation February:33–43, 1991

Boyeson MG, Feeney DM: The role of norepinephrine in recovery from brain injury (abstract). Society for Neuroscience Abstracts 10:68, 1984

Brain Injury Special Interest Group of the American Academy of Physical Medicine and Rehabilitation: Practice parameter: antiepileptic drug treatment of posttraumatic seizures. Arch Phys Med Rehabil 79:594–597, 1998

Breen R, Goldman CR: Response to "Evaluation of brain injury related behavioral disturbances in community mental health centers." Community Ment Health J 33:359–364, 1997

Brown KW, Sloan RL, Pentland B: Fluoxetine as a treatment for post-stroke emotionalism. Acta Psychiatr Scand 98:455–458, 1998

Burke JG, Dursun SM, Reveley MA: Refractory symptomatic schizophrenia resulting from frontal lobe lesion: response to clozapine. J Psychiatry Neurosci 24:456–461, 1999

Busto R, Dietrich WD, Globus MY, et al: Extracellular release of serotonin following fluid-percussion brain injury in rats. J Neurotrauma 14:35–42, 1997

Buysse DJ, Reynolds CF III: Insomnia, in Handbook of Sleep Disorders. Edited by Thorpy MJ. New York, Marcel Dekker, 1990, pp 373–434

Calatayud M, Calatayud V, Perez JB, et al: Effects of CDP-choline on the recovery of patients with head injury. J Neurol Sci 103 (suppl):S15–S18, 1991

Cardenas DD, McLean A, Farrell-Roberts L, et al: Oral physostigmine and impaired memory in adults with brain injury. Brain Inj 8:579–587, 1994

Cassidy JW: Fluoxetine: a new serotonergically active antidepressant. J Head Trauma Rehabil 4:67–69, 1989

Catsman-Berrevoets CE, Harskamp FV: Compulsive pre-sleep behavior and apathy due to bilateral thalamic stroke: response to bromocriptine. Neurology 38:647–649, 1988

Chandler MC, Barnhill JL, Gualtieri CT: Amantadine for the agitated head-injury patient. Brain Inj 2:309–311, 1988

Chemelli RM, Willie JT, Sinton CM, et al: Narcolepsy in Orexin knockout mice: molecular genetics of sleep regulation. Cell 98:437–451, 1999

Ciallella JR, Yan HQ, Ma X, et al: Chronic effects of traumatic brain injury on hippocampal vesicular acetylcholine transporter and M$_2$ muscarinic receptor protein in rats. Exp Neurol 152:11–19, 1998

Clark AF, Davison K: Mania following head injury: a report of two cases and a review of the literature. Br J Psychiatry 150:841–844, 1987

Clifton GL, Ziegler MG, Grossman RG: Circulating catecholamines and sympathetic activity after head injury. Neurosurgery 8:10–14, 1981

Corbett JA, Trimble MR, Nichol TC: Behavioral and cognitive impairments in children with epilepsy: the long-term effects of anticonvulsant therapy. J Am Acad Child Psychiatry 24:17–23, 1985

Crisostomo EA, Duncan PW, Propst M, et al: Evidence that amphetamine with physical therapy promotes recovery of motor function in stroke patients. Ann Neurol 23:94–97, 1988

Crow S, Meller W, Christenson G, et al: Use of ECT after brain injury. Convuls Ther 12:113–116, 1996

Cummings JL, Mega M, Gray K, et al: The Neuropsychiatric Inventory: comprehensive assessment of psychopathology in dementia. Neurology 44:2308–2314, 1994

Davidson J: Seizures and bupropion: a review. J Clin Psychiatry 50:256–261, 1989

De Smet Y, Ruberg M, Serdaru M, et al: Confusion, dementia, and anticholinergics in Parkinson's disease. J Neurol Neurosurg Psychiatry 45:1161–1164, 1982

DeAngelis MM, Hayes RL, Lyeth BG: Traumatic brain injury causes a decrease in M_2 muscarinic cholinergic receptor binding in the rat brain. Brain Res 653:39–44, 1994

Dewar D, Graham DI: Depletion of choline acetyltransferase but preservation of M_1 and M_2 muscarinic receptor binding sites in temporal cortex following head injury: a preliminary human postmortem study. J Neurotrauma 13:181–187, 1996

Dikmen SS, Temkin NR, Miller B, et al: Neurobehavioral effects of phenytoin prophylaxis of posttraumatic seizures. JAMA 265:1271–1277, 1991

Dikmen SS, Machamer JE, Winn HR et al: Neuropsychological effects of valproate in traumatic brain injury: a randomized trial. Neurology 54:895–902, 2000

Dinan TG, Mobayed M: Treatment resistance of depression after head injury: a preliminary study of amitriptyline response. Acta Psychiatr Scand 85:292–294, 1992

Dixon CE, Bao J, Bergmann JS, et al: Traumatic brain injury reduces hippocampal high–affinity [^{3}H]choline uptake but not extracellular choline levels in rats. Neurosci Lett 180:127–130, 1994a

Dixon CE, Hamm RJ, Taft WC, et al: Increased anticholinergic sensitivity following closed skull impact and controlled cortical impact traumatic brain injury in the rat. J Neurotrauma 11:275–287, 1994b

Dixon CE, Liu SJ, Jenkins LW, et al: Time course of increased vulnerability of cholinergic neurotransmission following traumatic brain injury in the rat. Behav Brain Res 70:125–131, 1995

Dixon CE, Ma X, Marion DW: Effects of CDP-choline treatment on neurobehavioral deficits after TBI and on hippocampal and neocortical acetylcholine release. J Neurotrauma 14:161–169, 1997a

Dixon CE, Ma X, Marion DW: Reduced evoked release of acetylcholine in the rodent neocortex following traumatic brain injury. Brain Res 749:127–130, 1997b

Donnemiller E, Brenneis C, Wissel J, et al: Impaired dopaminergic neurotransmission in patients with traumatic brain injury: a SPECT study using 123I–beta–CIT and 123I–IBZM. Eur J Nucl Med 27:1410–1414, 2000

Dreifuss FE, Santilli N, Langer DH, et al: Valproic acid hepatic fatalities: a retrospective review. Neurology 37:379–385, 1987

Dubois B, Pillon B, Lhermitte F, et al: Cholinergic deficiency and frontal dysfunction in Parkinson's disease. Ann Neurol 28:117–121, 1990

Dubovsky SL: Psychopharmacological treatment in neuropsychiatry, in The American Psychiatric Press Textbook of Neuropsychiatry, 2nd Edition. Edited by Yudofsky SC, Hales RE. Washington, DC, American Psychiatric Press, 1992, pp 663–701

Dubovsky SL, Franks RD, Allen S: Verapamil: a new antimanic drug with potential interactions with lithium. J Clin Psychiatry 48:371–372, 1987

Eames P: The use of Sinemet and bromocriptine. Brain Inj 3:319–320, 1989

Eames P: Feeling cold: an unusual brain injury symptom and its treatment with vasopressin. J Neurol Neurosurg Psychiatry 62:198–199, 1997

Eames P, Sutton A: Protracted post-traumatic confusional state treated with physostigmine. Brain Inj 9:729–734, 1995

Echiverri HC, Tatum WO, Merens TA, et al: Akinetic mutism: pharmacologic probe of the dopaminergic mesencephalofrontal activating system. Pediatr Neurol 4:228–230, 1988

Eghwrudjakpor PO, Miyake H, Kurisaka M, et al: Central nervous system bioaminergic responses to mechanical trauma: an experimental study. Surg Neurol 35:273–279, 1991

Elovic E: Use of Provigil for underarousal following TBI. J Head Trauma Rehabil 15:1068–1071, 2000

Evans RW, Gualtieri CT, Patterson D: Treatment of chronic closed head injury with psychostimulant drugs: a controlled case study and an appropriate evaluation procedure. J Nerv Ment Dis 175:106–110, 1987

Expert Consensus Panel for Agitation in Dementia: Treatment of agitation in older persons with dementia. Postgrad Med Spec No:1–88, 1998

Fann JR, Uomoto JM, Katon WJ: Sertraline in the treatment of major depression following mild traumatic brain injury. J Neuropsychiatry Clin Neurosci 12:226–232, 2000

Fann JR, Uomoto JM, Katon WJ: Cognitive improvement with treatment of depression following mild traumatic brain injury. Psychosomatics 42:48–54, 2001

Feeney DM, Westerberg VS: Norepinephrine and brain damage: alpha noradrenergic pharmacology alters functional recovery after cortical trauma. Can J Psychol 44:233–252, 1990

Feeney DM, Gonzalez A, Law WA: Amphetamine, haloperidol, and experience interact to affect rate of recovery after motor cortex injury. Science 217:855–857, 1982

Feldman H, Crumrine P, Handen BL, et al: Methylphenidate in children with seizures and attention-deficit disorder. Am J Dis Child 143:1081–1086, 1989

Ferraro L, Tanganelli S, O'Connor WT, et al: The vigilance promoting drug modafinil decreases GABA release in the medial preoptic area and in the posterior hypothalamus of the awake rat: possible involvement of the serotonergic 5-HT_3 receptor. Neurosci Lett 220:5–8, 1996

Ferraro L, Antonelli T, O'Connor WT, et al: The antinarcoleptic drug modafinil increases glutamate release in thalamic areas and hippocampus. Neuroreport 8:2883–2887, 1997a

Ferraro L, Antonelli T, O'Connor WT, et al: Modafinil: an antinarcoleptic drug with a different neurochemical profile to d-amphetamine and dopamine uptake blockers. Biol Psychiatry 42:1181–1183, 1997b

Gallassi R, Morreale A, Lorusso S, et al: Carbamazepine and phenytoin: comparison of cognitive effects in epileptic patients during monotherapy and withdrawal. Arch Neurol 45:892–894, 1988

Glenn MB: Methylphenidate for cognitive and behavioral dysfunction after traumatic brain injury. J Head Trauma Rehabil 13:87–90, 1998

Glenn MB, Wroblewski B, Parziale J, et al: Lithium carbonate for aggressive behavior or affective instability in ten brain-injured patients. Am J Phys Med Rehabil 68:221–226, 1989

Goldberg E, Gerstman LJ, Hughes JE, et al: Selective effects of cholinergic treatment on verbal memory in posttraumatic amnesia. J Clin Neuropsychol 4:219–234, 1982

Goldstein LB, Davis JN: Clonidine impairs recovery of beam-walking after a sensorimotor cortex lesion in the rat. Brain Res 508:305–309, 1990

Grimsley SR, Jann MW, Carter JG, et al: Increased carbamazepine plasma concentration after fluoxetine coadministration. Clin Pharmacol Ther 50:10–15, 1991

Grossman R, Beyer C, Kelly P, et al: Acetylcholine and related enzymes in human ventricular and subarachnoid fluids following brain injury. Proceedings of the 5th Annual Meeting for Neuroscience 76:3:506, 1975

Gualtieri CT: Buspirone for the behavior problems of patients with organic brain disorders. J Clin Psychopharmacol 11:280–281, 1991a

Gualtieri CT: Buspirone: neuropsychiatric effects. J Head Trauma Rehabil 6:90–92, 1991b

Gualtieri CT, Evans RW: Stimulant treatment for the neurobehavioural sequelae of traumatic brain injury. Brain Inj 2:273–290, 1988

Gualtieri CT, Chandler M, Coons TB, et al: Amantadine: a new clinical profile for traumatic brain injury. Clin Neuropharmacol 12:258–270, 1989

Gupta SR, Mlcoch AG: Bromocriptine treatment of nonfluent aphasia. Arch Phys Med Rehabil 73:373–376, 1992

Halliday AL: Pathophysiology, in Traumatic Brain Injury. Edited by Marion DW. New York, Thieme, 1999, pp 29–38

Hamill RW, Woolf PD, McDonald JV, et al: Catecholamines predict outcome in traumatic brain injury. Ann Neurol 21:438–443, 1987

Hibbard MR, Uysal S, Sliwinski M, et al: Undiagnosed health issues in individuals with traumatic brain injury living in the community. J Head Trauma Rehabil 13:47–57, 1998

Hoare P: The development of psychiatric disorder among schoolchildren with epilepsy. Dev Med Child Neurol 26:3–13, 1984

Hornstein A, Seliger G: Cognitive side effects of lithium in closed head injury. J Neuropsychiatry Clin Neurosci 1:446–447, 1989

Hornstein A, Lennihan L, Seliger G, et al: Amphetamine in recovery from brain injury. Brain Inj 10:145–148, 1996

Horsfield SA, Rosse RB, Tomasino V, et al: Fluoxetine's effects on cognitive performance in patients with traumatic brain injury. Int J Psychiatry Med 32:337–344, 2002

Hovda DA, Sutton RL, Feeney DM: Haloperidol blocks amphetamine-induced recovery of binocular depth perception after bilateral visual cortex ablation in cat. Proc West Pharmacol Soc 28:209–211, 1985

Hurley RA, Taber KH: Emotional disturbances following traumatic brain injury. Curr Treat Options Neurol 4:59–76, 2002

Jalil P: Toxic reaction following the combined administration of fluoxetine and phenytoin: two case reports. J Neurol Neurosurg Psychiatry 55:414–415, 1992

Johnston JA, Lineberry CG, Ascher JA, et al: A 102-center prospective study of seizure in association with bupropion. J Clin Psychiatry 52:450–456, 1991

Jorge R, Robinson RG: Mood disorders following traumatic brain injury. Int Rev Psychiatry 15:317–327, 2003

Kaelin DL, Cifu DX, Matthies B: Methylphenidate effect on attention deficit in the acutely brain-injured adult. Arch Phys Med Rehabil 77:6–9, 1996

Kant R, Smith-Seemiller L, Zeiler D: Treatment of aggression and irritability after head injury. Brain Inj 12:661–666, 1998

Kant R, Coffey CE, Bogyi AM: Safety and efficacy of ECT in patients with head injury: a case series. J Neuropsychiatry Clin Neurosci 11:32–37, 1999

Karakucuk EI, Pasaoglu H, Pasaoglu A, et al: Endogenous neuropeptides in patients with acute traumatic head injury, II: changes in the levels of cerebrospinal fluid substance P, serotonin and lipid peroxidation products in patients with head trauma. Neuropeptides 31:259–263, 1997

Kaye NS, Townsend JB III, Ivins R: An open-label trial of donepezil (Aricept) in the treatment of persons with mild traumatic brain injury. J Neuropsychiatry Clin Neurosci 15:383–384, 2003

Khouzam HR, Donnelly NJ: Remission of traumatic brain injury-induced compulsions during venlafaxine treatment. Gen Hosp Psychiatry 20:62–63, 1998

Kmeciak-Kolada K, Felinska W, Stachura Z, et al: Concentration of biogenic amines and their metabolites in different parts of brain after experimental cerebral concussion. Pol J Pharmacol Pharm 39:47–53, 1987

Kraus MF: Neuropsychiatric sequelae of stroke and traumatic brain injury: the role of psychostimulants. Int J Psychiatry Med 25:39–51, 1995

Kraus MF, Maki PM: Effect of amantadine hydrochloride on symptoms of frontal lobe dysfunction in brain injury: case studies and review. J Neuropsychiatry Clin Neurosci 9:222–230, 1997

Lal S, Merbitz CP, Grip JC: Modification of function in head-injured patients with Sinemet. Brain Inj 2:225–233, 1988

Lauterbach EC, Schweri MM: Amelioration of pseudobulbar affect by fluoxetine: possible alteration of dopamine-related pathophysiology by a selective serotonin reuptake inhibitor. J Clin Psychopharmacol 11:392–393, 1991

Lawson IR, MacLeod DM: The use of imipramine ("Tofranil") and other psychotropic drugs in organic emotionalism. Br J Psychiatry 115:281–285, 1969

Levin HS: Treatment of postconcussional symptoms with CDP-choline. J Neurol Sci 103:S39–S42, 1991

Levin HS, Peters BH, Kalisky S, et al: Effects of oral physostigmine and lecithin on memory and attention in closed head-injured patients. Cent Nerv Syst Trauma 3:333–342, 1986

Levin HS, High WM, Goethe KE, et al: The neurobehavioural rating scale: assessment of the behavioural sequelae of head injury by the clinician. J Neurol Neurosurg Psychiatry 50:183–193, 1987

Levy NA, Janicak PG: Calcium channel antagonists for the treatment of bipolar disorder. Bipolar Disord 2:108–119, 2000

Lewin J, Sumners D: Successful treatment of episodic dyscontrol with carbamazepine. Br J Psychiatry 161:261–262, 1992

Lieberman JA, Kane JM, Johns CA: Clozapine: guidelines for clinical management. J Clin Psychiatry 50:329–338, 1989

Lin L, Faraco J, Li R, et al: The sleep disorder canine narcolepsy is caused by a mutation in the hypocretin (Orexin) receptor 2 gene. Cell 98:365–376, 1999

Lipper S, Tuchman MM: Treatment of chronic post-traumatic organic brain syndrome with dextroamphetamine: first reported case. J Nerv Ment Dis 162:266–371, 1976

Livingston S, Pauli LL: Dextroamphetamine for epilepsy. JAMA 233:278–279, 1975

Lucki I, Rickels K, Geller AM: Chronic use of benzodiazepines and psychomotor and cognitive test performance. Psychopharmacology 88:426–433, 1986

Marangell LB, Silver JM, Goff DC, et al: Psychopharmacology and electroconvulsive therapy, in American Psychiatric Press Textbook of Clinical Psychiatry, 4th Edition. Edited by Hales RE, Yudofsky SC. Washington, DC, American Psychiatric Press, 2003, pp 1047–1149

Marin RS, Fogel BS, Hawkins J, et al: Apathy: a treatable syndrome. J Neuropsychiatry Clin Neurosci 7:23–30, 1995

Martin R, Kuzniecky R, Ho S, et al: Cognitive effects of topiramate, gabapentin, and lamotrigine in healthy young adults. Neurology 52:321–327, 1999

Masanic CA, Bayley MT, vanReekum R: Open-label study of donepezil in traumatic brain injury. Arch Phys Med Rehabil 82:896–901, 2001

Massagli TL: Neurobehavioral effects of phenytoin, carbamazepine, and valproic acid: implications for use in traumatic brain injury. Arch Phys Med Rehabil 72:219–226, 1991

Massey EW, Folger WN: Seizures activated by therapeutic levels of lithium carbonate. South Med J 77:1173–1175, 1984

McCauley SR, Levin HS, Vanier M, et al: The Neurobehavioural Rating Scale—Revised: sensitivity and validity in closed head injury assessment. J Neurol Neurosurg Psychiatry 71:643–651, 2001

McDowell S, Whyte J, D'Esposito M: Differential effect of a dopaminergic agonist on prefrontal function in traumatic brain injury patients. Brain 121:1155–1164, 1998

McIntosh TK, Juhler M, Raghupathi R, et al: Secondary brain injury: neurochemical and cellular mediators, in Traumatic Brain Injury. Edited by Marion DW. New York, Thieme, 1999, pp 39–54

Meador KJ, Loring DW, Ray PG, et al: Differential cognitive effects of carbamazepine and gabapentin. Epilepsia 40:1279–1285, 1999

Meythaler JM, Depalma L, Devivo MJ, et al: Sertraline to improve arousal and alertness in severe traumatic brain injury secondary to motor vehicle crashes. Brain Inj 15:321–331, 2001

Michals ML, Crismon ML, Roberts S, et al: Clozapine response and adverse effects in nine brain-injured patients. J Clin Psychopharmacol 13:198–203, 1993

Monji A, Yoshida A, Koga H, et al: Brain injury-induced rapid-cycling affective disorder successfully treated with valproate. Psychosomatics 40:448–449, 1999

Morey CE, Cilo M, Berry J, et al: The effect of Aricept in persons with persistent memory disorder following traumatic brain injury: a pilot study. Brain Inj 17:809–816, 2003

Morrison JH, Molliver ME, Grzanna R: Noradrenergic innervation of cerebral cortex: widespread effects of local cortical lesions. Science 205:313–316, 1979

Muller U, Murai T, Bauer-Wittmund T, et al: Paroxetine versus citalopram treatment of pathological crying after brain injury. Brain Inj 13:805–811, 1999

Murdoch I, Perry EK, Court JA, et al: Cortical cholinergic dysfunction after human head injury. J Neurotrauma 15:295–305, 1998

Nahas Z, Arlinghaus KA, Kotrla KJ, et al: Rapid response of emotional incontinence to selective serotonin reuptake inhibitors. J Neuropsychiatry Clin Neurosci 10:453–455, 1998

Newburn G, Edwards R, Thomas H, et al: Moclobemide in the treatment of major depressive disorder (DSM–3) following traumatic brain injury. Brain Inj 13:637–642, 1999

Nickels JL, Schneider WN, Dombovy ML, et al: Clinical use of amantadine in brain injury rehabilitation. Brain Inj 8:709–718, 1994

Nieves AV, Lang AE: Treatment of excessive daytime sleepiness in patients with Parkinson's disease with modafinil. Clin Neuropharmacol 25:111–114, 2002

Nizamie SH, Nizamie A, Borde M, et al: Mania following head injury: case reports and neuropsychological findings. Acta Psychiatr Scand 77:637–639, 1988

Obrenovitch TP, Urenjak J: Is high extracellular glutamate the key to excitotoxicity in traumatic brain injury? J Neurotrauma 14:677–698, 1997

Ojemann LM, Baugh-Bookman C, Dudley DL: Effect of psychotropic medications on seizure control in patients with epilepsy. Neurology 37:1525–1527, 1987

Olincy A, Ross RG, Harris JG, et al: The P50 auditory event-evoked potential in adult attention-deficit disorder: comparison with schizophrenia. Biol Psychiatry 47:969–977, 2000

Oliver AP, Luchins DJ, Wyatt RJ: Neuroleptic-induced seizures: an in vitro technique for assessing relative risk. Arch Gen Psychiatry 39:206–209, 1982

Pachet A, Friesen S, Winkelaar D, et al: Beneficial behavioural effects of lamotrigine in traumatic brain injury. Brain Inj 17:715–722, 2003

Panzer MJ, Mellow AM: Antidepressant treatment of pathologic laughing or crying in elderly stroke patients. J Geriatr Psychiatry Neurol 4:195–199, 1992

Pappius HM: Involvement of indoleamines in functional disturbances after brain injury. Prog Neuropsychopharmacol Biol Psychiatry 13:353–361, 1989

Parks RW, Crockett DJ, Manji HK, et al: Assessment of bromocriptine intervention for the treatment of frontal lobe syndrome: a case study. J Neuropsychiatry Clin Neurosci 4:109–110, 1992

Parmelee DX, O'Shanick GJ: Carbamazepine-lithium toxicity in brain-damaged adolescents. Brain Inj 2:305–308, 1988

Persinger MA: Subjective improvement following treatment with carbamazepine (Tegretol) for a subpopulation of patients with traumatic brain injuries. Percept Mot Skills 90:37–40, 2000

Pinder RM, Brogden RN, Speight TM, et al: Maprotiline: a review of its pharmacological properties and therapeutic efficacy in mental states. Drugs 13:321–352, 1977

Pleak RR, Birmaher B, Gavrilescu A, et al: Mania and neuropsychiatric excitation following carbamazepine. J Am Acad Child Adolesc Psychiatry 27:500–503, 1988

Plenger PM, Dixon CE, Castillo RM, et al: Subacute methylphenidate treatment for moderate to moderately severe traumatic brain injury: a preliminary double-blind placebo-controlled study. Arch Phys Med Rehabil 77:536–540, 1996

Poeck K: Pathological laughter and crying, in Handbook of Clinical Neurology. Edited by Fredericks JAM. 45:219–225, 1985

Pope HG Jr, McElroy SL, Satlin A, et al: Head injury, bipolar disorder, and response to valproate. Compr Psychiatry 29:34–38, 1988

Porch B, Wyckes J, Feeney DM: Haloperidol, thiazides and some antihypertensives slow recovery from aphasia (abstract). Society for Neuroscience Abstracts 11:52, 1985

Porta M, Bareggi SR, Collice M, et al: Homovanillic acid and 5-hydroxyindole-acetic acid in the CSF of patients after a severe head injury, II: ventricular CSF concentrations in acute brain post-traumatic syndromes. Eur Neurol 13:545–554, 1975

Post RM: Transduction of psychosocial stress into the neurobiology of recurrent affective disorders. Am J Psychiatry 149:999–1010, 1992

Prevey ML, Delaney RC, Cramer JA, et al: Effect of valproate on cognitive functioning: comparison with carbamazepine. The Department of Veterans Affairs Epilepsy Cooperative Study 264 Group. Arch Neurol 53:1008–1016, 1996

Prigatano GP, Stahl ML, Orr WC, et al: Sleep and dreaming disturbances in closed head injury patients. J Neurol Neurosurg Psychiatry 45:78–80, 1982

Rammohan KW, Rosenberg JH, Lynn DJ, et al: Efficacy and safety of modafinil (Provigil) for treatment of fatigue in multiple sclerosis: a two centre phase 2 study. J Neurol Neurosurg Psychiatry 72:179–183, 2002

Rao N, Jellinek HM, Woolston DC: Agitation and closed head injury: haloperidol effects on rehabilitation outcome. Arch Phys Med Rehabil 66:30–34, 1985

Reinhard DL, Whyte J, Sandel ME: Improved arousal and initiation following tricyclic antidepressant use in severe brain injury. Arch Phys Med Rehabil 77:80–83, 1996

Reynolds EH, Trimble MR: Adverse neuropsychiatric effects of anticonvulsant drugs. Drugs 29:570–581, 1985

Rivinus TM: Psychiatric effects of the anticonvulsant regimens. J Clin Psychopharmacol 2:165–192, 1982

Robinson RG, Parikh RM, Lipsey JR, et al: Pathological laughing and crying following stroke: validation of a measurement scale and a double-blind treatment study. Am J Psychiatry 150:286–293, 1993

Robinson RG, Schultz SK, Castillo C, et al: Nortriptyline versus fluoxetine in the treatment of depression and in short-term recovery after stroke: a placebo-controlled, double-blind study. Am J Psychiatry 157:351–359, 2000

Rosebush P, Stewart T: A prospective analysis of 23 episodes of neuroleptic malignant syndrome. Am J Psychiatry 146:717–725, 1989

Rosebush PI, Stewart T, Mazurek MF: The treatment of neuroleptic malignant syndrome: are dantrolene and bromocriptine useful adjuncts to supportive care? Br J Psychiatry 159:709–712, 1991

Roth T, Hartse KM, Saab PG, et al: The effects of flurazepam, lorazepam, and triazolam on sleep and memory. Psychopharmacology 70:231–237, 1980

Rothman KJ, Funch DP, Dreyr NA: Bromocriptine and puerperal seizures. Epidemiology 1:232–238, 1990

Ruedrich I, Chu CC, Moore SI: ECT for major depression in a patient with acute brain trauma. Am J Psychiatry 140:928–929, 1983

Saija A, Robinson SE, Lyeth BG, et al: The effects of scopolamine and traumatic brain injury on central cholinergic neurons. J Neurotrauma 5:161–170, 1988

Sandel ME, Olive DA, Rader MA: Chlorpromazine-induced psychosis after brain injury. Brain Inj 7:77–83, 1993

Sandyk R, Gillman MA: Nomifensine for emotional incontinence in the elderly. Clin Neuropharmacol 8:377–378, 1985

Saran AS: Depression after minor closed head injury: role of dexamethasone suppression test and antidepressants. J Clin Psychiatry 46:335–338, 1985

Sayal K, Ford T, Pipe R: Case study: bipolar disorder after head injury. J Am Acad Child Adolesc Psychiatry 39:525–528, 2000

Schallert T, Hernandez TD, Barth TM: Recovery of function after brain damage: severe and chronic disruption by diazepam. Brain Res 379:104–111, 1986

Schiff HB, Sabin TD, Geller A, et al: Lithium in aggressive behavior. Am J Psychiatry 139:1346–1348, 1982

Schiffer RB, Herndon RM, Rudick RA: Treatment of pathologic laughing and weeping with amitriptyline. N Engl J Med 312:1480–1482, 1985

Schmidt RH, Grady MS. Loss of forebrain cholinergic neurons following fluid-percussion injury: implications for cognitive impairment in closed head injury. J Neurosurg 83:496–502, 1995

Schmitt JA, Kruizinga MJ, Riedel WJ: Non-serotonergic pharmacological profiles and associated cognitive effects of serotonin reuptake inhibitors. J Psychopharmacol 15:173–179, 2001

Schreiber S, Klag E, Gross Y, et al: Beneficial effect of risperidone on sleep disturbance and psychosis following traumatic brain injury. Int Clin Psychopharmacol 13:273–275, 1998

Secades JJ, Frontera G: CDP-choline: pharmacological and clinical review. Methods Find Exp Clin Pharmacol 17 (suppl B):1–54, 1995

Seliger GM, Hornstein A, Flax J, et al: Fluoxetine improves emotional incontinence. Brain Inj 6:267–270, 1992

Showalter PE, Kimmel DN: Stimulating consciousness and cognition following severe brain injury: a new potential clinical use for lamotrigine. Brain Inj 14:997–1001, 2000

Silver JM, Anderson K: Vasopressin treats the persistent feeling of coldness after brain injury. J Neuropsychiatry Clin Neurosci 11:248–252, 1999

Silver JM, Yudofsky SC: The Overt Aggression Scale: overview and clinical guidelines. J Neuropsychiatry Clin Neurosci 3 (suppl):S22–S29, 1991

Silver JM, Hales RE, Yudofsky SC: Psychopharmacology of depression in neurologic disorders. J Clin Psychiatry 51 (suppl 1):33–39, 1990

Silver JM, Yudofsky SC, Hales RE: Depression in traumatic brain injury. Neuropsychiatry Neuropsychol Behav Neurol 4:12–23, 1991

Simantov R: Gamma-aminobutyric acid (GABA) enhances glutamate cytotoxicity in a cerebellar cell line. Brain Res Bull 24:711–715, 1990

Sloan RL, Brown KW, Pentland B: Fluoxetine as a treatment for emotional lability after brain injury. Brain Inj 6:315–319, 1992

Smith DB: Cognitive effects of antiepileptic drugs. Adv Neurol 55:197–212, 1991

Smith KR Jr, Goulding PM, Wilderman D, et al: Neurobehavioral effects of phenytoin and carbamazepine in patients recovering from brain trauma: a comparative study. Arch Neurol 51:653–660, 1994

Sovner R, Davis JM: A potential drug interaction between fluoxetine and valproic acid (letter). J Clin Psychopharmacol 11:389, 1991

Speech TJ, Rao SM, Osmon DC, et al: A double-blind controlled study of methylphenidate treatment in closed head injury. Brain Inj 7:333–338, 1993

Stanislav SW: Cognitive effects of antipsychotic agents in persons with traumatic brain injury. Brain Inj 11:335–341, 1997

Starkstein SE, Boston JD, Robinson RG: Mechanisms of mania after brain injury: 12 case reports and review of the literature. J Nerv Ment Dis 176:87–100, 1988

Starkstein SE, Mayberg HS, Berthier ML, et al: Mania after brain injury: neuroradiological and metabolic findings. Ann Neurol 27:652–659, 1990

Stewart JT, Hemsath RH: Bipolar illness following traumatic brain injury: treatment with lithium and carbamazepine. J Clin Psychiatry 49:74–75, 1988

Sutton RL, Feeney DM: Yohimbine accelerates recovery and clonidine and prazosin reinstate deficits after recovery in rats with sensorimotor cortex ablation (abstract). Society for Neuroscience Abstracts 13:913, 1987

Sutton RL, Weaver MS, Feeney DM: Drug-induced modifications of behavioral recovery following cortical trauma. J Head Trauma Rehabil 2:50–58, 1987

Tang YP, Noda Y, Nabeshima T: Involvement of activation of dopaminergic neuronal system in learning and memory deficits associated with experimental mild traumatic brain injury. Eur J Neurosci 9:1720–1727, 1997

Taverni JP, Seliger G, Lichtman SW: Donepezil mediated memory improvement in traumatic brain injury during post acute rehabilitation. Brain Inj 12:77–80, 1998

Teitelman E: Off-label uses of modafinil. Am J Psychiatry 158:1341, 2001

Temkin NR, Dikmen SS, Wilensky AJ, et al: A randomized, double-blind study of phenytoin for the prevention of posttraumatic seizures. N Engl J Med 323:497–502, 1990

Temkin NR, Dikmen SS, Anderson GD, et al: Valproate therapy for prevention of posttraumatic seizures: a randomized trial. J Neurosurg 91:593–600, 1999

Tsuiki K, Takada A, Nagahiro S, et al: Synthesis of serotonin in traumatized rat brain. J Neurochem 64:1319–1325, 1995

Udaka F, Yamao S, Nagata H, et al: Pathologic laughing and crying treated with levodopa. Neurology 41:1095–1096, 1984

Van Reekum R, Bayley M, Garner S, et al: N of 1 study: amantadine for the amotivational syndrome in a patient with traumatic brain injury. Brain Inj 9:49–53, 1995

Van Woerkom TCAM, Teelken AW, Minderhoud JM: Difference in neurotransmitter metabolism in frontotemporal-lobe contusion and diffuse cerebral contusion. Lancet 1:812–813, 1977

Varney NR, Martzke JS, Roberts RJ: Major depression in patients with closed head injury. Neuropsychology 1:7–9, 1987

Vecht CJ, Van Woerkom TCAM, Teelken AW, et al: Homovanillic acid and 5-hydroxyindoleacetic acid cerebrospinal fluid levels. Arch Neurol 32:792–797, 1975

Vincent FM, Zimmerman JE, Van Haren J: Neuroleptic malignant syndrome complicating closed head injury. Neurosurgery 18:190–193, 1986

Walburga van Laar M, Volkeerts ER, van Willigenburg APP: Therapeutic effects and effects on actual driving performance of chronically administered buspirone and diazepam in anxious outpatients. J Clin Psychopharmacol 12:86–95, 1992

Weinstein GS, Wells CE: Case studies in neuropsychiatry: posttraumatic psychiatric dysfunction—diagnosis and treatment. J Clin Psychiatry 42:120–122, 1981

Weller M, Kornhuber J: A rationale for NMDA receptor antagonist therapy of the neuroleptic malignant syndrome. Med Hypotheses 38:329–333, 1992

Whelan FJ, Walker MS, Schultz SK: Donepezil in the treatment of cognitive dysfunction associated with traumatic brain injury. Ann Clin Psychiatry 12:131–135, 2000

Whitlock JA: Brain injury, cognitive impairment, and donepezil. J Head Trauma Rehabil 1:424–427, 1999

Whyte J: Neurologic disorders of attention and arousal: assessment and treatment. Arch Phys Med Rehabil 73:1094–1103, 1992

Whyte J, Hart T, Schuster K, et al: Effects of methylphenidate on attentional function after traumatic brain injury: a randomized, placebo-controlled trial. Am J Phys Med Rehabil 76:440–450, 1997

Wilkinson R, Meythaler JM, Guin-Renfroe S: Neuroleptic malignant syndrome induced by haloperidol following traumatic brain injury. Brain Inj 13:1025–1031, 1999

Wolf B, Grohmann R, Schmidt LG, et al: Psychiatric admissions due to adverse drug reactions. Compr Psychiatry 30:534–545, 1989

Woolf PD, Hamill RW, Lee LA, et al: The predictive value of catecholamines in assessing outcome in traumatic brain injury. J Neurosurg 66:875–882, 1987

Wroblewski BA, McColgan K, Smith K, et al: The incidence of seizures during tricyclic antidepressant drug treatment in a brain-injured population. J Clin Psychopharmacol 10:124–128, 1990

Wroblewski BA, Guidos A, Leary J, et al: Control of depression with fluoxetine and antiseizure medication in a brain-injured patient. Am J Psychiatry 149:273–273, 1992a

Wroblewski BA, Leary JM, Phelan AM, et al: Methylphenidate and seizure frequency in brain-injured patients with seizure disorders. J Clin Psychiatry 53:86–89, 1992b

Wroblewski B, Glenn MB, Cornblatt R, et al: Protriptyline as an alternative stimulant medication in patients with brain injury: a series of case reports. Brain Inj 7:353–362, 1993

Wroblewski BA, Joseph AB, Cornblatt RR: Antidepressant pharmacotherapy and the treatment of depression in patients with severe traumatic brain injury: a controlled, prospective study. J Clin Psychiatry 57:582–587, 1996

Yassa R, Nair V, Schwartz G: Tardive dyskinesia and the primary psychiatric diagnosis. Psychosomatics 25:135–138, 1984a

Yassa R, Nair V, Schwartz G: Tardive dyskinesia: a two-year follow-up study. Psychosomatics 25:852–855, 1984b

Yudofsky SC, Hales RE: The reemergence of neuropsychiatry: definition and direction. J Neuropsychiatry Clin Neurosci 1:1–6, 1989

Zeilig G, Drubach DA, Katz-Zeilig M, et al: Pathological laughter and crying in patients with closed traumatic brain injury. Brain Inj 10:591–597, 1996

Zhang L, Plotkin RC, Wang G, et al: Cholinergic augmentation with donepezil enhances recovery in short-term memory and sustained attention after traumatic brain injury. Arch Phys Med Rehabil 85:1050–1055, 2004

Zifko UA, Rupp M, Schwarz S, et al: Modafinil in treatment of fatigue in multiple sclerosis: results of an open-label study. J Neurol 249:983–987, 2002

Zwil AS, McAllister TW, Price TRP: Safety and efficacy of ECT in depressed patients with organic brain disease: review of a clinical experience. Convuls Ther 8:103–109, 1992

Zwil AS, McAllister TW, Cohen I, et al: Ultra-rapid cycling bipolar affective disorder following a closed–head injury. Brain Inj 7:147–152, 1993

35 Psychotherapy

Irwin W. Pollack, M.D., M.A.

THERE CONTINUES TO be some disagreement among mental health professionals about whether the use of psychotherapeutic techniques in cases of depression and schizophrenia adds significantly to the known therapeutic effects of selected pharmacological agents. However, in the case of patients who have sustained traumatic brain injuries (TBIs), there is no doubt that drug treatment, although important in many cases, is not sufficient alone to bring about meaningful improvement in patients' life situations. Every TBI of any consequence causes some disturbance in a number of systems integral to the individual, including those responsible for motor, cognitive, and emotional function. For this reason, no single approach to treatment is sufficient. During the course of rehabilitation, a range of treatment approaches must be used, and among these, psychotherapy should be included to assist the patient with his or her efforts to reestablish an acceptable sense of self. Despite this need for a range of approaches, for the most part psychiatrists have limited their transactions with patients who have sustained TBIs to the prescription and management of medications. There are several factors that may be contributing to this state of affairs.

Possibly because in most medical schools little time and attention are devoted to the study of TBIs, many psychiatrists trained in these institutions are reluctant to accept a person with a history of brain injury for psychotherapy. Indeed, possibly because of their limited exposure to persons with TBI during the course of their training, many psychiatrists see no role in the rehabilitation process for psychotherapy, at least as it has been traditionally practiced.

Certainly, people with significant brain injuries do not fit the usual image of an appropriate candidate for this form of treatment. The traditional approach to psychotherapy is based on the assumption that the primary source of a person's emotional problems resides within that person and not in the outside world. Provided that a person possesses certain abilities, it is assumed that he or she has the potential to function more effectively and to gain greater satisfaction from life—a potential that can be actualized through the therapeutic process. A list of those requisite abilities includes the capacity for abstract thinking, a degree of self-awareness and the ability to self-monitor, the ability to tolerate frustration and anxiety, memory that is intact enough to recall significant information both within and across therapy sessions, and the ability to transfer what is learned in the treatment environment to other life situations. These abilities are rarely found in people with significant brain injuries (Bennett 1989; Ludwig 1980; Miller 1991). Rather, far more commonly, these individuals may be impulsive, emotionally labile, and only minimally able to tolerate anxiety and frustration. They may be unable to assume an abstract attitude and may have a limited ability to profit from experience. They may not self-monitor effectively and as a result may fail to recognize the existence of significant problems, even when those problems are quite obvious to others (Conboy et al. 1986; Eames 1988; Goldstein 1952; Prigatano 1987). When one contrasts this list of deficits with the aforementioned list of abilities that are assumed to be necessary for a successful psychotherapeutic experience, the reasons for the lingering doubts regarding the use of psychotherapy with TBI patients are better understood.

But the life experiences of persons with brain injuries are not so different from those of noninjured persons to justify limiting their treatment options on an a priori basis. After their accidents, people with brain injuries, like noninjured persons, may struggle with unresolved internalized conflicts; operate on irrational assumptions about themselves and their world; demonstrate anxiety, depression, phobias, and obsessions; feel alienated and devoid of feeling; and face confrontation by environmental circumstances that threaten to overwhelm them. All of these conditions are known to respond to psychotherapeutic intervention. Within limits, the fact that a person has sustained a TBI should not change this assessment. The problem is not that persons who have sustained brain injuries do not respond to psychotherapy but rather that every aspect of their being and their sense of self has been affected in ways that cannot be managed successfully by any single approach to therapy (Fordyce 1983; Weddell et al. 1980).

The Psychotherapeutic Process

The primary goal of psychotherapy in the treatment of a person with a brain injury is the same as that of the other therapeutic modalities involved in the rehabilitation process: to enable the injured person to reestablish an acceptable sense of self (Banja 1988; Condeluci and Gretz-Lasky 1987; Pollack 1994).

To accomplish this goal, the downhill course leading to social isolation and loneliness must be stopped and then reversed; however, all too often the physical, cognitive, and emotional residuals of the brain injury and their social consequences compromise the injured person's ability to regain the initiative without professional help. This is no less the case for many people who have sustained mild brain injuries who, over time, have become too bewildered and demoralized to put their lives back together without help.

Starting Point

To enable patients with brain injuries to breach the walls of their isolation and to begin to relate to other people effectively again, therapists and their patients must find areas of shared meaning (Stuewe-Portnoff 1988). The therapist and the patient must come to share an understanding of the nature of the problem as it is experienced by the patient (Cicerone 1989; Pollack 1989; Prigatano 1989). Prigatano (1989) expressed the view that a therapist working with an individual who has sustained a brain injury needs symbols, concepts, or analogies that adequately represent—for both the therapist and the patient—what it is like to have a damaged brain. The model thus developed provides a base from which a series of other shared experiences can evolve, eventually culminating in the reestablishment of the injured person's sense of self. In most cases, initially it is the therapist who must provide a rationale for what has happened to the patient as a result of his or her injury.

If the patient is competent enough to understand, he or she should be reassured that it is the brain injury, not a neurotic or psychotic process, that is causing his or her disturbances. As much as possible, specific complaints should be taken up and their relationship to the injury should be explained in nontechnical language. The pa-

tient should be told that although the final outcome of the injuries is not wholly predictable, some improvement in physical and cognitive abilities is to be expected, and the degree of this improvement often can be enhanced through rehabilitation activities. The patient should be forewarned that his or her efforts will be of the greatest importance because therapy of any kind will not be fruitful without this active participation, and that even under the best of circumstances, positive changes will be slow in coming, so great patience will be required. The patient should be discouraged from returning to his or her regular routine prematurely—that is, before relevant abilities have progressed to the point at which success can be reasonably expected. It is extremely important to avoid unnecessary failures and the demoralization that results.

In the case of a severely impaired person, the explanation of the effects of brain injury should be brief, concrete, and directed specifically at clarifying the most significant of the patient's complaints.

Importance of a Historical Perspective

Although the importance of obtaining an adequate history is emphasized in all areas of medical practice, in therapeutic work with people who have sustained a brain injury, it is the sine qua non. Not only must the therapist acquire in-depth information about the circumstances surrounding the injury and the patient's preinjury personality and postinjury symptoms, abilities, and behaviors, but the therapist must also know about that person's preinjury level of physical and social development, interests and values, school and work experiences, cultural background, and friendships and family relationships as they existed both before and after the brain injury (Cicerone 1989; Ellis 1989; Prigatano 1989). Events surrounding the injury can have far-reaching experiential and symbolic significance for the injured person, and the disinhibition that frequently follows as a consequence of brain injury can result in the reemergence of previously resolved psychological issues dating back to childhood (Bennett 1989; Silver et al. 1992). These factors all contribute to an injured person's vulnerabilities and predispositions; therefore, it is important to distinguish symptoms that are associated with one or another of these factors from those associated with the brain injury itself, because these distinctions affect the therapeutic approach (Prigatano 1989).

Patient Changeability: The Need for Therapist Flexibility

To paraphrase Heraclitus, for the therapist in the early stages of his or her attempts to understand the patient's postinjury behaviors, the only unchanging characteristic is change itself. As noted by Gardner (1976),

> I have never seen a brain damaged individual, with the possible exception of those either completely demented or virtually recovered, who did not display sizable variations in performance from day to day, if not across hours or minutes.... No skill seems to be completely destroyed or wholly intact; rather, each seems to be in a partial state of disrepair, and, depending upon such factors as the surrounding conditions, the extent of fatigue, the events of the preceding minutes, motivation at the given moment, the degree of alertness or attentiveness, the patient may succeed strikingly or fail dismally on a given set of tasks. This variability is all important because it precludes a ready foolproof description of the patient—as most consulting physicians soon learn, one must speak of the patient at-a-given-moment-in-time, or in particular circumstances, rather than as a fixed set of mechanized routines always performing at the same level. (p. 431)

Not only their behaviors but the entire beings of people with brain injuries are in a state of flux. Most are rather young when they are injured—in their adolescence or early adulthood—and still in the process of evolving both physically and psychosocially (Lewis and Rosenberg 1990). Additionally, over time, people with brain injuries usually show a progressive improvement in their physical and cognitive capacities, thereby enhancing their ability to analyze and comprehend the significance of their subjective experiences (Stein 1988). Successful psychotherapeutic work with people who have experienced a TBI usually requires that the therapist use several different approaches to treatment. It is most common for a therapist to begin the treatment process with an approach that is almost entirely under his or her control: taking a medical and social history, educating the patient and family members about the effects of a brain injury, and consulting with other members of the rehabilitation team, employers and teachers, and the staff of involved social agencies.

After arriving at a mutual understanding of what has happened to the patient as a result of the brain injury, therapeutic efforts should focus on selected concrete problems. Preferably, these issues should be raised by the client and pursued even if they are not considered to be important by the therapist. The patient should be assisted in attaining a clear picture of the problem as it affects both the patient and the family. At first, therapeutic efforts should be focused on the here and now, even when it is

clear that the patient's preinjury personality is playing a significant role. Therapist and patient together should determine how best to modify ineffectual responses, although at times, direct suggestions and advice are necessary. Often, a second or even a third approach to treatment is indicated, such as the addition of behavioral, group, or family therapy. In addition, environmental manipulation may be indicated, and for this reason the family, employer, and/or friends may need to be brought into the therapeutic situation.

The psychiatrist should emphasize the patient's remaining assets and help the patient see how these can be used to manage present problems. Success should be rewarded with acknowledgment and praise; failure should be addressed with acknowledgment and support. Emphasis should be placed on what the patient can learn from each experience, and the therapist must recognize that, for the most part, it is the process that is therapeutic, not the patient's insights.

As the therapeutic relationship develops and the patient makes additional gains in cognitive abilities, the approach to therapy should gradually shift to one that places greater demands on the patient (e.g., rational or even insight-oriented therapy). However, as noted earlier in this section, because of the patient's extreme changeability, the psychiatrist may need to shift the approach from treatment session to treatment session or even within a single treatment session.

Because a truly empathic relationship between the therapist and his or her TBI patient is often impossible to achieve, psychodynamic interpretations should be made rarely and, even then, tentatively. On the other hand, decisiveness is most appropriate when offering guidance. Cicerone (1989) suggests that interpretations should be used to make explicit connections that the patient has been unable to make.

The need for therapist flexibility is clear, because no single therapeutic approach suffices. The psychiatrist must be prepared to shift tactics as dictated by the patient's change in state and/or by the behaviors present at the moment; only through these measures can the ensuing transactions between therapist and patient be effective in promoting further recovery.

The therapist must be aware that if a patient with a brain injury is placed in a demanding situation in which information or concepts are presented too rapidly or are too complex for him or her to process effectively, a catastrophic response may be precipitated, thereby causing the patient to leave the therapeutic situation.

The course of recovery from even a mild brain injury is slow and uneven, whereas the impact on the life of the injured person and family and friends is immediate. Because loss of morale and increased anxiety and depression are continuing threats to each patient's successful rehabilitation, the psychotherapist must make every effort to instill hope in the patient and the family without making insubstantial predictions of a successful rehabilitation outcome (Prigatano 1986). Moreover, implicit in all contacts with even a moderately impaired person is a quality of uncertainty that tends to engender a level of anxiety in anyone (e.g., family and friends) who desires or needs to maintain a close relationship with the injured individual. A therapist can allay this anxiety most effectively through the sharing of information about the nature of the brain injury, the problems that can be expected, and the progress that the injured person is making in his or her therapy.

Goal-Directed Activities: Vehicles for Reconstituting a Sense of Self

The rebuilding of an acceptable sense of self cannot be achieved through talk alone. It requires action both by the members of the therapeutic team and the injured person. Only through the patient's actions that lead to a desired effect can a new sense of self begin to be acquired. Often, the most effective staff members in this patient–staff joint effort are those who are activity oriented (e.g., occupational therapists, recreation specialists, dancers and movement specialists, actors and drama specialists, artists and art therapists) (McKenna and Haste 1999; Stensrud et al. 1987) Unfortunately, for the most part, the therapeutic activities of this group of therapists are not considered to be significant enough to warrant reimbursement by patients' insurance carriers.

The therapeutic tactics described in the preceding sections are summarized in Table 35–1.

Treatment Goals and Outcome Measures

Most individuals who have sustained more than a mild TBI neither die nor fully recover. They are left with some degree of impairment, most often involving several areas of function. As a result, they are less effective in dealing with the everyday demands of the world around them. Many people who were employed before they were injured will never again be able to perform satisfactorily in the same position, regardless of the progress that they make in their rehabilitation programs. Although a significantly injured person may voice some concern about his or her financial future, this concern, when examined closely, appears to be

contributing relatively little to the intensity of that person's distress. This is understandable when one considers the degree of concern and anxiety that the individual feels about confronting the many other more pressing issues of immediate significance, not the least of which is the task of reestablishing a workable and acceptable sense of self. On the other hand, people with less significant brain injuries do appear to feel great concern and anxiety about the possibility that they will no longer be able to perform satisfactorily in the positions that they held before their injuries. Often, after treatment is concluded, many of these less impaired individuals are able to return to their preinjury jobs, and others are able to work successfully in new and less-challenging positions.

In both of the above cases, it appears that concern about the loss of income is less significant to a person with a brain injury than is the loss of the status and identity that are associated with having a job. The question "Who are you?" most often is answered by naming one's occupation (e.g., "I am a plumber," [or a physician, a housewife, a house painter, an actor, etc.]). To have no occupation is to have a hole in one's identity—a further assault on the injured person's sense of self.

When we consider that even after participating in an excellent rehabilitation program, many patients are still left with some permanent disability, agreement about what constitutes a satisfactory treatment outcome becomes even more important. Indeed, in the case of patients who have sustained a TBI, there is a lack of agreement among the experts over what outcome to measure (Rice-Oxley and Turner-Stokes 1999).

An often-used outcome measure is improvement in neuropsychological test performance. But improved test scores may have little or no relationship with a person's ability to manage real-life challenges successfully.

Two other measures often used by researchers to describe a satisfactory treatment outcome are "independent living" (McColl et al. 1999) and "community reentry." But both of these "measures" are poorly defined. For example, *independent* is defined in *Merriam-Webster's Collegiate Dictionary* as "not requiring or relying on something else.... not requiring or relying on others (as for care or livelihood)." But no one lives or can live without relying, at least to some degree, on someone else. Nor would that be a desirable condition, even if it were possible. So if total independence is neither possible nor desirable, what degree of independence is enough to be considered a satisfactory treatment outcome?

In considering community reentry as an outcome measure, we are left with the problem of deciding which community we are considering. Is it an inner-city community, a suburban community, a rural community, a con-

TABLE 35–1. Suggested tactics for the psychotherapeutic process

Tactic	Description
Gain a historical perspective.	Obtain information from family, friends, employers, and teachers concerning preinjury growth and development, health, education, occupation, personality, interests, values, goals, and impediments.
Find areas of shared meaning.	Determine what having a brain injury means to the patient and how he or she perceives its effects. At first, the psychiatrist may have to take the initiative, explaining the mechanism of traumatic brain injury in simple terms, relating the patient's difficulties to the injury, and describing the problems, events, and so on that can be expected in the future.
Encourage the patient to take the lead.	Concentrate on the concrete "real life" difficulties that the injury has caused the patient. Early in treatment, focus on the "here and now," avoid discussing the past (it requires good memory, and it is over), avoid discussing the future (it requires the ability to abstract, and at this point it is beyond comprehension).
Help the patient develop simple coping strategies.	For example, suggest that the patient keep a notebook, follow a sequence of predetermined steps, rest before becoming too fatigued, request that a confusing message be repeated slowly and in simpler terms, set up priorities for a series of necessary tasks.
Manipulate aspects of the environment to enable the patient to function more effectively.	For example, suggest organizing household equipment, utensils, dishes, and so on in a systematic fashion; labeling drawers and closets; using an alarm or calendar watch.
Mobilize assistance.	Mobilize the assistance of family members, employers, teachers, and friends to help keep the social and work demands as noncomplex and as manageable as possible.
Build on the patient's assets.	Build on the patient's remaining assets and avoid focusing on the residual deficits. Do not make every task seem like a test.
Engage the patient in meaningful goal-directed activities.	Use members of professional groups that are action oriented such as actors, dancers, and artists in addition to the more traditional rehabilitation staff.
Recognize that the patient's world may differ from that of the psychiatrist.	Interpret the meaning of behavior with caution. Provide guidance to improve inappropriate behavior with authority.
Maintain flexibility.	Many patients are adolescents or young adults in various stages of development; for most of these patients, some improvement in physical condition and cognitive function can be expected over time. Remember that a patient's abilities and emotional state can vary from moment to moment depending on preceding events, the character of the task, the degree of alertness and motivation, and the environmental conditions.
The approach to therapy should change as the patient changes.	This should happen both within and across treatment sessions. Ideally, the treatment approach should move gradually from one that is concerned primarily with the management of concrete, here-and-now, practical problems to one that places greater demands on the patient to consider psychodynamic issues.
Instill hope.	Instill hope in the patient and family without expressing unwarranted optimism.

servative community, a liberal community, a large community, a small community, a poor community, a wealthy community, a supportive community, a remote community, a community with many resources, or a community with few resources? In addition, we need to know whether the patient will be living with family, with friends, with some sort of organized support, or unsupported and alone. Clearly, the level of competence that is required of a patient is related directly to the amount and nature of the resources and support that are available and accessible to him or her.

If it is agreed that the most effective brain injury treatment program is one that is tailored as much as possible to the needs of the individual patient, it follows that the success or failure of a treatment program can be determined only in regard to that particular patient. The improvement resulting from the treatment program should make possible a lifestyle that is both acceptable to the patient and manageable without undue stress on the resources, both human and material, that are available to him or her. That is the only reasonable measure of a successful treatment outcome.

Mild Brain Injury

A number of animal and human studies have demonstrated that there is a continuum of neurological damage and functional impairment from mild to severe brain injury (Eisenberg and Levin 1989; Genarelli 1981; Rutherford 1989). The cognitive impairments that result from mild brain injuries are essentially the same as many of those that are seen after major brain trauma, although they are more subtle, at times becoming obvious only on neuropsychological testing. Commonly, these impairments include decrements in attention, concentration, short-term memory, and rapid and/or complex mental processing (Conboy et al. 1986; Rimel et al. 1981). For some individuals, the overall impact of these seemingly low-level deficits can be devastating, in large part because the quality of their combined effect is difficult to define and almost impossible to communicate effectively. As a result, the person with a mild brain injury often is seen as overreacting and neurotic. In such circumstances the individual, feeling misunderstood, maligned, and without support, can become confused, frightened, and angry.

Lezak, calling on her extensive experience in evaluating and treating patients with mild brain injuries, described a triad of subtle sequelae: perplexity, distractibility, and fatigue (Lezak 1978, 1989). Perplexity is reflected in the individual's distrust of his or her own abilities and in doubts regarding the validity of his or her thought processes. In interpersonal situations, perplexity is expressed as confusion, uncertainty, and self-doubt (Piotrowski 1937). Distractibility results when an individual cannot screen out unwanted or irrelevant stimulation. Because of the subtlety of this problem, it is quite common for the individual not to recognize that it exists. He or she is aware only of feeling uncomfortable when in contact with groups of people and of an intolerance of noise and random activity.

Unusual fatigability is found routinely after any brain injury. The injured person tires more easily, probably because formerly automatic activities and functions now require concentrated and sustained effort.

These subtle consequences of mild head injury, which are difficult to recognize and even more difficult to comprehend, can engender secondary feelings of confusion, anxiety, anger, and depression in both the injured person and members of his or her family. These painful emotions tend to cause the person with mild brain injury to overestimate the degree of his or her cognitive and physical impairments. Unlike many persons with profound brain injuries who do not complain, tending rather to deny the seriousness of their deficits, individuals who have experienced a mild brain injury frequently complain of their symptoms and mourn the loss of their former competencies.

Although some subtle impairments may be lifelong, most people who have experienced mild brain injuries are able to resume the key aspects of their lives within a period of 3–6 months. Symptoms that persist beyond 6 months usually are fueled by an interplay of the neurological damage, the person's premorbid personality traits, and his or her psychological response to the trauma (Levin et al. 1989). Lishman (1973) reported that psychological difficulties are more likely to follow mild brain injuries when the premorbid personality was characterized by insecurity and feelings of inadequacy.

Case Example

Mrs. D, a 40-year-old married bank officer, was seen for neuropsychiatric evaluation 3 years after she had been involved in a minor automobile accident. At the time, she experienced a very brief loss of consciousness, no more than 1 or 2 minutes in duration. A neurological evaluation done in the local hospital emergency room was described as essentially normal, and Mrs. D was discharged to her home after being advised to return if any one of a prescribed list of symptoms should appear. Over the next several months, Mrs. D began to notice difficulties in a number of areas of function that tended to reduce her effectiveness both at home and at work. She noticed that her short-term memory and her ability to concentrate had deteriorated, and she described having problems finding the appropriate words to express her thoughts. She frequently became distracted during business discussions and often felt so fatigued when she arrived home in the evening that she was unable to meet her family obligations.

Over the next 3 years, Mrs. D was evaluated by a number of physicians whom she saw either at her own initiative or at the request of her insurance company. The various consultants, most of whom were neurologists or psychiatrists, agreed on two points: first, there was no evidence of residual neurological damage; and second, Mrs. D appeared to be overreacting to ordinary life stresses. In Mrs.

D's opinion, she had received neither understanding nor relief as a result of her various contacts with members of the medical profession. As time passed, Mrs. D became increasingly confused and overwhelmed by her continuing problems. The quality of her work at the bank slipped badly, and her position there was in jeopardy. At home, the quality of her interactions with her husband and children deteriorated so far that she feared that her husband was about to leave her.

During our initial meeting, Mrs. D described the effect of her brain injury in the following manner: "Since my injury, I feel that there is not enough of me to cope. Everywhere I look I have a sense of 'not me.' It seems like I've been fractured internally [pointing to her head]. I have panic attacks! Something is terribly wrong!"

After completing the remainder of the evaluation, Mrs. D was assured that her complaints were those that typically follow a mild brain injury. A simplified explanation of what occurs in the brain when the head is forcefully impacted was presented to her, and some strategies that could help her manage her workload more effectively were suggested.

When Mrs. D returned the following week for her second appointment, she reported that the strategies had worked and that she was feeling less anxious and confused and more in control than at any time since her accident. Obviously, this was not the end of Mrs. D's problems, but an alliance had been forged that would support her further recovery.

In every case of mild brain injury, the best treatment is prevention—prevention of the secondary troubled emotional responses that are most disabling. The injured person and that person's family should be warned that the aftereffects of even a mild brain injury take time to clear. To prevent unnecessary and demoralizing failures during the early recovery period, the injured person's activities should be limited, the immediate environment should be structured and predictable, and the demands on his or her time and effort should be minimal.

As soon as possible after the injury, both the injured person and the family should be made aware of the nature of the problems that frequently follow a mild brain injury, and a simple explanation of the pathophysiology involved should be presented. Strategies to reduce stress and increase coping ability should be developed cooperatively with the participation of the injured person, that person's family, and the injured person's employer or teachers

when indicated (Conboy et al. 1986). Frequently, these preventive measures are sufficient to ensure an uneventful recovery. When the expected progress fails to occur, more formal psychotherapeutic intervention is indicated.

Special Therapeutic Problems

Transference and Countertransference Issues

Any significant threat to the integrity of a person's sense of self, whether caused by brain injury, abnormal brain chemistry, or some catastrophic environmental or human event, precipitates anxiety. In an effort to alleviate this anxiety, a person with a brain injury who has a compromised ability to adapt may attempt to modify or structure elements in the surrounding physical environment to increase its orderliness and therefore its predictability, thus reducing the probability that unexpected and/or unmanageable demands will arise.

For the same reason—that is, to reduce anxiety—interpersonal transactions may be managed, manipulated, interpreted, and evaluated in terms of the level of emotional stress that they provoke or alleviate. Under these circumstances, the brain-injured patient's evaluation of others' behavior during interpersonal transactions will be almost entirely based on the level of comfort that is experienced by the patient at that moment rather than reflective of the true character and motives of the other person or persons involved in these transactions. Accordingly, it should be expected that the injured person's specific attitudes and responses will stem, in most part, from earlier interpersonal experiences—that is, transference phenomena—rather than from the present circumstances. Because people who have survived a significant brain injury frequently have limited self-awareness and impaired self-monitoring abilities, potentially orienting and corrective interpersonal experiences may not be attended to or may be misinterpreted and discounted.

Psychotherapists who work with people who have had a brain injury must be alert to the fact that countertransference forces, both positive and negative, lie just below the surface of every encounter (Goldstein 1952). Such forces can lead a therapist to underestimate the severity of the patient's disabilities and overestimate the degree of recovery that reasonably can be expected after treatment. As a result, a therapist may encourage his or her patient to incorporate impossible personal goals and adopt social values that are in conflict with those of the community to which the patient eventually must return, thereby setting the stage for the patient's eventual failure.

Although it is common for the positive changes that result from *any* psychotherapeutic process to be slow in coming, an unusual level of patience is required of the psychotherapist in the treatment of patients with brain injuries because of their memory problems, inflexibility, and impaired comprehension.

Not infrequently, a patient appears to comprehend the relevance of a therapeutic exchange, but because of frontal cortex damage, he or she fails to initiate an appropriate action or, indeed, any action at all. Because the patient initially appeared to understand that there was a need to act and had repeatedly expressed his or her good intentions, inactivity and/or other "inappropriate" behaviors may be interpreted by the therapist as a lack of motivation or even as an act of rebelliousness and sabotage. When the patient does not meet the therapist's expectations, feelings of frustration and anger emerge and the quality of the therapeutic alliance begins to deteriorate. When the therapist gradually becomes aware of the wish to abandon the patient, feelings of guilt become the only "glue that"—for a short period—prevents the relationship from coming apart.

At the same time, the patient, as might be expected, is feeling hurt and confused. If expressions of pain and anger fail to communicate to the psychiatrist the depth of the patient's despair, and no improvement in the quality of the relationship is forthcoming, the patient's angry feelings can change to hate. Hate directed toward the therapist can serve as evidence for the patient that some sort of relationship continues to exist, thereby defending the patient against the possibility that he or she actually is alone (Gan 1983).

Unless the therapist can clarify what has been transpiring and can begin to redirect the process, the alliance inevitably dissolves. To avoid this state of affairs, the psychiatrist, from the very first, must work to moderate the transference–countertransference effects. Positive aspects of the transference relationship may be nurtured, but the boundaries between patient and therapist must be kept well defined. The negative aspects of both transference and countertransference reactions must be confronted and tested against reality to preserve the therapeutic alliance.

Denial

Perhaps the most striking of the many phenomena associated with brain injury is the capacity of many seriously impaired people to deny the existence of their impairments. In almost every case, several interacting factors contribute to the patient's distorted view of his or her abilities and limitations.

It is widely recognized that denial can be the direct result of brain injury. In this instance, denial is characterized by a lack of awareness or recognition of the presence and/or significance of functional impairments. This phenomenon, termed anosognosia by Babinski (1914), is reported most frequently in stroke patients who appear to be unaware of their hemiplegia and/or hemianopsia. Denial also is found in patients with cortical blindness and people with amnestic conditions (Heilman et al. 1985; McGlynn and Schacter 1989).

Many people who have experienced a TBI deny their memory deficits and the changes in their personalities (Bond 1984). In fact, people with brain injuries frequently exhibit some awareness of their physical and intellectual deficits while at the same time denying the existence of the changes in their temperament that are described by relatives and friends (Cicerone 1989; Fahy et al. 1967; Thomsen 1974). It is important to recognize that organically mediated denial is not motivated and serves no known defensive purpose for the injured person. On the other hand, so-called psychological denial is known to occur in the absence of brain injury. This kind of denial is mobilized either consciously or unconsciously in an effort to allay anxiety and/or other unpleasant affects that can arise when an individual's integrity is threatened (Beisser 1979; Cicerone 1989; Rosen 1986; Weinstein and Kahn 1955). It is probable that motivated unawareness (psychological denial) always plays some role in a patient's effort to cope with the effects of brain injury.

Although at times denial may disrupt the treatment process, several investigators have pointed out that frequently there are discrepancies between what patients say and what they do. Despite verbally denying the significance of their deficits, many patients continue to participate appropriately in prescribed treatment activities (Fordyce 1983; Tyerman and Humphrey 1984).

It is important for the therapist to distinguish between the neurogenic and psychogenic aspects of the patient's denial, and in this way to discriminate between those components that the patient is unable to change from those that he or she is unwilling to change. The management of denial is one of the most difficult problems confronting a psychiatrist who is working with TBI patients. As a rule, direct confrontation of the patient's denial is ineffective and may negatively affect the therapeutic relationship. Beisser (1979) advised that "if the physician takes an adversary stance to the patient's view, there is a risk either of the patient's compliance at the risk of his or her own integrity or opposition in the service of maintaining his or her integrity" (p. 1029). Modification of the therapeutic environment so that it supports reality in a consistent but nonthreatening manner is perhaps the most effective intervention in a situation where denial is hampering a patient's progress (Cicerone 1989; Rosen 1986).

When denial is not an immediate impediment to the patient's progress, therapy should concentrate on enabling the patient to recognize and strengthen his or her preserved assets. When the patient's sense of competence increases and self-esteem improves, the need for the protection afforded by denial will be reduced and perhaps eventually may even be eliminated. Beisser (1979) noted that "if the integrity of the person is respected, the person is more likely to move toward those aspects of reality which will serve his or her needs" (p. 1029).

Catastrophic Conditions

A person who has had a significant brain injury tends to limit both the range of his or her activities and the physical and social situations in which these activities are carried out for the purpose of keeping them manageable. If for any reason the individual's efforts to keep the elements of his or her world contained are not successful and a task must be confronted that is beyond his or her present capabilities, a catastrophic condition occurs (Goldstein 1952; Miller 1991; Prigatano 1988). The catastrophic condition was described by Goldstein (1952) in the following way:

> When the patient is unable to fulfill a task set before him…the overt behaviors [that result] appear very much the same as [they do in] a person in a state of anxiety…. In the catastrophic condition, the patient not only is incapable of performing a task which exceeds his impaired capacity but he also fails for a longer or shorter period in performances which he is able to carry out in the ordered state. (p. 255)

By a process of selective modification of behaviors and routines, people with TBI may be able to eliminate, or at least to decrease, the number of catastrophic episodes that they experience. For example, when they are threatened with the possibility of being overwhelmed, they may withdraw to reduce the number and intensity of stimuli affecting them, show a lack of interest or involvement in the task at hand or deny its relevance to their situation, question the competence and/or motives of a therapist, and ridicule other patients who have willingly worked on the same task. Usually, an injured person's defensive maneuvers are confined to words and avoidance behaviors but can escalate to physical assault if other tactics fail to reduce the stress. Therefore, as a first priority, psycho-

therapists working with this exceedingly vulnerable group of patients must strive to avoid precipitating a catastrophic condition. In particular, open-ended, anxiety-provoking comments and questions must be avoided. New concepts should be introduced gradually and in as simple a form as possible so they can be processed effectively. It is most important to avoid presenting each new task as though it constitutes another test of the injured person's abilities. If the onset of a catastrophic condition appears to be imminent, active manipulation of one or more aspects of the therapeutic situation many avert a crisis. For example, the psychiatrist can rephrase a question or a comment and/or give additional information to further clarify and simplify the patient's task. Or the patient can be presented with several possible solutions or alternative strategies that would permit the given task to be pursued more effectively. At times, it can be useful for the psychiatrist to acknowledge to the patient that explanations may have been unclear or expectations may have been unreasonably high for that point in the recovery process. Obviously, the therapist should not assume responsibility for the patient's growing anxiety unless he or she actually believes this to be the case. Ultimately, the best way to manage a catastrophic condition is to prevent it in the first place, because patients have few assets available to assist them in reestablishing their equilibrium once it has been disturbed.

Guilt, Shame, and Punishment

It is not uncommon for a person who survives significant brain trauma to experience distressing feelings of guilt and shame. If that person was the driver of a vehicle involved in a collision, and especially if he or she was drinking beforehand, the occurrence of these feelings is quite understandable. If a passenger in the vehicle was seriously injured or killed as a result of that collision, these feelings certainly are appropriate. Often, however, even when an injury is caused by a series of unavoidable events, intense feelings of guilt and shame add their weight to the injured person's already-heavy burden.

Robert Murphy, an anthropologist who was profoundly impaired as the result of a spinal cord tumor, wrote about guilt, shame, and punishment as they are experienced by seriously disabled people. What he has to say applies as well to persons who have had a significant TBI:

> The usual formula is that a wrongful act leads to a guilty conscience; if the guilt becomes publicly known, then shame must be added to the sequence, followed by punishment…. A fascinating aspect of

disability is that it dramatically and completely reverses the progression, while preserving every step. The sequence of the person damaged in body goes from punishment (the impairments) to shame, to guilt and finally to the crime. This is not a real crime but a self-delusion that lurks in our fears and fantasies; in the never articulated question, "What did I do to deserve this?" (Murphy 1987, p. 93)

This pressing question deserves a meaningful answer—one that is possible for the patient to find through the process of psychotherapy.

Stigmatization and Marginality: Society's Response to Disability

The classic model of psychotherapy starts with the assumption that the patient's problems arise from early life experiences and that, within limits, the character of the current outside world has limited impact on the patient's potential for recovery. This certainly is not the case for people who have been disabled by a TBI. They do not have a benign or even a neutral physical and social environment with which to contend during their struggle toward recovery. In effect, TBI, at one and the same time, is a condition of the injured person's body and an aspect of his or her social identity. The process is set in motion by the physical insult but is given definition and meaning by society (Murphy 1987; Thomsen 1984; Weddell et al. 1980). In fact, "very often, social relations between [people with brain injuries] and their non-injured peers are tense, awkward and problematic" (Murphy 1987, p. 86). In our society, brain injury is a condition that is deeply discrediting and stigmatizing (Goffman 1963). "By definition, the person with stigma is not quite human [and] on this assumption all varieties of discrimination are practiced through which the [injured] person's life choices are effectively reduced" (Murphy 1987, p. 6). Survivors of brain injuries may be treated as incompetent, stupid, or crazy. Frequently, they are held responsible for their conditions, for example, "He drove too fast," "She wasn't paying attention to the road conditions," or "He should have known that it is dangerous to drink and drive." In fact, many persons who have had a brain injury exist in a kind of marginal state—neither in society nor fully out of it, not sick nor entirely well—a fact that is reflected in the confusion over how they should be categorized: patient, client, or survivor? People who cannot be categorized neatly and whose behaviors are therefore not predictable tend to provoke anxiety in others (Murphy 1987; Murphy et al. 1988). Both of these qualities—not being easily cat-

egorized and being unpredictable—frequently cause people with brain injuries to be demeaned or ignored. This is an inescapable fact of life for a person with a brain injury, and its significance must not be excluded from the psychotherapeutic process.

Loneliness

Almost every person who survives a TBI, including many whose injuries are characterized as "mild," experiences periods of significant loneliness. This is not the sort of loneliness that is brought on by the breakup of a marriage, the absence of friends, or the unavailability of rewarding social activities, although certainly these situations occur with dismaying frequency after brain injury. Rather, the condition of loneliness considered here has a far more profound impact on the injured person and his or her family and friends. After a TBI, impaired cognitive function and alterations in emotional responsiveness can interfere with the injured person's ability to interact empathically with others. As a result, the injured person begins to experience the world in ways that are significantly different from those of other people. With the continued loss of meaningful interpersonal relationships, the individual begins to lose faith in the validity of his or her sense of self. In fact, the condition of intense loneliness is tantamount to a suspension in the very fashioning of identity (Becker 1962). In an understandable effort to maintain consistency in their world as well as control over it, exceedingly lonely people, brain injury survivors included, attempt to construct plausible explanations for their unhappy lives. In these efforts, there is a tendency to develop inaccurate or distorted standards for acceptable social relationships that are impossible for others to meet in a consistent fashion (Peplau et al. 1982). Then, to explain the reasons for the recurring disappointments while denying the possible sources in themselves, lonely individuals tend to evaluate the motives of others negatively, and from this paranoid thinking can follow. Psychiatrists working with survivors of a TBI who have become socially isolated should keep in mind that a sense of profound loneliness cannot be communicated verbally. Fromm-Reichmann (1959) related that "unlike other non-communicable emotional experiences, it [loneliness] cannot even be shared empathetically perhaps because the other person's empathetic abilities are obstructed by the anxiety arousing quality of its emanations" (p. 5). Lonely people, especially those who have had a brain injury, can communicate and be communicated with only in the most concrete terms; therefore, at least in its earliest phase, psychotherapy should emphasize behavior rather than words.

Meaningful communication with a lonely brain injury patient is not possible at all until some degree of that patient's isolation is breached. This may be accomplished by the psychiatrist's mere presence in the room without making demands, expecting nothing more than to be eventually accepted as a person who is there. To progress from that point, because the sense of profound loneliness is so difficult for the patient to communicate, it may be necessary for the psychiatrist to take the initiative and open the discussion about it (Fromm-Reichmann 1959).

The special therapeutic problems and the suggested therapist responses that were discussed in the preceding sections are summarized in Table 35–2.

Further Suggestions for Effective Psychotherapy

The psychotherapist must be responsive. An effective therapeutic relationship is one in which the patient's words and actions elicit appropriate and overt responses. There is no place for therapeutic passivity, open-ended questions, or nondirective comments in the treatment of individuals who have experienced significant brain injuries; nor is there room for intrusiveness or authoritarianism. Psychiatrists must be careful not to force their values and life goals on patients who, threatened as they are with further disruption of their identities, are quite vulnerable and therefore more likely to accept the therapist's values, no matter how inappropriate they may be.

The patient must be encouraged to lead the way. Whenever possible, the therapeutic endeavor should be guided by the present concerns of the patient and by what he or she believes is relevant or can accept as relevant, not by what the therapist thinks will be of greater significance for the patient at some future date. For most people, whether they have a brain injury or not, the ability to sustain attention is limited when they feel forced to attend to tasks that conflict with their present intentions in order to secure some future goal (Lichtenberg and Norton 1970). In the words of one of my own patients, "I hate it when I hear, 'It's for your own good!'" In treating patients who have experienced a brain injury, psychotherapists are limited in their ability to "tune in" fully to or empathize deeply with their patients because psychotherapists experience the world differently from their patients. For these reasons, therapists must follow the leads of their patients; only in this way can they come to understand the world in which their patients exist.

The need to follow the patient's lead applies also to practical issues such as the frequency and duration of therapy sessions and the length of the total psychotherapeutic endeavor. For example, many patients cannot attend effec-

tively for more than 15 or 20 minutes. As the information that they must process increases, they become more and more confused and fatigued. In these circumstances, patients absorb very little at best, and at worst, they may be threatened with the onset of a catastrophic condition. Usually, with improvement in their cognitive abilities, patients are able to work productively for longer periods. However, the psychiatrist must be aware of the possibility that a shift in topic or even termination of a treatment session may be necessary if such is indicated by the moment-to-moment evaluation of the patient's ability to cope.

The frequency of therapy sessions should be determined not only by the psychiatrist's appraisal of the emergent nature of the patient's problems but also by an evaluation of the patient's new learning ability. A patient with significant short-term memory difficulties may initially have to be scheduled on a daily basis to ensure carryover from treatment session to treatment session.

The length of the total therapeutic endeavor depends in large part on the patient's goals. Indeed, a significant part of the treatment involves helping the patient set appropriate goals—goals that are fashioned after the patient has become aware of both strengths and liabilities and has accepted and incorporated a new sense of self.

Group experiences are important. Every treatment program for TBI patients should include both formal and informal group experiences in addition to individual psychotherapy, because "the real world" with which they hope to reengage is composed of groups—large groups, small groups, quartets, triads, and pairs. In "the real world," no one functions in isolation; there are always others present, if only in one's memory and imagination (Pollack 1989).

People who have experienced significant brain injuries process information slowly and have difficulty attending to more than one thing at a time; consequently, high levels of anxiety can be generated when they engage in group activities. To avoid the onset of a catastrophic condition, the injured person may withdraw from the group or, if that is not possible, may express distress in an immoderate fashion. Controlled and graduated group experiences can assist patients with brain injuries in expressing their feelings appropriately and communicating their ideas effectively.

Family members should be involved in the patient's treatment. In every case of brain injury, the impact of the injury is "infectious." It affects not only the patient but also the patient's family, disrupting its integrity, disturbing the interrelatedness of its members, and tending to isolate them from each other as well as from the community at large (Brooks 1991; Lezak 1986; Thomsen 1984).

TABLE 35–2.   Special therapeutic problems and management issues

Condition	Description	Therapist response
Transference and countertransference reactions	*Transference:* Loss or threat to sense of self, limited adaptability, intolerance of anxiety; all promote the rapid development of intense transference relationships, both positive and negative in nature. *Countertransference:* Therapists' overidentification, overoptimism, impatience, inflexibility, and lack of awareness of the cognitive and emotional effects of brain injury stimulate countertransference reactions. Patients' slow progress, apparent lack of involvement and motivation, changeability, and emotional dyscontrol also contribute.	Be aware of the probability of some disruptive transference and countertransference reactions; negative transference reactions in the patient and all countertransference reactions in the psychiatrist must be confronted and resolved without delay; positive transference reactions may be supported, but the boundaries between psychiatrist and patient must be kept well defined.
Denial	Determined by several interacting factors, including the direct effect of the injury, feelings of shame and/or guilt, family attitudes, and the unconscious defenses against threats to the person's integrity (i.e., psychological denial).	Emphasize preserved intellectual and psychological assets to improve self-esteem and structure the therapeutic environment in ways that support reality; direct confrontation rarely succeeds because it further threatens the injured person's integrity (sense of self).
Catastrophic conditions	Intense anxiety occurs when patients are confronted by situations that are beyond their capacities to manage. Patients respond with withdrawal and other self-defensive measures, including reduced involvement in therapy, increased denial, and verbal—and at times physical—aggression.	Prevention is the best therapy: avoid open-ended, anxiety-provoking comments and questions; introduce new tasks or concepts gradually and in as simple a form as possible; if a catastrophic condition is imminent, provide additional information and structure; further simplify the task or discontinue the activity.
Guilt, shame, and punishment	Common responses to TBI, even when patients are entirely without responsibility for the event.	Consider the question "Why did this happen to me?" only after a stable therapeutic alliance has developed. Early reassurances are not helpful and may disturb the developing relationship.
Stigmatization and marginality	Brain injury patients are neither sick nor well, neither in society nor entirely out; their postinjury behaviors are difficult to understand and categorize; their responses may appear to be unpredictable, causing anxiety and even fear in others who tend to discredit and devalue the source of their discomfort.	Patients must be helped with dealing with the realities of an often hostile world.
Loneliness	Most common long-term residual of TBI; TBI patients have impaired abilities to respond to others empathically. Subsequent losses of meaningful relationships contribute to the further disruption of their already-disturbed sense of self; failed attempts to comprehend what has happened to their relationships and their impaired self-monitoring abilities lead to negative evaluations of the motives of other people and subsequently to paranoia.	Recognize that the sense of profound loneliness is difficult to communicate; a consistent supportive approach and a patient, nondemanding attitude can help breach the isolation. Provide practical, concrete assistance, and avoid dealing with abstract concepts.

Frequently, family members are confronted by old needs that were long thought to be outgrown and new demands that they can neither comprehend nor fulfill. In this situation, family members may feel guilty and responsible for events over which they have little control. They may then direct their anger inwardly and become self-punitive and depressed, or they may direct their feelings of frustration outwardly, seeking others in the family to blame for their pain, including the one with brain injury (Mwaria 1990).

Because the support of the family is crucial for the successful rehabilitation of the patient, each member of the therapeutic team must work to encourage ongoing healthy family interactions, not only in reference to the impaired family member but also with respect to the other members of the family and to the community.

Reasonable risk taking should be encouraged. Finally, therapists must be prepared to encourage reasonable risk taking by their patients. For this to happen, therapists must be prepared to allow and accept failure by their patients and by themselves, because the road that brain injury patients must travel to reestablish an acceptable sense of self is uncertain and therefore cannot be risk free. Without the possibility of failure, a person can never achieve true independence and the right to make choices on his or her own behalf (Banja 1988; Dybwad 1964).

References

Babinski MJ: Contribution to the study of mental disturbance in organic cerebral hemiplegia (anosognosia). Revue Neurologique 12:845–848, 1914

Banja JD: Independence and rehabilitation: a philosophic perspective. Arch Phys Med Rehabil 69:381–382, 1988

Becker E: The Birth and Death of Meaning. New York, Macmillan, 1962

Beisser AR: Denial and affirmation in illness and health. Am J Psychiatry 136:1026–1030, 1979

Bennett TL: Individual psychotherapy and minor head injury. Cognitive Rehabilitation 7:10–16, 1989

Bond M: The psychiatry of closed head injury, in Closed Head Injury. Edited by Brooks N. Oxford, England, Oxford University Press, 1984, pp 148–178

Brooks DN: The head injured family. J Clin Exp Neuropsychol 13:155–188, 1991

Cicerone KD: Psychotherapeutic interventions with traumatically brain injured patients. Rehabil Psychology 34:105–114, 1989

Conboy TJ, Barth J, Boll TJ: Treatment and rehabilitation of mild and moderate head trauma. Rehabil Psychology 31:203–215, 1986

Condeluci A, Gretz-Lasky S: Social role valorization: a model for community re-entry. J Head Trauma Rehabil 2:49–56, 1987

Dybwad G: Challenges in Mental Retardation. New York, Columbia University Press, 1964

Eames P: Behavior disorders after severe head injury: their nature and causes and strategies for management. J Head Trauma Rehabil 3:1–6, 1988

Eisenberg HM, Levin HS: Computed tomography and magnetic resonance imaging in mild to moderate head injury, in Mild Head Injuries. Edited by Levin HS, Eisenberg HM, Benton AL. New York, Oxford University Press, 1989, pp 217–228

Ellis DW: Neuropsychotherapy, in Neuropsychological Treatment After Brain Injury. Edited by Ellis DW, Christensen AL. Boston, MA, Kluwer Academic, 1989, pp 241–269

Fahy TJ, Irving MH, Millac P: Severe head injuries: a six-year follow-up. Lancet 2:475–479, 1967

Fordyce WE: Denial of disability in spinal cord injury: a behavioral perspective. Paper presented at the 91st Annual Convention of the American Psychological Association, Anaheim, CA, 1983

Fromm-Reichmann F: Loneliness. Psychiatry 22:1–15, 1959

Gan JS: Hate in the rehabilitation setting. Arch Phys Med Rehabil 64:176–179, 1983

Gardner H: The Shattered Mind: The Person After Brain Damage. New York, Knopf, 1976

Genarelli TA: Cerebral concussion and diffuse brain injuries, in Head Injury. Edited by Cooper PR. Baltimore, MD, Williams and Wilkins, 1981, pp 83–97

Goffman E: Stigma. Englewood Cliffs, NJ, Prentice-Hall, 1963

Goldstein K: The effect of brain damage on the personality. Psychiatry 15:245–260, 1952

Heilman KM, Watson RT, Valenstein E: Neglect and related disorders, in Clinical Neuropsychology, 2nd Edition. Edited by Heilman KM, Valenstein E. New York, Oxford University Press, 1985, pp 243–284

Levin HS, Eisenberg HM, Benton AL (eds): Mild Head Injuries. New York, Oxford University Press, 1989

Lewis L, Rosenberg S: Psychoanalytic psychotherapy with brain-injured adult psychiatric patients. J Nerv Ment Dis 178:69–77, 1990

Lezak MD: Subtle sequelae of brain damage: perplexity, distractibility and fatigue. Am J Phys Med 57:9–15, 1978

Lezak MD: Psychological implications of traumatic brain damage for the patient's family. Rehabil Psychology 31:241–250, 1986

Lezak MD: The walking wounded of head injury: when subtle deficits can be disabling. Trends in Rehabilitation 3:4–9, 1989

Lichtenberg P, Norton DG: Cognitive and Mental Development in the First Five Years of Life: A Review of the Recent Literature. Rockville, MD, National Institutes of Mental Health, 1970

Lishman WA: The psychiatric sequelae of head injury: a review. Psychol Med 3:304–318, 1973

Ludwig AM: Principles of Clinical Psychiatry. New York, The Free Press, 1980, pp 424–425

McColl MA, Davies D, Carlson P, et al: Transitions to independent living after ABI. Brain Inj 13:311–330, 1999

McGlynn SM, Schacter DL: Unawareness of deficits in neuropsychological syndromes. J Clin Exp Neuropsychol 11:143–205, 1989

McKenna P, Haste E: Clinical effectiveness of dramatherapy in the recovery from neuro-trauma. Disabil Rehabil 21:162–174, 1999

Miller L: Psychotherapy of the brain-injured patient: principles and practices. Cognitive Rehabil 9:24–30, 1991

Murphy RF: The Body Silent. New York, Henry Holt, 1987, pp 6, 85–110

Murphy RF, Scheer J, Murphy Y, et al: Physical disability and social liminality: a study in the rituals of adversity. Soc Sci Med 26:235–242, 1988

Mwaria CB: The concept of self in the context of crisis: a study of families of the severely brain injured. Soc Sci Med 30:889–893, 1990

Peplau LA, Miceli M, Morasch B: Loneliness and self-evaluation, in Loneliness: A Source Book of Current Theory, Research, and Therapy. Edited by Peplau LA, Perlman D. New York, Wiley, 1982, pp 135–151

Piotrowski Z: The Rorschach ink blot method in organic disturbances of the central nervous system. J Nerv Ment Dis 86:525–537, 1937

Pollack IW: Traumatic brain injury and the rehabilitation process: a psychiatric perspective, in Neuropsychological Treatment After Brain Injury. Edited by Ellis DW, Christensen AL. Boston, MA, Kluwer Academic, 1989, pp 105–125

Pollack IW: Reestablishing an acceptable sense of self, in Educational Dimensions of Acquired Brain Injury. Edited by Savage RC, Wolcott GE. Austin, TX, Pro Ed, 1994, pp 303–317

Prigatano GP: Neuropsychological Rehabilitation After Brain Injury. Baltimore, MD, Johns Hopkins University Press, 1986

Prigatano GP: Neuropsychological deficits, personality variables and outcome, in Community Re-Entry for Head Injured Adults. Edited by Ylvisaker M, Gobble ER. Boston, MA, College Hill, 1987, pp 1–23

Prigatano GP: Emotion and motivation in recovery and adaptation after brain damage, in Brain Injury and Recovery. Edited by Finger S, Levere TE, Almi CR, et al. New York, Plenum, 1988, pp 335–350

Prigatano GP: Work, love and play after brain injury. Bull Menninger Clin 53:414–431, 1989

Rice-Oxley M, Turner-Stokes L: Effectiveness of brain injury rehabilitation. Clin Rehabil 13 (suppl 1):7–24, 1999

Rimel RW, Giordani B, Barth JT, et al: Disability caused by minor head injury. Neurosurgery 9:221–228, 1981

Rosen M: Denial and the head trauma client: a developmental formulation and treatment plan. Cognitive Rehabil 4:20–22, 1986

Rutherford W: Post concussional symptoms, in Mild Head Injuries. Edited by Levin HS, Eisenberg HM, Benton AL. New York, Oxford University Press, 1989, pp 217–228

Silver JM, Hales RE, Yudofsky SC: Neuropsychiatric aspects of traumatic brain injury, in American Psychiatric Press Textbook of Neuropsychiatry, 2nd Edition. Edited by Yudofsky SC, Hales RE. Washington, DC, American Psychiatric Press, 1992, pp 363–395

Stein DG: In pursuit of new strategies for understanding recovery from brain damage: problems and perspectives, in Clinical Neuropsychology and Brain Function. Edited by Boll T, Bryant B. Washington, DC, American Psychological Association, 1988, pp 9–55

Stensrud C, Mishkin L, Craft C, et al: The use of drama techniques in cognitive rehabilitation. Therapeutic Recreation Journal 21:2nd Quarter, 1987

Stuewe-Portnoff G: Loneliness: lost in the landscape of meaning. J Psychol 122:545–555, 1988

Thomsen IV: The patient with severe head injury and his family. Scand J Rehabil Med 6:180–183, 1974

Thomsen IV: Late outcome of very severe head trauma: 10–15 year second follow-up. J Neurol Neurosurg Psychiatry 47:260–268, 1984

Tyerman A, Humphrey M: Changes in self-concept following severe head injury. Int J Rehabil Res 7:11–23, 1984

Weddell R, Oddy M, Jenkins D: Social adjustment after rehabilitation: a two year follow-up of patients with severe head injury. Psychol Med 10:257–263, 1980

Weinstein EA, Kahn RL: Denial of Illness. Springfield, IL, Charles C Thomas, 1955

36 Cognitive Rehabilitation

Wayne A. Gordon, Ph.D.

Mary R. Hibbard, Ph.D.

What Is Cognitive Rehabilitation?

Many terms are used to describe treatments provided to individuals with brain injury to ameliorate their cognitive deficits. For example, *cognitive remediation*, *cognitive rehabilitation*, and *cognitive retraining* commonly are used to describe interventions focused on post–brain injury cognitive impairments. However, the distinctive and different meanings of these terms are not always recognized or maintained. Diller and Gordon (1981b) and Gordon (1987) define cognitive remediation as a "constellation of procedures that are used by a neuropsychologist to provide patients with skills and strategies needed for the performance of tasks that are difficult and/or impossible for them to complete because of the existence of cognitive deficits." In contrast, they describe cognitive rehabilitation as the delivery of the wide array of services provided to a person with a brain injury by the rehabilitation team. The implications of these definitional distinctions are several:

- The primary focus of rehabilitation efforts in working with people with brain injury is the improvement of cognitive function. Thus, cognitive remediation is a component of cognitive rehabilitation, because it is an intervention delivered by one or more members of the rehabilitation team.
- Cognitive remediation is an intervention that is individualized to fit the specific needs of each patient.
- Cognitive remediation is a service that is usually delivered by a clinical neuropsychologist or a rehabilitation

psychologist. However, other members of the rehabilitation team (e.g., speech pathologists and occupational therapists) can provide this service.

Klonoff et al. (1989) defined cognitive retraining as "those activities that improve a brain-injured person's higher cerebral functioning or help patients to better understand the nature of those difficulties while teaching him or her methods of compensation." Although in reality little difference exists between the terms (and practice) of cognitive remediation and cognitive retraining, only cognitive remediation has been assigned a Current Procedural Terminology code, and, as a result, it has become the primary descriptor of this type of service.

Mateer and Raskin (1999) have further added to the nomenclature by suggesting that cognitive interventions can be classified as environmental modifications, compensatory approaches, or direct interventions. They describe environmental modifications as interventions that alter the person's external world, not involving any changes in the "individual's underlying capacities." They cite as examples the provision of extra time to complete a task or the use of external cue systems. Compensatory approaches are those that require the acquisition of new behaviors or skills. For example, learning the use of organizers and list keeping are examples of this category of cognitive interventions. Mateer and Raskin define direct interventions as procedures designed to improve an underlying cognitive ability. Attention Process Training (Sohlberg and Mateer 1989) is an example of this latter approach. The relative effectiveness of these three cate-

The preparation of this manuscript was supported in part by grant #H133B980013 from the National Institute on Disability and Rehabilitation Research, U.S. Department of Education.

gories of treatment has not been well studied. Thus, although these distinctions between approaches to cognitive intervention may be of some theoretical or heuristic value, because the goal of such interventions is ultimately the restoration of impaired cognitive function, their differentiation may be of little functional utility.

In this discussion of labels and definitions, the point must also be addressed that cognitive remediation and rehabilitation are sometimes confused with cognitive therapy. Cognitive therapy is a form of psychotherapy developed by Beck and his colleagues (Beck et al. 1979), which was designed to treat affective disorders such as depression and anxiety in individuals without cognitive impairments. This approach, called *cognitive-behavioral therapy* (CBT), has been adapted for use with individuals who are post-stroke (Hibbard et al. 1990a, 1990b). The efficacy of CBT has not been systematically examined in individuals with traumatic brain injury (TBI). In adapting CBT to individuals who are post-stroke, Hibbard et al. (1990a, 1990b) suggest that cognitive remediation should be incorporated as a component of treatment so that the person's cognitive deficits do not interfere with his or her ability to profit from this form of psychotherapeutic treatment.

Does Cognitive Remediation Work?

The variety of interventions to treat specific post–brain injury cognitive deficits was developed on the basis of research that began early in the 1970s. These studies provided documentation that individuals who are post-stroke are able to relearn cognitive tasks and that their learning style is lawful and not different from individuals without a brain injury (Ben-Yishay et al. 1971, 1974). Studies on the efficacy of treatment programs for specific cognitive deficits began appearing in the late 1970s (see Diller and Gordon 1981a, 1981b, for a discussion of this literature). In addition, several review papers have been published on this topic (Ben-Yishay and Diller 1993; Gordon 1990; Gordon and Hibbard 1991, 1992; Gordon et al. 1989; Mateer and Raskin 1999; Prigatano 1999). The rapid development of brain injury rehabilitation programs mirrored the development of this new form of rehabilitation therapy. Indeed, by the early 1990s, 95% of brain injury rehabilitation programs were providing some form of cognitive rehabilitation or remediation (Mazmanian et al. 1993).

Approaches have been developed to remediate the most commonly recognized cognitive difficulties experienced by individuals with brain injury: in attention and concentration, memory, executive functions, visual per-

ception, and language abilities and pragmatics. Two reviews have been published on the evaluation of these interventions (Carney et al. 1999; Cicerone et al. 2000). Carney et al. reviewed 32 studies on the efficacy of cognitive rehabilitation. Although their review did not specifically examine the impact of interventions on the specific domains of cognitive function being treated, the authors concluded, in general, that "compensatory strategies…improve the functional abilities of individuals with traumatic brain injury" and that cognitive interventions must be delivered within the context of a broader program. Cicerone et al. reviewed 171 papers that were classified into one of the following groups: 1) prospective, randomized controlled trials; 2) prospective cohort studies, retrospective case-control studies, or well-designed clinical studies; or 3) clinical studies without concurrent control subjects or studies with appropriate single-case methodology. They concluded that "Overall, support exists for the effectiveness of several forms of cognitive rehabilitation for persons with stroke and traumatic brain injury." Specific program efficacy was found for programs focused on remediation of language deficits after left hemisphere stroke, visual perceptual problems after right hemisphere stroke, and problems with attention, memory, functional communication, and executive deficits after TBI.

In their review, Cicerone et al. (2000) provided specific recommendations on the utility of various techniques that have been developed to improve function in each of the cognitive domains reviewed (e.g., visual perception, attention and concentration, and memory). Computer-based training was not recommended as a means of improving unilateral inattention or memory. Gordon and Hibbard (1991) have discussed several reasons why the outcomes of computer-assisted or computer-provided programs of cognitive remediation may be less than desired, including stimuli not being sufficiently compelling to engage adults; inflexibility of the programs, in terms of either the speed of stimulus presentation or the participant's speed of response; limitations in the number of training trials at each level of task difficulty; the absence of human interaction in the provision of treatment and feedback; and the lack of generalization of computer skills to everyday functional activities.

More recently, Park and Ingles (2001) published a meta-analysis of research on the effectiveness of attention training for individuals with acquired brain injury. A unique aspect of this review is that it separately examines the studies seeking to improve impaired cognitive function versus those attempting to teach specific functional skills. Sohlberg and Mateer's Attention Process Training (1989) is cited as an example of the former type of training, and Kewman et al.'s (1985) study of driver training is cited as an example of the latter. Park and Ingles found that skill training was more effective than training designed to improve cognitive function. They note further that the extent of the impact of skill training is equivalent to that associated with the effects of psychotherapy (i.e., approximately two-thirds of those receiving treatment improve, and about one-third of those not receiving treatment improve as well). The authors observe that learning does not generalize to tasks that are dissimilar to the skill being trained. In addition, they coined the phrase "neuropsychological scaffolding" to describe the layering of competencies needed to acquire complex skills and the division of complex tasks and skills into their simpler components. Thus, they were echoing the suggestions of others, several years earlier (Ben-Yishay et al. 1985; Diller and Gordon 1981b; Gordon and Hibbard 1992; Whyte 1986).

Does Time Since Injury Play a Role in the Efficacy of Cognitive Remediation?

A question frequently asked about cognitive remediation is whether length of time since injury plays a role in the person's ability to profit from intervention. Most research on cognitive remediation has involved individuals at least 1 year postinjury, when they are expected to be neurologically stable. The approach of focusing on individuals many months or years postinjury has been taken so that potential effects of spontaneous recovery of function is eliminated as a possible alternative explanation for functional improvement. Hence, the issue of duration post-TBI has not been directly examined in any of the studies in the literature.

Indeed, given the lack of empirical evidence, there is no reason based in theory to expect that cognitive remediation provided early in the course of recovery would be any more or less effective than intervention provided at a later point. In other words, cognitive remediation is not expected to augment or otherwise interact with the process of spontaneous neurological recovery.

Because length of time since injury has not been related theoretically or concretely to a person's ability to profit from treatment, time since injury should not be a barrier to a person's receiving services, even if the person is several years postinjury. Indeed, it has been our experience that people who initiate treatment many years postinjury improve, because perhaps, like the rest of us, they never stop learning. However, those who initiate treatment many years postinjury might be more difficult to engage because they may need to unlearn "bad habits"

that may have been picked up along the way, and they are likely to be less aware of the pervasive impact of brain injury on everyday function.

Does Severity of Injury Play a Role in the Efficacy of Cognitive Remediation?

The nature of the interaction between severity of brain injury and the ability to profit from cognitive remediation, although not specifically studied, may be inferred from research and clinical experience:

- Ben-Yishay et al. (1970) found that the number of cues required to pass previously failed block designs was related to initial competence. Thus, it takes as many cues for a person who passes four designs to pass the fifth as it does for a person who passes nine designs to pass the tenth. Ability to profit from retraining was not related to the person's initial level of impairment.
- Comprehensive outpatient rehabilitation programs are designed primarily for individuals who sustain moderate to severe brain injuries. The fact that these types of programs have been found to be effective suggests that positive outcomes of treatment are not limited by the severity of injury.
- The rate at which a person is able to relearn or acquire new information is affected by the severity of injury because the brain mediates all learning. Thus, one would expect that individuals with more severe injuries would have a slower rate of learning, thus necessitating longer periods of treatment.

Why Is a Neuropsychological Evaluation a Key Component of Cognitive Remediation?

Neuropsychological evaluation forms the basis for cognitive remediation because it provides information that describes the nature and extent of the impairment across domains of cognitive function (i.e., what domains of function are impaired and how impaired they are). It can validate the patient's self-report of functional difficulties experienced in everyday activities. Statements about the extent of impairment are based on normative data for each test as well as estimates of the person's level of function before the onset of the brain injury. The neuropsychological assessment provides the diagnostic rationale, hierarchy, and scope for the planned intervention. For example, if a person has both attention and memory disturbances, the attention difficulty would be treated first because it may be the basis for the observed memory deficit (i.e., information that is not encoded cannot be recalled). Similarly, when designing treatment for a memory disorder, the neuropsychological evaluation helps determine if memory skills across visual and verbal domains are uniform and how the nature of the stimulus (e.g., simple or complex, contextual or noncontextual) affects the person's ability to learn and recall new information. Finally, neuropsychological evaluation provides a means of describing the efficacy or the outcome of the intervention.

Do Patients Maintain Gains That They Have Made After Treatment Has Ended?

An issue that was not addressed in the literature is whether gains made in treatment are maintained over time. It has been our clinical experience that "booster treatments" are essential to help the patient maintain and use cognitive skills and techniques accrued during the course of treatment. Any number of life events suggest the need for booster sessions For example, changes in the environment (loss of a job, starting a new job, promotion, demotion, marriage, divorce, birth of a child) or psycho-stressors (increase in depression or anxiety, health changes) are typical times when patients need a brief series of sessions to help them adapt to life changes. After achieving some success in community reentry, some patients begin to think that they are "all better" and no longer need to use the compensatory strategies that they have learned. These individuals begin to fail and often return to treatment to confront (again) their losses, rekindle their use of compensatory tools, and once again rebuild their lives. Thus, individuals completing treatment need to be informed of the common need for brief follow-up sessions and encouraged to contact their therapist should there be a significant change in their home or community situation and/or social support. In our day-treatment program, we have initiated a monthly session that is open (without cost) to current and former participants in our program. The program is a huge success, with anywhere from 20–40 patients attending the group-sharing session each month. We use these booster sessions as a way of helping patients maintain social contact with other graduates, but, more important, for staff to "take the pulse" of the graduates and evaluate their community reentry levels. These follow-up meetings also serve as a reminder to past and present participants that staff members are there "for the duration" as well as a source of encouragement to maintain use of compensatory tools in the community.

Are Holistic or Comprehensive Rehabilitation Programs Successful?

In the 1980s, Ben-Yishay et al. (1985) developed a day-treatment program for individuals with TBI. Prigatano (1999) refers to this type of program as a *Holistic Neuropsychological Rehabilitation Program*, which is characterized by a combination of individual and group treatments, interweaving cognitive remediation and psychotherapeutic interventions. Individual treatments often include psychotherapy, cognitive remediation, and speech therapy. Group treatments focus on psychotherapy as well as on cognitive and social skill-building sessions designed to increase awareness, improve cognitive function, and increase self-acceptance and pragmatics (i.e., understanding social communication and improving overall communication skills). The programs often are operated as therapeutic communities and include vocational rehabilitation as a major component. Typically, comprehensive programs meet four to five times a week for several hours each day. The duration of participation in these programs ranges from several months to years.

A number of studies have examined the efficacy of these programs. Prigatano et al. (1984) reported that individuals with TBI participating in a holistic program were more likely to return to work and were more emotionally stable than a group of similar patients in an untreated control group. On 1-year follow-up, Ben-Yishay et al. (1985) reported that 50% of the program participants had returned to work, a finding in sharp contrast to those of Scherzer (1986), who reported that 69% of program participants were unemployed at follow-up. Prigatano (1999) suggests that these paradoxical findings are the result of insufficient amounts of individual and group psychotherapy received by patients in Scherzer's program. As a result, participants had insufficient opportunity to examine and work through their awareness and adjustment issues. More recently, Salazar et al. (2000) reported that a comprehensive day-treatment program facilitated the return to active military duty of the most severely brain-injured participants in their program. Similarly, Malec (2001) reported that participation in a comprehensive day-treatment program was more likely to have a positive impact on staff perceptions of program participants' social participation than of their cognitive function. Given these findings, it is not surprising that the review by Cicerone et al. (2000) of these holistic programs concluded that they resulted in a reduction in disability and improvements in both neuropsychological and psychosocial function.

Why Are Comprehensive Programs Effective?

Several reasons may be suggested to explain the effectiveness of these programs. First, comprehensive programs begin with a neuropsychological evaluation that forms the basis of individualized interventions provided, including cognitive remediation and all psychotherapeutic services. The assessment delineates the person's pattern of strengths and weaknesses, relating this constellation of findings to the day-to-day functioning of the person assessed. A neuropsychological evaluation is crucial to determining the cognitive deficits that need to be treated, the order of treatment, and the way a given treatment regimen should be tailored to meet the person's interests and background. Thus, each person is provided an individualized program of remediation that is consistent with his or her particular pattern of deficits as well as with the context of the person's values and concerns.

A second reason that comprehensive rehabilitation programs are successful is that treatment is provided hierarchically. Park and Ingles (2001) referred to this as the "neuropsychological scaffolding" of treatment. This approach to learning has been previously described by Whyte (1986) and Gordon (1990) and is based on the premise that learning proceeds in a logical fashion and that more complex forms of learning are based on an individual's achieving a solid foundation of interrelated skills at a less complex level. In other words, learning higher-level skills is introduced into treatment only after a foundation has been reestablished by the successful acquisition of more basic skills.

A third reason these programs are successful is because they include as integral components intensive individual and group psychotherapy. Psychotherapeutic interventions are needed in a comprehensive program to educate the person about his or her behavioral and cognitive challenges and, most important, to enhance the person's awareness of how these difficulties interfere with interpersonal relationships and everyday functioning. Psychotherapeutic interventions create an environment in which the person is able to confront issues of depression, agitation, aggression, disinhibition, perseveration, and other behavioral disturbances as they emerge, facilitating adjustment and increasing awareness. Thus, in people with (or without) brain injury, awareness of the

difficulties being treated is an essential element in any intervention aimed at a specific difficulty. Cognitive remediation in isolation of psychotherapy is doomed to failure if the person lacks adequate awareness of the day-to-day manifestations of his or her post-TBI cognitive and behavioral impairments and, instead, does an "end run" by viewing such problems as a normal aspect of daily life. Thus, cognitive remediation and psychotherapy must proceed hand in hand for either to be effective.

In individuals without brain injury, psychotherapy is often a long-term process; in individuals with brain injury, reduced cognitive function, in concert with the person's self-protective defense mechanisms, make this process even longer. Imagine how reduced memory, attention, processing speed, and executive functions wreak havoc with psychotherapy's assumption of the accumulation of session-to-session insights. Instead, for awareness to take hold, a constant repetition of information is required. Thus, the need for increasing awareness while simultaneously treating the cognitive and behavioral manifestations of brain injury translates to holistic treatment being a long-term process, lasting several months or even years. In sum, several factors make holistic programs effective:

- Holistic programs individualize the process of cognitive remediation and focus on the generalization of learning to relevant situations in the person's environment.
- They include long-term psychoeducation designed to increase the person's knowledge of the brain and how the person's brain injury interacts with his or her day-to-day function.
- Individual and group psychotherapy is a key component, designed to increase the person's self-awareness as well as to address other interpersonal issues.

Not all patients need the services provided by holistic programs, and not all facilities can afford to provide these programs. In these situations, individualized treatment programs should be provided to patients. The review paper by Cicerone et al. (2000) provides references for programs that have been effective in treating the range of cognitive impairments (e.g., visual perception, memory, and attention). Review of this material will provide the practitioner with information needed to implement the appropriate treatment program. When implementing these programs, clinicians need to be sure that they take into account the three factors (summarized in the preceding list) that are crucial to the effectiveness of holistic programs: focus on generalization to real-life situations and include psychoeducation and psychotherapy. These elements are crucial to the success of any program of cognitive remediation, be it holistic or one-to-one.

Conclusion

Both cognitive rehabilitation and cognitive remediation are relatively new options that have been added to the array of rehabilitation services offered to individuals with brain injury. To be successful, they must be embedded in an appropriate context, be delivered systematically and creatively, and be individualized to fit the unique cognitive and psychotherapeutic needs of each individual. The process of treatment is intense, lengthy, and demanding of both the program participant and the rehabilitation team. However, the benefits are clear, both in evaluation studies and in anecdotes, that these services are helping persons to regain lives by remediating deficits, building on strengths, and helping them adjust to the many challenges of living with a TBI.

References

Beck AT, Rush AJ, Shaw BF, et al: Cognitive Therapy of Depression. New York, Guilford, 1979

Ben-Yishay Y, Diller L: Cognitive remediation in traumatic brain injury: update and issues. Arch Phys Med Rehabil 74:204–213, 1993

Ben-Yishay Y, Diller L, Gerstman L, et al: Relationship between initial competence and ability to profit from cues in brain damaged individuals. J Abnorm Psychol 75:248–259, 1970

Ben-Yishay Y, Diller L, Mandelberg I, et al: Similarities and differences in block design performance between older normal and brain injured persons: a task analysis. J Abnorm Psychol 78:17–25, 1971

Ben-Yishay Y, Diller L, Mandelberg I, et al: Differences in matching persistence behavior during block design performance between older normal and brain-damaged persons: a process analysis. Cortex 10:121–132, 1974

Ben-Yishay Y, Rattok J, Lakin P, et al: Neuropsychological rehabilitation: quest for a holistic approach. Semin Neurol 5:252–258, 1985

Carney N, Chesnut RM, Maynard H, et al: Effect of cognitive rehabilitation on outcomes for persons with traumatic brain injury: a systematic review. J Head Trauma Rehabil 14:277–307, 1999

Cicerone KD, Dahlberg C, Kalmar K, et al: Evidence-based cognitive rehabilitation: recommendations for clinical practice. Arch Phys Med Rehabil 81:1596–1614, 2000

Diller L, Gordon WA: Interventions for cognitive deficits in brain-injured adults. J Consult Clin Psychol 49:822–834, 1981a

Diller L, Gordon WA: Rehabilitation and clinical neuropsychology, in Handbook of Clinical Neuropsychology. Edited by Filskov S, Boll T. New York, Wiley, 1981b, pp 702–733

Gordon WA: Methodological considerations in cognitive remediation, in Neuropsychological Rehabilitation. Edited by Meir M, Diller L, Benton A. London, England, Churchill Livingston, 1987, pp 111–131

Gordon WA: Cognitive remediation: an approach to the amelioration of behavioral disorders, in Neurobehavioral Sequelae of Traumatic Brain Injury. Edited by Wood RL. London, England, Taylor and Francis, 1990, pp 175–193

Gordon WA, Hibbard MR: The theory and practice of cognitive remediation, in Cognitive Rehabilitation for Persons With Traumatic Brain Injury. Edited by Kreutzer JS, Wehman P. Baltimore, MD, Paul Brooks, 1991, pp 13–22

Gordon WA, Hibbard MR: Critical issues in cognitive remediation. Neuropsychology 6:361–370, 1992

Gordon WA, Hibbard MR, Kreutzer JS: Cognitive remediation: issues in research and practice. J Head Trauma Rehabil 4:76–84, 1989

Hibbard MR, Grober SE, Gordon WA, et al: Cognitive therapy and the treatment of post-stroke depression. Topics in Geriatric Rehabilitation 5:43–55, 1990a

Hibbard MR, Grober SE, Gordon WA, et al: Modification of cognitive psychotherapy for the treatment of post-stroke depression. The Behavior Therapist 1:15–17, 1990b

Kewman DG, Seigerman C, Kinter H, et al: Simulation training of psychomotor skills: teaching the brain-injured to drive. Rehabil Psychol 30:11–27, 1985

Klonoff PS, O'Brien KP, Prigatano GP, et al: Cognitive retraining after traumatic brain injury. J Head Trauma Rehabil 4:37–45, 1989

Kreutzer JS, Gordon WA, Wehman P: Cognitive remediation following traumatic brain injury. Rehabil Psychol 34:117–129, 1989

Malec JF: Impact of comprehensive day treatment on societal participation for persons with acquired brain injury. Arch Phys Med Rehabil 82:885–895, 2001

Mateer CA, Raskin S: Cognitive rehabilitation, in Rehabilitation of the Adult and Child With Traumatic Brain Injury. Edited by Rosenthal M, Griffith E, Kreutzer JS, Pentland B. Philadelphia, PA, FA Davis, 1999, pp 254–270

Mazmanian PE, Kreutzer JS, Devany CW, et al: A survey of accredited and other rehabilitation facilities: education, training and cognitive rehabilitation in brain injury programmes. Brain Inj 7:319–331, 1993

Park NW, Ingles JL: Effectiveness of attention rehabilitation after an acquired brain injury: a meta-analysis. Neuropsychology 15:199–210, 2001

Prigatano GP: Principles of Neuropsychological Rehabilitation. New York, Oxford University Press, 1999

Prigatano GP, Fordyce DJ, Zeiner HK, et al: Neuropsychological rehabilitation after closed head injury in young adults. J Neurol Neurosurg Psychiatry 47:505–513, 1984

Salazar AM, Warden DL, Schwab K, et al: Cognitive rehabilitation for traumatic brain injury: a randomized trial. JAMA 283:3075–3081, 2000

Scherzer BP: Rehabilitation following severe head trauma: results of a three-year program. Arch Phys Med Rehabil 67:366–374, 1986

Sohlberg MM, Mateer C: Introduction to Cognitive Rehabilitation: Theory and Practice. New York, Guilford, 1989

Whyte J: Outcome evaluation in the remediation of attention and memory deficits. J Head Trauma Rehabil 1:64–71, 1986

37 Behavioral Treatment

Patrick W. Corrigan, Psy.D.

Patricia A. Bach, Ph.D.

IN ADDITION TO the various neuropathological, cognitive, personality, and mood changes that follow traumatic brain injury (TBI), severe and acute insult to the central nervous system typically results in discrete behavioral problems that often wreak major disruption on a person's quality of life. Behavior problems prevent some persons with a TBI from returning to work and home, engaging in recreational and leisure activities, and initiating and maintaining positive social relationships (Lovell and Starratt 1994). Some of these behavior problems spontaneously remit as the immediate impact of the injury subsides. Other behavioral problems diminish because alternate treatment modalities (e.g., neurosurgery and psychopharmacology) are effective in remediating the pronounced cognitive and physical sequelae of TBI. Some behavior problems may arise or be maintained, or both, by the treatment environment itself. Persons with TBI may experience disorientation and confusion and subsequently find the treatments and procedures used in the rehabilitation setting confusing and aversive. The person with TBI may then attempt to avoid and escape procedures, and such avoidance behaviors are viewed negatively and interfere with treatment (Mozzoni and Hartnedy 2000). Whatever their origin, many behavior problems observed in persons with TBI do not ameliorate easily and therefore require use of strategic behavioral interventions. The form of these behavioral problems and appropriate intervention strategies are outlined in this chapter.

Behavioral Problems of TBI

Although anatomical, physiological, psychophysiological, and cognitive consequences of TBI have been well documented, few studies have examined the behavioral and psychosocial correlates of brain injury. Several investigations have shown that the greatest postinjury deficits occur in the psychosocial domains (Adams et al. 1985; Klonoff et al. 1986; Tellier et al. 1990; Thomsen 1984). Applied behavior management has been shown to be effective in ameliorating behavioral problems in a variety of settings (Benson Yody et al. 2001) and populations, including children and adults with serious mental illness, developmental disabilities, skills deficits, and brain injuries. However, research on behavioral interventions with individuals with TBI is lacking because of difficulty establishing internal validity of treatments, experimental control, and subject homogeneity. Nevertheless, research suggests that clinical methods based on sound behavioral principles are transferable across settings and populations. Furthermore, case studies and single-subject research designs (Ducharme 2000) suggest strategies that can be used to understand behavioral difficulties in persons with TBI. Behavioral interventions applied after thorough assessment are individualized and strategies for increasing or decreasing a particular behavior are developed. Intervention strategies are developed ideographically on the basis of the function of a particular behavior rather than being determined by the more global description of a particular problem, disorder, or condition.

Behavioral problems have been represented dichotomously, either as a significant decrease in the frequency of appropriate target behaviors or as an increase in inappropriate behaviors. Using this distinction, the range of behavioral deficits that an individual with TBI might show is outlined in Table 37–1. Patients with large prosocial and self-care skill deficits as well as pronounced antisocial behaviors experience a more tortuous route to recovery, including longer stays in the hospital.

TABLE 37–1.   Behavioral deficits in individuals with traumatic brain injury

Aggressive behaviors

    Biting

    Spitting

    Yelling

    Harming self

    Scratching

    Swearing

    Hitting or kicking others

Self-care skills

    Diminished sleeping

    Diminished eating

    Does not wash

    Does not brush teeth

    Does not comb hair

    Does not feed self

    Does not clean clothes

    Does not make bed

    Does not keep area clean

Interpersonal skills

    Poor basic conversation skills

    Poor assertion skills

    Inability to complete tasks in a timely manner

    Lethargic and disinterested

    Unmotivated

Coping skills

    Refusing medications

    Unable to problem solve

    Poor response to stressors

Cognitive-related skills

    Poor attention and concentration

    Poor memory and learning

    Poor social comprehension

    Diminished reading and writing skills

Lack of Awareness of Behavioral Problems

Despite the breadth and severity of behavioral problems, research has shown that individuals with TBI often overestimate their behavioral competency compared with reports from their relatives (Prigatano 1999; Prigatano and Altman 1990; Sunderland et al. 1983; Sunderland et al. 1984; see Chapter 19, Awareness of Deficits). In fact, unawareness of deficits is a problem shown by 40% of patients after severe TBI (Oddy et al. 1985). Although some individuals are completely unaware of their deficits, others may be partially aware of their impairments but unable to describe exactly how their functioning has changed. The vague sense that something is wrong can lead to frustration and confusion, which may impede treatment compliance.

The cause of this deficit in awareness is unclear. Findings from two investigations have suggested that neglect of deficits is related to extent and severity of injury (Levin et al. 1982; Prigatano and Altman 1990). Family members also tend to initially deny the seriousness of some problems (Miller and Borden 1994) and may be more supportive when the injured individual ignores his or her injury and reports, "I will be back to my old self soon."

Research suggests a reciprocal relationship between problem unawareness and treatment outcome (McGlynn 1990). Individuals demonstrating an unawareness syndrome show diminished motivation and interest in treatment (Prigatano and Fordyce 1986), are less likely to comply with behavioral prescriptions (Cicerone and Tupper 1986), and frequently set unrealistic therapy goals (Ben-Yishay et al. 1985). To diminish problems related to treatment compliance, Fordyce and colleagues (Fordyce and Roueche 1986; Prigatano and Fordyce 1986) tested an awareness training program that targets appreciation of the consequences of injury. Awareness training includes 1) education regarding the impact of TBI, 2) self-monitoring of behaviors that staff believe have been affected by the injury, and 3) videotaped feedback of targeted inappropriate behaviors. Results of an evaluation of awareness training showed that approximately one-half of a sample of individuals with TBI who were misperceiving their level of deficits significantly improved awareness after participating in the training program (Fordyce and Roueche 1986).

Models of Behavioral Rehabilitation

Several models of behavioral rehabilitation have been developed to treat individuals with neuropsychiatric disorders and are summarized in Table 37–2. Most of these models have not been tested in terms of treatment outcome per se. Rather, they serve as heuristic guidelines for the development and future evaluation of rehabilitation programs. The integrative model situates behavioral rehabilitation among relatively disparate professional

TABLE 37–2. Conceptual models of behavioral rehabilitation for the individual with traumatic brain injury

Model (study)	Strengths
Integrative (Diller and Gordon 1981)	Combines strategies of neuropsychological assessment, neurological laboratory tests, and behavior intervention
Evaluative (Glasgow et al. 1977; Lewinsohn et al. 1977)	Uses neuropsychological data to develop and evaluate behavioral treatment plans
Recovery (Gazzaniga 1974)	Defines impact of behavioral intervention in terms of neurological models of recovery
Two-phase developmental (Passler 1987)	Combines strategies used for developmentally delayed patients with behavior modification
Process (Corrigan et al. 1990)	Bases interventions on processes that might cause behavioral deficits and excesses

perspectives that define the problems of individuals with TBI differently; the neurologist's definition of trauma is in terms of neuroanatomical foci and physiological sequelae, the neuropsychologist's perspective is based on test results that point to behavioral and cognitive deficits associated with the injury, and the behaviorist's treatment plan is based on targeting behavior problems (Diller and Gordon 1981). The integrative view developed out of the professional consensus regarding the need for blending what had previously been the independent domains of each profession (Horton and Miller 1984; Horton and Sautter 1986; Horton and Wedding 1984). According to this view, optimal behavioral plans are those that include insights into the localization of the brain injury and the cognitive and emotional sequelae of the localized insult.

Lewinsohn and colleagues developed a similar model of behavioral rehabilitation (Lewinsohn et al. 1977; Glasgow et al. 1977). According to the evaluative model, the information from neuropsychological assessment was used as a template for developing behavioral plans. Subsequent evaluations then served as feedback information to help determine successes and failures of the behavioral plan vis-à-vis this template and to titrate individual strategies accordingly. The behavioral plan and evaluative feedback loop began in a well-controlled laboratory setting and were transferred to the "real world" as limitations to the generalizability of treatment strategies were worked out.

Gazzaniga (1974, 1978) believed that behavioral strategies augmented remaining neural and cognitive pro-

cesses that led to the individual's recovery; his view was based on anatomical and physiological evidence regarding the natural recovery process after injury. Hence, behavioral strategies served as prosthetics that the individual with TBI might adopt to perform everyday interpersonal and self-care skills. For example, just as individuals without a leg are able to walk with the assistance of artificial limbs and crutches, so persons who have difficulty resolving interpersonal conflicts are able to reconcile these difficulties by using a behavioral aid such as the steps of problem solving (D'Zurilla 1986).

Many studies (Warschausky et al. 1999) have likened the behavioral deficits of many individuals with TBI to the problems of developmentally delayed individuals. On the basis of this similarity, Passler (1987) proposed a two-phase developmental rehabilitation program, with the first phase focusing on an individual's developmental limitations as assessed with, for example, the Kaufman Developmental Scale (Kaufman 1975). A developmental stimulation program based on the Kaufman Developmental Scale outlined a series of graded tasks that were progressively more demanding in developmental abilities. For example, tasks for an initial developmental profile for gross motor activity included jumping off the ground in place, jumping from a 1-ft level, balancing on one foot for one second, and broad jumping. Similarly, fine motor tasks might include copying a circle, tracing a line, drawing a cross by imitation, drawing a six-part human figure, and exhibiting motor control with dots. As these tasks were mastered, the frustrations commensurate with developmental limitations were diminished and individuals with TBI were more receptive to the second phase, typical behavioral interventions.

Unlike the other models that yielded behavioral strategies in terms of the descriptive paradigms of neurology and neuropsychology, the process model defined behavioral strategies by the more generic, dynamic, and interlocking processes that accounted for the original formation or subsequent maintenance, or both, of behavioral problems. This model was first developed to explain behavioral rehabilitation for severely mentally ill populations (Corrigan et al. 1988, 1990) but is easily adaptable to the disabilities of individuals with TBI. It includes the following four component processes:

1. *Acquisition*: Individuals with severe mental illness may lack interpersonal or self-care skills because they did not acquire these behaviors during their tumultuous premorbid adolescence. Rather than never having acquired the skills, those with TBI may have lost prosocial skills that were previously in their repertoire as a result of brain damage or may need to acquire new

compensatory skills to accommodate specific disabilities. Skills training strategies help both groups to (re)acquire necessary skills. In addition, individuals with TBI may learn symptom management skills and other behavioral prosthetics (e.g., stress management and problem-solving skills) that will help them manage life stressors associated with wide-ranging disabilities.

2. *Performance*: A person who has acquired a skill may not perform it if there are few incentives to performance or if barriers prevent performance. Several factors impede reinforcing conditions that provide patients with incentive to use their limited prosocial skills. For example, cognitively impaired individuals with TBI may be relatively insensitive to many of the normal social reinforcers that maintain interpersonal skills. Moreover, friends and family members may be unwilling to provide sufficient reinforcers for what they consider "meager" behaving. Incentive strategies such as contingency management and token economies facilitate skill performance.

3. *Generalization*: Even if those with TBI learn a range of skills and perform them in the training milieu, these skills frequently do not generalize outside of the treatment setting or are not maintained over time. Transfer training skills (e.g., homework, in vivo practice, and training the family) foster situational and response generalization.

4. *Cognition*: The cognitive deficits common to brain injury diminish the other component processes. For example, memory deficits that hamper learning may impair skill acquisition. Patients with attentional deficits may neglect reinforcers meant to govern the performance of certain behaviors. Furthermore, lack of sensitivity to the way in which real-world situations are similar to the training environment may hamper generalization. Cognitive rehabilitation strategies help individuals with TBI overcome problems like these and are reviewed in Chapter 36, Cognitive Rehabilitation. Points relevant to this model are discussed throughout the remainder of this chapter.

The process model is useful for rehabilitation of individuals with TBI because treatment strategies are clearly wedded to the specific, deficient process in question (i.e., to the phenomena that brought about the behavioral excess and deficit and to the phenomena that maintain these disabilities). When combined with the neuropsychiatrist's and neuropsychologist's perspective, the process model yields a potent programmatic approach to the treatment of behavioral excesses and deficits. The manner in which the first three component processes organize a behavioral rehabilitation program is outlined in the following sections.

Acquisition

Skill deficits may lead to confusion and frustration as someone with a TBI attempts to manage his or her environment. Persons with TBI have the same goals as other members of society and may find disruptive behavior their only option for managing the environment when social, instrumental, or other skills are impaired. Most people use the simplest and most effective means of attaining important goals. Disruptive behaviors will continue as long as they provide the easiest access to reinforcers. When individuals are taught adaptive skills for managing the environment, maladaptive behaviors are no longer needed. The acquisition of new skills provides the individual with ways to manage the environment and reduces the need for external control by others (Ducharme 2000).

Skills training methods are the primary strategy for facilitating acquisition. Typically, skills training is conducted in psychoeducational modules with one or two trainers and five to ten participants. Trainers rely on several learning activities presented in sequential order to facilitate skill acquisition. Through verbal instructions, the key learning points of the skill are presented. For example, in an assertiveness module, the trainer might say, "Today we are going to learn how to say 'No' using the broken record technique. When someone asks you for a dollar and you want to keep it, say, 'No, I do not want to give you my dollar.' If he or she persists, say the same message again, 'No, I do not want to give you the dollar,' like a broken record. Keep repeating the same message until the person stops asking."

After being introduced to the learning points, trainees observe a model demonstrating the skill. This can be done either by using prepackaged videotaped vignettes or by having the trainer model the targeted skills.

Next, trainees are encouraged to practice the skill in predesigned role plays. "Now Jim, I want you to practice saying 'No' when Harry asks you for a dollar." Trainers offer corrective feedback after the role play, especially focusing on successful approximations to the targeted behavior. Liberal rewards are handed out at the end of the session for participating in the module. After trainees have shown some mastery of the skill in the training milieu, they are given homework for practice in the real world to facilitate generalization and maintenance.

These learning activities may be used to improve skill acquisition in several domains of functioning, including self-care, interpersonal, and coping skills (Schade et al. 1990; Spiegler and Agigian 1977). Self-care skills encompass activities for daily living such as grooming, home maintenance skills, shopping, and money management.

Interpersonal skill deficits include poor conversation and assertion skills. Deficits in these domains represent a loss in functioning and therefore require a reintroduction to skills. Coping skills are "new" behaviors that individuals must learn to manage their illness; they include medication management (knowing the therapeutic and side effects of medication and how to talk with the physician when there are problems with these drugs), symptom management (identifying problem behaviors and coping techniques when these behaviors flare up), and stress management (behavioral strategies to handle recurrent tensions).

What accounts for the therapeutic effects of skills training? The operant and social learning components of skills training may yield a direct learning effect. Despite cognitive deficits, individuals with TBI are able to acquire the targeted skills. Alternately, learning points taught in skills training modules may serve as behavioral prosthetics, much as Gazzaniga (1978) believed. Instead of acquiring skills as they appear in the real world, individuals with TBI have learned manageable behavioral steps to help them with the skill domains.

Research on the effects of skills training in individuals with a brain injury, although limited mostly to single-case designs, has provided some interesting findings. Self-monitoring has been added to the traditional package of learning activities to improve the heterosexual conversation skills of four men (Gajar et al. 1984; Schloss et al. 1984). In self-monitoring, patients are instructed to keep track of the frequency of specific, jointly defined behaviors. The positive effects of this study were found to generalize to settings outside the training milieu. Similarly, the aggressive behaviors of another individual were significantly reduced as he acquired basic self-care skills (Godfrey and Knight 1988). Results were more limited in a fourth study, however (Brotherton et al. 1988). Training for four individuals with severe brain injury was more useful in the micro components of basic social behaviors (e.g., eye contact and posture) than in the macro skill (e.g., conversation) actually required to interpersonally relate.

Performance

Individuals who have experienced TBI often have low motivation that interferes with the completion of rehabilitation tasks (Feinstein 1999). It is important that treatment providers manage these motivational reactions and not be punitive when individuals resist rehabilitation activities (Prigatano 1999). Motivational interviewing is one approach that has been effective in helping individuals with a variety of psychiatric and other behavior problems, including individuals with cognitive deficits, identify incentives for changing their behavior (Miller and Rollnick 1991). Although motivational interviewing has not been studied in persons with TBI, research has been conducted in a variety of medical settings (Resinecow et al. 2002). Also, Bombardier et al. (1997), in a study of the readiness of persons with TBI to change alcohol drinking habits, concluded that motivational interviewing may be a useful approach with this population.

In motivational interviewing, the clinician facilitates increased motivation to change by helping the person identify and compare the costs and benefits of changing versus not changing behaviors. This can be accomplished by having the individual identify his or her goals and by linking specific behavior change to goal attainment. It is especially important that treatment providers focus on specific behavior change rather than general readiness for change. Ideally, the clinician will target behaviors to be increased in frequency rather than attempting to decrease problematic behaviors (Corrigan et al. 2001). Until fully motivated to change, however, individuals with TBI may initially require social and material rewards as incentives to incorporate relearned or newly acquired social, coping, and self-care skills into their everyday behavioral repertoire.

The law of effect from operant psychology describes the impact of incentives on behaviors; according to this law, behaviors that are reinforced in specific situations are more likely to occur again in those situations, whereas punished behaviors are less likely to be observed in the punished environment (Skinner 1953). Two treatment strategies are based on the law and have been widely used for treatment of individuals with TBI: contingency contracts and token economies. Contingency contracts are defined by if–then rules; if patients perform a targeted response, then they receive desired reinforcers. Targeted responses in research with individuals with TBIs have included verbal abilities, awareness, attention, motivation, social responsiveness, and participation in group activities (Ben-Yishay et al. 1980; Blackerby 1988; Burke and Lewis 1986; Ince 1976; McGlynn 1990; Mueller and Atlas 1972; Prigatano and Altman 1990; Turner et al. 1978; Wehman et al. 1990). Self-care functions such as feeding, bed making, personal hygiene, and clothes maintenance have also been included in these programs (Murphy 1976).

Contingency contracts (for that matter, any reinforcement program) are as effective as the rewards chosen as consequences. Consumables such as coffee or food; activities, including one-to-one attention from staff; and privileges such as use of a staff telephone are used as reinforcers. However, what is reinforcing for one person may be aversive for another. Several strategies exist for helping clinicians identify reinforcers. Patients can be instructed to identify reinforcing commodities and activities from several self-report surveys (Cautela and Lynch 1983). The reticent patient's reinforcer may be identified by providing a smorgasbord of commodities and opportunities to see what the person selects. Finally, according to principles of operant psychology, any behavior that a person does at a high rate is by definition reinforcing (Premack 1962). For example, hand washing or sitting in a favorite chair—responses not normally considered to be reinforcers—may be potent rewards for some individuals' behavior. Therefore, observing rates of various behaviors may provide clues to behavioral reinforcers.

There are also several rules about the manner in which rewards are handed out that affect their reinforcing potential. When the patient is first learning a behavior, rewards should be given immediately after the response has been performed. Staff passing out the rewards should offer verbal congratulations for meeting the goal by pointing out specifics of the goal that were demonstrated (e.g., "Nice job, Harry. You made your bed well by tucking in your sheets and straightening out your blanket. Here's the reward we talked about.").

Contingency contracts are sometimes ineffective because the targeted behavior is beyond the individual's response capabilities. For example, someone with a recent TBI who is restless will not be able to sit for an hour in skills training sessions. Therefore, clinicians should shape behaviors toward performance of "macro" targets—in this case, sitting still for an hour—by reinforcing successive approximations to the goals. During the first week of training, the target is 5 minutes of sitting. When this is accomplished, the goal is increased to 10 minutes and then slowly increased by 10-minute increments until the hour goal is reached. In one case study (Watson et al. 2001), the use of incentives along with gradual increases in expectations was effective in reducing aggressive behavior of an individual 10 years after he sustained a TBI.

Token economies are formalized and programmatic forms of contingency contracting that derive their potency from the law of effect and the law of association by contiguity (Skinner 1953). According to the second law, previously neutral stimuli (e.g., tokens) when presented frequently with reinforcing stimuli (e.g., consumables) become reinforcing in their own right. Unlike contingency contracts, token economies are typically set up for all members of an inpatient or outpatient program. Three steps are necessary to carry this out. First, behaviors that everyone in the treatment program is expected to demonstrate are identified (e.g., daily showering, clean bedroom, and talk with peers at meals). Next, token contingencies for accomplishing these behaviors are specified (e.g., "If you make your bed by 8:00 A.M., then you will receive 10 tokens.").

The frequency of inappropriate behaviors can be diminished by specifying response costs for these behaviors (e.g., "If you smoke in your bedroom, then you will lose 10 tokens."). Finally, exchange rules for turning in tokens should be outlined. When and where does someone swap his or her tokens for primary reinforcers like consumables, hygiene products, clothes, and reading material? How many tokens do individual commodities cost?

Token economies have been used extensively in the treatment of those with TBI to increase interpersonal and coping skills or to decrease maladaptive behaviors (Burke and Lewis 1986; Gajar et al. 1984; Horton and Howe 1981; Kushner and Knox 1973; Lira et al. 1983; Mueller and Atlas 1972; Webster and Scott 1983; Wood and Eames 1981). In some token economies, the frequency of inappropriate behaviors has been diminished successfully by fining patients for performing these behaviors. Inappropriate responses have included interpersonal aggression, treatment noncompliance, and alcohol consumption (Blackerby and Baumgarten 1990; Franzen and Lovell 1987; Horton and Howe 1981; Kushner and Knox 1973; Lira et al. 1983; McGlynn 1990; Wood and Eames 1981). Despite these successes, several limitations to the technology have been found, including poor generalization from a highly structured treatment setting to the real world (Kazdin and Bootzin 1972). For example, activities of daily living (ADLs) and basic conversation skills in the patient's home setting are not normally maintained by immediate receipt of tokens. Transfer training strategies help to improve the generalization of these effects.

Generalization

Despite great gains in facilitating acquisition and performance of social, coping, and self-care skills, generalization of skills to settings outside the treatment milieu and to behaviors other than those specifically targeted by the behavioral intervention has been lacking (Corrigan et al. 1993a). Generalization of behaviors improved in programs for individuals with TBI has been especially limited (McGlynn 1990). These negative findings may result from dominance of an older behavioral perspective that has viewed generalization as a naturally occurring phenomenon (i.e., some time after key learning events, performance of the skill transfers to similar situations [stimulus generalization] and behaviors [response generalization] in gradient fashion) (Skinner 1953). As a result, clinicians have passively sat back waiting for skills to appear in new settings. Others have argued that generalization only happens when actively introduced into the rehabilitation program (Corrigan and Basit 1997; Kazdin 1982; Stokes and Baer 1977; Stokes and Osnes 1989; Wesolowski and

Zencius 1994). Hence, use of generalization strategies significantly enhances transfer effects of token economies and skills training programs.

Generalization includes maintenance, situational or stimulus generalization, and response generalization. Maintenance occurs when skills are remembered and correctly performed over time. Stimulus generalization occurs when skills learned in the training setting are performed in the natural environment. Response generalization takes place when one is able to perform variations of the trained skill. Practices that facilitate generalization include fading reinforcers, teaching self-management strategies, assigning homework, including significant others in the generalization program, and cognitive rehabilitation (Corrigan and Basit 1997).

Repeated practice of newly learned skills increases the probability that targeted responses will be performed in situations similar to the practice milieu. However, repeating the same task many times is boring and discourages individuals from complying with the task. Multiple training approaches avoid this pitfall by providing different tasks to facilitate skills acquisition. Acquisition of conversational skills can be increased by role play activities within a skills training module, special practice sessions between therapist and patient, and token economy contingencies that provide rewards for performing the skill.

Skills transfer more readily from psychoeducational programs when they are practiced in settings other then the training milieu. While the individual is an inpatient, skills training sessions include in vivo tasks in which participants might be bused to relevant community settings and assigned a skill-relevant problem (Benson Yody et al. 2001; Liberman and Corrigan 1993). For example, individuals might be instructed at a shopping mall to go to a store, pick out a set of clothes, and determine the cost for the ensemble. Rehabilitation staff accompany the participants and offer prompts and feedback through the task. As trainees demonstrate competence, they are given homework assignments to complete independently.

For generalization to occur, the individuals must be sensitive to the stimulus similarities that define training situations and the rest of the world. TBI patients with cognitive deficits are likely to have diminished sensitivity to social cues and therefore are less likely to readily generalize newly learned skills from treatment programs. Therefore, attention-focusing techniques that improve patients' perception of interpersonal skills should enhance the transfer of skills. Similarly, trainers might enhance generalization by pointing out cues present outside the training environment that are similar to cues that signal the skill in the training environment. For example, the trainer may want to point out similarities between the

hospital cafeteria and the neighborhood diner so that the patient is vigilant to the waitress's statements. As a result, the patient will be ready to give a lunch order, a skill that he or she has repeatedly practiced at the hospital.

As suggested in the section Performance, newly learned behaviors maintained by a token economy do not generalize well to settings outside the hospital. Soon after discharge, individuals with TBI may discover that natural contingencies are not as specific or fruitful as economy-defined consequences, and the frequency of targeted behaviors quickly diminishes. Several strategies can be used to help avoid this pitfall. As targeted behaviors within the hospital approach "normal" rates, schedules are changed from continuous reinforcement (given tokens immediately after the behavior) to intermittent contingencies, especially variable-ratio or variable-interval schedules, which are more resistant to extinction (Skinner 1953). Staff successfully used a variation on this approach in a study of three persons with TBI who had difficulty participating in treatment for long periods and took frequent unauthorized breaks from scheduled rehabilitation activities. The intervention consisted of giving participants a short break every hour for 1 month. During this time, unauthorized breaks decreased, and subjects were eventually able to follow the program's less frequent break schedule (Wesolowski et al. 1999).

Generalization effects of both token economies and individual interventions can be enhanced by extending the program to the community. Family or other caregivers can be trained to continue specific contingencies at home or in vocational training settings (Falloon et al. 1984; Tharp and Wetzel 1969), and staff can, where possible, provide treatment in community as well as rehabilitation settings (Benson Yody et al. 2001). Interpersonal and instrumental skills vary in terms of their reinforcement value. Generalization of token economies to situations outside the treatment unit can be facilitated by targeting those skills that are "naturally" reinforced (Ayllon and Azrin 1968; Tharp and Wetzel 1969). For example, individuals are more likely to be reinforced in their community for talking politely and showing good hygiene than for demonstrating insight into their injuries or being able to speak about hidden conflicts. Staff must target behaviors in the token economy that are necessary for successful community living, as illustrated in the following case example.

Joe, a 30-year-old married bus driver, was hospitalized after a major car accident while driving home from work on the expressway. Joe was unconscious for several hours after the accident and experienced injuries to both hemispheres. After a brief hospitalization to manage acute injuries, Joe underwent intensive treatment at a rehabilitation facility for 6 months. Significant physical sequelae related to the injury had remitted at discharge from this facility.

Despite regaining most physical capabilities, Joe continued to exhibit cognitive and behavioral difficulties at home that prevented him from returning to work. His wife reported that he seemed less interested in people; for example, he was no longer golfing with his friends or fishing with his family, activities in which he had participated regularly. He would tend to sit uncomfortably in a corner during most social functions. "Joe was always such a friendly guy. It's like he doesn't know what to do when he's around others," his wife said. Family members reported that his grooming had diminished severely and that Joe did little to help keep the house clean. The patient did not remember to take his medications as prescribed and would frequently skip meals if not prompted. In addition to being frustrated about Joe's loss in social and self-care skills, the family expressed anger at his seeming lack of concern about his change in functioning.

Joe was referred to a behavioral day hospital that specialized in treatment of neuropsychological disorders. Interventions included in the treatment plan that was developed for Joe addressed the processes maintaining the behavioral problems. Joe was enrolled in several psychoeducational classes to help him better understand the course of his disorder as well as some fundamental skills he might use to cope with day-to-day problems. For example, Joe attended medication management and basic conversation skills modules each day. The medication management module offered exercises emphasizing the benefits of drugs, self-administration, side effects, and medication schedules for adaptation of his medication regimen at the program, at home, and, eventually, at the workplace. Participation in the basic conversation skills class helped Joe to relearn verbal and nonverbal communications as well as active listening skills. Modules incorporated cognitive rehabilitation strategies to help circumvent information processing deficits that might impede learning targeted skills.

The day-treatment program used token reinforcement to provide incentive for participants to use newly reacquired skills. Joe was observed to separate himself from peers during social gather-ings in the day hospital, so his case manager made receipt of 10 tokens contingent on having a friendly talk with a peer in the program for 5 minutes. Because of Joe's highly social premorbid history and his success in the basic conversation skills classes, he quickly met criterion on the 5-minute program, so the case manager raised the goal to 10 minutes. Program participants were also reinforced for completing responsibilities that helped to keep the facilities clean; Joe was assigned to lunch cleanup. His case manager instructed him on the specifics of his duties and offered prompts and provided cue cards to guide him through his work. Joe was able to earn his tokens on this job after a short time.

Despite the significant change in prosocial behaviors at the day program, family members reported that Joe was still asocial and unconcerned at home. The case manager arranged problem-focused family treatment to educate family members regarding Joe's limits. The goal of family treatment, however, was not to have family members accept Joe's prognosis but rather to teach them discrete strategies to help Joe improve his behaviors at home. Treatment was conducted over 6 months in 90-minute sessions that took place in the family home and decreased in frequency from initial biweekly sessions to once-monthly sessions. The family learned the basics of problem solving (identify the problem, brainstorm solutions, evaluate each solution, implement one or more, monitor the solution's effectiveness, and modify as needed) through practice with the therapist and were encouraged to follow the steps when a management problem occurred outside of the session. Family members were also taught the basics of contingency contracting through modeling and practice so that the rate of particularly recalcitrant behaviors (Joe would not make the bed no matter how they prompted him) could be modified by manipulating key reinforcers (Joe could watch the morning talk show only after he made the bed).

After several months of participation in the program, Joe's social skills were observed to have increased significantly, both at the day program and at home. Family members still reported times each day when Joe was tired and seemed to withdraw from his wife and children. However, overall his level of interaction was improved, and grooming and housekeeping had improved significantly as well. At a recent treatment meeting, Joe, his wife, and the treatment team had agreed that Joe was ready to try a work retraining program to prepare for reentry into the work force.

Joe's case is a composite of the behavioral problems that an individual with TBI might experience. Even though life-threatening aspects of the injury had been resolved and the patient was left with no significant physical disabilities, Joe and his family experienced enduring psychiatric problems that resulted from the accident. Typically, clinicians conducting behavioral programs are involved when physical symptoms have diminished and interpersonal problems are more apparent. Significant impact on these problems was realized by enrolling the patient in a comprehensive psychoeducational milieu and by involving significant others in carrying out the treatment plan. Resolution of behavioral problems is not usually as dramatic as treatments that address physical sequelae of the disease. Behavioral clinicians talk about reductions of inappropriate behaviors or increases of prosocial responses instead of remissions and cures. However, changing the rate of these behaviors can improve the individual's quality of life significantly.

Management of Aggression and Other Disruptive Behaviors

Aggressive behaviors present a special problem and may require behavioral interventions that are not subsumed by a process-based rehabilitation program. Aggressive responses are fairly common in psychiatric patients in general (Tardiff and Sweillam 1982) and after brain injury in particular (Silver and Yudofsky 1987). Aggressive behaviors may include verbal outbursts, damage to property, and physical assault. The form of aggression varies across individuals and, for the same individual, across situations. Aggressive behavior may spontaneously remit during recovery, but there are frequently behavioral sequelae in the postacute phase of treatment after medical stabilization. Factors related to brain injury, psychological sequelae, environmental contexts, and premorbid behavior can play a role in maintaining aggressive behavior (Ducharme 2000). A stress vulnerability model can be used to identify factors that may explain and remediate aggressive behavior. According to the stress vulnerability model, biological factors interact with environmental stressors to produce aggression (Corrigan and Mueser 2000). Hence, the most effective treatments combine psychopharmacological interventions and behavioral strategies for managing environmental antecedents to aggression (Corrigan et al. 1993b; Franzen and Lovell 1987).

Factors that may cause or exacerbate aggressive behavior include overarousal, cognitive deficits, social skills deficits, and lack of social support (Corrigan and Mueser 2000). Frequently, aggressive behaviors occur because individuals with TBI are more easily frustrated by everyday interpersonal demands. Hence, if they regain some interpersonal and self-care skills, or as they learn various behavioral prosthetics, the frequency of violent behaviors diminishes. However, many aggressive behaviors are of sufficient severity that treatment teams cannot wait for relatively slow skill acquisition processes to occur.

The range of alternative strategies that diminish overaggressiveness has been divided into "aggression replacement" strategies and "decelerative techniques" and is reviewed in Table 37–3 (Lennox et al. 1988; Liberman and Wong 1984). Many disruptive behaviors can be conceptualized as outgrowths of specific skill deficits (Ducharme 2000). Aggressive behaviors might be replaced with other, functionally equivalent, socially adaptive behaviors such as assertion. Assertion training uses the methods and rules of skills training reviewed in the section Models of Behavioral Rehabilitation. Content areas include saying no, making a complaint, and expressing appreciation (Douglas and Mueser 1990).

Persons with TBI may find ADLs aversive; thus, rehabilitation activities often occasion aggressive behavior (Proulx 1999). Skills training in performing ADLs may lead to reduced aggression as the individual with TBI masters the skills and finds them less aversive. Graduated introduction of frustrating situations may also reduce aggressive behavior. For example, one might begin with training in the least frustrating task, with a systematic introduction of more demanding activities, or begin with small time intervals that are gradually increased as the individual's distress tolerance increases (Ducharme 2000).

Consequence management strategies, another replacement method that helps to decrease aggressive behaviors without using aversive stimuli, may include differential reinforcement, extinction, and/or response costs (Wesolowski and Zencius 1994). When using differential reinforcement of other behavior (DRO) for decreasing agitation, staff reinforces all behaviors except the aggressive target. In practice, the patient's day is divided into discrete time periods (e.g., 20-minute increments); for each period in which the patient does not show the violent behavior, he or she receives the reward. For example, Hegel and Ferguson (2000) and Hollon (1973) combined a DRO procedure for nonaggressive behavior with planned ignoring of disruptive behavior in two patients with brain injuries. Within a few weeks, the disruptive behaviors decreased significantly, and more prosocial behaviors began to appear. Crewe (1980) found similar

TABLE 37–3.   Behavioral treatment of aggression

Strategies	Special considerations
Aggression replacement strategies	
Assertiveness training (for patients who become angry when they are unable to have their needs met)	Must work well in skills training groups.
Differential reinforcement schedule (a nonpunishing strategy to decrease the rate of previolent behaviors)	Resource requirements may be costly. Can diminish this problem by identifying suitable interfering behavior.
Decelerative techniques	
Social extinction (useful for previolent patients who respond to social reinforcers)	May not work with patients with schizophrenia.
Contingent observation (provides opportunity for violent responders to model self-control from peers)	Must be sufficiently organized to accurately perceive models.
Self-controlled time-out (advantages of time-out)	May diminish risky attempts to seclude or restrain.
Overcorrection (useful learning experience for relatively docile patients)	Stop if patient struggles with guided practice.
Contingent restraint (the last resort for violent patients who do not comply with self-controlled time-out and are resistant to guided practice)	Decreases inadvertent reinforcement of behaviors that covary with seclusion and restraint.

results using availability of nurses' attention as the differential reinforcer. However, DRO schedules are relatively costly interventions requiring the constant availability of staff to reinforce the relative infinity of patients' nonaggressive responses. Differential reinforcement of incompatible behaviors (DRI) offers a more efficient alternative in which only behaviors that are incompatible with the undesired target are reinforced (e.g., a patient might be reinforced each time she says "No" rather than yelling angrily at a peer who is begging for a dollar). Skills training is preferred over the DRO and DRI procedures because skill enhancement is nonpunitive, leads to greater generalization, and provides the individual with skills that may be useful in managing many life situations (Ducharme 2000).

Despite the increase in prosocial, nonhostile behaviors that results from aggression replacement strategies, assaultive incidents may still occur and should be ad-

dressed. Decelerative techniques rely on principles of operant psychology to decrease previolent behaviors (i.e., behaviors consistent with being irritable or grumpy that signal impending physical outbursts) and to diminish aggressive episodes when they occur. One such method, social extinction, is effective for individuals who actively seek staff approval. These individuals are told that acting out aggressively is unacceptable to the milieu and that they will be ignored when they do so again. Effective extinction requires all staff to ignore the designated patient during the intervention. The impact of extinction can be augmented by token fines that are levied for antisocial behavior (Horton and Howe 1981).

Although social extinction removes some previolent behaviors, the intervention strategy does not include a learning opportunity by which patients can acquire replacement behaviors. Clinicians using contingent observation tell patients who are acting out to sit quietly for a predefined time at the edge of the group (Porterfield et al. 1976). While sitting alone, patients are instructed to watch peers and staff carefully and observe alternative responses they might use to avoid future angry responses in the situation. Time-out from reinforcement is an operant technique in which socially inappropriate behaviors can be decreased by short-term removal of patients from overstimulating (and perhaps reinforcing) situations (Wood 1982; Wood and Eames 1981). A time-out chair in a quiet corner of the day room is a place where patients quickly learn to go when prompted by staff. Compared with seclusion, self-controlled time-out will probably not evoke as negative a reaction because patients have some control over the process. In this way, time-out offers a less restrictive alternative to seclusion and restraints, engenders less humiliation, and involves diminished risk of injury to patients, staff, and bystanders (Glynn et al. 1989). Overcorrection combines time-out and an effort requirement to reduce the rate of offensive behaviors by forcefully replacing these behaviors with more prosocial alternatives (Marholin et al. 1980; Matson and Stephens 1977). The effort requirement compels patients to restore the disturbed situation to a vastly improved condition. For example, after a patient who threw his tray at lunch calmed down in the time-out chair, he was instructed to clean up not only his table but several other tables in the cafeteria as well.

The replacement and decelerative interventions described above to target aggressive behaviors are equally effective in the management of other disruptive behaviors. Sexually inappropriate behaviors, constant disruptive or perseverative talking, and other intrusive behaviors are sometimes observed in individuals with TBI and may also be managed by using consequence management,

DRO, DRI, skills training, social extinction, contingent observation, time-out from reinforcement, and overcorrection. For example, contingent observation may be used with an individual who frequently interrupts a group activity; extinction may be used to address sexually inappropriate speech that is reinforced by attention; and both types of behaviors may be reduced by teaching replacement behaviors through skills training.

Some individuals are aggressive in response to physical properties of the environment such as noise, activity level, and other stimulating features of the milieu. Minimizing sources of agitation in the environment is an effective way to reduce aggressive behavior in some individuals. In a case study, Fluharty and Glassman (2001) found that reducing environmental stimuli antecedent to aggression both reduced aggression and increased the individual's participation in social activities. The only caveats for modifying the environment to reduce aggression are that it may not always be possible to control the amount of stimulation in the environment and, as in extinction procedures, the person with TBI is not taught alternative behaviors. Although many interventions are effective for a wide range of target behaviors, seclusion and restraint should be used only in response to aggressive behavior that is severe enough to threaten the safety of the environment and is unresponsive to less restrictive interventions.

Patients who are unresponsive to all other decelerative techniques may need to be secluded and physically restrained. However, staff should be aware of local and institutional statutes, regulations, and policies because there is a nationwide trend toward limiting the use of physical seclusion and restraint (Bernay and Devitt 2000). Where permissible, these techniques should always be regarded as a last resort when aggression replacement and other decelerative techniques have failed to decrease aggression. Restraint should never be used with individuals who are medically unstable. It should not be used as punishment, as a substitute for treatment, for staff convenience, or when it is positively reinforcing and therefore likely to increase aggression (Fisher 1994). Restraint is indicated to prevent harm to individuals in the treatment environment or damage to the environment itself, to decrease the stimulation an individual receives, to prevent serious disruptions of the treatment of others, and for treatment as part of an ongoing behavioral treatment plan (Bernay and DeVitt 2000). Contingent restraint may be part of a behavioral treatment plan. It is operationally similar to conventional restraining methods; however, it demands immediate and consistent administration of restraint after each severe violent episode. Staff do not interact verbally with patients during the application of re-

straints so as not to reinforce the maladaptive behavior inadvertently (Corrigan and Mueser 2000).

Behavioral Treatment of Emotional Reactions to TBI

The effects of the original injury, the resulting emergency care and hospitalization, the reaction of family members and friends, and the cognitive and behavioral sequelae of the injury are frequently upsetting for the patient. As a result, some individuals with TBI experience anxiety and panic with their new-found inabilities, anger with the frustration that comes with these inabilities, and depression as the road to recovery becomes difficult. In one sample of 60 postacute individuals with TBI, 50% reported significant anxiety and 70% reported depression (Linn et al. 1994). Although there is much empirical support for the management of behavior problems associated with TBI, there is a dearth of research on psychosocial interventions for managing emotional reactions to TBI (Warschausky et al. 1999).

Lira et al. (1983) used elements of stress inoculation training (SIT) (Meichenbaum 1975) to improve the frustration tolerance and diminish the anger of individuals with TBI. Treatment consisted of three phases: 1) education about the phenomenon of anger and appropriate ways to express it, 2) training in cognitive reappraisal of anger-evoking situations and countering with positive statements, and 3) application training to use skills hierarchically. Results of their study showed that after 4 weeks of treatment, hostile episodes decreased from 2.75 incidents per week to 0. Moreover, no hostile outbursts were reported at 5-month follow-up.

Environmental modifications can also ameliorate anxiety and depression. Caregivers may inadvertently create stress for individuals with TBI when demands exceed their capabilities (Miller and Borden 1994). Careful monitoring of demand situations, evaluation of stress tolerance, and use of appropriate prostheses and compensatory behaviors can increase independence and decrease anxiety and depression.

Results from studies on patients with multiple sclerosis (MS) have implications for some individuals with TBI. In one study, SIT was used to address depression in 20 patients with MS; another group of 20 patients with MS were randomly assigned to "current available care" as a control group (Foley et al. 1987). After six treatment sessions, the SIT group was significantly less anxious, distressed, and depressed than the control group. Results from a second study were similar; MS subjects in a cognitive-behavioral therapy group were significantly less depressed than MS subjects in a waiting-list control (Larcombe and Wilson 1984). Cognitive-behavioral therapy in the second study combined Lewinsohn et al.'s (1976) techniques to increase the number of patients' positive life experiences with Beck et al.'s (1979) strategies to decrease damaging cognitions. To improve the number of positive life experiences, individuals were taught to identify pleasurable activities, schedule them into their daily lives, and evaluate the efficacy of their schedules. To decrease damaging cognitions, they were also taught to identify negative self-statements, to recognize the connection between these self-statements and depression, to examine the evidence against negative statements, and to develop counters to the statements. Most subjects in the cognitive-behavioral therapy group maintained the therapeutic benefits of treatment at a 1-month follow-up. These findings suggest that, in addition to the behavioral rehabilitation goals of increasing lost skills and diminishing antisocial behaviors, clinicians must be sensitive to the emotional reactions to TBI.

Staff Management Issues

Despite the abundance of well-validated behavioral strategies that ameliorate the deficits and excesses that result from TBI, rehabilitation programs for this population are lacking (Bleiberg et al. 1991). Treatment approaches are often fragmented and focused on topographical assessment rather than functional assessment of behavior. That is, staff attend to the topography or form of the behavior (e.g., aggressive outbursts or refusal to participate in rehabilitation programming) rather than consider what function the behavior has for the individual (e.g., receiving attention, managing anxiety, or getting others to perform tasks for him or her). Thorough functional assessment increases the chance that staff will develop and implement effective behavioral interventions (Benson Yody et al. 2001; Ducharme 2000).

Treatment team members often have only partial knowledge about illness experienced by the individual with TBI, are not familiar with the disorder under consideration, have little awareness of what treatment is being provided by team members in other disciplines (Mills and Alexander 1999), and tend to use aversive strategies to manage disruptive behavior and to have little knowledge of behavior management strategies (Ducharme 2000). Every member of the treatment team requires education on what disorders will be treated, treatment provided by each discipline, development of treatment plans and goals, use of assessment and treatment approaches within the fiscal realities of the program, and routine evaluation

of the clinical relevance and effectiveness of different treatments (Mills and Alexander 1999).

Investigators have identified barriers to disseminating and implementing behavioral interventions in inpatient psychiatric settings, in the hope of identifying strategies for increasing the quantity and quality of behaviorally based mental health programs (Corrigan et al. 1992, 1994, 2001). Although the typical individual with TBI is treated at a rehabilitation hospital, many of the insights from these studies are applicable to decisions regarding introduction and implementation of behavioral innovations for brain-injured populations. The barriers include a lack of necessary supervisory structures to support these programs, insufficient monetary resources to maintain them, and little collegial support to implement them.

Barriers to dissemination are educational and organizational. Service providers often lack the knowledge to assimilate new practices. This barrier is compounded when organizational practices undermine the treatment team's ability to implement and maintain new approaches. Strategies that foster dissemination include providing education to treatment providers, packaging evidence-based practices so they are more accessible to providers, and removing organizational barriers that impede innovation (Corrigan et al. 2001).

One way to overcome barriers to implementation of behavior therapy is to establish training and incentive programs that manage staff behaviors. Training staff members in behavior therapy principles and practices has been shown to improve clinical performance markedly (Carsrud et al. 1980; Milne 1982, 1984; Watson and Uzell 1980). Training helps inexperienced staff who work with individuals with TBI acquire the necessary skills to implement behavior therapy and keeps the skills of experienced workers sharp. For training to be successful, hospital administrators must provide sufficient time for staff to learn behavioral strategies. Moreover, the administration must contract with well-trained behavioral consultants who can provide didactic sessions colored with real-life vignettes (Bernstein 1983; Tharp and Wetzel 1969). The curriculum for the training program should reflect the unique interventions that have been found useful to ameliorate the behavioral problems of individuals with TBI in the specific treatment setting.

Even if trainees learn behavioral strategies well, there is little guarantee that they will use the skills on the unit itself, especially after training has ceased (Bernstein 1979, 1983; Braukman et al. 1975). Just as behavioral clinicians provide support, guidance, and incentive for individuals with TBI to maintain newly acquired behaviors, so unit supervisors need to manage the behaviors of the clinicians charged with daily patient care. Regular clinical supervision assists these professionals and paraprofessionals in maintaining competent levels of behavioral intervention. Clinical supervision includes support and guidance, feedback and ongoing individualized training, and inspiration to continue working with individuals who define a tough treatment population.

Interactive staff training (IST) is an approach to teach psychiatric rehabilitation teams to deliver better psychiatric rehabilitation programs. IST combines educational and organizational strategies to increase the knowledge and skills of team members and foster administrative support, group cohesion, and leadership. Training takes place in the rehabilitation setting with the treatment team, and training content is based on a needs assessment completed by all members of the team. IST encourages the development of user-friendly programs because the needs assessment assures that training content is relevant to the needs of the team, takes place on the unit with all team members present, and is provided by outside consultants familiar with empirically validated treatments. Newly learned treatment strategies are thus likely to be implemented with integrity and monitored for ongoing relevance and effectiveness, and to be modified as needed to maintain a quality program (Corrigan and McCracken 1999). Although the effectiveness of IST has not yet been studied in the rehabilitation of persons with TBI, its emphasis is on training staff in service delivery skills at the individual and programmatic level. Different rehabilitation settings may emphasize different target populations; however, to the degree that they share the features of interdisciplinary teams of health care providers treating individuals with a variety of functional impairments using a variety of behavioral, pharmacological, and medical interventions, IST should be applicable in any rehabilitation treatment setting.

Returning to the Community

After initial intensive rehabilitation and stabilization, individuals with TBI may be placed in residential treatment settings or live independently or with family members. Many may participate in ongoing outpatient treatment after discharge from the rehabilitation hospital. Rehabilitation treatment providers must plan for this transition as early as possible, emphasizing both linkage to community services and generalization training so skills acquired in the rehabilitation program generalize to the community. This can be accomplished through discharge planning that includes participation with the injured individual as well as caregivers and significant others who will be interacting with him or her after discharge.

Where possible, rehabilitation staff can facilitate generalization by allowing the individual with TBI to practice skills through role-play activities in the rehabilitation setting as well as through practice in the community that can be planned, carried out, and evaluated. For example, an individual might make a weekend visit home or spend a day at a future outpatient treatment site before discharge from the rehabilitation facility. Such generalization activities allow the individual with TBI and his or her treatment providers to evaluate how effective the treatment program is, how well newly learned skills are being performed and generalizing, and whether new skills need to be acquired before discharge. Such planning should begin as early as feasible to promote a smooth transition from a rehabilitation treatment facility to the community.

Although it is preferable that discharge planning begin early and that the family and caregivers be involved in skills training, there is much that can be done to facilitate generalization of skills to community settings in cases in which the discharge setting is not known and/or family and discharge caregivers do not participate in the individual's treatment. Skills are more readily transferred to the community when practiced in settings other than the training milieu (Corrigan et al. 1993a); thus, staff might create opportunities to practice skills in the community by planning community outings. Also, staff can maximize the use of natural reinforcers by focusing on decreasing behaviors likely to be punished and increasing behaviors likely to be reinforced no matter what the eventual discharge setting (e.g., appropriate hygiene and social skills are likely to be reinforced in any setting an individual might be discharged to). That said, it is always preferable that future caregivers and significant others be involved in treatment as early as possible.

Although some individuals with TBI live independently or in residential facilities, many return home to their families. The independence and social integration of persons with TBI depend on successful family involvement (Proulx 1999). Thus, treatment providers should include the family in the rehabilitation process (Wesalowski and Zencius 1994). Research demonstrates that family intervention helps individuals with TBI become more cooperative and insightful (Prigatano 1999), facilitates family involvement in the rehabilitation program, and promotes recovery after TBI. In spite of these positive findings, many family members do not request or make use of available family support services (Miller and Borden 1994).

Family members often do not understand the role of psychology in rehabilitation or the role of behavior management strategies in the successful rehabilitation of persons with TBI (Iverson and Osman 1998). Although physical disabilities often require the most physical assistance, cognitive and behavioral deficits are often more difficult for family members to manage (Wesalowski and Zencius 1994). Family members of individuals with TBI tend to overestimate the individual's behavioral competencies (Miller and Borden 1994) and may become frustrated or punitive when he or she fails to live up to their expectations. Family members may also fail to maintain behavioral programming initiated in the rehabilitation setting, thereby reducing the likelihood of generalization and maintenance of newly learned adaptive behaviors. Education about TBI, stressing the importance of ongoing social support, and instruction in communication and problem-solving skills and behavior management and generalization techniques are key family interventions.

Most family support programs involve some form of education on diagnosis, course, treatment of conditions, and specific coping and behavior management strategies. This type of education can prevent negative emotional reactions to the TBI survivor. For example, education may prevent family members from blaming or criticizing the individual with TBI (Feinstein 1999) when they learn that the individual appears indifferent because he or she does not perceive the extent of the impairments rather than because he or she is unmotivated (Prigatano 1999).

Family members also benefit from instruction in behavior management skills to cope with both cognitive and behavioral deficits. For example, it is not uncommon for family members to have difficulty communicating with the cognitively impaired individual with TBI, to unwittingly promote dependence by completing tasks for the individual that he or she is able to complete without assistance (Wesolowski and Zencius 1994), or to perpetuate maladaptive behavior by reinforcing disruptive behaviors. Research suggests that training in communication skills and maximizing contextual support reduces confusion (Feinstein 1999). Giving family members explicit rehabilitative tasks to perform prevents them from placing unrealistic demands on the injured individual and, perhaps, also from doing too much for the individual. Family behaviors that promote independence have additional benefits in that persons with a greater activity level and more control have better memory and decision-making skills (Feinstein 1999). Instruction in extinction procedures is also beneficial for family members (Ducharme 2000) to make certain that maladaptive responses are not inadvertently reinforced. Overall, family training to maintain behavior programs begun in the rehabilitation setting is associated with patient adaptation and adjustment (Miller and Borden 1994).

Training in generalization techniques is also essential for the continued recovery of the TBI survivor. Without family training treatment, gains made by the individual will usually not be maintained over time once the individual is discharged to the home. Generalization does not occur automatically; it must be programmed (Wesolowski and Zencius 1994). Treatment providers must plan for generalization from the outset, identifying natural reinforcers present in the environment. Family members must be familiar with generalization from the rehabilitation setting to the individual's home environment and must be mindful of taking a long-term perspective and periodically reevaluating the effectiveness of behavior management strategies to assure lasting functional outcomes (Mills and Alexander 1999).

Finally, family members also benefit from information about family support services and instruction in communication and problem-solving skills (Liberman 1988; Mueser 1996). The level of family support is predictive of family stress. Those who receive more emotional and instrumental support report less stress, and training in problem-solving skills as outlined in the section Models of Behavioral Rehabilitation is associated with diminished family burden and improved psychological well-being (Miller and Borden 1994). Families are important allies in the rehabilitation process (Mueser and Glynn 1995) and must be regarded as consumers of rehabilitation services to promote the fullest possible family integration, attainment of the highest level of independence, and achievement of positive functional outcomes for the TBI survivor.

Summary

The model of behavioral treatment outlined in this chapter focuses on rehabilitation (i.e., facilitating the recovery of social and independent living skills so that individuals with TBI can meet everyday interpersonal and functional needs). As these individuals become competent in meeting life demands, frustrations and concomitant behavioral problems diminish in frequency. Clinicians who use a process model for setting up behavioral rehabilitation programs have a comprehensive outline for behavioral recovery. Skills training strategies facilitate acquisition of necessary skills. Contingency management and transfer training methods foster the performance and generalization of newly (re)acquired skills. Cognitive rehabilitation methods help those with TBI overcome learning deficits so they may profit from the program.

The process-based rehabilitation program is proactive in nature. Individuals are taught ways not only to cope with current problems but also to avoid future stressors. Behavioral programs must augment these programs with strategies that address patient aggression and extreme emotional responses. Replacement and decelerative strategies are ways to control aggression. Cognitive-behavioral interventions can be used to address the emotional reactions to TBI. When combined with judicious use of medications and physical rehabilitation, behavioral rehabilitation and therapy have significant effects on the individual with TBI.

References

Adams JH, Graham DI, Gennarelli TA: Contemporary neuropathological considerations regarding brain damage in head injury, in Central Nervous System Trauma Report. Edited by Becker DP, Povlishock JT. Prepared for the National Institute of Neurological and Communicative Disorders and Stroke, National Institutes of Health, Washington, DC, 1985, pp 65–67

Ayllon T, Azrin NH: The Token Economy: A Motivational System for Therapy and Rehabilitation. New York, Appleton-Century-Crofts, 1968

Beck AT, Rush AJ, Shaw BF, et al: Cognitive Therapy of Depression. New York, Guilford, 1979

Benson Yody B, Schaub C, Conway J, et al: Applied behavior management and acquired brain injury: approaches and assessment. J Head Trauma Rehabil 15:1041–1060, 2001

Ben-Yishay Y, Rattok Y, Ross B, et al: A remedial "module" for the systematic amelioration of basic disturbances in head trauma patients: working approaches to remediation of cognitive deficits in brain damaged persons. Rehabilitation monograph No. 61. New York, University Medical Center, Institute of Rehabilitation Medicine, 1980, pp 71–127

Ben-Yishay Y, Rattok J, Lakin P, et al: Neuropsychologic rehabilitation: quest for a holistic approach. Semin Neurol 5:252–259, 1985

Bernay LJ, Devitt JE: Managing acutely violent inpatients, in Understanding and Treating Violent Psychiatric Patients: Progress in Psychiatry #60. Edited by Crowner ML. Washington, DC, American Psychiatric Press, 2000, pp 49–68

Bernstein GS: Behavior analysis, professionalization, and deprofessionalization: issues and implications. Behavior Therapist 2:2–25, 1979

Bernstein GS: Training behavioral change agents. Behavior Therapist 13:1–23, 1983

Blackerby WF: Practical token economies. J Head Trauma Rehabil 3:33–45, 1988

Blackerby WF, Baumgarten A: A model treatment program for the head-injured substance abuser: preliminary findings. J Head Trauma Rehabil 5:47–59, 1990

Bleiberg J, Ciulla R, Katz B: Psychological components of rehabilitation programs for brain-injured and spinal-cord injured patients, in Clinical Psychology in Medical Settings. Edited by Sweet JJ, Rozensky RH, Tovian SM. New York, Academic Press, 1991, pp 122–149

Bombardier CH, Ehde D, Kilmer J: Readiness to change alcohol drinking habits after traumatic brain injury. Arch Phys Med Rehabil 78:592–596, 1997

Braukman CJ, Fixsen DL, Kirigan KA, et al: Achievement place: the training and certification of teaching parents, in Issues in Evaluating Behavior Modification. Edited by Woods WS. Champaign, IL, Research Press, 1975, pp 157–184

Brotherton FA, Thomas LL, Wisotzek IE, et al: Social skills training in the rehabilitation of patients with traumatic closed head injury. Arch Phys Med Rehabil 69:827–832, 1988

Burke WH, Lewis FD: Management of maladaptive social behavior of a brain injured adult. Int J Rehabil Res 9:335–342, 1986

Carsrud AL, Carsrud KB, Dodd BG: Randomly monitored staff utilization of behavior modification techniques: long term effects on clients. J Consult Clin Psychol 48:704–710, 1980

Cautela JR, Lynch E: Reinforcement survey schedules: scoring, administration, and completed research. Psychol Rep 53:447–465, 1983

Cicerone KD, Tupper DE: Cognitive assessment in the neuropsychological rehabilitation of head-injured adults, in Clinical Neuropsychology of Intervention. Edited by Uzzell BP, Gross Y. Boston, MA, Martinus Nijhoff, 1986, pp 155–173

Corrigan PW, Basit A: Generalization of social skills training for persons with severe mental illness. Cognitive and Behavioral Practices 4:191–206, 1997

Corrigan PW, McCracken SG: Interactive Staff Training: Rehabilitation Teams That Work. New York, Plenum, 1999

Corrigan PW, Mueser KT: Behavior therapy for aggressive psychiatric patients, in Treating Violent Psychiatric Patients: Progress in Psychiatry #60. Edited by Crowner ML. Washington, DC, American Psychiatric Press, 2000, pp 69–85

Corrigan PW, Davies-Farmer RM, Lome HB: A curriculum-based, psychoeducational program for the mentally ill. Psychosocial Rehabilitation Journal 12:71–73, 1988

Corrigan PW, Davies-Farmer RM, Lightstone R, et al: An analysis of the behavior components of psychoeducational treatment of persons with chronic, mental illness. Rehabil Couns Bull 33:200–211, 1990

Corrigan PW, Kwartarini WY, Pramana W: Barriers to the implementation of behavior therapy. Behav Modif 16:132–144, 1992

Corrigan PW, Schade ML, Liberman RP: Social skills training, in Rehabilitation of the Psychiatrically Disabled. Edited by Liberman RP. New York, Plenum, 1993a, pp 78–106

Corrigan PW, Yudofsky SC, Silver JM: Pharmacological and behavioral treatments for aggressive psychiatric inpatients. Hosp Community Psychiatry 44:125–133, 1993b

Corrigan PW, MacKain SJ, Liberman RP: Skills training modules: a strategy for dissemination and utilization of a rehabilitation innovation, in Intervention Research. Edited by Rothman J, Thomas E. Chicago, IL, Haworth, 1994, pp 317–352

Corrigan PW, Steiner L, McCracken SG, et al: Strategies for disseminating evidence-based practices to staff who treat people with serious mental illness. Psychiatr Serv 52:1598–1606, 2001

Crewe NM: Sexually inappropriate behavior, in Behavioral Problems and the Disabled: Assessment and Management. Edited by Bishop DS. Baltimore, MD, Williams & Wilkins, 1980, pp 120–141

Diller L, Gordon WA: Rehabilitation and clinical neuropsychology, in Handbook of Clinical Neuropsychology. Edited by Filskov SB, Boll TJ. New York, Wiley, 1981, pp 702–733

Douglas MS, Mueser KT: Teaching conflict resolution skills to the chronically mentally ill: social skills training groups for briefly hospitalized patients. Behav Modif 14:519–547, 1990

Ducharme JM: Treatment of maladaptive behavior in acquired brain injury: remedial approaches in postacute settings. Clin Psychol Rev 20:405–426, 2000

D'Zurilla TJ: Problem-Solving Therapy: A Social Competence Approach. New York, Springer, 1986

Falloon IRH, Boyd JL, McGill C: Family Care of Schizophrenia. New York, Guilford, 1984

Feinstein A: Mood and motivation in rehabilitation, in Cognitive Neurorehabilitation. Edited by Stuss DT, Winocour G. New York, Cambridge University Press, 1999, pp 230–239

Fisher WA: Restraint and seclusion: a review of the literature. Am J Psychiatry 151:1584–1591, 1994

Fluharty G, Glassman N: Use of antecedent control to improve the outcome of rehabilitation for a client with frontal lobe injury and intolerance for auditory and tactile stimuli. Brain Inj 15:995–1002, 2001

Foley FW, Bedell JR, LaRocca NG, et al: Efficacy of stress-inoculation training in coping with multiple sclerosis. J Consult Clin Psychol 55:919–922, 1987

Fordyce DJ, Roueche JR: Changes in perspectives of disability among patients, staff, and relatives during rehabilitation of head injury. Rehabil Psychol 31:217–229, 1986

Franzen MD, Lovell MR: Behavioral treatments of aggressive sequelae of brain injury. Special issue: treatment of aggressive disorders. Psychiatr Ann 17:389–396, 1987

Gajar AH, Schloss PJ, Schloss CN, et al: Effects of feedback and self-monitoring on head trauma youths' conversation skills. J Appl Behav Anal 17:353–358, 1984

Gazzaniga MS: Determinants of cerebral recovery, in Plasticity and Recovery of Function in the Central Nervous System. Edited by Stein DG, Rosen JJ, Butters N. New York, Academic Press, 1974, pp 203–216

Gazzaniga MS: Is seeing believing? Notes on clinical recovery, in Recovery from Brain Damage: Research and Theory. Edited by Finger S. New York, Plenum, 1978, pp 409–414

Glasgow RE, Zeiss RA, Barrera M, et al: Case studies on remediating memory deficits in brain damaged individuals. J Clin Psychol 33:1049–1054, 1977

Glynn SM, Bowen LL, Marshall BD, et al: Compliance with less restrictive aggression-control procedures. Hosp Community Psychiatry 40:82–84, 1989

Godfrey HPD, Knight RG: Memory training and behavioral rehabilitation of a severely head-injured adult. Arch Phys Med Rehabil 69:458–460, 1988

Hegel MT, Ferguson RJ: Differential reinforcement of other behavior (DRO) to reduce aggressive behavior following traumatic brain injury. Behav Modif 24:94–101, 2000

Hollon TH: Behavior modification in a community hospital rehabilitation unit. Arch Phys Med Rehabil 54:65–68, 1973

Horton AM, Howe NR: Behavioral treatment of the traumatically brain-injured: a case study. Percept Mot Skills 53:349–350, 1981

Horton AM, Miller WG: Brain damage and rehabilitation, in Current Topics in Rehabilitation Psychology. Edited by Golden CJ. New York, Grune & Stratton, 1984, pp 77–105

Horton AM, Sautter SW: Behavioral neuropsychology: behavioral treatment for the brain-injured, in The Neuropsychology Handbook: Behavioral and Clinical Perspective. Edited by Wedding A, Horton AM, Webster J. New York, Springer, 1986, pp 259–277

Horton AM, Wedding D: Clinical and Behavioral Neuropsychology. New York, Praeger, 1984

Ince LP: Behavior Modification in Rehabilitation Medicine. Springfield, IL, Charles C Thomas, 1976

Iverson G, Osman A: Behavioral interventions for children and adults with brain injuries: a guide for families. The Journal of Cognitive Rehabilitation 16:14–23, 1998

Kaufman H: Kaufman Developmental Scale. Chicago, IL, Stoetling, 1975

Kazdin AE: The token economy: a decade later. J Appl Behav Anal 15:431–445, 1982

Kazdin AE, Bootzin RR: The token economy: an evaluation review. J Appl Behav Anal 5:1–30, 1972

Klonoff PS, Snow WG, Costa LD: Quality of life in patients 2 to 4 years after closed head injury. Neurosurgery 19:735–743, 1986

Kushner H, Knox A: Application of the utilization technique to the behavior of a brain-injured patient. J Commun Disord 6:151–154, 1973

Larcombe NA, Wilson PH: An evaluation of cognitive-behavior therapy for depression in patients with multiple sclerosis. Br J Psychiatry 145:366–371, 1984

Lennox DB, Miltonberger RG, Sprengler P, et al: Decelerative treatment practices with persons who have mental retardation: a review of five years of the literature. Am J Ment Retard 92:492–501, 1988

Levin HS, Benton AL, Grossman RG: Neurobehavioral Consequences of Closed Head Injury. New York, Oxford University Press, 1982

Lewinsohn PM, Biglan BG, Zeiss AM: Behavioral treatment of depression, in Progress in Behavior Modification, Vol 1. Edited by Hersen M, Eisler RM, Miller PM. New York, Pergamon, 1976, pp 184–189

Lewinsohn PM, Danaher BG, Kikel S: Visual imagery as a mnemonic aid for brain injured persons. J Consult Clin Psychol 45:717–723, 1977

Liberman RP: Social skills training, in Psychiatric Rehabilitation of Chronic Mental Patients. Edited by Liberman RP. Washington, DC, American Psychiatric Press, 1988, pp 132–161

Liberman RP, Corrigan PW: Designing new psychosocial treatments for schizophrenia. Psychiatry 56:119–124, 1993

Liberman RP, Wong SE: Behavioral analysis and therapy procedures related to seclusion and restraint, in The Psychiatric Uses of Seclusion and Restraint. Edited by Tardiff K. Washington, DC, American Psychiatric Press, 1984, pp. 216–241

Linn RT, Allen K, Willer BS: Affective symptoms in the chronic stage of traumatic brain injury: a study of married couples. Brain Inj 8:135–147, 1994

Lira FT, Carne W, Masri AM: Treatment of anger and impulsivity in a brain damaged patient: a case study applying stress inoculation. Clin Neuropsychol 5:159–160, 1983

Lovell MR, Starratt C: Cognitive rehabilitation and behavior therapy of neuropsychiatric disorders, in Synopsis of Neuropsychiatry. Edited by Yudofsky SC, Hales RE. Washington, DC, American Psychiatric Press, 1994, pp 561–570

Marholin DH, Luiselli JK, Townsend NM: Overcorrection: An examination of its rationale and treatment effectiveness, in Progress in Behavior Modification, Vol 10. Edited by Hersen M, Eisler RM, Miller P. M. New York, Academic Press, 1980, pp 56–69

Matson JL, Stephens RM: Overcorrection of aggressive behavior in a chronic psychiatric patient. Behav Modif 1:559–564, 1977

McGlynn SM: Behavioral approaches to neuropsychological rehabilitation. Psychol Bull 108:420–441, 1990

Meichenbaum D: A self-instructional approach to stress management: a proposal for stress inoculation training, in Stress and Anxiety, Vol 1. Edited by Spielberger C, Sarasen I. New York, Wiley, 1975, pp 237–263

Miller FE, Borden W: Family caregivers of persons with neuropsychiatric illness: a stress and coping perspective, in Synopsis of Neuropsychiatry. Edited by Yudofsky SC, Hales RE. Washington, DC, American Psychiatric Press, 1994, pp 571–582

Miller WR, Rollnick S: Motivational Interviewing: Preparing People to Change Addictive Behavior. New York, Guilford, 1991

Mills VM, Alexander MP: Cognitive rehabilitation: leadership and management of the clinical programme, in Cognitive Neurorehabilitation. Edited by Stuss DT, Winocour G. New York, Cambridge University Press, 1999, pp 175–187

Milne DL: A comparison of two methods of teaching behaviour modification to mental handicap nurses. Behavioural Psychotherapy 10:54–64, 1982

Milne DL: The development and evaluation of structured learning format introduction to behavior therapy for psychiatric nurses. Br J Clin Psychol 23:175–185, 1984

Mozzoni MP, Hartnedy S: Escape and avoidance hypothesis testing using an alternative treatment design. Behavioral Interventions 15:269–277, 2000

Mueller DJ, Atlas L: Resocialization of regressed elderly residents: a behavioral management approach. J Gerontol 27:390–392, 1972

Mueser KT: Helping families manage severe mental illness. Psychiatric Rehabilitation Skills 1:21–42, 1996

Mueser KT, Glynn SM: Behavioral Family Therapy for Psychiatric Disorders. Boston, MA, Allyn & Bacon, 1995

Murphy ST: The effects of a token economy program on self-care behaviors of neurologically impaired inpatients. J Behav Ther Exp Psychiatry 7:145–147, 1976

Oddy M, Coughlan T, Tyerman A, et al: Social adjustment after closed head injury: a further follow-up seven years after injury. J Neurol Neurosurg Psychiatry 48:564–568, 1985

Passler MA: A two-phase treatment approach for traumatically brain-injured patients: a case study. Rehabil Psychol 32:215–226, 1987

Porterfield JK, Herbert-Jackson E, Risley TR: Contingent observation: an effective and acceptable procedure for reducing disruptive behavior of young children in a group setting. J Appl Behav Anal 9:55–64, 1976

Premack D: Reversibility of the reinforcement relation. Science 136:255–257, 1962

Prigatano GP: Motivation and awareness in cognitive neurorehabilitation, in Cognitive Neurorehabilitation. Edited by Stuss DT, Wincour J. New York, Cambridge University Press, 1999, pp 240–251

Prigatano GP, Altman IM: Impaired awareness of behavioral limitations after traumatic brain injury. Arch Phys Med Rehabil 71:1058–1064, 1990

Prigatano GP, Fordyce DJ: The neuropsychological rehabilitation program at Presbyterian Hospital, in Neuropsychological Rehabilitation After Brain Injury. Edited by Prigatano GP. Baltimore, MD, Johns Hopkins University Press, 1986, pp 96–118

Proulx GB: Family education and family partnership in cognitive rehabilitation, in Cognitive Neurorehabilitation. Edited by Stuss DT, Winocour G. New York, Cambridge University Press, 1999, pp 252–259

Reniscow K, DiIorio C, Soet JE, et al: Motivational Interviewing in medical and public health settings, in Motivational Interviewing: Preparing People for Change, 2nd Edition. Edited by Miller WR, Rollnick S. New York, Guilford, 2002, pp 251–269

Schade ML, Corrigan PW, Liberman RP: Comprehensive psychiatric rehabilitation. New Dir Ment Health Serv 45:3–17, 1990

Schloss PJ, Schloss CN, Gajar AH: Efficacy of four ratios of questions to text in computer assisted instruction modules. Journal of Computer Based Instruction 11:103–106, 1984

Silver JM, Yudofsky SC: Documentation of aggression in the assessment of the violent patient. Psychiatr Ann 17:375–384, 1987

Skinner BF: Science and Human Behavior. New York, Macmillan, 1953

Spiegler MD, Agigian H: Community Training Center: An Educational-Behavioral-Social Systems Model for Rehabilitating Psychiatric Patients. New York, Bruner/Mazel, 1977

Stokes TF, Baer DM: An implicit technology of generalization. J Appl Behav Anal 10:349–367, 1977

Stokes TF, Osnes PG: An operant pursuit of generalization. Behav Ther 20:337–355, 1989

Sunderland A, Harris JE, Baddeley AD: Do laboratory tests predict everyday memory? A neuropsychological study. Journal of Verbal Learning and Verbal Behavior 22:341–347, 1983

Sunderland A, Harris JE, Gleave J: Memory failures in everyday life following severe head injury. J Clin Neuropsychol 6:127–142, 1984

Tardiff K, Sweillam A: Assaultive behavior among chronic inpatients. Am J Psychiatry 139:212–215, 1982

Tellier A, Adams KM, Walker AE, et al: Long-term effects of severe penetrating head injury on psychosocial adjustment. J Consult Clin Psychol 58:531–537, 1990

Tharp R, Wetzel R: Behavior Modification in the Natural Environment. New York, Academic Press, 1969

Thomsen IV: Late outcome of very severe blunt head trauma: a 10–15 year second follow-up. J Neurol Neurosurg Psychiatry 48:21–28, 1984

Turner SM, Hersen M, Bellack AS: Social skills training to teach prosocial behavior in an organically impaired and retarded patient. J Behav Ther Exp Psychiatry 9:253–258, 1978

Warschausky S, Kewman D, Kay J: Empirically supported psychological and behavioral therapies in pediatric rehabilitation of TBI. J Head Trauma Rehabil 14:373–383, 1999

Watson C, Rutterford NA, Shortland D, et al: Reduction of chronic aggressive behavior 10 years after brain injury. Brain Inj 15:1003–1015, 2001

Watson LS, Uzell R: A program for teaching behavior modification skills to institutional staff. App Res Ment Retard 1:41–53, 1980

Webster JS, Scott RR: The effects of self-instructive training on attention deficits following head injury. Clin Neuropsychol 5:69–74, 1983

Wehman PH, Kreutzer JS, West MD, et al: Return to work for persons with traumatic brain injury: a supported employment approach. Arch Phys Med Rehabil 71:1047–1052, 1990

Wesolowski MD, Zencius AH: A Practical Guide to Head Injury Rehabilitation: A Focus on Postacute Residential Treatment. New York, Plenum, 1994

Wesolowski M, Zencius AH, Rodriquez IM: Mini-breaks: the use of escape on a fixed-time schedule to reduce unauthorized breaks from vocational training sites for individuals with brain injury. Behavioral Interventions 14:163–170, 1999

Wood R: Behavioural disturbance and behavioural management, in New Directions in the Neuropsychology of Severe Blunt Head Injury Symposium. Paper presented at the meeting of the International Neuropsychological Society, Deauville, FR, 1982

Wood RL, Eames PG: Application of behaviour modification in the rehabilitation of traumatically brain-injured patients, in Applications of Conditioning Theory. Edited by Davey G. New York, Methuen, 1981, pp 81–101

38 Alternative Treatments

Richard P. Brown, M.D.

Patricia L. Gerbarg, M.D.

HERBS, NUTRIENTS, AND nootropics are capturing the attention of researchers and clinicians interested in new treatments for patients with brain injury. Nootropics are compounds that enhance learning and memory and increase the resistance of learning functions. Alternative treatments encompass herbs, nutrients, and foreign medications that are not in general use by physicians in the United States, although they may be widely used in other countries and cultures. Many of these cross the threshold of acceptance and become mainstream treatments; for example, the herbalists' snowdrop, renamed galantamine for its debut as a cholinergic agent.

The number of human studies using alternative treatments in traumatic brain injury (TBI) per se is limited. Therefore, our review of the literature took advantage of overlaps in the pathophysiology of TBI with Alzheimer's dementia (AD), age-associated memory impairment (AAMI), poststroke, and animal models of trauma and ischemia. Because TBI is often complicated by secondary ischemia, patients may benefit from compounds used to treat ischemia (Chen et al. 1998; Zauner and Bullock 1995). Controlled clinical studies are available for many agents, but for some there are only animal studies, open trials, and clinical experience. In general, the deficiency of controlled studies may not reflect the usefulness of these agents, but rather the lack of financial incentive to invest in costly clinical trials for products that are inexpensive or not patentable.

Patients seek alternative treatments when prescription medications are ineffective or cause intolerable side effects. Alternative agents may have fewer side effects and may ameliorate fatigue, cognitive dysfunction (memory, attention, concentration, executive functions), affective disorders, aphasias, and postconcussion symptoms. They

can be integrated with conventional medications and cognitive rehabilitation to optimize recovery.

In our experience, the treatments described in this chapter appear to be helpful in some patients with TBI. Additional controlled studies are needed to confirm the efficacy and the clinical applications of alternative treatments.

Framework of Pathophysiological Mechanisms

The probable mechanisms by which alternative agents improve brain function can be placed within a pathophysiological framework using four constructs: neurotransmitter hypotheses, biochemical and metabolic derangements, neuroanatomy, and brain wave patterns.

Neurotransmitter abnormalities after TBI include abnormalities of the cholinergic system (acetylcholine [Ach]) (Arciniegas 2001), catecholamines (dopamine [DA] and norepinephrine) (Hayes and Dixon 1994), indoleamine (serotonin [5-HT]), and N-methyl-D-aspartate–glutamate receptor systems. Cholinergic deficits have been found in rat brain after brain injury (Schmidt and Grady 1995) and in TBI patients postmortem (Murdoch et al. 1998). Animal studies have demonstrated involvement of glutamate and DA systems in recovery after TBI. Human TBI studies of DA agonists, such as amantadine, methylphenidate, and bromocriptine, report improvements in brain function. Biochemical and metabolic derangements thought to be involved in brain injury include decreases in cellular energy (mitochondrial) production, presence of free radicals (Long et al. 1996), hypoxia, secondary ischemia, nerve membrane alterations, decreased calcium channel conductance, presence of nitric oxide (Sinz et al. 1999), and blood-brain barrier (BBB) damage (Hayes and Dixon 1994). A study of pericontusional edematous areas in patients with mild TBI (Glasgow Coma Scale [GCS] score of 13–15) showed significant cell loss and ischemic changes on magnetic resonance spectroscopy (Son et al. 2000). After TBI in rats, there is an increase in neurotrophic factors such as nerve growth factor, which attenuates cholinergic deficits (Dixon et al. 1997).

The areas most sensitive to traumatic injury in rodents are the hippocampus, ventromedial cortex, ventrobasal forebrain, cingulate gyrus, and reticular system (Murdoch et al. 1998; Schmidt and Grady 1995). Hippocampal cells in the CA3 region also decline during aging, with concomitant decreased neuronal firing, increased lipid peroxidation, and increased lipofuscin (accumulated membrane fragments of damaged proteins and fatty acids). Stimulation of CA3 fibers induces longterm potentiation of synaptic transmission, critical for memory and learning. Information transfer across the corpus callosum is also essential for learning and memory. Computerized electroencephalographic maps of patients with TBI show excess slow wave activity and/or decreased beta or alpha waves, similar to individuals after stroke (Rozelle et al. 1995). Cognitive activating agents decrease slow wave activity and increase alpha and beta waves (Itil et al. 1998).

General Principles in the Use of Alternative Treatments in TBI

The psychopharmacological principles for understanding the use of alternative medicines are essentially the same as those for conventional drugs, with some qualifications. As with prescription medications, in fragile patients, one begins with low doses and increases slowly. One titrates doses according to a balance of benefits and side effects. Adverse reactions to properly prescribed U.S. Food and Drug Administration–approved medications were the third leading cause of death in the United States in 1997 (100,000 deaths) (Starfield 2000). In contrast, few deaths have been attributed to properly administered alternative compounds, even in Germany where statistics of adverse reactions are carefully maintained by the National Health Service. For example, a Phase IV, postmarketing, 2-year study of S-adenosylmethionine (SAMe) in more than 20,000 arthritis patients documented a low incidence of mild side effects (Berger and Nowak 1987). There has never been a comparable postmarketing study of any prescription psychotropic medication in the United States.

Raw natural compounds often contain multiple bioactive constituents, which may have therapeutic, antagonistic, synergistic, and toxic properties. Advances in biochemistry (e.g., high-pressure liquid chromatography) have enabled substantial progress in identifying active therapeutic components and in removing toxic compounds. Each agent must be assessed for purity and interactions with other drugs. Although, on the one hand, there are fewer data on combination treatments, the paucity of side effects and the understanding in many cases of the probable mechanisms of action permit recognition of the need for caution with certain combinations (e.g., combining two agents when both have cholinergic effects) and the safety and synergistic benefits of other combinations. Some alternative agents have dramatic effects, but most are mild and gradual. However, in cases of TBI, even modest effects may lead to significant clinical improvements. Combining two or more agents with subtle action may enhance the patient's quality of life. The use of combined agents is discussed for those treatments that, in our experience, have been effective without serious adverse events.

Recovery from brain injury requires adequate vitamins and nutrients. Patients with TBI are often too ill, and patients with postconcussion syndromes too inattentive, to maintain a good diet. Therefore, particular attention must be given to vitamins and nutrients that sustain and enhance neuronal functions.

Space limitations preclude a detailed review of the in vitro and in vivo (predominantly animal) studies that indicate probable mechanisms of action for each compound. Refer to Table 38–1 for a summary of this research. Table 38–2 presents treatment guidelines, clinical indications, doses, and side effects. Figure 38–1 is a clinical decision-making flow sheet for target symptoms.

Specific Alternative Compounds With Neurological Benefits

Cholinergic Enhancing Agents

Galantamine

Galantamine, a tertiary alkaloid extracted from snowdrop (*Galanthus nivalus*), was used by the long-lived people of the Province of Georgia for centuries to enhance memory in old age. It was available in Eastern Europe and Russia for 40 years before being released in the United States as a prescription drug for AD (Riemann et al. 1994). Galantamine is a nicotinic allosteric modulator and a weak

TABLE 38–1. Putative mechanisms of action for alternative compounds

Compound	Neurotransmitters				Receptors	Cell energy	Antioxidant	Cell membrane
	Choline	Norepinephrine	Dopamine	Serotonin				
Galantamine	+				Nicotinic-Chol			
Huperzine	+							
Centrophenoxine	+					+	+	+
Acetyl-L-carnitine	+		+		NMDA	+++	+++	++
Citicholine	+	+	+	+		++	++	++
S-adenosylmethionine	+	+	+	+	β-NE Chol GABA	++	+++	+++
Pyritinol	+					+	++	+
Idebenone	½+		+	+		++	++	
Vinpocetine					Glutamate			+
Rhodiola rosea	+	+	+	+		+++	++	
Ginkgo			+	+			+	
Ginseng		+	+	?	GABA			
Pyrrolidones (racetams)	+	+	+	+	NMDA-glutamate (muscarinic-Chol)	++		+
L-Deprenyl		+	+	+	Protects		++	++
B vitamins (Bio-Strath)							++	+

(continued)

TABLE 38–1. Putative mechanisms of action for alternative compounds *(continued)*

Compound	↓ Hypoxia	↓ Secondary ischemia	Blood flow	Blood-brain barrier	Nerve growth factor	Lipofuscin	Long-term potentiation	Transcallosal	Cognitive activator
Galantamine									++
Huperzine									++
Centrophenoxine	+	+		+		+		+	++
Acetyl-L-carnitine	++	++	+	+		+			++
Citicholine	+	++		++					+
S-adenosylmethionine		++							+
Picamilon		++	+++						+
Pyritinol	+	+	+						+
Idebenone	+	+	?		+		+	+	+
Vinpocetine		+	+++				+		+
Rhodiola rosea	+								+++
Ginkgo	+	+							+
Ginseng	+	+	?						+
Pyrrolidones (racetams)	+	+					+	++	+
L-Deprenyl					+++				+
B vitamins (Bio-Strath)									+

Note. Chol=cholinergic; GABA=γ-aminobutyric acid; NMDA=*N*-methyl-D-aspartate; β-NE=β-adrenergic; GABA=γ-aminobutyric acid; +=some effect; ++=moderate effect; +++=strong effect; ?=possible effect; ↓=decreases; blank=no information available.

TABLE 38–2. Treatment guidelines

Alternative agent	Clinical indications	Dose	Side effects and drug interactions
Galantamine	AD	16–32 mg/day	Mild nausea, GI upset.
Huperzine	AD, TBI	100–400 µg/day	Rare: mild nausea.
Centrophenoxine	AD, TBI	500–2,000 mg/day	Minimal. When combined with other cholinergic agents: headache, muscle tension, insomnia, irritability, agitation, facial tics.
Acetyl-L-carnitine	AD (slowed progression), TBI, and CVA	1,500 mg bid	Mild GI upset. Take with food.
Citicholine	TBI	1,000–3,000 mg/day	None significant.
S-adenosylmethionine	AD, dementia	800–1,600 mg/day	Mild, occasional GI upset, agitation, anxiety, insomnia; rare palpitations. Mania in bipolar patients.
	TBI	400–4,000 mg/day	Take 30 minutes before breakfast and lunch.
Picamilon	TBI, CVA, toxic brain lesions	50 mg bid up to 100 mg tid	High dose: hypotension. No allergenic, carcinogenic, or teratogenic effects in 6-month test.
Pyritinol	CVD, AD, TBI	900–1,200 mg/day	Minimal, skin reactions.
Idebenone	CVD, AD, TBI	270–900 mg/day	GI upset, anxiety, insomnia, headache, tachycardia, ↓ platelet aggregation.
Vinpocetine	CVD, TBI	10 mg tid	Rare: nausea, low BP.
Rhodiola rosea	Cognitive enhancement	150–600 mg/day	Activation, agitation, insomnia, jitteriness, mania. Rare: ↑ BP, angina, bruising. Avoid in bipolar I patients.
	TBI	300–600 mg/day	Take 20 minutes before breakfast and lunch.
Ginkgo biloba	Age-associated memory impairment, AD, CVD	120–240 mg/day	Minimal, headache, ↓ platelet aggregation.
Ginseng	Dementia, neurasthenia	400–800 mg/day	Activation.
Racetams	Poststroke aphasia, dyslexia	Aniracetam, 1,500 mg/day	Minimal. Rare: anxiety, insomnia, agitation, irritability, headache.
L-Deprenyl	TBI	10–15 mg/week	Take 2.5 mg 5 days a week.
B vitamins (Bio-Strath)	TBI	B_{12}, 1,000 µg/day B-complex	None.

Note. AD=Alzheimer's dementia; BP=blood pressure; CVA=cardiovascular accident; CVD=cardiovascular disease; GI=gastrointestinal; TBI=traumatic brain injury; ↑=increases; ↓=decreases.

inhibitor of acetylcholinesterase (the enzyme that degrades Ach at cholinergic synapses). For treatment of AD, it is comparable to other cholinesterase inhibitors in short-term trials (5–6 months), and improvement continues beyond 6 months—that is, better than the delayed rate of deterioration seen with other cholinesterase inhibitors such as donepezil (Tariot et al. 2000; Wilcock et al. 2000). In our clinical experience, an herbal extract of *Galanthus nivalis* combined with *Rhodiola rosea* has been more

tolerable and effective in patients who could not tolerate galantamine or donepezil.

Huperzine-A

For patients who cannot tolerate any of the cholinergic agents, Huperzine-A is a useful alternative with fewer side effects. This alkaloid extract of Chinese club moss (*Huperzia serrata*) is a potent selective acetylcholinesterase inhibitor. Chinese researchers found that it enhanced

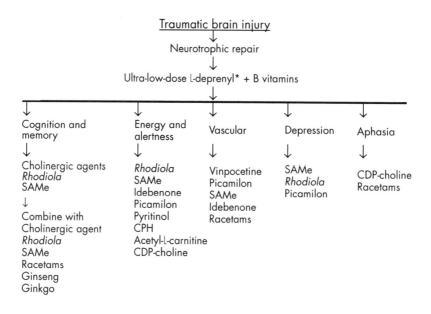

FIGURE 38–1.   Clinical decision making for target symptoms.

*Ultra low-dose L-deprenyl: 10–15 mg/week.

Abbreviations: SAMe=S-adenosylmethionine; CPH=centrophenoxine; CDP-choline=citicholine.

learning and memory in animals, including primates (Tang 1996; Xu et al. 1995). In a double-blind, randomized, placebo-controlled (DBRPC) multicenter (MC) study of Alzheimer's disease, 50 patients were given Huperzine, 0.2 mg bid, and 53 patients were given placebo for 8 weeks (Xu et al. 1995). All patients were evaluated with the Wechsler Memory Scale, the Hasegawa Dementia Scale, the Mini-Mental State Examination (MMSE), an activity of daily living scale, and the Treatment Emergent Symptom Scale. Approximately 58% (29/50) of patients treated with Huperzine showed improvements in memory ($P<0.01$), cognitive ($P<0.01$), and behavioral ($P<0.01$) functions compared with placebo (36%, 19/53; $P<0.05$). No severe side effects occurred (Xu et al. 1995).

Centrophenoxine (Meclofenoxate)

Centrophenoxine (CPH), or meclofenoxate, widely used in Europe (brand name, Lucidril), is a composite of dimethylaminoethanol (DMAE) and parachlorophenoxyacetic acid. DMAE is a byproduct of choline metabolism. Humans cannot produce enough choline by de novo synthesis to meet the body's needs. Although no optimal daily choline intake has been recommended, in 1998, the Food and Drug Board of the Institute of Medicine in Washington, DC, advised approximately 0.5 g/day of choline as the adequate intake level to prevent liver disease (Raloff 2001). The amount needed for wellness and recovery from tissue damage is probably higher. Changes

in contemporary diets tend to reduce consumption of foods that are highest in choline: 3 oz beef liver=452 mg choline, one large egg (yolk)=280 mg, 3 oz cooked beef=59 mg, 2 Tbsp peanut butter=26 mg, and 8 oz whole milk=10 mg. CPH supplementation elevates brain choline levels (Wood and Peloquin 1982). Parachlorophenoxyacetic acid is a synthetic version of plant growth hormones.

Zs-Nagy (1994), promoting the membrane hypothesis of aging, attributes the effects of CPH to the rapid delivery of DMAE to the brain for incorporation into nerve cell membranes as phosphatidyl-DMAE, an avid scavenger of OH-radicals. Rapidly acting OH-radicals cause a high rate of damage to membranes, with loss of permeability, increased intracellular density, accumulation of cross-linked proteins and lipofuscin, slowed RNA synthesis, and decreased protein turnover and repair. In aged rats, CPH increased acetylcholinesterase activity in the hippocampus and brainstem, reversed age-related microstructural deterioration of synapses, and reduced lipofuscin and lipid peroxidation (Sharma and Singh 1995). Ginkgo biloba (Egb-761) increased the effect of meclofenoxate in reducing membrane lipid peroxidation and increased the measure of free radical scavenging in the brain and heart of aged rats (al-Zuhair et al. 1998). Electroencephalographic data in aged rats show sustained increases in neuronal activity, even with hypoxia, via stimulation of the reticular formation (Nandy 1978). Reviewing the extensive research, Zs-Nagy and colleagues (Schneider et al. 1994; Zs-Nagy 1994) described its use in TBI, poststroke, and senility. However, there are no placebo-controlled (PC) trials of CPH in TBI. In our experience, CPH has been synergistic with racetams and ginkgo.

Acetyl-L-Carnitine

Forty years of research on acetyl-L-carnitine (ALCAR) have been reviewed (Anonymous 1999; Kelly 1998). ALCAR is an ester of L-carnitine, a trimethylated amino acid synthesized in brain, liver, and kidney. Animal studies indicate that ALCAR substantially enhances the cholinergic system (Pettegrew et al. 2000). It facilitates uptake of acetylcoenzyme A into mitochondria during fatty acid oxidation. ALCAR protected brain cells after stroke in rats and improved recovery (Calvani and Arrigoni-Martelli 1999; Lolic et al. 1997). In a 1-year DBRPC study of 431 patients with probable AD, Thal et al. (2000) found no difference between those given ALCAR, 3 g/day, versus placebo using the Alzheimer's Disease Assessment Scale (ADAS), the MMSE, and the Washington University Clinical Dementia Rating Scale. However, in their review of Thal's data, Pettegrew et al. (2000) noted that patients younger than 65 years showed less deterioration with ALCAR than with placebo using the ADAS-cognitive subscale (ADAS-cog) and the Washington University Clinical Dementia Rating Scale measures. Furthermore, multiple regression analysis of Thal's data by Brooks et al. (1998) found a significant age×drug interaction. Younger patients benefited more from ALCAR than older patients in slowing the progression of AD (Brooks et al. 1998). Pettegrew et al. (2000) concluded that "ALCAR could be more beneficial in presenile AD than in senile AD." Shortcomings of the Thal study included lack of apolipoprotein E genotyping, family histories, and information on statistical differences between test centers. ALCAR improved reaction time, memory, and cognitive performance in a double-blind, crossover, PC study of 12 elderly subjects with cerebral vascular disease. It caused no side effects (Arrigo et al. 1990). Rosadini et al. (1990) found increased regional cerebral blood flow in 8 out of 10 men with brain ischemia 1 hour after a dose of ALCAR, 1,500 mg intravenously. In our clinical experience, TBI patients often have improvement in energy and cognitive function within a week or two of beginning to take ALCAR.

Citicholine

Citicholine (CDP-choline), or cytidine 5-diphosphocholine (CDPc), readily crosses the BBB and dissociates into choline, an Ach precursor, and cytidine, a ribonucleoside. Animal studies suggest that CDP-choline helps restore structural integrity to nerve cell membrane damaged by numerous insults, including TBI. It also enhances incorporation of the choline moiety into phospholipids, synthesis of phospholipids, and cerebral mitochondrial lipid metabolism (Petkov et al. 1992). In addition to increasing phospholipid synthesis, CDPc improves the regulation of cellular energy charge and the function of neurotransmitters and receptors by increasing the ability of adenosine triphosphatase to break down adenosine triphosphate (ATP) (to generate energy in the mitochondria) and improving the function of Na^+/K^+-adenosine triphosphatase (to maintain cellular membrane potential), which is crucial for cell membrane integrity and electrical transmission (Galletti et al. 1991). The choline moiety is partially converted into betaine, a methyl donor to homocysteine, yielding methionine, which is incorporated into proteins.

CDPc has been used in Europe and Japan to treat stroke, dementia, and TBI. CDPc exerted a dose-dependent neuroprotective effect in the cerebral cortex and hippocampus by decreasing brain edema and BBB breakdown in rat cortical impact studies (Baskaya et al. 2000). In a Phase III DBRPC MC 6-week study, 899 patients were given either CDP-choline, 1,000 mg orally bid, or placebo within 24 hours of stroke. On the basis of the primary measure, the National Institutes of Health Stroke Scale scores, there were no significant differences between the two groups. However, post hoc analysis suggested a modest treatment effect using standard "excellent recovery" and other measures (Clark et al. 2001). The subgroup of patients with baseline National Institutes of Health Stroke Scale scores of 8 or higher showed a higher rate of full recovery, 33% of patients taking CDP-choline versus 21% taking placebo (Clark et al. 1999). In a DBRPC trial of 30 patients with mild to moderate AD and with the epsilon 4 allele of the apolipoprotein E (Global Deterioration Scale: stages 3–6), patients treated with 1,000 mg/day of CDPc for 12 weeks showed improved cognitive performance compared with patients given placebo. The comparison between the two groups showed an ADAS difference=−3.2±1.3 and ADAS-cog difference=−2.3±1.5. Patients with milder dementia (Global Deterioration Scale score <5) showed an even more pronounced improvement after taking CDPc. Transcranial Doppler recordings from both hemispheres and diastolic velocity in the left middle cerebral artery showed increased cerebral blood flow in patients treated with CDP-choline. CDPc also increased alpha and beta waves, while it decreased theta-type waves. There were no adverse effects (Alvarez et al. 1999). Warach et al. reported significant dose-related reduction in the average increase in infarct volume (as measured on magnetic resonance imaging) in a double-blind, PC (DBPC) 6-week trial of CDPc in 214 patients with middle cerebral artery strokes (Mitka 2002).

Spiers and Hochanadel (1999) reviewed the literature and reported positive results in two cases using CPDc, 1,000 mg bid, for TBI. Studies of CDPc done in the 1970s and 1980s found significant clinical and electroencephalographic improvements in TBI patients using measures available at the time. Limitations of early studies include less precise measures of coma level, fewer neuropsychological measures, use of subtherapeutic doses, and nonrandomization. In a double-blind, randomized series of 50 comatose patients (32 post-TBI) with coma levels ranging from I to IV, CDPc-treated patients recovered consciousness more rapidly compared with another series of similar patients receiving customary treatment (De La Herran et al. 1978). A double-blind study of 43 children with "altered levels of consciousness" secondary to TBI eliminated severe cases and cases requiring surgery (Carcassonne and LeTourneau 1979). The study group of children treated with CDPc showed accelerated recovery of normal consciousness, resolution of neuropsychic disorders, and improvements on electroencephalography compared with control subjects. One DBPC study of 46 patients found significantly more rapid recovery of consciousness in patients with less severe coma given low doses (250 mg/day intravenously) of CDP-choline compared with placebo. In more severe comas, recovery of consciousness was slow (>15 days) in 31% of patients and mortality rate was 12.5% in the CDPc-treated patients compared with slow recovery in 75.2% and mortality of 31% in those taking placebo (Espagno et al. 1979). Cohadon and Richer (1985) studied 60 comatose TBI patients given either CDPc or placebo for 90 days. The CDPc group had shorter duration of coma, improved motor deficits, and faster recovery of the ability to walk. In a DBRPC pilot study, 14 consecutively admitted patients with mild to moderate brain injury (GCS score of 13–15) were randomly assigned to receive 1,000 mg/day of CDP-choline or placebo. Patients were not started on treatment until they had come out of coma (1 month or more postinjury). CDP-choline produced significantly more improvement in postconcussion symptoms (especially dizziness) and recognition memory for designs. Better results might have been obtained if treatment had been started earlier (Levin 1991). In a single-blind, randomized study, 216 patients with moderate to severe brain injury (GCS score of 5–10) were given CDPc or conventional treatment. Those taking CDPc showed more cognitive, motor, and psychic improvements and shorter mean stays in the intensive care unit (ICU) (Calatayud Maldonado et al. 1991). Thirty-nine TBI patients with initial GCS scores of 5–7 and no intracranial pathol-

ogy requiring surgery were treated with continuous infusion of CDP-choline, 3–6 g/day, for the first 2 weeks. A comparison group with similar characteristics and similar General Cognitive Index scores received only standard treatment. Computed tomography scans at baseline and 2 weeks showed significantly greater development of cerebral edema in the control group ($P<0.005$). Average length of hospital stay for the CDPc group was 28.7 ± 21.6 days versus 37.3 ± 35.2 days for the placebo group ($P<0.001$). Differences in scores on the Glasgow Outcome Scale did not reach statistical significance, possibly because of the small number of cases. Limitations of this study included lack of double blinding, randomization, and placebo (Lozano 1991).

Leon-Carrion et al. (2000) conducted two studies of patients with severe persistent memory deficits after TBI 6 months after hospital discharge. All patients had GCS scores less than 8 during the acute phase and scores below 60% of expected memory capacity for age on Luria's Memory Words—Revised. In the first study, regional cerebral blood flow in seven patients showed hypoperfusion of the inferoposterior temporal lobe (a region associated with memory) during rest. An infusion of 1 g of CDPc 1 hour before inhalation of xenon-133 increased the average blood flow from 88.5% to 96.15% in area T3L. The second study of 10 patients given 3 months of ecological neuropsychological memory rehabilitation randomized 5 patients to CDPc, 1 g/day, and 5 to placebo. The placebo group had no statistically significant improvements. In contrast, the CDPc-treated group improved in attention, vigilance, and the Benton Visual Retention Test, but improvements reached statistical significance in verbal fluency and Luria's Memory Words—Revised ($P<0.05$) (Leon-Carrion et al. 2000). In these studies, the correlation between improved inferoposterior temporal perfusion and enhancement of neuropsychological training in TBI patients with severe memory deficits is reduced to an inference because two different groups of patients were used. A larger DBRPC follow-up study using positron emission tomography (PET) scans of the patients engaged in neuropsychological rehabilitation would provide stronger support for the benefits of CDPc.

Nutrients

S-*Adenosylmethionine*

SAMe, a naturally occurring condensation of the amino acid methionine and ATP, is crucial for methylation in the body. As a methyl donor, SAMe helps maintain cellular membrane integrity (repairing damaged proteins) and the fluidity of the lipid bilayer in nerve cell membrane (via formation of phosphatidyl choline) and generates glutathione, the body's major antioxidant (Brown et al. 2000). In primates, SAMe, 20–30 mg/kg/day intramuscularly, reduced impairments and facilitated recovery from lesions in motor cortex and dorsolateral prefrontal cortex. Data also suggest that SAMe enhanced migration of tissue, repairing macrophages to lesion sites (Takahashi et al. 1986, 1987). SAMe improved the status of the cholinergic system and reduced learning deficits in aged rats (Pavia et al. 1997). SAMe, 10 mg/kg/day, given subcutaneously to rats resulted in nearly 50% decreased free radical production, 50% increased glutathione levels, and nearly 100% increased glutathione peroxidase and transferase (De La Cruz et al. 2000).

In rat models, SAMe reduced infarct size up to 50% better than placebo when given within 2 hours of the onset of focal cerebral ischemia. Forty-one patients enrolled in a DBPC study within 24 hours of ischemia or hemorrhagic strokes were randomized to either SAMe, 2,400 mg/day intravenously or 3,200 mg/day intravenously, or placebo for 14 days. There was a significant difference in mortality: five patients died while taking placebo; one died while taking SAMe, 2,400 mg/day; and none died while taking SAMe, 3,200 mg/day (Monaco et al. 1996). In a DBPC 1-month study of postconcussion syndrome, 30 patients were given either placebo or low-dose parenteral SAMe, 150 mg/day (equivalent to 300 mg/day orally) for 1 month. Postconcussion symptoms, including headache, vertigo, depressed mood, cognitive slowing (slowed thought, speech, and decreased concentration), and other symptoms were rated for severity on a scale from 0 (none) to 4 (most severe or incapacitating). Patients who received SAMe showed a 77% decrease in mean clinical scores of postconcussion symptoms compared with a 49% decrease in the placebo group. The difference between SAMe and placebo was significant, with a 95% level of confidence (Bacci Ballerini et al. 1983). It would be of interest to study SAMe in postconcussion treatment using larger doses and current neuropsychiatric outcome measures.

We have found the butanedisulfonate form of SAMe to be somewhat more effective with fewer side effects than the tosylate forms. Also, vitamin B_{12} and folate may enhance response to SAMe.

Picamilon

Picamilon, a synthetic combination of two natural compounds, γ-aminobutyric acid and the B vitamin niacin, decreases cerebral blood vessel tone and increases cerebral blood flow in animal studies (Mirzoian and Gan'shina 1989). Despite its mild tranquilizing action (decreases motivated aggression in animals), it has mild stimulative properties and improves cognition. Although clinical trials in Russia using Picamilon for stroke,

dementia, and TBI have reported positive results, those studies were not available for our evaluation. In our clinical experience, Picamilon may improve alertness and symptoms of anxiety and depression in patients with cerebral vascular impairment and TBI.

Pyritinol

Pyritinol, a derivative of vitamin B_6 (pyridoxine) with no B_6 activity, has been used to treat TBI, dementia, cerebrovascular disorders, and dyslexia. Preclinical research indicates that it enhances cerebral glucose utilization, neuronal Ach release, cortical and striatal Ach levels, striatal and hippocampal high-affinity choline uptake, and cortical cyclic guanine monophosphate (presumed second messenger for Ach). Pyritinol prevented the learning deficits because of chronic mild hypoxia in a postnatal rat model. This may be relevant to the protective effect (reduced brain damage and seizures) of pyritinol in a human study of high-risk newborns (Lun et al. 1989). Numerous studies indicate positive effects in organic brain syndromes and dementia (Fischhof et al. 1992; Herrmann et al. 1986; Knezevic et al. 1989; Tazaki et al. 1980). In three TBI studies, pyritinol improved postoperative recovery and rehabilitation. In a small open pilot study, five ICU patients with severe TBI and apallic syndrome responded to prolonged intravenous pyritinol treatment with increased vigilance and reactivity to stimuli (Wild et al. 1976). Dalle Ore et al. (1980) compared 68 patients with TBI and coma admitted to an ICU and treated with intravenous pyritinol within 24 hours of admission with 68 TBI patients admitted to the same clinic with similar neurological conditions given intravenous glucose. Patients were divided into four groups: light coma, moderate coma, deep coma, and coma depasse. They were classified as follows: A (hemispheric syndrome), $n=33$; B (central syndrome), $n=4$; C (uncal syndrome), $n=1$; D (mesencephalic), $n=6$; E (pons/medulla oblongata), $n=1$; O (no neurological signs), $n=1$. Prolonged coma occurred in 22 patients, including 20 with apallic syndrome and 2 with akinetic mutism. The overall mortality rate with pyritinol was 35.3% versus 54.2% with placebo. For those with prolonged coma, mortality rate was 22.7% with pyritinol and 46.1% with placebo. The most significant and rapid positive effect of pyritinol was the recovery of consciousness (usually at doses of 800–1,600 mg), even before other neurological signs improved. Concomitant improvements in vigilance and electroencephalographic patterns (decreased diffuse slow waves and increased alpha waves) were noted. Effects on other neurological signs were relatively weak (Dalle Ore et al. 1980). Kitamura (1981) reported a PC MC study of 270 patients with TBI 1 month or more prior. The group included 70 postsurgical patients, 46 patients with concussion without loss of consciousness, 82 patients with transient (6 hours or less) loss of consciousness, 90 patients with contusion cerebri, 47 patients with intracranial hematomas, and 5 patients of uncertain class. After 6 weeks, 70% of those patients given pyritinol, 600 mg/day, improved significantly on the final global improvement rating versus 56% of those taking placebo. Patient subjective ratings of improvement showed 66% feeling better while taking pyritinol versus 53% taking placebo. The pyritinol group had greater improvement in somatic symptoms, cognitive function, and headache than the placebo group (Kitamura 1981). Side effects include rash, pruritus, and dizziness. Further studies using current neuropsychiatric measures would be useful.

Idebenone

Gillis et al. (1994) reviewed the extensive literature on idebenone, a variant of coenzyme Q10, that enhances the ATP-producing mitochondrial electron transport chain and exerts antioxidant effects in vitro and in animal models (Amano et al. 1995; Cardoso et al. 1998, 1999; Matsumoto et al. 1998; Mordente et al. 1998). Idebenone improved cognitive function in animals with lesions of the basal forebrain cholinergic system and with cerebral ischemia. It protected rat astrocytes against reperfusion injury (Takuma et al. 2000), augmented the action of vinpocetine on long-term potentiation in guinea pig hippocampal slices (Ishihara et al. 1989), and improved transcallosal response (Okuyama and Aihara 1988). Three hundred two patients with mild to moderate AD were given 270–360 mg/day of idebenone in a DBRPC MC 2-year study. Patients had statistically significant dose-dependent improvement (comparable to improvement with cholinesterase inhibitors) on the primary efficacy measure (ADAS-Total) and on all secondary efficacy measures (ADAS-cog, ADAS-noncognitive subscale, Clinical Global Impression [CGI] Scale, and the Nurses' Observation Scale for Geriatric Patients [NOSGER]). During the second year, further improvement occurred with no loss of efficacy. Safety and tolerability were comparable to placebo (Gutzmann and Hadler 1998). Controlled studies are needed in TBI. We have noted that sluggish, psychomotor-retarded patients tend to benefit the most. The cost of idebenone is prohibitive for many patients.

Herbal Alternative Treatments

Vinpocetine

Vinpocetine, a semisynthetic alkaloid derivative of periwinkle (*Vinca minor*), has been used in Eastern Europe since the 1980s for cerebral vascular disorders. In vitro and in vivo studies show neuroprotection by inhibiting calcium/calmodulin–dependent cyclic guanosine monophosphate-phosphodiesterase 1, enhancing intracellular cyclic guanosine monophosphate levels in vascular smooth muscle (van Staveren et al. 2001), and reducing resistance of cerebral blood vessels and increasing blood flow (Bonoczk et al. 2000). Vinpocetine inhibits the molecular cascade caused by the rise of intracellular calcium. In a DBPC study of 84 patients with "chronic cerebral dysfunction" of presumed vascular origin and cognitive impairment, 42 subjects were given vinpocetine for 60 days; the other 42 received placebo. Patients on vinpocetine scored significantly better on the CGI and MMSE, and on all but the affect factor of the Sandoz Clinical Assessment–Geriatric scale (Balestreri et al. 1987). Radiological evidence of cerebrovascular disease was not presented. Hindmarch et al. (1991) evaluated 203 patients with mild to moderate organic brain syndromes, including dementia in a DBRPC MC study. Compared with placebo, the vinpocetine-treated patients showed statistically significant improvements after 16 weeks on CGI and ratings of severity of illness and quality of life (Hindmarch et al. 1991). Limited information on the diagnoses of subjects is a weakness of this study. Feigin et al. (2001) treated 30 consecutive patients with computed tomography–verified diagnoses of acute ischemic stroke within 72 hours of stroke onset in a DBPC pilot study with low-molecular-weight dextran alone (*n*=15) or dextran plus vinpocetine (*n*=15). In the vinpocetine group, the relative risk reduction of poor outcome at 3 months was 30%. The National Institutes of Health–National Institute of Neurological Disorders and Stroke Scale score was marginally significantly better at 3 months in the vinpocetine group, suggesting that a full-scale randomized trial would be warranted (Feigin et al. 2001). A review of PET scan studies of 12 patients found that vinpocetine improved cerebral glucose kinetics and blood flow in the peristroke area (Bonoczk et al. 2000). In clinical practice, we observe that vinpocetine helps patients with single-photon emission computed tomography or PET scan evidence of blood flow abnormalities.

Rhodiola rosea (Golden Root, Arctic Root, or Roseroot)

Rhodiola rosea has a long history in folk medicines of Russia, Scandinavia, and other countries. Forty years of *Rhodiola* research was hidden in classified documents by the former Soviet Union. Despite their recent declassification, many documents are difficult to obtain. The following discussion draws on a comprehensive review, Rhodiola rosea: *A Valuable Medicinal Plant* (Saratikov and Krasnov 1987c), on the basis of translations by Zakir Ramazanov (Z. Ramazanov, personal communication, July 2001). The reader is referred to more accessible reviews (Brown and Gerberg 2002; Furmanowa et al. 1995; Petkov et al. 1986). Of the 30 species identified in the *Rhodiola* genus, *R. rosea* has been the most extensively studied in animals and humans (Brown and Gerberg 2002). Root extracts of *R. rosea* have been approved for medicinal uses and listed in the Russian Pharmacopoeia since the late 1960s and in pharmaceutical texts in Scandinavian countries. Since the 1960s, animal and human *R. rosea* studies by Soviet scientists had identified complex effects on brain function: cognitive stimulation with emotional calming, and enhanced learning and memory. *R. rosea* was the most powerful plant adaptogen studied (it protected every organism tested, from snails to humans, against physical and mental stresses, extreme exertion, toxins, and mental fatigue). *Rhodiola* species contain many compounds that scavenge superoxide and hydroxyl radicals (Furmanowa et al. 1998). It acts on the brainstem reticular formation and cerebral hemispheres, increasing the efficiency of energy metabolism. In animal studies, *R. rosea* increases and maintains higher levels of ATP and creatine in brain, muscle, liver, and blood (Furmanowa et al. 1998; Kurkin and Zapesochonaya 1986; Saratikov and Krasnov 1987a). In rat studies, *R. rosea* improved learning and memory in the maze model and "staircase training." It also increased brain norepinephrine, DA, and 5-HT (Petkov et al. 1986).

In healthy individuals, *R. rosea* enhanced intellectual work capacity, abstract thinking, and reaction time. Proofreading tests (Anfimov's tables) administered to 27 students, doctors, and scientists given *R. rosea*, 100 mg bid, showed an 88% reduction in the number of mistakes over time, compared with an 84% increase in mistakes by those given placebo (Saratikov and Krasnov 1987d). One hundred twenty college students were repeatedly tested for symbol correction at 1, 4, 6, and 8 hours. Those given *R. rosea* had 56% fewer errors at 4 hours and less than 5% more errors at 6 and 8 hours. Those given placebo had 37% more errors at 4 hours, 88% more errors at 6 hours, and 180% more errors at 8 hours (Saratikov and Krasnov 1987d). In a DBPC study of 60 first-year college students under stress, those given low-dose *R. rosea* (100 mg/day) showed significant improvement in mental fatigue, psychomotor function, overall well-being (self-evaluation), physical work capacity, and heart rate. The average final examination grade in the *R. rosea* group was 3.47; in the placebo group, it was 3.2 (Spasov et al. 2000). Soviet investigators observed therapeutic effects in posttraumatic and vascular lesions of the brain, especially in early postinjury stages. *R. rosea* improved cognitive function better in conjunction with piracetam. Patients with hysterical, volatile, or euphoric symptoms needed tranquilizers and antidepressants combined with *R. rosea* (Saratikov and Krasnov 1987b). Many of these early observations were based on open studies using outdated methodologies. Nevertheless, such extensive study and clinical observation coupled with some more recent evidence deserve further investigation using modern controlled research techniques. The translation of research documents may provide the impetus for wider medical use and clinical research.

In patients with brain injury, *R. rosea* has a mild stimulant effect while being emotionally calming. No significant drug interactions have been reported. In our experience, *R. rosea*, particularly combined with ginseng or ginkgo, can be beneficial for memory and cognition in TBI, AAMI, stroke, and dementia. Response takes 2–8 weeks. *R. rosea* should be given 20 minutes before breakfast and lunch, starting with 150 mg/day and increasing by 150 mg every 3–7 days. Elderly, medically ill, or anxious patients should start by taking one-fourth to one-half of a capsule per day dissolved in tea or juice and increased slowly.

Ginkgo Biloba

As a neuroprotectant, ginkgo biloba improves membrane fluidity and resistance to oxidative damage (Drieu et al. 2000). A review by Wong et al. (1998) discusses ischemia and reperfusion protective effects and benefits in AAMI, vascular dementia, and AD. Diamond et al. (2000) reviewed 22 controlled ginkgo studies with standardized outcome measures in cerebrovascular disease, memory impairment, cognitive impairment, dementia (Alzheimer's and multi-infarct), subarachnoid hemorrhage, aging, hypoxia, and vestibular disorder and 2 studies in healthy volunteers. Despite the complexity of the data, they found that clinically meaningful (though subtle) improvements had been found in a number of studies. Le Bars et al. (1997) conducted a 52-week DBRPC MC study of ginkgo biloba extract EGb 761 in patients with multi-infarct dementia and AD. One hundred twenty-two AD patients in severity stratum 1 (MMSE score >23) and 114 with AD in stratum 2 (MMSE score <24) were given either 120 mg/day EGb or placebo. The stratum 1 placebo group showed no change at 52 weeks, whereas the EGb group improved 1.7 points on the ADAS-cog and 0.09 on the Geriatric Evaluation by Relatives Rating Instrument (GERRI). In the stratum 2 placebo group, scores worsened on the ADAS-cog by 4.1 points and on the GERRI by 0.18. The stratum 2 EGb group had 60% less decline on the ADAS-cog (2.5 points) and no change on the GERRI (Le Bars et al. 1997). Our clinical experience is that ginkgo is best used to augment CPH and racetams in patients with TBI because its effects alone are mild. Because ginkgo can reduce platelet aggregation, it should not be given with coumadin, and it should be discontinued 2 weeks before surgery.

Ginseng (Panax, Korean)

Ginseng contains many compounds that exert complex effects in animal models. It increased production of nitric oxide by endothelial cells (crucial for blood flow and oxygen delivery) in the rabbit (Kang et al. 1995). Danish researchers randomized healthy volunteers older than 40 years: 55 received ginseng, 400 mg/day, and 56 received placebo for 8 weeks. The ginseng group showed significantly better abstract thinking and reaction time. However, there were no significant differences in memory or concentration (Sorensen and Sonne 1996).

Nootropics and Vitamins

Pyrrolidones (Racetams)

Piracetam increases nerve cell membrane fluidity and normalizes hyperactive platelet aggregation. In animal learning models and aged rodents with memory deficits, the effect is modest (Vernon and Sorkin 1991). However, it is considerably potentiated by CDP-choline, idebenone, vinpocetine, and deprenyl (Gouliaev and Senning 1994). Piracetam enhanced the antihypoxic effect of CPH by protecting cell membranes from phospholipid peroxidation (Fischer et al. 1984). Although racetams activated electroencephalographs and improved memory in patients with dementia (Itil et al. 1986), studies in mild dementia and AAMI give only weak support. Oxiracetam, aniracetam, and pramiracetam show greater benefits than piracetam (Flicker et al. 2001). Human studies combining racetams with CDP-choline and cholinesterase inhibitors are needed.

Large DBPC studies support racetam benefits in poststroke aphasia and dyslexia (Huber et al. 1997). With speech therapy, piracetam enhanced language recovery when given within 7 hours of stroke (De Deyn et al. 1997; Orgogozo 1999) and improved task-related blood flow in left hemisphere speech areas on PET scan (Kessler et al. 2000). In studies of patients with dyslexia, piracetam improved reading rates, accuracy, word retrieval, writing, and comprehension (Wilsher 1986). Significant effects occur with 3,300 mg/day or more given for at least 12 weeks. Piracetam activates the left hemisphere preferentially in dyslexic patients (Ackerman et al. 1991; Tallal et al. 1986).

In a DBPC randomized study of 60 patients with postconcussion syndrome of 2–12 months, piracetam, 4,800 mg/day for 8 weeks, reduced the severity of symptoms, especially vertigo and headache (Hakkarainen et al. 1978). A case series of 903 patients with concussion reported that piracetam hastened recovery of function and normal electroencephalograph, and decreased length of hospitalization (Cicerchia et al. 1985). The lack of a placebo control group renders this study merely tantalizing. Methodological problems also limit the significance of a study of 36 patients with postconcussion syndrome: one group was treated with 3,000 mg/day oxiracetam intramuscularly; the other group was simply observed. Oxiracetam accelerated recovery (Russello et al. 1990). Studies of dyslexia, AAMI, and aphasia show significant enhancement of cognitive retraining: ginkgo improved attention and perception, whereas piracetam improved learning (Enderby et al. 1994).

L-Deprenyl (Eldepryl, Selegiline)

Although L-deprenyl is a prescription drug in the United States, we consider it an alternative agent because most physicians are not familiar with its use in brain injury. Data suggest mechanisms of action different from its monoamine oxidase inhibitor effect when used in very low doses. Animal studies implicate the boosting of antioxidants and neurotrophic factors in protecting catecholaminergic and cholinergic neurons (Kitani et al. 2000; Maruyama and Naoi 1999). In a rat TBI model, L-deprenyl improved cognitive function and neuroplasticity, particularly in the hippocampus (Zhu et al. 2000). Joseph Knoll, the discoverer of L-deprenyl, described a novel mechanism of action at a receptor site for an endogenous enhancer, which selectively improves impulse propagation–mediated release of catecholamines and 5-HT in the brain, most markedly in the hippocampus (Knoll 2000). In response to stimulation of this receptor, glial cells and astrocytes secrete higher amounts of nerve growth factors (J. Knoll, personal communication, July 2001). Our clinical experience is that L-deprenyl has a modest place in treatment of TBI in ultra low doses (that do not cause monoamine oxidase inhibition) using 5-mg tablets, giving half a pill 5 days of the week. We use it hoping to enhance neuronal repair (as seen in animal TBI models [Zhu et al. 2000]) and response to other treatments. Liquid L-deprenyl citrate may be more effective and tolerable, but no comparative studies have been done. L-deprenyl has significant neuroprotective properties and deserves further study.

B Vitamins and Bio-Strath

The methylation pathways that maintain cellular proteins, membranes, and antioxidants depend on B vitamins and folate as cofactors. B vitamin and folate deficiencies are associated with abnormalities of mood, memory, and cognition (Bottiglieri 1996; Hassing et al. 1999). Supplementation with B vitamins improves mood and cognitive function in healthy subjects (Benton et al. 1997). Bio-Strath, a

TABLE 38–3.   How to obtain quality alternative compounds

Compound	Brand/company	Source
Galantamine/*Rhodiola*	A/P Formula/Ameriden	888-405-3336; http://www.ameriden.com
Huperzine-A	GNC (General Nutrition Centers)	http://www.gnc.com
Centrophenoxine	Lucidril/International Antiaging Systems (IAS)	http://www.antiaging-systems.com; Fax: 011-44-870-151-4145
Acetyl-L-carnitine	Life Extension Foundation (LEF)	800-544-4440; http://www.lef.org
Citicholine	Smart Nutrition (SN); LEF	http://www.smart-nutrition.net
S-adenosylmethionine	Donnamet/IAS	See above
	NatureMade (tosylate and butanedisulfonate)	http://www.naturemade.com, pharmacies, chain stores, buyer's clubs, Costco, BJs
	LEF	See above
Pyritinol	SN	800-479-2107; http://www.smart-nutrition.net
Idebenone	SN; Thorne Research	800-932-2953 (Thorne)
Vinpocetine	LEF; SN; Intensive Nutrition	See above
Rhodiola rosea	Rosavin/Ameriden	888-405-3336; http://www.ameriden.com
	Energy Kare/Kare-N-Herbs	http://www.Kare=N-herbs.com
	Rodax/Pinnacle	GNC
	Rhodiola Force/New Chapter	Health food stores or online
Ginkgo	Ginkgold/Nature's Way	Health food stores, pharmacies
	Ginkoba/Pharmaton	
Ginseng (Panax/Korean)	Hsu's Ginseng	800-388-3818; http://www.hsuginseng.com
	Power Max 4x/Action Labs	800-932-2953
Piracetam (all racetams)	IAS	See above
L-Deprenyl	Jumex tabs, Cyprenil (liquid)/IAS	
	Deprenyl, Selegiline, Eldepryl	By prescription from U.S. pharmacies
B vitamins	Bio-Strath/Nature's Answer	800-681-7099 or health food stores

Note.   This list of specific brands is not comprehensive. It simply represents easily available brands that we have used and found to be consistently of good quality. Because brands and companies may change, the physician should reevaluate each product over time. See Table 38–4 for independent evaluations of many brands and check www.consumerlab.com or www.supplementwatch.com.

B-vitamin supplement at double the usual adult dose, was given to 75 patients age 55–85 years with mild dementia in a 3-month DBRPC trial. The placebo group deteriorated. In contrast, the Bio-Strath group showed improvement in short-term memory with physical and emotional benefits at 3 months (Pelka and Leuchtgens 1995). The relationship between B vitamins and cognitive function persuades us to treat brain-injured patients with B vitamins.

Homeopathy

A pilot study (at Spaulding Rehabilitation Hospital in Boston) of 50 patients with mild TBI found that homeopathic treatment significantly reduced the intensity of patients' symptoms ($P=0.01$) and reduced difficulty functioning ($P=0.0008$) (Chapman et al. 1999). Limitations of this study include the small number of patients, the variety of symptoms, duration of treatment, the use of different combinations of multiple homeopathic preparations in different patients, and questions about the validity and reliability of the measures used (Chapman 2001). Nevertheless, the finding of statistically significant differences in this PC study is intriguing. The investigators acknowledged the need for a larger collaborative MC study to validate these findings, but such a study has not been funded as of this date. It is not possible to place this study within

TABLE 38–4. Resources for information on alternative medicine

The Desktop Guide to Complementary and Alternative Medicine: An Evidence Based Approach. Edited by Edzard Ernst. New York, Mosby, 2001

Focus on Alternative and Complementary Therapies, Pharmaceutical Press, P.O. Box 151, Wallingford, OX10 8QU, UK; Phone: +44 1491 829272; Fax: +44 1491 829292; rpsgb@cabi.org

Martindale: The Complete Drug Reference. Pharmaceutical Press, 1 Lambeth High St., London SE1 7JN, UK

American Botanical Council, P.O. Box 144345, Austin, TX, 78714; Phone: 512-926-4900; http://www.herbalgram.org

ConsumerLab, http://www.ConsumerLab.com

FDA MedWatch, http://www.fda.gov/medwatch

Herb Research Foundation, 1007 Pearl St., Suite 200, Boulder, CO 80302; Phone: 303-449-2265; http://www.herbs.org

Natural Medicines Comprehensive Database, Therapeutic Research Facility, 3120 W. March Lane, PO Box 8190, Stockton, CA 95208; Phone: 209-472-2244; Fax: 209-472-2249; Mail@NaturalDatabase.com; http://www.NaturalDatabase.com

Supplement Watch, http://www.supplementwatch.com

the framework of the other treatments in this chapter because the pathophysiological basis of homeopathy is unproven. Biological effects are inferred from observations of change after treatment is administered. For a discussion of the state of homeopathic research, we refer the reader to *Alternative and Complementary Treatment in Neurological Illness* (Weintraub 2001).

Summary

Doctors and consumers are concerned about the quality of herbs and nutrients. Advances in biochemistry have improved the purity and stability of many products (Wagner 1999). Although the publication of specific brands is not the norm in a text of this kind, in the field of alternative medicine it is particularly important to choose products that have proven to be of good quality. To help clinicians find their way through the morass of unreliable, ineffective lookalikes, Table 38–3 lists brands that we have investigated. The following compounds in the brands we have listed are pharmaceutical grade, regulated by European governmental agencies: centrophenoxine, acetyl-L-carnitine, citicholine, *S*-adenosylmethionine (SAMe), Picamilon, pyritinol, idebenone, vinpocetine, racetams,

and L-deprenyl. The brands of the herbs, ginkgo, and ginseng have been assessed by independent laboratories as reported by ConsumerLab.com. The authors have personally contacted the manufacturers of *Rhodiola rosea*, galantamine, and SAMe to obtain adequate information regarding standardization, content, purity, and batch testing procedures (including shelf life) to be reasonably assured of the quality and reliability of these products. Invariably, some products and companies will change over time. Physicians should stay current by using unbiased sources of product evaluation and rigorous studies. Table 38–4 provides resources for those interested in reliable information on alternative compounds. Anyone interested in an alternative product may contact the manufacturer and request information about content, purity, testing, and quality control, as well as consulting independent sources of evaluation when available.

Alternative compounds can offer significant benefits with few side effects in some patients with TBI. Certain agents may help repair the nervous system and enhance plasticity. In practice, it often requires several attempts to design an effective combination of treatments. Many patients and families can participate in the development of an alternative treatment regimen.

References

Ackerman PT, Dykman RA, Holloway C, et al: A trial of piracetam in two subgroups of students with dyslexia enrolled in summer tutoring. J Learn Disabil 24:542–549, 1991

al-Zuhair H, Abd el-Fattah A, el-Sayed MI: The effect of meclofenoxate with ginkgo biloba extract or zinc on lipid peroxide, some free radical scavengers and the cardiovascular system of aged rats. Pharmacol Res 38:65–72, 1998

Alvarez XA, Mouzo R, Pichel V, et al: Double-blind placebo-controlled study with citicoline in APOE genotyped Alzheimer's disease patients: effects on cognitive performance, brain bioelectrical activity and cerebral perfusion. Methods Find Exp Clin Pharmacol 21:633–644, 1999

Amano T, Terao S, Imada I: Effects of 6-(10-hydroxydecyl)-2,3-dimethoxy-5-methyl-1,4-benzoquinone (idebenone) and related benzoquinones on porcine pancreas phospholipase A_2 activity. Biol Pharm Bull 18:779–781, 1995

Anonymous: Acetyl-L-carnitine. Altern Med Rev 4:438–441, 1999

Arciniegas DB: Traumatic brain injury and cognitive impairment: the cholinergic hypothesis. Neuropsychiatry Reviews 17–20, 2001

Arrigo A, Casale R, Buonocore M, et al: Effects of acetyl-L-carnitine on reaction times in patients with cerebrovascular insufficiency. Int J Clin Pharmacol Res 10:133–137, 1990

Bacci-Ballerini F, Lopez-Anguera A, Accarezy N, et al: Tratiamiento del sindrome posconmocional con SAMe. Med Clin (Barc) 80:161–164, 1983

Balestreri R, Fontana L, Astengo F: A double-blind placebo controlled evaluation of the safety and efficacy of vinpocetine in the treatment of patients with chronic vascular senile cerebral dysfunction. J Am Geriatr Soc 35:425–430, 1987

Baskaya MK, Dogan A, Rao AM, et al: Neuroprotective effects of citicoline on brain edema and blood-brain barrier breakdown after traumatic brain injury. J Neurosurg 92:448–452, 2000

Benton D, Griffiths R, Haller J: Thiamine supplementation, mood and cognitive functioning. Psychopharmacology 129:66–71, 1997

Berger R, Nowak H: A new medical approach to the treatment of osteoarthritis: report of an open phase IV study with ademetionine (Gumbaral). Am J Med 83(5A):84–88, 1987

Bonoczk P, Gulyas B, Adam-Vizi V, et al: Role of sodium channel inhibition in neuroprotection: effect of vinpocetine. Brain Res Bull 53:245–254, 2000

Bottiglieri T: Folate, vitamin B_{12}, and neuropsychiatric disorders. Nutr Rev 54:382–390, 1996

Brooks JO, Yesavage JA, Carta A, et al: Acetyl-L-carnitine slows decline in younger patients with Alzheimer's disease: a re-analysis of a double-blind, placebo-controlled study using the trilinear approach. International Psychogeriatrics 10:193–203, 1998

Brown RP, Gerbarg PL, Bottiglieri T: S-Adenosylmethionine (SAMe) in the clinical practice of psychiatry, neurology, and internal medicine. Clinical Practice of Alternative Medicine 1:230–241, 2000

Brown RP, Gerbarg PG: *Rhodiola rosea*: a phytomedical overview. Herbalgram, 56:40–52, 2002

Calatayud Maldonado V, Calatayud Perez JB, Aso Escario J: Effects of CDP-choline on the recovery of patients with head injury. J Neurol Sci 103 (suppl):S15–18, 1991

Calvani M, Arrigoni-Martelli E: Attenuation by acetyl-L-carnitine of neurological damage and biochemical derangement following brain ischemia and reperfusion. Int J Tissue React 21:1–6, 1999

Carcassonne M, LeTourneau JN: Etude double insu du Rexort en neuro-traumatologie infantile (French). La Vie Medicale 12:1007, 1979

Cardoso SM, Pereira C, Oliveira CR: The protective effect of vitamin E, idebenone and reduced glutathione on free radical mediated injury in rat brain synaptosomes. Biochem Biophys Res Commun 246:703–710, 1998

Cardoso SM, Pereira C, Oliveira R: Mitochondrial function is differentially affected upon oxidative stress. Free Radic Biol Med 26:3–13, 1999

Chapman EH: Homeopathy, in Alternative and Complementary Treatment in Neurological Illness. Edited by Weintraub MI. Series Medical Guides to Complementary and Alternative Medicine. Series Edited by Micozzi MS. New York and London, Churchill Livingstone, 2001, pp 51–67

Chapman EH, Weintraub RJ, Milburn MA, et al: The homeopathic treatment of mild traumatic brain injury: a randomized, double-blind, placebo controlled clinical trial. J Head Trauma Rehabil 14:521–542, 1999

Chen Y, Shohami E, Constantini S, et al: Rivastigmine, a brain-selective acetylcholinesterase inhibitor, ameliorates cognitive and motor deficits induced by closed-head injury in the mouse. J Neurotrauma 15:231–237, 1998

Cicerchia G, Santucci R, Palmieri M: [Use of piracetam in the treatment of cranial injuries. Observations on 903 cases] (Italian). Clin Ter 114:481–487, 1985

Clark WM, Williams BJ, Selzer KA, et al: A randomized efficacy trial of citicoline in patients with acute ischemic stroke. Stroke 30:2592–2597, 1999

Clark WM, Wechsler LR, Sabounjian LA, et al: A phase III randomized efficacy trial of 2000 mg citicoline in acute ischemic stroke patients. Neurology 57:1595–1602, 2001

Cohadon F, Richer E: CDP-choline in severe traumatic coma: a double blind study, in Novel Biochemical, Pharmacological and Clinical Aspects of Cytidinediphosphocholine. Edited by Zappia V, Kennedy EP, Nilsson BI, Galletti P. New York, Elsevier, 1985, pp 299–303

Dalle-Ore G, Bricolo A, Alexandre A: The influence of the administration of pyritinol on the clinical course of traumatic coma. J Neurosurg Sci 24:1–8, 1980

De Deyn PP, Reuck JD, Deberdt W, et al: Treatment of acute ischemic stroke with piracetam: members of the Piracetam in Acute Stroke Study (PASS) Group. Stroke 28:2347–2352, 1997

De La Cruz JP, Pavia J, Gonzalez-Correa JA, et al: Effects of chronic administration of S-adenosyl-L-methionine on brain oxidative stress in rats. Naunyn Schmiedebergs Arch Pharmacol 361:47–52, 2000

De La Herran J, Cortina J, Salazar J, et al: Utilización del citidindifosfato de colina en las lesiones encefálicas graves (Spanish). Actas Luso-Espanolas de neurologia, Psiquiatria y Ciencias Afines 6:3–12, 1978

Diamond BJ, Shiflett SC, Feiwel N, et al: Ginkgo biloba extract: mechanisms and clinical indications. Arch Phys Med Rehabil 81:668–678, 2000

Dixon CE, Flinn P, Bao J, et al: Nerve growth factor attenuates cholinergic deficits following traumatic brain injury in rats. Exp Neurol 146:479–490, 1997

Drieu K, Vranckx R, Benassayad C, et al: Effect of the extract of Ginkgo biloba (EGb 761) on the circulating and cellular profiles of polyunsaturated fatty acids: correlation with the anti-oxidant properties of the extract. Prostaglandins Leukot Essent Fatty Acids 63:293–300, 2000

Enderby P, Broeckx J, Hospers W, et al: Effect of piracetam on recovery and rehabilitation after stroke: a double-blind, placebo-controlled study. Clin Neuropharmacol 17:320–331, 1994

Espagno J, Tremoulet M, Gigaud M, et al: Etude de l'action de la CDP-choline dans les troubles de la vigilance post-traumatique (French). La Vie Medicale 3:195–196, 1979

Feigin VL, Doronin BM, Popova TF, et al: Vinpocetine treatment in acute ischaemic stroke: a pilot single-blind randomized clinical trial. Eur J Neurol 8:81–85, 2001

Fischer HD, Schmidt J, Wustmann C: On some mechanisms of antihypoxic actions of nootropic drugs. Biomed Biochim Acta 43:541–543, 1984

Fischhof PK, Saletu B, Ruther E, et al: Therapeutic efficacy of pyritinol in patients with senile dementia of the Alzheimer type (SDAT) and multi-infarct dementia (MID). Neuropsychobiology 26:65–70, 1992

Flicker L, Grimley-Evans G: Piracetam for dementia or cognitive impairment (Cochrane Review). Cochrane Database Syst Rev 2:CD0010112001

Furmanowa M, Oledzka H, Michalska M, et al: *Rhodiola rosea* L. (Roseroot): in vitro regeneration and the biological activity of roots, in Biotechnology in Agriculture and Forestry, Vol 33, in Medicinal and Aromatic Plants VIII. Edited by Bajaj YPS. Berlin and Heidelberg, Germany, Springer-Verlag, 1995, pp 412–426

Furmanowa M, Skopinska-Rozewska E, Ragola E, et al: *Rhodiola rosea* in vitro culture: phytochemical analysis and antioxidant action. Acta Societatis Botanicorum Poloniae 67:69–73, 1998

Galletti P, De Rosa M, Cotticelli MG, et al: Biochemical rationale for the use of CDPcholine in traumatic brain injury: pharmacokinetics of the orally administered drug. J Neurol Sci 103 (suppl):S19–25, 1991

Gillis JC, Benefield P, McTavish D: Idebenone: a review of its pharmacodynamic and pharmacokinetic properties, and therapeutic use in age-related cognitive disorders. Drugs Aging 5:133–152, 1994

Gouliaev AH, Senning A: Piracetam and other structurally related nootropics. Brain Res Brain Res Rev 19:180–222, 1994

Gutzmann H, Hadler D: Sustained efficacy and safety of idebenone in the treatment of Alzheimer's disease: update on a 2-year double-blind multicentre study. J Neural Transm Suppl 54:301–310, 1998

Hakkarainen H, Hakamies L: Piracetam in the treatment of post-concussional syndrome: a double-blind study. Eur Neurol 17:50–55, 1978

Hassing L, Wahlin A, Winblad B, et al: Further evidence of the effects of vitamin B_{12} and folate levels on episodic memory functioning: a population-based study of healthy very old adults. Biol Psychiatry 45:1472–1480, 1999

Hayes RL, Dixon CE: Neurochemical changes in mild head injury. Semin Neurol 14:25–31, 1994

Herrmann WM, Kern U, Rohmel J: On the effects of pyritinol on functional deficits of patients with organic mental disorders. Pharmacopsychiatry 19:378–385, 1986

Hindmarch I, Fuchs HH, Erzigkeit H: Efficacy and tolerance of vinpocetine in ambulant patients suffering from mild to moderate organic psychosyndromes. Int Clin Psychopharmacol 6:31–43, 1991

Huber W, Willmes K, Poeck K, et al: Piracetam as an adjuvant to language therapy for aphasia: a randomized double-blind placebo-controlled pilot study. Arch Phys Med Rehabil 78:245–250, 1997

Ishihara K, Katsuki H, Sugimura M, et al: Idebenone and vinpocetine augment long-term potentiation in hippocampal slices in the guinea pig. Neuropharmacology 28:569–573, 1989

Itil TM, Menon GN, Songar A, et al: CNS pharmacology and clinical therapeutic effects of oxiracetam. Clin Neuropharmacol 9 (suppl 3):S70–72, 1986

Itil TM, Eralp E, Ahmed I, et al: The pharmacological effects of ginkgo biloba, a plant extract, on the brain of dementia patients in comparison with tacrine. Psychopharmacol Bull 34:391–397, 1998

Kang SY, Kim SH, Schini VB, et al: Dietary ginsenosides improve endothelium-dependent relaxation in the thoracic aorta of hypercholesterolemic rabbit. Gen Pharmacol 26:483–487, 1995

Kelly GS: L-Carnitine: therapeutic applications of a conditionally essential amino acid. Altern Med Rev 3:345–360, 1998

Kessler J, Thiel A, Karbe H, et al: Piracetam improves activated blood flow and facilitates rehabilitation of poststroke aphasic patients. Stroke 31:2112–2116, 2000

Kitamura K: Therapeutic effect of pyritinol on sequelae of head injuries. J Int Med Res 9:215–221, 1981

Kitani K, Minami C, Maruyama W, et al: Common properties for propargylamines of enhancing superoxide dismutase and catalase activities in the dopaminergic system in the rat: implications for the life prolonging effect of (-)deprenyl. J Neural Transm Suppl (60):139–156, 2000

Knezevic S, Mubrin Z, Risberg J, et al: Pyritinol treatment of SDAT patients: evaluation by psychiatric and neurological examination, psychometric testing and rCBF measurements. Int Clin Psychopharmacol 4:25–38, 1989

Knoll J: Outlines of a drug strategy to slow brain aging. Neuropsychopharmacologia Hungarica 11:151–170, 2000

Kurkin VA, Zapesochnaya GG: Khimicheskiy sostav i farmakologicheskiye svoystva rasteniy roda *Rhodiola*. Obzor. [Chemical composition and pharmacological properties of *Rhodiola rosea*] (Russian). Khim-Farm Zh [Chemical and Pharmaceutical Journal Moscow] 20:1231–1244, 1986

Le Bars PL, Katz MM, Berman N, et al: A placebo-controlled, double-blind, randomized trial of an extract of *Ginkgo biloba* for dementia. North American EGb Study Group. JAMA 278:1327–1332, 1997

Leon-Carrion J, Dominguez-Roldan JM, Murillo-Cabezas F, et al: The role of citicholine in neuropsychological training after traumatic brain injury. NeuroRehabilitation 14:33–40, 2000

Levin HS: Treatment of postconcussional symptoms with CDP-choline. J Neurol Sci 103 (suppl):S39–42, 1991

Lolic MM, Fiskum G, Rosenthal RE: Neuroprotective effects of acetyl-L-carnitine after stroke in rats. Ann Emerg Med 29:758–765, 1997

Long DA, Ghosh K, Moore AN, et al: Deferoxamine improves spatial memory performance following experimental brain injury in rats. Brain Res 717:109–117, 1996

Lozano R: CDP-choline in the treatment of cranio-encephalic traumata. J Neurol Sci 103 (suppl):S43–47, 1991

Lun A, Gruetzmann H, Wustmann C, et al: Effect of pyritinol on the dopaminergic system and behavioural outcome in an animal model of mild chronic postnatal hypoxia. Biomed Biochim Acta 48:S237–242, 1989

Maruyama W, Naoi M: Neuroprotection by (-)-deprenyl and related compounds. Mech Ageing Dev 111:189–200, 1999

Matsumoto S, Mori N, Tsuchihashi N, et al: Enhancement of nitroxide-reducing activity in rats after chronic administration of vitamin E, vitamin C, and idebenone examined by an in vivo electron spin resonance technique. Magn Reson Med 40:330–333, 1998

Mirzoian RS, Gan'shina TS: [The new cerebrovascular preparation pikamilon] (Russian). Farmakol Toksikol 52:23–26, 1989

Mitka M: News about neuroprotectants for the treatment of stroke. JAMA 287:1253–1254, 2002

Monaco P, Pastore L, Rizzo S, et al: Safety and tolerability of adometionine (ADE) SD for inpatients with stroke: a pilot randomized, double-blind, placebo controlled study. Abstract presented at the Third World Stroke Conference and Fifth European Stroke Conference, Munich, Germany, Sept. 1996

Mordente A, Martorana GE, Minotti G, et al: Antioxidant properties of 2,3-dimethoxy-5-methyl-6-(10-hydroxydecyl)-1,4-benzoquinone (idebenone). Chem Res Toxicol 11:54–63, 1998

Murdoch I, Perry EK, Court JA, et al: Cortical cholinergic dysfunction after human head injury. J Neurotrauma 15:295–305, 1998

Nandy K: Centrophenoxine: effects on aging mammalian brain. J Am Geriatr Soc 26:74–81, 1978

Okuyama S, Aihara H: Action of nootropic drugs on transcallosal responses in rats. Neuropharmacology 27:67–72, 1988

Orgogozo JM: Piracetam in the treatment of acute stroke. Pharmacopsychiatry 32 (suppl 1):25–32, 1999

Pavia J, Martos F, Gonzalez-Correa JA, et al: Effect of S-adenosyl methionine on muscarinic receptors in young rats. Life Sci 60:825–832, 1997

Pelka RB, Leuchtgens H: Pre-Alzheimer study: action of a herbal yeast preparation (Bio-Strath) in a randomised double-blind trial. Ars Medici 85:1–5, 1995

Petkov VD, Yonkov D, Mosharoff A, et al: Effects of alcohol aqueous extract from Rhodiola rosea L. roots on learning and memory. Acta Physiol Pharmacol Bulg 12:3–16, 1986

Petkov VD, Mosharrof AH, Kehayov R, et al: Effect of CDP-choline on learning and memory processes in rodents. Methods Find Exp Clin Pharmacol 14:593–605, 1992

Pettegrew JW, Levine J, McClure RJ: Acetyl-L-carnitine physical-chemical, metabolic, and therapeutic properties: relevance for its mode of action in Alzheimer's disease and geriatric depression. Mol Psychiatry 5:616–632, 2000

Raloff J: Brain food: choline enters the limelight. Science News 160:282–284, 2001

Riemann D, Gann H, Dressing H, et al: Influence of the cholinesterase inhibitor galanthamine hydrobromide on normal sleep. Psychiatry Res 51:253–267, 1994

Rosadini G, Marenco S, Nobili F, et al: Acute effects of acetyl-L-carnitine on regional cerebral blood flow in patients with brain ischaemia. Int J Clin Pharmacol Res 10:123–128, 1990

Rozelle GR, Budzynski TH: Neurotherapy for stroke rehabilitation: a single case study. Biofeedback Self Regul 20:211–228, 1995

Russello D, Randazzo G, Favetta A, et al: [Oxiracetam treatment of exogenous post-concussion syndrome. Statistical evaluation of results] (Italian). Minerva Chir 45:1309–1314, 1990

Saratikov AS, Krasnov EA: Biochemical mechanisms of the stimulative effect of Rhodiola, in Rhodiola rosea Is a Valuable Medicinal Plant (Golden Root). Edited by Saratikov AS, Krasnov EA. Tomsk, Russia, Tomsk State University, 1987a, pp 91–149

Saratikov AS, Krasnov EA: Clinical studies of Rhodiola, in Rhodiola rosea Is a Valuable Medicinal Plant (Golden Root). Edited by Saratikov AS, Krasnov EA. Tomsk, Russia, Tomsk State University, 1987b, pp 216–227

Saratikov AS, Krasnov EA (eds): Rhodiola rosea Is a Valuable Medicinal Plant (Golden Root). Tomsk, Russia, Tomsk State University, 1987c

Saratikov AS, Krasnov EA: Stimulative properties of Rhodiola rosea, in Rhodiola rosea Is a Valuable Medicinal Plant (Golden Root). Edited by Saratikov AS, Krasnov EA. Tomsk, Russia, Tomsk State University, 1987d, pp 69–90

Schmidt RH, Grady MS: Loss of forebrain cholinergic neurons following fluid-percussion injury: implications for cognitive impairment in closed head injury. J Neurosurg 83:496–502, 1995

Schneider F, Popa R, Mihalas G, et al: Superiority of antagonic-stress composition versus nicergoline in gerontopsychiatry. Ann N Y Acad Sci 717:332–342, 1994

Sharma D, Singh R: Centrophenoxine activates acetylcholinesterase activity in hippocampus of aged rats. Indian J Exp Biol 33:365–368, 1995

Sinz EH, Kochanek PM, Dixon CE, et al: Inducible nitric oxide synthase is an endogenous neuroprotectant after traumatic brain injury in rats and mice. J Clin Invest 104:647–656, 1999

Son BC, Park CK, Choi BG, et al: Metabolic changes in pericontusional oedematous areas in mild head injury evaluated by 1H MRS. Acta Neurochir Suppl 76:13–16, 2000

Sorensen H, Sonne J: A double-masked study of the effects of ginseng on cognitive functions. Curr Ther Res 57:959–968, 1996

Spasov AA, Wikman GK, Mandrikov VB, et al: A double-blind, placebo-controlled pilot study of the stimulating and adaptogenic effect of Rhodiola rosea SHR-5 extract on the fatigue of students caused by stress during an examination period with a repeated low-dose regimen. Phytomedicine 7:85–89, 2000

Spiers PA, Hochanadel G: Citicoline for traumatic brain injury: report of two cases, including my own. J Int Neuropsychol Soc 5:260–264, 1999

Starfield B: Is US health really the best in the world? (commentary). JAMA 284:483–485, 2000

Takahashi J, Nishino H, Ono T: [Effect of S-adenosyl-L-methionine (SAMe) on disturbances in hand movement and delayed response tasks after lesion of motor or prefrontal cortex in the monkey] (Japanese). Nippon Yakurigaku Zasshi 87:507–519, 1986

Takahashi J, Nishino H, Ono T: S-adenosyl-L-methionine facilitates recovery from deficits in delayed response and hand movement tasks following brain lesions in monkeys. Exp Neurol 98:459–471, 1987

Takuma K, Yoshida T, Lee E, et al: CV-2619 protects cultured astrocytes against reperfusion injury via nerve growth factor production. Eur J Pharmacol 406:333–339, 2000

Tallal P, Chase C, Russell G, et al: Evaluation of the efficacy of piracetam in treating information processing, reading and writing disorders in dyslexic children. Int J Psychophysiol 4:41–52, 1986

Tang XC: Huperzine A (shuangyiping): a promising drug for Alzheimer's disease. Zhongguo Yao Li Xue Bao 17:481–484, 1996

Tariot PN, Solomon PR, Morris JC, et al: A 5-month, randomized, placebo-controlled trial of galantamine in AD. The Galantamine USA-10 Study Group. Neurology 54:2269–2276, 2000

Tazaki Y, Omae T, Kuromaru S, et al: Clinical effect of Encephabol (pyritinol) in the treatment of cerebrovascular disorders. J Int Med Res 8:118–126, 1980

Thal LJ, Calvani M, Amato A, et al: A 1-year controlled trial of acetyl-L-carnitine in early onset AD. Neurology 55:805–810, 2000

van Staveren WC, Markerink-van Ittersum M, Steinbusch HW, et al: The effects of phosphodiesterase inhibition on cyclic GMP and cyclic AMP accumulation in the hippocampus of the rat. Brain Res 888:275–286, 2001

Vernon MW, Sorkin EM: Piracetam: an overview of its pharmacological properties and a review of its therapeutic use in senile cognitive disorders. Drugs Aging 1:17–35, 1991

Wagner H: Phytomedicine research in Germany. Environ Health Perspect 107:779–781, 1999

Weintrab MI (ed): Alternative and Complementary Treatments in Neurological Illness (Medical Guides to Complementary and Alternative Medicine Series; Micozzi MS, series ed.). New York, Elsevier, 2001

Wilcock GK, Lilienfeld S, Gaens E: Efficacy and safety of galantamine in patients with mild to moderate Alzheimer's disease: multicentre randomised controlled trial. Galantamine International-1 Study Group. BMJ 321:1445–1449, 2000

Wild KV, Dolce G: Pathophysiological aspects concerning the treatment of the apallic syndrome. J Neurol 213:143–148, 1976

Wilsher CR: Effects of piracetam on developmental dyslexia. Int J Psychophysiol 4:29–39, 1986

Wong AH, Smith M, Boon HS: Herbal remedies in psychiatric practice. Arch Gen Psychiatry 55:1033–1043, 1998

Wood PL, Peloquin A: Increases in choline levels in rat brain elicited by meclofenoxate. Neuropharmacology 21:349–354, 1982

Xu SS, Gao ZX, Weng Z, et al: Efficacy of tablet Huperzine-A on memory, cognition, and behavior in Alzheimer's disease. Zhongguo Yao Li Xue Bao 16:391–395, 1995

Zauner A, Bullock R: The role of excitatory amino acids in severe brain trauma: opportunities for therapy: a review. J Neurotrauma 12:547–554, 1995

Zhu J, Hamm RJ, Reeves TM, et al: Postinjury administration of L-deprenyl improves cognitive function and enhances neuroplasticity after traumatic brain injury. Exp Neurol 166:136–152, 2000

PART VII

Prevention

39 Pharmacotherapy of Prevention

Saori Shimizu, M.D., Ph.D.

Carl T. Fulp, M.S.

Nicolas C. Royo, Ph.D.

Tracy K. McIntosh, Ph.D.

NEUROPATHOLOGICAL INVESTIGATIONS HAVE classified traumatic brain injury (TBI) as either focal or diffuse (Graham et al. 1995). Although focal injuries most often involve contusions and lacerations accompanied by hematoma (Gennarelli 1994), diffuse brain swelling, ischemic brain damage, and diffuse axonal injury are also considered to be major components of the diffuse injury profile (Adams et al. 1989; Graham et al. 1995; Maxwell et al. 1997). All TBIs can be further stratified into primary injury (encompassing the immediate, nonreversible mechanical damage to the brain), and secondary or delayed injury, which represents a potentially reversible process with a time of onset ranging from hours to days after injury that progresses for weeks or months (Graham et al. 1995). This secondary injury process is a complex and poorly understood cascade of interacting functional, structural, cellular, and molecular changes, including, but not limited to, impairment of energy metabolism, ionic dysregulation, breakdown of the blood–brain barrier (BBB), edema formation, activation and/or release of autodestructive neurochemicals and enzymes, changes in cerebral perfusion and intracranial pressure (ICP), inflammation, and pathologic/protective changes in intracellular genes and proteins (Figure 39–1). Although these events may lead to delayed cell death and/or neurological dysfunction, the delayed onset and reversibility of secondary damage offer a unique opportunity for targeted therapeutic pharmacological intervention to attenuate cellular damage and functional recovery during the chronic phase of the injury (McIntosh et al. 1998).

It is now well established that several clinically relevant experimental TBI models mimic many aspects of behavioral impairment and histopathological damage reported after human brain injury (for review see Laurer et al. 2000). Moreover, these experimental models provide us with the unique opportunity to both identify and investigate the pathophysiological changes triggered by TBI and target these pathways using new pharmacological strategies. As the pathophysiological sequelae of TBI are multifactorial, the development and characterization of new compounds remains extremely challenging. This chapter reviews some of the more promising neuroprotective strategies studied to date in clinical and preclinical settings.

Excitatory Amino Acid Antagonists

Pathologic release of the excitatory amino acid (EAA) neurotransmitters glutamate and aspartate and subsequent activation of specific glutamate receptors result in increased neuronal influx of cations (sodium and calcium) into the cell (Figure 39–2). This ionic influx may damage or destroy cells (i.e., excitotoxicity) through direct or indirect pathways (Olney et al. 1971). Both experimental and clinical brain injury induce an acute and potentially neurotoxic increase in extracellular glutamate concentrations (Faden et al. 1989; Globus et al. 1995; Katayama et

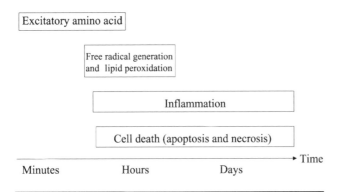

FIGURE 39–1. **Cascade of secondary damaging events in experimental traumatic brain injury.**

al. 1989, 1990; Nilsson et al. 1990; Palmer et al. 1993; Panter et al. 1992). Although most experimental studies have suggested that the posttraumatic rise in extracellular glutamate is of short duration, clinical studies have reported that glutamate concentrations are significantly elevated in the cerebrospinal fluid (CSF) of brain-injured patients for several days or perhaps weeks (Baker et al. 1993; Palmer et al. 1994).

Regional distribution of both *N*-methyl-D-aspartate (NMDA) and α-amino-3-hydroxy-5-methyl-4-isoxazole-propionate/kainic acid (AMPA/KA) receptors has been directly related to the selective vulnerability of specific brain regions caused by CNS injury (for review see Choi 1990). Miller et al. (1990) reported an acute decrease in NMDA but not AMPA/KA receptor binding in the hippocampal CA1 stratum radiatum, the molecular layer of the dentate gyrus, and the outer (1–3) and inner (5–6) layers of the neocortex within 3 hours after TBI in the rat. The hippocampus, which plays a prominent role in learning and memory, possesses a high density of glutamate receptors (Monaghan and Cotman 1986). Cognitive dysfunction, including a suppression of long-term potentiation and deficits in learning and memory, has been reported after TBI (for review see Albensi 2001). Sun and Faden (1995b) demonstrated that pretreatment with antisense oligodeoxynucleotides directed against the NMDA-R1 receptor subunit enhances survival and neurological motor recovery after TBI in rats. These studies un-

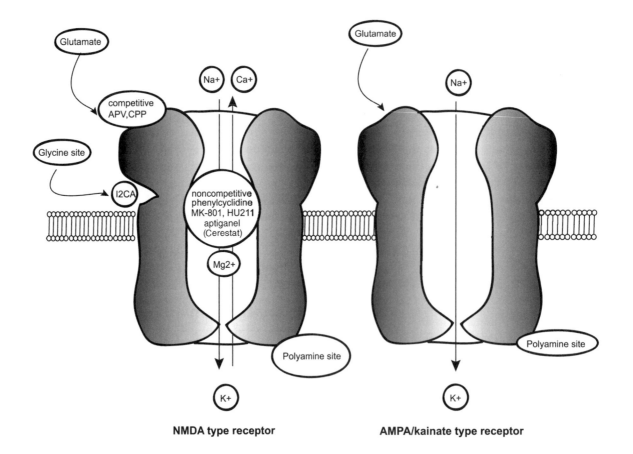

FIGURE 39–2. **Glutamate receptor subtypes: *N*-methyl-D-aspartate (NMDA) and α-amino-3-hydroxy-5-methyl-4-isoxazolepropionate (AMPA)/kainate.**

APV=2-amino-5-phosphovaleric acid; CPP=3-(2-carboxypiperizin-4yl)-propyl-1-phosphonic acid; I2CA=indole-2-carboxylic acid.

derscore the potentially important role of the NMDA receptor in mediating part of the pathological response to brain trauma (Table 39–1).

Although competitive NMDA receptor antagonists are logical candidates for the treatment of traumatic CNS injury, most of the early-generation compounds such as 2-amino-5-phosphovaleric acid (APV) and 3-(2-carboxypiperizin-4yl)-propyl-1-phosphonic acid (CPP) were strongly lipophobic and possessed poor BBB permeability, resulting in the necessity for direct CNS administration. Intracerebral administration of CPP was shown to improve neurological outcome (Faden et al. 1989), and intracerebroventricular APV administration was reported to reverse hypermetabolism after TBI in rats (Kawamata et al. 1992). In addition, CPP has recently been shown to increase apoptotic damage despite its ability to decrease excitotoxic cell damage in a model of TBI in the developing rat (Pohl et al. 1999).

More recently developed competitive NMDA antagonists such as Selfotel (CGS-19755 or cis-4-[phosphomethyl]-2-piperidine carboxylic acid), LY233053 ([1]-[2SR,4RS]-4-[1H-tetrazol-5-ylmethyl] piperidine-2-carboxylic acid), and CP101,606 ([1S, 29]-1-[4-hydroxyphenyl]-2-[hydroxy-4-phenylpiperidino]-1-propanol), an NR2B-selective NMDA receptor antagonist, have been shown to have greater BBB permeability than earlier generations of similar compounds (Menniti et al. 1995).

Although Selfotel has shown no beneficial effects on behavioral outcome, administration of this antagonist has been reported to reduce trauma-induced extracellular glutamate release in rats (Panter and Faden 1992). On the basis of this and other published data from experimental models of ischemia, a multicenter trial of Selfotel was initiated in the United States and Europe but was prematurely terminated because of side effects associated with competitive NMDA antagonism (Bullock 1995). Administration of CP101,606 and its stereoisomers has been shown to attenuate both cognitive dysfunction and regional cerebral edema in TBI in the rat (Okiyama et al. 1997, 1998). The CP101,606 compound is currently in Phase II trials in the United States and in Phase I trials in Japan for the potential treatment of brain injury and has been shown to be well tolerated and able to penetrate CSF and brain (Bullock et al. 1999; Merchant et al. 1999). In the initial pilot studies, mild to moderately head-injured patients did not exhibit differences in performance on the Neurobehavioral Rating Scale or Kurtzke Scoring (Merchant et al. 1999), whereas severely head-injured patients who were treated with the CP101,606 compound presented with, on average, better Glasgow Outcome Scores (Bullock et al. 1999).

Noncompetitive NMDA receptor antagonists also appear to have efficacy in the treatment of TBI. Hayes et al. (1988) first reported that pretreatment with the dissociative anesthetic and noncompetitive NMDA antagonist phencyclidine (PCP) attenuated neurological motor deficits after TBI in rats. Similar results were obtained with prophylactic treatment using dizocilpine (MK-801) (McIntosh et al. 1990). Treatment with MK-801 after TBI in rats also improved brain metabolic function and restored magnesium homeostasis (McIntosh et al. 1990), and administration of higher doses improved neurological motor deficits and reduced regional cerebral edema (Shapira et al. 1990). Pretreatment with MK-801 was found to attenuate the extracellular rise in glutamate associated with closed head injury followed by hypoxia in rats (Katoh et al. 1997) and enhance the recovery of spatial memory performance in animals subjected to combined TBI and entorhinal cortical lesions (Phillips et al. 1997). Administration of the noncompetitive NMDA antagonists dextrophan and dextromethorphan improved brain metabolic state, attenuated neurological motor deficits, and reduced the postinjury decline in brain magnesium concentrations observed after TBI in rats (Faden et al. 1989). Golding and Vink (1995) reported that dextromethorphan improved brain bioenergetic state and restored brain magnesium homeostasis after TBI in rats. Dextrophan also improved neurologic motor function and reduced edema after TBI in rats (Shohami et al. 1993). The NMDA-associated channel blocker ketamine has also been shown to improve posttraumatic cognitive outcome (Smith et al. 1993a), maintain both calcium and magnesium homeostasis (Shapira et al. 1993), and reduce expression of several immediate early genes (IEGs) induced in cerebral cortex and hippocampal dentate gyrus after TBI in rats (Belluardo et al. 1995). Gacyclidine, a more recently discovered phencyclidine derivative that acts as a noncompetitive NMDA antagonist (Hirbec et al. 2000), reduced lesion volume and improved neuronal survival and motor function when administered intraparenchymally after TBI (Smith et al. 2000). Although administration of the high-affinity, noncompetitive NMDA receptor antagonist CNS1102 (Aptiganel or Cerestat) was shown to attenuate contusion volume and hemispheric swelling after TBI in rats (Kroppenstedt et al. 1998), a clinical trial of this drug was prematurely terminated because of high mortality rates in an associated stroke trial. Although few studies have evaluated the potential neuroprotective effects of noncompetitive NMDA antagonists in models of brain trauma, Smith et al. (1997) reported that the NMDA receptor-associated ionophore blocker remacemide (2-amino-N-[1-methyl-1,2-diphenylethyl] acetamide hydrochloride) also signifi-

TABLE 39–1.   **Excitatory amino acid antagonists and agonists classified according to binding site**

	Compound	Type of research	Outcome	References
NMDA antagonist				
Competitive	APV	e	↓ glucose utilization	Kawamata et al. 1992
	CPP	e	↑ motor function, apoptotic damage; ↓ necrosis	Faden et al. 1989; Pohl et al. 1999
	Selfotel	e,c	↑ bioenergetic state, Mg^{2+} homeostasis	Bullock 1995; Juul et al. 2000; Morris et al. 1998; Panter et al. 1992
	CP101,606	e,c	↑ cognitive function; ↓ cell death, edema	Bullock et al. 1999; Merchant et al. 1999; Okiyama et al. 1997, 1998
Noncompetitive	Phencyclidine	e	↑ motor function	Hayes et al. 1988
	MK-801	e	↑ bioenergetic state, Mg^{2+} homeostasis, motor/ cognitive function; ↓edema, glutamate release	Katoh et al. 1997; McIntosh et al. 1990; Phillips et al. 1997; Shapira et al. 1990
	Dextrophan	e	↑ bioenergetic state, motor function, Mg^{2+} homeostasis; ↓ edema	Faden et al. 1989
	Dextromethorphan	e	↑ bioenergetic state, motor function, Mg^{2+} homeostasis	Faden et al. 1989; Golding et al. 1995
	Ketamine	e	↑ cognitive function, Mg^{2+},Ca^{2+} homeostasis; ↓ immediate early genes	Belluardo et al. 1995; Shapira et al. 1993; Smith et al. 1993a
	Gancyclidine	e	↑ motor function; ↓ cell death, lesion volume	Hirbec et al. 2001; Smith et al. 2000
	Cerestat	e,c	↓ edema, lesion volume; ↑ psychomotor side effect	Kroppenstedt et al. 1998; Muir et al. 1995
	Remacemide hydrochloride	e	↓ lesion volume	Smith et al. 1997
NMDA glycine site	I2CA	e	↑ motor/cognitive function; ↓ edema	Smith et al. 1993b
NMDA Mg^{2+} site	MgCl$_2$	e	↑ motor/cognitive function; ↓edema	Bareyre et al. 2000; Heath and Vink 1998; McIntosh et al. 1989; Okiyama et al. 1995; Saatman et al. 2001; Smith et al. 1993a
	MgSO$_4$	e	↑ motor/cognitive function; ↓ edema	Heath and Vink 1998; McIntosh et al. 1988
NMDA polyamine site	Ifenprodil	e	↓ edema, BBB breakdown	Okiyama et al. 1998
	Eliprodil	e	↑ cognitive function; ↓ lesion volume	Hogg et al. 1998
ODC inhibitor	DFMO	e	↑ cognitive function; ↓ edema, ODC	Baskaya et al. 1996
mGluR1 antagonist	AIDA	e	↑ motor/cognitive function; ↓ cell death, lesion volume	Faden et al. 2001; Lyeth et al. 2001

TABLE 39–1. Excitatory amino acid antagonists and agonists classified according to binding site *(continued)*

	Compound	Type of research	Outcome	References
mGluR1/2 antagonist	MCPG	e	↓ cell death	Gong et al. 1995; Mukhin et al. 1996
mGluR2 agonist	LY354740	e	↑ motor function	Allen et al. 1999
	DCG-IV	e	↓ cell death	Zwienenberg et al. 2001
mGluR3 agonist	CPPG	e	No effect	Zwienenberg et al. 2001
mGluR5 antagonist	MPEP	e	↑ motor/cognitive function; ↓ lesion volume	Movsesyan et al. 2001
Inhibition of Glu release	Lamotrigine	e,c	↓ glutamate release	Miller et al. 1986; Showalter and Kimmel 2000
	BW1003C87	e	↓ edema	Okiyama et al. 1995
	619C89	e,c	↑ motor/cognitive function; ↓ cell death, gliosis	Sun et al. 1995; Voddi et al. 1995
	Riluzole	e	↑ motor/cognitive function; ↓ edema, lesion volume, glutamate release	Bareyre et al. 1997; McIntosh et al. 1996; Stover et al. 2000; Wahl et al. 1997; Zhang et al. 1998
AMPA/KA antagonist	KYNA	e	↑ cognitive function; ↓ cell death, edema	Hicks et al. 1994; Smith et al. 1993b
Competitive	CNQX	e	↓ glucose utilization	Kawamata et al. 1990, 1992
	NBQX	e	↓ cell death	Bernert and Turski 1996; Ikonomidou and Turski 1996; Ikonomodou et al. 1996, 2000
Noncompetitive	GYKI-52466	e	↑ cognitive function; ↓ cell death	Hylton et al. 1995
	Talampanel	e	↓ cell death	Belayev et al. 2001

Note. BBB=blood–brain barrier; c=clinical trial; e=experimental study; NMDA = *N*-methyl-D-aspartate.

cantly reduced posttraumatic cortical lesion volume after TBI in rats.

The magnesium ion functions as a key endogenous modulator of the NMDA receptor, and its essential roles in many bioenergetic and cellular metabolic and genomic processes makes it an attractive candidate for use in the treatment of TBI. The loss of intracellular magnesium concentrations after experimental TBI (Shohami et al. 1993; Vink et al. 1996) suggests that replacement therapy using this ionic salt may have therapeutic value. Both pre- and postinjury treatment with magnesium salts ($MgCl_2$ or $MgSO_4$) has been demonstrated to improve neurological motor and cognitive deficits and decrease regional cerebral edema formation (Bareyre et al. 2000; McIntosh et al. 1988, 1989; Okiyama et al. 1995; Saatman et al. 2001; Shapira et al. 1993; Smith et al. 1993a). Because of this documented efficacy in experimental trauma models, a single-center National Institutes of Health–sponsored clinical trial in severely injured TBI patients has been initiated in the United States.

Other strategies to block NMDA-receptor associated neurotoxicity involve blockade or modulation of the NMDA receptor–associated glycine sites and/or polyamine binding sites. One selective glycine site antagonist, indole-2-carboxylic acid (I2CA), has been shown to improve behavioral outcome and reduce edema after TBI in rats (Smith et al. 1993b). Two broad-spectrum glutamate antagonists, kynurenate (KYNA) and 6-cyano-7-nitroquinoxaline-2,3-dione (CNQX), which antagonize both the glycine site and AMPA/KA receptors with varying affinity, have also been shown to be efficacious in reducing posttraumatic metabolic and neurobehavioral dysfunction in experimental TBI (Kawamata et al. 1992; Smith et al. 1993b). Postinjury administration of KYNA reduced the posttraumatic loss of hippocampal neurons after TBI in the rat (Hicks et al. 1994). Inhibition of the ornithine decarboxylase (ODC) enzyme using difluoromethylornithine (DFMO) has been shown to reduce regional cerebral edema after TBI in rats (Baskaya et al. 1996), and competitive antagonism of the NMDA-associated polyamine binding site by ifenprodil and its derivative eliprodil (SL 82.0715) has also been reported to exert beneficial effects after experimental TBI (Toulmond et al. 1993).

Although the NMDA receptor is implicated as playing an important role in mediating part of the pathological response to brain trauma, AMPA antagonists have also been used therapeutically with some success. Administration of 2,3-dihydroxy-6-nitro-7-sulfamoyl-benzo(f)quinoxaline (NBQX) has been shown to prevent hippocampal cell loss after brain trauma in adult but not immature rats (Bernert and Turski 1996; Ikonomidou and Turski 1996; Ikonomidou et al. 1996). The compound GYKI-52466 (1-[4-aminophenyl]-4-methyl-7,8-methylenedioixy-5H-2,3-benzodiazepine), a noncompetitive AMPA/KA antagonist, markedly improved cognitive function after TBI in the rat (Hylton et al. 1995). More recently, an orally active, noncompetitive AMPA antagonist, (R)-7-acetyl-5-(4-aminophenyl)-8,9-dihydro-8-methyl-7H-1,3-dioxolo(4,5-h)(2,3) benzodiazepine (Talampanel) has also been shown to significantly attenuate neuronal CA1 cell loss when administered after TBI (Belayev et al. 2001).

Elevated concentrations of extracellular glutamate after TBI activate metabotropic receptors (mGluRs), in addition to ionotropic receptors, and a number of recent studies implicate activation of mGluRs in acute TBI pathology (Faden et al. 1997; Gong et al. 1995, 1999; Mukhin et al. 1996, 1997). Eight mGluR subtypes have been classified, and these have been divided into three major classes on the basis of sequence homology, signal transduction pathways, and pharmacological sensitivity (Pin and Duvoisin 1995; Schoepp et al. 1999). A differential role for the different subgroups of mGluRs in posttraumatic cell death and survival has been proposed, and the blockade of group I or the activation of group II or group III receptors seems to be a beneficial strategy after TBI. On the basis of the use of antisense oligonucleotides and less selective group I antagonists such as (S)-α-methyl-4-carboxyphenylglycine (MCPG), a drug that acts as both a group I and group II antagonist, it has been suggested that mGluR1 activation contributes to traumatic cell death (Gong et al. 1995; Mukhin et al. 1996). Administration of (R,S)-1-aminoindan-1,5-dicarboxylic acid (AIDA), a selective mGluR1 antagonist, resulted in significant improvement in motor and cognitive function and reduction in the numbers of degenerating neurons and in lesion volume when administered after TBI (Faden et al. 2001; Lyeth et al. 2001). Although comparable re-

sults were obtained with administration of 2-methyl-6-(2-phenylethenyl)-pyridine (MPEP), a specific mGluR5 antagonist, it was suggested that the therapeutic utility of this drug may reflect its ability to modulate NMDA receptor activity rather than its ability to act as an mGluR5 agonist (Movsesyan et al. 2001). A number of laboratories have recently produced evidence that activation of group I mGluRs may reduce apoptotic cell death in models exhibiting neuronal apoptosis but increase necrotic cell death in vitro (Allen et al. 2000). The mechanism underlying the apparent dual neurotoxic/neuroprotective effects of group I mGluR activation remains unidentified.

With respect to group II and III mGluRs, postinjury administration of LY354740, a specific group II mGluR agonist, significantly improved neurological outcome after TBI in experimental animals with apparently fewer side effects and better tolerance than those associated with NMDA receptor antagonists (Allen et al. 1999). Administration of the group II mGluR2 agonist 2-(2',3')-dicarboxycyclopropylglycine (DCG-IV) directly into the hippocampus after TBI in rats resulted in a decrease in the number of degenerating neurons in the CA2 and CA3 regions (Zwienenberg et al. 2001), although hippocampal administration of (R,S)-alpha-cyclopropyl-4-phosphonophenylglycine (CPPG), a group III agonist, failed to protect CA2 or CA3 hippocampal neurons (Zwienenberg et al. 2001). A combination of MK-801 and the group III agonist L-(+)2 amino-4-phosphobutyric acid (L-AP4) provided enhanced neuroprotection compared with NMDA blockade alone after experimental TBI (Zwienenberg et al. 2001). Taken together, these data suggest that treatment with agents influencing the different subclasses of mGluRs may be beneficial after brain trauma.

Given the apparent failure of postsynaptic glutamate antagonist clinical trials, one novel strategy to attenuate glutamatergic neurotoxicity after brain trauma may be to use pharmacological agents that function presynaptically to inhibit glutamate release. The compound lamotrigine (3,5-diamino-6-[2,3-dichlorophenyl]-1,2,4-triazine) and its derivatives BW 1003C87 (5-[2,3,5-trichlorophenyl] pyrimidine-2,4-diamine ethane sulphonate), 619C89 (4-amino-2-[4-methyl-1-piperazinyl]-5-[2,3,5-trichlorophenyl] pyrimidine mesylate monohydrate), and riluzole all inhibit veratrine- but not potassium-stimulated glutamate release, presumably by reducing ion flux through voltage-gated sodium channels with subsequent attenuation of glutamate release (Miller et al. 1986). Preinjury treatment with 619C89 has been shown to reduce neuronal loss in CA1 and CA3 hippocampal pyramidal cells after TBI in rats (Sun and Faden 1995a), whereas postinjury treatment with BW1003C87 can attenuate regional cerebral edema and improve neurobehavioral function (Okiyama et al. 1995; Voddi et al. 1995). Treatment with riluzole after TBI significantly attenuated both cognitive and motor deficits (McIntosh et al. 1996), reduced cerebral edema (Bareyre et al. 1997; Stover et al. 2000a), and reduced posttraumatic lesion volume (Wahl et al. 1997; C. Zhang et al. 1998). The use of presynaptic inhibitors of glutamate release, such as riluzole, in clinical brain injury may present a possible alternative to the use of postsynaptic glutamate antagonists, which are known to be associated with neurotoxicity and psychomimetic side effects.

Inhibition of Lipid Peroxidation

Oxidative damage has been implicated in many of the pathological changes that occur after TBI (Ercan et al. 2001; Hsiang et al. 1997). Oxidative damage in the CNS manifests itself primarily as lipid peroxidation because the brain is rich in peroxidizable fatty acids and possesses relatively few antioxidant defense systems (for review see Floyd 1999). After TBI, alterations in regional cerebral blood flow (CBF) and reductions in substrate delivery likely combine to produce intracellular arachidonic acid cascade metabolites and reactive oxygen species (ROS) (Ikeda and Long 1990; Kontos and Povlishock 1986). The genesis of ROS after TBI has also been related to nonischemic events, including the increase in intracellular calcium concentrations that induces ROS release from mitochondria (Tymianski and Tator 1996). Other endogenous ROS also occur from enzymatic processes, monoamine oxidase, cyclooxygenase (COX), nitric oxide synthase (NOS), and nicotine adenine dinucleotide phosphate oxidase, as well as macrophages and neutrophils. Excessive glutamate release can also generate high levels of ROS (Dugan and Choi 1994). These ROS cause peroxidative destruction of the lipid bilayer cell membrane, oxidize cellular proteins and nucleic acids, and attack the cerebrovasculature, thereby affecting the BBB integrity and/or vascular reactivity. Several regulatory mechanisms can be affected by ROS, including activation of cytokine or growth factor–mediated signal transduction pathways, induction of IEGs, and disruption of calmodulin-regulated gene transcription (Yao et al. 1996). Free reactive iron, a catalyst for the formation of ROS, may also be involved in trauma-induced peroxidative tissue damage.

Several studies have indirectly demonstrated the early generation of superoxide radicals in injured brains, which subsequently resulted in secondary damage to the brain microvasculature (Povlishock and Kontos 1992). Some

investigators have used spin trap probes of salicylate trapping methods to demonstrate an early posttraumatic formation of hydroxyl radicals in injured brains (Hall et al. 1993) that also correlated with the development of BBB disruption (Smith et al. 1994). Still others have used cyclic-voltammetry techniques to measure the production of low-molecular-weight antioxidants (LMWAs) by the injured brain as another indirect indication of ROS production after brain trauma (Beit-Yannai et al. 1997; Shohami et al. 1997b). These studies suggest that LMWAs are mobilized from brain cells to the extracellular space (Moor et al. 2001). More stable molecules such as 3,4-dihydroxybenzoic acid (3,4-DHBA) have been used to detect an increase in ROS with microdialysis after TBI (Marklund et al. 2001a). Recently, isoprostanes have been used as specific markers to detect lipid peroxidation after TBI (Tyurin et al. 2000); in one study, $8,12$-iso-IPF$_{2\alpha}$-VI levels increased in brain and blood between 1 and 24 hours after TBI (Pratico et al. 2002).

Posttraumatic alterations in intracellular calcium precipitate an attack on the cellular cytoarchitecture via activation of calpains and lipases and also induce the formation of ROS that attack the cell membrane. Trauma-induced activation of phospholipases A_2 (PLA2) and C (PLC) results in the release of free fatty acids, diacylglycerol (DAG), thromboxane B_2, and leukotrienes, whereas accumulation of free arachidonic acid itself may affect membrane permeability (for a review see Bazan et al. 1995). TBI-induced DAG formation is associated with posttraumatic cerebral edema (Dhillon et al. 1994, 1995), and DAG activates protein kinase C, which may modulate other signal transduction pathways. Protein kinase C increases over time in the cortex and hippocampus after TBI in the rat (Sun and Faden 1994). Homayoun et al. (1997) reported that TBI in rats induces a delayed and sustained activation of phospholipase-mediated signaling pathways, leading to membrane phospholipid degradation that targets docosahexaenoyl phospholipid-enriched membranes.

Compounds that block various steps in the arachidonate cascade have been shown to be somewhat effective in experimental models of TBI (Table 39–2). The nonselective COX inhibitors ibuprofen and indomethacin have been shown to improve neurologic function and to decrease mortality after TBI (Hall 1985; Kim et al. 1989). Head-injured patients who have received intravenous indomethacin present with reduced ICP and CBF and increased cerebral perfusion pressure (Slavik and Rhoney 1999). COX-2 levels have been shown to be elevated in injured cortex and in the ipsilateral hippocampus after experimental TBI in rats (Dash et al. 2000). Although administration of selective COX-2 inhibitors 4-(5-[4-

TABLE 39–2.   Antioxidant, antiinflammatory, and neurotrophic factors

Type of agent	Compound	Type of research	Outcome	References
COX inhibitor	Indomethacin	e,c	↓ ICP	Slavik et al. 1999
COX-2 inhibitor	Celecoxib	e	↑ cognitive function; ↓ motor function	Dash et al. 2001
	Nimesulide	e	↑ motor/cognitive function	Cernak et al. 2001
	SC 58125	e	↓ antioxidants	Tyurin et al. 2000
Iron chelator	Deferoxamine	e	↑ motor function; ↓ tissue SOD	Panter et al. 1992
	Desferal	e	↑ motor/cognitive function; ↓ edema	Ikeda et al. 1989; Zhang et al. 1998
Antioxidant	U-101033E	e	↓ mitochondria dysfunction	Xiong et al. 1997
	SOD	e	↓ edema	Shohami et al. 1997
	PEG-SOD	e,c	↑ motor function, BBB penetration; ↓ ARDS	Hamm et al. 1996; Muizelaar et al. 1993; Young et al. 1996
	PC-SOD	e	↓ edema	Yunoki et al. 1997
	PBN	e	↑ cognitive function; ↓ lesion volume, tissue loss	Marklund et al. 2001
	S-PBN	e	↓ tissue loss	Marklund et al. 2001
	LY341122	e	↓ cell death, lesion volume	Wada et al. 1999
21-aminosteroid	Freedox	e	↑ motor function, metabolism; ↓ edema, mortality	Hall et al. 1988, 1994; McIntosh et al. 1992; Sanada et al. 1993
	U-743896	e	↓ axonal injury	Marion and White 1996
NOS inhibitor	BN 80933	e	↑ sensory/motor function	Chabrier et al. 1999
ICAM-1 inhibitor	1A29	e	No change	Isaksson et al. 2001
Leukocyte adherence inhibition	Prostacyclin	e	↓ cell death	Allan et al. 2001
IL-1ra	IL-1ra	e	↑ cognitive function; ↓ cell death	Knoblach et al. 2000; Sanderson et al. 1999; Toulmond et al. 1995
Tetracycline	Minocycline	e	↑ motor function; ↓ lesion volume	Fink et al. 1999; Sanchez Mejia et al. 2001
IL-10	IL-10	e	↑ motor function; ↓ TNF expression	Knoblach et al. 1998
Immunosuppressant	Pentoxifylline	e	↑ motor function; ↓ edema	Shohami et al. 1996
Kallikrein-kinin	CP-0127	e,c	↑ GCS; ↓ edema, mortality	Marmarou et al. 1999; Narotam et al. 1998;
B_2 receptor antagonist	Lf-16-068Ms	e	↓ edema	Stover et al. 2000a, 2000b
Endocannabinoid	2-AG	e	↓ edema	Panikashvili et al. 2001
	Dexabinol	c	↓ ICP/CPP	Pop 2000
Neutrophic factors	NGF	e	↑ cognitive function, cholinergic reinnervation; ↓ cell death	Philips et al. 2001

TABLE 39–2.   Antioxidant, antiinflammatory, and neurotrophic factors *(continued)*

Type of agent	Compound	Type of research	Outcome	References
	BDNF	e	No change	Blaha et al. 2000
	GDNF	e	↓ cell death, lesion volume	Hermann et al. 2001; Kim et al. 2001
	bFGF	e	↑ cognitive function; ↓ cell death	Dietrich et al. 1996; McDermott et al. 1997; Yang et al. 2000
	IGF-1	e,c	↑ motor/cognitive function	Hatton et al. 1997; Saatman et al. 1997

Note.   ARDS=adult respiratory distress syndrome; BBB=blood–brain barrier; BDNF=brain-derived neurotrophic factor; bFGF=basic fibroblast growth factor; c=clinical trial; COX=cyclooxygenase; CPP=cerebral perfusion pressure; e=experimental study; FGF= fibroblast growth factor; GDNF=glial cell-line–derived neurotrophic factor; ICAM-1=intercellular adhesion molecule-1; ICP=intracranial pressure; IGF=insulin-like growth factor; IL=interleukin; NGF=nerve growth factor; NOS=nitric oxide synthase; PC-SOD=lecithinized superoxide dismutase; PEG-SOD=polyethylene glycol superoxide dismutase; SOD = superoxide dismutase; TNF = tumor necrosis factor.

methylphenyl]-3-[trifluoromethyl]-1H-pyrazol-1-yl) benzenesulfonamide (celecoxib) and nimesulide was shown to improve cognitive function after TBI, its effect on motor function remains controversial (Hurley et al. 2002). The COX-2 inhibitor SC 58125 prevented depletion of antioxidants after TBI in rats (Tyurin et al. 2000). Although COX-2 induction after TBI may result in selective beneficial responses, chronic COX-2 production may actually potentiate free radical–mediated cellular damage, vascular dysfunction, and alterations in cellular metabolism (Strauss et al. 2000).

Experimental work suggests that ROS scavengers may confer some neuroprotection in experimental models of TBI (Hensley et al. 1997; Shohami et al. 1997a). Antioxidants such as α-tocopherol (vitamin E) have been shown to be beneficial in TBI (Clifton et al. 1989; Stein et al. 1991; Conte et al. 2004). Conversely, Stoffel and colleagues (1997) have reported that increasing plasma vitamin E levels had no effect on posttraumatic vasogenic brain edema. It has been reported that systemic levels of two major antioxidants, vitamin E and ascorbic acid (vitamin C), were significantly reduced in injured rats after TBI and that these reductions inversely correlated with isoprostane levels (Pratico et al. 2002).

Panter et al. (1992) reported that administration of the iron chelator dextran-deferoxamine, which protects brain tissue by terminating radical-chain reactions and removing intracellular superoxide, improved neurological impairment after TBI in mice, suggesting that brain injury is associated with significant iron-dependent ROS-induced lipid peroxidation. Desferal, another potent chelator of redox-active metals, has been shown to attenuate brain edema and improve neurological recovery after TBI in rats (Ikeda et al. 1989; R. Zhang et al. 1998). Administration of the novel antioxidant pyrolopyrimidine (U-101033E) after TBI in the rat was also shown to reduce mitochondrial dysfunction.

The use of stable nitroxide radicals as antioxidant therapy in CNS injury has also been attempted. Nitroxides, which are cell-permeable, nontoxic, stable radicals, have been shown to prevent ROS-induced lipid peroxidation (Krishna et al. 1996; Pogrebniak et al. 1991). Administration of these compounds markedly improved neurological recovery, reduced edema, and protected the impaired BBB after TBI in rats (Beit-Yannai et al. 1996). Administration of nitrone radical scavengers, another class of potent ROS, has been evaluated for neuroprotective efficacy after TBI. Administration of α-phenyl-*tert*-N-butyl nitrone (PBN) or 2-sulfo-phenyl-N-*tert*-butyl nitrone (S-PBN) in rats significantly reduced ROS formation, cognitive impairment, and lesion volume after TBI (Marklund et al. 2001b, 2001c, 2001d). Other ROS scavengers that recently have been demonstrated to exert neuroprotective effects in experimental TBI include the second-generation azulenyl nitrone stilbazulenyl nitrone (STAZN) (Belayev et al. 2002), melatonin (Sarrafzadeh et al. 2000), a superoxide radical scavenger (OPC-14117) (Aoyama et al. 2002; Mori et al. 1998) 2-(3,5-di-*t*-butyl-4-hydroxyphenyl)-4-(2-[4-methylethylaminomethyl-phenyloxy]ethyl)oxazole LY341122 (Wada et al. 1999), and citicoline, an endogenous intermediate of phosphatidylcholine synthesis reported to stabilize the cell membrane integrity and free fatty acid formation (Baskaya et al. 2000).

Administration of the antioxidant enzyme SOD was reported to have beneficial effects on survival and neurological recovery (Shohami et al. 1997a). The conjugation of polyethylene glycol to SOD (PEG-SOD, Dismutec), thereby improving BBB penetration and increasing SOD's plasma half-life, has been shown to reduce motor deficits (Hamm et al. 1996). DeWitt et al. (1997) have shown that PEG-SOD administration reverses cerebral hypoperfusion after TBI in rats, and others have reported that administration of lecithinized SOD (PC-SOD) reduced brain edema after weight-drop brain injury in rats (Yunoki et al. 1997). A multicenter clinical trial of Dismutec was conducted in the United States. Although initial Phase II studies were compelling (Muizelaar et al. 1993), the results of the larger Phase III trials in severely head-injured patients were disappointing (Muizelaar et al. 1995; Young et al. 1996).

High-dose glucocorticoids stabilize membranes and also reduce ROS-induced lipid peroxidative injury (Braughler et al. 1987; Hall et al. 1987). Although many early clinical studies reported that high-dose steroid treatment is without effect in TBI (Braakman et al. 1983; Cooper et al. 1979; Gudeman et al. 1979), a few tantalizingly positive studies have been published. Giannotta et al. (1984) reported that high-dose methylprednisolone significantly reduced mortality in severely head-injured patients. In a multicenter trial conducted in Germany, treatment of severely head-injured patients with the synthetic corticosteroid triamcinolone significantly reduced mortality and improved long-term neurological outcome (Grumme et al. 1995). The CRASH (Corticosteroid Randomization After Significant Head Injury) trial has been designed to determine the effects of short-term steroid treatment on death and disability after severe brain injury in more than 7,000 patients in the United Kingdom (Roberts 2001).

A group of 21-aminosteroid compounds have been developed that lack true glucocorticoid activity while maintaining the ability to scavenge ROS and inhibit lipid peroxidation (Braughler and Pregenzer 1989). The most widely evaluated member of this group of compounds, tirilazad mesylate (Freedox), has been shown to enhance neurological recovery and survival (Hall et al. 1988), attenuate posttraumatic edema, reduce mortality (McIntosh et al. 1992), improve motor function (Sanada et al. 1993), and increase metabolism of nonedematous tissue adjacent to contusion (Hall et al. 1994) after experimental TBI in rodents. Freedox appears to exert its antilipid peroxidative action through two mechanisms: free radical scavenging and membrane stabilization (Fernandez et al. 1997; Kavanagh and Kam 2001). Treatment of TBI with the Freedox-like 21-aminosteroid U-743896, or moder-

ate hypothermia, or a combination of both significantly reduces axonal injury, although the 21-aminosteroid therapy was more effective when treatment was initiated 40 minutes after injury (Knoblach et al. 1999). The lipophilicity of these 21-aminosteroids, coupled with their potent inhibition of lipid peroxidation over a wide dose-response range and the positive data collected from a wide variety of animal models of CNS injury generated momentum to launch a multicenter clinical trial of Freedox in the treatment of severely brain-injured patients in the United States and Europe. However, the results of these studies were largely negative (Marshall and Marshall 1995). Future studies enrolling patients with mild and moderate severity of brain trauma may demonstrate clinical use of this class of compounds.

An overproduction of the free radical nitric oxide (NO) and its derivative anion peroxynitrite is also thought to play an active role in the pathophysiology of TBI. Although pharmacological intervention with both nonselective inhibitors of NOS and selective inhibitors of neuronal and inducible NOS isoforms have proven effective in experimental TBI (Gahm et al. 2002; Khaldi et al. 2002), further preclinical work is necessary to clarify the therapeutic potential of these compounds, particularly because NO can be either neuroprotective or destructive, depending on its spatiotemporal distribution and concentration. A novel agent linking an antioxidant to a selective inhibitor of neuronal NOS (BN 80933) has been shown to be neuroprotective in models of both TBI and cerebral ischemia (Chabrier et al. 1999). The inhibition of NOS-induced cellular damage may confer neuroprotection to the injured brain, and future studies should emphasize the evaluation and development of pathway-specific compounds.

Anti-Inflammatory Strategies

Although CNS inflammation was long believed to be a catastrophic event leading to sustained functional impairment and even death, there is increasing evidence that inflammatory pathways may be of importance for initiation of regenerative response. Posttraumatic edema formation is associated with complex cytotoxic events and vascular leakage after the breakdown of the BBB (Baskaya et al. 1997; Unterberg et al. 1997), and a profound disruption of the BBB has been observed in a variety of experimental TBI models (Barzo et al. 1996; Fukuda et al. 1995; Soares et al. 1992) as well as in human TBI (Csuka et al. 1999; Morganti-Kossmann et al. 1999; Pleines et al. 1998). As such, infiltration and accumulation of polymorphonuclear leukocytes into brain parenchyma occurs in the acute posttraumatic period, reaching a peak by 24 hours postinjury (Soares et al. 1995; Stahel et al. 2000b). Alterations in bloodborne immunocompetent cells have been described in head-injured patients (Hoyt et al. 1990; Piek et al. 1992; Quattrocchi et al. 1992). Immunocytochemical studies have further demonstrated the presence of macrophages, natural killer cells, helper T cells, and T cytotoxic suppressor cells as early as 2 days postinjury (Holmin et al. 1995). The entry of macrophages into brain parenchyma has been shown to be maximal by 24–48 hours after TBI in rats and humans (Holmin et al. 1995, 1998; Soares et al. 1995). A recent study of severe TBI patients suggested that the activated cell population after CNS trauma appears to be composed predominantly of the macrophage/microglia lineage, as opposed to the T-cell lineage (Lenzlinger et al. 2001). Both macrophages and microglia have been proposed as key cellular elements in the progressive tissue necrosis—presumably associated with the release of cytotoxic molecules that may be involved in mediating the local inflammatory response to trauma and the phagocytosis of debris from dying cells—that occurs after CNS trauma (Morganti-Kossmann et al. 2001).

Zhuang et al. (1993) have suggested a relationship between cortical polymorphonuclear leukocyte accumulation and secondary brain injury, including lowered CBF, increased edema, and elevated ICP. The migration of leukocytes into damaged tissue typically requires the adhesion of these cells to the endothelium, which is mediated by the expression of the intercellular adhesion molecule-1 (ICAM-1). An upregulation of ICAM-1 has been described in a variety of experimental TBI models (Carlos et al. 1997; Isaksson et al. 1997; Rancan et al. 2001), suggesting a role for leukocyte adhesion in the pathobiology of posttraumatic cell infiltration in the brain. In humans, soluble ICAM-1 (sICAM-1) in CSF has been associated with the breakdown of the BBB after severe TBI (Pleines et al. 1998). However, treatment with the anti-ICAM-1 antibody 1A29 failed to significantly improve the learning deficits or histopathological damage after severe TBI in rats (Isaksson et al. 2001) (see Table 39–2). Recently, prostacyclin, which is known to inhibit leukocyte adherence and aggregation and platelet aggregation, was shown to reduce neocortical neuronal death in rats after TBI (Bentzer et al. 2001). Besides the expression of adhesion molecules, leukocyte transmigration appears to require the production of chemokines that activate and guide leukocytes to the injured area.

The specific cytokines and growth factors that have been implicated in the posttraumatic inflammatory cascade include the interleukin (IL) and tumor necrosis factor (TNFα) families of peptides (for review see Allan and Rothwell 2001). Alterations in systemic and intrathecal concentrations of these cytokines have been reported to occur in human patients after severe brain injury, and regional mRNA and protein concentrations have been shown to increase markedly in the acute posttraumatic period after experimental brain trauma in the rat (Allan and Rothwell 2001). IL-1α and IL-1β, two IL-1 agonists, and IL-1 receptor antagonist (IL-1ra), a naturally occurring physiological IL-1 antagonist, are produced as precursors. While pro-IL-1α and pro-IL-1ra are active, pro-IL-1β is activated when it is cleaved by IL-1 converting enzyme (ICE or caspase-1). IL-1 has been implicated in an array of pathological and nonpathological processes, including apoptotic cell death (Friedlander et al. 1996), leukocyte-endothelial adhesion (Bevilacqua et al. 1985), BBB disruption (Quagliarello et al. 1991), edema (Yamasaki et al. 1992), astrogliosis and neovascularization (Giulian et al. 1988), and synthesis of neurotrophic factors (DeKosky et al. 1996). IL-1, in turn, stimulates other inflammatory mediators, such as phospholipase A_2, COX-2, prostaglandins, NO, and matrix metalloproteinases (Basu et al. 2002; Rothwell and Luheshi 2000). A significant increase in pro-IL-1β mRNA in the injured hemisphere as early as 1 hour and remaining up to 6 hours postinjury has been reported after experimental TBI (Fan et al. 1995). A similar acute increase in IL-1 activity and mature IL-1β protein levels after TBI has been reported (Taupin et al. 1993), which can be directly correlated to the severity of injury in experimental models of TBI (Kinoshita et al. 2002).

Caspase-1 mRNA is increased in ipsilateral cortex and hippocampus between 24 and 72 hours after TBI in rats (Sullivan et al. 2002; Yakovlev et al. 1997) although increased cleavage of caspase-1 is observed after human brain injury (Clark et al. 1999). Intracerebroventricular administration of IL-1ra results in improved cognitive function without motor improvement (Sanderson et al. 1999), and administration of recombinant IL1-ra resulted in reduced neuronal damage after TBI in rodents (Toulmond and Rothwell 1995). Despite the inability to readily detect caspase-1 activity in the injured rat brain, administration of a selective inhibitor of caspase-1 (e.g., acetyl-Tyr-Val-Ala-Asp-chloromethyl-ketone [AcYVAD-cmk] or the tetracycline derivative minocycline) before TBI significantly reduces lesion volume and attenuates motor deficits (Fink et al. 1999; Sanchez Mejia et al. 2001).

The pleiotropic cytokine IL-6 has been implicated in a variety of physiological as well as pathological processes including induction of nerve growth factor (NGF) expression (Frei et al. 1989; Gruol and Nelson 1997; Marz et al. 1999; Nieto-Sampedro et al. 1982). Elevated levels of IL-6 have been detected in the CSF and the serum of patients with severe TBI over a period of up to 3 weeks after trauma

(Hans et al. 1999a; Kossmann et al. 1995). The higher concentration of IL-6 reported in the CSF of TBI patients suggests an intrathecal production of this factor, which has been reported to occur in several models of experimental TBI (Woodroofe et al. 1991). Hans and coworkers (1999b) demonstrated that IL-6 mRNA was upregulated in cortical and thalamic neurons as well as in infiltrating macrophages as early as 1 hour postinjury, whereas IL-6 immunoreactivity and protein levels in rat CSF peaked within the first 24 hours after TBI. In a study by Kossmann et al. (1996), a temporal relationship between high CSF concentrations of IL-6 and the detection of NGF in CSF was noted in brain-injured patients. In vitro experiments using CSF from these patients showed that IL-6 stimulated cultured primary mouse astrocytes to produce NGF, an effect which could be significantly attenuated by preincubation with anti-IL-6 antibodies (Kossmann et al. 1996). IL-6 released in the CNS has also been shown to be associated with the systemic acute phase response after severe TBI in humans (Kossmann et al. 1995), indicating that centrally released immune mediators may evoke a substantial systemic response to trauma, with profound implications for the outcome of TBI patients.

In a study subjecting IL-6 knockout mice and their wild-type (WT) littermates to a cortical freeze lesion, Penkowa and colleagues (1999) found that the lack of IL-6 greatly reduced reactive astrogliosis and the appearance of brain macrophages around the lesion site. IL-6 deficiency also caused greater lesion-induced neuronal cell loss. These observations highlight the dual role that this pleiotropic cytokine may play in the posttraumatic cascade. Conversely, a recent study using IL-6 knockout mice subjected to TBI showed that these animals were not significantly different from their WT littermates in their response to TBI in several outcome measures, such as neurologic motor function, BBB permeability, intracerebral neutrophil infiltration, and neuronal cell loss (Stahel et al. 2000b). Therefore, IL-6 appears to promote an inflammatory response to trauma but at the same time also seems to enhance neuronal survival. The exact nature, severity, and type of the CNS injury as well as the timing of IL-6 release may be decisive for either a detrimental or a beneficial effect of this factor after TBI.

IL-10 is an anti-inflammatory cytokine that inhibits a variety of macrophage responses and is also a potent suppressor of T-cell proliferation and cytokine response by blocking expression of TNF and IL-1 (Benveniste et al. 1995; Chao et al. 1995) and enhancing synthesis and secretion of their endogenous antagonists (Cassatella et al. 1994; Joyce et al. 1994). IL-10 also reduces leukocyte–endothelial interactions that promote procoagulation (Jungi et al. 1994) and extravasation of blood cells (Krakauer

1995; Perretti et al. 1995). Subcutaneous or intravenous administration of IL-10 before or after TBI in rats significantly reduced TNF expression in the injured cortex and enhanced neurological recovery (Knoblach and Faden 1998). Although a combination of IL-10 systemic administration and hypothermia was expected to exhibit increased neuroprotection after TBI, this combination therapy resulted in adverse effects when compared with hypothermia alone after TBI (Kline et al. 2002).

TNF-α, a proinflammatory cytokine with cytotoxic properties, has been detected in the CSF and the serum of patients with TBI (Goodman et al. 1990; Ross et al. 1994). Csuka and coworkers (1999) found increased patterns of TNF-α concentrations among 28 TBI patients over a 3-week study period. These observations together with the detection of TNF-α mRNA and protein in the injured rodent brain suggest that this cytokine is markedly and acutely unregulated in brain tissue after TBI (Fan et al. 1996; Shohami et al. 1994). Increases in TNF-α expression were immunohistochemically localized primarily to neurons and to a much lesser extent to astrocytes after TBI in rats (Knoblach et al. 1999). The upregulation of TNF-α therefore appears to be an endogenous response of the brain parenchyma to trauma, as opposed to being the result of a nonspecific invasion of the brain by peripheral blood leukocytes. TNF-α may mediate secondary damage after TBI through several different mechanisms (for a review see Shohami et al. 1999). This cytokine is known to affect BBB integrity, leading to cerebral edema and infiltration of blood leukocytes, and it has been shown to induce expression of the receptor for the potent secondary inflammatory mediator anaphylatoxin (or C5a) on neurons (Stahel et al. 2000a). Furthermore, TNF can induce both apoptosis and necrosis via intracellular signaling pathways (Reid et al. 1989).

On the basis of the above evidence, it is not surprising that both direct and indirect inhibition of TNF-α activity has been shown to be beneficial in experimental TBI studies. Administration of the immunosuppressive pentoxifylline as well as of TNF-α binding protein, a physiological inhibitor of TNF-α activity, has been shown to significantly diminish edema formation and enhance motor function recovery after experimental TBI (Shohami et al. 1996). These studies suggest a detrimental effect of TNF-α in the sequelae of TBI. However, more recent investigations in genetically engineered animals point again toward a dual role of this cytokine after TBI. Mice deficient in both subtypes of TNF receptors have been shown to be more vulnerable to TBI than WT animals, suggesting a neuroprotective role for TNF-α in the pathological sequelae of brain injury (Sullivan et al. 1999). Moreover, brain-injured TNF-deficient (–/–) mice show an early benefit from the lack of TNF, with neurologic motor scores initially better than brain-injured WT controls. However, this trend is reversed from 1–4 weeks after injury: the injured WT animals recover while the TNF –/– mice do not (Scherbel et al. 1999). Taken together, these data suggest that a differential role of this cytokine may be dependent on the temporal profile of its release within the posttraumatic cytokine cascade. These data suggest that antagonism of TNF activity may be beneficial for the injured brain in the acute posttraumatic period but may prove deleterious if extended into the chronic phase, when it may be essential for initiating a regenerative response. Alternatively, another possibility allows that the expression of TNF receptor subtypes may change over the acute and chronic postinjury phases, and recent evidence suggests that neuronal death or survival in response to TNF-α may depend on the particular subtype that is predominantly expressed (Yang et al. 2002).

The role of the kallikrein–kinin system in inflammation and pain has led to the development of bradykinin B_2 receptor antagonists. In a multicenter clinical trial, Bradycor (CP-0127) was found to be neuroprotective in severely brain-injured patients (Marmarou et al. 1999), and a recently developed nonpeptide B_2 receptor antagonist (LF-16–0687Ms) was shown to reduce TBI-induced brain vasogenic edema in rats (Stover et al. 2000b). Inhibition of the posttraumatic inflammatory cascade continues to be a viable avenue of development of neuroprotective compounds.

Recently, several groups have implicated modulation of the endocannabinoid system, including the arachidonoylethanolamide (anandamide), 2-arachidonyl glyceryl ether, and 2-arachidonoyl glycerol (2-AG) ligands and their cognate CB_1 and CB_2 receptors, as a possible therapeutic paradigm after TBI. Cannabinoid receptor agonists have been shown to inhibit glutamatergic synaptic transmission (Shen et al. 1996) and protect neurons from excitotoxicity in vitro (Shen and Thayer 1998). It has also been suggested that cannabinoid receptor agonists can counteract the vasoconstrictory effects of endothelin-1 (Chen and Buck 2000), a molecule that may play a role in TBI-induced ischemia. Gallily et al. (2000) have reported that 2-AG suppresses formation of ROS and have noted lower levels of TNF-α in the serum of LPS-treated mice after administration of 2-AG (Gallily et al. 2000). Most recently, it has been demonstrated that levels of anandamide (Hansen et al. 2001; Panikashvili et al. 2001) and 2-AG (Panikashvili et al. 2001) are significantly elevated after TBI, and if this response is further augmented by administration of synthetic 2-AG, injured animals exhibit a significant reduction in brain edema, reduced lesion volume, and quicker recovery of neurological

function (Panikashvili et al. 2001). Collectively, these data provide a rationale for the use of cannabinoids in the treatment of TBI. Indeed, dexanabinol (HU-211), a nonpsychotropic cannabinoid, has been reported to have a significant neuroprotective role after TBI. In a randomized, placebo-controlled Phase II clinical trial, patients with severe closed head injury receiving an intravenous injection of dexanabinol showed significantly better ICP, cerebral perfusion pressure, and clinical outcome (Knoller et al. 2002).

Neurotrophic Factors

The peptide growth factors, including NGF, basic fibroblast growth factor (bFGF), ciliary neurotrophic factor (CNTF), brain-derived neurotrophic factor (BDNF), insulinlike growth factor (IGF-1), neurotrophin-3 (NT-3), neurotrophin-4/5 (NT-4/5), and glial-derived neurotrophic factor (GDNF), all function in the normal brain to support neuronal survival, induce sprouting of neurites (neuronal plasticity), and facilitate the guidance of neurons to their proper target sites during development (for a review see Huang and Reichardt 2001) (Figure 39–3). Several recent studies suggest that some of these neurotrophic factors are altered after brain injury, perhaps as a response designed to facilitate neuronal repair and reestablish functional connections in the injured brain. DeKosky and colleagues (1994) observed a marked increase in NGF mRNA and protein expression in the acute posttraumatic period after both weight-drop and TBI in rats, whereas a significant reduction in NGF p75^{NTR} receptor was observed in the chronic postinjury period after TBI in rats (Leonard et al. 1994). Goss et al. (1997) observed an increase in the antioxidant enzyme glutathione peroxidase and catalase concentrations over a time course that reflected the temporal increase in NGF and hypothesized that the upregulation of NGF after TBI serves as a mediator of oxidative homeostasis by inducing the production of ROS. The same authors suggested that astrocytes are the major source of NGF upregulation after TBI in the rat (Goss et al. 1998). Using models of TBI, several laboratories reported that intraparenchymal administration of NGF can attenuate cognitive but not neurobehavioral motor deficits or hippocampal cell loss after TBI in rats (Dixon et al. 1997; Sinson et al. 1995, 1996) (see Table 39–2). Follow-up studies demonstrated that central NGF administration can reduce the extent of apoptotic cell death in septal cholinergic neurons after TBI (Sinson et al. 1997) and can reverse the trauma-induced reductions in scopolamine-evoked acetylcholine release (Dixon et al. 1997). Recently, both rat- and hippocampal-

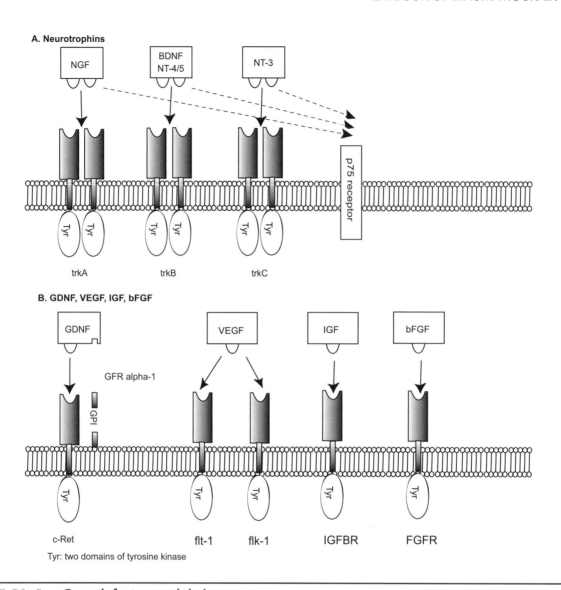

FIGURE 39–3. **Growth factors and their cognate receptors.**

BDNF = brain-derived neurotrophic factor; bFGF = basic fibroblast growth factor; FGFR = FGF receptor; GDNF = glial-derived neurotrophic factor; GFR = GDNF family receptor; IGF = insulin-like growth factor; IGFBR= IGF receptor; NGF = nerve growth factor; NT-3 = neurotrophin-3; VEGF = vascular endothelial growth factor.

derived precursor (HiB5) cells and human NT2M neurons, transfected to express NGF and transplanted into the injured cortex, have been shown to improve cognitive and neurological motor function and reduce CA3 neuronal cell death when transplanted into the injured cortex at 24 hours after TBI in rats (Longhi et al., in press; Philips et al. 2001).

BDNF, a member of the neurotrophin family of trophic factors, has almost 50% homology with NGF (Leibrock et al. 1989), although BDNF is more abundant in the adult brain than NGF (Maisonpierre et al. 1990). BDNF has two receptors: the high-affinity receptor TrkB and the low-affinity receptor p75^{NTR} (Table 39–3). A second ligand, NT-4/5, also binds to TrkB with high affinity and is expressed ubiquitously within the adult rodent brain (Timmusk et al. 1993); however, changes in NT-

4/5 expression have not been evaluated to date in an experimental model of TBI, nor has its therapeutic value after TBI been evaluated and documented. BDNF and its primary receptor, the TrkB tyrosine kinase, are found in many areas of the brain, including the hippocampal CA3 and the dentate hilus regions (Nawa et al. 1995; Yan et al. 1997a, 1997b) (see Table 39–3). BDNF regulates the generation and differentiation of neurons during development, axon growth and growth cone mobility, and synaptic plasticity (Lu and Chow 1999; McAllister et al. 1999; Schinder and Poo 2000), and it was recently shown to promote neurogenesis from adult stem cells in vivo (Benraiss et al. 2001; Pencea et al. 2001).

Initial observations suggested that a rapid increase in BDNF mRNA levels occurs in injured brain as early as 1

TABLE 39–3. Neurotrophic receptor families and endogenous ligands in the central nervous system

Types of receptors and neurotrophic factor family	Neurotrophic factors as ligand
Tyrosine kinase receptors	—
NGF receptor family	Neurotrophins (NGF, BDNF, NT-3, NT-4/5)
FGF receptor family	FGF-2
Ret receptor family	GDNF, neurturin, artemin, persephin
Insulin receptor family	Insulin, IGF-1
VEGF receptor family	—

Note. BDNF=brain-derived neurotrophic factor; FGF=fibroblast growth factor; GDNF=glial cell-line–derived neurotrophic factor; IGF=insulin-like growth factor; NGF=nerve growth factor; NT-3=neurotrophin 3; NT-4/5=neurotrophin 4/5; VEGF=vascular endothelial growth factor.

hour after TBI and persists for days (Griesbach et al. 2002; Hicks et al. 1997; Oyesiku et al. 1999; Truettner et al. 1999) with a concomitant acute increase in trkB mRNA levels within the hippocampus (Hicks et al. 1998; Mudo et al. 1993). Animals in which milder injuries are induced exhibit unilateral, rather than bilateral, increases in BDNF and trkB mRNA levels (Hicks et al. 1999b). Another study reported significantly decreased levels of BDNF mRNA in the injured cortex at 72 hours and increased levels in other adjacent cortical areas from 3–24 hours postinjury (Hicks et al. 1999a). This apparent discrepancy in observations could be a function of difference of injury models, the time points chosen for observation if expression levels prove to be biphasic, or differences in the sensitivity of assays used to measure the reported changes. In one of the few treatment studies, administration of BDNF directly into injured brain parenchyma failed to attenuate behavioral deficits or histological damage after TBI in rats (Blaha et al. 2000). Although there are many possible explanations of why BDNF administration failed to confer neuroprotection after TBI, one interesting possibility is that injury selectively upregulated the truncated form of trkB rather than the full-length form.

The neurotrophic factors GDNF, neurturin, persephin, and artemin are included among the TGF-β superfamily (for a review see Airaksinen et al. 1999) (see Table 39–3). The GDNF family ligands signal via a two-component receptor complex that includes c-Ret, a protooncogene and tyrosine kinase receptor (Durbec et al. 1996; Trupp et al. 1996), and GDNF family receptor-α (GFR-

α), a glycosyl-phosphatidylinositol-anchored protein that is devoid of an associated kinase activity (Baloh et al. 1997; Jing et al. 1996) (see Table 39–3). The GDNF transcript has been detected in all major brain regions (Schaar et al. 1993), including those regions vulnerable to TBI, and GDNF and neurturin exert neurotrophic effects in a wide spectrum of neuronal populations (Arenas et al. 1995; Henderson et al. 1994; Kotzbauer et al. 1996; Lin et al. 1993; Mount et al. 1995). GDNF appears to reduce NMDA-induced calcium influx via the activation of the mitogen-activated protein kinase pathway and as a result attenuates NMDA-induced excitotoxic cell death (Nicole et al. 2001). Such activity suggests that GDNF may be an especially attractive candidate for reducing excitotoxic neuronal death after TBI if administered at acute time points when excitotoxicity is predominant (see above).

To date, little evidence exists documenting changes in expression of GDNF or its receptors after TBI. A single preliminary report suggests that GDNF protein levels, as measured by quantitative enzyme-linked immunosorbent assay (ELISA), increase approximately 2.5 times in the injured cortex after TBI in rats (Shimizu et al. 2002). When GDNF or artificial CSF is infused continuously for 7 days into the lateral ventricle after TBI in rats, a significant decrease was observed in injury-induced CA2 and CA3 cell loss (Kim et al. 2001). Likewise, when an adenovirus engineered to confer GDNF expression was injected into the sensorimotor cortex 24 hours before freeze-lesion injury in rats, a significant reduction in lesion volume and the number of cells immunopositive for iNOS, activated caspase-3, and TUNEL was observed (Hermann et al. 2001).

The polypeptide FGF-2 (also known as bFGF) is a member of the FGF family, which currently includes seven members (for a review see Gimenez-Gallego and Cuevas 1994), all of which possess the ability to stimulate fibroblast growth with the notable exception of FGF-7. FGF-2 binds to four cell surface receptors that are expressed as a number of splice variants (for a review see Nugent and Iozzo 2000), of which FGFR1 is the high-affinity receptor (for a review see (Stachowiak et al. 1997) (see Table 39–3). FGF-2 and FGFR1 proteins, as well as their mRNAs, have been demonstrated to be expressed in both the developing and the adult brain (for a review see Unsicker et al. 1991). FGF-2 has been implicated as a neurotrophin, a neurite branching factor, an enhancer of synaptic transmission, and a neural inducer (Abe and Saito 2001).

Initial reports demonstrated an increase in FGF-2 protein after TBI at the lesion periphery in cells with morphological features consistent with reactive astrocytes (Finklestein et al. 1988). Further analysis resulted in the observation that FGF-2 mRNA, FGF-2 protein, FGFR1 mRNA, and FGFR1 protein were increased as early as hours postinjury and persisted for at least 2 weeks postinjury (Frank and Ragel 1995; Reilly and Kumari 1996; Yang and Cui 1998). Furthermore, at acute time points, FGF-2 co-localized with MAC-1 immunopositive microglial/macrophages, whereas at later time points FGF-2 co-localized with reactive astrocytes (Frautschy et al. 1991; Reilly and Kumari 1996), neurons, and vascular endothelial cells (Logan et al. 1992; Yang and Cui 1998). Given the early expression patterns and the localization of the FGF-2 ligand and its receptors, these data collectively suggest that one of the roles of FGF-2 induction after TBI may be in stimulating astrogliosis. Additionally, recent evidence suggests that FGF-2 is necessary and sufficient to stimulate proliferation and differentiation of neuroprogenitor cells in the adult hippocampus after various brain insults (Yoshimura et al. 2001) and may regulate postlesional sprouting (Ramirez et al. 1999). Dietrich et al. (1996) reported that acute administration of FGF-2 could attenuate cortical cell loss after TBI in rats, whereas McDermott et al. (1997) demonstrated that delayed intraparenchymal administration of FGF-2, beginning 24 hours after TBI, can significantly improve posttraumatic cognitive deficits in the rat. Exogenous FGF-2 was also shown to reduce hippocampal cell death after diffuse brain injury (Yang and Cui 2000). Furthermore, the combination of FGF with hypothermia (Yan et al. 2000) may increase the magnitude of the protective effect.

IGF-I is polypeptide hormone that shares several structural features with insulin (Isaksson et al. 1991) and is produced in many tissues in the body including the brain (Bondy and Lee 1993; Rotwein et al. 1988; Werther et al. 1990). In rodents, expression of mRNA for IGF-I is highest during the development of the nervous system, but it is also expressed in many regions of the adult rat brain (Bondy and Lee 1993). IGF-I readily crosses the BBB and as a result the brain is influenced by the concentration of circulating IGF-I (Armstrong et al. 2000; Carro et al. 2000; Pulford and Ishii 2001). IGF-I exerts its actions primarily via the type I IGF receptor, although interactions with the insulin receptor have been reported (Butler et al. 1998; Lamothe et al. 1998) (see Table 39–3). IGF binding proteins (IGFBPs) modulate the interaction of IGF-I with its receptor (Ocrant et al. 1990). IGFBP-2, IGFBP-4, and IGFBP-5 are the predominant binding proteins in the brain and can bind IGF-I, thus rendering it biologically inactive (Dore et al. 2000). However, there is also evidence suggesting that some IGFBPs potentiate the effect of IGF-I, possibly by presenting IGF-I more efficiently to its receptor, protecting IGF-I from degradation, or transporting IGF-I to regions of injury (Beilharz et al. 1998; Guan et al. 2000).

Initial reports of IGF-I expression after TBI localized expression to reactive astrocytes from acute time points to 1 month after injury (Garcia-Estrada et al. 1992). In a different model of TBI, a dramatic increase in the expression of IGFBP-2 and IGFBP-4 mRNA was observed between 24 hours and 7 days within injured cortex, whereas increased expression of IGF-1 mRNA peaked at 3 days postinjury (Sandberg Nordqvist et al. 1996). This increase in IGFBP-4 mRNA is completely blocked by administration of the NMDA antagonist MK-801, and injury-induced IGF-1 mRNA expression is blocked by both MK-801 and the AMPA antagonist CNQX (Nordqvist et al. 1997), suggesting that activation of glutamatergic systems may influence IGF expression or function in the setting of brain injury. In contrast, another study provided evidence that MK-801 reversed a measured decrease in IGF-II mRNA levels after injury (Giannakopoulou et al. 2000). Further studies using IGFBP-1 overexpressing transgenic mice observed that reactive astrogliosis, reflected by morphology and glial fibrillary acidic protein expression in astrocytes in response to a mechanical lesion, was substantially less in transgenic compared with WT mice (Ni et al. 1997), suggesting that IGF-I may play a role in astrogliosis.

Saatman and colleagues (1997) showed that continuous subcutaneous administration of IGF-I for 7 days dramatically accelerated neurological motor recovery and attenuated cognitive deficits after TBI in rats. A Phase II clinical trial demonstrated that continuous intravenous IGF-I in moderate to severe TBI patients resulted in greater weight gain, higher glucose concentrations and nitrogen outputs, and moderate to good Glasgow Outcome Scale scores at 6 months (Hatton et al. 1997). Taken together, the above data suggest that systemic IGF-I therapy should be further evaluated as a potential candidate for neuroprotection after clinical brain injury.

The VEGF family currently includes six known members. VEGF, or VEGF-A as it is now designated, was the first member of the VEGF family to be discovered and is also the best-characterized member (for a review see Neufeld et al. 1999). VEGF-A is established as a major inducer of endothelial cell proliferation, migration, sprouting, neural tube formation, and permeability during embryonic vasculogenesis and in physiological and pathological angiogenesis. These effects are mediated mainly by the VEGF receptor VEGFR-2 (see Table 39–3). More recently, VEGFR-1 was suggested to be an important mediator of stem cell recruitment (Eriksson and Alitalo 2002; Jin et al. 2002). A role of VEGF in BBB breakdown and angiogenesis/repair has been reported in rats after a freeze lesion, needle-stick lesion, or stab lesion to the cerebral cortex (Nag et al. 1997; Papavassiliou et al. 1997; Salhia et al. 2000). Increased VEGF immunoreactivity has also been observed in various postmortem tissues isolated from head-injured patients (Salhia et al. 2000). Other studies observed that a majority of VEGF-immunoreactive cells were also immunoreactive for the astrocytic marker GFAP and reported a similar time course for the observed increase in VEGF immunoreactivity after TBI (Papavassiliou et al. 1997; Salhia et al. 2000). Recent studies suggest that inhibition of VEGF after TBI fails to ameliorate the cognitive or functional deficits after injury, although attenuation of brain edema was observed (Hoover et al. 2001; Lenzlinger et al. 2004). These results likely occurred because of the ability of the inhibitor to inhibit presumptive protective activities (e.g., neurogenesis [Jin et al. 2002], angiogenesis, migration, sprouting [vide supra]), as well as the pathological disruption of the BBB.

Conclusion

Although the number of novel and promising pharmacological compounds and the elucidation of the multiple pathophysiological cascades associated with TBI remain challenges for scientists and clinicians, continued work in this area using clinically relevant experimental models of TBI is a requirement for the development of future therapies. The studies outlined in this chapter identify several promising potential targets for the treatment of the secondary or delayed damage occurring after TBI. However, pharmacological intervention in TBI must be placed in the perspective of a combination of interventions including intensive care, surgery, and rehabilitation. These factors should be incorporated into the design of rational and efficacious treatment strategy for TBI. Combination or polypharmacological therapies involving timed administration of several targeted compounds will likely contribute to improved treatment of TBI patients.

References

Abe K, Saito H: Effects of basic fibroblast growth factor on central nervous system functions. Pharmacol Res 43:307–312, 2001

Adams JH, Doyle D, Ford I, et al: Diffuse axonal injury in head injury: definition, diagnosis and grading. Histopathology 15:49–59, 1989

Airaksinen MS, Titievsky A, Saarma M: GDNF family neurotrophic factor signaling: four masters, one servant? Mol Cell Neurosci 13:313–325, 1999

Albensi BC: Models of brain injury and alterations in synaptic plasticity. J Neurosci Res 65:279–283, 2001

Allan SM, Rothwell NJ: Cytokines and acute neurodegeneration. Nat Rev Neurosci 2:734–744, 2001

Allen JW, Ivanova SA, Fan L, et al: Group II metabotropic glutamate receptor activation attenuates traumatic neuronal injury and improves neurological recovery after traumatic brain injury. J Pharmacol Exp Ther 290:112–120, 1999

Allen JW, Knoblach SM, Faden AI: Activation of group I metabotropic glutamate receptors reduces neuronal apoptosis but increases necrotic cell death in vitro. Cell Death Differ 7:470–476, 2000

Aoyama N, Katayama Y, Kawamata T, et al: Effects of antioxidant, OPC-14117, on secondary cellular damage and behavioral deficits following cortical contusion in the rat. Brain Res 934:117–124, 2002

Arenas E, Trupp M, Akerud P, et al: GDNF prevents degeneration and promotes the phenotype of brain noradrenergic neurons in vivo. Neuron 15:1465–1473, 1995

Armstrong CS, Wuarin L, Ishii DN: Uptake of circulating insulin-like growth factor-I into the cerebrospinal fluid of normal and diabetic rats and normalization of IGF-II mRNA content in diabetic rat brain. J Neurosci Res 59:649–660, 2000

Baker AJ, Moulton RJ, MacMillan VH, et al: Excitatory amino acids in cerebrospinal fluid following traumatic brain injury in humans. J Neurosurg 79:369–372, 1993

Baloh RH, Tansey MG, Golden JP, et al: TrnR2, a novel receptor that mediates neurturin and GDNF signaling through Ret. Neuron 18:793–802, 1997

Bareyre F, Wahl F, McIntosh TK, et al: Time course of cerebral edema after traumatic brain injury in rats: effects of riluzole and mannitol. J Neurotrauma 14:839–849, 1997

Bareyre FM, Saatman KE, Raghupathi R, et al: Postinjury treatment with magnesium chloride attenuates cortical damage after traumatic brain injury in rats. J Neurotrauma 17:1029–1039, 2000

Barzo P, Marmarou A, Fatouros P, et al: Magnetic resonance imaging-monitored acute blood-brain barrier changes in experimental traumatic brain injury. J Neurosurg 85:1113–1121, 1996

Baskaya MK, Rao AM, Puckett L, et al: Effect of difluoromethylornithine treatment on regional ornithine decarboxylase activity and edema formation after experimental brain injury. J Neurotrauma 13:85–92, 1996

Baskaya MK, Rao AM, Dogan A, et al: The biphasic opening of the blood-brain barrier in the cortex and hippocampus after traumatic brain injury in rats. Neurosci Lett 226:33–36, 1997

Baskaya MK, Dogan A, Rao AM, et al: Neuroprotective effects of citicoline on brain edema and blood-brain barrier breakdown after traumatic brain injury. J Neurosurg 92:448–452, 2000

Basu A, Krady JK, O'Malley M, et al: The type 1 interleukin-1 receptor is essential for the efficient activation of microglia and the induction of multiple proinflammatory mediators in response to brain injury. J Neurosci 22:6071–6082, 2002

Bazan NG, Rodriguez de Turco EB, Allan G: Mediators of injury in neurotrauma: intracellular signal transduction and gene expression. J Neurotrauma 12:791–814, 1995

Beilharz EJ, Russo VC, Butler G, et al: Co-ordinated and cellular specific induction of the components of the IGF/IGFBP axis in the rat brain following hypoxic-ischemic injury. Brain Res Mol Brain Res 59:119–134, 1998

Beit-Yannai E, Zhang R, Trembovler V, et al: Cerebroprotective effect of stable nitroxide radicals in closed head injury in the rat. Brain Res 717:22–28, 1996

Beit-Yannai E, Kohen R, Horowitz M, et al: Changes of biological reducing activity in rat brain following closed head injury: a cyclic voltammetry study in normal and heat-acclimated rats. J Cereb Blood Flow Metab 17:273–279, 1997

Belayev L, Alonso OF, Liu Y, et al: Talampanel, a novel noncompetitive AMPA antagonist, is neuroprotective after traumatic brain injury in rats. J Neurotrauma 18:1031–1038, 2001

Belayev L, Becker DA, Alonso OF, et al: Stilbazulenyl nitrone, a novel azulenyl nitrone antioxidant: improved neurological deficit and reduced contusion size after traumatic brain injury in rats. J Neurosurg 96:1077–1083, 2002

Belluardo N, Mudo G, Dell'Albani P, et al: NMDA receptor-dependent and -independent immediate early gene expression induced by focal mechanical brain injury. Neurochem Int 26:443–453, 1995

Benraiss A, Chmielnicki E, Lerner K, et al: Adenoviral brain-derived neurotrophic factor induces both neostriatal and olfactory neuronal recruitment from endogenous progenitor cells in the adult forebrain. J Neurosci 21:6718–6731, 2001

Bentzer P, Mattiasson G, McIntosh TK, et al: Infusion of prostacyclin following experimental brain injury in the rat reduces cortical lesion volume. J Neurotrauma 18:275–285, 2001

Benveniste EN, Tang LP, Law RM: Differential regulation of astrocyte TNF-alpha expression by the cytokines TGF-beta, IL-6 and IL-10. Int J Dev Neurosci 13:341–349, 1995

Bernert H, Turski L: Traumatic brain damage prevented by the non-N-methyl-D-aspartate antagonist 2,3-dihydroxy-6-nitro-7-sulfamoylbenzo[f] quinoxaline. Proc Natl Acad Sci U S A 93:5235–5240, 1996

Bevilacqua MP, Pober JS, Wheeler ME, et al: Interleukin 1 acts on cultured human vascular endothelium to increase the adhesion of polymorphonuclear leukocytes, monocytes, and related leukocyte cell lines. J Clin Invest 76:2003–2011, 1985

Blaha GR, Raghupathi R, Saatman KE, et al: Brain-derived neurotrophic factor administration after traumatic brain injury in the rat does not protect against behavioral or histological deficits. Neuroscience 99:483–493, 2000

Bondy CA, Lee WH: Patterns of insulin-like growth factor and IGF receptor gene expression in the brain: functional implications. Ann N Y Acad Sci 692:33–43, 1993

Braakman R, Schouten HJ, Blaauw-van Dishoeck M, et al: Megadose steroids in severe head injury: results of a prospective double-blind clinical trial. J Neurosurg 58:326–330, 1983

Braughler JM, Hall ED, Means ED, et al: Evaluation of an intensive methylprednisolone sodium succinate dosing regimen in experimental spinal cord injury. J Neurosurg 67:102–105, 1987

Braughler JM, Pregenzer JF: The 21-aminosteroid inhibitors of lipid peroxidation: reactions with lipid peroxyl and phenoxy radicals. Free Radic Biol Med 7:125–130, 1989

Bullock MR, Merchant RE, Carmack CA, et al: An open-label study of CP-101,606 in subjects with a severe traumatic head injury or spontaneous intracerebral hemorrhage. Ann N Y Acad Sci 890:51–58, 1999

Bullock R: Strategies for neuroprotection with glutamate antagonists: extrapolating from evidence taken from the first stroke and head injury studies. Ann N Y Acad Sci 765:272–278, 1995

Butler AA, Yakar S, Gewolb IH, et al: Insulin-like growth factor-I receptor signal transduction: at the interface between physiology and cell biology. Comp Biochem Physiol B Biochem Mol Biol 121:19–26, 1998

Carlos TM, Clark RS, Franicola-Higgins D, et al: Expression of endothelial adhesion molecules and recruitment of neutrophils after traumatic brain injury in rats. J Leukoc Biol 61:279–285, 1997

Carro E, Nunez A, Busiguina S, et al: Circulating insulin-like growth factor I mediates effects of exercise on the brain. J Neurosci 20:2926–2933, 2000

Cassatella MA, Meda L, Gasperini S, et al: Interleukin 10 (IL-10) upregulates IL-1 receptor antagonist production from lipopolysaccharide-stimulated human polymorphonuclear leukocytes by delaying mRNA degradation. J Exp Med 179:1695–1699, 1994

Cernak I, O'Connor C, Vink R: Activation of cyclo-oxygenase-2 contributes to motor and cognitive dysfunction following diffuse traumatic brain injury in rats. Clin Exp Pharmacol Physiol 28:922–925, 2001

Chabrier PE, Auguet M, Spinnewyn B, et al: BN 80933, a dual inhibitor of neuronal nitric oxide synthase and lipid peroxidation: a promising neuroprotective strategy. Proc Natl Acad Sci U S A 96:10824–10829, 1999

Chao CC, Hu S, Sheng WS, et al: Tumor necrosis factor-alpha production by human fetal microglial cells: regulation by other cytokines. Dev Neurosci 17:97–105, 1995

Chen Y, Buck J: Cannabinoids protect cells from oxidative cell death: a receptor-independent mechanism. J Pharmacol Exp Ther 293:807–812, 2000

Choi DW: Methods for antagonizing glutamate neurotoxicity. Cerebrovasc Brain Metab Rev 2:105–147, 1990

Clark RS, Kochanek PM, Chen M, et al: Increases in Bcl-2 and cleavage of caspase-1 and caspase-3 in human brain after head injury. FASEB J 13:813–821, 1999

Clifton GL, Lyeth BG, Jenkins LW, et al: Effect of D, alpha-tocopheryl succinate and polyethylene glycol on performance tests after fluid percussion brain injury. J Neurotrauma 6:71–81, 1989

Conte V, Uryu K, Fujimoto S, et al: Vitamin E reduces amyloidosis and improves cognitive function in T82576 mice following repetitive concussive brain injury. J Neurochem 90:758–764, 2004

Cooper PR, Moody S, Clark WK, et al: Dexamethasone and severe head injury: a prospective double-blind study. J Neurosurg 51:307–316, 1979

Csuka E, Morganti-Kossmann MC, Lenzlinger PM, et al: IL-10 levels in cerebrospinal fluid and serum of patients with severe traumatic brain injury: relationship to IL-6, TNF-α, TGF-β1 and blood-brain barrier function. J Neuroimmunol 101: 211–221, 1999

Dash PK, Mach SA, Moore AN: Regional expression and role of cyclooxygenase-2 following experimental traumatic brain injury. J Neurotrauma 17:69–81, 2000

DeKosky ST, Goss JR, Miller PD, et al: Upregulation of nerve growth factor following cortical trauma. Exp Neurol 130:173–177, 1994

DeKosky ST, Styren SD, O'Malley ME, et al: Interleukin-1 receptor antagonist suppresses neurotrophin response in injured rat brain. Ann Neurol 39:123–127, 1996

DeWitt DS, Smith TG, Deyo DJ, et al: L-arginine and superoxide dismutase prevent or reverse cerebral hypoperfusion after fluid-percussion traumatic brain injury. J Neurotrauma 14:223–233, 1997

Dhillon HS, Donaldson D, Dempsey RJ, et al: Regional levels of free fatty acids and Evans blue extravasation after experimental brain injury. J Neurotrauma 11:405–415, 1994

Dhillon HS, Carbary T, Dose J, et al: Activation of phosphatidylinositol bisphosphate signal transduction pathway after experimental brain injury: a lipid study. Brain Res 698:100–106, 1995

Dietrich WD, Alonso O, Busto R, et al: Posttreatment with intravenous basic fibroblast growth factor reduces histopathological damage following fluid-percussion brain injury in rats. J Neurotrauma 13:309–316, 1996

Dixon CE, Flinn P, Bao J, et al: Nerve growth factor attenuates cholinergic deficits following traumatic brain injury in rats. Exp Neurol 146:479–490, 1997

Dore S, Kar S, Zheng WH, et al: Rediscovering good old friend IGF-I in the new millenium: possible usefulness in Alzheimer's disease and stroke. Pharm Acta Helv 74:273–280, 2000

Dugan LL, Choi D: Excitotoxicity, free radicals, and cell membrane changes. Ann Neurol 35 (suppl):S17–S21, 1994

Durbec P, Marcos-Gutierrez CV, Kilkenny C, et al: GDNF signalling through the Ret receptor tyrosine kinase. Nature 381:789–793, 1996

Ercan M, Inci S, Kilinc K, et al: Nimodipine attenuates lipid peroxidation during the acute phase of head trauma in rats. Neurosurg Rev 24:127–130, 2001

Eriksson U, Alitalo K: VEGF receptor 1 stimulates stem-cell recruitment and new hope for angiogenesis therapies. Nat Med 8:775–777, 2002

Faden AI, Demediuk P, Panter SS, et al: The role of excitatory amino acids and NMDA receptors in traumatic brain injury. Science 244:798–800, 1989

Faden AI, Ivanova SA, Yakovlev AG, et al: Neuroprotective effects of group III mGluR in traumatic neuronal injury. J Neurotrauma 14:885–895, 1997

Faden AI, O'Leary DM, Fan L, et al: Selective blockade of the mGluR1 receptor reduces traumatic neuronal injury in vitro and improves outcome after brain trauma. Exp Neurol 167:435–444, 2001

Fan L, Young PR, Barone FC, et al: Experimental brain injury induces expression of interleukin-1 beta mRNA in the rat brain. Mol Brain Res 30:125–130, 1995

Fan L, Young PR, Barone FC, et al: Experimental brain injury induces differential expression of tumor necrosis factor-alpha mRNA in the CNS. Mol Brain Res 36:287–291, 1996

Fernandez MP, Belmonte A, Meizoso MJ, et al: Desmethyl tirilazad reduces brain nitric oxide synthase activity and cyclic guanosine monophosphate during cerebral global transient ischemia in rats. Res Commun Mol Pathol Pharmacol 95:33–42, 1997

Fink KB, Andrews LJ, Butler WE, et al: Reduction of post-traumatic brain injury and free radical production by inhibition of the caspase-1 cascade. Neuroscience 94:1213–1218, 1999

Finklestein SP, Apostolides PJ, Caday CG, et al: Increased basic fibroblast growth factor (bFGF) immunoreactivity at the site of focal brain wounds. Brain Res 460:253–259, 1988

Floyd RA: Antioxidants, oxidative stress, and degenerative neurological disorders. Proc Soc Exp Biol Med 222:236–245, 1999

Frank E, Ragel B: Cortical basic fibroblast factor expression after head injury: preliminary results. Neurol Res 17:129–131, 1995

Frautschy SA, Walicke PA, Baird A: Localization of basic fibroblast growth factor and its mRNA after CNS injury. Brain Res 553:291–299, 1991

Frei K, Malipiero UV, Leist TP, et al: On the cellular source and function of interleukin 6 produced in the central nervous system in viral diseases. Eur J Immunol 19:689–694, 1989

Friedlander RM, Gagliardini V, Rotello RJ, et al: Functional role of interleukin 1 beta (IL-1 β) in IL-1 β–converting enzyme-mediated apoptosis. J Exp Med 184:717–724, 1996

Fukuda K, Tanno H, Okimura Y, et al: The blood-brain barrier disruption to circulating proteins in the early period after fluid percussion brain injury in rats. J Neurotrauma 12:315–324, 1995

Gahm C, Holmin S, Mathiesen T: Nitric oxide synthase expression after human brain contusion. Neurosurgery 50:1319–1326, 2002

Gallily R, Breuer A, Mechoulam R: 2-Arachidonylglycerol, an endogenous cannabinoid, inhibits tumor necrosis factor-alpha production in murine macrophages, and in mice. Eur J Pharmacol 406:R5–R7, 2000

Garcia-Estrada J, Garcia-Segura LM, Torres-Aleman I: Expression of insulin-like growth factor I by astrocytes in response to injury. Brain Res 592:343–347, 1992

Gennarelli TA: Animate models of human head injury. J Neurotrauma 11:357–368, 1994

Giannakopoulou M, Mansour M, Kazanis E, et al: NMDA receptor mediated changes in IGF-II gene expression in the rat brain after injury and the possible role of nitric oxide. Neuropathol Appl Neurobiol 26:513–521, 2000

Giannotta SL, Weiss MH, Apuzzo ML, et al: High dose glucocorticoids in the management of severe head injury. Neurosurgery 15:497–501, 1984

Gimenez-Gallego G, Cuevas P: Fibroblast growth factors, proteins with a broad spectrum of biological activities. Neurol Res 16:313–316, 1994

Giulian D, Woodward J, Young DG, et al: Interleukin-1 injected into mammalian brain stimulates astrogliosis and neovascularization. J Neurosci 8:2485–2490, 1998

Globus MY, Alonso O, Dietrich WD, et al: Glutamate release and free radical production following brain injury: effects of posttraumatic hypothermia. J Neurochem 65:1704–1711, 1995

Golding EM, Vink R: Efficacy of competitive vs noncompetitive blockade of the NMDA channel following traumatic brain injury. Mol Chem Neuropathol 24:137–150, 1995

Gong QZ, Delahunty TM, Hamm RJ, et al: Metabotropic glutamate antagonist, MCPG, treatment of traumatic brain injury in rats. Brain Res 700:299–302, 1995

Gong QZ, Phillips LL, Lyeth BG: Metabotropic glutamate receptor protein alterations after traumatic brain injury in rats. J Neurotrauma 16:893–902, 1999

Goodman JC, Robertson CS, Grossman RG, et al: Elevation of tumor necrosis factor in head injury. J Neuroimmunol 30:213–217, 1990

Goss JR, Taffe KM, Kochanek PM, et al: The antioxidant enzymes glutathione peroxidase and catalase increase following traumatic brain injury in the rat. Exp Neurol 146: 291–294, 1997

Goss JR, O'Malley ME, Zou L, et al: Astrocytes are the major source of nerve growth factor upregulation following traumatic brain injury in the rat. Exp Neurol 149:301–309, 1998

Graham DI, Adams JH, Nicoll JA, et al: The nature, distribution and causes of traumatic brain injury. Brain Pathol 5: 397–406, 1995

Griesbach GS, Hovda DA, Molteni R, et al: Alterations in BDNF and synapsin I within the occipital cortex and hippocampus after mild traumatic brain injury in the developing rat: reflections of injury-induced neuroplasticity. J Neurotrauma 19:803–814, 2002

Grumme T, Baethmann A, Kolodziejczyk D, et al: Treatment of patients with severe head injury by triamcinolone: a prospective, controlled multicenter clinical trial of 396 cases. Res Exp Med (Berl) 195:217–229, 1995

Gruol DL, Nelson TE: Physiological and pathological roles of interleukin-6 in the central nervous system. Mol Neurobiol 15: 307–339, 1997

Guan J, Beilharz EJ, Skinner SJ, et al: Intracerebral transportation and cellular localisation of insulin-like growth factor-1 following central administration to rats with hypoxic-ischemic brain injury. Brain Res 853:163–173, 2000

Gudeman SK, Miller JD, Becker DP: Failure of high-dose steroid therapy to influence intracranial pressure in patients with severe head injury. J Neurosurg 51:301–306, 1979

Hall ED: Beneficial effects of acute intravenous ibuprofen on neurologic recovery of head-injured mice: comparison of cyclooxygenase inhibition with inhibition of thromboxane A2 synthetase or 5-lipoxygenase. Cent Nerv Syst Trauma 2:75–83, 1985

Hall ED, McCall JM, Chase RL, et al: A nonglucocorticoid steroid analog of methylprednisolone duplicates its high-dose pharmacology in models of central nervous system trauma and neuronal membrane damage. J Pharmacol Exp Ther 242:137–142, 1987

Hall ED, Yonkers PA, McCall JM, et al: Effects of the 21-aminosteroid U74006F on experimental head injury in mice. J Neurosurg 68:456–461, 1988

Hall ED, Andrus PK, Yonkers PA: Brain hydroxyl radical generation in acute experimental head injury. J Neurochem 60:588–594, 1993

Hall ED, Andrus PK, Yonkers PA, et al: Generation and detection of hydroxyl radical following experimental head injury. Ann N Y Acad Sci 738:15–24, 1994

Hamm RJ, Temple MD, Pike BR, et al: The effect of postinjury administration of polyethylene glycol- conjugated superoxide dismutase (pegorgotein, Dismutec) or lidocaine on behavioral function following fluid-percussion brain injury in rats. J Neurotrauma 13:325–332, 1996

Hans VH, Kossmann T, Joller H, et al: Interleukin-6 and its soluble receptor in serum and cerebrospinal fluid after cerebral trauma. Neuroreport 10:409–412, 1999a

Hans VH, Kossmann T, Lenzlinger PM, et al: Experimental axonal injury triggers interleukin-6 mRNA, protein synthesis and release into cerebrospinal fluid. J Cereb Blood Flow Metab 19:184–194, 1993b

Hansen HH, Schmid PC, Bittigau P, et al: Anandamide, but not 2-arachidonoylglycerol, accumulates during in vivo neurodegeneration. J Neurochem 78:1415–1427, 2001

Hatton J, Rapp RP, Kudsk KA, et al: Intravenous insulin-like growth factor-I (IGF-I) in moderate-to-severe head injury: a phase II safety and efficacy trial. J Neurosurg 86:779–786, 1997

Hayes RL, Jenkins LW, Lyeth BG, et al: Pretreatment with phencyclidine, an N-methyl-D-aspartate antagonist, attenuates long-term behavioral deficits in the rat produced by traumatic brain injury. J Neurotrauma 5:259–274, 1988

Heath DL, Vink R: Neuroprotective effects of MgSO4 and MgCl2 in closed head injury: a comparative phosphorus NMR study. J Neurotrauma 15:183–189, 1998

Henderson CE, Phillips HS, Pollock RA, et al: GDNF: a potent survival factor for motoneurons present in peripheral nerve and muscle. Science 266:1062–1064, 1994

Hensley K, Carney JM, Stewart CA, et al: Nitrone-based free radical traps as neuroprotective agents in cerebral ischaemia and other pathologies. Int Rev Neurobiol 40:299–317, 1997

Hermann DM, Kilic E, Kugler S, et al: Adenovirus-mediated glial cell line-derived neurotrophic factor (GDNF) expression protects against subsequent cortical cold injury in rats. Neurobiol Dis 8:964–973, 2001

Hicks RR, Smith DH, Gennarelli TA, et al: Kynurenate is neuroprotective following experimental brain injury in the rat. Brain Res 655:91–96, 1994

Hicks RR, Numan S, Dhillon HS, et al: Alterations in BDNF and NT-3 mRNAs in rat hippocampus after experimental brain trauma. Brain Res Mol Brain Res 48:401–406, 1997

Hicks RR, Zhang L, Dhillon HS, et al: Expression of trkB mRNA is altered in rat hippocampus after experimental brain trauma. Brain Res Mol Brain Res 59:264–268, 1998

Hicks RR, Li C, Zhang L, et al: Alterations in BDNF and trkB mRNA levels in the cerebral cortex following experimental brain trauma in rats. J Neurotrauma 16:501–510, 1999a

Hicks RR, Martin VB, Zhang L, et al: Mild experimental brain injury differentially alters the expression of neurotrophin and neurotrophin receptor mRNAs in the hippocampus. Exp Neurol 160:469–478, 1999b

Hirbec H, Gaviria M, Vignon J: Gacyclidine: a new neuroprotective agent acting at the N-methyl-D-aspartate receptor. CNS Drug Rev 7:172–198, 2001

Hirbec H, Privat A, Vignon J: Binding properties of [3H]gacyclidine in the rat central nervous system. Eur J Pharmacol 388:235–239, 2000

Hogg S, Perron C, Barneoud P, et al: Neuroprotective effect of eliprodil: attenuation of a conditioned freezing deficit induced by traumatic injury of the right parietal cortex in the rat. J Neurotrauma 15:545–553, 1998

Holmin S, Mathiesen T, Shetye J, et al: Intracerebral inflammatory response to experimental brain contusion. Acta Neurochir (Wien) 132:110–119, 1995

Holmin S, Soderlund J, Biberfeld P, et al: Intracerebral inflammation after human brain contusion. Neurosurgery 42:291–298, 1998

Homayoun P, Rodriguez de Turco EB, Parkins NE, et al: Delayed phospholipid degradation in rat brain after traumatic brain injury. J Neurochem 69:199–205, 1997

Hoover RC, Lenzlinger PM, Cheney JA, et al: The vascular endothelial growth factor (VEGF) inhibitor BSF476921 reduces edema following experimental traumatic brain injury. J Neurotrauma 18:1170, 2001

Hoyt DB, Ozkan AN, Hansbrough JF, et al: Head injury: an immunologic deficit in T-cell activation. J Trauma 30:759–766, 1990

Hsiang JN, Wang JY, Ip SM, et al: The time course and regional variations of lipid peroxidation after diffuse brain injury in rats. Acta Neurochir (Wien) 139:464–468, 1997

Huang EJ, Reichardt LF: Neurotrophins: roles in neuronal development and function. Annu Rev Neurosci 24:677–736, 2001

Hurley SD, Olschowka JA, O'Banion MK: Cyclooxygenase inhibition as a strategy to ameliorate brain injury. J Neurotrauma 19:1–15, 2002

Hylton C, Perri BR, Voddi MD, et al: NMDA antagonist GYKI 52466 enhances spatial memory after experimental brain injury. J Neurotrauma 12:124, 1995

Ikeda M, Nakazawa T, Abe K, et al: Extracellular accumulation of glutamate in the hippocampus induced by ischemia is not calcium dependent: in vitro and in vivo evidence. Neurosci Lett 96:202–206, 1989

Ikeda Y, Long DM: The molecular basis of brain injury and brain edema: the role of oxygen free radicals. Neurosurgery 27:1–11, 1990

Ikonomidou C, Turski L: Prevention of trauma-induced neurodegeneration in infant and adult rat brain: glutamate antagonists. Metab Brain Dis 11:125–141, 1996

Ikonomidou C, Qin Y, Labruyere J, et al: Prevention of trauma-induced neurodegeneration in infant rat brain. Pediatr Res 39:1020–1027, 1996

Isaksson OG, Ohlsson C, Nilsson A, Isgaard J, Lindahl A: Regulation of cartilage growth by growth hormone and insulin-like growth factor I. Pediatr Nephrol 5:451–453, 1991

Isaksson J, Lewen A, Hillered L, et al: Up-regulation of intercellular adhesion molecule 1 in cerebral microvessels after cortical contusion trauma in a rat model. Acta Neuropathol (Berl) 94:16–20, 1997

Isaksson J, Hillered L, Olsson Y: Cognitive and histopathological outcome after weight-drop brain injury in the rat: influence of systemic administration of monoclonal antibodies to ICAM-1. Acta Neuropathol (Berl) 102:246–256, 2001

Jin K, Zhu Y, Sun Y, et al: Vascular endothelial growth factor (VEGF) stimulates neurogenesis in vitro and in vivo. Proc Natl Acad Sci U S A 99:11946–11950, 2002

Jing S, Wen D, Yu Y, et al: GDNF-induced activation of the ret protein tyrosine kinase is mediated by GDNFR-alpha, a novel receptor for GDNF. Cell 85:1113–1124, 1996

Joyce DA, Gibbons DP, Green P, et al: Two inhibitors of proinflammatory cytokine release, interleukin-10 and interleukin-4, have contrasting effects on release of soluble p75 tumor necrosis factor receptor by cultured monocytes. Eur J Immunol 24:2699–2705, 1994

Juul N, Morris GF, Marshall SB, et al: Intracranial hypertension and cerebral perfusion pressure: influence on neurological deterioration and outcome in severe head injury. The Executive Committee of the International Selfotel Trial. J Neurosurg 92:1–6, 2000

Jungi TW, Brcic M, Eperon S, et al: Transforming growth factor-beta and interleukin-10, but not interleukin-4, downregulate procoagulant activity and tissue factor expression in human monocyte-derived macrophages. Thromb Res 76:463–474, 1994

Katayama Y, Cheung MK, Alves A, et al: Ion fluxes and cell swelling in experimental traumatic brain injury: the role of excitatory amino acids, in Intracranial Pressure, Vol VII. Edited by Hoff JT, Betz AL. Berlin, Springer-Verlag, 1989, pp 584–588

Katayama Y, Becker DP, Tamura T, et al: Massive increases in extracellular potassium and the indiscriminate release of glutamate following concussive brain injury. J Neurosurg 73:889–900, 1990

Katoh H, Sima K, Nawashiro H, et al: The effect of MK-801 on extracellular neuroactive amino acids in hippocampus after closed head injury followed by hypoxia in rats. Brain Res 758:153–162, 1997

Kavanagh RJ, Kam PC: Lazaroids: efficacy and mechanism of action of the 21-aminosteroids in neuroprotection. Br J Anaesth 86:110–119, 2001

Kawamata T, Katayama Y, Hovda DA, et al: Administration of excitatory amino acid antagonists via microdialysis attenuates the increase in glucose utilization seen following concussive brain injury. J Cereb Blood Flow Metab 12:12–24, 1992

Khaldi A, Chiueh CC, Bullock MR, et al: The significance of nitric oxide production in the brain after injury. Ann N Y Acad Sci 962:53–59, 2002

Kim BT, Rao VL, Sailor KA, et al: Protective effects of glial cell line-derived neurotrophic factor on hippocampal neurons after traumatic brain injury in rats. J Neurosurg 95:674–679, 2001

Kim HJ, Levasseur JE, Patterson JL Jr, et al: Effect of indomethacin pretreatment on acute mortality in experimental brain injury. J Neurosurg 71:565–572, 1989

Kinoshita K, Chatzipanteli K, Vitarbo E, et al: Interleukin-1β messenger ribonucleic acid and protein levels after fluid-percussion brain injury in rats: importance of injury severity and brain temperature. Neurosurgery 51:195–203, 2002

Kline AE, Bolinger BD, Kochanek PM, et al: Acute systemic administration of interleukin-10 suppresses the beneficial effects of moderate hypothermia following traumatic brain injury in rats. Brain Res 937:22–31, 2002

Knoblach SM, Faden AI: Interleukin-10 improves outcome and alters proinflammatory cytokine expression after experimental traumatic brain injury. Exp Neurol 153:143–151, 1998

Knoblach SM, Fan L, Faden AI: Early neuronal expression of tumor necrosis factor-alpha after experimental brain injury contributes to neurological impairment. J Neuroimmunol 95:115–125, 1999

Knoller N, Levi L, Shoshan I, et al: Dexanabinol (HU-211) in the treatment of severe closed head injury: a randomized, placebo-controlled, phase II clinical trial. Crit Care Med 30:548–554, 2002

Kontos HA, Povlishock JT: Oxygen radicals in brain injury. Cent Nerv Syst Trauma 3:257–263, 1986

Kossmann T, Hans VH, Imhof HG, et al: Intrathecal and serum interleukin-6 and the acute-phase response in patients with severe traumatic brain injuries. Shock 4:311–317, 1995

Kossmann T, Hans V, Imhof HG, et al: Interleukin-6 released in human cerebrospinal fluid following traumatic brain injury may trigger nerve growth factor production in astrocytes. Brain Res 713:143–152, 1996

Kotzbauer PT, Lampe PA, Heuckeroth RO, et al: Neurturin, a relative of glial-cell-line-derived neurotrophic factor. Nature 384:467–470, 1996

Krakauer T: IL-10 inhibits the adhesion of leukocytic cells to IL-1-activated human endothelial cells. Immunol Lett 45:61–65, 1995

Krishna MC, Russo A, Mitchell JB, et al: Do nitroxide antioxidants act as scavengers of $O_2-\cdot$ or as SOD mimics? J Biol Chem 271:26026–26031, 1996

Kroppenstedt SN, Schneider GH, Thomale UW, et al: Protective effects of aptiganel HCl (Cerestat) following controlled cortical impact injury in the rat. J Neurotrauma 15:191–197, 1998

Lamothe B, Baudry A, Christoffersen CT, et al: Insulin receptor-deficient cells as a new tool for dissecting complex interplay in insulin and insulin-like growth factors. FEBS Lett 426:381–385, 1998

Laurer HL, Lenzlinger PM, McIntosh TK: Models of traumatic brain injury. Eur J Trauma 26:95–110, 2000

Leibrock J, Lottspeich F, Hohn A, et al: Molecular cloning and expression of brain-derived neurotrophic factor. Nature 341:149–152, 1989

Lenzlinger PM, Hans VH, Joller-Jemelka HI, et al: Markers for cell-mediated immune response are elevated in cerebrospinal fluid and serum after severe traumatic brain injury in humans. J Neurotrauma 18:479–489, 2001

Lenzlinger PM, Saatman KE, Hoover RC, et al: Inhibition of vascular endothelial growth factor receptor (VEGFR) signaling by BSF476921 attenuates regional cerebral edema following traumatic brain injury in rats. Restor Neurol Neurosci 22:73–79, 2004

Leonard JR, Maris DO, Grady MS: Fluid percussion injury causes loss of forebrain choline acetyltransferase and nerve growth factor receptor immunoreactive cells in the rat. J Neurotrauma 11:379–392, 1994

Lin LF, Doherty DH, Lile JD, et al: GDNF: a glial cell line-derived neurotrophic factor for midbrain dopaminergic neurons. Science 260:1130–1132, 1993

Logan A, Frautschy SA, Gonzalez AM, et al: A time course for the focal elevation of synthesis of basic fibroblast growth factor and one of its high-affinity receptors (flg) following a localized cortical brain injury. J Neurosci 12:3828–3837, 1992

Longhi L, Watson DJ, Saatman KE, et al: Ex vivo gene therapy using targeted engraftment of NGF-expressing human NT2N neurons attenuates cognitive deficits following TBI in mice. J Neurotrauma (in press)

Lu B, Chow A: Neurotrophins and hippocampal synaptic transmission and plasticity. J Neurosci Res 58:76–87, 1999

Lyeth BG, Gong QZ, Shields S, et al: Group I metabotropic glutamate antagonist reduces acute neuronal degeneration and behavioral deficits after traumatic brain injury in rats. Exp Neurol 169:191–199, 2001

Maisonpierre PC, Belluscio L, Friedman B, et al: NT-3, BDNF, and NGF in the developing rat nervous system: parallel as well as reciprocal patterns of expression. Neuron 5:501–509, 1990

Marion DW, White MJ: Treatment of experimental brain injury with moderate hypothermia and 21-aminosteroids. J Neurotrauma 13:139–147, 1996

Marklund N, Clausen F, Lewander T, et al: Monitoring of reactive oxygen species production after traumatic brain injury in rats with microdialysis and the 4-hydroxybenzoic acid trapping method. J Neurotrauma 18:1217–1227, 2001a

Marklund N, Clausen F, Lewen A, et al: α-Phenyl-*tert*-N-butyl nitrone (PBN) improves functional and morphological outcome after cortical contusion injury in the rat. Acta Neurochir (Wien) 143:73–81, 2001b

Marklund N, Clausen F, McIntosh TK, et al: Free radical scavenger posttreatment improves functional and morphological outcome after fluid percussion injury in the rat. J Neurotrauma 18:821–832, 2001c

Marklund N, Lewander T, Clausen F, et al: Effects of the nitrone radical scavengers PBN and S-PBN on in vivo trapping of reactive oxygen species after traumatic brain injury in rats. J Cereb Blood Flow Metab 21:1259–1267, 2001d

Marmarou A, Nichols J, Burgess J, et al: Effects of the bradykinin antagonist Bradycor (deltibant, CP-1027) in severe traumatic brain injury: results of a multi-center, randomized, placebo-controlled trial. American Brain Injury Consortium Study Group. J Neurotrauma 16:431–444, 1999

Marshall LF, Marshall SB: Pharmacologic therapy: promising clinical investigations. New Horiz 3:573–580, 1995

Marz P, Heese K, Dimitriades-Schmutz B, et al: Role of interleukin-6 and soluble IL-6 receptor in region-specific induction of astrocytic differentiation and neurotrophin expression. Glia 26:191–200, 1999

Maxwell WL, Povlishock JT, Graham DL: A mechanistic analysis of nondisruptive axonal injury: a review. J Neurotrauma 14:419–440, 1997

McAllister AK, Katz LC, Lo DC: Neurotrophins and synaptic plasticity. Annu Rev Neurosci 22:295–318, 1999

McDermott KL, Raghupathi R, Fernandez SC, et al: Delayed administration of basic fibroblast growth factor (bFGF) attenuates cognitive dysfunction following parasagittal fluid percussion brain injury in the rat. J Neurotrauma 14:191–200, 1997

McIntosh TK, Faden AI, Yamakami I, et al: Magnesium deficiency exacerbates and pretreatment improves outcome following traumatic brain injury in rats: ^{31}P magnetic resonance spectroscopy and behavioral studies. J Neurotrauma 5:17–31, 1988

McIntosh TK, Vink R, Yamakami I, et al: Magnesium protects against neurological deficit after brain injury. Brain Res 482:252–260, 1989

McIntosh TK, Vink R, Soares H, et al: Effect of noncompetitive blockade of N-methyl-D-aspartate receptors on the neurochemical sequelae of experimental brain injury. J Neurochem 55:1170–1179, 1990

McIntosh TK, Thomas M, Smith D, et al: The novel 21-aminosteroid U74006F attenuates cerebral edema and improves survival after brain injury in the rat. J Neurotrauma 9:33–46, 1992

McIntosh TK, Smith DH, Voddi M, et al: Riluzole, a novel neuroprotective agent, attenuates both neurologic motor and cognitive dysfunction following experimental brain injury in the rat. J Neurotrauma 13:767–780, 1996

McIntosh TK, Saatman KE, Raghupathi R, et al: The Dorothy Russell Memorial Lecture: the molecular and cellular sequelae of experimental traumatic brain injury: pathogenetic mechanisms. Neuropathol Appl Neurobiol 24:251–267, 1998

Menniti JE, Collins MA, Chenard BL, et al: CP-101,606, a potent and selective antagonist of forebrain NMDA receptors: in vitro neuroprotective activity. Soc Neurosci Abstr 21:72, 1995

Merchant RE, Bullock MR, Carmack CA, et al: A double-blind, placebo-controlled study of the safety, tolerability and pharmacokinetics of CP-101,606 in patients with a mild or moderate traumatic brain injury. Ann N Y Acad Sci 890:42–50, 1999

Miller AA, Sawyer DA, Roth B: Lamotrigine, in New Anticonvulsant Drugs. Edited by Meldrum BS, Porter RJ. London, John Libbey, 1986, pp 165–177

Miller LP, Lyeth BG, Jenkins LW, et al: Excitatory amino acid receptor subtype binding following traumatic brain injury. Brain Res 526:103–107, 1990

Monaghan DT, Cotman CW: Identification and properties of N-methyl-D-aspartate receptors in rat brain synaptic plasma membranes. Proc Natl Acad Sci U S A 83:7532–7536, 1986

Moor E, Kohen R, Reiter RJ, et al: Closed head injury increases extracellular levels of antioxidants in rat hippocampus in vivo: an adaptive mechanism? Neurosci Lett 316:169–172, 2001

Morganti-Kossmann MC, Hans VH, Lenzlinger PM, et al: TGF-beta is elevated in the CSF of patients with severe traumatic brain injuries and parallels blood-brain barrier function. J Neurotrauma 16:617–628, 1999

Morganti-Kossmann MC, Rancan M, Otto VI, Stahel PF, Kossmann T: Role of cerebral inflammation after traumatic brain injury: a revisited concept. Shock 16: 165–177, 2001

Mori T, Kawamata T, Katayama Y, et al: Antioxidant, OPC-14117, attenuates edema formation, and subsequent tissue damage following cortical contusion in rats. Acta Neurochir Suppl (Wien) 71:120–122, 1998

Morris GF, Juul N, Marshall SB, et al: Neurological deterioration as a potential alternative endpoint in human clinical trials of experimental pharmacological agents for treatment of severe traumatic brain injuries. Executive Committee of the International Selfotel Trial. Neurosurgery 43:1369–1372, 1998

Mount HT, Dean DO, Alberch J, et al: Glial cell line-derived neurotrophic factor promotes the survival and morphologic differentiation of Purkinje cells. Proc Natl Acad Sci U S A 92:9092–9096, 1995

Movsesyan VA, O'Leary DM, Fan L, et al: mGluR5 antagonists 2-methyl-6-(phenylethynyl)-pyridine and (E)-2-methyl-6-(2-phenylethenyl)-pyridine reduce traumatic neuronal injury in vitro and in vivo by antagonizing N-methyl-D-aspartate receptors. J Pharmacol Exp Ther 296:41–47, 2001

Mudo G, Persson H, Timmusk T, et al: Increased expression of trkB and trkC messenger RNAs in the rat forebrain after focal mechanical injury. Neuroscience 57:901–912, 1993

Muir KW, Grosset DG, Lees KR: Clinical pharmacology of CNS 1102 in man. Ann N Y Acad Sci 765:336–337, 1995

Muizelaar JP, Marmarou A, Young HF, et al: Improving the outcome of severe head injury with the oxygen radical scavenger polyethylene glycol-conjugated superoxide dismutase: a phase II trial. J Neurosurg 78:375–382, 1993

Muizelaar JP, Kupiec JW, Rapp LA: PEG-SOD after head injury. J Neurosurg 83:942, 1995

Mukhin A, Fan L, Faden AI: Activation of metabotropic glutamate receptor subtype mGluR1 contributes to posttraumatic neuronal injury. J Neurosci 16:6012–6020, 1996

Mukhin AG, Ivanova SA, Faden AI: mGluR modulation of posttraumatic neuronal death: role of NMDA receptors. Neuroreport 8:2561–2566, 1997

Nag S, Takahashi JL, Kilty DW: Role of vascular endothelial growth factor in blood-brain barrier breakdown and angiogenesis in brain trauma. J Neuropathol Exp Neurol 56:912–921, 1997

Narotam PK, Rodell TC, Nadvi SS, et al: Traumatic brain contusions: a clinical role for the kinin antagonist CP-0127. Acta Neurochir (Wien). 140:793–802; discussion, 802–803, 1998

Nawa H, Carnahan J, Gall C: BDNF protein measured by a novel enzyme immunoassay in normal brain and after seizure: partial disagreement with mRNA levels. Eur J Neurosci 7:1527–1535, 1995

Neufeld G, Cohen T, Gengrinovitch S, et al: Vascular endothelial growth factor (VEGF) and its receptors. FASEB J 13:9–22, 1999

Ni W, Rajkumar K, Nagy JI, et al: Impaired brain development and reduced astrocyte response to injury in transgenic mice expressing IGF binding protein-1. Brain Res 769:97–107, 1997

Nicole O, Ali C, Docagne F, et al: Neuroprotection mediated by glial cell line-derived neurotrophic factor: involvement of a reduction of NMDA-induced calcium influx by the mitogen-activated protein kinase pathway. J Neurosci 21:3024–3033, 2001

Nieto-Sampedro M, Lewis ER, Cotman CW, et al: Brain injury causes a time-dependent increase in neuronotrophic activity at the lesion site. Science 217:860–861, 1982

Nilsson P, Hillered L, Ponten U, et al: Changes in cortical extracellular levels of energy-related metabolites and amino acids following concussive brain injury in rats. J Cereb Blood Flow Metab 10:631–637, 1990

Nordqvist AC, Holmin S, Nilsson M, et al: MK-801 inhibits the cortical increase in IGF-1, IGFBP-2 and IGFBP-4 expression following trauma. Neuroreport 8:455–460, 1997

Nugent MA, Iozzo RV: Fibroblast growth factor-2. Int J Biochem Cell Biol 32:115–120, 2000

Ocrant I, Fay CT, Parmelee JT: Characterization of insulin-like growth factor binding proteins produced in the rat central nervous system. Endocrinology 127:1260–1267, 1990

Okiyama K, Smith DH, Gennarelli TA, et al: The sodium channel blocker and glutamate release inhibitor BW1003C87 and magnesium attenuate regional cerebral edema following experimental brain injury in the rat. J Neurochem 64:802–809, 1995

Okiyama K, Smith DH, White WF, et al: Effects of the novel NMDA antagonists CP-98,113, CP-101,581 and CP-101,606 on cognitive function and regional cerebral edema following experimental brain injury in the rat. J Neurotrauma 14:211–222, 1997

Okiyama K, Smith DH, White WF, et al: Effects of the NMDA antagonist CP-98,113 on regional cerebral edema and cardiovascular, cognitive, and neurobehavioral function following experimental brain injury in the rat. Brain Res 792:291–298, 1998

Olney JW, Ho OL, Rhee V: Cytotoxic effects of acidic and sulphur containing amino acids on the infant mouse central nervous system. Exp Brain Res 14:61–76, 1971

Oyesiku NM, Evans CO, Houston S, et al: Regional changes in the expression of neurotrophic factors and their receptors following acute traumatic brain injury in the adult rat brain. Brain Res 833:161–172, 1999

Palmer AM, Marion DW, Botscheller ML, et al: Traumatic brain injury-induced excitotoxicity assessed in a controlled cortical impact model. J Neurochem 61:2015–2024, 1993

Palmer AM, Marion DW, Botscheller ML, et al: Increased transmitter amino acid concentration in human ventricular CSF after brain trauma. Neuroreport 6:153–156, 1994

Panikashvili D, Simeonidou C, Ben Shabat S, et al: An endogenous cannabinoid (2-AG) is neuroprotective after brain injury. Nature 413:527–531, 2001

Panter SS, Faden AI: Pretreatment with NMDA antagonists limits release of excitatory amino acids following traumatic brain injury. Neurosci Lett 136:165–168, 1992

Panter SS, Braughler JM, Hall ED: Dextran-coupled deferoxamine improves outcome in a murine model of head injury. J Neurotrauma 9:47–53, 1992

Papavassiliou E, Gogate N, Proescholdt M, et al: Vascular endothelial growth factor (vascular permeability factor) expression in injured rat brain. J Neurosci Res 49:451–460, 1997

Pencea V, Bingaman KD, Wiegand SJ, et al: Infusion of brain-derived neurotrophic factor into the lateral ventricle of the adult rat leads to new neurons in the parenchyma of the striatum, septum, thalamus, and hypothalamus. J Neurosci 21:6706–6717, 2001

Penkowa M, Moos T, Carrasco J, et al: Strongly compromised inflammatory response to brain injury in interleukin-6-deficient mice. Glia 25:343–357, 1999

Perretti M, Szabo C, Thiemermann C: Effect of interleukin-4 and interleukin-10 on leucocyte migration and nitric oxide production in the mouse. Br J Pharmacol 116:2251–2257, 1995

Philips MF, Mattiasson G, Wieloch T, et al: Neuroprotective and behavioral efficacy of nerve growth factor-transfected hippocampal progenitor cell transplants after experimental traumatic brain injury. J Neurosurg 94:765–774, 2001

Phillips LL, Lyeth BG, Hamm RJ, et al: Effect of prior receptor antagonism on behavioral morbidity produced by combined fluid percussion injury and entorhinal cortical lesion. J Neurosci Res 49:197–206, 1997

Piek J, Chesnut RM, Marshall LF, et al: Extracranial complications of severe head injury. J Neurosurg 77:901–907, 1992

Pin JP, Duvoisin R: The metabotropic glutamate receptors: structure and functions. Neuropharmacology 34:1–26, 1995

Pleines UE, Stover JF, Kossmann T, et al: Soluble ICAM-1 in CSF coincides with the extent of cerebral damage in patients with severe traumatic brain injury. J Neurotrauma 15:399–409, 1998

Pogrebniak H, Matthews W, Mitchell J, et al: Spin trap protection from tumor necrosis factor cytotoxicity. J Surg Res 50:469–474, 1991

Pohl D, Bittigau P, Ishimaru MJ, et al: N-methyl-D-aspartate antagonists and apoptotic cell death triggered by head trauma in developing rat brain. Proc Natl Acad Sci U S A 96:2508–2513, 1999

Pop E: Dexanabinol Pharmos. Cur Opin Investig Drugs 1:494–503, 2000

Povlishock JT, Kontos HA: The role of oxygen radicals in the pathobiology of traumatic brain injury. Hum Cell 5:345–353, 1992

Pratico D, Reiss P, Tang LX, et al: Local and systemic increase in lipid peroxidation after moderate experimental traumatic brain injury. J Neurochem 80:894–898, 2002

Pulford BE, Ishii DN: Uptake of circulating insulin-like growth factors (IGFs) into cerebrospinal fluid appears to be independent of the IGF receptors as well as IGF-binding proteins. Endocrinology 142:213–220, 2001

Quagliarello VJ, Wispelwey B, Long WJ Jr, et al: Recombinant human interleukin-1 induces meningitis and blood-brain barrier injury in the rat: characterization and comparison with tumor necrosis factor. J Clin Invest 87:1360–1366, 1991

Quattrocchi KB, Miller CH, Wagner FC Jr, et al: Cell-mediated immunity in severely head-injured patients: the role of suppressor lymphocytes and serum factors. J Neurosurg 77:694–699, 1992

Ramirez JJ, Finklestein SP, Keller J, et al: Basic fibroblast growth factor enhances axonal sprouting after cortical injury in rats. Neuroreport 10:1201–1204, 1999

Rancan M, Otto VI, Hans VH, et al: Upregulation of ICAM-1 and MCP-1 but not of MIP-2 and sensorimotor deficit in response to traumatic axonal injury in rats. J Neurosci Res 63:438–446, 2001

Reid TR, Torti FM, Ringold GM: Evidence for two mechanisms by which tumor necrosis factor kills cells. J Biol Chem 264:4583–4589, 1989

Reilly JF, Kumari VG: Alterations in fibroblast growth factor receptor expression following brain injury. Exp Neurol 140:139–150, 1996

Roberts I: The CRASH trial: the first large-scale, randomised, controlled trial in head injury. Crit Care 5:292–293, 2001

Ross SA, Halliday MI, Campbell GC, et al: The presence of tumour necrosis factor in CSF and plasma after severe head injury. Br J Neurosurg 8:419–425, 1994

Rothwell NJ, Luheshi GN: Interleukin 1 in the brain: biology, pathology and therapeutic target. Trends Neurosci 23:618–625, 2000

Rotwein P, Burgess SK, Milbrandt JD, et al: Differential expression of insulin-like growth factor genes in rat central nervous system. Proc Natl Acad Sci U S A 85:265–269, 1988

Saatman KE, Contreras PC, Smith DH, et al: Insulin-like growth factor-1 (IGF-1) improves both neurological motor and cognitive outcome following experimental brain injury. Exp Neurol 147:418–427, 1997

Saatman KE, Bareyre FM, Grady MS, et al: Acute cytoskeletal alterations and cell death induced by experimental brain injury are attenuated by magnesium treatment and exacerbated by magnesium deficiency. J Neuropathol Exp Neurol 60:183–194, 2001

Salhia B, Angelov L, Roncari L, et al: Expression of vascular endothelial growth factor by reactive astrocytes and associated neoangiogenesis. Brain Res 883:87–97, 2000

Sanada T, Nakamura T, Nishimura MC, et al: Effect of U74006F on neurologic function and brain edema after fluid percussion injury in rats. J Neurotrauma 10:65–71, 1993

Sanchez Mejia RO, Ona VO, Li M, et al: Minocycline reduces traumatic brain injury-mediated caspase-1 activation, tissue damage, and neurological dysfunction. Neurosurgery 48:1393–1399, 2001

Sandberg Nordqvist AC, von Holst H, Holmin S, et al: Increase of insulin-like growth factor (IGF)-1, IGF binding protein-2 and -4 mRNAs following cerebral contusion. Brain Res Mol Brain Res 38:285–293, 1996

Sanderson KL, Raghupathi R, Saatman KE, et al: Interleukin-1 receptor antagonist attenuates regional neuronal cell death and cognitive dysfunction after experimental brain injury. J Cereb Blood Flow Metab 19:1118–1125, 1999

Sarrafzadeh AS, Thomale UW, Kroppenstedt SN, et al: Neuroprotective effect of melatonin on cortical impact injury in the rat. Acta Neurochir (Wien) 142:1293–1299, 2000

Schaar DG, Sieber BA, Dreyfus CF, et al: Regional and cell-specific expression of GDNF in rat brain. Exp Neurol 124:368–371, 1993

Scherbel U, Raghupathi R, Nakamura M, et al: Differential acute and chronic responses of tumor necrosis factor-deficient mice to experimental brain injury. Proc Natl Acad Sci U S A 96:8721–8726, 1999

Schinder AF, Poo M: The neurotrophin hypothesis for synaptic plasticity. Trends Neurosci 23:639–645, 2000

Schoepp DD, Jane DE, Monn JA: Pharmacological agents acting at subtypes of metabotropic glutamate receptors. Neuropharmacology 38:1431–1476, 1999

Shapira Y, Yadid G, Cotev S, et al: Protective effect of MK801 in experimental brain injury. J Neurotrauma 7:131–139, 1990

Shapira Y, Lam AM, Artru AA, et al: Ketamine alters calcium and magnesium in brain tissue following experimental head trauma in rats. J Cereb Blood Flow Metab 13:962–968, 1993

Shen M, Thayer SA: The cannabinoid agonist Win55,212–2 inhibits calcium channels by receptor-mediated and direct pathways in cultured rat hippocampal neurons. Brain Res 783:77–84, 1998

Shen M, Piser TM, Seybold VS, et al: Cannabinoid receptor agonists inhibit glutamatergic synaptic transmission in rat hippocampal cultures. J Neurosci 16:4322–4334, 1996

Shimizu S, Royo NC, Saatman KE, et al: Evaluation of the temporal and regional alterations in endogenous GDNF expression after experimental traumatic brain injury. J Neurotrauma 19:1344, 2002

Shohami E, Novikov M, Mechoulam R: A nonpsychotropic cannabinoid, HU-211, has cerebroprotective effects after closed head injury in the rat. J Neurotrauma 10:109–119, 1993

Shohami E, Novikov M, Bass R, et al: Closed head injury triggers early production of TNF alpha and IL-6 by brain tissue. J Cereb Blood Flow Metab 14:615–619, 1994

Shohami E, Bass R, Wallach D, et al: Inhibition of tumor necrosis factor alpha (TNFα) activity in rat brain is associated with cerebroprotection after closed head injury. J Cereb Blood Flow Metab 16:378–384, 1996

Shohami E, Beit-Yannai E, Horowitz M, et al: Oxidative stress in closed-head injury: brain antioxidant capacity as an indicator of functional outcome. J Cereb Blood Flow Metab 17:1007–1019, 1997a

Shohami E, Gallily R, Mechoulam R, et al: Cytokine production in the brain following closed head injury: dexanabinol (HU-211) is a novel TNF-alpha inhibitor and an effective neuroprotectant. J Neuroimmunol 72:169–177, 1997b

Shohami E, Gati I, Beit-Yannai E, et al: Closed head injury in the rat induces whole body oxidative stress: overall reducing antioxidant profile. J Neurotrauma 16: 365–376, 1999

Showalter PE, Kimmel DN: Stimulating consciousness and cognition following severe brain injury: a new potential clinical use for lamotrigine. Brain Inj 14:997–1001, 2000

Sinson G, Voddi M, McIntosh TK: Nerve growth factor administration attenuates cognitive but not neurobehavioral motor dysfunction or hippocampal cell loss following fluid-percussion brain injury in rats. J Neurochem 65:2209–2216, 1995

Sinson G, Voddi M, McIntosh TK: Combined fetal neural transplantation and nerve growth factor infusion: effects on neurological outcome following fluid-percussion brain injury in the rat. J Neurosurg 84:655–662, 1996

Sinson G, Perri BR, Trojanowski JQ, et al: Improvement of cognitive deficits and decreased cholinergic neuronal cell loss and apoptotic cell death following neurotrophin infusion after experimental traumatic brain injury. J Neurosurg 86:511–518, 1997

Slavik RS, Rhoney DH: Indomethacin: a review of its cerebral blood flow effects and potential use for controlling intracranial pressure in traumatic brain injury patients. Neurol Res 21:491–499, 1999

Smith DH, Okiyama K, Gennarelli TA, et al: Magnesium and ketamine attenuate cognitive dysfunction following experimental brain injury. Neurosci Lett 157:211–214, 1993a

Smith DH, Okiyama K, Thomas MJ, et al: Effects of the excitatory amino acid receptor antagonists kynurenate and indole-2-carboxylic acid on behavioral and neurochemical outcome following experimental brain injury. J Neurosci 13:5383–5392, 1993b

Smith DH, Perri BR, Raghupathi R, et al: Remacemide hydrochloride reduces cortical lesion volume following brain trauma in the rat. Neurosci Lett 231:135–138, 1997

Smith JS, Fulop ZL, Levinsohn SA, et al: Effects of the novel NMDA receptor antagonist gacyclidine on recovery from medial frontal cortex contusion injury in rats. Neural Plast 7:73–91, 2000

Smith SL, Andrus PK, Zhang JR, et al: Direct measurement of hydroxyl radicals, lipid peroxidation, and blood-brain barrier disruption following unilateral cortical impact head injury in the rat. J Neurotrauma 11:393–404, 1994

Soares HD, Thomas M, Cloherty K, et al: Development of prolonged focal cerebral edema and regional cation changes following experimental brain injury in the rat. J Neurochem 58:1845–1852, 1992

Soares HD, Hicks RR, Smith D, et al: Inflammatory leukocytic recruitment and diffuse neuronal degeneration are separate pathological processes resulting from traumatic brain injury. J Neurosci 15:8223–8233, 1995

Stachowiak MK, Moffett J, Maher P, et al: Growth factor regulation of cell growth and proliferation in the nervous system. A new intracrine nuclear mechanism. Mol Neurobiol 15:257–283, 1997

Stahel PF, Kariya K, Shohami E, et al: Intracerebral complement C5a receptor (CD88) expression is regulated by TNF and lymphotoxin-alpha following closed head injury in mice. J Neuroimmunol 109:164–172, 2000a

Stahel PF, Shohami E, Younis FM, et al: Experimental closed head injury: analysis of neurological outcome, blood-brain barrier dysfunction, intracranial neutrophil infiltration, and neuronal cell death in mice deficient in genes for pro-inflammatory cytokines. J Cereb Blood Flow Metab 20:369–380, 2000b

Stein DG, Halks-Miller M, Hoffman SW: Intracerebral administration of alpha-tocopherol-containing liposomes facilitates behavioral recovery in rats with bilateral lesions of the frontal cortex. J Neurotrauma 8:281–292, 1991

Stoffel M, Berger S, Staub F, et al: The effect of dietary alpha-tocopherol on the experimental vasogenic brain edema. J Neurotrauma 14:339–348, 1997

Stover JF, Beyer TF, Unterberg AW: Riluzole reduces brain swelling and contusion volume in rats following controlled cortical impact injury. J Neurotrauma 17:1171–1178, 2000a

Stover JF, Dohse NK, Unterberg AW: Bradykinin 2 receptor antagonist LF 16–0687Ms reduces posttraumatic brain edema. Acta Neurochir Suppl 76:171–175, 2000b

Strauss KI, Barbe MF, Marshall RM, et al: Prolonged cyclooxygenase-2 induction in neurons and glia following traumatic brain injury in the rat. J Neurotrauma 17:695–711, 2000

Sullivan PG, Bruce-Keller AJ, Rabchevsky AG, et al: Exacerbation of damage and altered NF-kappaB activation in mice lacking tumor necrosis factor receptors after traumatic brain injury. J Neurosci 19:6248–6256, 1999

Sullivan PG, Keller JN, Bussen WL, et al: Cytochrome c release and caspase activation after traumatic brain injury. Brain Res 949:88–96, 2002

Sun FY, Faden AI: N-methyl-D-aspartate receptors mediate post-traumatic increases of protein kinase C in rat brain. Brain Res 661:63–69, 1994

Sun FY, Faden AI: Neuroprotective effects of 619C89, a use-dependent sodium channel blocker, in rat traumatic brain injury. Brain Res 673:133–140, 1995a

Sun FY, Faden AI: Pretreatment with antisense oligodeoxynucleotides directed against the NMDA-R1 receptor enhances survival and behavioral recovery following traumatic brain injury in rats. Brain Res 693:163–168, 1995b

Taupin V, Toulmond S, Serrano A, et al: Increase in IL-6, IL-1 and TNF levels in rat brain following traumatic lesion: influence of pre- and post-traumatic treatment with Ro5 4864, a peripheral-type (p site) benzodiazepine ligand. J Neuroimmunol 42:177–185, 1993

Timmusk T, Belluardo N, Metsis M, et al: Widespread and developmentally regulated expression of neurotrophin-4 mRNA in rat brain and peripheral tissues. Eur J Neurosci 5:605–613, 1993

Toulmond S, Rothwell NJ: Interleukin-1 receptor antagonist inhibits neuronal damage caused by fluid percussion injury in the rat. Brain Res 671:261–266, 1995

Toulmond S, Serrano A, Benavides J, et al: Prevention by eliprodil (SL 82.0715) of traumatic brain damage in the rat: existence of a large (18 h) therapeutic window. Brain Res 620:32–41, 1993

Truettner J, Schmidt-Kastner R, Busto R, et al: Expression of brain-derived neurotrophic factor, nerve growth factor, and heat shock protein HSP70 following fluid percussion brain injury in rats. J Neurotrauma 16:471–486, 1999

Trupp M, Arenas E, Fainzilber M, et al: Functional receptor for GDNF encoded by the c-ret proto-oncogene. Nature 381:785–789, 1996

Tymianski M, Tator CH: Normal and abnormal calcium homeostasis in neurons: a basis for the pathophysiology of traumatic and ischemic central nervous system injury. Neurosurgery 38:1176–1195, 1996

Tyurin VA, Tyurina YY, Borisenko GG, et al: Oxidative stress following traumatic brain injury in rats: quantitation of biomarkers and detection of free radical intermediates. J Neurochem 75:2178–2189, 2000

Unsicker K, Grothe C, Otto D, et al: Basic fibroblast growth factor in neurons and its putative functions. Ann N Y Acad Sci 638:300–305, 1991

Unterberg AW, Stroop R, Thomale UW, et al: Characterisation of brain edema following "controlled cortical impact injury" in rats. Acta Neurochir Suppl (Wien) 70:106–108, 1997

Vink R, Heath DL, McIntosh TK: Acute and prolonged alterations in brain free magnesium following fluid-percussion induced brain trauma in rats. J Neurochem 66:2477–2483, 1996

Voddi MD, Perri BR, Perlman KG, et al: The use-dependent sodium channel antagonist 619C89 attenuates memory disfunction following experimental brain injury. J Neurotrauma 12:146, 1995

Wada K, Alonso OF, Busto R, et al: Early treatment with a novel inhibitor of lipid peroxidation (LY341122) improves histopathological outcome after moderate fluid percussion brain injury in rats. Neurosurgery 45:601–608, 1999

Wahl F, Renou E, Mary V, et al: Riluzole reduces brain lesions and improves neurological function in rats after a traumatic brain injury. Brain Res 756:247–255, 1997

Werther GA, Abate M, Hogg A, et al: Localization of insulin-like growth factor-I mRNA in rat brain by in situ hybridization: relationship to IGF-I receptors. Mol Endocrinol 4:773–778, 1990

Woodroofe MN, Sarna GS, Wadhwa M, et al: Detection of interleukin-1 and interleukin-6 in adult rat brain, following mechanical injury, by in vivo microdialysis: evidence of a role for microglia in cytokine production. J Neuroimmunol 33:227–236, 1991

Xiong Y, Peterson PL, Muizelaar JP, et al: Amelioration of mitochondrial function by a novel antioxidant U-101033E following traumatic brain injury in rats. J Neurotrauma 14:907–917, 1997

Yakovlev AG, Knoblach SM, Fan L, et al: Activation of CPP32-like caspases contributes to neuronal apoptosis and neurological dysfunction after traumatic brain injury. J Neurosci 17:7415–7424, 1997

Yamasaki Y, Suzuki T, Yamaya H, et al: Possible involvement of interleukin-1 in ischemic brain edema formation. Neurosci Lett 142:45–47, 1992

Yan HQ, Yu J, Kline AE, et al: Evaluation of combined fibroblast growth factor-2 and moderate hypothermia therapy in traumatically brain injured rats. Brain Res 887:134–143, 2000

Yan Q, Radeke MJ, Matheson CR, et al: Immunocytochemical localization of TrkB in the central nervous system of the adult rat. J Comp Neurol 378:135–157, 1997a

Yan Q, Rosenfeld RD, Matheson CR, et al: Expression of brain-derived neurotrophic factor protein in the adult rat central nervous system. Neuroscience 78:431–448, 1997b

Yang L, Lindholm K, Konishi Y, et al: Target depletion of distinct tumor necrosis factor receptor subtypes reveals hippocampal neuron death and survival through different signal transduction pathways. J Neurosci 22:3025–3032, 2002

Yang SY, Cui JZ: Expression of the basic fibroblast growth factor gene in mild and more severe head injury in the rat. J Neurosurg 89:297–302, 1998

Yang S, Cui J: Study on the value of exogenous bFGF in the treatment of brain injury. Chin J Traumatol 3:131–135, 2000

Yao Y, Yin D, Jas GS, et al: Oxidative modification of a carboxyl-terminal vicinal methionine in calmodulin by hydrogen peroxide inhibits calmodulin-dependent activation of the plasma membrane Ca-ATPase. Biochemistry 35:2767–2787, 1996

Yoshimura S, Takagi Y, Harada J, et al: FGF-2 regulation of neurogenesis in adult hippocampus after brain injury. Proc Natl Acad Sci U S A 98:5874–5879, 2001

Young B, Runge JW, Waxman KS, et al: Effects of pegorgotein on neurologic outcome of patients with severe head injury: a multicenter, randomized controlled trial. JAMA 276:538–543, 1996

Yunoki M, Kawauchi M, Ukita N, et al: Effects of lecithinized superoxide dismutase on traumatic brain injury in rats. J Neurotrauma 14:739–746, 1997

Zhang C, Raghupathi R, Saatman KE, et al: Riluzole attenuates cortical lesion size, but not hippocampal neuronal loss, following traumatic brain injury in the rat. J Neurosci Res 52:342–349, 1998

Zhang R, Shohami E, Beit-Yannai E, et al: Mechanism of brain protection by nitroxide radicals in experimental model of closed-head injury. Free Radic Biol Med 24:332–340, 1998

Zhuang J, Shackford SR, Schmoker JD, et al: The association of leukocytes with secondary brain injury. J Trauma 35:415–422, 1993

Zwienenberg M, Gong QZ, Berman RF, et al: The effect of groups II and III metabotropic glutamate receptor activation on neuronal injury in a rodent model of traumatic brain injury. Neurosurgery 48:1119–1126, 2001

40 Prevention

Elie Elovic, M.D.

Ross Zafonte, D.O.

PREVENTABLE INJURY IS one of the most significant health care issues in the United States. Estimates place the annual cost in the United States to be $260 billion, and 30% of all life years lost before age 75 years are a result of injury. The Centers for Disease Control and Prevention (CDC) estimates that during 1995, 2.6 million hospital discharges and more than 36 million emergency department visits occurred as a result of injury (Centers for Disease Control and Prevention 2001). At the more serious end of the spectrum, injury is the cause of 150,000 deaths every year and is the leading source of death for Americans ages 1–44 years (Nguyen et al. 2001).

Looking specifically at traumatic brain injury (TBI), the figures are only slightly less daunting, with TBI one of the leading causes of death and disability for children and young adults in the United States. The CDC estimates that in the United States between 1 million and 1.5 million people seek medical attention secondary to TBI. In addition, there are 230,000 hospitalizations and 80,000–90,000 people who develop disability secondary to TBI every year (Centers for Disease Control and Prevention 2001; McDeavitt 2001; Thurman et al. 1999). TBI also accounts for more than 50,000 deaths annually, which constitutes one-third of all injury-related deaths. Current estimates place the number of Americans who have some disability as a result of TBI at roughly 5.3 million (Centers for Disease Control and Prevention 2001). Schootman and Fuortes (2000) reported that during the years 1994–1997, 1.4 million people in the United States sought care either at a doctor's office or the emergency department secondary to TBI, whereas Guerro et al. (2000) reported TBI incidence between 392 and 444 per 100,000 population when emergency department visits are included. These numbers suggest a much higher incidence of TBI than those based on deaths and hospital admissions.

Looking at deaths and hospital admissions, TBI incidence is close to 100 per 100,000 (Thurman et al. 1999). This is a drop of 50% from previous reports of rates of 200 per 100,000 during the 1970s and 1980s (Annegers et al. 1980; Centers for Disease Control and Prevention 2001; Jagger et al. 1984; Kraus et al. 1984). The decrease may in part be a result of insurance's influence on admission decisions, in addition to prevention efforts. This is in contrast to TBI mortality, because a reduction in the incidence is more likely a result of prevention efforts. In 1980, the rate of TBI-related mortality in the United States was 24.7 per 100,000. This had fallen 20% by 1994 to a rate of 19.8. Motor vehicle–related mortality showed the greatest decline. With the advent of air bags, seat belts, and child safety seats, mortality dropped 38% from 11.1 to 6.9 per 100,000 between 1980 and 1994 (Thurman et al. 1999).

TBI Versus Other Disabling Conditions

TBI has often been called the silent or invisible epidemic (Centers for Disease Control and Prevention 2001), the stepchild that has only received minimal public awareness and dedication of financial resources to its treatment and prevention. To obtain a better perspective on this statement, one can compare TBI incidence to other conditions that have greater notoriety despite a lower incidence. The Brain Injury Association of America has made substantial effort to spread the word and inform the lay and scientific public about TBI incidence. The association has a Web site that actively deals with the issue (Brain Injury Association of America 2001b). At this time, the annual incidence of TBI is greater than that of the more widely known conditions of spinal cord injury, breast cancer, multiple sclerosis, and human immunodeficiency virus (HIV) (Figure 40–1).

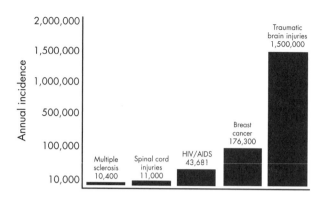

FIGURE 40–1. **A comparison of traumatic brain injury and leading injuries or diseases: annual incidence.**

AIDS=acquired immunodeficiency syndrome; HIV=human immunodeficiency virus.

Source. Brain Injury Association of America, March 2001. Available at: http://www.biausa.org/word.files.to.pdf/good.pdfs/2002.Fact.Sheet.tbi.incidence.pdf. Accessed March 22, 2004. Used with permission.

The magnitude of TBI-related mortality as compared with these other conditions is quite striking. As compared with the 50,000 deaths that occur each year as a result of TBI, the number of HIV-related deaths during 1999 was 16,273 (U.S. Department of Health and Human Services 2001), whereas 43,700 people died during 1999 from breast cancer (American Cancer Society 2001). What may be most striking for HIV information is that the mortality rate in 1999 is a substantial drop from the 1995 high of 50,610 HIV-related deaths (U.S. Department of Health and Human Services 2001). With dedication to prevention, treatment, and increased public awareness, a similar drop in the personal suffering and economic loss of TBI may also be possible.

Economics of TBI and Its Prevention

Because TBI often occurs in the very young, the cost to society in lost years of productivity and years of dependent care can be enormous. Estimates of work years lost because of TBI run as high as 2.6 million, which accounts for 58% of all injury-related losses reported (McDeavitt 2001). Max et al. (1991) reported that the cost associated with TBI in 1988 dollars was $44 billion. With the enormous personal suffering, loss of life, and economic hardship on society, the fact that many of these often catastrophic events are preventable only compounds this tragedy.

With the competition for dollars in today's world, the cost-benefit ratio of preventive efforts is an issue of some

importance. Some prevention techniques are widely accepted in society today, such as childhood vaccinations and flu vaccine, as they have proven to be efficacious both financially and as a vehicle for health maintenance. This has been proven to be true with injury prevention as well. Pediatricians who administer injury prevention counseling to families with children younger than 4 years have demonstrated a 13 to 1 benefit to cost ratio (Miller and Galbraith 1995). Bicycle helmets for children ages 4–15 years have also shown great benefit. For every $1 spent on bicycle helmets, society saves $2 in direct medical costs, $6 in future earnings, and $17 in quality of life. The use of child safety seats for children younger than 4 years has also proven to be of substantial benefit to society. If child safety seats are used, the savings in direct medical costs, future earnings, and quality of life are $2, $6, and $25, respectively (Miller et al. 2000). Finally, Graham et al. (1997) demonstrated that the use of seat belts and air bags demonstrated a cost effectiveness that matched any other prevention effort that addressed any medical or public health issues.

What Is Prevention?

People use the word *prevention* for many activities. Speed limits, highway barriers, and highway designs to lessen the number of motor vehicle accidents (MVAs) are clearly aimed at injury prevention. So too are seat belts and air bags, for though they do not play a major role in accident prevention, they minimize personal injury to passengers in the car once an accident occurs. The development of advanced trauma care to mitigate further injury is also a form of prevention. Although all three of these examples are geared toward injury prevention, they clearly have differences. As a result, the distinction between primary, secondary, and tertiary prevention has been made. Primary prevention efforts are directed to prevent the injury from occurring. Other examples of primary prevention include fall-proofing homes, traffic laws and their enforcement, salting of ice-covered roads, and education about drinking and driving. In contrast, secondary efforts lessen an injury's effect once it has occurred, with helmets, automobile design, and air bags examples of secondary prevention. Development of advanced trauma care and emergency management services are examples of tertiary prevention (Nguyen et al. 2001).

Injury Control Theory

Originally, the general belief was that TBI was a result of accidents, which implied that all persons had equal probability of sustaining injury (Elovic and Antoinette 1996;

Guyer and Gallagher 1985). Any discussion of TBI epidemiology, such as the one in Chapter 1, Epidemiology, clearly demonstrates the fallacy of this position. There are certain people who are at higher risk of sustaining injury. As a result, there has been substantial work devoted to the identification of people at risk and to developing effective preventive countermeasures (Elovic et al. 1996; Teutsch 1992), with a substantial increase in the science of injury control theory since the 1950s.

The relationship between infectious pathogens and their related illness has been investigated since the time of Louis Pasteur, more than 100 years ago. More than 50 years ago, Gordon first raised the idea that injury can be studied in the same fashion as infectious illness (Gielen and Girasek 2001). In 1961, James Gibson introduced the idea that the energy that induced injury could be studied as a causative agent similar to an infectious agent (Gielen and Girasek 2001). Baker (1975) compared the concept of the epidemiologic model of injury to that of illness by describing the etiologic agent as one that demonstrates a negative effect on a host in a particular environment.

Haddon Matrix

Further work on the study of injury prevention was carried out by Haddon, resulting in the construction of the Haddon Matrix (Haddon 1968). With this model, injury is divided into three separate areas. First is the host; the second is the vector, or injuring agent; and the third is the environment that the first two interact within. The environment is further divided into two separate components, physical and social. In addition, the matrix model divides the injury using temporal factors; preinjury, injury, and postinjury. This is comparable to the primary, secondary, and tertiary prevention efforts mentioned in the section What Is Prevention? (Nguyen et al. 2001). Using these sets of variables, a table can be created in which each cell represents an area and a temporal component. All factors related to injury can be placed into one of the table's cells. An example of this would be the decreased balance and vision of an elderly person who sustained a fall. In the Haddon Matrix, these items would be placed in the host, preinjury cell. The contribution of the shag rug that caused the fall would be classified as preinjury, physical environment. The vector in falls is the energy that is transmitted to the brain tissue. Head height is a source of potential injury before an event. Clearly, by standing on a ladder there is greater potential energy, which places the host at greater risk. The energy is converted to kinetic energy during a fall that is transmitted to the brain tissue at impact. The distortion of brain tissue and bleeding that result from the energy transfer can be considered the postinjury vector component.

Passive Versus Active Strategies

There are two general approaches to the promotion of injury prevention, passive and active. A passive strategy is one that the host takes no action to use (Gielen et al. 2001) and may as a result be more effective than active interventions. By nature, passive strategies offer protection to a larger percentage of the population (Karlson 1992). Some examples of these include air bags, road barriers, fingerprint-based gun locks, and car safety engineering. A system that would not let a driver start his or her car if he or she could not pass a Breathalyzer test is another example of a passive strategy that would prevent the host from driving while intoxicated. Active strategies are ones that require some action on the host's part. The donning of a seat belt, avoiding driving when under the influence, motorcycle helmet usage, and car seats are just some examples of active prevention. Although these items may be more effective than passive approaches, their distinct disadvantage is that somehow society must convince the host to use them.

As a result, there is some controversy as to how injury prevention resources should be applied. It is general knowledge that changing human behavior is a challenging endeavor, and passive interventions aimed at the vector and environment may be the most effective in reducing death and injury (Haddon 1970). That does not negate the potential benefit of using a combined approach, because the use of one method does not exclude the use of another. An example of this is, of course, the use of seat belts in combination with air bags. Each prevention method has shown its benefit; however, using both together has been shown to be more effective than either one by itself. As a result, there is evidence that a combined approach of active and passive interventions should be used in a comprehensive approach.

Facilitating Active Strategies to Develop Comprehensive Injury Control

How can society develop a comprehensive approach to injury control? Also, how can society influence the host that can be potentially injured to act according to its wishes? These important questions must be answered to maximize the benefit of an injury control program.

The first of these questions can only be answered once one defines what components are critical to the development of a comprehensive program. Clearly, engineering solutions are important components of passive interventions such as energy-absorbing car bodies, road barriers, and air bags. What methods should be used for the active strategies? Education is an important component, both at the individual and community level (Nguyen et al. 2001). However, there is a problem if education is performed alone without giving the listener some incentive to change his or her behavior on the basis of the information presented. An example of this was the early public service announcements that used fear as a potential motivator for increased seat belt usage, but they were largely ineffective (Roberston et al. 1974). Education prevention counseling by health care professionals in a clinical setting has been proven to be much more effective. DiGuiseppi and Roberts (2000), after reviewing many clinical trials, reported that education counseling was effective in encouraging the use of automobile restraints.

A method to facilitate a host's compliance with safer behaviors is to connect them to incentives. This can be accomplished with legislative intervention and appropriate enforcement. Community-based intervention programs combining education with legislative options has been shown to be effective in increasing bicycle helmet usage (Klassen et al. 2000). Work performed in three separate Maryland counties explored the issue of children's bicycle helmet usage under three separate conditions. In one county, legislation and education were undertaken, and helmet use increased from 4% to 47%. Another county used education alone and experienced a small, statistically insignificant increase in usage from 8% to 19%. The third county, which did nothing, actually demonstrated a decreased rate of helmet usage from 19% to 4%.

The third piece of the puzzle to facilitate active interventions is enforcement of legislation. Passing laws without proper enforcement leads to only minimal benefits, with seat belts being an example. By 1984, all passenger cars were required to have seat belts. However, rates of usage were only 15%. This rate increased to 42% by 1987 with a combination of educative efforts and seat belt legislation. By 1992, when secondary enforcement laws were enacted for nonuse of seat belts, usage increased to 62%. A secondary enforcement law is one that allows the giving of a citation when the driver has been pulled over for another traffic offense. This 62% usage rate persisted through 1998 in the states that used secondary enforcement laws. In states that have enacted primary enforcement legislation, which allowed ticketing when seat belt nonuse was the only infraction, usage rates increased to 79% (National Highway Traffic Safety Administration 1999). In summary, facilitation of active prevention requires a combination approach. Education, both at a community and individual level, must be included with appropriate legislation and its enforcement. Standing in the way of many of these changes is the idea that preventive legislation infringes on personal freedoms. The op-

position to gun control by the National Rifle Association and to helmet laws by motorcycle clubs are just two examples of this problem. However, with the great cost to society, both financially and emotionally, of TBI the government has not only the right, but also the obligation, to deal effectively with these issues.

TBI Prevention and Motor Vehicles

As the discussion is turned to more specific issues of TBI prevention, it is appropriate to begin with efforts that involve motor vehicles. The reasons for this are twofold. First, MVAs are the leading cause of TBI in the United States (Centers for Disease Control and Prevention 2001), with data from state registries reporting that transportation accounted for 48.9% of TBIs reported (Thurman et al. 1999). Second, there is evidence that prevention efforts aimed at reduction of transportation-related mortality have been efficacious. There was a 38% decrease in motor vehicle–related deaths from 1980 to 1994 (Centers for Disease Control and Prevention 2001). Transportation-related TBI prevention efforts can be approached by looking at both passive and active methods, as well as using the Haddon Matrix discussed in an earlier section.

Air Bags and Seat Belts

Air bags are a classic example of passive prevention that exerts its influence at the time of incident. Jagger (1992) has strongly advocated their use and has stated that installing them as standard equipment in the front seats of passenger cars would have a greater effect on TBI than any other prevention method. She estimated that 25% of patients admitted to a hospital secondary to TBI had sustained an injury that air bags are designed to protect against.

Air bags are automatic protection systems that are designed to protect during a frontal collision. They are designed to deploy when a car hits a similarly sized vehicle at 20–30 miles an hour, or a brick wall at 15 miles an hour. They provide a protective cushion between occupants and the car's interior, slowing the energy transfer that occurs at impact. This occurs within $1/20$ of a second after impact, and deflation begins within $4/20$ of a second, with the entire cycle completed within 1 second. This allows the driver to maintain control of the car and avoids trapping of passengers (National Highway Traffic Safety Administration 2002).

With the exception of some recently designed side-impact bags, air bags have not been engineered to protect the occupants from side impact, rear, or rollover events. One of the major sources of crash mortality is ejection from the vehicle, and this is another event that air bags are not designed to protect against. In addition, during a rollover, car occupants can be thrown against hard objects such as the steering wheel that can cause further injury. Instead, it is the seat belt that is most protective for these events, and air bags should not be considered as a solo item, but should be used in conjunction with seat belts. The combined utilization of seatbelts and air bags has been proven to be the most protective. In the National Highway Safety Administration's Third Report to Congress in 1996, air bags were reported to reduce fatalities in pure frontal crashes, excluding rollovers, by 34% and 18% in near-frontal collisions. In this analysis, the fatality rate using air bags alone ws reduced by 13%, taking all crashes into consideration. This is in comparison with a 45% reduction rate using lap-shoulder belts alone and a 50% reduction using both modalities (National Highway Traffic Safety Administration 2002).

The information gathered by the National Highway Traffic Safety Administration's National Accident Sampling System's Crashworthiness Data System regarding the effect of air bag and seat belt use on moderate and severe injuries is eye opening (National Highway Traffic Safety Administration 2002). A moderate injury was defined as having a Maximum Abbreviated Injury Score of 2 or greater, and a severe injury was defined as one with a Maximum Abbreviated Injury Score of 3 or greater. On the basis of information collected on two car crashes, the effect of air bags alone was not statistically significant, with a reported reduction of 18% and 7% in moderate and severe injuries, respectively. In contrast, the use of a lap-shoulder belt system alone resulted in a 49% and 59% reduction in moderate and severe injuries, respectively. A 60% reduction was found when used in combination. Before one draws the incorrect conclusion that air bags have little value, one must remember that all body systems are not equally important when discussing injury severity. Gennarelli et al. (1989) reported that TBI is the major source of mortality in multiple trauma patients. Therefore, a system that has its greatest effect on head and brain injury may play an important role. The combination of manual lap-shoulder belt and air bag reduced moderate and severe brain injuries 83% and 75%, respectively. This compares to 59% and 38% reductions in moderate and severe brain injuries, respectively, when a lap-shoulder belt was used alone. Although the data suggest that lap-shoulder belts provide a greater level of protection than air bags, the reader must of course be aware that the key phrase is "when used"; the passive nature of the air bag system clearly underscores its importance, whereas the greater protection afforded by the lap-shoulder belt means society must encourage its use.

Although both air bags and seat belts have a net positive benefit from an injury prevention standpoint, there are problems associated with their use. Seat belts have been associated with various injuries, especially when used improperly. Some of the injuries reported include spinal injuries; brachial plexopathy; liver lacerations; small bowel tears; traumatic hernias; aortic and other vascular, ocular, and facial injuries; neck sprains; cardiac injuries; kidney injuries; neck injuries; sternal fracture; lung perforation; chest injuries; and placental and fetal injury (Agran et al. 1987; Appleby and Nagy 1989; Arajarvi et al. 1987; Blacksin 1993; Bourbeau et al. 1993; Chandler et al. 1997; Hall et al. 2001; Holbrook and Bennett 1990; Immega 1995; Johnson and Falci 1990; Kaplan and Cowley 1991; Lubbers 1977; May et al. 1995; Restifo and Kelen 1994; Santavirta and Arajarvi 1992; Shoemaker and Ose 1997; Verdant 1988; Warrian et al. 1988; Yarbrough and Hendey 1990). In particular, injuries to children have prompted development of car seats and booster seats that are discussed in the section Car Seats and Air Bags. Like seat belts, air bags have also been shown to be a potential source of injury. Problems with air bags have included skull fracture and facial injury (Bandstra and Carbone 2001; Murphy et al. 2000; Rozner 1996), ocular trauma (Ghafouri et al. 1997; Lueder 2000; Ruiz-Moreno 1998; Stein et al. 1999; Zabriskie et al. 1997), burn injuries (Conover 1992; Ulrich et al. 2001; White et al. 1995), extremity fracture (Kirchhoff and Rasmussen 1995; Ong and Kumar 1998), chest injuries, spinal injury (Giguere et al. 1998; Traynelis and Gold 1993), ear injury and hearing loss (Beckerman and Elberger 1991; Kramer et al. 1997; Morris and Borja 1998), and reflex sympathetic dystrophy (Guarino 1998; Shah and Weinstein 1997). Children, in particular, are at greatest risk of injury from air bag deployment ("Air-bag-associated" 1995; From the Centers for Disease Control and Prevention 1995; "Update" 1996; From the Centers for Disease Control and Prevention 1997; Giguere et al. 1998; Marshall et al. 1998; McCaffrey et al. 1999; Totten et al. 1998). Properly and improperly positioned children have sustained severe and sometimes fatal injuries from air bag deployment (Angel and Ehlers 2001; "Air-bag-associated" 1995; from the Centers for Disease Control and Prevention 1995; "Update" 1996; from the Centers for Disease Control and Prevention 1997; Giguere et al. 1998; Lueder 2000; Marshall et al. 1998; McCaffrey et al. 1999; Morrison et al. 1998; Willis et al. 1996). As a result, special efforts have been directed to ensure the safe coexistence of children and air bags.

Motorcycles

Motorcycles account for 6% of all transportation accidents in the United States, but may be the most dangerous form of transportation (Flint 2001). From 1979 through 1986, more than 15,000 motorcycle deaths were associated with brain injury (Elovic et al. 1996), and from 1989 through 1991, almost 10,000 people died in the United States as a result of a motorcycle accident ("Head injuries" 1994). This is also true in New Zealand as documented by Begg et al. (1994) who reported that between 1978 and 1987 the incidence of motorcycle-related injury hospitalization was 80.4 per 100,000 whereas the mortality rate was 3.6 per 100,000. A study from Connecticut (Braddock et al. 1992) reported a lower fatality rate of 1.2 per 100,000 and a hospitalization rate of 24.7 per 100,000, with 22% of those injuries occurring in the head, brain, or spinal area.

In 1994, some of the factors that were linked to motorcycle-related fatal trauma included driver error (76%), with excessive speed found commonly (Elovic et al. 1996), and elevated blood alcohol levels and a failure to use a helmet. Alcohol is a major problem, and the highest rate of alcohol use among all methods of transportation is in motorcycle drivers (Peek-Asa and Kraus 1996) who also have the highest rate of legal intoxication of any group.

Helmet usage is another critical item that plays a major part in brain injury and mortality prevention. In 1982, Heilman et al. reported that helmetless riders were 2.3 times as likely to have a head, neck, or facial injury than those wearing a helmet, and they were also 3.19 times as likely to have a fatal injury. Bachulis et al. (1988) reported similar results, with the rate of brain injury twice as likely and severe brain injury six times more likely when helmets were not worn. Reporting on data from Colorado, Gabella et al. (1995) reported that the risk of brain injury was 2.5 times as high when helmets were not worn. Ferrando et al. (2000) demonstrated a 25% reduction in motorcycle-related fatalities after implementation of a mandatory helmet law in Spain, whereas Chiu et al. (2000) reported a 33% reduction in brain injuries, better outcomes, shorter hospital lengths of stay, as well as decease in injury severity in Taiwan after implementation of a mandatory helmet law. Many other investigators around the world have demonstrated similar results after the implementation of mandatory helmet laws. The rate of overall fatalities, TBI-related fatalities, overall TBI injury severity (Chiu et al. 2000; Ferrando et al. 2000; Fleming and Becker 1992; Kraus et al. 1994; Muelleman et al. 1992; Rowland et al. 1996; Sosin et al. 1990; Tsai and Hemenway 1999), length of hospitalization (Muelleman et al. 1992; Rowland et al. 1996), and overall cost to society (Muelleman et al. 1992; Rowland et al. 1996; Vaca and Berns 2001) are all decreased as a result of helmet law legislation.

Despite the strength of the evidence, motorcycle helmet laws are not pervasive in the United States. As of November 2000, only 20 states had legislation that required all motorcycle riders to wear helmets, whereas another 27 states had laws that required them for teenagers. Three states had no legislation at all (Vaca and Berns 2001). This is a step backward from the 1970s.

In 1967, the federal government through the Department of Transportation required that all states pass a motorcycle helmet law. If a state did not comply, it would be punished by a loss of federal safety funds. As a result, by 1975 47 states had mandatory helmet laws. However, in 1975 Congress rescinded the requirement. Within 3 years, more than one-half of the states with mandatory helmet laws repealed them (Vaca et al. 2001). Opponents argued that adults have the right of choice in this country, and the government has no right to interfere, but the simple facts do not support this position. First, helmet use has been shown to decrease with the abolition of mandatory helmet laws. In Texas and Arkansas, where the helmet rate was at 97% before legislation repeal, usage rate dropped to 66% and 52%, respectively, within 9 months of the repeal. Data from the Arkansas Trauma Registry demonstrated that there was also an increase in overall injuries and brain injuries, and a larger proportion of motorcyclists injured had brain injuries (Vaca et al. 2001). Recent work from Miami Dade County by Hotz et al. (2002) demonstrated decreased helmet use and increased incidence of brain injury and lethality post repeal of mandatory helmet laws. The authors noted that helmet use dropped from 83% to 56%, whereas the number of fatalities and brain injuries increased substantially.

There is also the financial cost that is borne by society when helmet laws are repealed. In Texas, as a result of the repeal of the motorcycle helmet laws, the cost of motorcycle-related TBI increased 75% to more than $32,000, whereas the median cost increased 300% to $22,531. These numbers are greater than the required insurance coverage of the majority of these riders, and therefore society has been forced to pick up this cost (National Highway Traffic Safety Administration 2000). The riders' freedom to choose has resulted in increased cost borne by the society in general.

Finally, the issue of alcohol and motorcycle driving is an important one. Alcohol has a tremendous effect on all motor vehicle–related trauma. This may be even truer for motorcycle-related trauma because the handling of a motorcycle requires greater coordination and judgment than driving a car. Sun et al. (1998) demonstrated that although many of the drivers of both cars and motorcycles brought into the trauma center are under the influence, motorcyclists have a lower level as compared with other drivers. As a result, it may be warranted to set an even lower level for acceptable blood alcohol levels for motorcycle drivers.

Falls

Falls have been identified as the second most common source of TBI in numerous studies (Annegers et al. 1980; Cooper et al. 1983; Jagger et al. 1984; Kraus et al. 1984; Sosin et al. 1989; Tiret et al. 1990; Whitman et al. 1984). The greatest number of falls occurs in young children younger than age 5 years and in the elderly (Elovic et al. 1996). A survey from Switzerland (Addor and Santos-Eggimann 1996) demonstrated that 66% of all injuries that occurred to preschoolers were as a result of a fall, whereas the work of Benoit et al. (2000) demonstrated that falls accounted for 41% of admissions to a suburban hospital for children ages 0–14 years. Among older adults, more than 60% of fall-related deaths occur in people older than 75 years (National Center for Injury Prevention and Control 2002). A study from New Zealand demonstrated that falls were far more likely to be the cause of injury for elderly patients admitted to the intensive care unit as compared with young patients (Safih et al. 1999). Fatalities as a result of TBI are most common in those older than age 75 years, and falls are the number one cause of TBI in the elderly (Centers for Disease Control and Prevention 2001). Overall, the economic impact of falls can be enormous. In 1994, the estimated cost in the United States from falls approached $20.2 billion (Koplan and Thacker 2000).

Efforts at fall prevention are clearly critical and have shown efficacy in Sweden (Bjerre and Schelp 2000) as well as in an American urban neighborhood (Davidson et al. 1994; Durkin et al. 1998). Because the pattern of those injured secondary to fall is bimodal, so must be the prevention efforts. For children, issues such as protective surfaces on playgrounds (Consumer Product Safety Commission 2001a); having a safe, 12-inch border of a soft material such as wood chips, sand, or rubber around play areas (Consumer Product Safety Commission 2001b); adult supervision; and equipment maintenance and age appropriateness are beneficial ("Playground Safety" 1999). Educational efforts directed at both children and communities have also shown possible benefits (Gresham et al. 2001; Jeffs et al. 1993). Certainly, with falls from windows accounting for 11% of falls in a suburban neighborhood (Benoit et al. 2000), safety devices can be helpful.

Falls involving the elderly require different solutions. Miller et al. (2000) mentioned four common issues that have been implicated in an increased risk of falls in the elderly. They are 1) postural hypotension, 2) gait and balance instability, 3) polypharmacy, and 4) the use of sedating medications. Other host-related factors that have been associated with falls in the elderly include musculo-skeletal or neurological abnormalities, visual disturbances, dementia (National Center for Injury Prevention and Control 2001), and frailty (Speechley and Tinetti 1991). The environment plays an important part in falls of the elderly. The National Bureau of Standards has estimated that 18%–50% of falls are a result of highly waxed floors, loose rugs, sharp furniture, poor lighting, or problems with tubs and showers (Elovic et al. 1996). Some of the fall-prevention ideas for the elderly become quite obvious. The elderly should work on areas of physical conditioning; review medications with their pharmacist or physicians; wear comfortable, gripping shoes; and modify their environment (Brain Injury Association of America 2001a). A study by Plautz et al. (1996) demonstrated that 10 hours of nonskilled time and $93 of supplies per person were all that was needed to make an elderly person's environment substantially safer. When the environment was modified, the rate of falls decreased by 60%, from an annual rate of 0.81 falls per person per year to just 0.33 falls.

Sports and Recreational Injury

Recreation and sports are an important part of many people's lives; however, they can also be a significant cause of injury, including TBI (Annegers et al. 1980; Elovic et al. 1996; Kraus et al. 1984; Whitman et al. 1984). The majority of these injuries are, of course, concussions. Unlike musculoskeletal events, the brain cannot be conditioned to withstand the energy assault that is the cause of concussion (Johnston et al. 2001). Therefore, the emphasis must instead be directed at efforts to design equipment and structure the individual sports to minimize the likelihood of sustaining a TBI. This includes proper equipment design such as helmets for contact sports, sport rules that discourage dangerous activities, and training and educational efforts for coaches and participants.

The importance of dealing with the issue of bicycle-related trauma and TBI becomes obvious once one looks at the statistics. In 1996, more than 500,000 visits to the emergency department were as a result of bicycle-related injuries; almost three-fourths of those injured were younger than 21 years. In 1997, 817 people riding bicycles were killed in an accident between them and a motor vehicle. Almost one-third of them were children younger than 16 years, and only 3% of those killed were wearing a bicycle helmet (Koplan et al. 2000). In patients admitted to a hospital secondary to a brain injury, the risk of death is 20 times higher for those who did not wear a helmet (Think First Foundation 2004). The use of helmets would reduce fatalities by more than 500 and reduce the number of nonfatal injuries by up to 151,000 every year. Financially, the cost of nonfatal bicycle injuries in children younger than 14 years approaches $113 million every year (Koplan et al. 2000).

Thompson et al. (2000) performed an extensive review of the literature to analyze the reduction of risk for cyclists when they are wearing helmets. They found that helmet use was beneficial in the reduction of head, brain, and severe brain injury in all age groups. This was true with both bicycle versus motor vehicle as well as other types of crashes. The reduction in risk in both instances approached 70%. These estimates are conservative when compared with the numbers suggested by work sponsored by the CDC, which reported a risk difference of 85% for brain injury and 88% for TBI (Koplan et al. 2000). Clearly, helmet usage is a major health issue and, as discussed in the section Facilitating Active Strategies to Develop Comprehensive Injury Control in regards to the Maryland experience, legislation and enforcement are important factors in helmet usage. Still, only one-fourth of riders younger than 14 years wear helmets, whereas it is closer to zero for high school students. The goal of Healthy Person 2010 (an initiative sponsored by the U.S. Department of Health and Human Services to promote health) is to increase those rates up to 50% (Koplan et al. 2000).

Helmet usage is only one part of the solution. Modifying cyclists' behavior can also play an important part in prevention. Counseling children to avoid swerving into traffic, riding against traffic flow, and ignoring traffic regulations can also play a part (Koplan et al. 2000). In one study from Iowa (Spence et al. 1993), the behavior of the cyclist was considered the cause of the accident in 70% of fatal cases. Finally, passive strategies must also be used, including road engineering such as bicycle lanes and speed bumps (Koplan et al. 2000).

The incidence of TBI obviously varies depending on the sport being discussed. As expected, the sport of boxing, in which the participants attempt to give each other concussions, has the highest rate. Atha et al. (1985) compared the blow thrown by a top-quality heavyweight boxer to a 13-pound mallet swung at 20 miles an hour. Jordan (2000) reported the incidence of TBI in professional boxers to be approximately 20%. Risk factors that increased its likelihood included career length, number of bouts, poor showings in the ring, and apolipoprotein E genotype. Ryan (1987) performed a review of boxing at both the professional and amateur level between 1918 through 1985 and noted that there was a substantial number of fatalities at both levels. He reported that changes to increase ring safety and improved monitoring of the fighters by the referee and ringside physician have re-

sulted in decreased mortality. However, Ryan thought that these actions were unlikely to affect TBI incidence and that there should be some fundamental rule changes, such as forbidding blows to the head. Public awareness of this issue has been increased with the illness of Muhammad Ali; however, efforts up to this point have not eliminated this substantial source of TBI. Leclerc and Herrera (1999) have suggested that physicians must take an active role in educating the public regarding the risks of boxing. Their statement, "a watchful agnostic position among sport physicians is no longer justifiable" is a call to arms for health care providers to work diligently to educate the public concerning the dangers of boxing. Although abolishing boxing may be an ultimate, but unrealistic, goal, physicians must at a minimum strongly advocate for even greater safety measures (Elovic et al. 1996).

Football is another popular sport that places its participants at risk of sustaining a TBI. In 1974, Blyth and Mueller reported that although TBI accounted for only 5% of overall football injuries, it accounted for 70% of the fatalities, with 75% of them occurring during tackling. At a national level, the estimates for football-related TBI are up to 250,000 concussions and 8 fatalities every year. Furthermore, up to 20% of high school football players sustain one concussion per season played (Kelly et al. 1991; Nguyen et al. 2001; Wilberger 1993). Mueller (1998) reported that TBI and spinal cord injury accounted for 85% of football-related fatalities from 1945 to 1994. The vast majority of the fatalities occurred while tackling or being tackled. As Porter (1999) stated, "players of football will suffer injury." If clinicians have any fantasy of banning boxing, they should have no such illusions regarding football, which is considered by many to be as sacred as a religious icon. Therefore, injury prevention for those who participate and removing the players at greatest risk become the key issues.

Injury prevention methods in football are effective, and the issue of legislation and enforcement as well as passive and active strategies can again be revisited. With immediate punishment and consequences for illegal plays called by the officials, dangerous plays can be discouraged and their incidence greatly reduced. Rule changes prohibiting head butting and face tackling in combination with tougher helmet laws resulted in a significant reduction in football-related fatalities (Mueller and Blyth 1987). Many other prevention efforts are important for TBI associated with football. These include preseason conditioning, safe use of equipment, and training for proper technique (Porter 1999). In addition, proper fitting of helmets and physician evaluation postinjury are also key components of any prevention program (Elovic et al. 1996).

Although found in other sports with the risk of concussion, the issue of second impact syndrome (SIS) is especially critical when dealing with football. SIS is a potentially fatal complication that can result from repeated injuries before recovery from a previous injury that may appear to be relatively minor, with massive cerebral edema, resultant brainstem compression, and possible death (McCrory and Berkovic 1998). The authors caution that SIS is overreported and that there is little strong evidence that is helpful to clinicians regarding warning signs. As a result, the guidelines published by the Colorado Medical Society regarding return to play postconcussion offer the best guidance that physicians have regarding return to play (Kelly et al. 1991).

Another major sport that can account for significant TBI is soccer, or football to the rest of the non-North American world. With estimates of more than 200 million active participants in soccer around the world, injuries that can be caused by playing the sport can become extremely significant even if the rate of injury may be lower than that of other higher contact sports (Dvorak and Junge 2000). Estimates of injury incidence as high as 35 per 1,000 game hours have been reported, with 4%–22% of injuries related to TBI (Nguyen et al. 2001). In Sweden, soccer is the number one source of recreational-related injury, with a rate of 39% reported (Lindqvist et al. 1996). A similar finding was identified in Norway, where an 8-year study demonstrated that soccer accounted for 45% of all sports-related brain injuries (Ytterstad 1996). A survey of athletic trainers looked at the incidence of mild TBI in high school athletes (Powell and Barber-Foss 1999). As expected, football was the largest culprit, implicated in 63% of cases. However, only football had a higher incidence of TBI than soccer, because when injuries to males and females were combined, nearly 13% of all mild TBI resulted from soccer. The incidence for mild TBI per 100 player seasons was 1.14 and 0.92, respectively, for girls and boys high school soccer players (Powell and Barber-Foss 1999). Dvorak et al. (2000) have worked out both a risk analysis for prediction of injuries and a prevention program that addresses issues pertinent to the activities of the trainers, medical professionals, players, and others. They made recommendations for structured training, better medical supervision, improvement of player reaction time (minimizing distractions and personal stress), and improvement in rule design and enforcement that can all lead to less injuries overall.

It is controversial whether or not heading of the ball plays a part in the development of soccer-associated TBI (Nguyen et al. 2001). Soccer is the only sport that has as a major component the intentional use of one's head to redirect a projectile (Kirkendall et al. 2001). Head gear that has been designed to protect soccer players has been of limited value (McIntosh and McCrory 2000). A review of the literature has suggested that heading plays a small part in soccer-related TBI; instead, accidental, unplanned contact against goal posts, head-to-head contact, elbow contact, and a ball kicked directly at the head are more likely to be the source of problems (Kirkendall et al. 2001; Nguyen et al. 2001).

Injury prevention efforts in soccer, therefore, are directed in a means similar to that of American football, including improved training techniques, keeping the players at risk on the sidelines, medical supervision postinjury, enforcement and rule design that minimizes unintentional head contact, and development of better head protection (Kirkendall et al. 2001).

Hockey is one of the roughest and fastest of all sports (Biasca et al. 1995) and places its participants at risk for sustaining TBI. Occasionally, these injuries are potentially lethal, but the vast majority of them are concussive in nature. These injuries occur throughout the spectrum of competition, including small children, high school, college, and the elite professional teams (Honey 1998). These injuries can be potentially career ending because repeated concussions may force a player to retire prematurely. Reid and Losek (1999) surveyed children who presented to an emergency department with ice hockey–related injuries and noted that 57% of all injuries resulted from checking and that 58% of injuries caused by checking were considered significant. They also found a substantial level of ignorance among these children, because 45% of them reported that they could not sustain a brain injury with their protective equipment on. What was most promising was the near 100% compliance with mandatory safety equipment requirements. On the other hand, what may be most frightening is that 32% of the injured children said they would check illegally to win, and 6% said they would intentionally injure an opposing player.

What can be done to lessen the rate of injury from ice hockey? LaPrade et al. (1995) reported that mandatory face masks reduced both facial injuries and TBI. Voaklander et al. (1996) confirmed this in adult recreational hockey players as well, with a decrease in injuries reported when facial masks were used. Honey (1998) reported that mandatory helmet usage also reduced the incidence of TBI. Education of players regarding the risk of TBI as well as examining the pressures to win at the junior level (Reid and Losek 1999) may also play a part in injury prevention. At the youth level, the attitude of the parents must also be examined, with the recent tragic death as a result of a fight between two hockey parents highlighting this issue. Conditioning may also play a part. Pinto et al. (1999) demonstrated that more injuries occur early in the season, late in the periods, and in the final period of games, suggesting that conditioning may assist in injury prevention. The majority of injuries occur during checking, both legal and illegal (Dryden et al. 2000; Reid and Losek 1999). Reduction or at least tighter regulation of checking may also help in injury prevention efforts. Although tough talk is always present with professional hockey teams, analysis shows that in the Stanley Cup finals the teams with the fewest penalties secondary to violent behavior win the majority of the series (McCaw and Walker 1999).

In summary, for all sports-related activities, the formula for reducing TBI and all other injuries is quite simple. Education, better safety equipment, better officiating, improved training, and rule modifications to minimize potential injuries are all critical at all levels but certainly at the amateur level. Society should look at the priorities in regards to competitive sports. How much has society evolved since the Roman gladiators? That is a question that society has to answer.

Violence and Suicide

Concerns over violent injuries have been raised to the highest level of national attention. In the 1990s, violence-related injuries reached epidemic proportions in the United States. In 1987, 89 persons per day were killed by gun violence (Centers for Disease Control and Prevention 1997). Gunshot wounds are a rising cause of brain injuries. Approximately 90% of all persons who sustain a gunshot wound to the head die, many of those before even reaching the emergency department (Kaufman et al. 1986). The percentage of gunshot injuries that are self-inflicted has varied in studies from 11% to 50%, with an unclear number of the self-inflicted injuries being accidental (Krieger et al. 1995; Nagib et al. 1986). In a multicenter study of outcomes after violent injury, Harrison-Felix et al. (1998) have reported that the majority of gunshot wound victims are young males from minority backgrounds.

Gun Control

Dresang (2001) evaluated gun deaths in urban and rural settings. He noted a higher percentage of shotgun and rifle injuries, suicides, and accidents in rural areas, with handguns accounting for more than 50% of gun deaths. Physicians and public policy makers have long struggled with the issue of handgun control, with recent high-profile shootings in the United States causing the issue to come under greater scrutiny. The likelihood of homicide is increased by threefold and suicide by fivefold among those with a gun in the home (Kellermann et al. 1992, 1993). However, the problem is complex because signifi-

cant lobbies exist on both sides of the issue. Thus, policies aimed at handgun control have been attempted but have met with varying success. Sales of firearms at gun shows still occur outside of the realm of regulation (Rodriguez and Gorovitz 1999). Organizations advocating for state gun control laws have typically used media, public education, and legislative lobbying as tactics. Zakocs et al. (2001) have noted that only legislative lobbying has been linked to organizational resources. Although Rodriguez and Gorovitz (1999) stated that only the power of litigation will bring some response to these issues, handgun public policy can make a difference. This was evidenced even in Columbia, a country with a history of handgun violence (Villaveces et al. 2000). Villaveces et al. (2000) noted that a 2-week ban on handguns in Cali and Bogota, Columbia, was associated with a reduction in homicide rates in both cities.

Traditionally, there has been strong opposition in the state legislatures and Congress to enacting gun control laws (Rodriguez and Gorovitz 1999). Howard et al. (1999) reported that 29% of respondents surveyed thought that gun ownership made their homes safer. These individuals tend to be young males who have completed 12 or fewer years of education and have low trust of the police. An additional concern is that no single government agency can compel changes in gun design flaws and complete gun recalls.

Gun Safety

Extrinsic gun safety locks have been the center of debate on gun safety. More than 20 separate types of available locks exist and include trigger locks (the most common), lock boxes, chamber locks, cable locks, hammer locks, barrel locks, grip safeties, and magazine disconnectors (Milne and Hargarten 1999b). The user of any type of safety device should think about the types of injuries the device is designed to prevent and be aware of its limitations (Milne and Hargarten 1999a). Community-based education programs have had some success in encouraging proper storage of firearms (Coyne-Beasley et al. 2001). Gun turn-in programs appear most effective when some tangible reward is offered and among those persons who simply do not desire to have a gun any longer. New technology has allowed for personalized handguns, which may only be discharged by the registered owner. However, demand for such products has been limited.

Other Sources of Violent Injury

The rate of blunt assaults in the United States continues to grow, and this problem is focused in urban areas. Fists, baseball bats, bricks, and bottles are typical instruments of blunt assault (Zafonte et al. 1997). No significant functional outcome differences were noted between survivors of blunt assault and those with nonviolence-related injury. Little has been done in the way of public policy to focus on prevention of blunt assault. Stab wound injuries are common in other parts of the world, and the rate is quite high in South Africa (Campbell et al. 1997).

Depression, Suicide, and TBI

In a study of 2,637 adults sustaining TBI, gender, minority status, age, substance abuse, and residence in a zip code with a low average income were associated with intentional TBI (Wagner et al. 2000). The most highly predictive factors were noted to be minority status and substance abuse. An additional concern is the risk of suicide among those with TBI. Mackenzie and Popkin (1987) reported that suicide risk is greater among patients with physical illness than among the general population. Head trauma has been associated with twice the risk of suicide when compared with the general population. Kishi et al. (2001b) performed a study of several disability groups and noted 25% of patients had major depression and 7.3% reported clinically significant suicidal ideation. Of interest, 11.5% of patients developed such ideation during the rehabilitation phase of care (Kishi et al. 2001a). Several studies have described the fact that among those with major depression, suicidal plans are often not detected (Kishi et al. 2001b). Many patients with brain injury are at risk of developing depressive and suicidal disorders. Clinical evaluation should include an active screening component, and future research should be performed regarding prognostic factors and developing protocols to identify high-risk patients. (See Chapter 11, Psychotic Disorders.)

Drugs and Alcohol

The problem of TBI has been greatly complicated by the additional problem of drugs and alcohol. In 1988, the white paper produced by the National Head Injury Foundation Substance Abuse Task Force stated, "neither age, nor occupation, nor any other factors place an individual at a greater risk of a TBI than does alcohol" (National Head Injury Foundation Professional Council Substance Abuse Task Force 1988). Rivara et al. (1993) reported that the presence of intoxication at the time of trauma admission made the likelihood of a repeat admission for trauma within the next 2 years 2.5 times more likely. Shults et al. (2001) reported that in 1999 there were 15,786 deaths and 300,000 injuries as a result of alcohol-related MVAs. Legal intoxication has been reported in up to 51% of people involved in TBI, whereas up to two-

thirds have some history of drug or alcohol abuse (Corrigan 1995). Cornwell et al. (1998), reporting on data from a level I trauma center, found that 71% of victims tested positive for either drugs or alcohol, with 52% testing positive for alcohol and 42% for other illicit drugs. Madan et al. (1999) reported a similar result, with 70% of trauma patients testing positive for drugs or alcohol. Andersen et al. (1990) reported that 51% of nonbelted passengers involved in MVAs had alcohol on board, whereas Everett et al. (2001) reported that in 1997, 37% of high school students would ride with a driver who had been drinking, and 17% would drive after they had been drinking. Evidence from crashes involving motorcycles indicates a rate of driver alcohol intoxication of 42% (Peek-Asa and Kraus 1996), which is comparable with the numbers in the other studies quoted.

As expected, alcohol problems have an effect on injury occurrence, even when driving is not involved. Hingson et al. (2001) reported that those who started drinking alcohol before age 17 years were four times more likely to be involved in a fight after drinking than those who started drinking after age 21 years. Kolakowsky-Hayner et al. (1999) examined the incidence of alcoholism in both TBI and spinal cord injury patients and found that in both groups premorbid alcohol use was high. The rates were 81% and 96%, respectively, for the two groups, whereas the rate for heavy drinking was 42% and 57%.

There is some question as to whether alcohol has any effect on patient outcome when those who used alcohol premorbidly are compared with others with equivalent injuries who did not use alcohol. In 1992, Gurney et al. reported that acute intoxication at time of injury resulted in an increased risk of pulmonary complications, including aspiration, pneumonia, and respiratory distress, and patients were more likely to require intubation. However, the work of Cornwell et al. (1998) did not support the notion that alcohol increased acute problems. Relative to rehabilitation outcomes, there has been evidence that alcohol may negatively affect outcome. Sparedo and Gill (1989) reported a correlation between acute intoxication and lower functional levels at discharge and a longer duration of agitation, whereas Kaplan and Corrigan (1992) reported that it was correlated with longer acute hospitalization and a longer period of posttraumatic amnesia. Tate et al. (1999) reported that the presence of alcohol on admission screen to the trauma hospital has been correlated with decreases in verbal memory and visuospatial function.

Trauma patients are not always tested for the presence of alcohol (Corrigan 1995), with some studies reporting less than one-half of trauma patients being tested. This information is critical for both clinical and academic purposes, and it is tragic that it is not being collected. A possible reason for the reluctance to obtain this information is to protect the patient. Evidence of legal intoxication or the presence of illicit drugs may result in either legal prosecution or denial of insurance coverage. This lack of information may compromise both clinical care and further research efforts.

The numbers speak for themselves and are a confirmation of the National Head Injury Foundation's White Paper from 1988. Prevention efforts must clearly be designed that will minimize and mitigate the effects that alcohol and drugs have on both the incidence and severity of trauma. Passive efforts at injury prevention related to alcohol such as Breathalyzer, mental status, or coordination testing before individuals are allowed to start a car have been discussed for years but have not become a reality. In other words, efforts at purely passive strategies have been quite limited.

One possible intervention that remains passive for the drinker is to modify the behavior of those who serve alcohol. This is partly based on the concept that many people drink and drive after consuming alcohol at bars, clubs, and restaurants (Shults et al. 2001). Past research has demonstrated that 40%–60% of those who drive under the influence have recently left a professional establishment that serves alcohol (Lang and Stockwell 1991; O'Donnell 1985). What possible interventions can be undertaken by servers? Slowing services for rapid drinkers, refusing service, careful screening of potential underage drinkers, and offering food to those drinking are all means to delay, minimize, and eliminate potential intoxication and driving under the influence (DUI). By early 2000, 11 states had mandatory and 10 others had voluntary programs addressing server education. These programs are not well standardized, but often include items such as education about the laws regarding intoxication and DUI and recognizing the signs of intoxication. Other items that are addressed include review of the liability issues that the establishment may be subject to on the basis of serving potential drivers who then drive under the influence and possibly have a severe accident. Knowledge of potential liability may assist the servers to be supported by their management structure (Shults et al. 2001).

These programs appear to be effective in several measures. The performance of the servers themselves was improved in rating for both appropriate and inappropriate actions (Gliksman et al. 1993) as well as demonstrating decreased levels of intoxication (Lang et al. 1998; Russ and Geller 1987; Saltz 1987). These interventions have been shown to be of some benefit, but how long is the effect maintained? Buka and Birdthistle (1999) have demonstrated efficacy for up to 15 months, with a gradual dropoff after that point. This suggests that some form of

a refresher or recertification program for the servers may be indicated.

What is gratifying about alcohol-related prevention efforts is that progress has been made. Since 1982, the rate of alcohol-related MVA fatalities has steadily dropped from a rate of 57%–38% (Shults et al. 2001). By the year 2000, alcohol-related MVA fatalities had dropped to a rate of 5.8 per 100,000. This is probably due to the combined work of numerous interventions, including public education, community involvement, legislation, and enforcement. Community programs such as Mothers Against Drunk Driving have been instrumental in having the legal drinking age raised to 21 years throughout the United States (Elovic et al. 1996).

Making alcohol "illegal" for teenagers has not totally eliminated alcohol as a problem for teenage drivers. Alcohol has clearly been found in adolescents involved in trauma (Spain et al. 1997). In addition, when asked, 41% of college students report having been binge drinking during the previous 2 weeks (National Center for Alcohol and Drug Information 1999), and in 1997, 21% of those killed while driving intoxicated were 15–20 years old (Koplan et al. 2000). Control of access clearly is not enough to address the problem of alcohol-related MVA because literature has shown that people can obtain an agent even if it is against the law. For teenagers and those older than the age of 21 years, it has to be illegal to drive under the influence of alcohol, and the authorities must enforce these regulations.

It is estimated that there are more than 1.4 million DUI arrests every year in the United States, which is just a small number when compared with the estimated 126 million episodes of DUI that actually occur (Koplan et al. 2000). The original driving while intoxicated or under the influence laws set the legal blood alcohol level at 0.10 g/dL. In 1983, Utah and Oregon were the first two states that lowered the level to 0.08 g/dL. As of May 2001, there were 24 states that had passed laws that lowered the acceptable blood alcohol level to less than 0.08 g/dL for drivers 21 years old and older (Shults et al. 2001). For those 20 years old and younger, any evidence of blood alcohol is considered illegal and is subject to legal sanction (Brain Injury Association of America 2002; Shults et al. 2001).

What has been the result of the lower tolerated blood alcohol level? This question has been addressed in several studies (Apsler et al. 1999; Foss et al. 2001; Hingson et al. 1996, 2000; Johnson and Fell 1995; Research and Evaluation Associates 1991; Rogers 1995; Scopatz 1998; Voas et al. 2000), which have been reviewed by Shults et al. (2001). The reviewers reported that the overall rate of alcohol-related MVA fatalities dropped by 7% in the combined studies. Some of the data were difficult to interpret because of other changes in legal enforcement of DUI laws. In California and some of the other states, laws allowing immediate confiscation of licensure, called *administrative license revocation*, were also implemented. In an effort to isolate the effects, Hingson et al. (2000) looked at the effect of the blood alcohol concentration (BAC) change in states that already had administrative license revocation rules on the books and noted a 5% decrease in alcohol-related fatalities when the lower BAC rule was instituted. Voas et al. (2000) used multivariate analysis to demonstrate that the lowering of the BAC level accounted for 8% of the reduction in alcohol-related fatalities by itself. The states involved in these studies are culturally, demographically, and geographically diverse, including the states of California, Utah, Vermont, Maine, and Oregon. As a result, it is reasonable to assume that the results of these studies are likely to be representative of the United States as a whole (Shults et al. 2001). The U.S. Congress was impressed enough by the evidence that in 2000 legislation was passed that required all states to lower the BAC to 0.08 g/dL by October 2003 or they would lose federal highway funds (Department of Transportation and Related Agencies Appropriations Act of 2001 [P.L. 106-346]).

There is evidence that younger drivers partake in other risk-taking behaviors when they drive and are at greater risk of MVA than more experienced drivers. This may be an issue of decreased experience or a combination of other risk-taking behaviors that are associated with alcohol ingestion. As an example, in 1990 Andersen et al. demonstrated that more than one-half of non–seat-belt-wearing drivers involved in an MVA were positive for alcohol as compared with 22% of those wearing shoulder belts. In addition, those who ingest alcohol are less likely to use restraints. Spain et al. (1997) demonstrated that only 7% of adolescents involved in MVAs with positive alcohol screens were using a restraint system at the time of the accident as compared with 22% who had no alcohol found on screening. Also, Peek-Asa and Kraus (1996) demonstrated that motorcyclists involved in accidents who tested positive for alcohol were more likely to be speeding and not be wearing a helmet. Finally, Zador et al. (2000) estimated that a 16- to 20-year-old male with a BAC level between 0.08 and 0.1 g/dL has a 24 times greater chance of dying from an MVA as compared with a BAC of 0. Again mandated by the U.S. Congress' threat to withhold highway funding, by July 1998, all states had passed laws requiring a BAC level of less than 0.02 g/dL for all drivers younger than 21 years (Shults et al. 2001). The minimum drinking age (MDA) was first raised to 21 years in several states in the 1970s. By 1987, all 50 states had raised the MDA to 21 years (Shults et al.

2001). The review by Shults et al. demonstrated double-digit decreases in both fatal and nonfatal MVAs with the increase in the MDA.

Proper enforcement is required for legislative actions to be effective. As mentioned earlier, the number of DUI arrests is less than 1% of the actual violation. There is a need to improve enforcement efforts to give teeth to any legislative efforts. Sobriety checkpoints are one effective means of addressing this issue. There are two types of sobriety checkpoints. The first, using random breath testing (RBT), has been used with effect in Australia and some countries in Europe. RBT is not currently in use in the United States because of the issue of probable cause and legal searches. In the United States, only the second type of sobriety checkpoints, called *selective breath testing* (SBT), is in use. With SBT checkpoints, only when there is a suspicion of intoxication is breath testing performed. These checkpoints are used not so much to actually identify drivers who are DUI, but rather it is believed that the risk of testing for BAC can be a deterrent that will cause drivers to modify their behavior (Shults et al. 2001).

These SBT checkpoints have been shown to reduce fatal car crashes 20%–26% (Castle et al. 1995; Lacey et al. 1999) as well as to reduce overall crashes anywhere from 5% to 23% (Shults et al. 2001). RBT has been tested and has also been shown to be effective in reducing both fatal (Arthurson 1985; Henstridege et al. 1997; Hormel et al. 1988; Ross et al. 1981) and nonfatal crashes (Armour et al. 1985; Cameron et al. 1997; Dunbar et al. 1987; Hardes et al. 1985; Henstridege et al. 1997; Hormel et al. 1988; McLean et al. 1984; Ross et al. 1981). The studies of RBT showed a reduction in fatal crashes between 13% and 36% (Arthurson 1985; Henstridege et al. 1997; Hormel et al. 1988; Ross et al. 1981) and 11%–20% for all crashes (Armour et al. 1985; Cameron et al. 1997; Dunbar et al. 1987; Hardes et al. 1985; Henstridege et al. 1997; Hormel et al. 1988; McLean et al. 1984; Ross et al. 1981). There is also direct evidence that RBT can potentially modify drivers' behavior in regards to drinking and driving. One study from Australia reported a 13% drop in drivers with any detectable alcohol on board and a 24% decrease in BAC level greater than 0.08 g/dL with RBT (Henstridege et al. 1997). The literature has shown that both the selective and random method of testing has been useful in reducing crashes of all types. Although RBT is more sensitive than SBT relative to detecting elevated BAC, the literature has not demonstrated any difference in efficacy between the two methods relative to crash prevention (Shults et al. 2001). In addition, passive sensors that can sample for the presence of alcohol are being developed that may further increase the sensitivity of SBT by 50% (Voas et al. 1997).

Despite the apparent efficacy of these programs, there is some resistance to them. On the basis of possible violation of civil rights, many have objected to the use of sobriety checkpoints. The United States Supreme Court has ruled on the appropriateness of a properly performed brief sobriety check. The court's decision was based on the premise that the minor intrusion on human rights was more than balanced out by reducing DUI (*Michigan Department of State Police v. Sitz* [1990]). Another objection raised regarding the use of SBT is the economics of having police officers man these checkpoints. Miller et al. (1998) have looked at the economic benefit of SBT. They created a model for one community of 100,000 licensed drivers and assumed that the intervention would reduce accidents by 15%, a number that is reasonable after reviewing the literature on SBT. Incorporating all of the costs of alcohol-related MVA, including medical and property costs, their estimates were that $9.2 million would be saved, with an expenditure of $1.6 million (a ratio of nearly 6 to 1). An actual study from California was even more promising. Four communities introduced SBT for more than nine months at a relatively small cost of $165,000. The resultant savings were 23 times as large, with an estimated benefit of $3.86 million. This was in addition to a 20% reduction in alcohol-related car crashes during that time. RBT testing has also been shown to be of possibly even greater benefit than SBT from a financial standpoint. Work from Australia and New South Wales suggested that at an annual cost of $4 million per year, a savings of $228 million was realized as a result of accident prevention (Arthurson 1985). The efficacy of these programs, both from a financial as well as from crash prevention standpoints, warrants serious consideration. (See Chapter 29, Alcohol and Drug Disorders.)

Pediatric Brain Trauma

Brain trauma is one of the most common childhood injuries, resulting in more than 500,000 emergency department visits annually (Schutzman and Greenes 2001). The annual costs exceed $1 billion annually, and 29,000 children sustain permanent disabilities.

Child Abuse

In a survey of pediatric brain trauma, accidents accounted for 81% of cases and definite abuse for 19% (Reece and Sege 2000). The definite abuse group was noted to have a higher rate of subdural hematoma and subarachnoid hemorrhage, as well as retinal hemorrhages (Reece and Sege 2000). Of interest, retinal hemorrhage occurs rarely in accidental brain injury and appears to be associated with extraordinary force (Johnson et al. 1993). Cutaneous

and skeletal injuries were higher in the definite abuse group, whereas mortality rates were also higher in this group. Shaken baby syndrome results from aggressive movements of a child, with young infants particularly susceptible to injury because of their weak neck muscles, leaving them vulnerable to sustain subdural hematoma and shearing injuries. Injuries seen with shaken baby syndrome include cerebral axonal injury and occult cervical injury (Shannon et al. 1998). Coagulopathy is a common complication in the presence of abusive brain trauma with associated parenchymal damage (Hymel et al. 1997). Family and public education programs have begun to educate the community about the severe danger of shaking infants. Clinicians should be keenly aware of findings that point away from accidental injury and toward intentional trauma.

Car Seats and Air Bags

Motor vehicle crashes are the leading cause of death in children ages 5–14 years. Children placed in the front seat are at particular risk for injury. After a substantial public education campaign, the 1990s saw a decline in front seating of children in vehicles involved in fatal crashes (Wittenberg et al. 2001). However, children ages 6–12 years remained at high risk for being front seated (Wittenberg et al. 2001). Air bags systems pose a threat to the front-seated child passenger if deployed, with resultant cranial and cervical spine trauma (Marshall et al. 1998). Although low-powered systems are available, these systems remain potentially fatal to the front-seated child passenger because of the biomechanics at impact placing the child closer to the deploying air bag (Tyroch et al. 2000). Both the age and weight of the child determine the appropriate restraint system. Child restraint system use has been affected by legislation; however, the rate of correct usage of these devices is concerning (Kunkel et al. 2001). Programs focused on educating parents regarding the proper use of child restraint systems have met with mixed results.

Playground and Recreational Injuries

Between 1990 and 1994, more than 200,000 playground injuries were reported. The vast majority of these injuries are related to climbing activities (monkey bars, jungle gyms, swings, and slides), with some 25% of such injuries requiring hospitalization (Waltzman et al. 1999). Of all children hospitalized, some 62% were injured on a climbing apparatus, and swings are disproportionately associated with brain injuries (Waltzman et al. 1999). Of those children younger than age 5 years, 58% had head and cervical injuries (Lillis and Jaffe 1997). Adult supervision does not seem to influence the injury pattern, and a fall of just a few feet can result in serious consequences (Kotch et al. 1993). Kelley et al. (2001) have noted that 8% of sport- and recreation-related brain injuries are playground related. Several preventable sources of injury such as walking behind a moving swing and the use of equipment designed for younger children by older children have been identified. Falls from playground equipment offer some potential for prevention (Plunkett 2001). The design of safer playground sites has been pushed more by litigation than public policy. The role of multipurpose helmets in such a setting is not yet clear. Skateboards are a common source of brain injuries in the pediatric population. It appears that the rate of injury secondary to skateboards has surpassed that of bicyclists for those younger than 25 years (Illingworth et al. 1978). A significant portion of these injuries occur on the first day of skateboarding, and the role of helmets in preventing serious injury appears to be self-evident.

Summary

Great strides have been made in TBI prevention since the 1950s. Although much work still needs to be accomplished, the savings in life years, productive years, health resources, and human suffering have been enormous. Health care providers must continue to be vigilant to assist politicians and the lay public in recognizing the benefits of injury prevention. It is hoped that as technology improves, so will prevention efforts.

References

Air-bag-associated fatal injuries to infants and children riding in front passenger seats—United States. MMWR Morb Mortal Wkly Rep 44:845–847, 1995

Addor V, Santos-Eggimann B: Population-based incidence of injuries among preschoolers. Eur J Pediatr 155:130–135, 1996

Agran PF, Dunkle DE, Winn DG: Injuries to a sample of seatbelted children evaluated and treated in a hospital emergency room. J Trauma 27:58–64, 1987

American Cancer Society: Cancer facts and figures, selected cancers. Available at: http://www.cancer.org/statistics/cff99/selectedcancers.html. Accessed August 2, 2001.

Andersen JA, McLellan BA, Pagliarello G, et al: The relative influence of alcohol and seatbelt usage on severity of injury from motor vehicle crashes. J Trauma 30:415–417, 1990

Angel CA, Ehlers RA: Images in clinical medicine: atloido-occipital dislocation in a small child after air-bag deployment. N Engl J Med 345:1256, 2001

Annegers JF, Grabow JD, Kurland LT, et al: The incidence, causes, and secular trends of head trauma in Olmsted County, Minnesota, 1935–1974. Neurology 30:912–919, 1980

Appleby JP, Nagy AG: Abdominal injuries associated with the use of seatbelts. Am J Surg 157:457–458, 1989

Apsler R, Char AR, Harding WM, et al: The effects of .08 BAC laws. DOT HS 808 892. Washington, DC, U.S. Department of Transportation, National Highway Traffic Safety Administration, National Center for Statistics and Analysis, Community Preventive Services, 1999

Arajarvi E, Santavirta S, Tolonen J: Abdominal injuries sustained in severe traffic accidents by seatbelt wearers. J Trauma 27:393–397, 1987

Armour M, Monk K, South D, et al: Evaluation of the 1983 Melbourne random breath testing campaign: interim report, casualty accident analysis. N8–85. Melbourne, Australia, Victoria Road Traffic Authority, 1985

Arthurson RM: Evaluation of random breath testing. Sydney, Australia, Research Note RN 10/85, Traffic Authority of New South Wales, 1985

Atha J, Yeardon MR, Sandover J, et al: The damaging punch. BMJ 291:21–28, 1985

Bachulis BL, Sangster W, Gorrell GW, et al: Patterns of injury in helmeted and nonhelmeted motorcyclists. Am J Surg 155:708–711, 1988

Baker SP: Determinates of injury and opportunities for intervention. Am J Epidemiol 101:98–102, 1975

Bandstra RA, Carbone LS: Unusual basal skull fracture in a vehicle equipped with an air bag. Am J Forensic Med Pathol 22:253–255, 2001

Beckerman B, Elberger S: Air bag ear. Ann Emerg Med 20:831–832, 1991

Begg DJ, Langley JD, Reeder AI: Motorcycle crashes in New Zealand resulting in death and hospitalisation, I: introduction, methods and overview. Accid Anal Prev 26:157–164, 1994

Benoit R, Watts DD, Dwyer K, et al: Windows 99: a source of suburban pediatric trauma. J Trauma 49:477–481, 2000

Biasca N, Simmen HP, Bartolozzi AR, et al: Review of typical ice hockey injuries: survey of the North American NHL and Hockey Canada versus European leagues. Unfallchirurg 98:283–288, 1995

Bjerre B, Schelp L: The community safety approach in Falun, Sweden: is it possible to characterise the most effective prevention endeavours and how long-lasting are the results? Accid Anal Prev 32:461–470, 2000

Blacksin MF: Patterns of fracture after air bag deployment. J Trauma 35:840–843, 1993

Blyth CS, Mueller F: Football injury survey, Part 1: when and where players get hurt. Physician Sportsmed 9:45–52, 1974

Bourbeau R, Desjardins D, Maag U, et al: Neck injuries among belted and unbelted occupants of the front seat of cars. J Trauma 35:794–799, 1993

Braddock M, Schwartz R, Lapidus G, et al: A population-based study of motorcycle injury and costs. Ann Emerg Med 21:273–278, 1992

Brain Injury Association of America: Falls. Available at: http://www.biausa.org. Accessed August 2, 2001. 2001a.

Brain Injury Association of America: TBI incidence. Available at: http://www.biausa.org. Accessed August 2, 2001. 2001b.

Brain Injury Association of America: Understanding and preventing adolescent brain injury: the teenage years. Available at: http://www.biausa.org. Accessed October 7, 2002.

Buka SL, Birdthistle IJ: Long-term effects of a community-wide alcohol server training intervention. J Stud Alcohol 60:27–36, 1999

Cameron M, Diamantopolou K, Mullan N, et al: Evaluation of the country random breath testing and publicity program in Victoria, 1993–1994. Report 126. Melbourne, Australia, Monash University Accident Research Center, 1997

Campbell NC, Thomson SR, Muckart DJ, et al: Review of 1198 cases of penetrating cardiac trauma. Br J Surg 84:1737–1740, 1997

Castle SP, Thompson JD, Spataro JA: Early evaluation of a statewide sobriety checkpoint program, in 39th annual proceedings of the Association for the Advancement of Automotive Medicine. Chicago, IL, 1995

Centers for Disease Control and Prevention: Traumatic brain injury in the United States: a report to Congress. Available at: http://www.cdc.gov/ncipc/pub-res/tbicongress.htm. Accessed August 2, 2001.

Centers for Disease Control and Prevention. National Center for Health Statistics Division of Vital Statistics. National Center for Injury Prevention and Control. 1997

Chandler CF, Lane JS, Waxman KS: Seatbelt sign following blunt trauma is associated with increased incidence of abdominal injury. Am Surg 63:885–888, 1997

Chiu WT, Kuo CY, Hung CC, et al: The effect of the Taiwan motorcycle helmet use law on head injuries. Am J Public Health 90:793–796, 2000

Conover K: Chemical burn from automotive air bag. Ann Emerg Med 2:770, 1992

Consumer Product Safety Commission: Home playground safety tips. Available at: http://www.cpsc.gov/cpscpub/pubs/323.html. Accessed August 2, 2001. 2001a.

Consumer Product Safety Commission: Public playground safety checklist. Available at: http://www.cpsc.gov/cpscpub/pubs/327.html. Accessed August 2, 2001. 2001b.

Cooper K, Tabaddor K, Hauser WA, et al: The epidemiology of head injury in the Bronx. Neuroepidemiology 2:70–88, 1983

Cornwell EE III, Belzberg H, Velmahos G, et al: The prevalence and effect of alcohol and drug abuse on cohort-matched critically injured patients. Am Surg 64:461–465, 1998

Corrigan JD: Substance abuse as a mediating factor in outcome from traumatic brain injury. Arch Phys Med Rehabil 76:302–309, 1995

Coyne-Beasley T, Schoenbach VJ, Johnson RM: "Love our kids, lock your guns": a community-based firearm safety counseling and gun lock distribution program. Arch Pediatr Adolesc Med 155:659–664, 2001

Davidson LL, Durkin MS, Kuhn L, et al: The impact of the Safe Kids/Healthy Neighborhoods Injury Prevention Program in Harlem, 1988 through 1991. Am J Public Health 84:580–586, 1994

Department of Transportation and Related Agencies Appropriations Act of 2001. Pub. L. No. 106–346. 2000. (2002)

DiGuiseppi C, Roberts IG: Individual-level injury prevention strategies in the clinical setting. Future Child 10:53–82, 2000

Dresang LT: Gun deaths in rural and urban settings: recommendations for prevention. J Am Board Fam Pract 14:107–115, 2001

Dryden DM, Francescutti LH, Rowe BH, et al: Epidemiology of women's recreational ice hockey injuries. Med Sci Sports Exerc 32:1378–1383, 2000

Dunbar JA, Penttila A, Pikkarainen J: Drinking and driving: success of random breath testing in Finland. BMJ (Clin Res Ed) 295:101–103, 1987

Durkin MS, Olsen S, Barlow B, et al: The epidemiology of urban pediatric neurological trauma: evaluation of, and implications for, injury prevention programs. Neurosurgery 42:300–310, 1998

Dvorak J, Junge A: Football injuries and physical symptoms: a review of the literature. Am J Sports Med 28:S3–S9, 2000

Dvorak J, Junge A, Chomiak J: Risk factor analysis for injuries in football players. Am J Sports Med 28:S69–S74, 2000

Elovic E, Antoinette T: Epidemiology and primary prevention of traumatic brain injury, in Medical Rehabilitation of Traumatic Brain Injury. Edited by Horn LJ, Zasler ND. Philadelphia, PA, Hanley & Belfus, 1996, pp 1–28

Everett SA, Shults RA, Barrios LC, et al: Trends and subgroup differences in transportation-related injury risk and safety behaviors among high school students, 1991–1997. J Adolesc Health 28:228–234, 2001

Ferrando J, Plasencia A, Oros M, et al: Impact of a helmet law on two wheel motor vehicle crash mortality in a southern European urban area. Inj Prev 6:184–188, 2000

Fleming NS, Becker ER: The impact of the Texas 1989 motorcycle helmet law on total and head-related fatalities, severe injuries, and overall injuries. Med Care 30:832–845, 1992

Flint S: Prevention Matters. McLean, VA, Brain Injury Association of America, 2001

From the Centers for Disease Control and Prevention: Air-bag-associated fatal injuries to infants and children riding in front passenger seats—United States. JAMA 274:1752–1753, 1995

From the Centers for Disease Control and Prevention: Update: fatal air-bag-related injuries to children—United States, 1993–1996. JAMA 277:11–12, 1997

Foss RD, Stewart JR, Reinfurt DW: Evaluation of the effects of North Carolina's 0.08% BAC law. Available at: http://www.nhtsa.dot.gov/people/ncsa/nc08.html. Accessed August 2, 2001.

Gabella B, Reiner KL, Hoffman RE, et al: Relationship of helmet use and head injuries among motorcycle crash victims in El Paso County, Colorado, 1989–1990, Accid Anal Prev 27:363–369, 1995

Gennarelli TA, Champion HR, Sacco WJ, et al: Mortality of patients with head injury and extracranial injury treated in trauma centers. J Trauma 29:1193–1201, 1989

Ghafouri A, Burgess SK, Hrdlicka ZK, et al: Air bag–related ocular trauma. Am J Emerg Med 15:389–392, 1997

Gielen AC, Girasek DC: Integrating perspectives on the prevention of unintentional injuries, in Integrating Behavioral and Social Sciences With Public Health. Edited by Schneiderman NM, Speers A, Silva JM, Tomes H, Gentry JH. Washington, DC, American Psychological Association, 2001, pp 203–227

Giguere JF, St Vil D, Turmel A, et al: Airbags and children: a spectrum of C-spine injuries. J Pediatr Surg 33:811–816, 1998

Gliksman L, McKensie D, Single E, et al: The role of alcohol providers in prevention: an evaluation of a server intervention programme. Addiction 88:1195–1203, 1993

Graham JD, Thompson KM, Goldie SJ, et al: The cost-effectiveness of air bags by seating position. JAMA 278:1418–1425, 1997

Gresham LS, Zirkle DL, Tolchin S, et al: Partnering for injury prevention: evaluation of a curriculum-based intervention program among elementary school children. J Pediatr Nurs 16:79–87, 2001

Guarino AH: More on reflex sympathetic dystrophy syndrome following air-bag inflation. N Engl J Med 338:335, 1998

Guerrero JL, Thurman DJ, Sniezek JE: Emergency department visits associated with traumatic brain injury: United States, 1995–1996. Brain Inj 14:181–186, 2000

Gurney JG, Rivara FP, Mueller BA, et al: The effects of alcohol intoxication on the initial treatment and hospital course of patients with acute brain injury. J Trauma 33:709–713, 1992

Guyer B, Gallagher SS: An approach to the epidemiology of childhood injuries. Pediatr Clin North Am 32:5–15, 1992

Haddon W: The changing approach to the epidemiology, prevention, and amelioration of trauma: the transition to approaches etiologically rather than descriptively based. Am J Public Health 58:1431–1438, 1968

Haddon W: On the escape of tigers: an ecological note. MIT Tech Review 72:44–53, 1970

Hall CE, Norton SA, Dixon AR: Complete small bowel transection following lap-belt injury. Injury 32:640–641, 2001

Hardes G, Gibberd RW, Lam P, et al: Effects of random breath testing on hospital admissions of traffic-accident casualties in the Hunter Health Region. Med J Aust 142:625–626, 1985

Harrison-Felix C, Zafonte R, Mann N, et al: Brain injury as a result of violence: preliminary findings from the traumatic brain injury model systems. Arch Phys Med Rehabil 79:730–737, 1998

Head injuries associated with motorcycle use—Wisconsin, 1991. MMWR Morb Mortal Wkly Rep 43:423, 429–423, 431, 1994

Heilman DR, Weisbuch JB, Blair RW, et al: Motorcycle-related trauma and helmet usage in North Dakota. Ann Emerg Med 11:659–664, 1982

Henstridge J, Homel R, Mackay P: The long-term effects of random breath testing in four Australian states: a time series analysis, No. CR 162. Canberra, Australia, Federal Office of Road Safety, 1997

Hingson R, Heeren T, Winter M: Lowering state legal blood alcohol limits to 0.08%: the effect on fatal motor vehicle crashes. Am J Prev Med 86:1297–1299, 1996

Hingson R, Heeren T, Winter M: Effects of recent 0.08% legal blood alcohol limits on fatal crash involvement. Inj Prev 6:109–114, 2000

Hingson R, Heeren T, Zakocs R: Age of drinking onset and involvement in physical fights after drinking. Pediatrics 108:872–877, 2001

Holbrook JL, Bennett JB: Brachial plexus injury associated with chest restraint seatbelt: case report. J Trauma 30:1413–1414, 1990

Honey CR: Brain injury in ice hockey. Clin J Sport Med 8:43–46, 1998

Hormel R, Carseldine D, Kearns I: Drink-driving countermeasures in Australia. Alcohol Drugs Driving 4:113–144, 1988

Hotz GA, Cohn SM, Popkin C, et al: The impact of a repealed motorcycle helmet law in Miami-Dade County. J Trauma 52:469–474, 2002

Howard KA, Webster DW, Vernick JS: Beliefs about the risks of guns in the home: analysis of a national survey. Inj Prev 5:284–289, 1999

Hymel KP, Abshire TC, Luckey DW, et al: Coagulopathy in pediatric abusive head trauma. Pediatrics 99:371–375, 1997

Illingworth CM, Jay A, Noble D, et al: 225 skateboard injuries in children. Clin Pediatr (Phila) 17:781–789, 1978

Immega G: Whiplash injuries increase with seatbelt use. Can Fam Physician 41:203–204, 1995

Jagger J: Prevention of brain trauma by legislation, regulation and improved technology: a focus on motor vehicles. Neurotrauma 9S:313–316, 1992

Jagger J, Levine JI, Jane JA, et al: Epidemiologic features of head injury in a predominantly rural population. J Trauma 24:40–44, 1984

Jeffs D, Booth D, Calvert D: Local injury information, community participation and injury reduction. Aust J Public Health 17:365–372, 1993

Johnson D, Fell J: The impact of lowering the illegal BAC limit to .08 in five states, in 39th Annual Proceedings, Association for the Advancement of Automotive Medicine, Chicago, IL, 1995

Johnson DL, Falci S: The diagnosis and treatment of pediatric lumbar spine injuries caused by rear seat lap belts. Neurosurgery 26:434–441, 1990

Johnson DL, Braun D, Friendly D: Accidental head trauma and retinal hemorrhage. Neurosurgery 33:231–234, 1993

Johnston KM, McCrory P, Mohtadi NG, et al: Evidence-based review of sport-related concussion: clinical science. Clin J Sport Med 11:150–159, 2001

Jordan BD: Chronic traumatic brain injury associated with boxing. Semin Neurol 20:179–185, 2000

Kaplan BH, Cowley RA: Seatbelt effectiveness and cost of noncompliance among drivers admitted to a trauma center. Am J Emerg Med 9:4–10, 1991

Kaplan CP, Corrigan JD: Effect of blood alcohol level on recovery from severe closed head injury. Brain Inj 6:337–349, 1992

Karlson TA: Injury control and public policy. Crit Rev Environ Contr 22:195–241, 1992

Kaufman HH, Makela ME, Lee KF, et al: Gunshot wounds to the head: a perspective. Neurosurgery 18:689–695, 1986

Kellermann AL, Rivara FP, Somes G, et al: Suicide in the home in relation to gun ownership. N Engl J Med 327:467–472, 1992

Kellermann AL, Rivara FP, Rushforth NB, et al: Gun ownership as a risk factor for homicide in the home. N Engl J Med 329:1084–1091, 1993

Kelly JP, Nichols JS, Filley CM, et al: Concussion in sports: guidelines for the prevention of catastrophic outcome. JAMA 266:2867–2869, 1991

Kelly KD, Lissel HL, Rowe BH, et al: Sport and recreation-related head injuries treated in the emergency department. Clin J Sport Med 11:77–81, 2001

Kirchhoff R, Rasmussen SW: Forearm fracture due to the release of an automobile air bag. Acta Orthop Scand 66:483, 1995

Kirkendall DT, Jordan SE, Garret WE: Heading and head injuries in soccer. Sports Med 31:369–386, 2001

Kishi Y, Robinson RG, Kosier JT: Suicidal ideation among patients during the rehabilitation period after life-threatening physical illness. J Nerv Ment Dis 189:623–628, 2001a

Kishi Y, Robinson RG, Kosier JT: Suicidal ideation among patients with acute life-threatening physical illness: patients with stroke, traumatic brain injury, myocardial infarction, and spinal cord injury. Psychosomatics 42:382–390, 2001b

Klassen TP, MacKay JM, Moher D, et al: Community-based injury prevention interventions. Future Child 10:83–110, 2000

Kolakowsky-Hayner SA, Gourley EV III, Kreutzer JS, et al: Pre-injury substance abuse among persons with brain injury and persons with spinal cord injury. Brain Inj 13:571–581, 1999

Koplan JP, Thacker SB: Working to prevent and control injury in the United States. Fact Book for the Year 2000. Centers for Disease Control and Prevention National Center for Injury Prevention and Control, 1999

Kotch JB, Chalmers DJ, Langley JD, et al: Child day care and home injuries involving playground equipment. J Paediatr Child Health 29:222–227, 1993

Kramer MB, Shattuck TG, Charnock DR: Traumatic hearing loss following air-bag inflation. N Engl J Med 337:574–575, 1993

Kraus JF, Black MA, Hessol N, et al: The incidence of acute brain injury and serious impairment in a defined population. Am J Epidemiol 119:186–201, 1984

Kraus JF, Peek C, McArthur DL, et al: The effect of the 1992 California motorcycle helmet use law on motorcycle crash fatalities and injuries. JAMA 272:1506–1511, 1994

Krieger MD, Levy ML, Apuzzo ML: Gunshot wounds to the head in an urban setting. Neurosurg Clin N Am 6:605–610, 1994

Kunkel NC, Nelson DS, Schunk JE: Do parents choose appropriate automotive restraint devices for their children? Clin Pediatr (Phila) 40:35–40, 2001

Lacey JH, Jones RK, Smith RG: Evaluation of checkpoint Tennessee: Tennessee's statewide sobriety checkpoint program. Washington, DC, U.S. Department of Transportation, National Highway Traffic Safety Administration, DOT HS 808 841, 1999

Lang E, Stockwell TR: Drinking locations of drink-drivers: an analysis of accident and non-accident cases. Accid Anal Prev 23:573–584, 1991

Lang E, Stockwell TR, Rydon P, et al: Can training bar staff in responsible serving practices reduce alcohol-related harm? Drug Alcohol Rev 17:39–50, 1998

LaPrade RF, Burnett QM, Zarzour R: The effect of the mandatory use of face masks on facial laceration and head and neck injuries in ice hockey. Am J Sports Med 23:773–775, 1995

Leclerc S, Herrera CD: Sport medicine and the ethics of boxing. Br J Sports Med 33:426–429, 1999

Lillis KA, Jaffe DM: Playground injuries in children. Pediatr Emerg Care 13:149–153, 1997

Lindqvist KS, Timpka T, Bjurulf P: Injuries during leisure physical activity in a Swedish municipality. Scand J Soc Med 24:282–292, 1996

Lubbers EJ: Injury of the duodenum caused by a fixed three-point seatbelt. J Trauma 17:960, 1977

Lueder GT: Air bag-associated ocular trauma in children. Ophthalmology 107:1472–1475, 2000

Mackenzie TB, Popkin MK: Suicide in the medical patient. Int J Psychiatry Med 17:3–22, 1987

Madan AK, Yu K, Beech DJ: Alcohol and drug use in victims of life-threatening trauma. J Trauma 47:568–571, 1999

Marshall KW, Koch BL, Egelhoff JC: Air bag-related deaths and serious injuries in children: injury patterns and imaging findings. AJNR Am J Neuroradiol 19:1599–1607, 1998

Max W, MacKenzie EJ, Rice DP: Head injuries: costs and consequences. J Head Trauma Rehabil 6:76–91, 1991

May AK, Chan B, Daniel TM, et al: Anterior lung herniation: another aspect of the seatbelt syndrome. J Trauma 38:587–589, 1995

McCaffrey M, German A, Lalonde F, et al: Air bags and children: a potentially lethal combination. J Pediatr Orthop 19:60–64, 1999a

McCaw ST, Walker JD: Winning the Stanley Cup final series is related to incurring fewer penalties for violent behavior. Tex Med 95:66–69, 1999

McCrory PR, Berkovic SF: Second impact syndrome. Neurology 50:677–683, 1998

McDeavitt JT: Preface: traumatic brain injury. Physical Medicine and Rehabilitation: State of the Art Reviews 15:ix–x, 2001

McIntosh AS, McCrory P: Impact energy attenuation performance of football headgear. Br J Sports Med 34:337–341, 2000

McLean AJ, Clark MS, Dorsch MM, et al: Random breath testing in South Australia: effects on drink-driving: HS 038 357. Adelaide, South Australia, NHMRC Road Accident Research Unit, University of Adelaide, 1984

Michigan Department of State Police v Sitz, 496 U.S. 444, 110 L. Ed. 2d 412, 1990 U.S. LEXIS 3144, 110 S. Ct. 2481, 58 U.S.L.W. 4781 (1990)

Miller KE, Zylstra RG, Standridge JB: The geriatric patient: a systematic approach to maintaining health. Am Fam Physician 61:1089–1104, 2000

Miller TR, Galbraith M: Injury prevention counseling by pediatricians: a benefit-cost comparison. Pediatrics 96:1–4, 1995

Miller TR, Galbraith MS, Lawrence BA: Costs and benefits of a community sobriety checkpoint program. J Stud Alcohol 59:462–468, 1998

Miller TR, Romano EO, Spicer RS: The cost of childhood unintentional injuries and the value of prevention. Future Child 10:137–163, 2000

Milne JS, Hargarten SW: The availability of extrinsic handgun locking devices in a defined metro area. WMJ 98:25–28, 1999a

Milne JS, Hargarten SW: Handgun safety features: a review for physicians. J Trauma 47:145–150, 1999b

Morris MS, Borja LP: Air bag deployment and hearing loss. Am Fam Physician 57:2627–2628, 1998

Morrison AL, Chute D, Radentz S, et al: Air bag–associated injury to a child in the front passenger seat. Am J Forensic Med Pathol 19:218–222, 1998

Muelleman RL, Mlinek EJ, Collicott PE: Motorcycle crash injuries and costs: effect of a reenacted comprehensive helmet use law. Ann Emerg Med 21:266–272, 1992

Mueller FO: Fatalities from head and cervical spine injuries occurring in tackle football: 50 years' experience. Clin Sports Med 17:169–182, 1998

Mueller FO, Blyth CS: Fatalities from head and cervical spine injuries occurring in tackle football: 40 years experience. Clin Sports Med 6:185–196, 1987

Murphy RX Jr, Birmingham KL, Okunski WJ, et al: The influence of airbag and restraining devices on the patterns of facial trauma in motor vehicle collisions. Plast Reconstr Surg 105:516–520, 2000

Nagib M, Rockswold G, Sherman R: Civilian gunshot wounds to the brain; prognosis and management. Neurosurgery 18:533–537, 1986

National Center for Alcohol and Drug Information: Traumatic brain injury and alcohol, tobacco and other drugs and the college experience. Washington, DC, U.S. Department of Health and Human Services, 1999

National Center for Injury Prevention and Control: Falls and hip fractures among older adults. Available at: http://www.cdc.gov/ncipc/factsheets/falls.htm. Accessed October 7, 2002.

National Head Injury Foundation Professional Council Substance Abuse Task Force: National Head Injury Foundation Professional Council Substance Abuse Task Force White Paper. Washington, DC, National Head Injury Foundation, 1988

National Highway Traffic Safety Administration: Third report to Congress: effectiveness of occupant protection systems and their use. National Highway Traffic Safety Administration. Available at: http://www.nhtsa.dot.gov/people/injury/airbags/208con2e.html. Accessed March 18, 2002.

National Highway Traffic Safety Administration: Standard enforcement saves lives: the case for strong seatbelt laws. Washington, DC, U.S. Department of Transportation, 1999

National Highway Traffic Safety Administration: Evaluation of motorcycle helmet law repeal in Arkansas and Texas. Washington, DC, U.S. Department of Transportation, 2000

Nguyen VQC, Cruz TH, McDeavitt JT: Traumatic brain injury and the science of injury control. State of the Art Reviews. Physical Medicine and Rehabilitation 15:213–227, 2001

O'Donnell MA: Research on drinking locations of alcohol-impaired drivers: implications for prevention policies. J Public Health Policy 6:510–525, 1985

Ong CF, Kumar VP: Colles fracture from air bag deployment. Injury 29:629–631, 1998

Peek-Asa C, Kraus JF: Alcohol use, driver, and crash characteristics among injured motorcycle drivers. J Trauma 41:989–993, 1996

Pinto M, Kuhn JE, Greenfield ML, et al: Prospective analysis of ice hockey injuries at the Junior A level over the course of one season. Clin J Sport Med 9:70–74, 1999

Plautz B, Beck DE, Selmar C, et al: Modifying the environment: a community-based injury-reduction program for elderly residents. Am J Prev Med 12:33–38, 1996

Playground safety—United States, 1998–1999. MMWR Morb Mortal Wkly Rep 48:329–332, 1999

Plunkett J: Fatal pediatric head injuries caused by short-distance falls. Am J Forensic Med Pathol 22:1–12, 2001

Porter CD: Football injuries. Phys Med Rehabil Clin N Am 10:95–115, 1999

Powell JW, Barber-Foss KD: Traumatic brain injury in high school athletes (see comments). JAMA 282:958–963, 1999

Reece RM, Sege R: Childhood head injuries: accidental or inflicted? Arch Pediatr Adolesc Med 154:11–15, 2000

Reid SR, Losek JD: Factors associated with significant injuries in youth ice hockey players. Pediatr Emerg Care 15:310–313, 1999

Research and Evaluation Associates: The effects following the implementation of an 0.08 BAC limit and administrative per se law in California. Washington, DC, U.S. Department of Transportation, National Highway Traffic Safety Administration, National Center for Statistics and Analysis, 1991

Restifo KM, Kelen GD: Case report: sternal fracture from a seatbelt. J Emerg Med 12:321–323, 1994

Rivara FP, Koepsell TD, Koepsell TD, et al: The effects of alcohol abuse on readmission for trauma. JAMA 270:1962–1964, 1993

Roberston LS, Kelley AB, O'Neill B, et al: A controlled study of the effect of television messages on safety belt use. Am J Public Health 64:1071–1080, 1974

Rodriguez MA, Gorovitz E: The politics and prevention of gun violence. West J Med 171:296–297, 1999

Rogers PN: The General Deterrent Impact of California's 0.08% Blood Alcohol Concentration Limit and Administrative per se License Suspension Laws, Vol 1. Sacramento, CA, California Department of Motor Vehicles, Research and Development Section, 1995

Ross HL, McCleary R, Epperlein T: Deterrence of drinking and driving in France: an evaluation of the law of July 12, 1978. Law Soc Rev 16:345–374, 1981

Rowland J, Rivara F, Salzberg P, et al: Motorcycle helmet use and injury outcome and hospitalization costs from crashes in Washington state. Am J Public Health 86:41–45, 1996

Rozner L: Air bag-bruised face. Plast Reconstr Surg 97:1517–1519, 1996

Ruiz-Moreno JM: Air bag-associated retinal tear. Eur J Ophthalmol 8:52–53, 1998

Russ NW, Geller ES: Training bar personnel to prevent drunken driving: a field evaluation. Am J Public Health 77:952–954, 1987

Ryan AJ: Intracranial injuries resulting from boxing: a review (1918–1985). Clin Sports Med 6:31–40, 1987

Safih MS, Norton R, Rogers I, et al: Elderly trauma patients admitted to the intensive care unit are different from the younger population. N Z Med J 112:402–404, 1999

Saltz RF: The role of bars and restaurants in preventing alcohol-impaired driving: an evaluation of server intervention. Eval Health Professions 10:5–27, 1987

Santavirta S, Arajarvi E: Ruptures of the heart in seatbelt wearers. J Trauma 32:275–279, 1992

Schootman M, Fuortes LJ: Ambulatory care for traumatic brain injuries in the US, 1995–1997. Brain Inj 14:373–381, 2000

Schutzman SA, Greenes DS: Pediatric minor head trauma. Ann Emerg Med 37:65–74, 2001

Scopatz RA: Methodological study of between-states comparisons, with particular application to .08% BAC law evaluation. Transportation Research Board 77th annual meeting, Washington, DC, 1–11–1998, 1998

Shah N, Weinstein A: Reflex sympathetic dystrophy syndrome following air-bag inflation. N Engl J Med 337:574, 1997

Shannon P, Smith CR, Deck J, et al: Axonal injury and the neuropathology of shaken baby syndrome. Acta Neuropathol (Berl) 95:625–631, 1998

Shoemaker BL, Ose M: Pediatric lap belt injuries: care and prevention. Orthop Nurs 16:15–22, 1997

Shults RA, Elder RW, Sleet DA, et al: Reviews of evidence regarding interventions to reduce alcohol-impaired driving. Am J Prev Med 21:66–88, 2001

Sosin DM, Sacks JJ, Smith SM: Head injury-associated deaths in the United States from 1979 to 1986 (see comments). JAMA 262:2251–2255, 1989

Sosin DM, Sacks JJ, Holmgreen P: Head injury-associated deaths from motorcycle crashes: relationship to helmet-use laws. JAMA 264:2395–2399, 1990

Spain DA, Boaz PW, Davidson DJ, et al: Risk-taking behaviors among adolescent trauma patients. J Trauma 43:423–426, 1997

Sparedo FR, Gill D: Effects of prior alcohol use on head injury recovery. J Head Trauma Rehabil 4:75–82, 1989

Speechley M, Tinetti M: Falls and injuries in frail and vigorous community elderly persons. J Am Geriatr Soc 39:46–52, 1991

Spence LJ, Dykes EH, Bohn DJ, et al: Fatal bicycle accidents in children: a plea for prevention. J Pediatr Surg 28:214–216, 1993

Stein JD, Jaeger EA, Jeffers JB: Air bags and ocular injuries. Trans Am Ophthalmol Soc 97:59–82, 1993

Sun SW, Kahn DM, Swan KG: Lowering the legal blood alcohol level for motorcyclists. Accid Anal Prev 30:133–136, 1998

Tate PS, Freed DM, Bombardier CH, et al: Traumatic brain injury: influence of blood alcohol level on post-acute cognitive function. Brain Inj 13:767–784, 1999

Teutsch SM: A framework for assessing the effectiveness of disease and injury prevention. MMWR Morb Mortal Wkly Rep 41:1–12, 1992

Think First Foundation: Think first fact sheet bicycle safety. Available at: http://www.thinkfirst.org/news/bikesafety.html. Accessed August 17, 2004.

Thompson DC, Rivara FP, Thompson R: Helmets for preventing head and facial injuries in bicyclists. Cochrane Database Syst Rev CD001855, 2000

Thurman DJ, Alverson C, Dunn KA, et al: Traumatic brain injury in the United States: a public health perspective. J Head Trauma Rehabil 14:602–615, 1999

Tiret L, Hausherr E, Thicoipe M, et al: The epidemiology of head trauma in Aquitaine (France), 1986: a community-based study of hospital admissions and deaths. Int J Epidemiol 19:133–140, 1990

Totten VY, Fani-Salek MH, Chandramohan K: Hyphema associated with air bag deployment in a pediatric trauma patient. Am J Emerg Med 16:102–103, 1998

Traynelis VC, Gold M: Cervical spine injury in an air-bag-equipped vehicle. J Spinal Disord 6:60–61, 1993

Tsai MC, Hemenway D: Effect of the mandatory helmet law in Taiwan. Inj Prev 5:290–291, 1999

Tyroch AH, Kaups KL, Sue LP, et al: Pediatric restraint use in motor vehicle collisions: reduction of deaths without contribution to injury. Arch Surg 135:1173–1176, 2000

Ulrich D, Noah EM, Fuchs P, et al: Burn injuries caused by air bag deployment. Burns 27:196–199, 2001

Update: fatal air bag-related injuries to children—United States, 1993–1996. MMWR Morb Mortal Wkly Rep 45:1073–1076, 1996

U.S. Department of Health and Human Services: HIV Aids Surveillance Reports. Available at: http://www.cdc.gov/hiv/stats/hasr1102.pdf. Accessed August 2, 2001.

Vaca F, Berns SD: National Highway Traffic Safety Administration. Motorcycle helmet law repeal: a tax assessment for the rest of the United States (commentary)? Ann Emerg Med 37:230–232, 2001

Vaca F, Berns SD, Harris JS, et al: National Highway Traffic Safety Administration. Evaluation of the repeal of motorcycle helmet laws. Ann Emerg Med 37:229–230, 2001

Verdant A: Abdominal injuries sustained in severe traffic accidents by seatbelt wearers. J Trauma 28:880–881, 1988

Villaveces A, Cummings P, Espitia VE, et al: Effect of a ban on carrying firearms on homicide rates in 2 Colombian cities. JAMA 283:1205–1209, 2000

Voaklander DC, Saunders LD, Quinney HA, et al: Epidemiology of recreational and old-timer ice hockey injuries. Clin J Sport Med 6:15–21, 1996

Voas RB, Holder HD, Gruenewald PJ: The effect of drinking and driving interventions on alcohol-involved traffic crashes within a comprehensive community trial. Addiction 92 (suppl 2):S221–S236, 1997

Voas RB, Tippets AS, Fell J: The relationship of alcohol safety laws to drinking drivers in fatal crashes. Accid Anal Prev 32:483–492, 2000

Wagner AK, Sasser HC, Hammond FM, et al: Intentional traumatic brain injury: epidemiology, risk factors, and associations with injury severity and mortality. J Trauma 49:404–410, 2000

Waltzman ML, Shannon M, Bowen AP, et al: Monkeybar injuries: complications of play. Pediatrics 103:e58, 1999

Warrian RK, Shoenut JP, Iannicello CM, et al: Seatbelt injury to the abdominal aorta. J Trauma 28:1505–1507, 1988

White JE, McClafferty K, Orton RB, et al: Ocular alkali burn associated with automobile air-bag activation. CMAJ 153:933–934, 1995

Whitman S, Coonley-Hoganson R, Desai BT: Comparative head trauma experiences in two socioeconomically different Chicago-area communities: a population study. Am J Epidemiol 119:570–580, 1984

Wilberger JE: Minor head injuries in American football: prevention of long term sequelae. Sports Med 15:338–343, 1993

Willis BK, Smith JL, Falkner LD, et al: Fatal air bag mediated craniocervical trauma in a child. Pediatr Neurosurg 24:323–327, 1996

Wittenberg E, Goldie SJ, Graham JD: Predictors of hazardous child seating behavior in fatal motor vehicle crashes: 1990 to 1998. Pediatrics 108:438–442, 2001

Yarbrough BE, Hendey GW: Hangman's fracture resulting from improper seat belt use. South Med J 83:843–845, 1990

Ytterstad B: The Harstad injury prevention study: the epidemiology of sports injuries: an 8 year study. Br J Sports Med 30:64–68, 1996

Zabriskie NA, Hwang IP, Ramsey JF, et al: Anterior lens capsule rupture caused by air bag trauma. Am J Ophthalmol 123:832–833, 1997

Zador PL, Krawchuk SA, Voas RB: Alcohol-related relative risk of driver fatalities and driver involvement in fatal crashes in relation to driver age and gender: an update using 1996 data. J Stud Alcohol 61:387–395, 2000

Zafonte RD, Mann NR, Millis SR, et al: Functional outcome after violence related traumatic brain injury. Brain Inj 11:403–407, 1997

Zakocs RC, Earp JA, Runyan CW: State gun control advocacy tactics and resources. Am J Prev Med 20:251–257, 2001

Index

Note: Page numbers followed by *f* refer to figures; numbers followed by *t* refer to tables.

Abstinence in substance abuse, 518
Abstract thought in personality disorders, 252
Abulia, 338
    bromocriptine in, 329
    conditions associated with, 343t
    treatment of, 345–346
Acceleration causing brain injury, 28, 28t
Accommodative dysfunction, 411
Acetaminophen in pain relief, 425t
    in headache, 389
N-Acetylaspartate labeled with hydrogen-1 in magnetic resonance spectroscopy, 125t
Acetyl-L-carnitine, 681t–682t, 683t, 685, 691t
Acetylcholine
    activity after brain injury, 40, 206, 615
    in aging brain, 498, 499t
    CSF levels in aggression, 264
    deficiency in delirium, 186, 187f
Acquisition of skills in process model of behavioral therapy, 663–665
ACTH, psychiatric side effects of, 611t, 612t
Activation studies
    PET scans in, 122–123
    SPECT imaging in, 117
Activities of daily living (ADL), 208
    aggression in, 669
    in vision problems, 409
Addiction Severity Index, 513
Addictive disorders. *See* Substance abuse
Adenosine triphosphate labeled with phosphorus-31 in magnetic resonance spectroscopy, 125t

S-Adenosylmethionine, 681t–682t, 683t, 686–687, 691t
Adjustment disorder in children, differential diagnosis of, 488
Adrenal disorders, 66, 66t
β-Adrenergic receptor blockers
    affecting sexual function, 440t
    in aggression, 272–273
    in headache, 389t
Advance directives, 587–588
Affective disorders after mild TBI, 291t
Affective lability
    medications in, 620–621
    in personality disorders, 251
2-AG compound, neuroprotection with, 706t, 711
Age. *See also* Elderly persons; Pediatric injuries
    and duration of posttraumatic amnesia, 186
    and mild brain injuries, 281, 281t
    and outcomes after injury, 495–498, 497t
    and risk of brain injury, 8–9, 10f, 14–15, 15f, 24
    and seizure development, 312t
Aggression, 259–274
    assessment of, 264–266
    behavioral therapy in, 274, 669–671, 670t
    clinical features of, 261
    common etiologies of, 265, 265t
    and depression after TBI, 203
    differential diagnosis of, 264–265
    documentation of, 266
    drugs associated with, 264–265
    medications in, 269–274, 630, 630t
    mood disorders with, 264, 264t

    neuroanatomy in, 261–263, 262t
    neuropsychiatric factors in, 267, 269f
    neurotransmitters in, 263–264
    in personality disorders, 251
    physiology of, 264
    prevalence of, 259–260, 260t
    treatment of, 266–274
        in acute aggression, 269–270, 273t
        in chronic aggression, 270–274, 273t, 630t
Agitated Behavior Scale, 266, 269f
    in delirium study, 177
Agitation
    in elderly persons, 503–504
    medications in, 24t, 194, 273t, 630
    neuropsychiatric factors in, 267, 269f
    posttraumatic, 177, 179, 259
        rating scales for, 182–184, 183t
    in substance abuse, 515–516
Agitation Behavior Scale (ABS), 183t
    and selection of antipsychotic drugs, 194
Agnosia, 354t
AIDA compound as NMDA receptor antagonist, 702t, 704
Air bag systems, 730–731
    affecting children, 740
Akinesia, differential diagnosis of, 339
ALCAR, 681t–682t, 683t, 685, 691t
Alcohol abuse. *See* Substance abuse
Alcoholics Anonymous (AA), 517, 517t
    letter to sponsor of member with TBI, 525–527
    original twelve steps of, 528
        written for TBI patients, 529
Alertness and orientation, testing of, 160–161
Almotriptan in headache, 390

Alprazolam in withdrawal from alcohol or drugs, 514t
Alternative treatments, 679–692
  cholinergic enhancing agents, 680–686, 681t
  decision making for target symptoms in, 684f
  guidelines for, 683t
  herbal, 688–690
  homeopathy, 691–692
  information resources, 692, 692t
  mechanisms of action, 681t–682t
  nootropics and vitamins, 690–691
  nutrients, 686–688
  pathophysiological framework for, 679–680
  principles in, 680
  sources for quality compounds, 691t, 692
Alzheimer's disease. *See also* Dementia
  acetyl-L-carnitine in, 685
  awareness deficits in, 356
  development after brain injury, 206, 500
  ginkgo biloba affecting, 689
  magnetic resonance spectroscopy in, 126
  medications in, 327
  novelty seeking in, 342
  PET scans in, 119
  SPECT imaging in, 111
Amantadine
  adverse effects of, 624
  in affective lability, 621
  and cognition in elderly persons, 504
  in cognitive dysfunction, 326t, 329, 622, 622t, 624
  in fatigue, 379, 627
  in mood disorders, 209
  in motivational loss, 348, 348t
  in personality disorders, 255, 255t
  psychiatric side effects of, 611t
American Academy of Neurology (AAN) Practice Parameters, 465
American Academy of Psychiatry and the Law, 596
American Medical Association's Guide to the Evaluation of Permanent Impairment, 599
Americans With Disabilities Act of 1990, 578
Amino acids, excitatory
  activity after brain injury, 41–42
  antagonists and agonists of, 699–705, 702t–703t
γ-Aminobutyric acid levels after brain injury, 264
α-Amino-3-hydroxy-5-methyl-4-isoxazole-propionate/kainic acid (AMPA/KA) receptors, antagonists and agonists of, 700, 703t, 703–704

21-Aminosteroid compounds, neuroprotection with, 706t, 708
Amitriptyline
  adverse effects of, 618
  in aggression, 272
  in cognitive impairment, 623
  in depression, 616–617
    in childhood, 489
  in headache, 389, 390
  in pain relief, 425t
Amnesia, posttraumatic (PTA), 63
  anterograde, 163
  attentional deficits in, 321
  clinical features of, 178–179
  and competency to stand trial, 591
  definition of, 175–176, 176f
  features related to outcome, 185–186
  functional neuroimaging in, 190–191
  memory studies in, 180, 323
  in mild TBI, 279, 280t, 281
  outcome in coma survivors, 185
  and posttraumatic stress disorder, 168, 180, 235–236
  rating scales for, 182–184, 183t
  and recovery of cognitive abilities, 180, 181f
  relation to coma and confusion, 176, 176f
  retrograde, 163
  and seizure development, 312t
  structural neuroimaging in, 189–190
Amobarbital
  in pain relief, 426
  in withdrawal from alcohol or drugs, 514t
AMPA/KA receptors, antagonists of, 700, 703t, 703–704
Amphetamines. *See also* Dextroamphetamine
  affecting sexual function, 440t
  and cognition in elderly persons, 504
  in mild TBI, 299
  psychiatric side effects of, 612t
Amygdala
  in aggression, 262
  kindling of, 264
  in motivational circuitry, 341
  in sexual function, 438
  in stress response, 237–238
β-Amyloid
  deposits in brain, 500
    increased after brain injury, 206
  precursor protein immunoreactivity in diffuse axonal injury, 35f, 36
Analgesia, patient-controlled, 427
Analgesics, 425, 425t
Anesthetics, local, 425t
Animal studies. *See* Experimental models
Aniracetam as alternative treatment, 690
Anisotropy, 94
  fractional, in maps of brain, 95, 95f

Anosmia, posttraumatic, 65, 65t
Anosodiaphoria, 354t, 360
Anosognosia, 354t
  in aphasia, 355–356
  hemiplegia and hemianopia with, 355
Anoxia
  anemic, 73
  anoxic, 73
  brain damage in, 73–74
  toxic, 73
Antianxiety medications in aggression, 270–271
Anticholinergics, psychiatric side effects of, 611t
Anticonvulsants
  in aggression, 271, 630t
  in anxiety, 241
  cognitive effects of, 631–632
  in pain relief, 425, 425t
  psychiatric side effects of, 611t
  in seizures with behavioral symptoms, 314–315, 315t
Antidepressants, 615–619
  affecting sexual function, 441t
  in affective lability, 620
  in aggression, 272, 630t
  in anxiety, 240–241
  in cognitive dysfunction, 326t, 330
  in depression after brain injury, 209, 210
  for elderly persons, 503
  in headache, 389, 389t
  interactions with other drugs, 619
  in mild TBI, 298
  in pain relief, 425, 425t
  psychiatric side effects of, 611t
  in seizures with behavioral symptoms, 315
Antidiuretic hormone secretion, inappropriate, after TBI, 66, 66t
Antihistamines, psychiatric side effects of, 611t
Antihypertensives
  in aggression, 272–273
  psychiatric side effects of, 611t
Anti-inflammatory agents
  neuroprotection with, 706t, 708–711
  nonsteroidal drugs in headaches, 389
Antioxidants, neuroprotection with, 706t, 707–708
Antipsychotic agents, 628–629
  adverse effects of, 628, 629
  in aggression, 269–270, 630t
  in anxiety, 241
  in delirium, 192–194
  for elderly persons, 503–504
  in posttraumatic psychosis, 225–226
Anton syndrome, awareness deficit in, 355
Anxiety, 231–241
  after mild TBI, 291t, 292–293
  and aggressive behavior, 264, 264t

in children, 485
cognitive and behavioral effects of, 231–232
and depression after TBI, 203
differential diagnosis of, 167
dizziness and balance problems in, 402
incidence after brain injury, 233–235, 235t
medications in, 240–241, 629–630
neurobiology of, 237–238
and posttraumatic stress disorder, 235–239
psychotherapy in, 239–240
relationship to brain injury, 233
in seizures after brain injury, 314t
somatic symptoms in, 232–233
SPECT imaging in, 110
in substance abuse, treatment of, 520–521
treatment of, 239–241
Apathy, 338. *See also* Motivation, impairment of
affective, 342
in children, treatment of, 489
cognitive, 342
conditions associated with, 343t
differential diagnosis of, 204
medications in, 626–627
motor, 342
treatment of, 345–346
Apathy Evaluation Scale (AES), 344, 345f
Aphasia, 165, 326
anosognosia in, 355–356
Broca, 165
conduction, 165
posttraumatic, 65, 65t
Wernicke, 165, 359
Aphasia Examination, 161t, 165
Apnea in sleep, 375
Apolipoprotein E ε4 allele linked to poor outcome, 456, 463–464, 500
Apomorphine affecting sexual function, 446
Apoptosis, brain injury affecting, 43
Aprosodia
differential diagnosis of, 339
motor or sensory, 253
Aptiganel as NMDA receptor antagonist, 701, 702t
APV compound as NMDA receptor antagonist, 701, 702t
Arachidonic acid cascade in brain injury, 40, 705
Arctic root (*Rhodolia*), 681t–682t, 683t, 688–689
Arithmetic skill after brain injury in children, 478–479
Arousal impairment, medications in, 622t, 622–623
Asparaginase, psychiatric side effects of, 611t, 612t

Aspartate activity after brain injury, 41
Assault-related brain injuries, 12, 12f
Assertiveness training in aggression, 669, 670t
Assessment procedures, 59–75, 159–170. *See also* Neuropsychiatric assessment
alertness and orientation in, 160–161
approaches to, 159–160
attentional processes in, 161t, 161–163
cognitive domains in, 160, 161t
in differential diagnosis of TBI, 166–170
in anxiety, 167
in attention-deficit/hyperactivity disorder, 169
in depression, 167
in learning disorders, 169–170
in obsessive-compulsive disorder, 168
in posttraumatic stress disorder, 168
in schizophrenia, 168–169
in estimation of premorbid functioning, 166–167
executive functioning in, 161t, 164
fixed battery approach, 160
flexible battery approach, 160
memory in, 161t, 163–164
motivation and malingering in, 165–166
motor processes in, 161t
role of neuropsychologist in, 159
screening instruments in, 166
speech and language in, 161t, 164–165
in sports injuries, 467–468
Asthma, headache in, 389t
Ataxia, posttraumatic, 65, 65t
Atomoxetine in attention-deficit/ hyperactivity disorder, 489
Atrophy of brain
clinical ratings of, 95–97, 96f
magnetic resonance images of corpus callosum, 86f, 90
frontal or temporal lobes, 89, 89f, 97
Attention-deficit/hyperactivity disorder (ADHD)
differential diagnosis of, 169, 487–488
treatment of, 489
Attention impairment, 321–323
in addicted persons with brain damage, 526
in delirium, 180
interaction of components in, 322t
in mild TBI, medications affecting, 298–299
in personality disorders, 251
testing in, 161t, 161–163
Attention Process Training, 655
Auditory Consonant Trigrams (ACT), 161t, 164

Auditory evoked potentials. *See* Evoked potentials
Auditory perception
problems in, 253
screening tests for, 397
Autism
after brain injury, 486
magnetoencephalography in, 126
Automated Neuropsychological Assessment Metric (ANAM) in sports injuries, 467–468
Automatisms as defense to criminal charge, 594
Automobile insurance
liability, 567
no-fault, 567
Automobile transport. *See* Motor vehicles
Autopsy studies, consent for, 28
Awareness impairment, 353–364
affecting motivation, 342
affecting treatment and rehabilitation, 361–363, 363t
after brain injury, 356–364
in Anton syndrome, 355
in aphasia, 355–356
assessment of, 363t
definition of, 353, 354t
dimensions of, 353–354
and functional outcome after brain injury, 357, 359t
hemiplegia and hemianopia with, 355
and intentional distortions by healthy individuals, 354
measurement of, 357–358, 358t
neuroanatomy in, 358–360, 360t
in neuropsychiatric disorders, 355–356
neuropsychological evaluation in, 363t
therapeutic alliance developed in, 362, 363t
Awareness Questionnaire, 358t
Axonal injury, 34f, 35f, 34–38
β-amyloid precursor protein immunoreactivity in, 35f, 36
axoplasmic transport in, 36–37
and delayed axotomy in mild brain injury, 282
grades of, 35–36
hemorrhage in, 34, 34t, 34f
histological appearance of, 34–35, 35f, 35t
mechanisms of, 36–37
primary axotomy in, 36
secondary axotomy in, 36
vegetative state in, 35, 35f
wallerian degeneration in, 36

B vitamins, 681t–682t, 683t, 690–691, 691t
Baclofen
affecting sexual function, 440t
psychiatric side effects of, 611t, 612t

Balance problems, 393–403. *See also*
    Dizziness and balance problems
Barbiturates
    in delirium, 194
    psychiatric side effects of, 611t
    in withdrawal from alcohol or drugs,
        514t
Barrow Neurological Institute Screen for
    Higher Cerebral Functions, 358t
Barthel Index, and postconcussive
    symptoms, 286
Beck Anxiety Inventory (BAI), 423t
Beck Depression Inventory-2, 423t
Behavioral problems, 61t
    affecting families, 535, 535t
    assessment of, 69–70
    in children with brain injury, 479
    in mild brain injury, 285–293
    PET scans in, 122
    related to clinical rating of MR scans,
        95–97, 97f
    in seizures after brain trauma,
        313–314, 314t
        treatment of, 314–316
    SPECT imaging in, 115–116
Behavioral treatment, 661–675
    in aggression, 274
    cognitive strategies in, 664
    in disruptive behaviors, 669–671, 670t
    in emotional reactions to injury,
        671–672
    evaluative model of, 663, 663t
    in fatigue, 380
    in headache, 389
    integrative model of, 663, 663t
    models of, 662–669, 663t
    in motivational loss, 346
    in pain relief, 428, 429t
    process model in, 663t, 663–669
    recovery process in, 663, 663t
    in return to community, 673–674
    skill deficits encountered in, 661, 662t
    in sleep disorders, 382
    staff management issues in, 672–673
        and interactive staff training, 673
    two-phase developmental program
        in, 663, 663t
    unawareness in, 662
Benton Visual Retention Test, 161t, 163
    and benefits of citicoline, 686
Benzodiazepines
    adverse effects of, 629
    in aggression, 270, 630t
    in anxiety, 240
    in delirium, 194
    in insomnia, 380
    in posttraumatic psychosis, 226
    psychiatric side effects of, 611t
    withdrawal from, 514, 515t
    in withdrawal from alcohol or drugs,
        514t

Berg Balance Scale, 398
Beta blockers. *See* β-Adrenergic receptor
    blockers
Bicycle injuries, 13, 13t, 459–460
    prevention of, 733–734
Bio-Strath, 681t–682t, 683t, 690–691
Biofeedback in pain management, 429t
Bipolar disorder
    headache in, 389t
    medications in, 619–620
Block Design Test, 161t
Blood alcohol level (BAL)
    in diagnosis of alcohol abuse,
        512–513
    and higher costs for medical care,
        516
    and motor vehicle accidents, 739
Blood-brain barrier disrupted in injured
    brains, 705
Blood flow, cerebral, posttraumatic
    reduction of, 37–38, 461–462
BN 80933 compound, neuroprotection
    with, 706t, 708
Booklet Category Test, 161t, 164
Boston Diagnostic Aphasia
    Examination, 161t, 165
Boston Naming Test, 161t
Boxing, injuries in, 455–457, 500
    prevention of, 734
Bradykinin B$_2$ receptor antagonist,
    neuroprotection with, 706t, 711
Brain. *See also* Neuroanatomy
    age-related changes in, 498–500,
        499t
    circuitry in unawareness, 360t
        and pathology after brain injury,
            361
    imaging of. *See* Imaging techniques
    location of lesions affecting mood
        disorders, 207
    motivational circuitry in, 339–342,
        340f
Brain-derived neurotrophic factor
    (BDNF), 707t, 712f, 712–713, 713t
Brain Injury Association of America,
    546, 555, 562, 571, 578, 727
Brain Trauma Foundation, 563–564
Breath testing at sobriety checkpoints,
    739–740
Brief Michigan Alcoholism Screening
    Test, 512, 513f
Brief Psychiatric Rating Scale
    in personality changes, 249
    in posttraumatic amnesia, 183
Brief Visuospatial Memory
    Test—Revised, 161t, 163
Broca aphasia, 165
Bromocriptine
    adverse effects of, 624
    affecting memory after mild TBI,
        298–299

affecting sexual function, 440t
    in cognitive dysfunction, 329, 622,
        622t, 623–624
    in motivational loss, 348t
    in personality disorders, 255, 255t
    psychiatric side effects of, 611t, 612t
Brown-Peterson test of memory, 164
Bulimia, organic, opiate antagonists in,
    255, 255t
Bupropion
    affecting sexual function, 441t
    in attention-deficit/hyperactivity
        disorder, 489
    in motivational loss, 347, 348t
    seizures from, 618–619
Burst lobe, 29, 32, 32f, 33
Buspirone
    in aggression, 270–271, 630t
    in anxiety, 241, 629
    in delirium, 194
Butabarbital in withdrawal from alcohol
    or drugs, 514t
Butalbital in withdrawal from alcohol or
    drugs, 514t
BW 1003C87 compound as NMDA
    receptor antagonist, 703t, 704

CAGE questionnaire for alcohol
    disorders, 512, 513f
Calcium
    channel agents in headache, 389t
    ion changes after brain injury, 42
California Verbal Learning Test
    (CVLT), 161t, 163, 165
Caloric stimulation, vestibuloocular
    reflex in, 399, 399t
Cannabinoid receptor agonists,
    neuroprotection with, 706t, 711
Cantu concussion grading guidelines,
    464, 464t, 466, 466t
Capgras syndrome, 220
Capsaicin in pain relief, 425t, 426
Captopril, psychiatric side effects of, 611t
Car seats for children, 740
Carbamazepine
    affecting sexual function, 440t
    in affective lability, 621
    in aggression, 271, 630t
    cognitive effects of, 631–632
    in delirium, 194
    early posttrauma use of, 310
    for elderly persons, 504
    in mania, 619–620
    in pain relief, 425t
    in personality change in children, 489
    psychiatric side effects of, 612t
    in seizures with behavioral
        symptoms, 314, 315t
Carbidopa
    in cognitive impairment, 622t, 623
    in fatigue, 379

in motivational loss, 348t
in personality disorders, 254, 255t
Carbon-11 in PET scans, 121t
Carbon monoxide poisoning, magnetic
    resonance spectroscopy in, 126
Care systems, 559–568
    accredited programs in, 562–563,
        563t
    acute care in, 563
    acute inpatient rehabilitation in, 563
    development of, 559–560
    funding and public policy aspects of,
        566–568
    individual outpatient therapy in, 564
    lifetime supported living services in,
        565
    mental health services in, 565–566
    neurobehavioral treatment in, 564
    outpatient day hospital or program
        in, 564
    professionals in, 560–562
    residential treatment in, 564
    settings in, 562f, 562–563
    special educational services in, 565
    subacute rehabilitation in, 563–564
    vocational services in, 564–565
Catastrophic conditions, and
    psychotherapy, 649, 652t
Catatonia, differential diagnosis of, 339
Catecholamine activity after brain
    injury, 40–41, 613–614
Catecholaminergic agents
    affecting memory after mild TBI,
        298–299
    in cognitive dysfunction, 326t,
        328–329
Category Test, 164
CDP-choline. See Cytidine 5'-
    diphosphocholine
Celecoxib as COX-2 inhibitor, 706t, 707
Cell death, programmed, brain injury
    affecting, 43
Cellular changes after brain injury, 43
Centers for Disease Control and
    Prevention, 6, 7, 12, 560, 727
    study of traumatic brain injury,
        574–575
Centers for Independent Living, 578
Centrophenoxine, 681t–682t, 683t,
    684–685, 691t
Cerebral blood flow
    in hypoxic-ischemic brain damage,
        37–38
    reduced in concussions, 461–462
Cerebral perfusion pressure monitoring
    in severe TBI, 53, 54t
Cerebrovascular accident, imaging in, 118
Cerestat as NMDA receptor antagonist,
    701, 702t
Chameleon-like effect of brain injury,
    personality changes in, 250

Childish behavior after brain injury,
    250–251
Children and adolescents. See Pediatric
    injuries
Children's Motivation Scale, 344
Chlordiazepoxide in withdrawal from
    alcohol or drugs, 514t
Chlorpromazine
    in headache, 390
    in posttraumatic psychosis, 225
Choline labeled with hydrogen-1 in
    magnetic resonance spectroscopy,
    125t
Cholinergic agents. See also
    Acetylcholine
    affecting memory after mild TBI,
        298–299
    alternative compounds, 680–686, 681t
    in cognitive dysfunction, 326t,
        327–328
Cholinesterase inhibitors
    and cognition in elderly persons, 504
    in cognitive impairment, 624–626
    in motivational loss, 347–348
Chronotherapy in sleep disorders, 382
Cimetidine, psychiatric side effects of,
    611t
Circadian rhythm sleep disorder, 376–377
    phototherapy in, 381–382
Citalopram
    in affective lability, 621
    in depression, 209, 616
Citicholine. See Cytidine 5'-
    diphosphocholine
Civil litigation, 595–596
Classification of brain damage, 27, 28t
Clinical Global Impression Scale (CGI),
    idebenone affecting, 688
Clonazepam
    in aggression, 271
    in insomnia, 380
    in pain relief, 425t
    in seizures with behavioral
        symptoms, 315t
    in withdrawal from alcohol or drugs,
        514t
Clonidine
    affecting sexual function, 440t
    in mania, 209, 620
    in mild TBI, 299
    in opiate withdrawal, 514
Clorazepate in withdrawal from alcohol
    or drugs, 514t
Closed-head injury, and posttraumatic
    psychosis, 218–219
Clozapine
    in aggression, 270
    in anxiety, 241
    in delirium, 193
    in psychosis, 225, 628
    seizures from, 629

Cluster headaches, 390
CNQX compound as AMPA/KA
    receptor antagonist, 703, 703t
CNS1102 as NMDA receptor
    antagonist, 701, 702t
CO-0127 compound, neuroprotection
    with, 706t, 711
Cobalt-55 in PET scans, 121t
Cocaine abuse. See Substance abuse
Codeine for pain relief, 426t
Cogniphobia Scale, 422t
Cognition
    "bedside" testing of, 69, 69t
    domains in assessment process, 160,
        161t
Cognitive activation paradigm, 122
Cognitive Coping Strategies Inventory,
    422t
Cognitive dysfunction, 61t
    in addicted persons with brain
        damage, 526–527
    after coronary artery bypass graft, 74
    after mild TBI, 283–285
        long-term effects in, 283–285
        short-term effects in, 283
    antidepressants in, 326t, 330
    in attention impairments, 321–323
    catecholaminergic agents in, 326t,
        328–329
    cholinergic agents in, 326t, 327–328
    in dizziness and balance problems, 398
    in elderly persons, 497, 501–502
        treatment of, 504
    in executive functions, 324t, 324–325
    in language and communication,
        325t, 325–326
    in learning and memory, 323t,
        323–324
    medications in, 621–626, 622t
    pain affecting, 420–421
    in personality disorders, 252
    posttraumatic, 179, 179f
    in posttraumatic stress disorder, 237
    in psychotic disorders, 219, 221, 222
    related to clinical rating of MR scans,
        95–97, 97f
    in substance abuse, 516
    treatment of, 326t, 326–331
        questions concerning, 331, 331t
        shortcomings in, 330t, 330–331
Cognitive rehabilitation, 655–660, 664
    definition of, 655
    effectiveness of, 659
    and length of time since injury, 657
    neuropsychological evaluation in,
        657–658
    severity of injury affecting, 657
Cognitive Test for Delirium (CTD), 183t
Cognitive therapy
    in emotional reactions to injury, 672
    in pain management, 429t

Coldness, medications in, 627–628
Collateral history in TBI, 60–62, 61t
Coma
    anatomic origins of, 37
    causes of, 73
    differential diagnosis of, 339
    duration of, and outcome of
        posttraumatic amnesia, 185
    electroencephalography in, 143
    prognostic factors in, 73, 74t
    relation to confusion and
        posttraumatic amnesia, 176, 176f
Commission on Accreditation of
    Rehabilitation Facilities, 562, 563t
Communication disorders, 325t,
    325–326
    in addicted persons with brain
        damage, 526
Communities
    family roles in, 545, 547–548
    outpatient day hospitals or programs
        in, 564
    support systems in, 548
Comparator region in monitoring of
    actions, 359, 360t
Compensation neurosis, 579
Competency, 583–584
    definition of, 584, 585
    to stand trial, 591
    task-specific, 586
Comprehensive Crime Control Act of
    1984, 592
Computed tomography, 79–84
    abnormalities related to outcome,
        80–81
    day of injury scan as baseline in,
        81–82, 83f, 93f
    in delirium, 189
    findings related to severity of injury,
        80, 81t, 82f
    indications for, 79–80
    limitations of, 82–84, 83f
    in mild TBI, 293–294, 294t
    rating scale in, 80, 81t, 82f
    in severe TBI, 52
    single-photon. See Single-photon
        emission computed tomography
        (SPECT)
    xenon-enhanced, 127, 127f,
        128f–129f
Computerized tests in assessment of
    sports injuries, 467–468
Concentration and attention, testing of,
    161t, 161–163
Concussion
    definition of, 464
    grading of, 279–280, 280t
    mild. See Mild traumatic brain injury
    neurophysiology of, 460–464
    severity measurements, 464t,
        464–465, 465t

Concussion Resolution Index (CRI) in
    sports injuries, 468
Conduction aphasia, 165
Confusion Assessment Method (CAM),
    183t
    for the Intensive Care Unit (CAM-
        ICU), 183t
Confusion related to coma and
    posttraumatic amnesia, 176, 176f
Congress of Neurological Surgeons,
    Committee on Head Injury
    Nomenclature, 464
Consent for treatment, informed,
    584–586, 585t
    options available for, 586, 586t
Consequences of brain injuries
    costs of, 22–23, 23f, 24f
    fatality rates, 6, 8f, 16–17, 18f
    long-term effects, 17
    in mild TBI, 17–19, 19f, 20f
    mood disorders affecting, 207–208
    prediction of, 19–20, 21f, 22f, 25
Conservators, 588
Contact causing brain lesions, 28, 28t
Contingency contracts in behavioral
    therapy, 665–666
Contingent observation in aggression,
    670, 670t
Contingent restraint in aggression, 670t,
    671
Continuous Performance Test, 161t, 163
Contraceptives, oral, psychiatric side
    effects of, 611t
Controlled Oral Word Association Test,
    161t
Contusion index, 30
Contusions
    acute, 29–30, 30f
    brain swelling with, 38, 39f
    MRI image of, 88, 89f
Coping Strategies Questionnaire, 422t
Coronary artery bypass graft surgery,
    cognitive problems after, 74
Corticosteroids
    in pain relief, 425, 425t
    psychiatric side effects of, 611t, 612t
Cortisol levels in stress response,
    237–238
Costs
    of head injuries, 22–23, 23f, 24f, 728
    of treatment
        in mild brain injuries, 281t, 282
        and role of compensation in
            postconcussive symptoms,
            287–289, 287t
        substance abuse affecting, 516
COX. See Cyclooxygenase
CP101,606 compound as NMDA
    receptor antagonist, 701, 702t
CPP compound as NMDA receptor
    antagonist, 701, 702t

CPPG compound as NMDA receptor
    antagonist, 703t, 704
Craniectomy, decompressive, in severe
    TBI, 57
Cranioelectrotherapy in pain relief,
    427–428
Creatine labeled with hydrogen-1 in
    magnetic resonance spectroscopy,
    125t
Criminal proceedings, 590–595
    and competency to stand trial, 591
    diminished capacity in, 593
    in exculpatory and mitigating
        disorders, 594–595
    guilty but mentally ill, 593–594
    insanity defense, 592–593
    level of intent in, 590–591
Crying, pathological, 204
    medications in, 620–621
Cultural background, and family
    reactions to disabilities, 554–555
6-Cyano-7-nitroquinoxaline as AMPA/
    KA receptor antagonist, 703, 703t
Cycling, injuries in, 13, 13t, 459–460
    prevention of, 733–734
Cyclobenzaprine, psychiatric side effects
    of, 611t
Cyclooxygenase (COX)
    in brain injury, 705
    inhibitors of, 705, 706t, 707
    in headache, 389
Cytidine 5'-diphosphocholine,
    681t–682t, 683t, 685–686, 691t
    in cognitive dysfunction, 326t, 327,
        626
Cytokine activity after brain injury, 41

DCG-IV compound as NMDA receptor
    antagonist, 703t, 704
DDAVP nasal spray in coldness, 628
Death row prisoners
    history of TBI in, 260
    posttraumatic psychosis in, 223
Deceleration causing brain injury, 28,
    28t
Decelerative techniques in aggression,
    670, 670t
Decompressive craniectomy in severe
    TBI, 57
Deferoxamine, neuroprotection with,
    706t, 707
Definitions
    amnesia, 175–176, 176f
    awareness impairment, 353, 354t
    cognitive rehabilitation, 655
    competency, 584, 585
    concussion, 464
    delirium, 175–178, 179, 353, 354t
    headache, 385
    incompetency, 584, 588–589
    mild TBI, 279–281, 280t

nootropics, 679
pain, 419
personality disorders, 246
psychosis, 214
Delirium, 175–195
causes of, 180–181, 181t, 191
in continuum of consciousness, 176, 177f
definitions of, 175–178, 179, 353, 354t
differential diagnosis of, 339
duration of, 186
encephalography in, 187–189
environmental manipulations in, 191–192
functional neuroimaging in, 190–191
hyperactive, 178, 179
affecting outcome, 185
hypoactive, 178
affecting outcome, 185
medications in, 192–194
motoric agitation in, 179
neuropathophysiology of, 186f, 186–191
rating scales for, 182–184, 183t
and recovery of cognitive abilities, 180, 181f
reversibility in elderly patients, 185
risk factors for, 181–182, 182t
severity and location of injury in, 184–185
signs and symptoms of, 178t, 178–180
structural neuroimaging in, 189–190
subclinical, 176–177
treatment of, 191–194
Delirium Rating Scale (DRS), 177, 183t, 184
Dementia
in Alzheimer's disease. See Alzheimer's disease
awareness deficits in, 356
differential diagnosis of, 339
in elderly persons, cholinesterase inhibitors affecting, 504
PET scans in, 119
pugilistica, 456, 500
SPECT imaging in, 110, 111
Demoralization as dysphoric state, 339
Denial of illness, 354t
organic, 246
and psychotherapy, 648–649, 652t
in substance abuse, 518
L-Deprenyl, 681t–682t, 683t, 690, 691t
in personality disorders, 254, 255t
Depression, 201–205, 208
and aggressive behavior, 203, 264, 264t
anxiety in, 203
apathy associated with, treatment of, 347
in children, 485
differential diagnosis of, 488
treatment of, 489

demographic variables in, 204t, 204–205, 205t
diagnosis of, 203
differential diagnosis, 167, 203–204
as dysphoric state, 339
in elderly persons, 502–503
functional MRI in, 124
headache in, 389t
medications in, 615–619
adverse effects of, 618–619
guidelines for, 610
in mild TBI, 290–292, 291t
medications in, 298
PET scans in, 119
with posttraumatic stress disorder, 237
prevalence of, 201–203, 202f
in seizures after brain injury, 314
SPECT imaging in, 110, 113
in substance abuse, treatment of, 520–521
suicide risk in, 737
treatment of, 208–209–210
Derogatis Interview of Sexual Function, 441
Desensitization in pain management, 430, 430t
Desferal, neuroprotection with, 706t, 707
Design Fluency Test, 161t
Desipramine
in cognitive impairment, 623
in depression, 209, 298, 617
in pain relief, 425t
Dexamethasone in pain relief, 425t
Dexanabinol, neuroprotection with, 706t, 711
Dextroamphetamine
adverse effects of, 624
in affective lability, 621
in attention-deficit/hyperactivity disorder, 489
in cognitive dysfunction, 328, 622t, 622–623
in fatigue, 379, 627
interaction with haloperidol, 631
in motivational loss, 348, 348t
in personality disorders, 254, 254t
Dextromethorphan
as NMDA receptor antagonist, 701, 702t
psychiatric side effects of, 611t
Dextrophan as NMDA receptor antagonist, 701, 702t
DFMO compound as NMDA receptor antagonist, 702t, 704
Diabetes insipidus after TBI, 66, 66t
Diacylglycerol formation in brain injury, 705
Diathermy in pain relief, 427

Diazepam
adverse effects of, 629
in delirium, 194
Differential diagnosis of TBI, 166–170
Differential reinforcement of other behaviors (DRO), 669–670, 670t
Diffuse injuries, 28, 28t, 34–38, 699
axonal, 34–38, 34f, 35f, 34t, 35t
experimental models of, 44
hypoxic-ischemic damage in, 37–38
multifocal vascular injury in, 38
secondary insults in, 38
Diffusion-tensor imaging, 94f, 94–95, 95f
Difluoromethylornithine (DFMO) as NMDA receptor antagonist, 702t, 704
Digit Span Test, 161t, 163
Digit Symbol Test, 161t, 163
Digitalis, psychiatric side effects of, 611t, 612t
Dihydroergotamine in headache, 390
Diminished capacity concept, 593
Disabilities
after mild TBI, 293
determined in civil litigation, 599
estimated new numbers of, 20–22, 22f
Disability insurance, 576–577
Disability Rating Scale (DRS), 81
Disorientation in delirium, 180
Distractibility, testing of, 163
Divalproex sodium for elderly persons, 504
Dix-Hallpike maneuver, 400
Dizocilpine (MK-801) as NMDA receptor antagonist, 701, 702t
Dizziness and balance problems, 393–403, 413
in benign positional paroxysmal vertigo, 400
common complaints in, 394–395, 395t
diagnostic procedures in, 394–399
drug-induced, 395, 397t
emotional factors in, 402–403
history of patient in, 394–395
laboratory tests in, 398–399, 399t
medications in, 401, 401t
in Ménière's disease, 400
outcomes in, 403
in perilymphatic fistula, 400
physical examination in, 395–398, 398t
physiology in, 394
prevalence of, 393–394
vestibular dysfunction in
central, 400–401
peripheral, 400
vestibular rehabilitation in, 402
Dizziness Handicap Inventory, 395, 396f

Do-not-resuscitate (DNR) orders, 587
Donepezil
    affecting memory in mild TBI, 299
    and cognition in elderly persons, 504
    in cognitive dysfunction, 326t,
        327–328, 622t, 625–626
    in delirium, 194
    in mood disorders, 209
    in motivational loss, 347, 348f
Dopamine systems
    activity in delirium, 186
    in aggression, 263
    in aging brain, 499, 499t
    agonists
        affecting cognition in elderly
            persons, 504
        affecting memory, 299
        in fatigue, 379
        in motivational loss, 347–348
        in personality disorders, 254–255,
            255t
    in diminished motivation, 343
    dysfunction after brain injury, 41,
        613–614
    and personality attributes, 248
Dopaminergic agents
    adverse effects of, 624
    in apathy, 627
    in cognitive impairment, 622t,
        622–624
Doxepin
    adverse effects of, 618
    affecting sexual function, 440t
Droperidol in delirium, 193
Drug abuse. See Substance abuse
Drug interactions with antidepressants,
    619
Drug therapy. See Medications
DSM-III diagnoses, depression after
    mild TBI, 291
DSM-III-R diagnoses, delirium, 177
DSM-IV diagnoses
    delirium, 177
    insomnia, 372
DSM-IV-TR diagnoses, 64, 64t
    alcoholism and drug addiction, 511,
        512t
    concussion, 280
    delirium, 178, 179t
    depression, 201, 203
    in forensic psychiatric evaluation,
        597
    learning disorders, 169
    manic syndromes, 205
    pain disorder with psychological
        factors, 419
    personality changes in medical
        conditions, 214t, 249t, 261t
    psychotic disorders, 214
Durable power of attorney, 587–588
Dynamic Gait Index, 398

Dynorphin activity after brain injury, 41
Dysarthria, 326

Eagle syndrome, 387, 387t, 390
Ear, anatomy of, 394
Edinburgh Rehabilitation Status Scale,
    and postconcussive symptoms, 286
Education. See also Psychoeducation
    for pain management, 429t
        programs for disabled children, 560,
            565
        and school problems after brain
            injury, 68, 478–479, 488
        and school relationship with parents,
            549–550
Eldepryl, 690
Elderly persons, 495–504
    age affecting outcomes after injury,
        495–498, 497t
    agitation and psychosis in, 503–504
    Alzheimer's disease in. See
        Alzheimer's disease
    apoE ε4 allele linked to poor
        outcomes, 500
    assessment of, 501–502
    clinical features of injuries in, 501
    cognitive dysfunction in, treatment
        of, 504
    cognitive outcome after injury, 497,
        501–502
    delirium reversibility in, 185
    depression in, 502–503
    falls in, 495, 496t, 733
    families of, 502
    functional outcome after injury,
        496–497, 501–502, 501f
    medications affecting, 502, 503t
    neurobiology of aging in, 498
    neurochemical changes in, 498–499,
        499t
    neuroimaging, 501
    population of, 495, 496t
    treatment of, 502–504
Electrical injuries, brain damage in, 74,
    75t
Electroconvulsive therapy
    in agitated delirium, 194
    in depression, 618
    in mania, 620
    in mood disorders, 209
Electroencephalography, 142–144
    burst-suppression ratio in, 144
    in delirium, 187–189
    in headache after trauma, 388
    in mild TBI, 296
    normal and trauma-related findings
        in, 142t, 142–144
    outcome predictions in, 144–145
    quantitative (QEEG), 144–147
        in delirium after brain injury,
            188–189

discriminant function scores in,
    145–147
    in mild TBI, 296–297
    in seizures, 311
    silence ratio in, 144
Electronystagmography, 398–399, 399t
Electrophysiology, 135–153
    abnormal rhythms in, 137
    alpha rhythm in, 136, 137f, 137t
    basic principles of, 136–137
    beta activity in, 136, 137f, 137t
    brain electrical activity mapping in
        (BEAM), 139, 141f
    delta activity in, 136, 137f, 137t
    dipoles in
        radially oriented, 138, 138f
        tangentially oriented, 138, 138f
    electrode placement in, 138, 139f
    electroencephalography. see
        Electroencephalography
    event-related potentials in, 147,
        149–152
    evoked potentials in, 147–152. See
        also Evoked potentials
    idling in, 136, 137
    intermixed slowing in, 137
    limitations of recordings in, 140
    magnetoencephalography, 152–153
        recording methods, 140–141
    in mild TBI, 296–297
    misinterpretation of data in, 139
    montages in, 138, 140f
    normal rhythms in, 136–137
    quantitative analyses in, 139
    reactivity diminished in, 137
    recording methods in, 137–141
    sharp waves in, 137
    slow waves in, 137
    spikes in, 137
    thalamic pacemaker neurons in, 136
    theta activity in, 136, 137f, 137t
Eletriptan in headaches, 390
Eliprodil as NMDA receptor antagonist,
    702t, 704
Emergency department workup in
    severe TBI, 51
Emotional disorders, 61t
    in addicted persons with brain
        damage, 527
    in children with brain injuries, 479
    dizziness and balance problems in,
        402–403
    environmental interventions in, 671
    medications in, 615–621
Emotional incontinence, 620
Employment after brain injury,
    574–576, 575f
    and vocational rehabilitation, 577–578
Encephalopathy in boxers, 456
Endocannabinoid system activity in
    brain injury, 711

Endocrine symptoms, 66, 66t
Environmental interventions
    in aggression, 671
    in delirium, 191–192
    for elderly persons, 502
    in emotional reactions to injury, 671
Epidemiology, 3–25
    case definitions and inclusion criteria,
        3–6, 4t–5t
    estimated annual injuries, 10f
    estimation of new disabilities, 20–22,
        22f
    exposures associated with injuries,
        12f, 12–13, 13f
    fatality rates, 6, 8f, 16–17, 18f
        in elderly patients, 496
    high-risk groups, 8–12
    hospital discharges, 14–15
        by diagnoses, 8, 9t, 14, 16f, 24
        sex- and age-specific, 15f, 24
    hospitalization rates, 7–8, 10f
    incidence studies, 6–8, 7f
    mild TBI, 281t, 281–282
    seizures, 309–311
    severity distribution of injuries,
        13–14, 14f
    types of lesions, 15–16, 17f
Epilepsy. *See* Seizures
Epinephrine activity after brain injury,
    40–41
Epworth Sleepiness Scale, 375, 376t
Equestrian sports, injuries in, 460
Erectile dysfunction, treatment of,
    446–447
Eriksonian stages
    and childish behavior after brain
        injury, 250, 250t
    clinical use of, 254
Estrogen, 439, 440t, 445t
    therapy affecting sexual function, 440t
Ethical issues, 583. *See also* Legal issues
    in sexual dysfunction, 447–448
Ethnicity or race
    and family reactions to disabilities,
        554–555
    and risk of brain injury, 9
Ethosuximide in seizures with
    behavioral symptoms, 315t
Evaluation of patient. *See* Assessment
    procedures
Evaluative model of behavioral therapy,
    663, 663t
Event-related potentials, 147, 149–152
    middle-latency, 149–150
    in mild TBI, 297
    N200 latency in, 151–152
    P300 latency in, 151–152
    in sensation-seeking behavior, 247
Evoked potentials, 147–152
    auditory mismatch negativity in
        (MMN), 151

contingent negative variation in
    (CNV), 151
    latency of, 147
    long-latency, 150
    middle-latency, 149–150
    in mild TBI, 297
    multimodal, 148
    N100 waveform in, 147, 147f
    P30 and P50 waveforms in, 147, 147f
    polarity of, 147
    postinjury P50 response to paired
        auditory stimuli, 149–150, 150f
    short-latency, 147–149
    somatosensory, in posttraumatic
        amnesia, 187–188
Executive functions
    in addicted persons with brain
        damage, 526–527
    changes related to clinical rating of
        MR scans, 95–97, 97f
    impairment of, 324t, 324–325
    in personality disorders, 252, 252t
    testing of, 161t, 164
Exercise in pain relief, 428
Experimental models
    diffuse brain injury, 44
    focal brain injury, 43–44
    mild brain injury, 282–283, 461
    seizures, 312
Expert Consensus Panel for Agitation in
    Dementia, 630
Extinction techniques in aggression,
    670, 670t
Eye problems. *See* Vision problems
Eysenck Personality Questionnaire, 535
Falls causing brain injuries, 12, 12f
    prevention of, 733
    risk in elderly persons, 495, 496t
Families, 533–555
    as advocates of patients, 578
    of children with psychiatric
        disorders, 482, 490
    community relationships of, 545,
        547–548
    cultural backgrounds of, 554–555
    differing perceptions in, 536
    of elderly persons, 502
    formal therapy for, 546
    guardianship arrangements, 588–589
    homeostasis and involvement in,
        533–534
    impact of TBI, 534–555
        on children, 537, 541
        clinical observations of, 538–539
        on extended family, 541–542
        on parents, 540–541
        phase I in, 534
        phase II in, 534
        phase III in, 534–535
        phase IV in, 535–538
        research on, 534–538, 535t

        on siblings, 541
        on spouses, 539–540
    individuality of, 555
    information and education for,
        545–546
    instruction in behavior management
        skills, 673–674
    interventions for, 538, 543–549, 544t
        acute care in, 546
        community reintegration in,
            547–548
        concentric circles of, 544f,
            544–545
        levels of, 545f, 545–546
        long-term issues in, 548–549
        rehabilitation in, 546–547
        stages of, 546–548, 547f
    involvement in patient's treatment,
        533–534, 651–652
    issues in mild TBI, 549
    legal issues in, 553–554
    long-term outcome in, 536
    Natural-Setting Behavior
        Management Program for, 538
    of patients with awareness deficits, 363
    of patients with motivational deficits,
        349
    proxy decision making, 589–590
    psychiatric symptoms in, 68, 68t
    relationship with school system,
        549–550
    sexual problems affecting, 447
    stages of adjustment in, 534, 542t,
        542–543
    structural and role changes in,
        539–542
    support, problem-solving, and
        restructuring for, 546
    translators for, 545
    unrealistic expectations of, 550–553
Family history of TBI patients, 67
    and posttraumatic psychosis, 219,
        221, 226
Fatality rates, 6, 8f, 16–17, 18f
    in elderly patients, 496
Fatigue and sleep problems, 369–382
    abnormal sleep-wake cycle in,
        376–377
    apnea in sleep, 375
    circadian rhythm sleep disorder,
        376–377
    clinical features of, 371–377
        in fatigue, 371–372
        in sleep disorders, 372–377
    evaluation of, 371–378
        in brain injury, 377t, 377–378
    hypersomnia, 375–376
    insomnia, 372–375
    medications in, 379–380, 627, 630
    narcolepsy, 375–376
    parasomnias, 377

Fatigue and sleep problems—*continued*
pathophysiology in, 370–371
relation to brain injury, 371, 371f
SPECT imaging in, 111, 113
treatment of, 378t, 378–382, 379t
in fatigue, 379–380
in sleep disorders, 380–382
Fatigue Impact Scale (FIS), 372, 373f–374f
Fatigue Severity Scale (FSS), 372
Females
sexual dysfunction in, 442
diagnostic testing in, 444, 445t
sports injuries in, 455
Fentanyl in pain relief, 426t
Fibroblast growth factor (FGF), 707t, 712f, 713t, 713–714
activity after brain injury, 42
Finger Tapping Test, 161t
Firearms causing brain injuries, 12, 12f
prevention of, 736
Flecainide in pain relief, 425t
Fluoride-18 in PET scans, 117, 121t
Fluoxetine
in affective lability, 620–621
in aggression, 272
in depression, 615–616
in childhood, 489
in pain relief, 425t
seizures from, 616, 618
Fluphenazine in anxiety, 241
Flurazepam in withdrawal from alcohol or drugs, 514t
Focal brain injuries, 28, 28t, 29–34, 699
blood vessels in, 33
cranial nerves in, 33
experimental models of, 43–44
hemorrhagic lesions in, 33–34
hypothalamus and pituitary in, 33
intracranial hematomas in, 30–33
intracranial pressure in, 33
pontomedullary junction tears in, 33
scalp, skull, and dura lesions in, 29
surface contusions and lacerations in, 29–30, 30f, 30t
Follicle-stimulating hormone, 439, 440t, 445t
Football, injuries in, 457, 472
prevention of, 734–735
Forensic psychiatric evaluations, 579, 591, 596–599
brain injury mimics in, 598–599
collateral sources of information in, 597–598, 598t
and disability determinations, 599
factors affecting test findings in, 598, 599t
index of suspicion for malingering in, 597, 598t
medications affecting, 599
mental status examination in, 598
no confidentiality in, 597

no doctor-patient relationship in, 597
standard diagnostic schema in, 597
team approach in, 597
Fractures. *See* Skull fractures
Freedox, neuroprotection with, 706t, 708
Fregoli syndrome, 220
Frontal lobe
"bedside" evaluation of function, 69t
executive function impairments, 324t, 324–325
syndromes, 247
aggression in, 261, 262
symptoms in, 64
Frovatriptan in headaches, 390
Functional Independence Measure (FIM), 81
Functional Self-Assessment Scale, 358t

g-force calculations of injury severity, 471
G-stop task, functional MRI in, 124
Gabapentin
in aggression, 271
in anxiety disorders, 241
in headache, 389t
in mania, 620
in pain relief, 425t
in seizures with behavioral symptoms, 314, 315t
Gacyclidine as NMDA receptor antagonist, 701, 702t
Gage, Phineas, 246
Galantamine, 680, 681t–682t, 683, 683t, 691t
in motivational loss, 347, 348f
Galveston Orientation and Amnesia Test (GOAT), 63, 70, 161, 162f
in delirium study, 177
in posttraumatic amnesia, 180, 182, 183t
Gender
and mild brain injuries, 281, 281t
and posttraumatic psychosis, 219
and risk of brain injury, 9, 11f, 15f, 24
General Rehabilitation Assessment Sexuality Profile, 443, 443t, 444t
Generalization of behaviors in process model of behavioral therapy, 664, 666–669
Genetic vulnerability
to anxiety disorders, 238
and bipolar illness after TBI, 292
and posttraumatic psychosis, 219, 221, 226
and response to neurotrauma, 299–300
Geniculate body, lateral, 408, 408f
Geriatric Evaluation by Relative's Rating Instrument (GERRI) scores affected by ginkgo biloba, 689
Ginkgo biloba, 681t–682t, 683t, 689–690, 691t
Ginseng, 681t–682t, 683t, 690, 691t

Glasgow Coma Scale, 5t, 5–6, 24–25, 60t, 70, 477
and assessment of older patients, 496, 501
and benefits of citicholine, 686
in mild TBI, 51, 279, 280t, 281
and postconcussive symptoms, 286
in posttraumatic amnesia, 182, 183t
relation to CT findings, 80, 82f
and return to work, 575, 576
and seizure development, 312, 312t
in severe TBI, 51
substance abuse affecting, 516
Glasgow Outcome Scale, 17
and postconcussive symptoms, 286
Glial-derived neurotrophic factor (GDNF), 707t, 712f, 713, 713t
Glucose levels, and diminished capacity concept, 593, 595
Glutamate activity after brain injury, 41–42
cerebrospinal fluid levels in, 206
Glutethimide in withdrawal from alcohol or drugs, 514t
Glycerol in withdrawal from alcohol or drugs, 514t
Goal-directed behavior
in awareness deficits, 362, 363
diminished motivation in, 338
Golden root, 681t–682t, 683t, 688–689
Gonadotropin-releasing hormone, 439, 440t
Grooved Pegboard Test, 161t
Group therapy
in awareness impairment, 363, 363t
in substance abuse, 518–519
Growth factors
activity after brain injury, 42, 706t–707t, 711–715
receptors for, 712f
Growth hormone, impaired release after TBI, 66
Guanfacine in mild TBI, 299
Guardianship, 588–589
Guilt experienced by patients, 649–650, 652t
Guilty but mentally ill, 593–594
Gunshot injuries, 12, 12f
prevention of, 736
GYKI-52466 compound as AMPA/KA receptor antagonist, 703t, 704

Habit reversal in pain management, 429t
Haddon Matrix, 729
Hair cells in ear, 394
Halazepam in withdrawal from alcohol or drugs, 514t
Hallpike-Dix maneuver, 400
Haloperidol
affecting sexual function, 440t
in aggression, 269–270

in anxiety, 241
in delirium, 192–193, 194
interaction with dextroamphetamine, 631
Halstead-Reitan Neuropsychological Test Battery (HRNB), 160
in sports injuries, 467
Hamilton Rating Scale for Depression after mild TBI, 291
Hasegawa Dementia Scale, Huperzine affecting, 684
Head Injury Behaviour Scale, 358t
Headache, posttraumatic, 385–390
assessment of, 386–388
causes of, 386–387, 387t
cluster, 390
complications of, 388
definitions of, 385
in life-threatening conditions, 386, 387t
natural history of, 388
pathophysiology in, 385–386
PET scans in, 119
prevalence of, 385
SPECT imaging in, 111, 112
tension-type, 385–386, 386t
treatment of, 388–390, 389t
Headache Disability Rating, 422t
Health care proxy, 587–588, 603–605
Health insurance policies, 567
Hearing problems, screening for, 397
Helmet use
bicycle, 459–460, 733–734
in equestrian events, 460
football, 472, 734
motorcycle, 732
skateboarding, 741
Hematoma
burst lobe in, 29, 32, 32f, 33
epidural, 31, 31f, 31t
in infancy and childhood, 39
in severe TBI, 54–55, 55f
xenon-enhanced computed tomography in, 129f
intracerebellar, 32–33
intracerebral, 32–33
swelling of brain with, 38
intracranial, 21f, 29–33, 31t, 32f, 32t
in skull fractures, 29
types and frequency of, 30t
intradural, 31–33
subarachnoid, 31–32
subdural, 29, 32, 32f
in infancy and childhood, 39
in severe TBI, 55f, 55–56, 56f
swelling of brain with, 38–39, 39f
Hemianopia, 411
awareness deficit with, 355
Hemiplegia, awareness deficit with, 355
Hemorrhage in diffuse axonal injury, , 34, 34f, 34t

Hendler Chronic Pain Screening Test, 422t
Hennebert sign in perilymphatic fistula, 400
Herbal alternative treatments, 688–690
in sleep disorders, 381
Herniations, intracranial, 33
Hexamethylpropyleneamine oxime labeled with technetium-99m in SPECT imaging, 112t
Hinckley, John, Jr., 592
Hippocampus in stress response, 237–238
History of patient, 59–60, 60t, 66–69
in dizziness and balance problems, 394–395
in prisoners on death row, 260
sexual history, 443–444
Hockey, prevention of injuries in, 735–736
Homeless people, posttraumatic psychosis in, 223
Homeopathy, 691–692
Hooper Visual Organization Test, 161t
Hopkins Verbal Learning Test, 161t, 163
in sports injuries, 467
Horseback riding, injuries in, 460
Hospitalization
discharges and diagnoses, 14–15, 15f, 16f
length of stay in, substance abuse affecting, 515
rates for brain injuries, 7–8, 9t, 10f
stresses in, 248, 249t
Huperzine, 681t–682t, 683t, 683–684, 691t
Hydrocodone in pain relief, 426t
Hydrogen-1 in magnetic resonance spectroscopy, 125, 125t
Hydromorphone in pain relief, 426t
Hydrotherapy in pain relief, 427
Hydroxyzine in headaches, 390
Hyperphagia, 66, 66t
Hypersexuality
in Klüver-Bucy syndrome, 438, 446
treatment of, 446
Hypersomnia, 375–376
Hypertension
headache in, 389t
intracranial. See Intracranial pressure
Hypnosis in pain management, 429t
Hypnotics, psychiatric side effects of, 612t
Hypoglycemia as defense to criminal charge, 595
Hypomania in children, 485
Hyposexuality, treatment of, 446
Hypothalamus, 66, 66t
in aggression, 262, 262t
dysregulation of, opiate antagonists in, 255, 255t
in focal brain injury, 33
in sexual function, 438

Hypoxic-ischemic brain damage, 37–38, 73
evoked potentials in, 148
in infants and children, 40

Ibuprofen
as COX inhibitor, 705
psychiatric side effects of, 611t
Idebenone, 681t–682t, 683t, 688, 691t
Ifenprodil as NMDA receptor antagonist, 702t, 704
Illness, denial of. See Denial of illness
Illness Behavior Questionnaire, 422t
Imagery and hypnosis, in pain management, 429t
Imaginary Processes Inventory, Sexual Imagery subscale of, 442
Imaging techniques. See also specific techniques
computed tomography, 79–84
xenon-enhanced, 127, 127f, 128f–129f
for elderly persons, 501
functional, 107–129
in delirium and posttraumatic amnesia, 190–191
frontal lobe in, 247
in mild TBI, 294t, 295, 296
magnetic resonance imaging, 84–92
functional, 108t, 123–125
magnetic resonance spectroscopy (MRS), 108t, 125–126
magnetoencephalography, 126–127
in mild TBI, 293–296, 294t
positron emission tomography (PET), 117–123
in posttraumatic stress disorder, 238–239
single-photon emission computed tomography (SPECT), 108–117
structural, 79–104
in delirium and posttraumatic amnesia, 189–190
Imipramine
adverse effects of, 618
in affective lability, 621
in premature ejaculation, 446
Immediate Post-Concussion Assessment and Cognitive Testing (ImPACT), 468
Immunohistochemistry in diffuse axonal injuries, 35f, 36
Immunosuppressants, neuroprotection with, 706t, 710
Impulse disorders, and insanity defense, 593
Inappropriate behavior after brain injury, 251
Incidence of brain injuries, 6–8, 7f, 24, 727–728, 728f
mild injuries in, 281, 281t

Incompetency, 586–587
  definition of, 584, 588–589
Individuals With Disabilities Education
    Act, 565
Indole-2-carboxylic acid (I2CA) as
    NMDA receptor antagonist, 702t,
    703
Indomethacin
  as COX inhibitor, 705, 706t
  psychiatric side effects of, 611t, 612t
Infancy, brain injuries in, 39–40
Infarction of brain tissue, 33
Informed consent, 584–586, 585t
  options available for, 586, 586t
Injury control theory, 728–729
Insanity defense, legal issues in, 592–593
Insight deficiency, 354t
  in brain injury and in psychotic
      disorders, 222
Insomnia, 372–375
Insulinlike growth factor-1, 707t, 712f,
    713t, 714
Insurance
  coverage for care of patients, 566–568
  disability, 576–577
Integrative model of behavioral therapy,
    663, 663t
Intelligence quotient (IQ), and
    posttraumatic psychosis, 219
Intelligence tests, 161
Interactive staff training (IST), 673
Interleukins
  activity in brain injury, 709–710
    IL-1, 41
    IL-6, 41
  neuroprotection with
    IL-1ra, 706t, 709
    IL-10, 706t, 710
International Classification of Diseases
    (ICD), 8, 9t, 14, 16
Intoxication as defense to criminal
    charge, 594
Intracranial pressure
  increased
    brain damage from, 33
      in hypoxia-ischemia, 37
    in children, 477
  monitoring in severe TBI, 53, 54t
  normal values, 33
Iodine-123–*N*-isopropyl-*p*-
    iodoamphetamine in SPECT
    imaging, 112t
Ion changes after brain injury, 42
Iron chelators, neuroprotection with,
    706t, 707
Irritability in personality disorders, 251
Ischemia, cerebral. *See* Hypoxic-
    ischemic brain damage
N-Isopropyl-*p*-iodoamphetamine
    labeled with iodine-123 in SPECT
    imaging, 112t

Jargon aphasia, 355–356
Judgment
  in addicted persons with brain
      damage, 526
  impairment after brain injury, 251
Judgment of Line Orientation Test, 161t
Julia Farr Centre PTA scale, 183, 183t

Kallikrein-kinin system in brain injury,
    711
Ketamine
  as NMDA receptor antagonist, 701,
      702t
  psychiatric side effects of, 611t, 612t
Ketorolac in pain relief, 426
Klüver-Bucy syndrome
  hypersexuality in, 438, 446
  violent behavior in, 590
Kynurenate (KYNA) as AMPA/KA
    receptor antagonist, 703, 703t

Lacerations, 29–30, 30t
  brain swelling with, 38, 39f
Lactate labeled with hydrogen-1 in
    magnetic resonance spectroscopy,
    125t
Lamotrigine
  in anxiety disorders, 241
  in cognitive dysfunction, 326t, 330, 623
  in mania, 620
  as NMDA receptor antagonist, 703t,
      704
  in pain relief, 425t
  in seizures with behavioral
      symptoms, 314, 315t
Language impairment, 65, 250, 250t,
    252–253, 325t, 325–326
  in addicted persons with brain
      damage, 526
  testing of, 161t, 164–165
Laughing, pathological, 204
  medications in, 620–621
Learning disorders, 323t, 323–324
  differential diagnosis of, 169–170
  testing in, 161t
Lecithin, and cognition in elderly
    persons, 504
Leeds scale in depression after mild
    TBI, 291
Legal issues, 287–289, 287t, 583–605
  advance directives, 587–588
  civil litigation, 595–596
    disability determinations in, 599
    expert testimony in, 595
    forensic experts in, 596. *See also*
        Forensic psychiatric
        evaluations
    treating clinician in, 595–596
  competency concept in, 583–584
  and competency to stand trial, 591
  criminal proceedings, 590–595

diminished capacity concept, 593
do-not-resuscitate (DNR) orders, 587
exculpatory and mitigating disorders,
    594–595
in family matters, 553–554
guardianship, 588–589
guilty but mentally ill, 593–594
health care decision making,
    584–590, 603–605
incompetent patients, 586–587
informed consent, 584–586, 585t
insanity defense, 592–593
litigation problems, 578–579
in mild TBI, 300
and public policy decisions, 571–574
in sexual dysfunction, 447–448
substituted judgment in proxy
    decision making, 589–590
Leukocyte adherence inhibitors,
    neuroprotection with, 706t, 709
Levetiracetam in pain relief, 425t
Levodopa
  affecting sexual function, 440t
  in affective lability, 621
  in cognitive dysfunction, 326t, 329,
      622t, 623
  in fatigue, 379
  in mild TBI, 299
  in motivational loss, 348t
  in personality disorders, 254, 255t
  psychiatric side effects of, 611t, 612t
LF-16-0687Ms compounds,
    neuroprotection with, 706t, 711
Lidocaine
  in pain relief, 425t
  in premature ejaculation, 446
Lifestyle
  adjustments in headache, 389
  and fatigue, 380
  and sleep disorders, 381
Lifetime supported living services in
    care system, 565
Limbic system
  in aggression, 262, 262t
  in motivational circuitry, 341
Lipid peroxidation after brain injury,
    42–43
Lithium
  in affective lability, 621
  in aggression, 271–272, 630t
  for elderly persons, 504
  in mania, 209–210, 619
Litigation problems, 578–579
Living wills, 587
Location of brain lesions
  and mood disorders, 207
  and psychosis, 218, 222–223
Loneliness of patients, 650–651, 652t
Lorazepam
  in delirium, 194
  in insomnia, 380

Loss of consciousness (LOC)
    in mild brain injury, 279, 280t, 281
    relation to CT findings, 80, 82f
    and severity of concussion, 464t,
        464–465, 465t
Lubeluzole as glutamate inhibitor, 206
Luria's Memory Words—Revised, and
    benefits of citicholine, 686
Luteinizing hormone, 439, 440t, 445t
LY341122 compound, neuroprotection
    with, 706t, 707
LY354740 compound as NMDA
    receptor antagonist, 703t, 704
Magnesium
    ion changes after brain injury, 42
    salts as NMDA receptor antagonists,
        702t, 703
Magnetic resonance imaging, 84–92
    anatomic specificity of, 84, 84f
    clinical rating of scans in, 95, 96f
        related to behavioral and
            cognitive function, 96–97,
            97f
    in corpus callosum atrophy, 86f, 90
    degenerative changes tracked in, 85,
        86f
    in delirium after brain injury, 189
    diffusion-tensor imaging in, 94f,
        94–95, 95f
    in dizziness and balance problems,
        398, 399t
    findings related to outcome, 90–92, 91f
    in focal brain injury, 33–34
    in follow-up of baseline CT images,
        87, 89f
    functional, 108t, 123–125
        abnormal findings in, 124
        blood oxygen level dependent
            (BOLD), 296
        in brain injury, 124
        indications for, 123
        limitations to, 123
        in mild TBI, 194t, 295, 296
        practical considerations in, 123
        in psychiatric disorders, 124
        recommendations for, 124–125
    image sequences in, 88, 88t
        diffusion-weighted (DW), 88, 88f
        fluid-attentuated inversion
            recovery (FLAIR), 88, 88f,
            189
        gradient recalled echo (GRE), 88,
            88f
        proton density (PD), 88, 88f
        T1 and T2, 88, 88f
    indications for, 85–87
    in mild TBI, 294t, 294–295
    quantitative image analysis in, 84,
        89–90, 103–104
    small but critical lesions in, 83f, 86f,
        89f, 92

SPECT imaging with, 92, 93f, 113,
    114f, 116f
    superiority of, 92, 93f
    typical lesions in, 87–89
        contusion, 88, 89f
        focal atrophy, 89, 89f
        shear, 86f, 88
        white matter abnormalities, 89,
            89f, 189
    ventricle to brain ratio (VBR) in, 85f,
        90, 91f
    in ventriculomegaly, 84, 85f
    voxel-based morphometry in, 87f
Magnetic resonance spectroscopy
    (MRS), 108t, 125–126
    in brain injury, 126
    indications for, 125
    limitations of, 126
    in mild TBI, 294t
    proton, in delirium after brain injury,
        189–190
    in psychiatric disorders, 126
    recommendations for, 126
    tracers used in, 125, 125t
Magnetic source imaging in brain
    injuries, 152–153, 294t
Magnetoencephalography, 126–127,
    152–153
    abnormal low-frequency magnetic
        activity in (ALFMA), 152–153
    recording methods in, 140–141
Malingering
    detection of, 579
    in litigation, 597, 598t
    postconcussive symptoms in,
        287–289
    testing for, 165–166
Mania
    after mild TBI, 291t, 292
    in children, 485
    differential diagnosis of, 205–206
    in elderly persons, 504
    medications in, 619–620
    in seizures after brain injury, 314
    treatment of, 209–210
Mannitol in intracranial hypertension,
    53, 54t
Maprotiline, seizures from, 618–619
Matrix Reasoning Test, 161t
Maximum Abbreviated Injury Scale
    (MAIS), 20, 25
MCPG compound as NMDA receptor
    antagonist, 703t, 704
Mechanisms of brain damage after
    injury, 27–28, 28t
Meclizine in dizziness and balance
    problems, 401, 401t
Meclofenoxate. See Centrophenoxine
Medicaid, 565, 567–568
    waiver programs in states, 574,
        574t

Medical disorders
    apathy in, 343t
    personality changes in, 214t, 249,
        249t, 261, 261t
    psychotic disorders in, 214, 214t
Medical history of TBI patients, 67
Medicare, 567
Medications
    affecting elderly persons, 502, 503t
    affecting neuropsychological test
        results, 599
    affecting sexual function, 439,
        440t–441t, 446–447
    aggression associated with, 265, 265t
    in anxiety, 240–241
    apathy from, 343t, 344
    in attention-deficit/hyperactivity
        disorder, 489
    in cognitive dysfunction, 326t,
        326–338
    in delirium, 192–194
    in depression, 615–619
        in children, 489
    in dizziness and balance problems,
        401, 401t
    drugs interacting with
        antidepressants, 619
    in fatigue and sleep problems,
        379–380, 627, 630
    in history of TBI patients, 67
    interactions of, 610, 613
    in mild TBI, 298–300
    in motivational loss, 347–349
    neuroleptics, 628–629. See also
        Neuroleptic medications
    overuse causing headaches, 387, 388
    for pain, 424–427, 425t, 426t
        issues involved with, 421, 423–424
    in personality disorders, 254t,
        254–255, 255t
    psychiatric side effects of, 611t–612t
    psychopharmacology, 609–632. See
        also Psychopharmacology
    psychotropic agents
        effects in brain injury patients,
            208–209
        in mild TBI, 298
    in substance abuse, 520–521
Medroxyprogesterone affecting sexual
    function, 441t
Melatonin in sleep disorders, 381
Memory
    in addicted persons with brain
        damage, 526
    declarative, 323, 323t
    and delayed recall, 163
    dysfunction of, 323t, 323–324
    episodic, 323, 323t
    functional MRI studies of, 124
    immediate, 163
    implicit, 323, 323t

Memory—*continued*
　metamemory deficits, 323
　in mild TBI, cholinergic and
　　catecholaminergic agents
　　affecting, 298–299
　in personality disorders, 252
　in posttraumatic stress disorder, 168
　prospective, 323
　recent, 163
　studies in posttraumatic amnesia, 180
　testing of, 161t, 163–164
　working, 323, 323t
　　dysfunction of, 323
Ménière disease, 400
Mens rea, 590
Menstrual disorders after TBI, 66, 66t
Mental health services in care system,
　565–566
Mental status examination, 69, 69t
Meperidine in pain relief, 426t
Meprobamate in withdrawal from
　alcohol or drugs, 514t
Metabolic disorders, and diminished
　capacity concept, 593, 595
Methadone in opiate withdrawal, 514
Methandrostenolone affecting sexual
　function, 440t
Methaqualone in withdrawal from
　alcohol or drugs, 514t
N-Methyl-D-aspartate (NMDA),
　699–700, 700f
　receptor antagonists and agonists,
　　700–704, 702t–703t
Methyldopa affecting sexual function, 440t
Methylphenidate
　adverse effects of, 624
　affecting memory after mild TBI,
　　298–299
　in affective lability, 621
　in attention-deficit/hyperactivity
　　disorder, 489
　and cognition in elderly persons, 504
　in cognitive dysfunction, 328, 622t,
　　622–623
　in depression, 617
　for elderly persons, 503
　in fatigue, 379, 627
　in motivational loss, 348, 348t
　in personality disorders, 254, 254t
　psychiatric side effects of, 611t
Methysergide
　in headache, 390
　psychiatric side effects of, 611t
Metoclopramide
　in headache, 390
　psychiatric side effects of, 611t
Mexiletine in pain relief, 425t
Michigan Alcoholism Screening Test
　(MAST), 512
Migraine
　PET scans in, 119

SPECT imaging in, 112
　treatment of, 390
Mild brain injury, 6
　amnesia in, 279, 280t, 281
　and anxiety disorders, 291f, 292–293
　behavioral sequelae in, 285–293
　cognitive sequelae in, 283–285
　definitions of, 279–281, 280t
　depression in, 290–292, 291t
　diffuse cerebral swelling in, 283
　disability in, 293
　electrophysiological studies in,
　　296–297
　epidemiology of, 281t, 281–282
　evaluation of, 297–298
　experimental studies, 461
　family issues in, 549
　Glasgow Coma Scale in, 51, 60t, 279,
　　281, 477
　indicators of, 280t
　loss of consciousness in, 279, 280t,
　　281
　and mania, 291t, 292
　medical-legal issues in, 300
　medications in, 298–300
　neuroimaging in, 293–296, 294t
　pathophysiology of, 282–283
　postconcussive symptoms in,
　　285–290, 300–301
　and posttraumatic stress disorder,
　　236–237, 291t, 292–293
　psychoeducation in, 300
　psychotherapy in, 646–647
　and psychotic disorders, 290, 291t
　second impact syndrome in, 283,
　　462–463
　in sports, 453–472
　treatment of, 297–300
Millon Behavioral Health Inventory,
　422t
Mini-Mental State Examination
　(MMSE), 69, 166
　in delirium, 184
　Ginkgo biloba affecting, 689
　Huperzine affecting, 684
　vinpocetine affecting, 688
Minnesota Multiphasic Personality
　Inventory (MMPI), 248, 423t
Minocycline, neuroprotection with,
　706t, 709
Mirtazapine
　affecting sexual function, 441t
　in depression, 616
Mitral valve prolapse, headache in, 389t
MK-801 compound as NMDA receptor
　antagonist, 701, 702t
Moclobemide in depression, 617–618
Modafinil
　in cognitive impairment, 622t
　in fatigue, 379–380, 627
　in motivational loss, 348, 348t

in narcolepsy, 381
　in personality disorders, 254t
Moderate brain injury, Glasgow Coma
　Scale in, 60t, 477
Monoamine oxidase
　in aging brain, 499
　inhibitors of
　　in depression, 617–618
　　in motivational loss, 347
Mood disorders after TBI, 201–210
　affecting patient outcome, 207–208
　depression, 201–205
　mania, 205–206
　physiological correlations in,
　　206–207
　treatment of, 208–210
Morphine in pain relief, 426t
Mortality rates, 6, 8f, 16–17, 18f
　in elderly patients, 496
Motivation
　brain circuitry in, 339–342, 340f
　description of, 337
　impairment of, 337–349. *See also*
　　Apathy
　　assessment of, 343–345
　　behavioral interventions in, 346
　　clinical pathogenesis of, 342
　　differential diagnosis of, 339
　　disorders in, 338–339
　　environmental interventions in, 346
　　medications in, 347–349
　　neurobehavioral mechanisms in,
　　　342–343
　　neurochemical mechanisms in,
　　　343
　　psychological prosthesis in,
　　　346–347
　　rating methods in, 344–345
　　recognition of, 338–339
　　treatment of, 345–349
　in test performance, 289
　testing of, 165
Motor processes
　in disabled intention system, 359
　dysfunction of, 65, 65t
　　agitation in, 179
　testing of, 161
Motor vehicles
　car seats for children, 740
　injuries in, 12, 510
　　prevention of, 730–732, 739
　insurance policy types, 567
Motorcycle accidents, injuries in, 13, 13f
　prevention of, 731–732, 739
MPEP compound as NMDA receptor
　antagonist, 703t, 704
Multiaxial Pain Inventory, 422t
Multilingual Aphasia Examination, 161t
Multiple sclerosis
　association with TBI, 65
　fatigue in, treatment of, 379, 380

Multiple Sleep Latency Test (MSLT), 378
Mutism, akinetic, 338
    conditions associated with, 343t
    treatment of, 345–346

Nadolol in aggression, 272, 273
Naproxen affecting sexual function, 440t
Naratriptan in headache, 390
Narcolepsy, 375–376
    modafinil in, 381
Narcotics
    addiction to. *See* Substance abuse
    psychiatric side effects of, 611t
Narcotics Anonymous (NA), 517, 517t
National Center for Catastrophic Sports
        Injury Research, 455
National Head Injury Foundation, 571,
        572
National Health Interview Survey
        (NHIS), 5t, 6, 7
National Highway Safety
        Administration, 731
National Hospital Ambulatory Medical
        Care Survey (NHAMCS), 5t, 6, 7
National Hospital Discharge Survey
        (NHDS), 5t, 6, 7, 14, 15, 16
National Institutes of Health, 560
    research and conference on traumatic
        brain injury, 572–573, 573t
    Stroke Scale scores affected by
        citicholine, 685
National Rehabilitation Association, 577
Natural-Setting Behavior Management
        Program for families, 538
NBQX compound as AMPA/KA
        receptor antagonist, 703t, 704
Nefazodone in depression, 616
Neglect, unilateral, 355
Neocortex in aggression, 262–263
Nerve growth factor, 706t, 711–712, 712f
    activity after brain injury, 42
    in aging brain, 498
Neuralgia syndromes, headache in, 387t
    treatment of, 390
Neuroanatomy
    in aggression, 261–263, 262t
    in dizziness and balance problems,
        394
    in pain, 420
    in personality change, 246–247
    in sexual functioning, 437–439, 438t
Neurobehavioral Cognitive Status
        Examination (NCSE), 70, 72f, 166
Neurobehavioral Rating Scale, 609
    in personality changes, 249
    in posttraumatic amnesia, 183, 183t
Neurobehavioral Rating Scale—Revised
        (NRS-R), 70
Neurobehavioral treatment in care
        system, 564

Neurobiology
    in aging, 498
    in anxiety disorders, 237–238
Neurochemical changes. *See also*
        Neurotransmitter changes after
        brain injury
    in aging, 498, 499t
    posttraumatic, 40–43
        acetylcholine levels, 40
        amino acids, excitatory, 41–42
        arachidonic acid cascade, 40
        catecholamine and monoamine
            neurotransmitters, 40–41
        cytokines, 41
        growth factors, 42
        ions, 41
        opioid peptides, endogenous, 41
        oxygen-free radicals and lipid
            peroxidation, 42–43
Neuroendocrine disorders in sexual
        dysfunction, 445–446, 445t
    treatment of, 446
Neuroimaging. *See* Imaging techniques
Neuroleptic malignant syndrome, 629
Neuroleptic medications, 628–629
    in aggression, 269–270
    in delirium, 192–193
    in posttraumatic psychosis, 225
    in seizures with behavioral
        symptoms, 315
Neurological disorders
    apathy in, 343t, 344
    and posttraumatic psychosis, 219
    symptoms in TBI, 65t, 65–66
Neuron-specific enolase in cerebrospinal
        fluid, after brain injury, 41
Neuropathology, 27–44
    brain swelling, 38–39, 39f
    cellular changes, 43
    classification of damage in, 27, 28t
    in fatal blunt head injury, 29–40
    in focal injury, 29–34
    in infancy and childhood, 39–40
    mechanisms of damage in, 27–28, 28t
    neurochemical changes in, 40–43
Neurophysiology
    in balance problems and dizziness, 394
    in concussion, 460–464
    in delirium, 186f, 186–191
Neuropsychiatric assessment, 59–75
    after coronary artery bypass graft, 74
    in anoxia/hypoxia, 73–74
    behavioral assessment in, 69–70
    behavioral disorders in, 61t
    biopsychosocial approach, 59–71
    classification of injury in, 60t
    cognitive disorders in, 61t
    in cognitive rehabilitation, 657–658
    collateral history in, 60–62, 61t
    current behavioral symptoms in, 62,
        62t

of elderly persons, 501–502
    in electrical injuries, 74, 75t
    emotional disorders in, 61t
    endocrine symptoms in, 66
    history of patient in, 59–60, 60t
        family history, 67
        medical history, 67
        medications used, 67
        preinjury disorders, 66–67
        psychiatric disorders, 66
        social functioning, 67–69
        substance abuse, 67
    mental status examination in, 69, 69t
    neurological symptoms in, 65t, 65–66
    in nontraumatic brain injuries, 71–74
    and PET scan results, 122
    physical examination in, 69
    physical symptoms in, 61t, 66
    psychiatric disorders in, 64t, 64–65
        preinjury disorders, 66
    Rancho Los Amigos Cognitive Scale
        in, 62, 63t
    results related to SPECT findings,
        116–117
    in severe TBI, 62–63
    in sports injuries, 467–468
    symptom checklist in, 60, 61t
    symptoms after TBI, 63–66
        DSM-IV-TR disorders in, 64, 64t
    in traumatic brain injuries, 59–71
    Web-based protocol in, 468
Neuropsychiatric disorders
    care systems in, 559–568
    in children, 479–490
    in elderly persons, management of,
        502–504
Neuropsychiatric Inventory, 344, 609
Neurosis, compensation, 579
Neurosurgical interventions, 51–58. *See
    also* Severe brain injury
Neurotransmitter changes after brain
        injury, 613–615. *See also*
        Neurochemical changes
    acetylcholine, 615
    in aggression, 263–264
    catecholamines, 613–614
    serotonin, 614–615
Neurotrophic factors, brain injury
        affecting, 42, 711–715
New York University Head Injury
        Family Interview, 537–538,
        538t
Newtonian formulas in mechanics of
        injury, 471–472
Nimesulide as COX-2 inhibitor, 706t,
        707
Nitric oxide synthase (NOS)
    in brain injury, 705
    inhibitors of, neuroprotection with,
        706t, 708
Nitrogen-13 in PET scans, 121t

NMDA receptors, 699–700, 700f
  antagonists and agonists of, 700–704,
    702t–703t
Nonfatal brain injuries, 6–8, 9t
Nonsteroidal anti-inflammatory drugs
    in headaches, 389
Nootropics, 690
  definition of, 679
Norepinephrine
  activity after brain injury, 40–41,
    613–614
    cerebrospinal fluid levels, 207
    serum levels in aggression, 263
  in aging brain, 498–499, 499t
North American Adult Reading Test, 167
Nortriptyline
  affecting sexual function, 440t
  in affective lability, 621
  in depression, 209, 617
  in pain relief, 425t
Novelty seeking, apathy affecting,
    342
Nucleus accumbens in motivational
    circuitry, 340f, 341
Nurses' Observation Scale for Geriatric
    Patients (NOSGER), idebenone
    affecting, 688
Nursing homes, neurobehavioral
    programs in, 566
Nutrients as alternative treatments,
    686–688
Nutrition
  in fatigue, 380
  in sleep disorders, 381
Nystagmus, 394, 395–396, 407t

Obsessive-compulsive disorder, 235, 235t
  in children, 485
  differential diagnosis of, 168
  PET scans in, 119
  SPECT imaging in, 111, 113
Occupational functioning of TBI
    patients, 68–69
Oculomotor problems, 410
Olanzapine
  affecting sexual function, 440t
  in aggression, 270
  in anxiety, 241
  in delirium, 193, 194
  for elderly persons, 504
  in posttraumatic psychosis, 225–226
Olfactory disorders, 253
  screening for, 397
Ophthalmology, 407
Opiates
  in pain relief, 426t
  patient agreement for use of, 427,
    435–436
  withdrawal from, 514
Opioid peptides
  activity after brain injury, 41

antagonists in personality disorders,
    255, 255t
Oppositional defiant disorder in
    children, 479, 484
  differential diagnosis of, 487
Optic tract, 408, 408f
Optometry, 407
Orientation
  disorders in delirium, 180
  testing of, 160–161
Orientation Log (O-Log), 70, 71f
Otoliths, 394
Outcomes of brain injuries. See
    Consequences of brain injuries
Outpatient therapy services, 564
Ovarian hormones in sexual function,
    439, 440t, 445t
Overcorrection in aggression, 670, 670t
Overt Aggression Scale (OAS), 259, 266,
    267f, 609
Overt Agitation Severity Scale, 183t,
    266, 268f
  and selection of antipsychotic drugs,
    194
Oxazepam in withdrawal from alcohol
    or drugs, 514t
Oxcarbazepine
  in aggression, 271
  in mania, 620
  in pain relief, 425t
Oxford PTA scale, 183, 183t
Oxiracetam as alternative treatment, 690
Oxybutynin affecting sexual function, 440t
Oxycodone in pain relief, 426t
Oxygen-15 in PET scans, 117, 121t
Oxygen reactive species formed after
    brain injury, 705

P30 and P50 evoked potentials, 147, 147f
  P50 nonsuppression in responses,
    626
Paced Auditory Serial Addition Task
    (PASAT), 161t, 163, 322
  in sports injuries, 467
Pain
  assessment of, 421, 422t–423t
    during examinations, 421, 424t
  behavioral therapy in, 428, 429t
  chronic, 419–430
  cognitive dysfunction in, 420–421
  definition of, 419
  desensitization model for
    interventions in, 430, 430t
  in headaches. See Headache
  and insomnia, 375
  medications in, 424–427, 425t, 426t
    issues involved with, 421, 423–424
    and "narcotics agreement" for
      patients, 427, 435–436
    neuroanatomy of, 420
    PET scans in, 119

physical agents for therapy in,
    427–428
SPECT imaging in, 111, 112–113
Panic disorder, 235, 235t
  dizziness and balance problems in,
    402
Paranoid symptoms in children,
    treatment of, 489
Parasomnias, 377
Parenchymal lesions in severe TBI, 56,
    57f
Parkinson disease, SPECT imaging in,
    111
Paroxetine
  adverse effects of, 618
  in affective lability, 621
  in depression, 209
  in pain relief, 425t
Patient Competency Rating Scale,
    358t
Patient education in pain management,
    429t
Patient Self-Determination Act, 587
PBN compound, neuroprotection with,
    706t, 707
PC-SOD enzyme, neuroprotection
    with, 706t, 708
Pediatric injuries, 39–40, 477–490
  adjustment disorder in, 488
  attention-deficit/hyperactivity
    disorder in, 479, 483–484
    differential diagnosis of,
      487–488
    treatment of, 489
  on bicycles, 13, 13t, 459–460
    prevention of, 733–734
  in child abuse, 740
  depression in
    differential diagnosis of, 488
    treatment of, 489
  educational services for, 565
  epidemiology of, 477
  etiology and pathophysiology,
    477–478
  falls in, 733
  and family functioning, 482, 537
  neurological sequelae of, 478
  oppositional defiant disorder in, 479,
    484
    differential diagnosis of, 487–488
  and parental relationship with school
    system, 549–550
  personality change in, 479, 482–483
    differential diagnosis of, 487–488
    treatment of, 488–489
  personality style changes in, 487
  postconcussion syndrome in,
    differential diagnosis of, 488
  posttraumatic stress disorder in,
    484–485
  prevention of, 490

prevention of brain trauma in, 740–741
psychiatric disorders in, 479–490
  adaptive function after, 486
  affecting family function, 482
  cognitive outcome in, 486
  differential diagnosis of, 486–488
  frequency of, 483t
  postinjury status in, 480
  predictors of, 480–482, 482t
  preinjury status in, 480
  studies of, 480, 481t
  treatment of, 488–489
psychosis after, 216–217, 224
psychosocial treatments in, 489–490
and schizophrenia development, 220
school failure in, 488
school programs in, 560
school sequelae of, 478–479
PEG-SOD enzyme, neuroprotection
  with, 706t, 708
Pemoline
  in fatigue, 379
  in personality disorders, 254
Penetrating injuries, and posttraumatic
  psychosis, 219
Penis
  biothesiometry of, 444
  innervation of, 439
Pentazocine, psychiatric side effects of,
  612t
Pentobarbital in withdrawal from
  alcohol or drugs, 514t
Pentoxifylline, neuroprotection with,
  706t, 710
Perceived Stress Scale (PSS), 423t
Perception problems in personality
  disorders, 253
Performance in process model of
  behavioral therapy, 664, 665–666
Pergolide
  in cognitive dysfunction, 326t, 329
  in motivational loss, 348t
  in personality disorders, 255, 255t
Personality
  assessment after brain injury,
    248–249
  changes in, 206
    affecting families, 535, 535t
    in children, 479, 482–483
      differential diagnosis of,
        487–488
      treatment of, 488–489
    compared with changes in
      personality style, 487
    in medical conditions, 249, 249t,
      261, 261t
  functional neuroimaging studies, 247
  localization in brain, 246–248
  neurochemical basis of, 248
  premorbid, and reactions to brain
    injury, 248

Personality disorders, 245–255
  abstract thought in, 252
  affective instability in, 251
  aggression and irritability in, 251
  assessment of, 253–254
  attention in, 251
  childish behavior in, 250–251
  clinical features of, 249–253
  definition of, 246
  inappropriate behavior in, 251
  language deficits in, 250, 250t,
    252–253
  medications in, 254t, 254–255, 255t
  memory in, 252
  perceptual problems in, 253
  psychotherapy in, 255
  in seizures, 314t
  treatment of, 253–255
Pharmacotherapy. See Medications
Phencyclidine as NMDA receptor
  antagonist, 701, 702t
Phenelzine
  in depression, 616–617
  psychiatric side effects of, 612t
Phenobarbital
  in aggression, 271
  in seizures with behavioral
    symptoms, 315t
  in withdrawal from alcohol or drugs,
    514t
Phenoxybenzamine
  affecting sexual function, 441t
  in premature ejaculation, 446–447
Phentolamine in erectile dysfunction,
  446
Phenytoin
  affecting sexual function, 440t
  in aggression, 271
  cognitive effects of, 631, 632
  early posttrauma use of, 310
  in pain relief, 425t
Phobias, 235t
Phospholipases, activation of, 705
Phosphorus-31 in magnetic resonance
  spectroscopy, 125, 125t
Photosensitivity, 411–412
Phototherapy in circadian rhythm sleep
  disorder, 381–382
Physical modalities in pain relief,
  427–428
Physical symptoms in TBI, 61t, 66
Physostigmine
  affecting memory in mild TBI, 299
  in cognitive dysfunction, 326t, 327,
    625
    in elderly persons, 504
  in delirium, 194
Picamilon, 681t–682t, 683t, 687
Pindolol in aggression, 272, 273
Piperidinedione in withdrawal from
  alcohol or drugs, 514t

Piracetam, 691t
  as alternative treatment, 690
Pittsburgh Sleep Quality Index, 375
Pituitary gland in TBI, 66, 66t
  in focal brain injury, 33
Pituitary hormones in sexual function,
  439, 445t
Playground injuries, prevention of, 733,
  740–741
Polysomnography, 378
Portland Digit Recognition Test, 165
Positron emission tomography (PET),
  108t, 117–123
  in activation studies, 122–123
  in behavioral disorders, 122
  capabilities of, 118, 120f, 121f
  compared to CT or MRI, 120–122
  in headache after trauma, 386, 388
  improvements in, 119f
  in mild TBI, 294t, 295–296
  in neuropsychological assessments,
    122
  normal adult brain in, 120f
  procedure in, 117, 118f
  in psychiatric disorders, 118–119
  recommendations for, 123
  tracers in, 117–118, 121t, 123
  in traumatic brain injury, 119–120,
    190–191
Postconcussion symptoms, 285–290, 388
  checklist for, 60, 61t. See also
    Symptomatologies
  in children, differential diagnosis of,
    488
  headache in, 385
  in immediate postinjury period,
    285–286
  in mild TBI, 300–301
    medications in, 298–299
  persistence of, 286–287
  role of compensation and litigation
    in, 287–289, 287t
Posterior fossa lesions in severe TBI, 56
Posttraumatic stress disorder, 235–239
  after brain injury with amnesia,
    235–236
  after mild TBI, 291t, 292–293
  in children, 484–485
  cognition in, 237
  depression with, 237
  differential diagnosis of, 168, 204
  incidence of, 235–236
  medications in, 629–630
  neurobiology in, 237–238
  neuroimaging in, 238–239
  relation to acute stress disorder,
    236–237
  relation to posttraumatic amnesia, 180
Posturography, 399, 399t
Potassium ion changes after brain injury,
  42

Prader-Willi syndrome, opiate
  antagonists in, 255, 255t
Pramipexole
  in cognitive dysfunction, 326t, 329
  in motivational loss, 348
  in personality disorders, 255, 255t
Pramiracetam as alternative treatment,
  690
Prazepam in withdrawal from alcohol or
  drugs, 514t
Prednisone in pain relief, 425t
Prehospital management in severe TBI,
  52
Prevention, 727–741
  antagonists of excitatory amino acids
    in, 699–705, 702t–703t
  anti-inflammatory agents in, 706t,
    708–711
  in bicycle riding, 733–734
  in boxing, 734
  in children, 740–741
  comprehensive approach to, 729–741
  in falling, 733
  in football, 734–735
  Haddon Matrix in, 729
  in hockey, 735–736
  and injury control theory, 728–729
  lipid peroxidation inhibition in,
    705–708
  in motor vehicles, 730–732
  neurotrophic factors in, 706t–707t,
    711–715
  passive versus active strategies in, 729
  pharmacotherapy in, 699–715
  in soccer, 735
  in sports and recreational injury,
    733–736
  in substance abuse, 737–740
  and suicide risk in depression, 737
  violent injuries, 736–737
Primary injuries, 27, 28t, 699
Primidone in seizures with behavioral
  symptoms, 315t
Prisoners on death row
  history of TBI in, 260
  posttraumatic psychosis in, 223
Process model of behavioral therapy,
  663t, 663–669
Prochlorperazine in dizziness and
  balance problems, 401, 401t
Progesterone, 439, 440t
Prolactin, 439, 440t, 445t
  serum levels in seizures, 311
Promethazine in dizziness and balance
  problems, 401, 401t
Propranolol
  in aggression, 272–273, 273t, 630t
  in agitation, 194
  in headache, 390
  psychiatric side effects of, 611t, 612t
Prosodic dysfunction, 252–253

Prostacyclin, neuroprotection with,
  706t, 709
Protein kinase C formation in brain
  injury, 705
Protriptyline
  adverse effects of, 618
  in cognitive impairment, 623
  in motivational loss, 348t
Proxy decision making for patients,
  589–590
Pseudobulbar affect, 620
Pseudodepression, 247
Psychiatric disorders
  in brain injury, 64t, 64–65
  mimicking brain injury, 598–599
  in substance abuse, 515
Psychiatrists in civil litigation
  procedures, 595–596
Psychoeducation
  after mild TBI, 300
  in awareness impairment, 362, 363t
  in fatigue, 380
  in motivational loss, 349
Psychogenic conditions
  balance disorders, 399
  PET scans in, 119
  SPECT imaging in, 113
Psychological factors in pain disorders,
  419
Psychological prosthesis in motivational
  loss, 346–347
Psychomotor retardation, differential
  diagnosis of, 339
Psychopharmacology, 609–632
  concerns about medications in,
    630–632
  in emotional disorders, 615–621
  evaluation of patients in, 609–610
  general principles of, 610, 612t, 613
  medications recommended,
    615–630
    in aggression and agitation, 630,
      630t
    in anxiety and posttraumatic
      stress, 629–630
    in apathy, 626–627
    in cognitive impairment,
      621–626, 622t
    in coldness, 627–628
    in depression, 615–619
    in emotional disorders, 615–621
    in fatigue, 627
    in mania, 619–620
    in psychosis, 628–629
    in sleep disorders, 630
  and neurotransmitter dysfunction
    after brain injury, 613–615
  and psychiatric side effects of
    neurological drugs, 611t–612t
Psychosexual Assessment Questionnaire,
  441

Psychosocial therapy in pediatric brain
  injuries, 489–490
Psychostimulants. See Stimulants
Psychotherapy, 641–653
  in anxiety, 239–240
  avoidance of childish responses in,
    250–251
  catastrophic conditions in, 649, 652t
  denial in, 648–649, 652t
  in depression after brain injury, 209
  for elderly persons, 502
  family involved in, 651–652
  in fatigue, 380
  flexibility needed in, 642–644
  goal-directed activities in, 644, 645t
  group experiences in, 651
  guilt, shame, and punishment in,
    649–650, 652t
  historical perspective in, 642
  loneliness in, 650–651, 652t
  in mild brain injury, 646–647
  outcome measures in, 644–646
  in personality disorders, 255
  risk-taking encouraged in, 653
  in sleep disorders, 382
  starting point in, 642
  and stigmatization of patients, 650,
    652t
  suggested tactics in, 5t, 644
  transference and countertransference
    issues in, 647–648, 652t
Psychotic disorders
  associated with epilepsy, 206,
    219–220, 314t
  in children, 485–486
  definition of, 214
  in elderly persons, 503–504
  in medical conditions, 214, 214t
  medications in, 225–226, 628–629
  posttraumatic, 213–226
    after mild TBI, 290, 291t
    atypical versus typical symptoms
      in, 220–221
    in children and teens, 216–217,
      224, 485–486
    cognition in, 221
    in death row prisoners, 223
    diagnosis of, 214–215
    follow-up studies, 215–216
    gender affecting, 219
    in homeless people, 223
    and inherent vulnerability to
      psychoses, 219, 221
    IQ/cognition affecting, 219, 221
    location of injury in, 218, 222–223
    presence of, versus absence of,
      in brain-injured patients,
      217–218
    prevention of, 226
    and prior neurological disorder,
      219

in schizophrenia patients, 220
severity of injury in, 218
socioeconomic status in, 219
and substance abuse, 219
treatment of, 225–226
type of injury in, 218–219
in vulnerable populations,
   223–224
schizophrenia development after
   childhood trauma, 220. *See also*
   Schizophrenia
in seizures after brain injury, 314t
Psychotropic agents. *See also*
   Neuroleptic medications
effects in brain injury patients,
   208–209
in mild TBI, 298
Public policy and legislation on
   traumatic brain injury, 571–574
state programs in, 571–572, 572t
Pudendal nerve, 439
Punch-drunk syndrome, 456, 500
Punishment experienced by patients,
   649–650, 652t
Pursuit deficits, ocular, 407t, 410
Pyritinol, 681t–682t, 683t, 687–688, 691t
Pyrrolidones, 681t–682t, 683t, 690

Quetiapine
   affecting sexual function, 440t
   in aggression, 270
   in anxiety, 241
   in delirium, 193
   for elderly persons, 504
   in posttraumatic psychosis, 225–226
Quinazolines in withdrawal from
   alcohol or drugs, 514t

Race or ethnicity
   and family reactions to disabilities,
      554–555
   and risk of brain injury, 9
Racetams, 681t–682t, 683t, 690, 691t
Raclopride in PET scans, 123
Radicals, oxygen-free, activity after
   brain injury, 42–43
Radiotracers
   in magnetic resonance spectroscopy,
      125, 125t
   in PET imaging, 117–118, 121t
   in SPECT SCANS, 109, 112T
Railway spine, 579
Rancho Los Amigos Cognitive Scale
   in delirium study, 177, 185
   in posttraumatic amnesia, 182–183,
      183t
   in recovery phase, 564
Ranitidine affecting sexual function,
   440t
Raynaud phenomenon, headache in,
   389t

Reaction times, slowing of, 322
Reading skills after brain injury in
   children, 478–479
Reasoning and judgment in addicted
   persons with brain damage, 526
Recovery process in behavioral therapy,
   663, 663t
Recreation, brain injuries in, 12, 12f
   prevention of, 733–736
Recurrent TBI, 10–11
Refraction, ocular, after brain injury,
   410–411
Rehabilitation
   acute, inpatient, 563
   awareness impairment affecting,
      361–363, 363t
   cognitive, 655–660, 664. *See also*
      Cognitive rehabilitation
   family focus in, 546
   subacute, 563–564
   systems of care in, 559–568. *See also*
      Care systems
   vestibular, 402
   vocational, 577–578
Rehabilitation Act of 1973, 577, 578
Reinforcers
   in behavioral therapy, 665–666
   and differential reinforcement of
      other behaviors (DRO),
      669–670, 670t
Relaxation techniques
   in headache, 389
   in pain management, 429t
Remacemide hydrochloride as NMDA
   receptor antagonist, 701–702, 702t
Repeatable Battery for the Assessment of
   Neuropsychological Status, 166
Residential treatment in care system,
   564
Restraints used in aggression, 670t, 671
Ret receptor family in central nervous
   system, 713, 713t
Rewards in behavioral therapy, 665–666
Rey 15-Item Memory Test, 165
Rey Auditory-Verbal Learning Test,
   161t, 163
   in sports injuries, 467
Rey-Osterrieth Complex Figure Test,
   161t, 163
Rhodiola rosea, 681t–682t, 683t, 688–689,
   691t
Riluzole
   as glutamate inhibitor, 206
   as NMDA receptor antagonist, 703t,
      705
Risk factors
   age in, 8–9, 10f, 14–15, 15f, 24
   for delirium, 181–182, 182t
   ethnicity or race in, 9
   for falls, 495, 496
   gender in, 9, 11f, 15f, 24

in high-risk groups, 8–12
socioeconomic status in, 11–12
substance abuse in, 9–10, 67
for suicide, 737
Risk-taking encouraged in
   psychotherapy, 653
Risperidone
   affecting sexual function, 440t
   in aggression, 270
   in anxiety, 241
   in delirium, 193
   for elderly persons, 504
   in personality change in children, 489
   in psychosis, 225–226, 628
Rivastigmine in motivational loss, 347,
   348f
Rivermead PTA Protocol, 183t,
   183–184
Rizatriptan in headaches, 390
Romberg testing, 397–398
Ropinirole
   in cognitive dysfunction, 326t, 329
   in personality disorders, 255, 255t
Roseroot, 681t–682t, 683t, 688–689
Rotatory (Barany) chair testing, 399,
   399t

S-100 protein in cerebrospinal fluid
   after brain injury, 41
S-PBN compound, neuroprotection
   with, 706t, 707
Saccades after brain injury, 407t, 410
Sandoz Clinical Assessment—Geriatric
   scale, vinpocetine affecting, 688
SC 58125 as COX-2 inhibitor, 706t, 707
Schedule for the Assessment of Negative
   Symptoms (SANS), 344
Schizophrenia
   awareness deficits in, 356
   in childhood, 220, 485–486
   cognitive features in common with
      brain injury, 222
   differential diagnosis of, 168–169
   functional MRI in, 124
   genetic vulnerability for, 219, 221
   magnetic resonance spectroscopy in,
      126
   PET scans in, 119
   SPECT imaging in, 111, 113
Schizophrenia-like psychosis (SLP), 169
School
   problems after brain injury, 68,
      478–479, 488
   programs for children with brain
      injuries, 560, 565
   relationship with parents, 549–550
Scopolamine
   affecting sexual function, 440t
   in dizziness and balance problems,
      401, 401t
Seat belts and air bags, 730–731

Secobarbital in withdrawal from alcohol or drugs, 514t

Second impact syndrome, 283, 462–463
  in football, 735

Secondary injuries, 27, 28t, 38, 51, 52t, 699, 700f

Sedatives
  in aggression, 270
  in insomnia, 380–381
  vestibular, 401

Seizures, 309–316
  aggression in, 265t, 265–266
  from antidepressants, 618–619
  from antipsychotic medications, 629
  in children, 478
  consequences of, 313, 313t
  diagnosis of, 311
  electroencephalography in, 143–144
  emotional impact of, 315–316
  epidemiology of, 309–311
  functional MRI in, 124
  headache in, 389t
  magnetoencephalography in, 126
  pathogenesis of, 311–312, 312t
  PET scans in, 118
  posttraumatic, 65t, 66
  and posttraumatic psychosis, 219–220
  prognosis of, 312–313
  prolactin levels in, 311
  psychopathology in, 313–314, 314t
    treatment of, 314–316
  psychosis associated with, 206
  in severe TBI, 53–54
  temporal lobe
    as defense to criminal charge, 594–595
    sexual problems in, 442, 446

Selegiline, 690
  in cognitive dysfunction, 326t, 329
  in motivational loss, 348t

Self, innate sense of, loss after brain injury, 249–250

Self-Awareness of Deficits Interview, 358t

Self-concept, brain injury affecting, 356–357

Self-controlled time-out in aggression, 670, 670t

Self-injurious behavior, opiate antagonists in, 255, 255t

Self/Other Rating Form, 358t

Selfotel as NMDA receptor antagonist, 701, 702t

Semicircular canals, 394

Sensory disorders, 65, 65t

Sensory gating, impairment of, 626

Serotonin
  activity after brain injury, 41, 614–615
  activity in aggression, 263
  in aging brain, 499, 499t

cerebrospinal fluid levels after brain injury, 207
  and personality attributes, 248
  selective reuptake inhibitors
    adverse effects of, 618
    affecting sexual function, 441t, 446
    in aggression, 272
    in anxiety, 240–241
    in cognitive dysfunction, 326t, 330
    in depression, 209, 615–616
    in motivational loss, 347
    in personality change in children, 489

Sertraline
  in aggression, 272
  in depression, 209, 298, 616
  in motivational loss, 347

Severe TBI, 51–58
  computed tomography in, 52
  decompressive craniectomy in, 57
  depressed skull fractures in, 56–57
  emergency department workup in, 52
  epidural hematoma in, 54–55, 55f
  Glasgow Coma Scale in, 51, 60t, 477
  in-hospital management of, 52–54
  intracranial pressure monitoring in, 53, 54t
  management guidelines, 51
    affecting patient outcome, 57–58, 58t
  parenchymal lesions in, 56, 57f
  posterior fossa lesions in, 56
  prehospital care, 52
  primary survey in, 53t
  prognosis of, 51, 57
  recovery stages in, 62–63
  resuscitation in, 53t
  secondary survey in, 53t
  seizures in, 53–54
  subdural hematoma in, 55f, 55–56, 56f
  surgery in, 54–57

Severity of injuries
  distribution of, 13–14, 14f
  and posttraumatic psychosis, 218

Sexual abuse, recognition of, 448

Sexual dysfunction, 66, 66t, 419–431
  clinical evaluation in, 443–444, 444t
  counseling issues in, 447–448
  diagnostic testing in, 444, 445t
  family issues in, 448
  genital, 446–447
  neuroanatomy in, 437–439, 438t
  neuroendocrine dysfunction in, 445–446, 445t
    treatment of, 446
  neurophysiology in, 439, 440t
  nongenital, 446
  physical examination in, 444

research literature, 439–443
  sexual history in, 443–444
  treatment of, 444–448
  in women, 442
    diagnostic testing in, 444, 445t

Shaken baby syndrome, 39–40

Shame experienced by patients, 649–650, 652t

Shearing injury
  diffuse white matter, 34
  MRI image of, 86f, 88
  triad of, 34

Shipley Institute of Living Scale, 166

Sickness Impact Profile, 422t

Sildenafil in erectile dysfunction, 446

Sinemet in cognitive impairment, 622t, 623

Single-photon emission computed tomography (SPECT), 108t, 108–117
  in activation studies, 117
  in behavioral problems, 115–116
  in brain injury, 110
  capabilities of, 109, 111f, 112f
  combined with structural imaging, 113–115
  computed tomography with, 113, 114f
  in headache after trauma, 386, 388
  improvements in, 109, 110f
  indications for, 110
  limitations of, 110
  in mild TBI, 294t, 295
  MRI integrated with, 92, 93f, 113, 114f, 116f
  in neuropsychological testing, 116–117
  normal adult brain in, 111f
  practical considerations in, 109–110
  procedure in, 109, 109f
  in psychiatric disorders, 110–113
  recommendations for, 117
  tracers in, 109, 112t
  in traumatic brain injury, 190
  in various patient populations, 117

619C89 compound as NMDA receptor antagonist, 703t, 704

Skateboarding, injuries in, 741

Skiing, injuries in, 459

Skills training
  in behavioral therapy, 664–665
  in pain management, 429t

Skull fractures
  in children, 477
  depressed, management of, 56–57
  and seizure development, 312t
  types of, 29t

SLAM model for concussion assessment, 457, 467, 471

Sleep
  disorders in. See Fatigue and sleep problems
  normal cycle in, 370, 370t